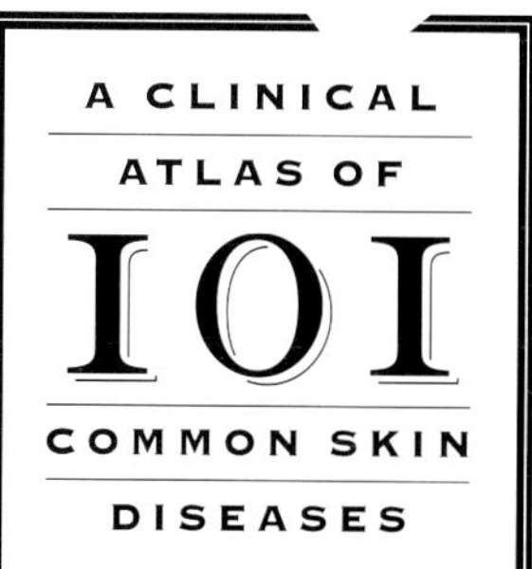
A CLINICAL
ATLAS OF
IOI
COMMON SKIN
DISEASES

A CLINICAL ATLAS OF 101 COMMON SKIN DISEASES

with Histopathologic Correlation

A. BERNARD ACKERMAN

HELMUT KERL

JORGE SÁNCHEZ

YING GUO · ANGELIKA HOFER

PAUL KELLY · TETSU KIMURA

GIOVANNI BORRONI · CHARLES
CRUTCHFIELD · VOLKER STEINKRAUS
WOLFGANG WEYERS

Ardor Scribendi
NEW YORK CITY

To the memory of those dermatologic forebears,

exemplified by Carl Truman Nelson, who were fascinated

by diseases of the skin, who advanced knowledge of those

diseases, and who cared for and about patients

and

to those dermatologists in situ *who will sustain that*

lofty tradition, among them Katrin Kerl and Julio Sánchez.

ACKNOWLEDGMENTS

THE IDEA FOR THIS ATLAS came from A. Bernard Ackerman, M.D., who also was its architect and its principal author. Collaborating with him closely, from beginning to end, were Jorge Sánchez and Helmut Kerl, who wrote the sections about "Therapy," and "Adjunctive Diagnostic Tests," and who were engaged fully and passionately in every one of the many sessions in which photographs were selected, legends were crafted, and ideas were forged, debated, and refined. They, too, read through draft after draft and page proof after galley. Bernie Ackerman and Jorge Sánchez were at the press in Indiana for three days in early February 2000, overseeing every detail of the work as it was being printed.

Wolfie Weyers made valuable additions to the Preface.

Angelika Hofer organized the entire project in regard to the more than 30,000 photographs that were screened initially, the deliberate process of narrowing choices, and, eventually, the selections with finality.

Helmut Kerl and his department of dermatology in Graz supplied more than two-thirds of the photographs that appear in the atlas. The rest were provided by Giovanni Borroni, Charles Crutchfield, Paul Kelly, Tetsu Kimura, Volker Steinkraus, and Wolfgang Weyers. Those coworkers also participated in several of the intensive working sessions during which the very best pictures were chosen. A few photographs were furnished by Bruce Bart, Helmut Hintner, Emmilia Hodak, Wilhelm Meigel, Luis Requeña, Martin Sangueza, and Norman Walton.

Most of the photographs were "shot" by Anton Sams and Werner Stieber of Graz, the remainder being by photographers and colleagues in Giessen, Hamburg, Los Angeles, Minneapolis, Pavia, and Sapporo.

Ying Guo took all of the photomicrographs.

The manuscript was typed and retyped many times by Christina Nyborg.

Sarah Fitz-Hugh did the copy editing.

Florence Nygaard was the proofreader.

Louise Fili and Mary Jane Callister created the design.

John Matey of Hollis Digital Imaging oversaw every aspect of the production process, including page composition by Wendy Voorhees of Painted Pony Typography Service.

CONTENTS

PREFACE

WHAT PROMPTED THE undertaking of this pocket atlas of dermatology? The reasons were several and varied, among them the following:

1. PICTURES ARE AND always have been an extraordinarily valuable vehicle in the study of clinical dermatology. The first textbook of modern dermatology by Robert Willan, titled *Description and Treatment of Cutaneous Diseases* and published more than 200 years ago in 1798, was the first to use pictures for purposes of teaching clinical attributes of skin diseases. That Willan understood well the importance of illustrations to the achievement of his purpose is apparent in his words: "In order to convey distinct ideas on the subject, I shall elucidate every genus by coloured engravings representing some of its most striking varieties. This method is new, and will be attended with many advantages. . . . " In his book, Willan was the first to classify skin diseases systematically, according to different appearances of their individual lesions—such as macules, papules, and pustules—a method that has remained the basis of diagnosis in dermatology to this day. The success of Willan's book, however, was largely attributable to the drawings housed in it.

Willan's use of pictures had an impact on all subsequent texts devoted to clinical dermatology. Hardly any textbook of skin diseases published in the ensuing 200 years was devoid of illustrations. Furthermore, the publication of pictures by Willan gave impetus, beginning in the middle third of the 19th century, to enthusiasm for publication of atlases that sought to portray skin diseases of all kinds as realistically and as beautifully as possible. This objective was achieved remarkably well by startlingly magnificent paintings in volumes like those of Jean-Louis Alibert, Erasmus Wilson, Ferdinand von Hebra, Salomon Ehrmann, Robert Taylor, Prince Morrow, and Radcliffe Crocker, and the riveting lifelike moulages shown in volumes like the ones by Eduard Jacobi and by Leopold Arzt and Karl Zieler. In the 20th century, photographs became the mode of recording diseases morphologically in atlases of dermatology. Some of those atlases, especially the one by Pierre de Graciansky and Stephane Boulle published in 1955, contained photographs of superb quality.

In general, however, the quality of photographs of skin diseases in atlases published in the last third of the 20th century has declined; they have failed to capture the character of skin lesions in a manner comparable to the paintings and moulages of the 19th century. Not only is that statement true of photographs printed in black and white, but also of those in the more recent past that have been exhibited in color. The atlases of the 19th century were art books that enabled students of skin diseases to appreciate lesions in their many hues and surface characteristics, as well as to learn something about the impact of those lesions on the human beings who bore them; the artists rendered facies in a remarkably poignant way that told of the anguish of metastatic carcinoma and conveyed the madness of factitious dermatitis. In this volume we have set out to produce an atlas of dermatology that is a work of art as well as a work of substance.

2. NEARLY ALL CONTEMPORARY atlases devoted to dermatology have portrayed particular skin diseases in but very few images, often only a single photograph or two or three at most per subject. As Willan acknowledged in the preface to his book, pictures of diseases cannot "extend to every minute circumstance in the course of a disease, being necessarily taken at some fixed period of it." We have sought deliberately to capture as many facets as possible of every disease under consideration here, and to do so by showing as many photographs as we deemed necessary to accomplish that purpose; in one case, no fewer than 88 are requisite for a single disease. We have chosen only images of impeccable quality and of incomparable teaching value; for every one photograph selected, scores were rejected. In short, we have tried diligently to teach clinical dermatology superbly through the pictures printed in the pages that follow.

3. VIRTUALLY EVERY ATLAS of dermatology has depicted lesions in the skin of Caucasians only. We have determined to produce an atlas with universal application, mandating thereby the showing of lesions in the skin of Africans, Asians, and Native Americans, as well as of Caucasians. And that is why the dermatologists who were responsible for selecting photographs for this atlas were recruited from all corners of the world.

4. THE TEACHING OF clinical dermatology has declined dramatically in recent years, as dermatology as a specialty has become increasingly a province of surgery and cosmetology and, concurrently, less and less a sovereign state of internal medicine. Coincident with that decline have been the effects on medicine in the United States of managed care, one of the results of which has been that more and more patients with skin diseases are being seen by gener-

alists, and fewer and fewer are being managed by dermatologists. But those physicians in addition to generalists who are actually caring for most patients with skin diseases—for example, pediatricians, gynecologists, and internists—are receiving less and less training in the diagnosis of skin diseases, and the instruction they are being given is of declining worth. We have sought in this atlas to compensate for the deterioration in the teaching of clinical dermatology by producing a volume that would be inordinately educational to those interested seriously in learning about common diseases of the skin, from medical students to residents in dermatology, from generalists to internists, from nurses to physician assistants. We hope that general pathologists and even seasoned dermatologists will profit from this work.

5. ALL TOO MANY atlases of dermatology are not really atlases; they are texts to which a few pictures have been added. We have been committed to preparing instead an authentic atlas in which the pictures do the teaching, and the text, including the legends to photographs, serves to complement them. If any picture in this atlas fails to convey compellingly an important aspect of a disease, we will have fallen short of our purpose.

6. ATLASES OF DERMATOLOGY extant do not, for the most part, strive to teach a method for diagnosis and, concurrently, a comprehension of skin diseases. We have endeavored to accomplish both ends by constructing each of the 101 chapters in a methodical way. Each chapter begins with a terse definition of the disease itself, followed by a photograph that portrays typical clinical features of a particular disease. Accompanying it are photomicrographs shot at low and high magnification that capture stereotypical histopathologic findings of the disease and serve as a vehicle to accomplish correlation with the gross findings. Thereafter, in sequence, is a schema just like the one a clinician should employ in examining an actual patient with a skin disease—namely, distribution of lesions, arrangement of lesions, configuration of lesions, and attributes of individual lesions. The sum of those findings, in algorithmic fashion, should lead an examiner to a specific, accurate diagnosis.

Comprehension of each disease is heightened, where appropriate, by showing, pictorially, the life of the lesions that constitute that disease, and the life of the disease in chronological sequence. Unconventional variations in clinical appearance also are shown. A statement about course is followed by a comment that seeks to integrate the morphologic findings, clinically and histopathologically, with the biologic course. Last, a few lines are devoted to practical, effective therapy, the rationale for which is predicated on a grasp of morphologic and biologic aspects of a particular disease.

7. MANY TEXTS AND atlases of dermatology represent a mere reshuffling of "knowledge"; the information is presented in a less than comprehensible way. Authors tend to copy from one another and to perpetuate clichés. Original ideas are in short supply. A critical perspective based on actual "hands on"experience with patients is missing all too often from those volumes.

We have sought to bring to bear on these pages our own considerable experience with patients and to convey it to those who use this atlas. We have done our best to accomplish that desideratum in a distinctive and instructive way. For example, we have scrupulously avoided the use of trite expressions that abound in dermatology, like "silvery scales" for psoriasis, "footprints in the snow" for lichen planopilaris of the scalp, and "salmon color" for pityriasis rosea. Those banalities are not helpful to an inquisitive, thoughtful student of diseases of the skin. For the most part, we make no reference in legends to photographs to the "stereotypical" color of lesions of diseases because those hues, too, are clichés, being applicable only to skin of lightly pigmented Caucasians; for just one example, pityriasis rosea in darkly pigmented Africans is not salmon colored!

We have also tried diligently to eschew incorrect concepts and to refrain from perpetuating them, such as the myth that three types of acanthosis nigricans exist—benign, pseudo-, and malignant; the typing of melanoma as lentigo maligna, superficial spreading, acral lentiginous, and nodular; and the idea of small-plaque parapsoriasis and large-plaque parapsoriasis as being something other than patches of mycosis fungoides. By avoiding clichés and erroneous concepts, and by striving to integrate the often many and varied morphologic expressions of a single disease, we have made a conscientious effort to elucidate subjects without oversimplifying them.

8. EVER SINCE INDIVIDUAL lesions of the skin were defined and given names, first by the Viennese physician Joseph Jakob Plenck, and then by London dermatologist Robert Willan, dermatologic terminology has suffered from inconsistencies that have hampered communication and, inevitably, have compromised teaching of the subject. Willan, for example, distinguished

three major types of papules without making clear their morphologic differences. In textbooks of the last 30 years, the definition of papules has varied considerably; they are defined as solid elevations smaller than 0.5 cm in diameter in the textbook by Braun-Falco et al., as solid elevations smaller than 1.0 cm in diameter in the textbook of Fitzpatrick et al., and as the size of a lentil in the textbook by Korting, notwithstanding the fact that the size of lentils varies greatly. In order to avoid such inconsistencies and to employ a language that is crisp and precise, we have set forth prior to the presentation of individual diseases our definition of individual skin lesions, which are the most important words and phrases we use in this atlas.

9. SIMPLIFICATION OF SUBJECTS was also meant to be enhanced by our decision to craft succinct legends to photographs. Toward that end, for example, we have made no mention of a particular anatomic site, e.g., the penis, if a glance at a picture makes obvious the site. An exception occurs when the anatomic site is crucial to clinical diagnosis, such as in photodermatitis. In such circumstances, particularly in the section of each chapter given to distribution of lesions, site is mentioned for the purpose of emphasis.

We have also made brief the definition of each of the 101 diseases that constitute the chapters of this volume. It encompasses only those attributes essential to the accurate characterization of each of them. Of course succinctness carries with it the risk of incompleteness, but our goal was not to write a textbook. It was to cut a pictorial swath so wide through common skin diseases that a novice could gain an understanding of those diseases, and an experienced practitioner could conceive of all diseases already well known to him or her in a fresh, novel, and more profound way.

10. ALTHOUGH THIS ATLAS emphasizes the clinical aspects of common skin diseases, we have attempted to correlate clinical and histopathologic features and to explain the findings by gross pathology—i.e., the clinical attributes—on the basis of the findings by conventional microscopy. That effort at correlation is exemplified not only at the outset of each chapter, where the clinical picture is joined by photomicrographs, but also near the end of each chapter in the section titled "Integration: Unifying Concept." Our major purpose in that section is to convey the gross pathologic aspects of skin disease in vivo—what clinicians encounter in their daily practice of medicine. Exposure to gross pathology is what practitioners need, not dizzying references to "retic-

ular alteration of the epidermis," "flame figures," and "Miescher's radial granulomas." Nonetheless, histopathologists, e.g., general pathologists, can profit greatly from this atlas because the surfeit of pictures it contains should enable them to begin to achieve what for many of them has been beyond attainment, to wit, clinicopathologic correlation of diseases they usually meet at their microscopes as sections of tissue from punched-out, shaved-off, and curetted specimens. It merits mention that each of the contributors to this atlas is a dermatologist as well as a dermatopathologist.

The organization of the diseases in this atlas is alphabetical (just as it was almost 100 years ago in a textbook titled *La Pratique Dermatologique* by the French dermatologists, Besnier, Brocq, and Jacquet). All other attempts to classify skin diseases clinically, e.g., "eczematous dermatitis," "disorders of cell kinetics," "benign neoplasms and hyperplasias," and "precancerous lesions and cutaneous carcinomas," have failed because they lack logic and, therefore, consistency.

The names given to the diseases in this work are the ones most dermatologists use. For example, we refer to Darier's disease rather than "keratosis follicularis," Grover's disease instead of "transient acantholytic dermatosis," and Mucha-Habermann disease in lieu of "pityriasis lichenoides et varioliformis acuta" and "pityriasis lichenoides chronica." Some diseases of particular importance, such as melanocytic nevi, melanoma, and mycosis fungoides, have been given more attention than diseases that are also important but less so, such as sebaceous gland hyperplasia, seborrheic dermatitis, and seborrheic keratosis. Parenthetically, the diagnosis of all neoplasms shown, including every melanoma, was verified by histopathologic examination of tissue from a biopsy specimen.

Because we have sought to limit the number of subjects in the atlas to the 101 most common ones, we have had to deviate from our original intention of including in the table of contents discrete specific conditions only, e.g., acne vulgaris, allergic contact dermatitis, and allergic vasculitis. Some subjects incorporated in the contents are more inclusive, to wit, alopecias, cysts and cystic hamartomas, drug eruptions, sclerodermas, viral exanthems, amyloidosis, atypical mycobacterial infections, deep fungal infections, epidermal nevi, connective tissue nevi, epidermolysis bullosa, fibromas, ichthyoses, lymphomas, and porokeratosis. Had we not adopted this system for organization, individual types of alopecia, cysts and cystic hamartomas, and drug eruptions alone would have made up nearly all of the 101 subjects of the book.

In actuality, however, many more than 101 diseases are incorporated in this work. As will become apparent on perusal of the atlas itself, and even the table of contents, more than one disease is covered in various chapters. For example, linear IgA dermatosis is discussed along with dermatitis herpetiformis, herpes gestationis with bullous pemphigoid, and phototoxic dermatitis with photoallergic dermatitis. Furthermore, all kinds of benign proliferations of melanocytes, including so-called blue nevi, are incorporated in the chapter about melanocytic nevi and melanotic macules, all kinds of ichthyoses in the chapter devoted to that subject, and all kinds of sclerodermas in the chapter concerning those conditions, to mention but three examples of the breadth of sweep. Last, wherever a skin lesion—be it a cherry hemangioma, a Miescher's nevus, or a seborrheic keratosis—is encountered as an incidental finding in a photograph, we call it to the reader's attention in the legend.

Some decisions about classification were arbitrary. For example, we chose to place varicella in a chapter with herpes simplex and zoster, rather than with the other viral exanthems, some of which also are vesicular, e.g., hand, foot, and mouth disease caused by Coxsackie A 5, 10, and 16.

The decision to make this atlas the size it is was prompted by our desire to produce a handy, ever-available companion that would be light in weight, but weighty in substance. It will fit neatly in a wide pocket, ready for use.

The team that put this atlas together was made up of close colleagues who also are friends. The co-captains were Bernie Ackerman (USA), Helmut Kerl (Austria), and Jorge Sánchez (Puerto Rico). The invaluable players were Ying Guo (Peoples Republic of China/USA), Angelika Hofer (Austria), a resident in the department of dermatology at the University of Graz, who was responsible for managing the team and organizing the material itself—a task that for more than five years she carried out splendidly and with good humor, Paul Kelly (USA), Tetsu Kimura (Japan), Giovanni Borroni (Italy), Charles Crutchfield (USA), Volker Steinkraus (Germany), and Wolfgang Weyers (Germany).

We earnestly hope that those who use our atlas will derive as much benefit and pleasure from it as we have had preparing it!

A. Bernard Ackerman, M.D.
Ackerman Academy of Dermatopathology
New York City
January, 2000

IN SEEKING A SPECIFIC subject, go first to the table of contents, where diseases are listed in alphabetical order. A common disorder may not at first glance be found therein because it may not be the first subject listed in the title. For example, herpes gestationis is treated in the chapter that also addresses bullous pemphigoid, to wit, BULLOUS PEMPHIGOID AND HERPES GESTATIONIS. Some subjects are not specified in a title; for example, insect bites and scabies are found in the chapter titled ARTHROPOD ASSAULTS. If a subject being sought is not discovered quickly in the table of contents, go directly to the index, where all the conditions pictured and discussed in the atlas are recorded alphabetically.

To use a particular chapter most effectively, be aware that photographs are grouped consistently according to distribution, arrangement, configuration, and morphologic attributes of individual lesions. Each chapter begins with the definition of a particular disease, proceeds to morphologic findings, and ends with sections devoted to adjunctive diagnostic tests, course, integration: unifying concept, and therapy.

PLANES *(flush with the level of skin)*

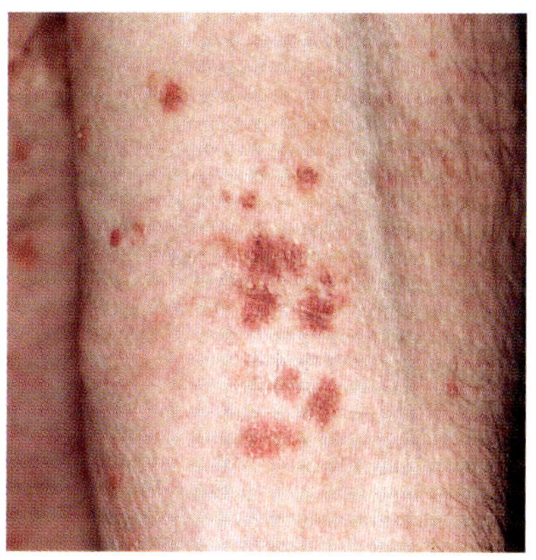

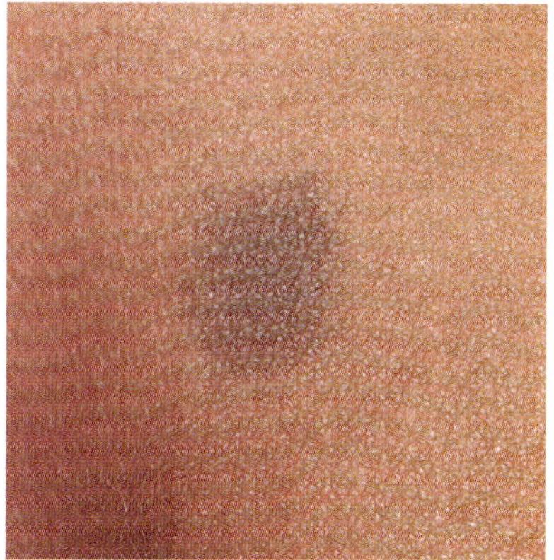

MACULE: *A lesion less than 1.0 cm in greatest dimension that is flush with the level of surrounding normal skin and whose color differs from that of the surrounding normal skin (example: traumatic "senile" purpura).*

PATCH: *A lesion 1.0 cm or larger in greatest dimension that is flush with the level of surrounding normal skin and whose color differs from that of the surrounding normal skin (example: "Mongolian spot").*

ELEVATIONS *(above the level of skin)*

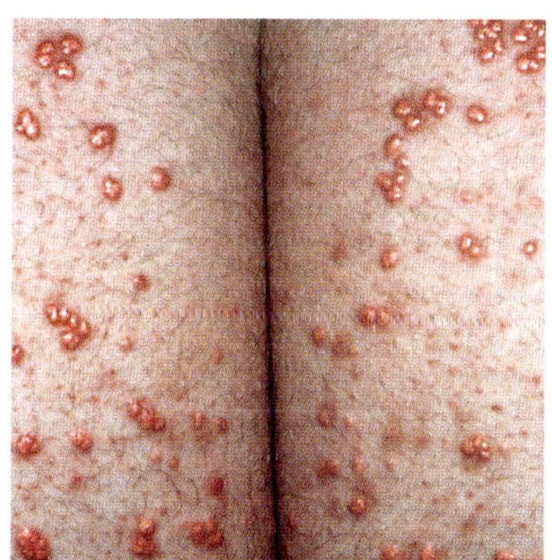

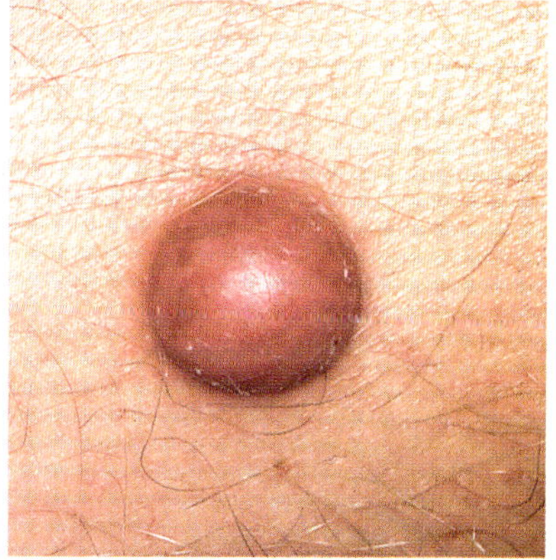

PAPULE: *A solid or cystic elevation less than 1.0 cm in diameter (example: eruptive xanthoma).*

NODULE: *A solid or cystic elevation 1.0 cm or more, but less than 2.0 cm, in diameter (example: dermatofibroma).*

ELEVATIONS *(above the level of skin)*

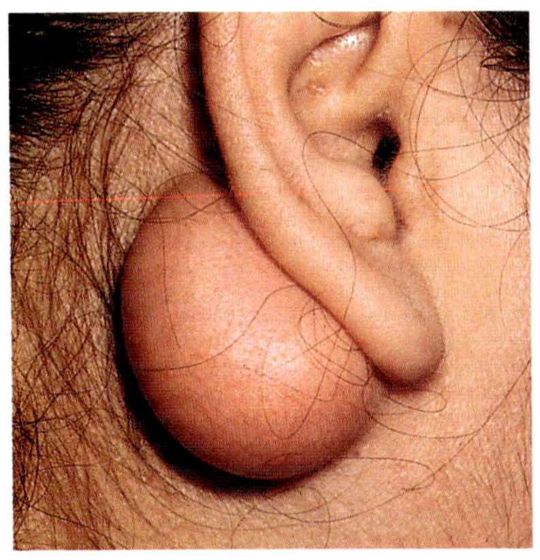

TUMOR: *A solid or cystic elevation 2.0 cm or more in diameter (example: follicular cyst, infundibular type).*

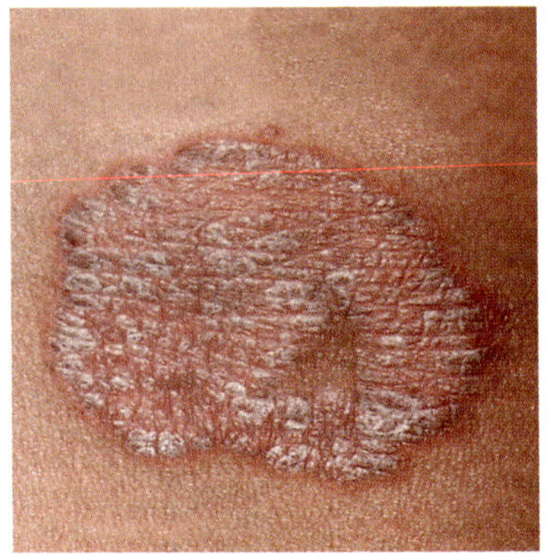

PLAQUE: *A lesion that rises slightly above the surface of the skin and is larger than 1.0 cm in greatest dimension (example: psoriasis).*

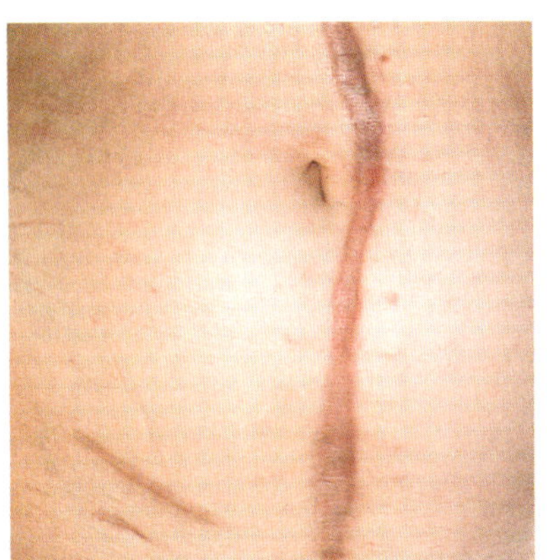

CORD: *A string-like or rope-like structure of variable length (example: hypertrophic scar).*

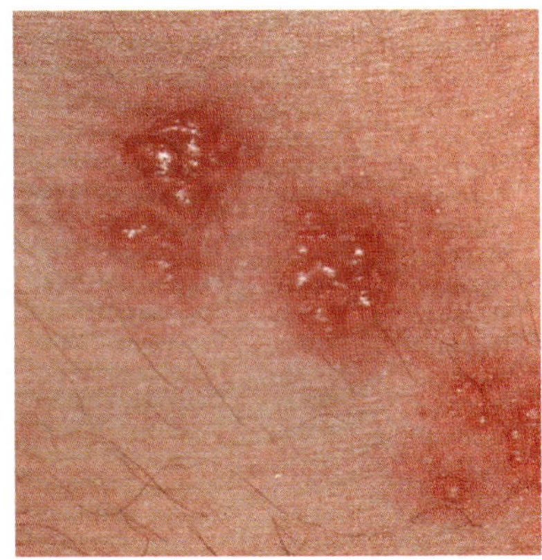

VESICLE: *A noncystic transparent fluid-filled elevation less than 1.0 cm in greatest dimension (example: herpes simplex).*

ELEVATIONS *(above the level of skin)*

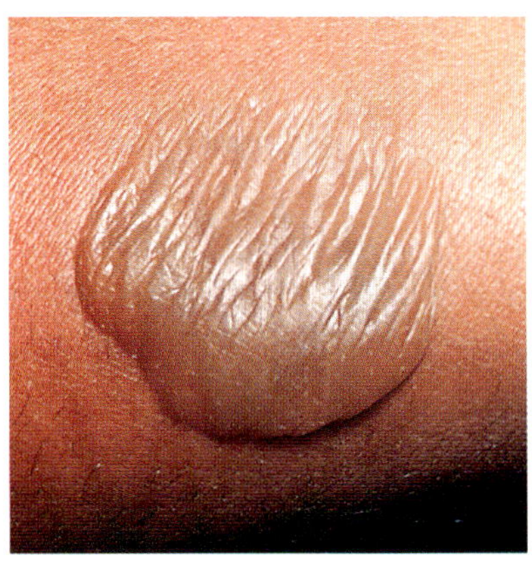

BULLA: *A noncystic, transparent, fluid-filled elevation 1.0 cm or larger in greatest dimension (example: bullous pemphigoid).*

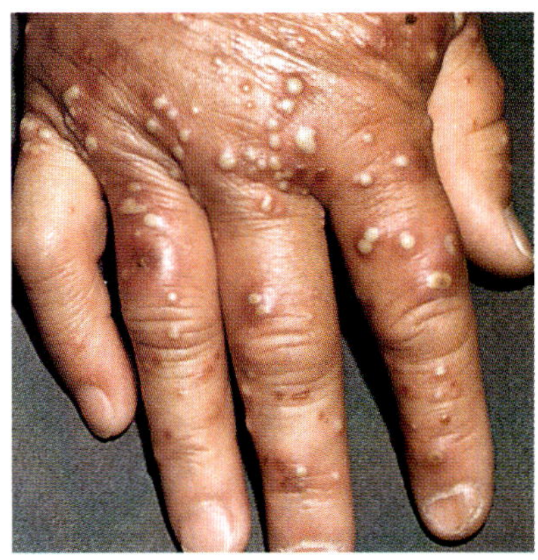

PUSTULE: *An elevation formed of pus (example: drug eruption).*

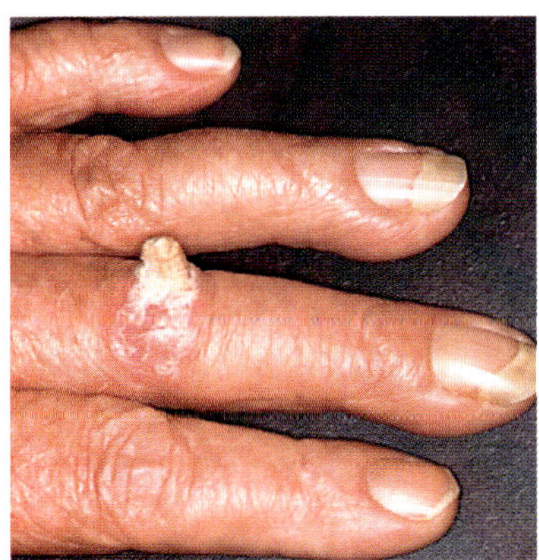

KERATOSIS: *A horny projection from the skin that often takes the form of a spike or spine (example: Bowen's disease).*

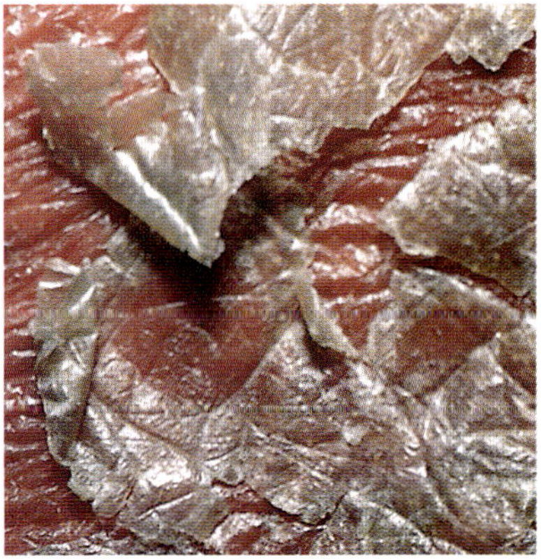

SCALE: *A collection of horn that is visible on the skin as a flake (example: psoriasis).*

ELEVATIONS
(above the level of skin)

DEPRESSIONS
(below the level of skin)

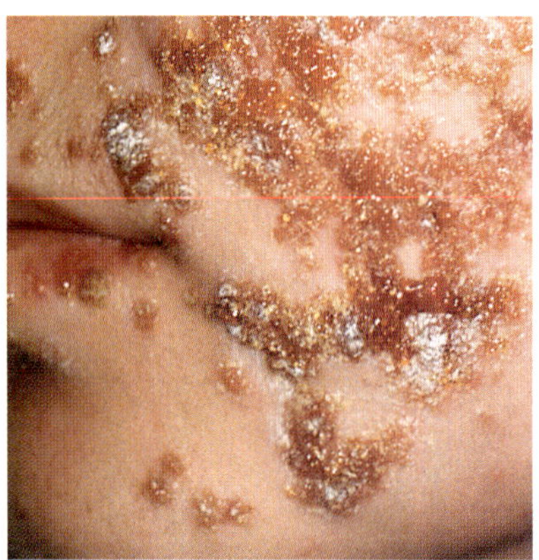

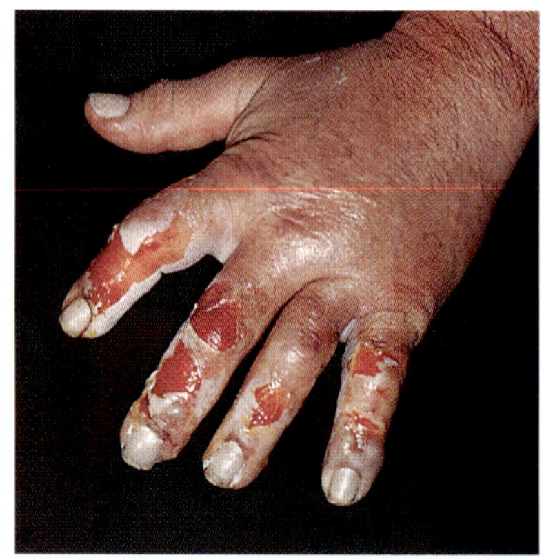

CRUST: *A heap composed of inspissated plasma that contains white blood cells, red blood cells, or both (example: impetigo).*

EROSION: *Loss of part or all of the epidermis (example: burn).*

DEPRESSIONS *(below the level of skin)*

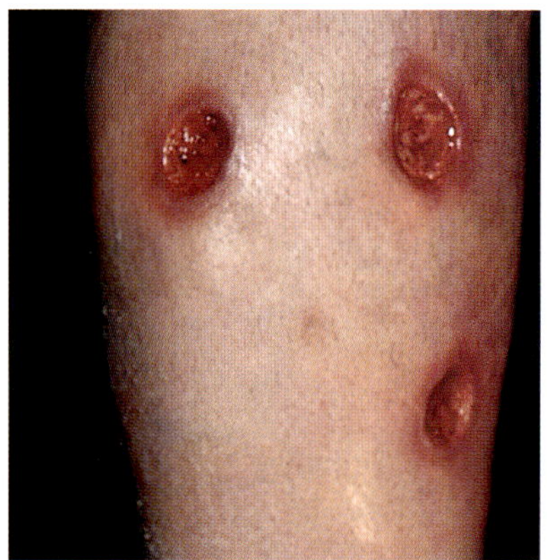

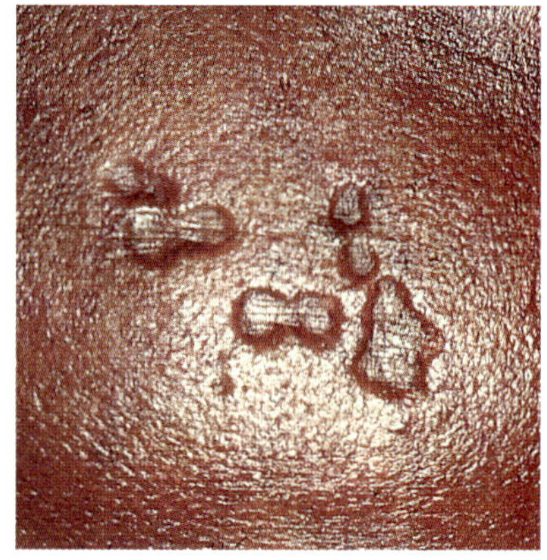

ULCER: *Loss of the entire epidermis and at least some of the dermis (example: ecthyma).*

DELL: *A slight depression or dimple less than 1.0 cm in diameter (example: atrophic scar).*

DEPRESSIONS *(below the level of skin)*

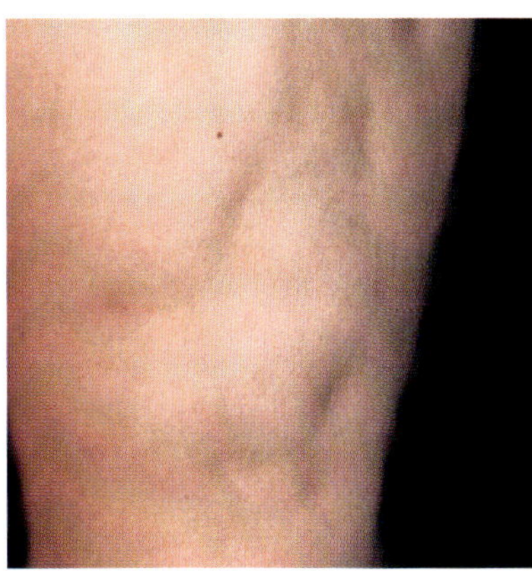

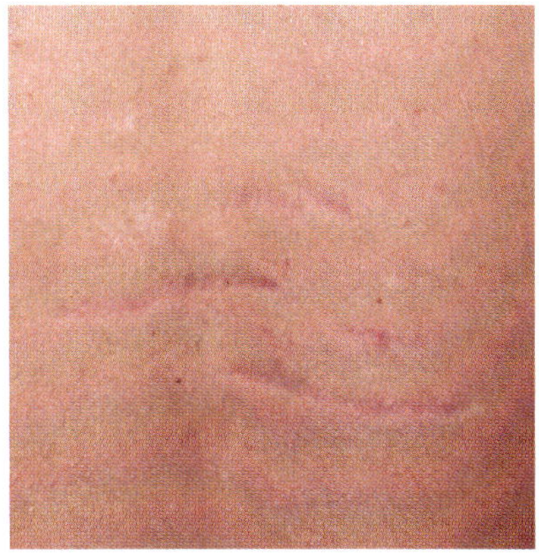

GULLY: *A deep depression, an exaggeration of a dell, greater than 1.0 cm in diameter (example: lupus profundus).*

TROUGH: *A shallow depression greater than 1.0 cm in diameter (example: stria atrophicans).*

OPENINGS *(a parting or break in the skin without loss of epidermis)*

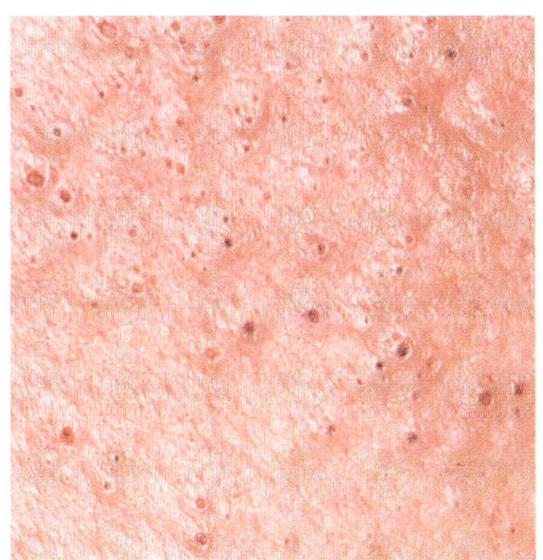

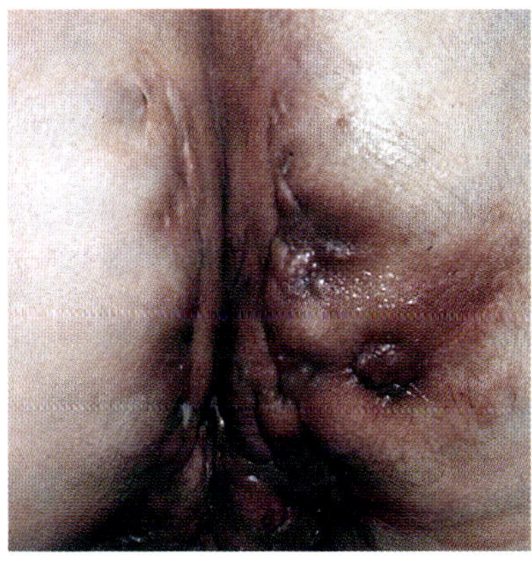

COMEDO: *A horn-filled dilated infundibulum (that also contains sebaceous material and microorganisms) expressing itself clinically as a "blackhead" (example: acne vulgaris).*

SINUS: *An epithelium-lined channel (example: hidradenitis suppurativa).*

OPENINGS *(a parting or break in the skin without loss of epidermis)*

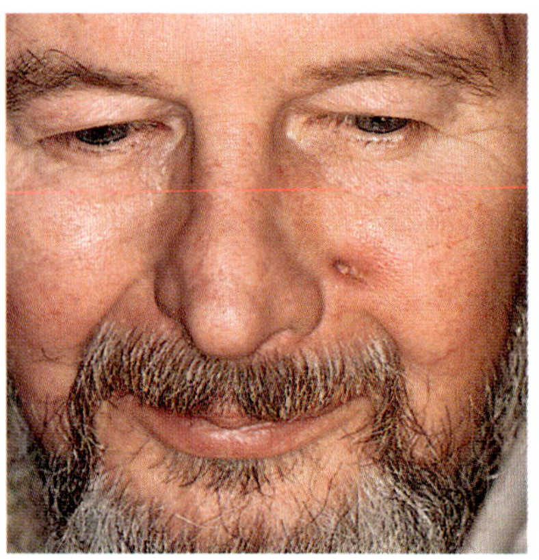

FISTULA: *An epithelium-lined channel that opens to the skin surface and that may originate in the skin or in a structure beneath it, such as an organ like a lymph node, a bone, or the gastrointestinal tract (example: from a periapical abscess).*

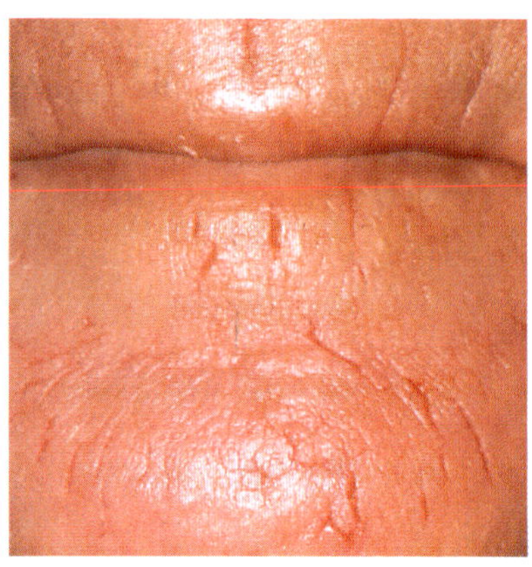

FISSURE: *A linear defect that extends from the surface of the skin to the dermis (example: lichen simplex chronicus).*

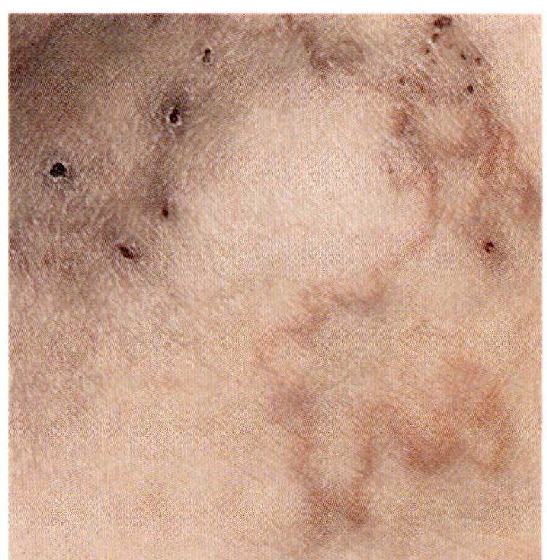

BURROW: *A tunnel fashioned by a parasite in the uppermost part of the skin (example: cutaneous larva migrans).*

DISEASES

DEFINITION Pigmented plaques formed by confluence of smooth-surfaced soft papules, some of which may become polypoid, traversed by accentuations of skin folds. This disease has a predilection for intertriginous regions. The condition may develop consequent to obesity, an endocrine disorder, or a malignant neoplasm in an internal organ. Morphologically, i.e., clinically and histopathologically, the appearance of the altered skin is the same, irrespective of cause.

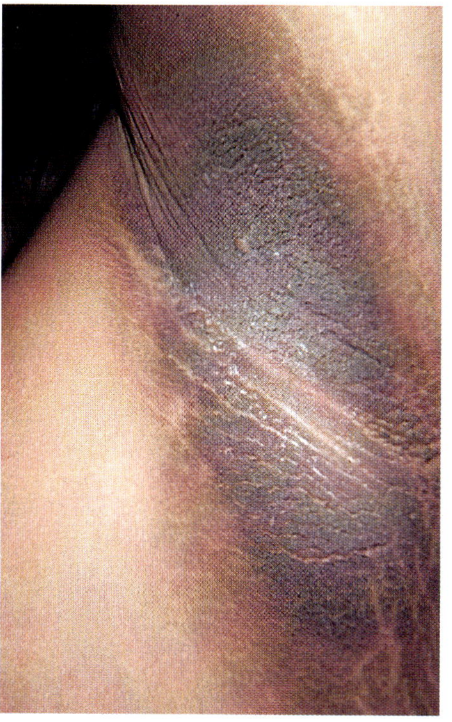

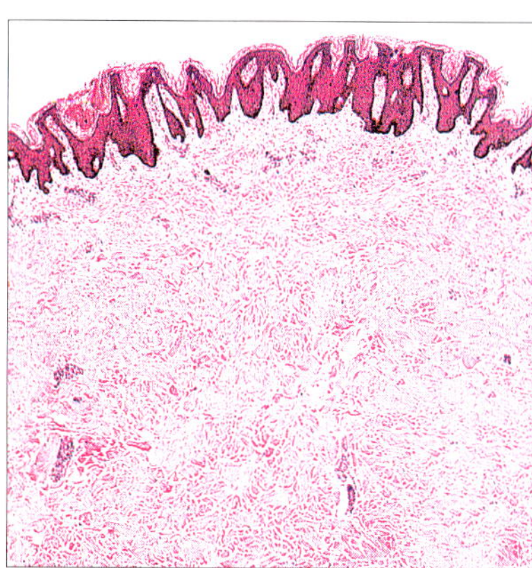

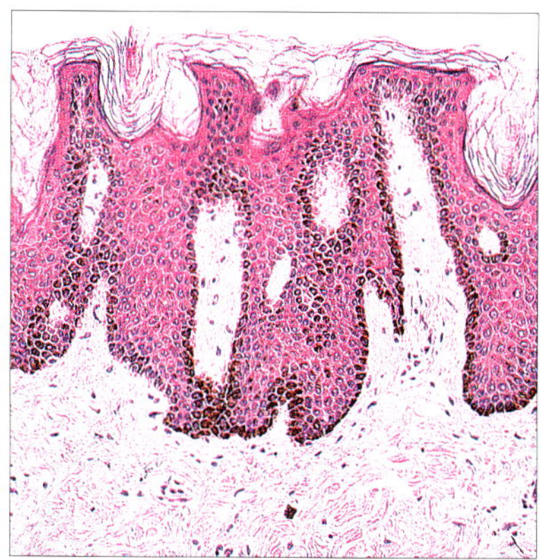

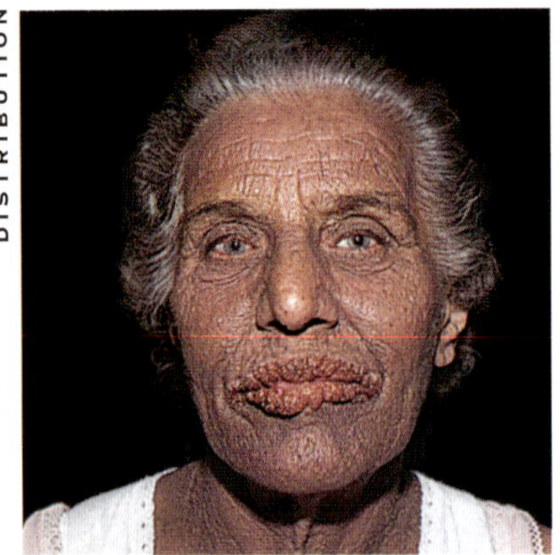

FIG. 1-1 *Widespread acanthosis nigricans. This implies concurrence of an internal malignancy.*

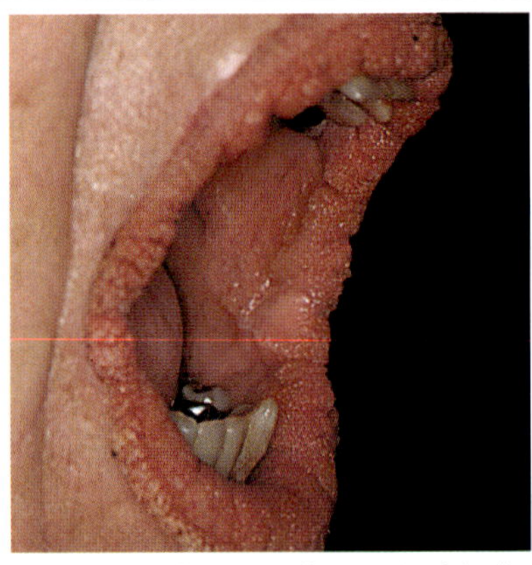

FIG. 1-2 *Confluent papillomatosis of the lips and buccal mucosa.*

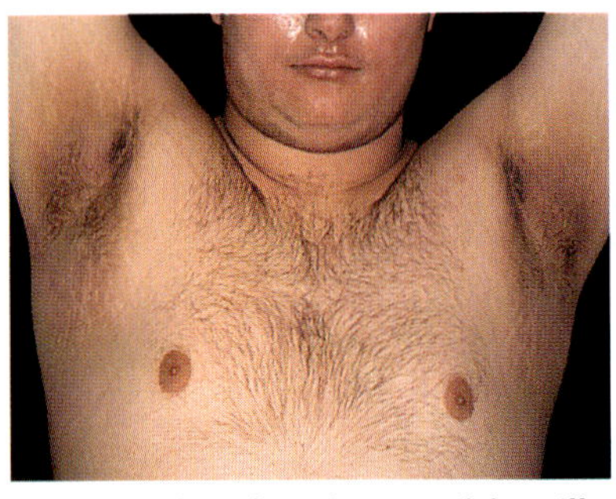

FIG. 1-3 *Bilateral involvement of the axillae in this obese young man with an endocrine disorder.*

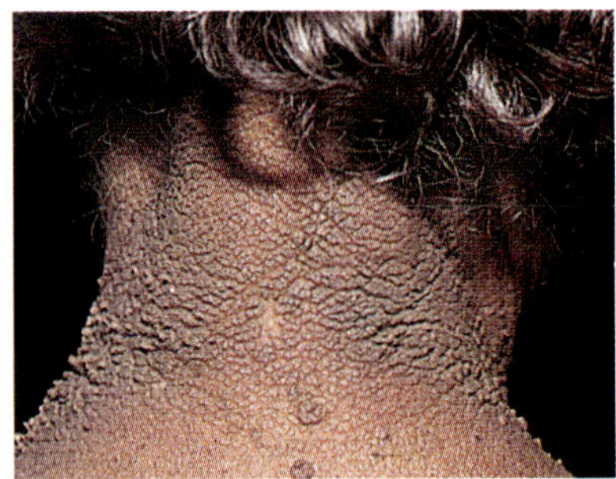

FIG. 1-4 *The neck is a favorite site.*

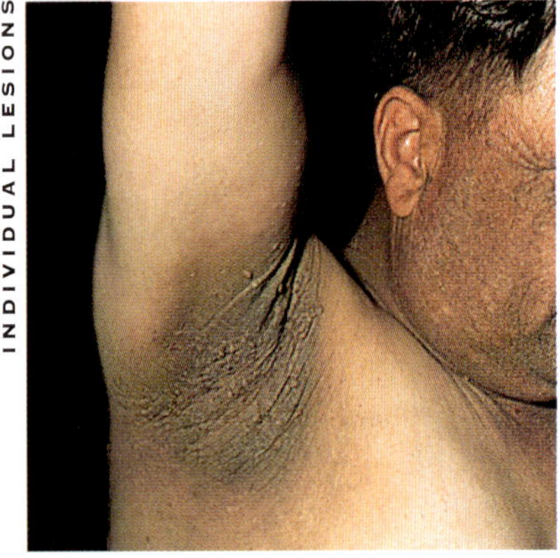

FIG. 1-5 *Closely set tiny papules in linear array.*

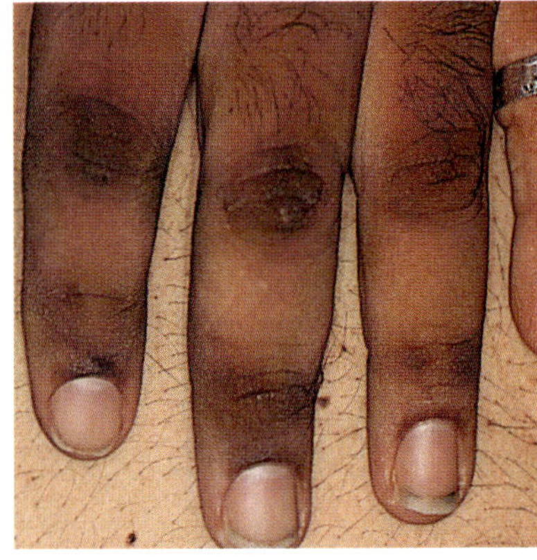

FIG. 1-6 *Lesions situated over joints. Note how dark are the fingers in contrast to the rest of the skin.*

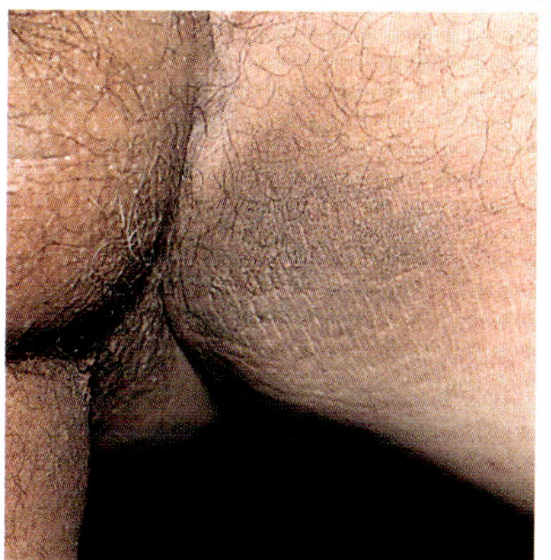

FIG. I-7 *Pigmented plaque with mammillated surface.*

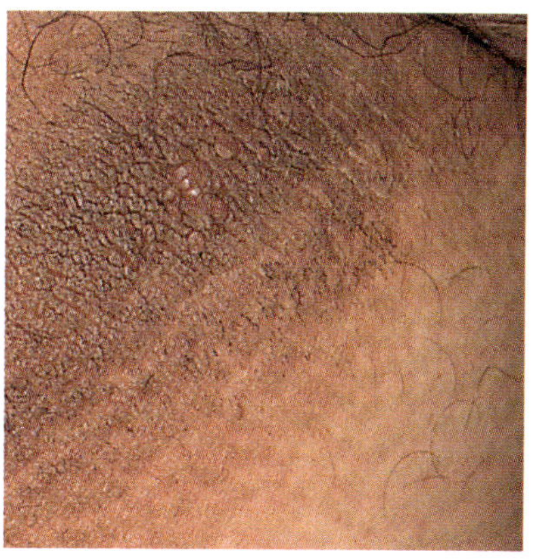

FIG. I-8 *Pigmented, slightly elevated plaque with a gently papillated smooth surface, in this instance punctuated by atrophic striae.*

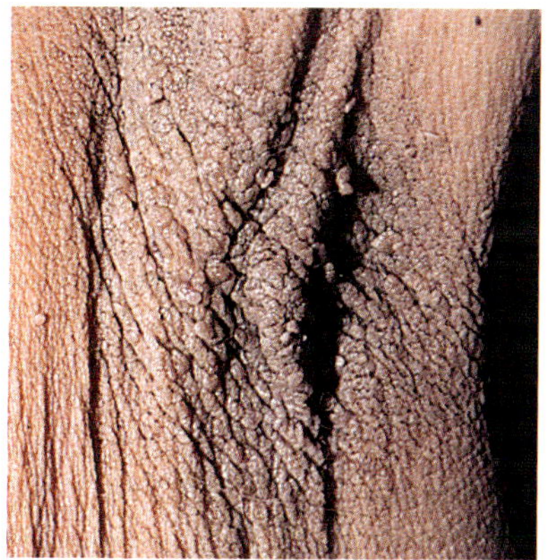

FIG. I-9 *Polypoid excrescences, as well as subtle papules. Grooves that traverse plaques represent accentuation of skin lines.*

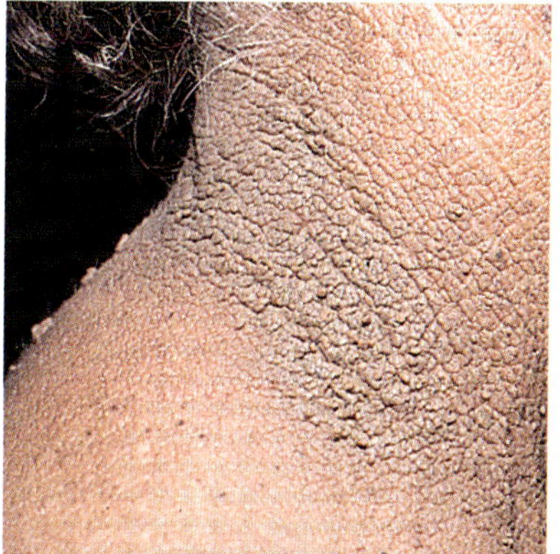

FIG. I-10 *Ill-defined plaque, thrown into folds, made up of prominent, smooth-surfaced papules, some of them polypoid.*

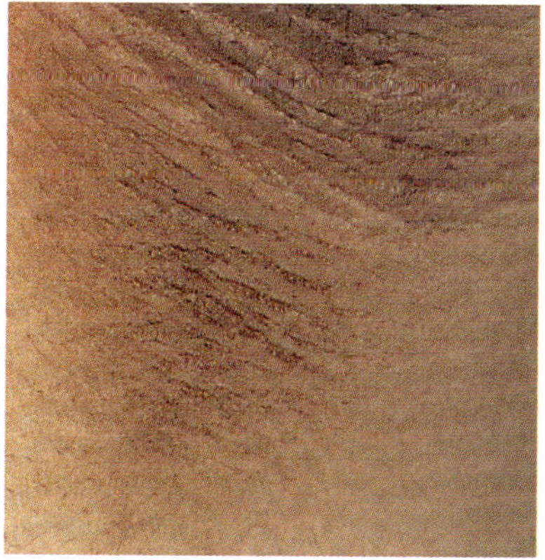

FIG. I-11 *Pigmented plaque in which skin folds are accentuated.*

COURSE Acanthosis nigricans tends to persist unless its cause is identified and corrected. For example, lesions of acanthosis nigricans secondary to an endocrine disorder, such as diabetes mellitus or hypothyroidism, disappear when that abnormality has been remedied by appropriate hormonal therapy. Lesions consequent to the effects of a malignant neoplasm in an internal organ, such as an adenocarcinoma of the stomach or the colon, may regress entirely after complete surgical extirpation of the inciting neoplasm, if that neoplasm has not yet metastasized.

INTEGRATION: UNIFYING CONCEPT Whether acanthosis nigricans is a consequence of an endocrine disorder or of a malignant neoplasm in an internal organ, the morphologic attributes are the same, clinically and histopathologically. When the cause of acanthosis nigricans is remedied, whether by treatment of the endocrine abnormality or by excision of a malignant neoplasm, the lesions of acanthosis nigricans wane and may disappear altogether.

The morphologic features of the confluent and reticulated papillomatosis of Gougerot and Carteaud seem to be those of a muted expression of acanthosis nigricans on an anterior aspect of the trunk.

The mechanism whereby acanthosis nigricans and its variants come to be formed is not known, but in some patients, evidence implicates insulin as an etiologic factor (insulin resistance). In patients with acanthosis nigricans who harbor an internal malignancy, humoral growth factors produced by the neoplastic cells may be important in the formation of the skin lesions.

THERAPY Treatment of lesions of acanthosis nigricans themselves is ineffective. Therapy must be directed at the pathologic process responsible for the development of acanthosis nigricans, such as obesity, an endocrinopathy, or an internal malignancy.

DEFINITION A disease of folliculosebaceous units, in particular infundibula, that may manifest itself solely as noninflammatory lesions, i.e., comedones and intact cysts, or as inflammatory lesions, i.e., papules, nodules, and pustules. The process may resolve without residua or with scars of different types, e.g., keloidal or atrophic, including cribriform. The condition usually affects adolescents, but may at times be seen in neonates and young adults.

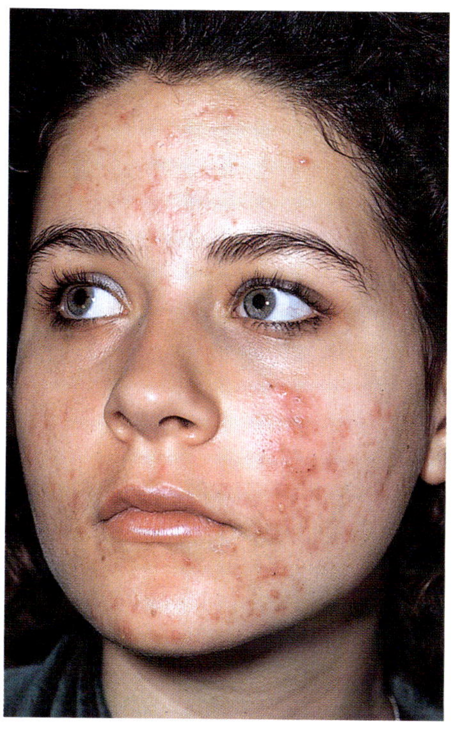

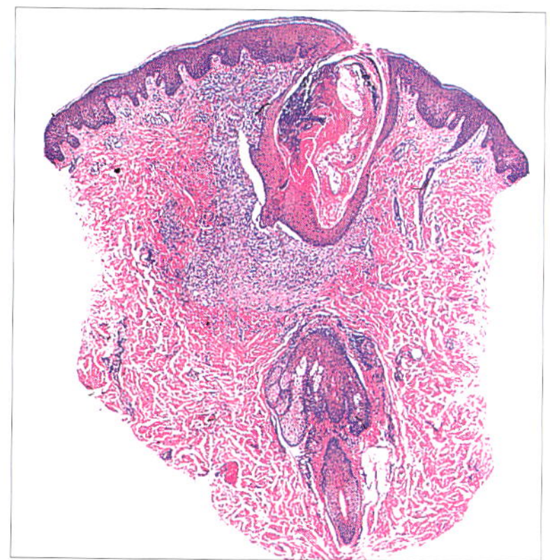

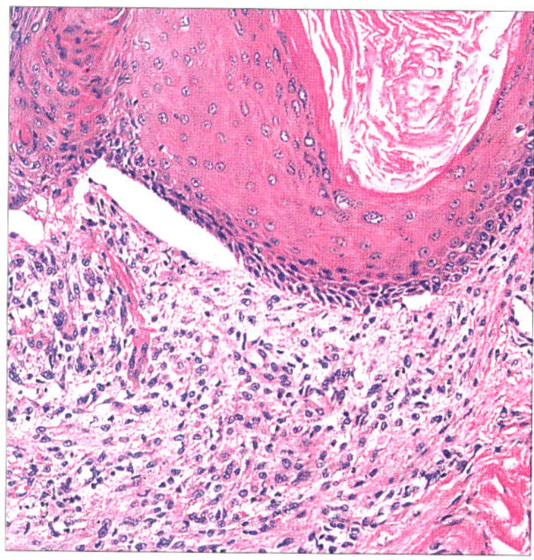

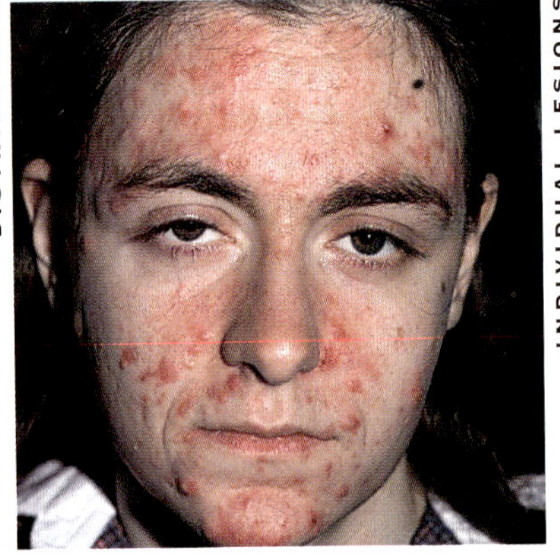

FIG. 2-1 *The face is the favored site.*

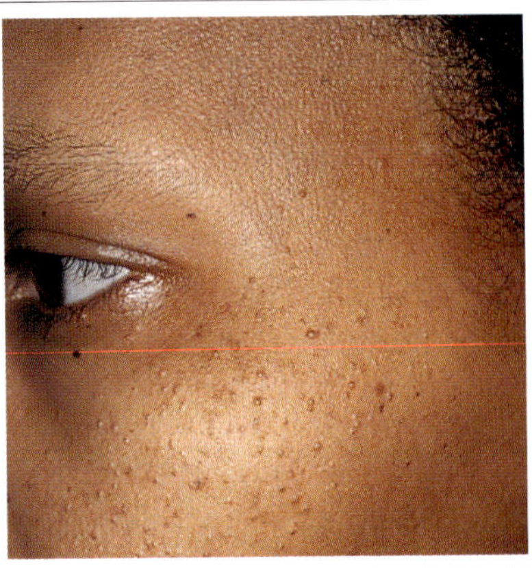

FIG. 2-2 *Comedones may be "open" (black) and "closed" (white).*

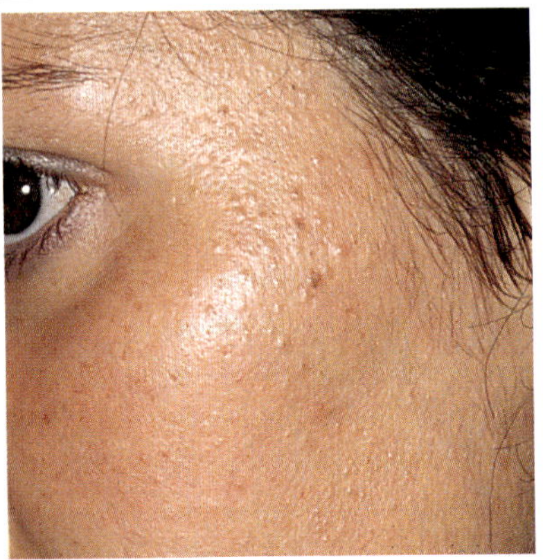

FIG. 2-3 *Comedones, "open" and "closed," the latter being synonymous with milia.*

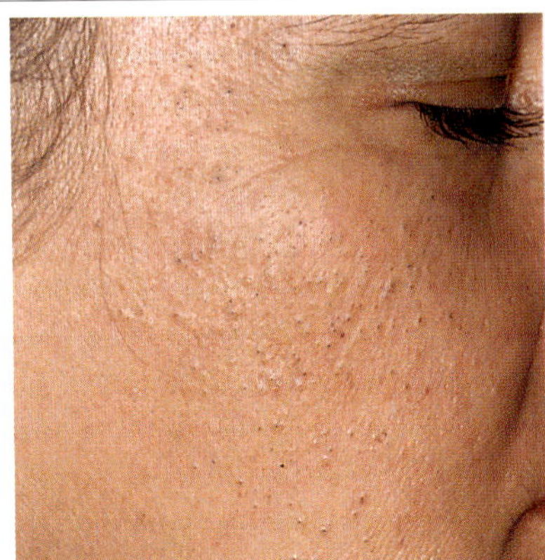

FIG. 2-4 *"Open" comedones are present mostly, but milia are, too.*

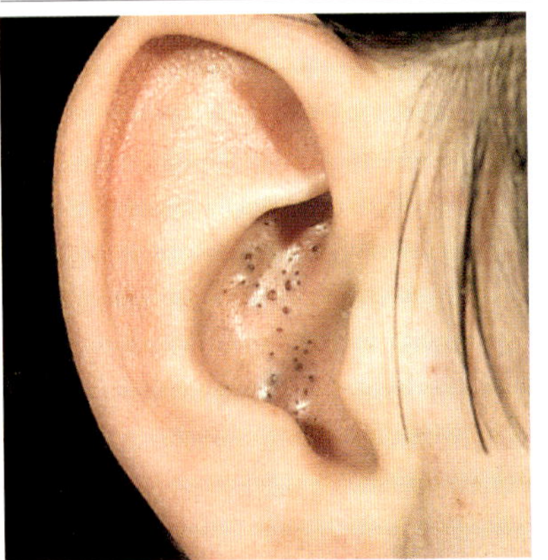

FIG. 2-5 *A cluster of comedones situated on an uncommon site.*

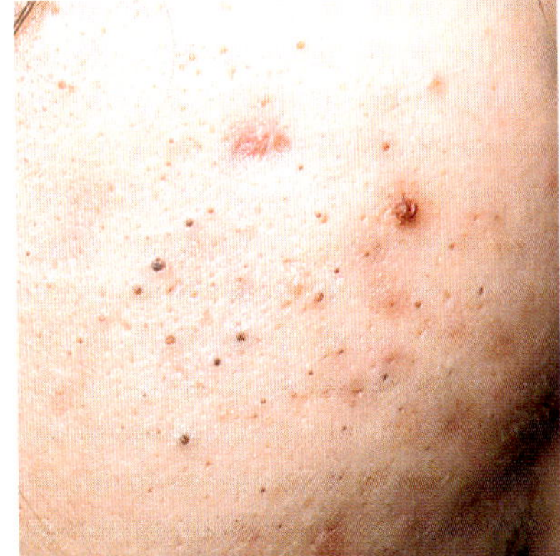

FIG. 2-6 *Comedones, inflamed papules, and tiny atrophic scars.*

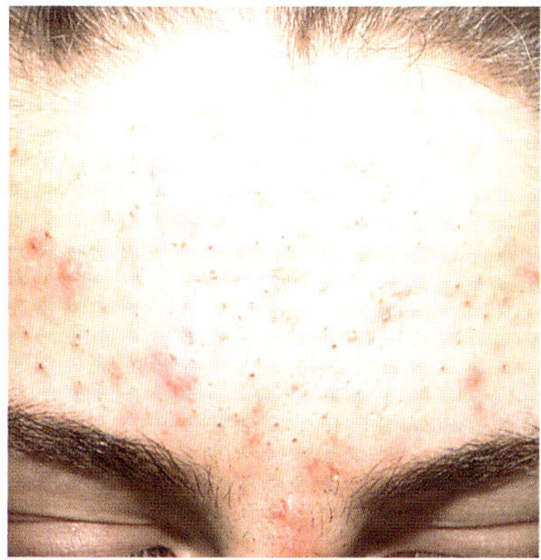

FIG. 2-7 *Comedones, inflamed papules, and tiny pitted scars.*

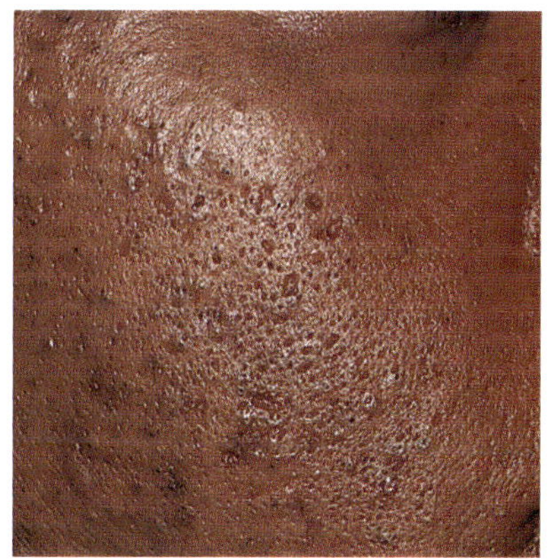

FIG. 2-8 *Comedones, patulous follicles, and small atrophic scars.*

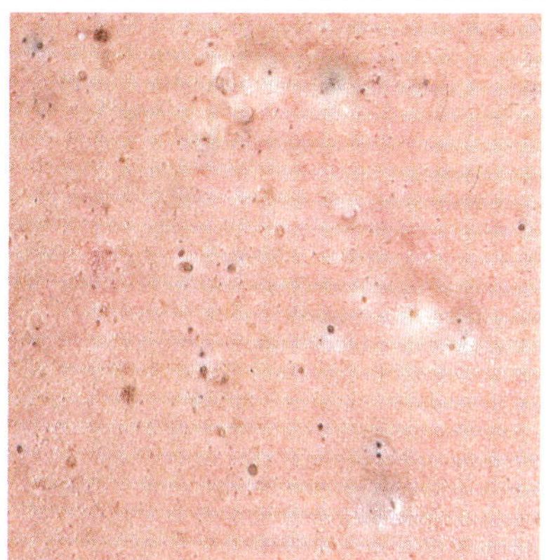

FIG. 2-9 *Comedones, patulous follicles, and tiny atrophic scars.*

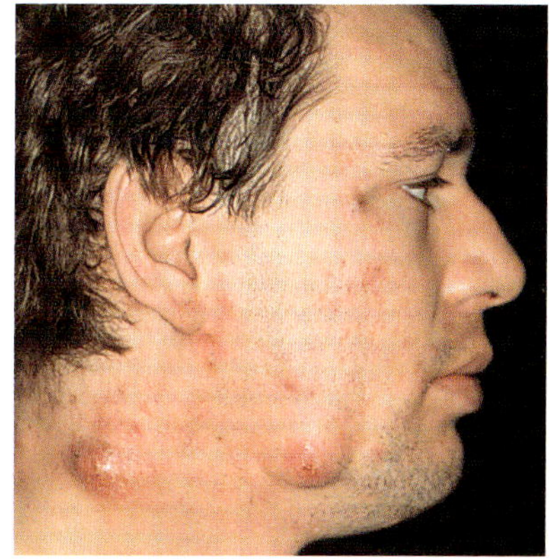

FIG. 2-10 *Inflamed papules and nodules, as well as scars. The nodules represent the effects of rupture of follicular cysts.*

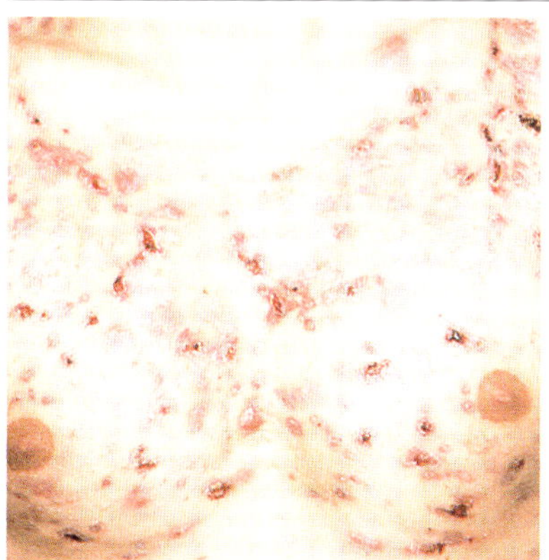

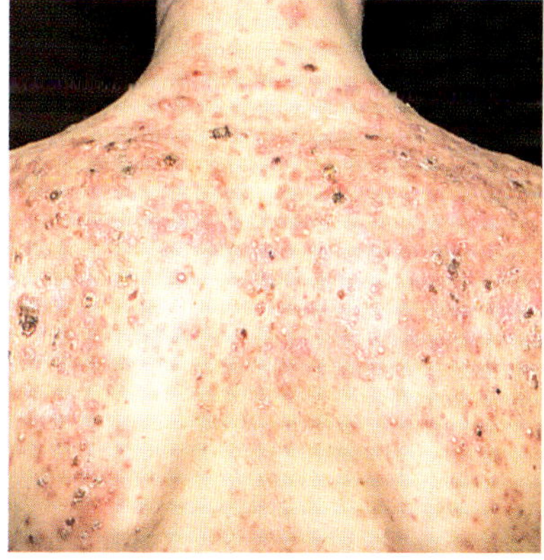

FIG. 2-11 (A, B) *The upper part of the chest is a common site, as is the upper part of the back.*

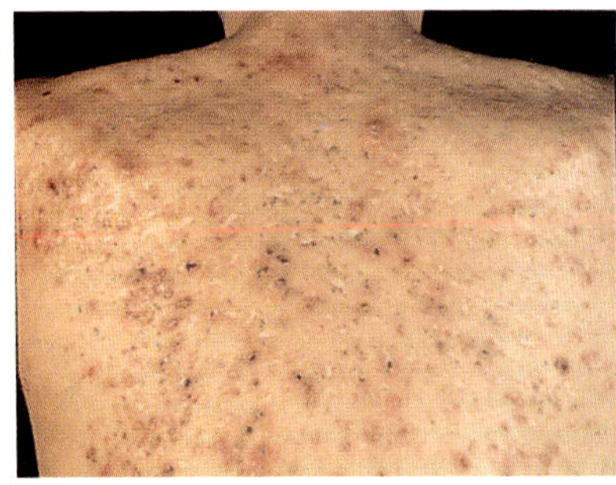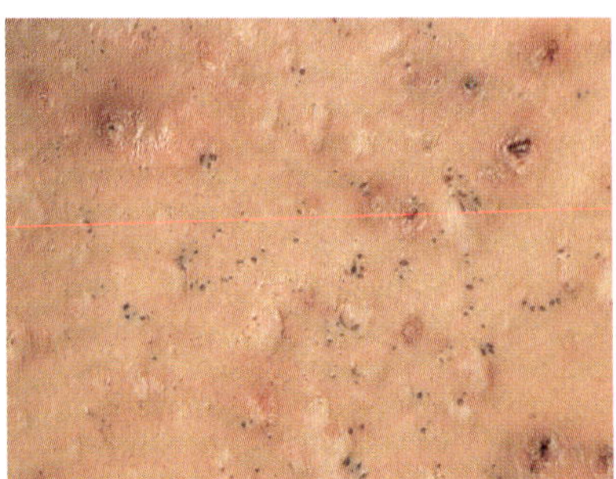

FIG. 2-12 (A, B) *Comedones, patulous follicles, inflamed papules, pustules, hemorrhagic crusts, and scars; (b) closeup view of (a).*

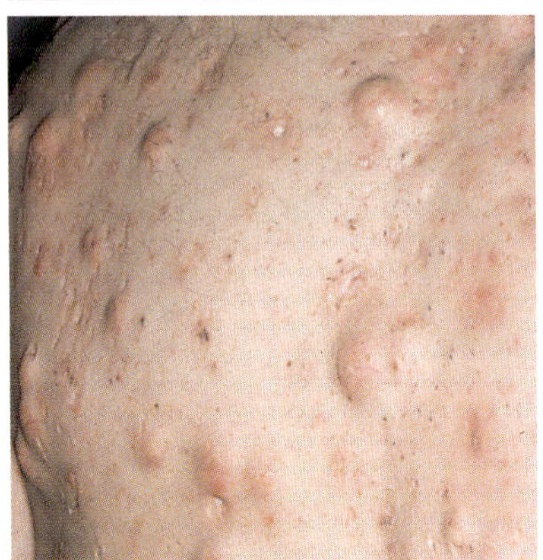

FIG. 2-13 *Comedones, patulous ostia of follicles, inflamed papules, inflamed nodules (ruptured infundibular cysts), and scars.*

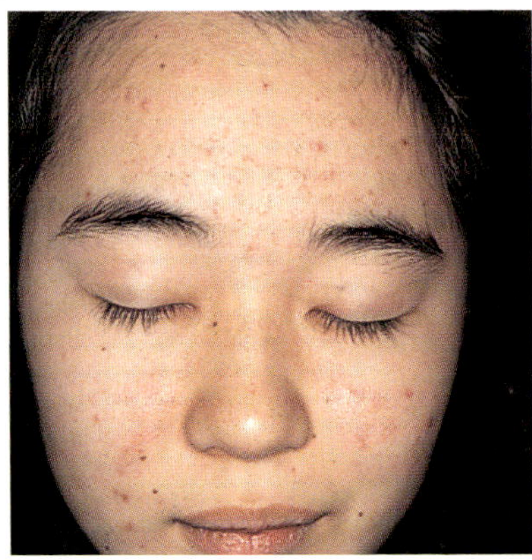

FIG. 2-14 *Inflamed papules, some of them excoriated ("acne excoriée des jeunes filles" because it occurs mostly in young girls).*

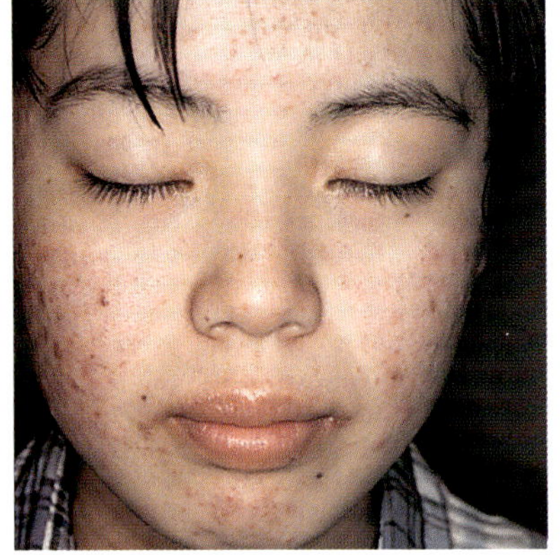

FIG. 2-15 *Comedones, inflamed papules (some of them excoriated), and scars.*

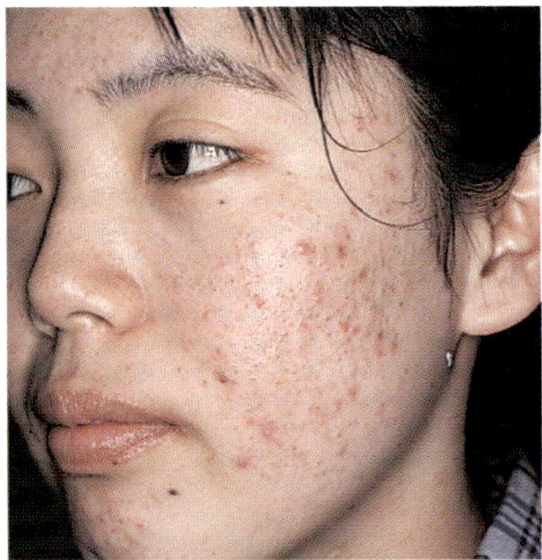

FIG. 2-16 *Comedones, inflamed papules, and a few pustules.*

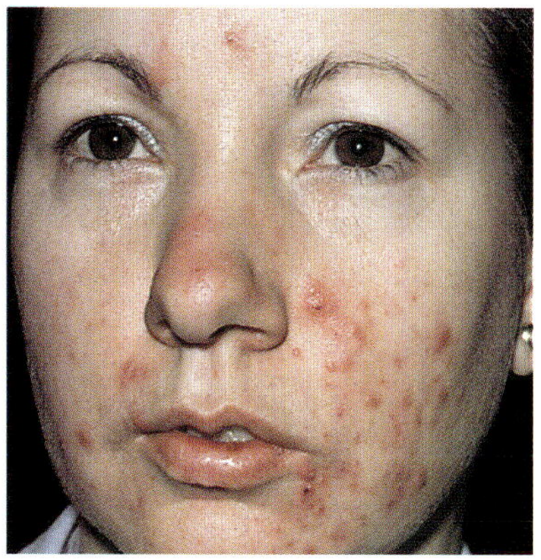

FIG. 2-17 *Inflamed papules and papulopustules.*

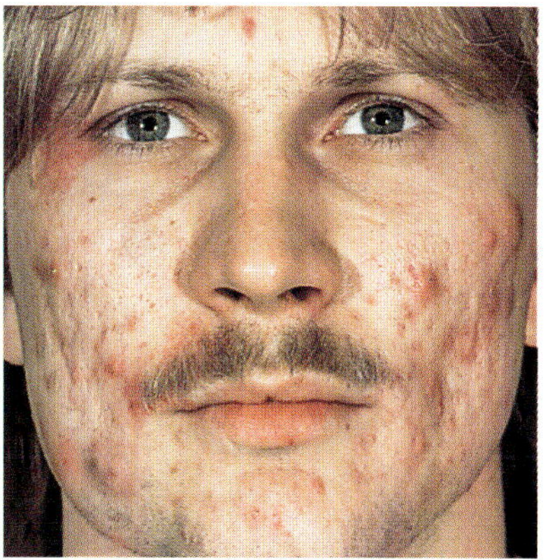

FIG. 2-18 *Patulous ostia of follicles, inflamed papules, pustules, and scars.*

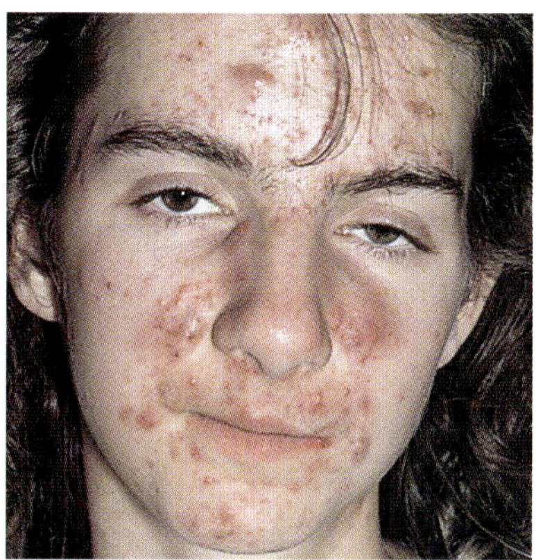

FIG. 2-19 *Inflamed papules and nodules, as well as papulopustules, patulous ostia, and scars.*

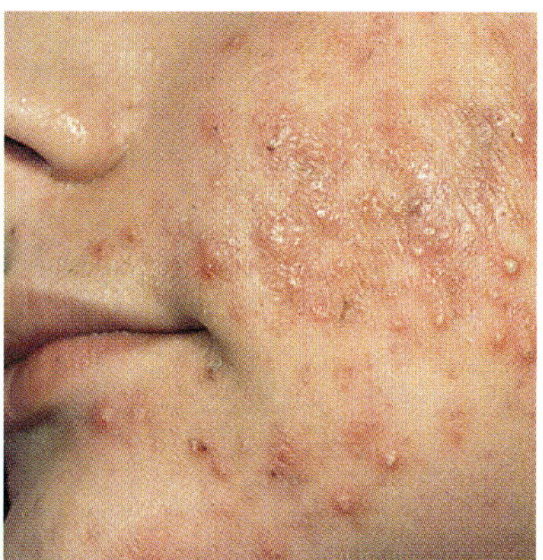

FIG. 2-20 *Patulous ostia of follicles, inflamed papules, pustules, and scars.*

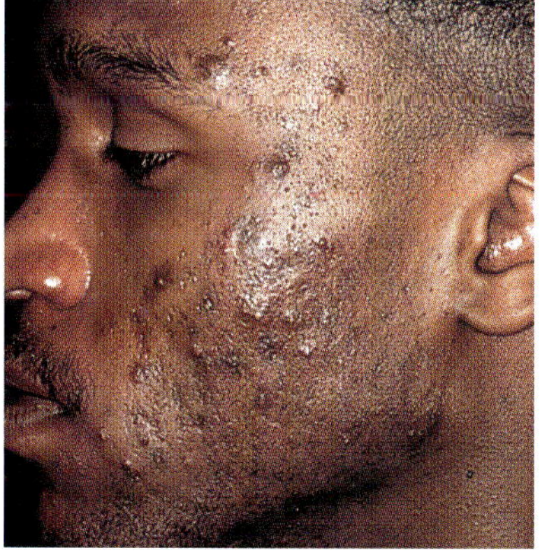

FIG. 2-21 *Inflamed papules and papulopustules, and residual hyperpigmented atrophic scars.*

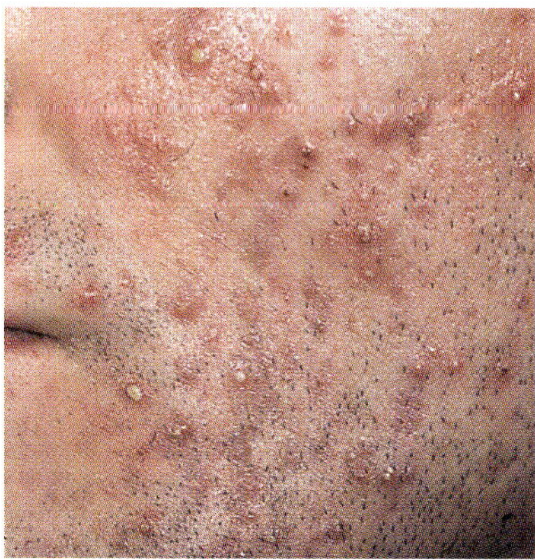

FIG. 2-22 *Inflamed papules, papulopustules, pustules, and crusts.*

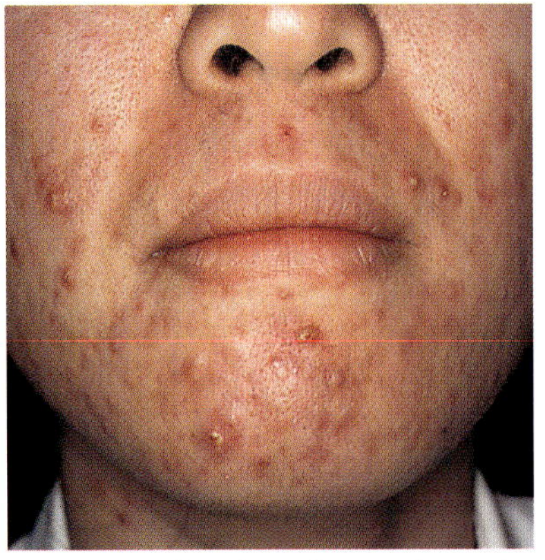

FIG. 2-23 *Inflamed papules, papulopustules, and pustules.*

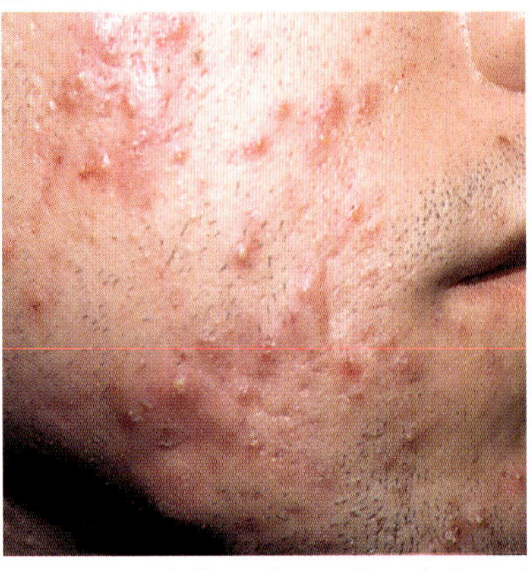

FIG. 2-24 *Inflamed papules, inflamed nodules, and papulopustules.*

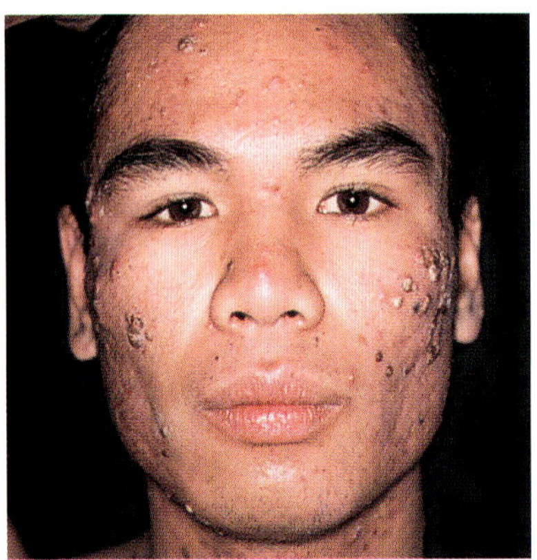

FIG. 2-25 *Inflamed papules, pustules, and crusts.*

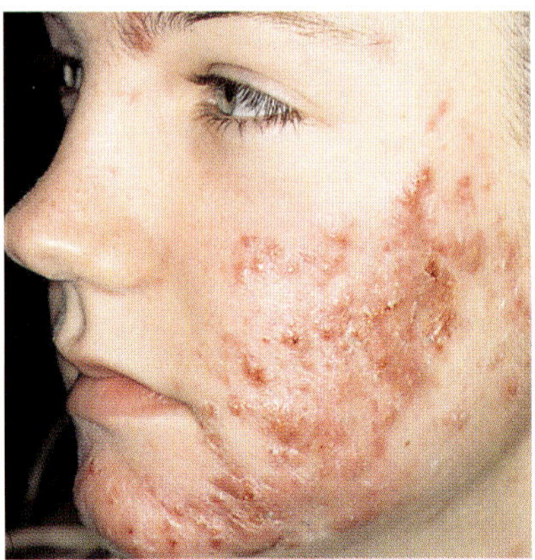

FIG. 2-26 *Inflamed papules, papulopustules, erosions, and hemorrhagic crusts. The erosions are secondary to excoriation.*

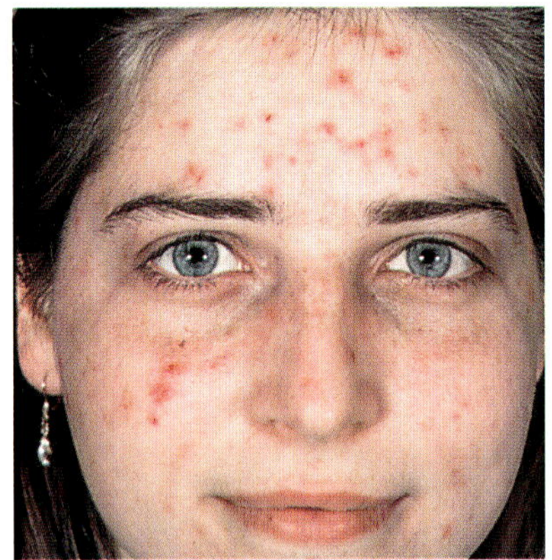

FIG. 2-27 *Excoriated papules.*

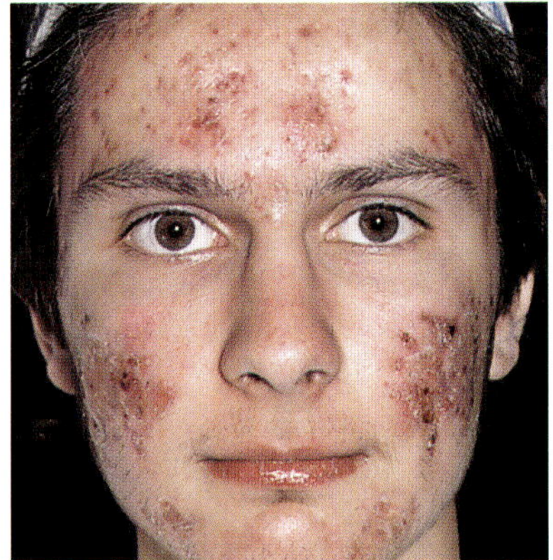

FIG. 2-28 *Inflamed papules and plaques, erosions, hemorrhagic crusts, and scars.*

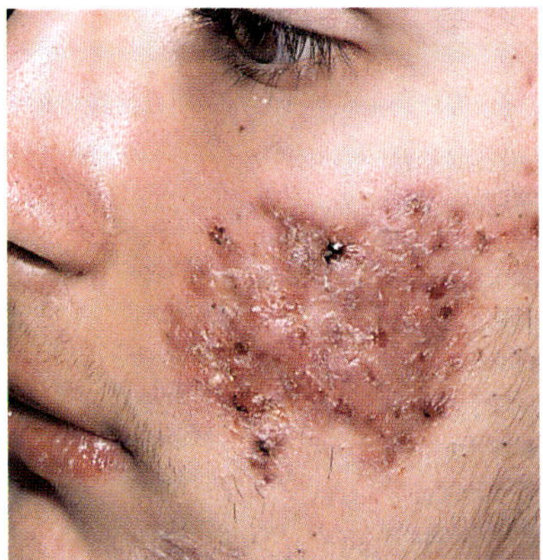

FIG. 2-29 *Inflamed plaque, erosions, hemorrhagic crusts, and pustules.*

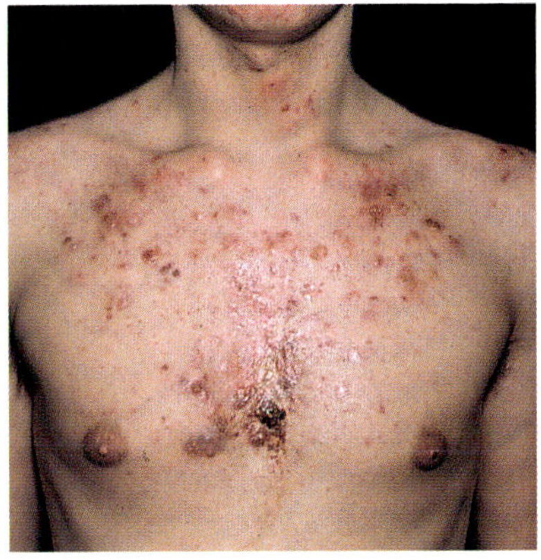

FIG. 2-30 *Inflamed papules and plaques, hemorrhagic crusts, and scars.*

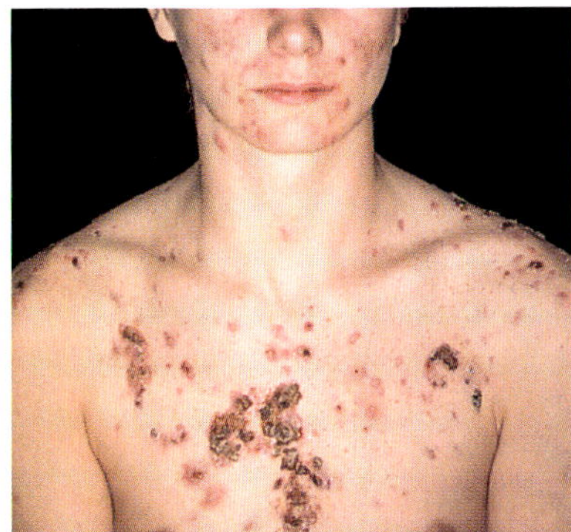

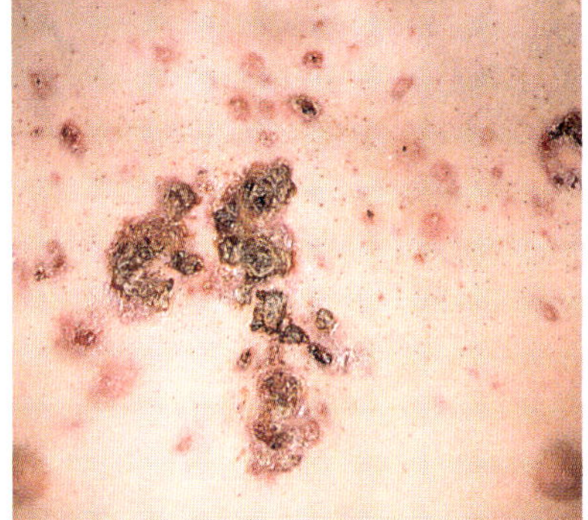

FIG. 2-31 (A, B) *Inflamed papules, erosions, large vegetative hemorrhagic crusts, and scars.*

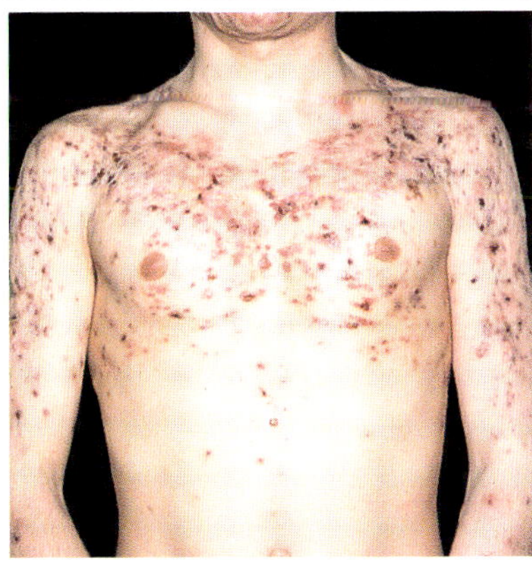

FIG. 2-32 *Papules, nodules, scars, and crusts.*

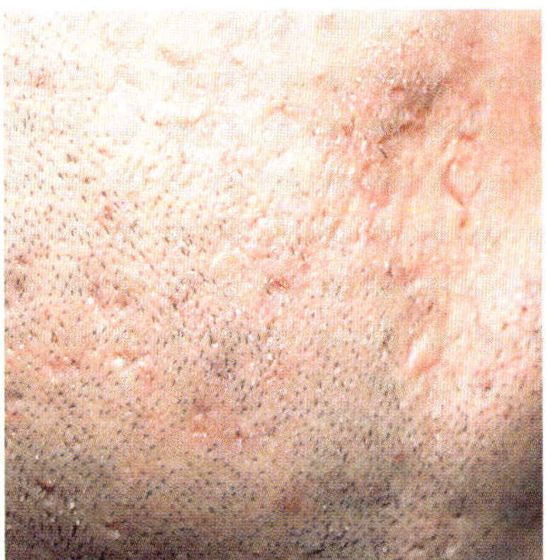

FIG. 2-33 *Pitted scars.*

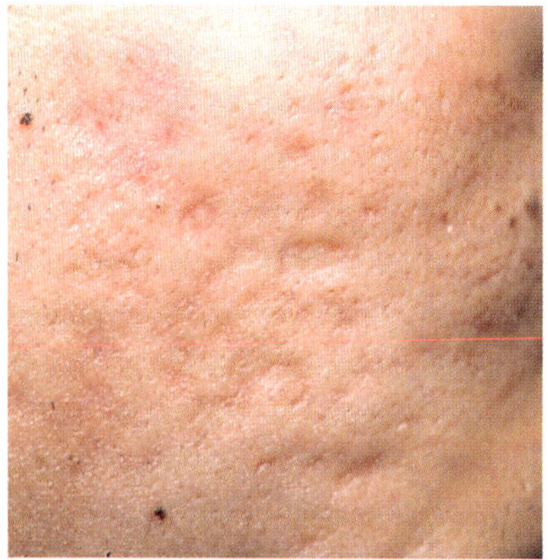

FIG. 2-34 *Atrophic scars.*

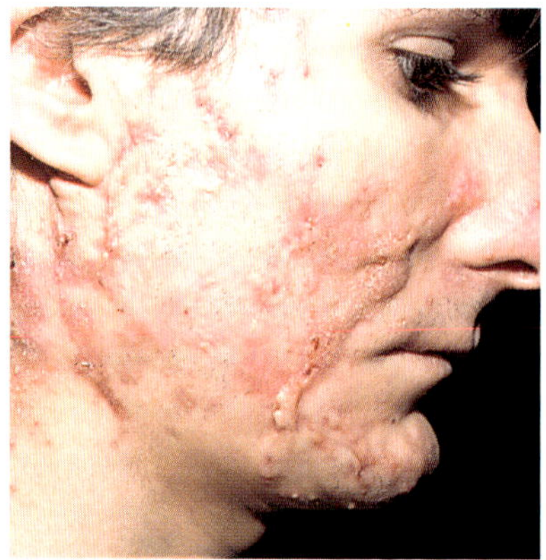

FIG. 2-35 *Atrophic and hypertrophic scars.*

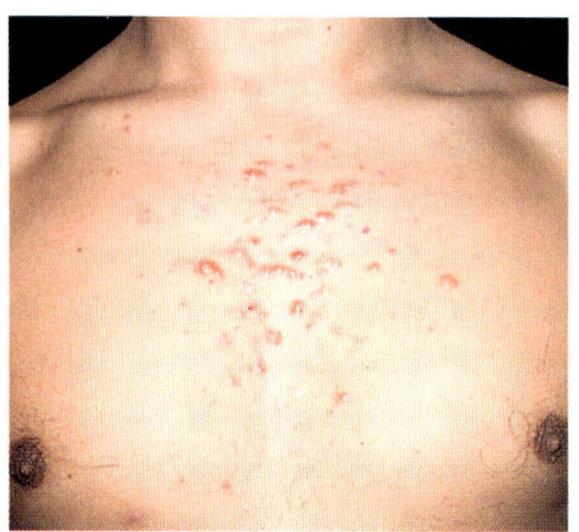

FIG. 2-36 *Many small keloids.*

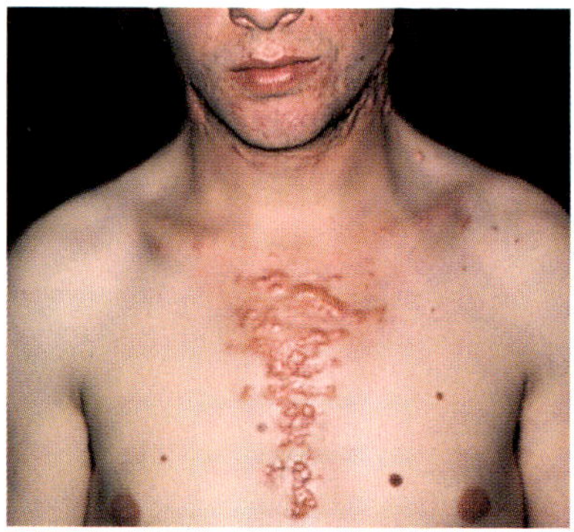

FIG. 2-37 *Large keloids on the chest, and inflamed papules and scars on the face.*

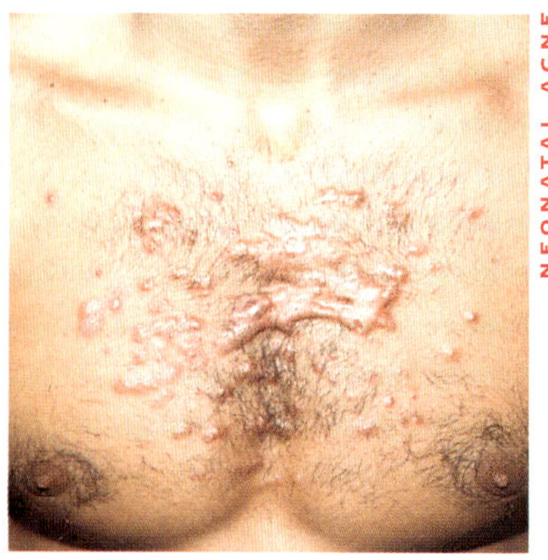

FIG. 2-38 *Keloids.*

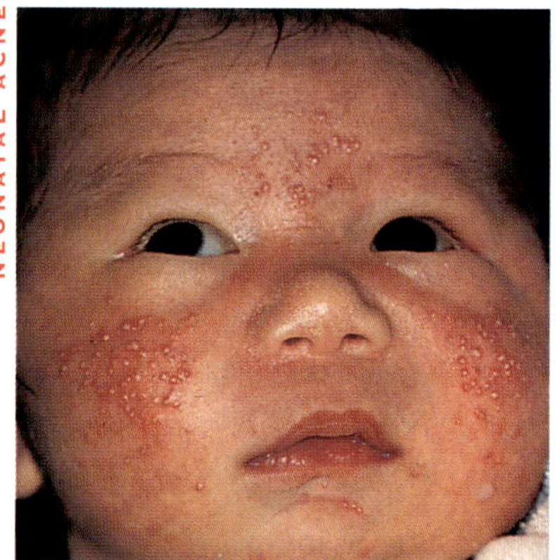

FIG. 2-39 *Papulopustules and pustules.*

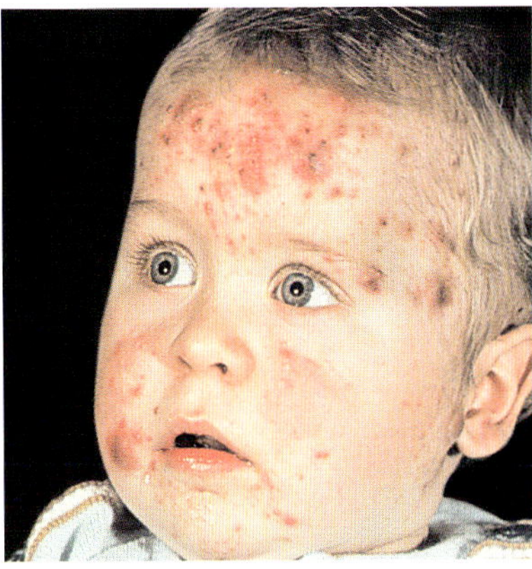

FIG. 2-40 *Inflamed papules (some of them purpuric) and papulopustules.*

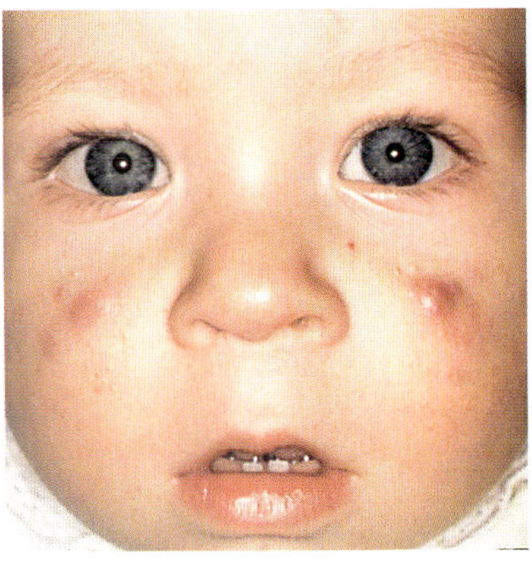

FIG. 2-41 *Inflamed papules and milia.*

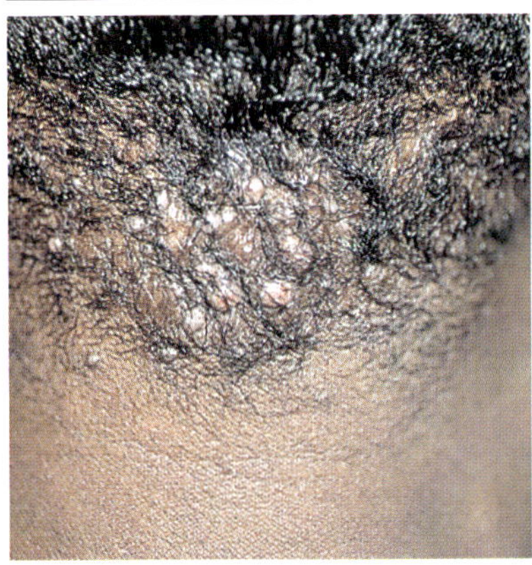

FIG. 2-42 *Follicular pustules and keloidal papules.*

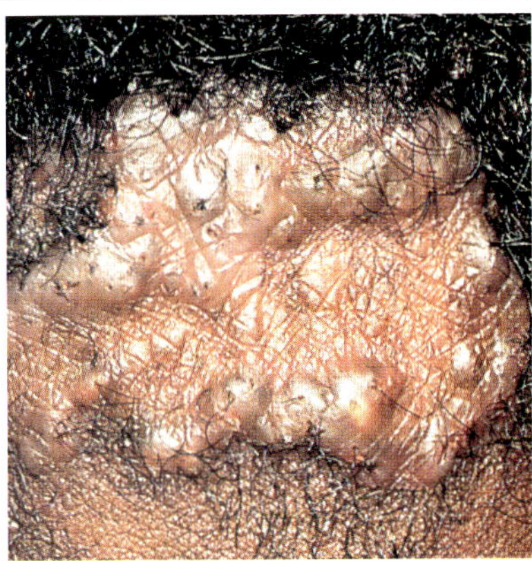

FIG. 2-43 *Comedones, infundibular cysts, pustules, and keloids.*

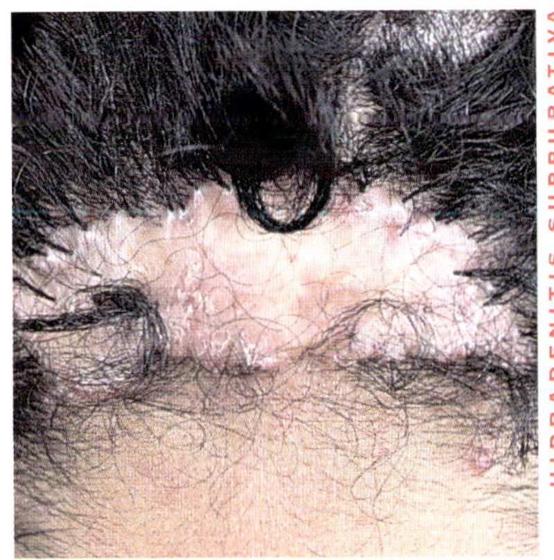

FIG. 2-44 *Keloids with tufted hairs.*

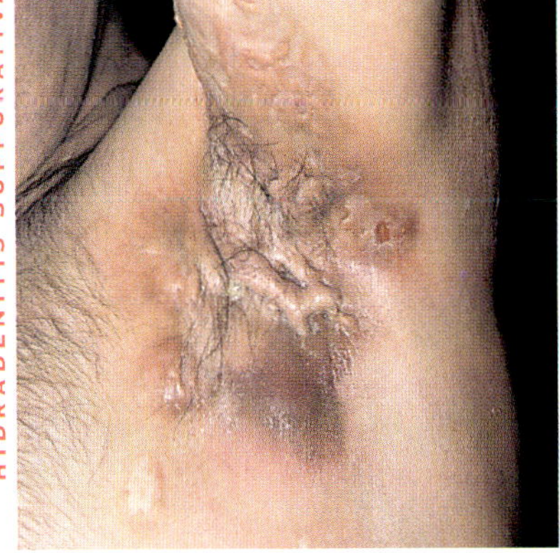

FIG. 2-45 *Patulous ostia of follicles, pus at ostia of sinus tracks, noninflamed and inflamed nodules, an ulcer, and linear scars.*

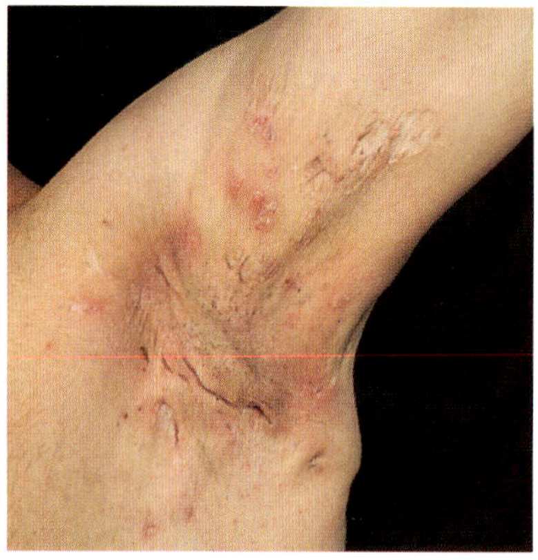

FIG. 2-46 *Markedly patulous ostia of follicles, some representing the opening of sinuses, papules, nodules, and scars.*

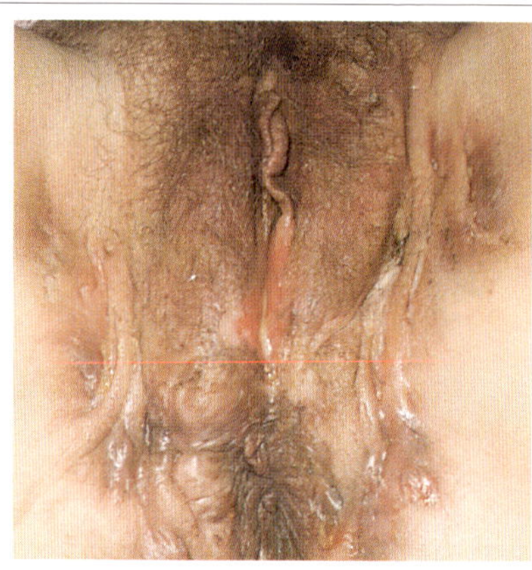

FIG. 2-47 *Patulous ostia of sinuses, some having discharged pus, nodules, and hypertrophic scars.*

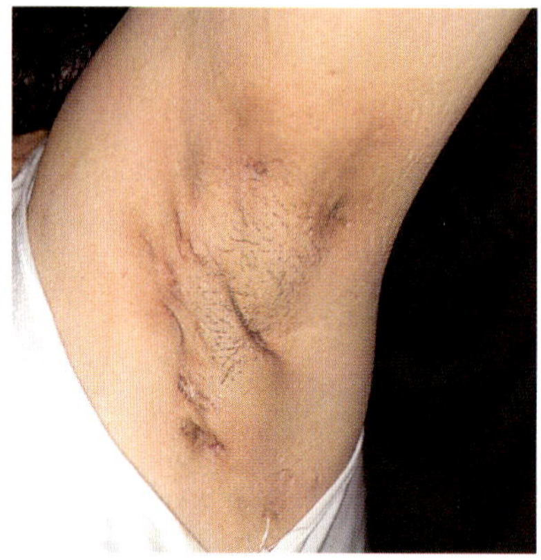

FIG. 2-48 *Scars at sites of sinuses.*

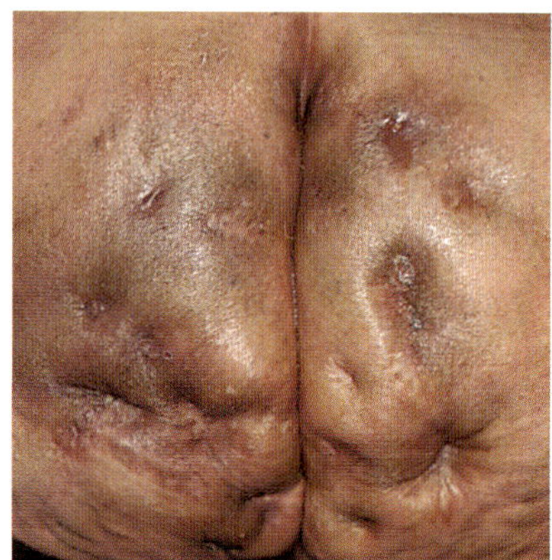

FIG. 2-49 *Patulous ostia of sinuses and depressed hyperpigmented scars.*

STEROID ACNE

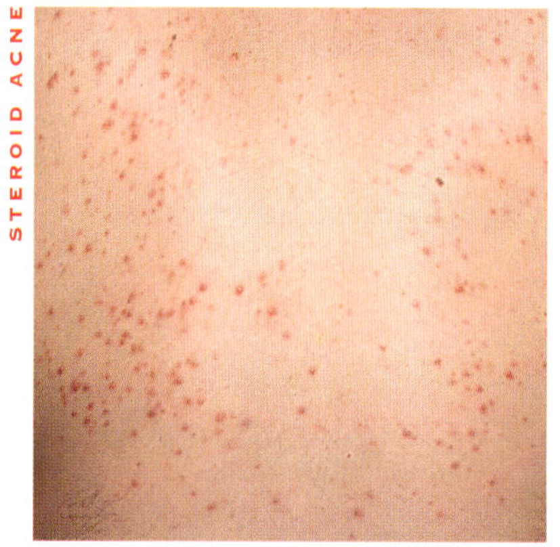

FIG. 2-50 *Monomorphous follicular papules.*

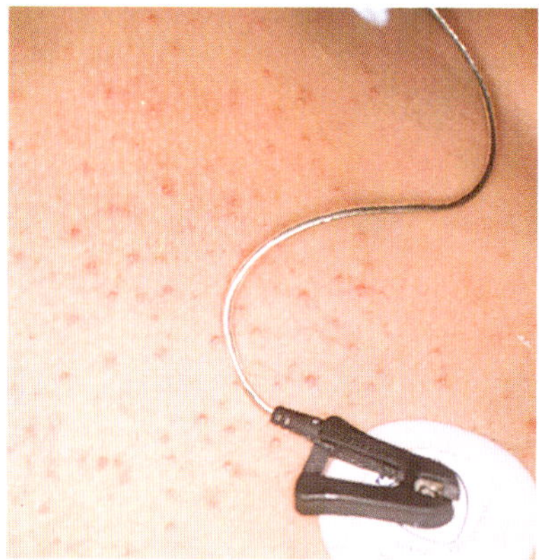

FIG. 2-51 *Monomorphous follicular papules in a patient in intensive care.*

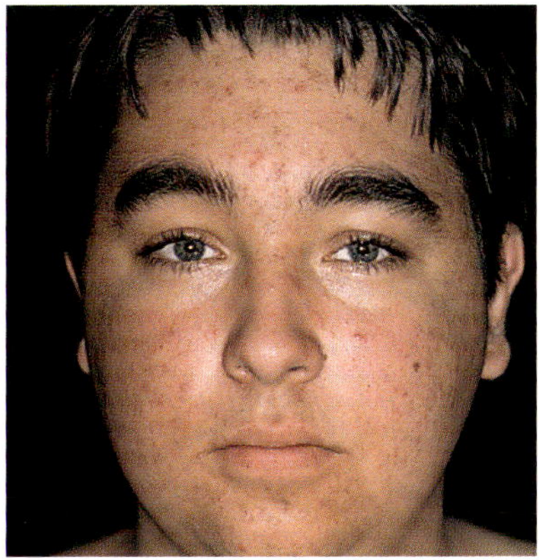
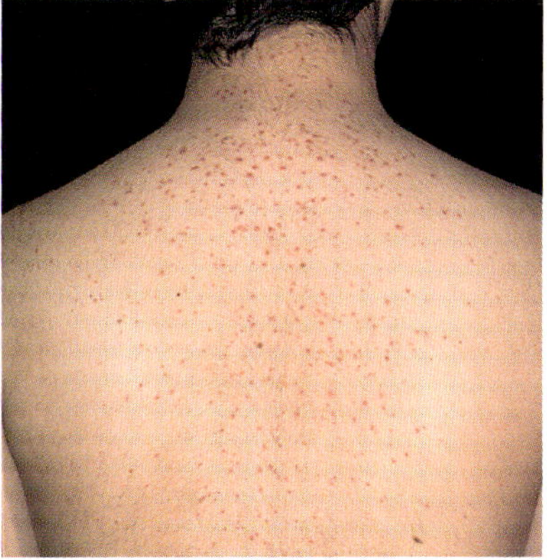

FIG. 2-52 (A, B) *Monomorphous follicular papules and papulopustules.*

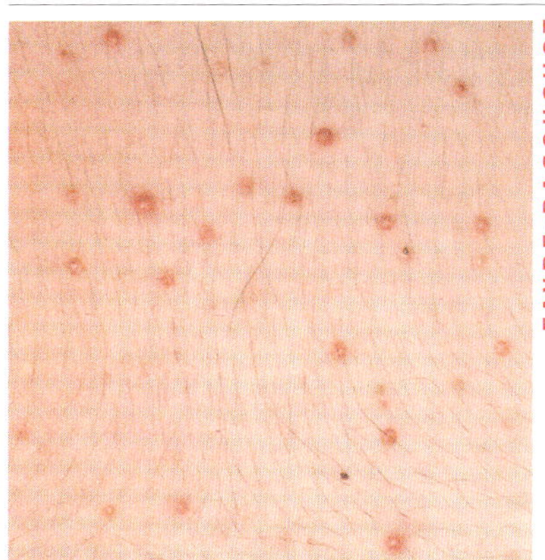
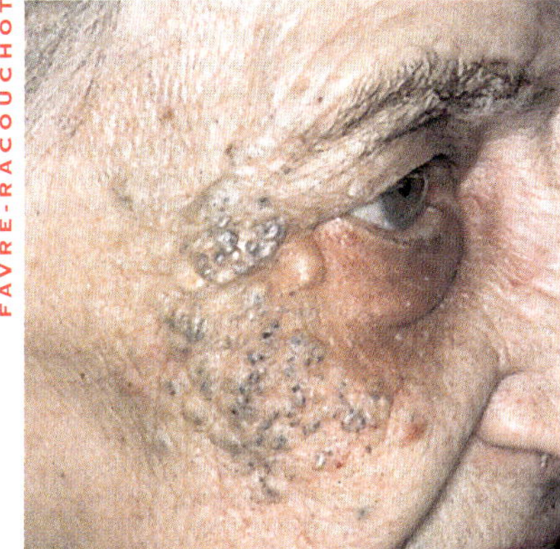

FIG. 2-52 (C) *Widespread discrete papules and papulopustules are all folliculocentric.*

FIG. 2-53 *Cluster of comedones and infundibular cysts on sun-damaged skin.*

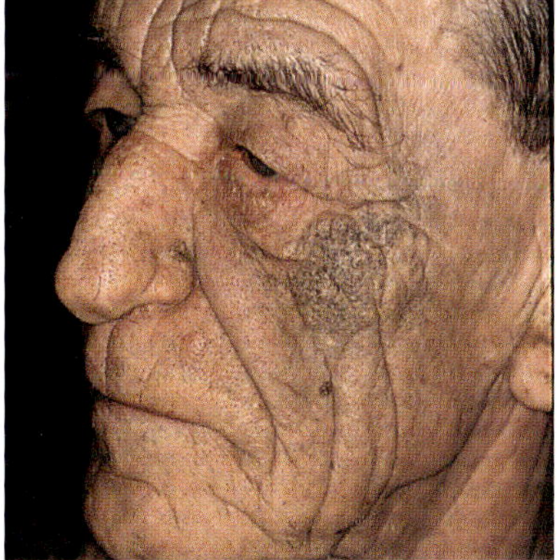
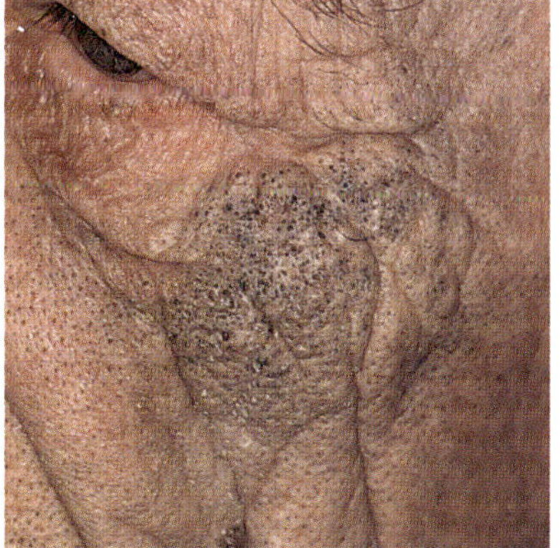

FIG. 2-54 (A, B) *Numerous comedones and infundibular cysts of different sizes in clusters on skin injured badly by sunlight.*

Virtually every adolescent is affected by acne vulgaris, if only in a mild form. In adolescents and young adults it may persist for years, whereas in neonates it usually lasts for weeks or a few months. The most severe expressions of acne occur in males.

COURSE Beginning with the flow of androgens at puberty, typical lesions of mild to moderately severe acne vulgaris in adolescents come and go for several years, usually disappearing completely and without residua, except at times for patulous follicles on the nose and malar region. Episodically, the process is more fulminant and prolonged, conglobate lesions being long lasting and healing with unsightly atrophic scars. New lesions of acne keloidalis on a nape may continue to appear as the inflammatory process smoulders well into adulthood. Severe acne that occurs especially on the back in males often resolves with a type of anetoderma that presents itself as atrophic papules, and that is incorrectly designated "macular atrophy."

A comedo may become progressively larger and eventually be gigantic. In time, the ever-expanding plug of cornified cells causes the wall of an infundibulum to become so thin that eventually it is breached, spewing into the dermis cornified cells, sebaceous secretion, and microorganisms. This event sets in motion an inflammatory reaction marked initially by suppuration, then by granulomatous inflammation, and, in time, by fibrosis. A pustule situated within an infundibulum, in a fashion comparable to a comedo, may become so large that its contents are disgorged into the dermis where they inevitably induce granulomatous inflammation and, sometimes, fibrosis.

If the focus of suppuration in the reticular dermis (and, at times, the subcutaneous fat) becomes very large, a huge abscess forms and the destructive effects of products of the neutrophils that compose it lead invariably to extensive fibrosis. When the epithelium of infundibula and eccrine ducts then proliferates (pseudocarcinomatous hyperplasia) in an attempt to "wall off" the abscess, sinus tracts may come into being. If several contiguous abscesses have formed, each being positioned at the site of a follicle, the result may be sinus tracks that are interconnected. That phenomenon resolves with extensive fibroplasia.

Acne vulgaris may consist only of comedones, but in most patients, comedones are joined by reddish papules and pustules. That very common expression of acne vulgaris does not, as a rule, resolve with scars. If, however, abscesses form and especially if the process eventuates in draining sinuses, severe scarring is a certainty. Whereas pustules of acne vulgaris may begin to wane in days, abscesses that are followed by granulomatous inflammation and fibrosis may not resolve completely for many months.

INTEGRATION: UNIFYING CONCEPT The follicle-centered acne vulgaris and variants of it seem to be a single pathologic process. The spectrum of its severity ranges from comedones and inflamed papules that resolve without residua to fluctuant and draining sinuses that heal with ugly scars. But whether the condition is called acne vulgaris, acne conglobata, acne keloidalis, hidradenitis suppurativa, or dissecting cellulitis of the scalp (perifolliculitis capitis abscedens et suffodiens), the process is fundamentally the same.

Inflammatory cells, neutrophils chief among them, appear first around and then within infundibula. If the collection of neutrophils is confined to an infundibulum, the lesion is a pustule. If the process is more florid and the collection of neutrophils is so great that it obscures a follicle, pseudocarcinomatous hyperplasia develops in an attempt to contain it. The result is one or more of a constellation of acne conglobata, acne keloidalis, dissecting cellulitis of the scalp, and hidradenitis suppurativa. The legitimacy of the concept that acne is basically a single pathologic process seems to be verified by the fact that all of its manifestations—among them, vulgaris, conglobata, keloidalis, dissecting cellulitis, and hidradenitis suppurativa—may be present in one person. For acne, in any of its expressions, to come into being requires the play of androgens on the folliculosebaceous unit.

THERAPY Administration of topical vitamin A acid, benzoyl peroxide, and azelaic acid cream, or a combination thereof, is effective for mostly "comedonal acne"; topical antibiotics and oral antibiotics, such as tetracycline, may be added for mostly "pustular acne," and oral administration of retinoids (isotretinoin) for severe, recalcitrant nodular acne and "conglobate acne." Antiandrogen taken orally may be beneficial in women. Laser therapy may be efficacious for scars.

DEFINITION Allergic contact dermatitis is an inflammatory process induced by direct contact of the skin of a sensitized individual to an allergen. Within hours, red macules or patches develop that usually evolve quickly, sometimes through an intermediate stage of urticarial papules or plaques, into vesicles that may become bullae. Because the lesions, i.e., macules, papules, vesicles, and bullae, are not in themselves specific, diagnosis clinically is made by virtue of distinctive distribution that reflects the manner in which a particular allergen was contacted.

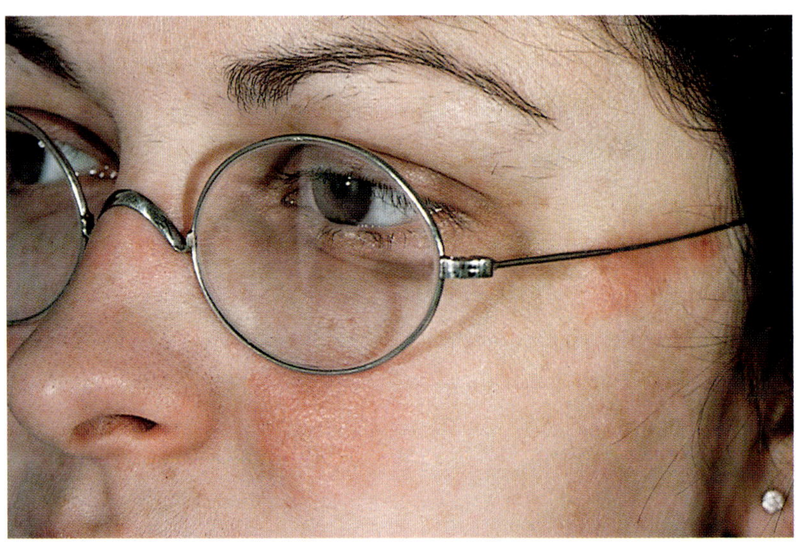

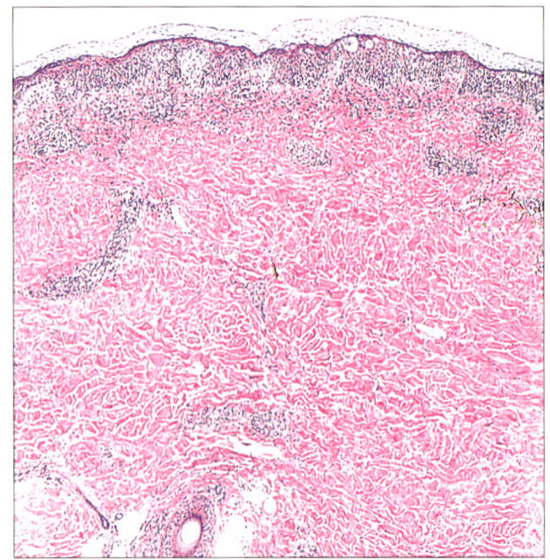

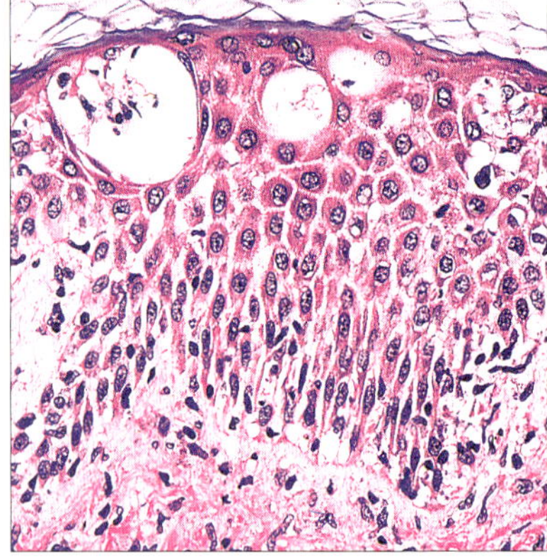

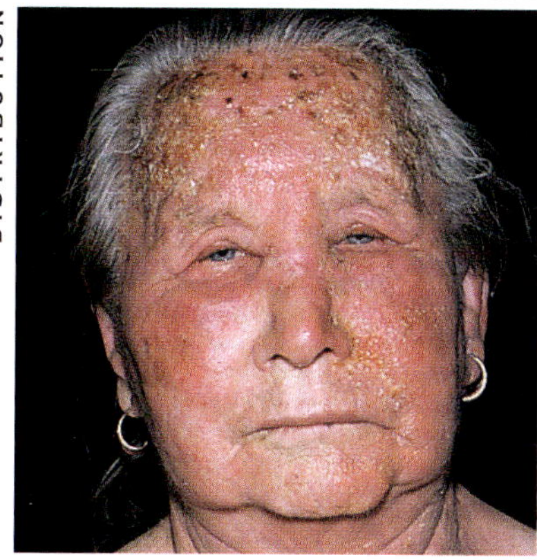

FIG. 3-1 *The patient's face and neck are affected by erythema, edema, vesicles, and yellow crusts.*

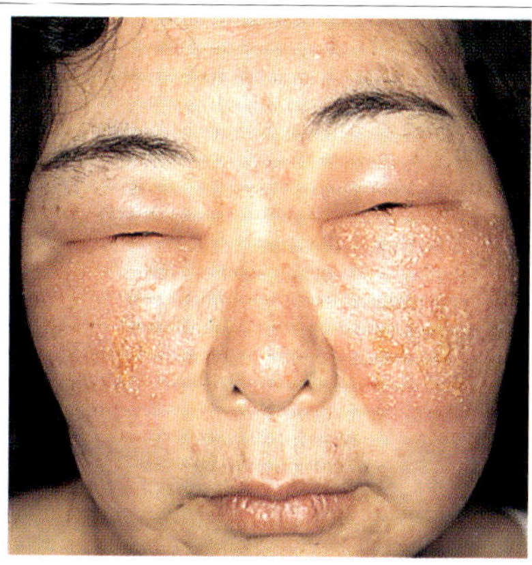

FIG. 3-2 *Edema, erythema, papules, pustules, and crusts. The bridge of the nose and paranasal folds have been spared.*

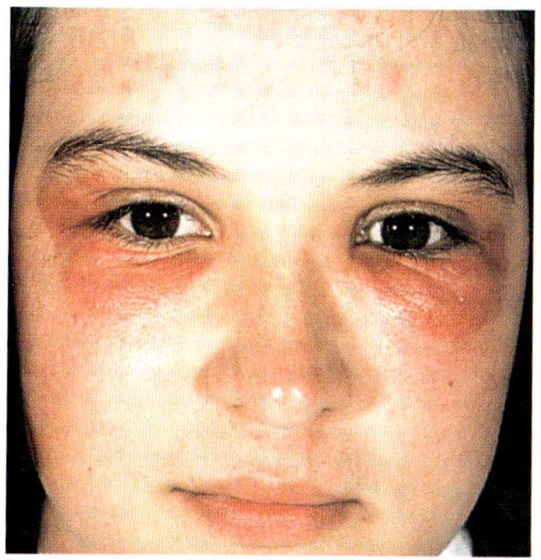

FIG. 3-3 *Erythematous patches, papules, and plaques distributed in symmetrical fashion.*

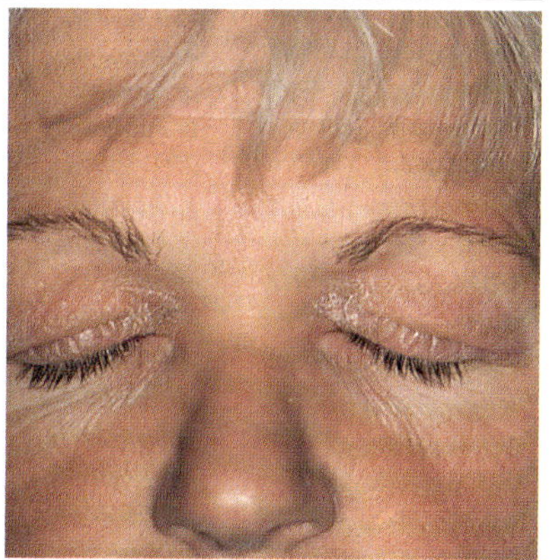

FIG. 3-4 *The upper eyelids show edema, erythema, and scales.*

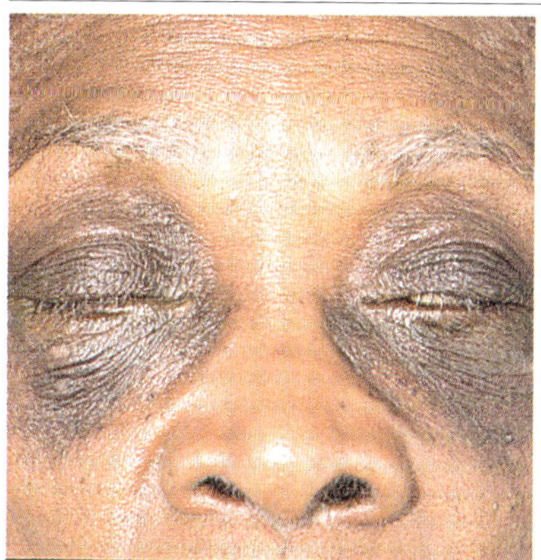

FIG. 3-5 *Lichenification and hyperpigmentation of eyelids. The allergic contactant was sulfa in eye drops.*

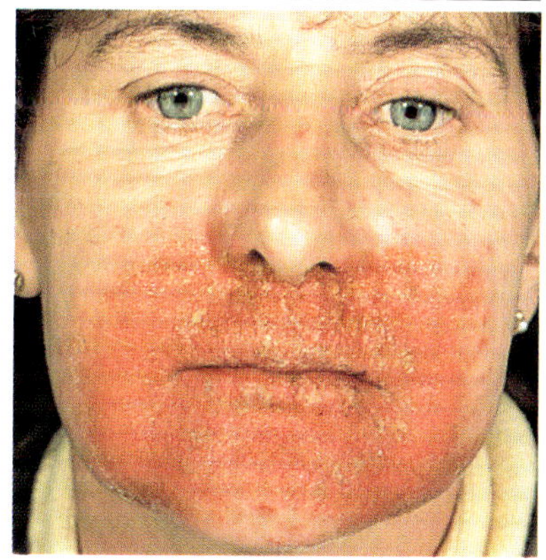

FIG. 3-6 *Perioral region displaying erythematous papules and plaques, crusts, scales, and fissures.*

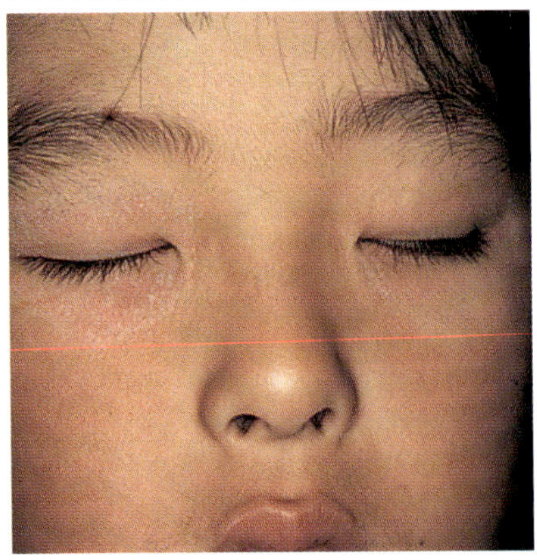 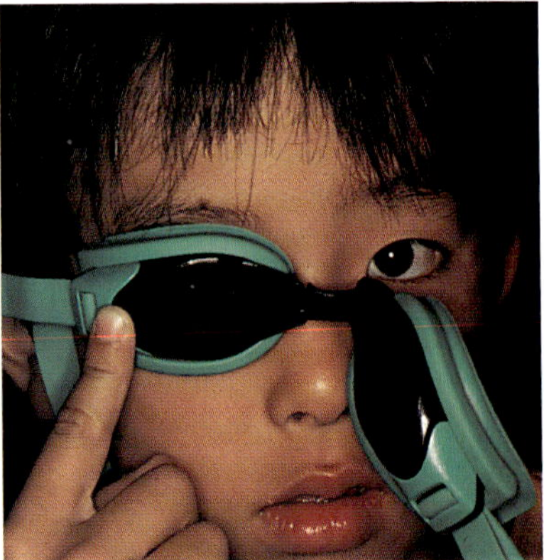

FIG. 3-7 (A, B) *Periocular, erythematous papules. The cause was rubber in goggles.*

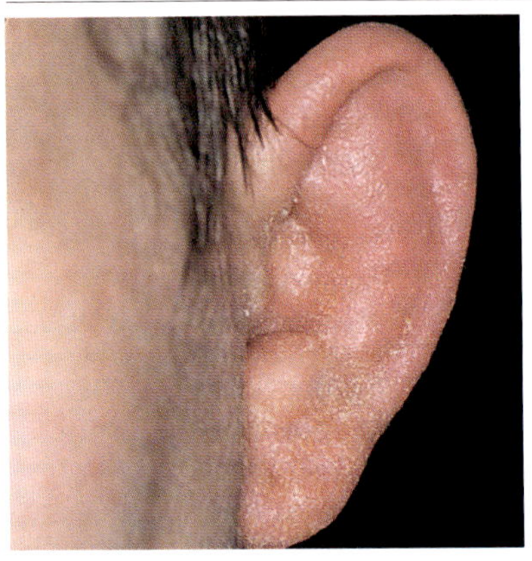 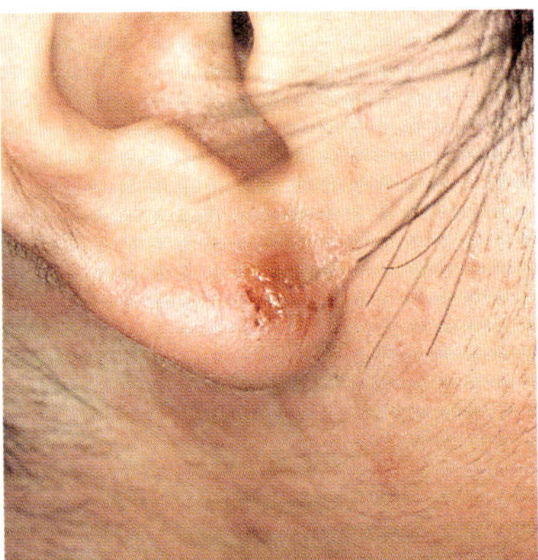

FIG. 3-8 *Ear with edema, erythema, crusts, and scales.*

FIG. 3-9 *Erosion on an earlobe and plaques on the neck and face.*

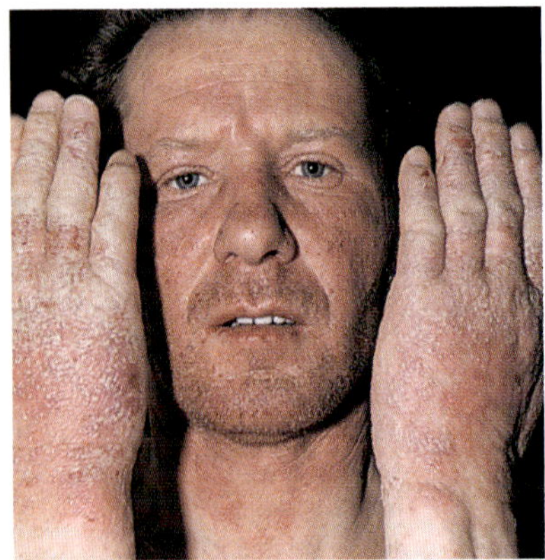 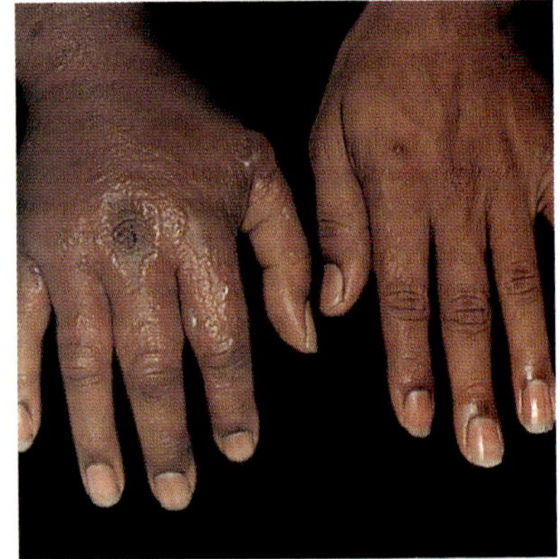

FIG. 3-10 *Face, neck, and dorsa of hands and wrists with edema, erythema, scales, and erosions.*

FIG. 3-11 *Dorsa of hands with tense vesicles and a bulla.*

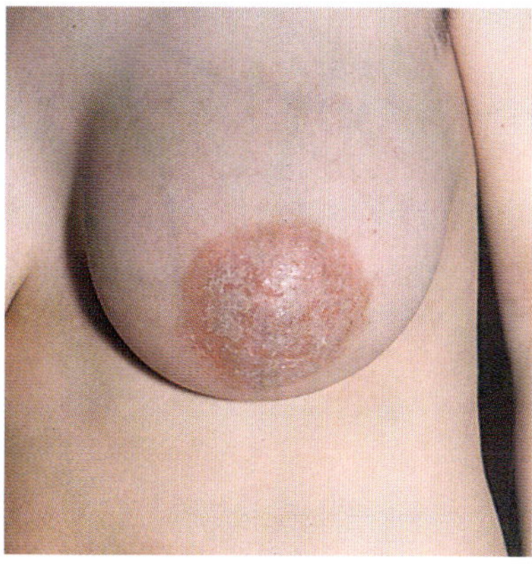

FIG. 3-12 *Nipple and areola altered by a scaly plaque.*

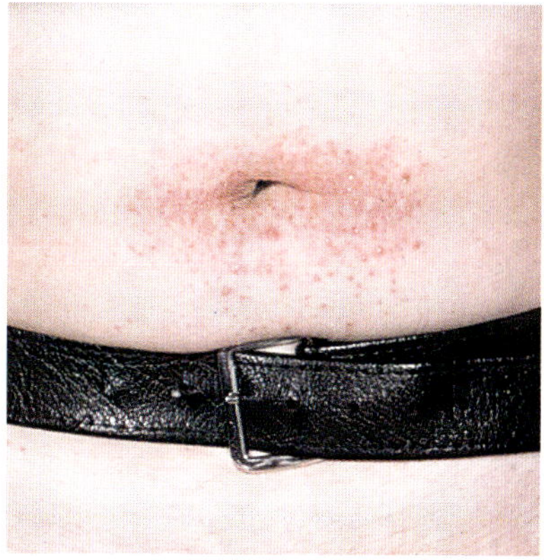

FIG. 3-13 *Scales, erosions, and discrete and confluent erythematous papules. The cause was nickel in the belt buckle.*

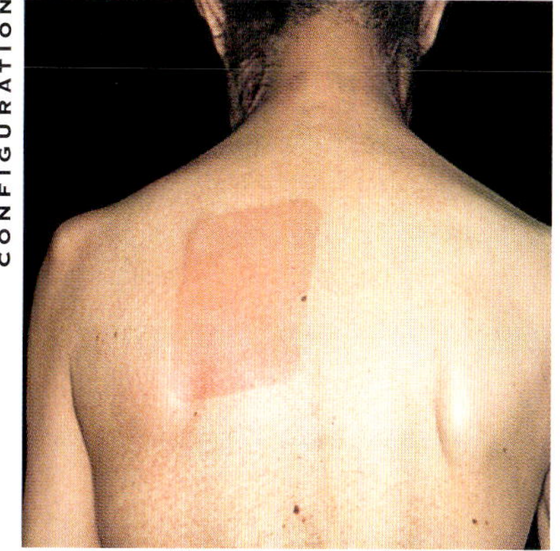

FIG. 3-14 *A rectangular zone of erythema is artificial indicating external cause, a plaster containing an herb.*

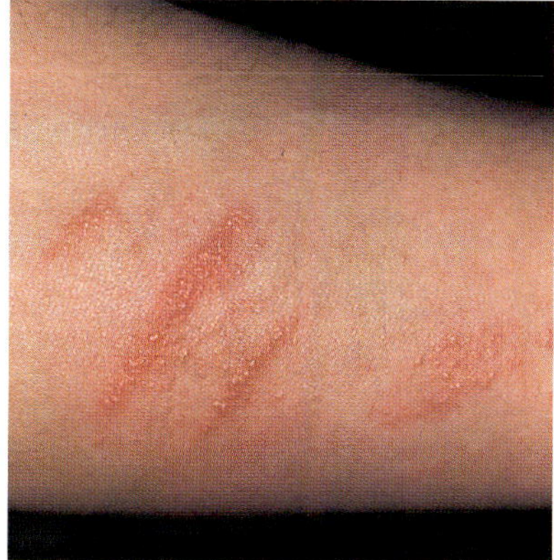

FIG. 3-15 *A line of erythematous papules and vesicles of Rhus dermatitis.*

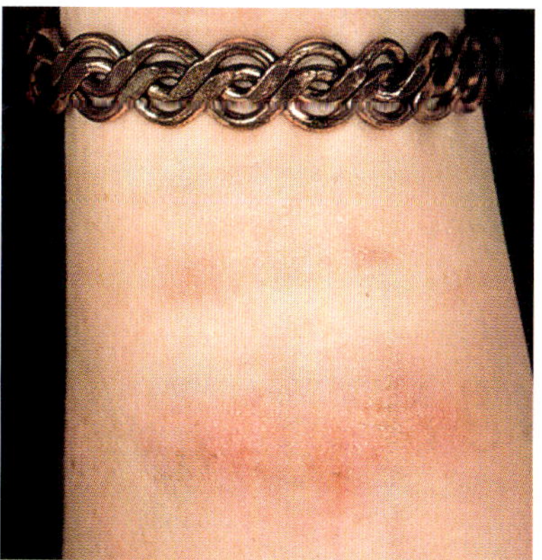

FIG. 3-16 *A line of erythematous macules, papules, and scales induced by sensitivity to nickel in a bracelet.*

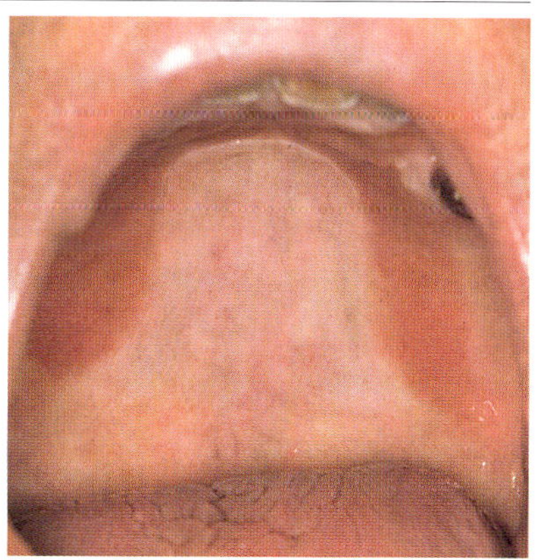

FIG. 3-17 *Arciform lesion of the hard palate secondary to a sensitizer in a prosthesis.*

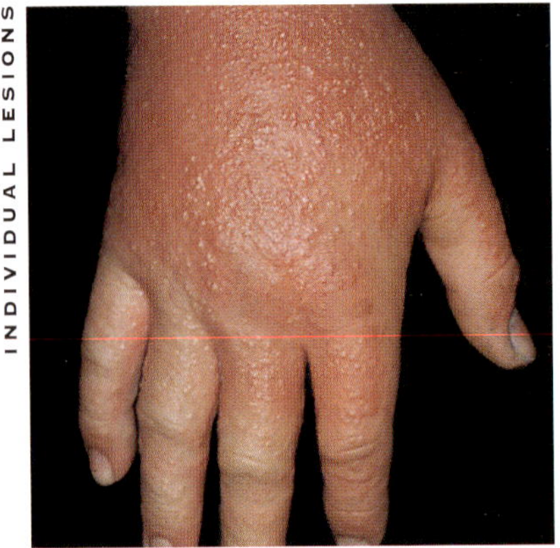

FIG. 3-18 *Marked edema, diffuse erythema, papules, and vesicles.*

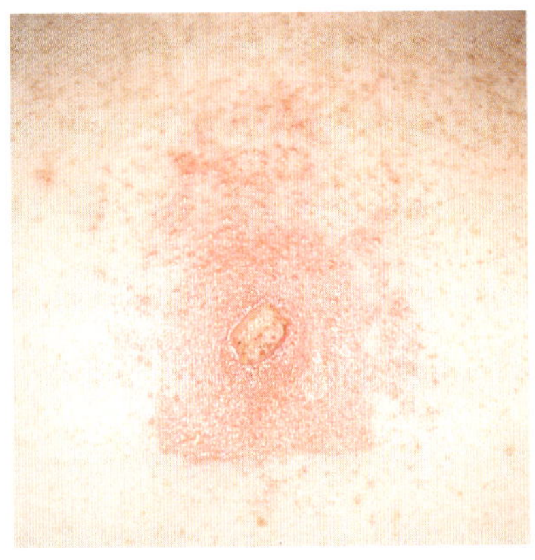

FIG. 3-19 *Closely-set papules and papulovesicles around an ulcer that had been treated by neomycin.*

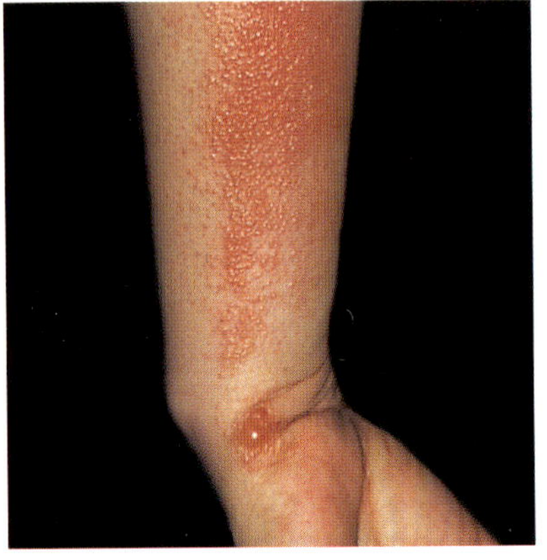

FIG. 3-20 *Diffuse erythema, papules, vesicles, and a bulla.*

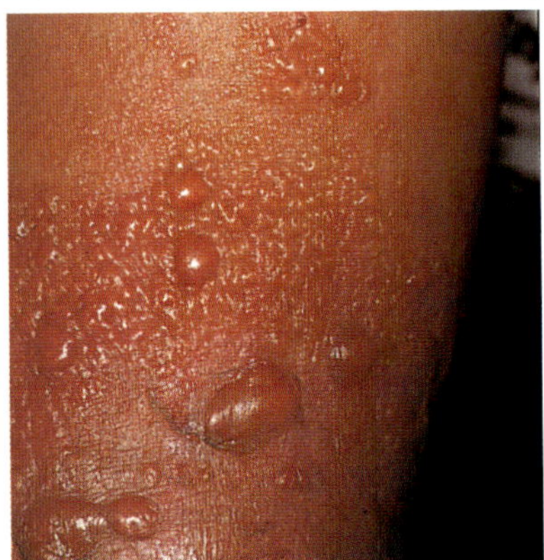

FIG. 3-21 *Clusters of vesicles and scattered bullae on a red base.*

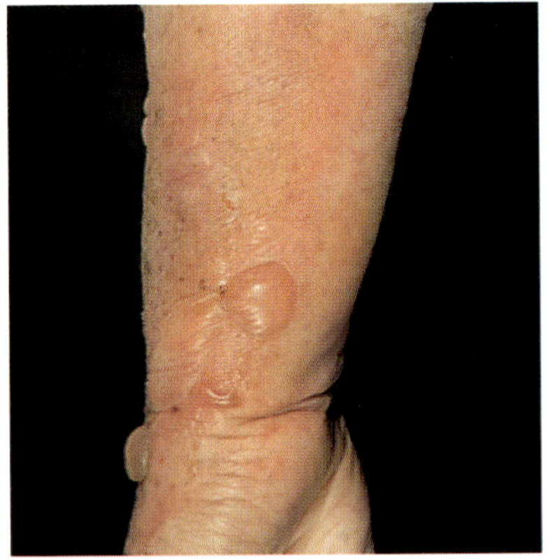

FIG. 3-22 *Vesicles and bullae on a base of erythema.*

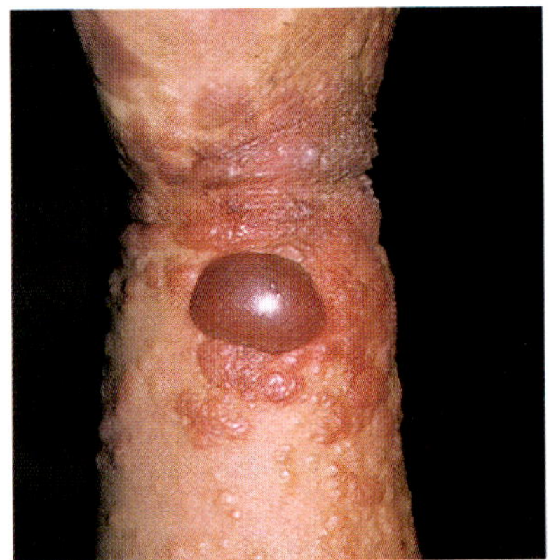

FIG. 3-23 *Skin-colored and pink papules, and hemorrhagic vesicles and bullae.*

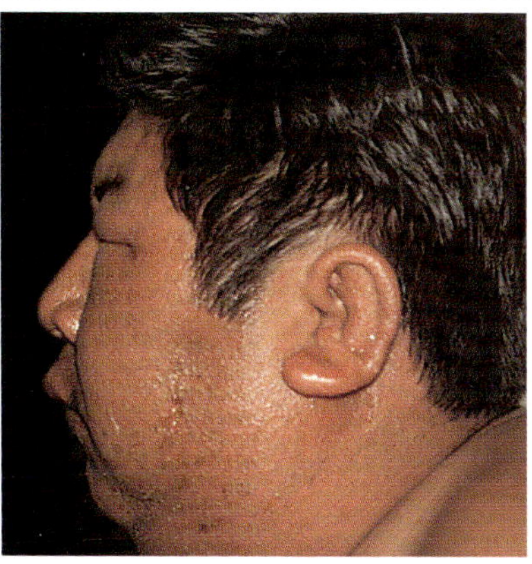

FIG. 3-24 *Extensive edema of the entire face, including eyelids, cheeks, lips, and ear, with oozing and scale-crusts.*

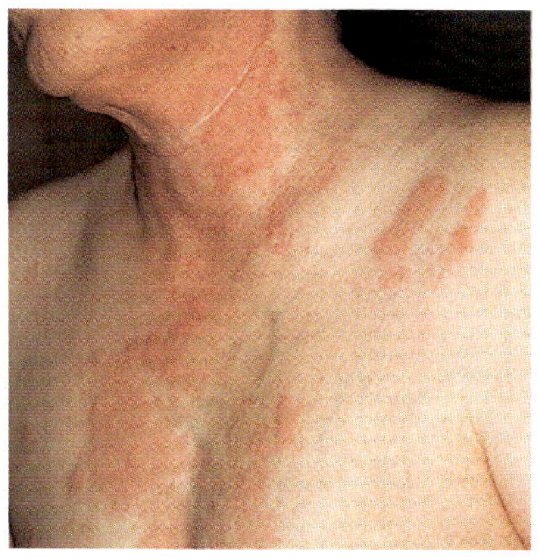

FIG. 3-25 *Erythematous macules and urticarial papules and plaques called forth by a sensitizer in a hair dye.*

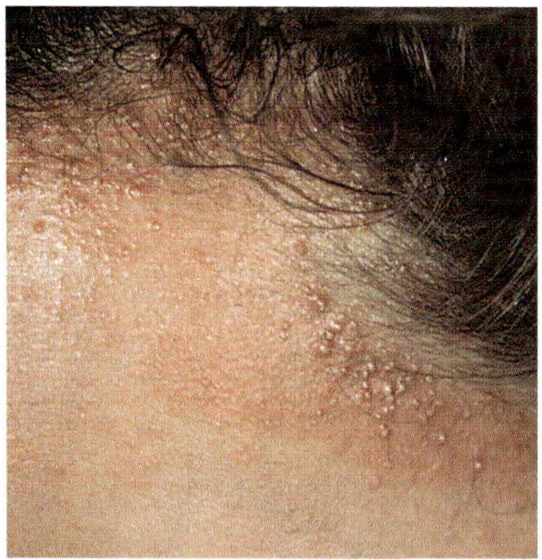

FIG. 3-26 *Clusters of pustules on an erythematous base consequent to an allergen in a hair dye.*

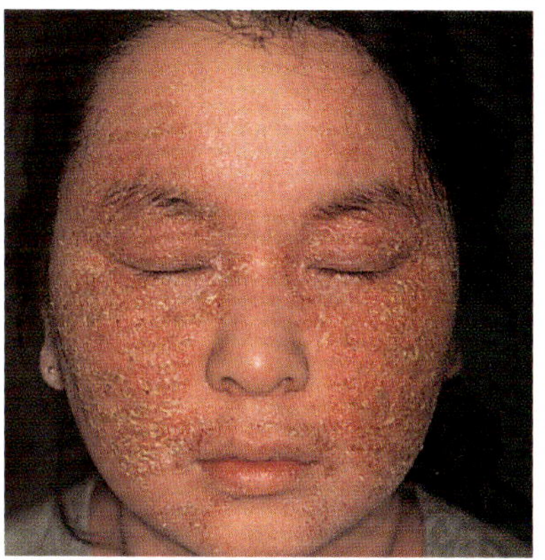

FIG. 3-27 *Scale-crusts, erosions, and fissures in an edematous face.*

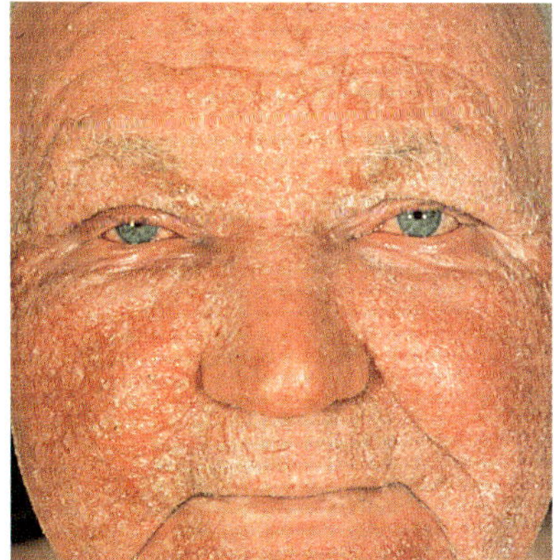

FIG. 3-28 *Scale-crusts and fissures, as well as erythematous urticarial papules and plaques.*

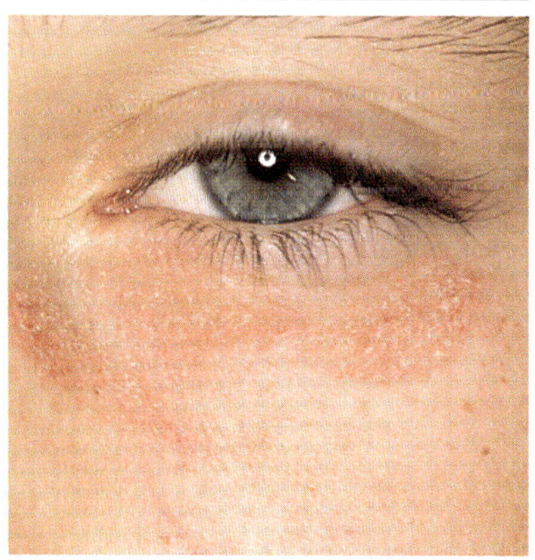

FIG. 3-29 *Scales and erosions on an erythematous base secondary to an allergen in fingernail polish.*

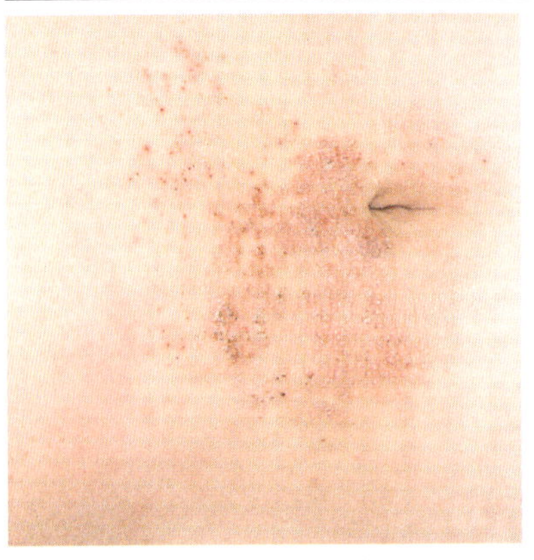

FIG. 3-30 *Erythematous papules, some excoriated, and others lichenified secondary to vigorous rubbing.*

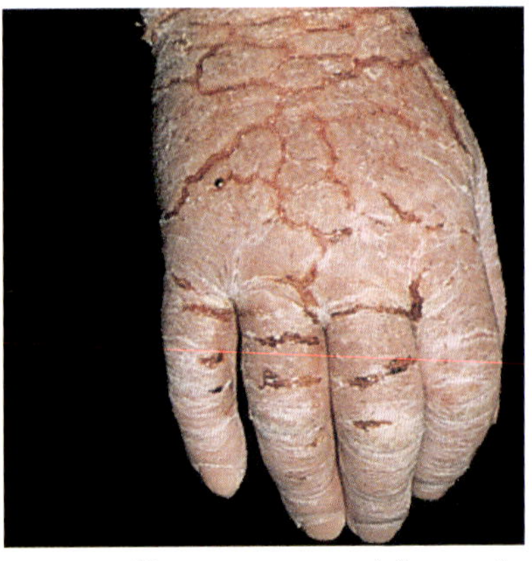

FIG. 3-31 *Keratoses, crusts, and fissures of a markedly edematous hand.*

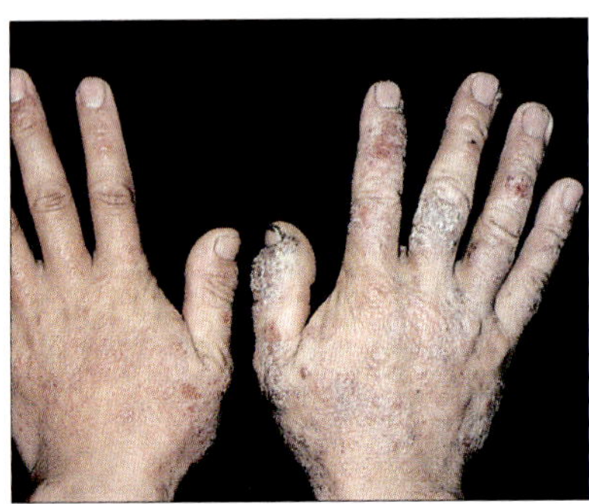

FIG. 3-32 *Diffuse erythema, keratoses, scales, and erosions.*

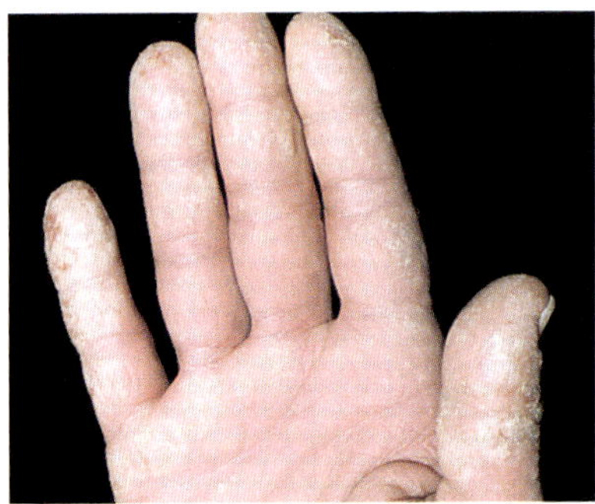

FIG. 3-33 *Slightly erythematous papules, some of them lichenified, verrucous keratoses, scales, and erosions.*

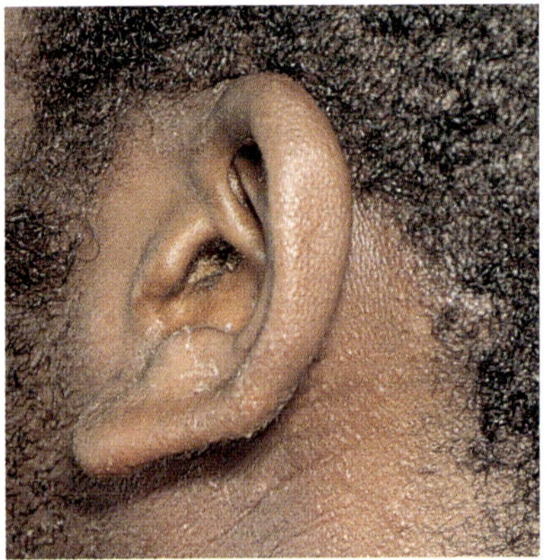

FIG. 3-34 *Papules and vesicles.*

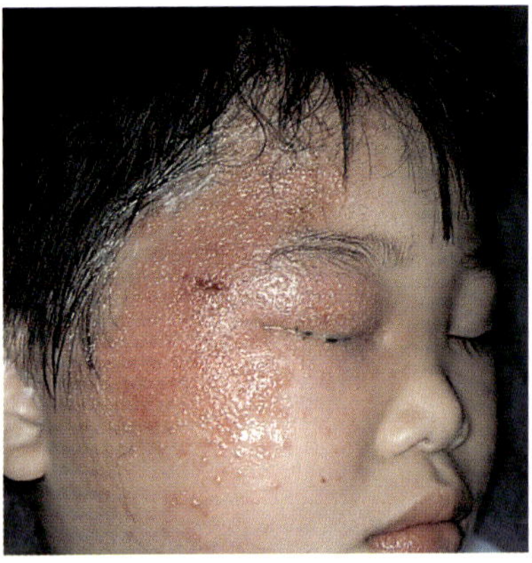

FIG. 3-35 *Vesicles, crusts, and extensive periorbital edema.*

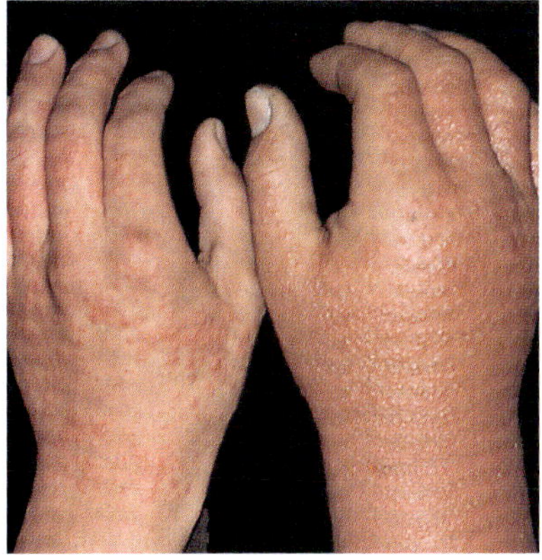

FIG. 3-36 *Tense vesicles on an edematous right hand and red papules on the left one.*

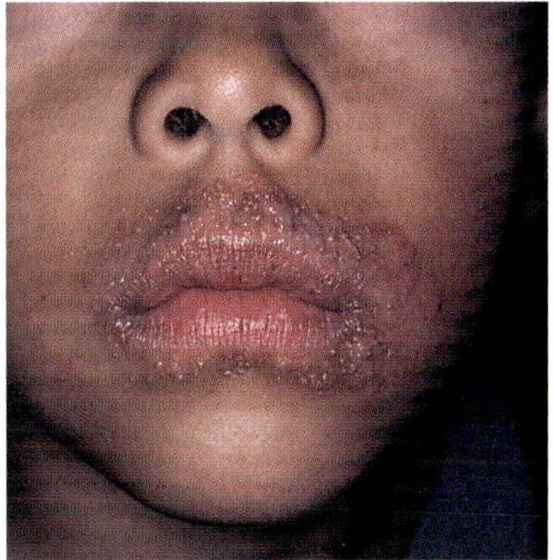

FIG. 3-37 *Papules and vesicles on edematous lips.*

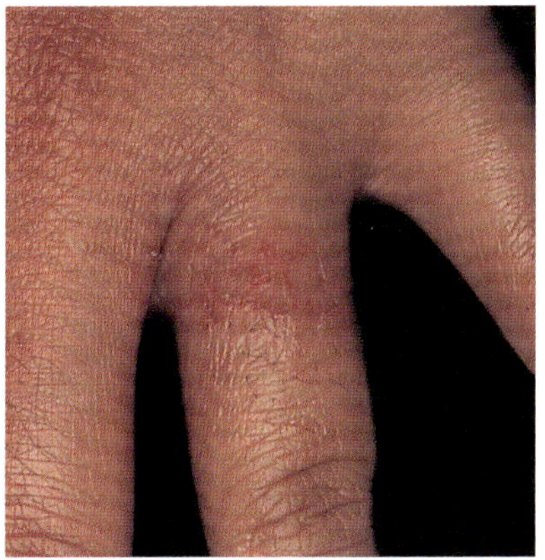

FIG. 3-38 *Papules and papulovesicles at the site of a ring.*

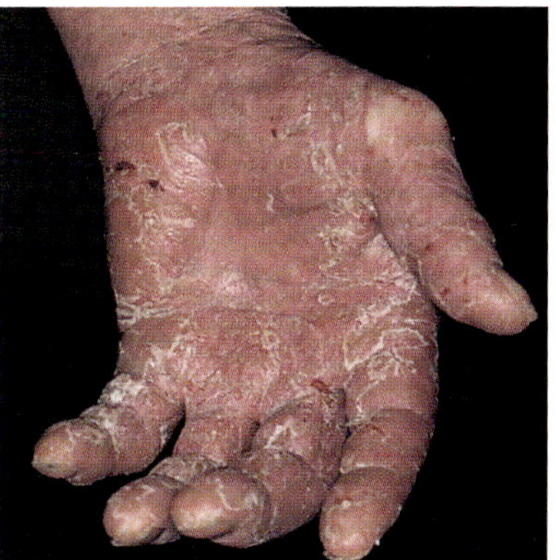

FIG. 3-39 *Scales, crusts, lichenification, and fissures secondary to rubber in gloves.*

Examples of common allergic contactants are Rhus toxicodendron ("poison ivy"), nickel, thiurames in rubber, parabens in ointments, and chemicals in fragrances, whereas agents commonly responsible for irritant contact dermatitis are acids, alkaloids, machine oils, organic solvents, and oxidants.

ADJUNCTIVE DIAGNOSTIC TEST The most effective method for diagnosis with surety of allergic contact dermatitis is the patch test. Red macules, papules, or tense vesicles that arise at a site where the suspected causative agent has been applied confirm the diagnosis of allergic contact dermatitis.

COURSE Within hours after the skin of a sensitized person has come into contact with a particular allergen, red macules or patches develop that usually evolve quickly, sometimes through an intermediate stage of urticarial papules or plaques, into vesicles that may become bullae. Sometimes, however, allergic contact dermatitis may present itself only as reddish papules or papulovesicles, but more often as tense vesicles as well. Episodically, depending on the patient's degree of hypersensitivity, bullae may come into being. If the offending agent is removed, lesions of allergic contact dermatitis, no matter how widespread or severe, resolve, even without therapy, within a matter of weeks at most. If, however, the allergen continues to come into contact with the skin, the process may persist for years. In that latter situation, annoying pruritus leads to persistent rubbing, which causes lichen simplex chronicus to be imposed on the effects of longstanding allergic contact dermatitis.

The same general principles that apply to allergic contact dermatitis apply equally to irritant contact dermatitis, the earliest stage being red macules or patches that very soon are surmounted by vesicles or bullae, or both. In the case of irritant-induced blisters, however, the roof of the lesions often has a gray cast, a consequence of the epidermis having become necrotic secondary to the effects of the irritant. Although both allergic contact dermatitis and irritant contact dermatitis result from direct contact of the skin with an offending agent, the two mechanisms are completely different; allergic contact dermatitis results from immunologic mechanisms, whereas irritant contact dermatitis does not.

INTEGRATION: UNIFYING CONCEPT What has been written about clinical diagnosis of allergic contact dermatitis applies in principle to irritant contact dermatitis. Distribution, in addition to character of individual lesions, is decisive.

Irritant contact dermatitis is unrelated to hypersensitivity and is inducible in every human being by virtue of the intrinsically damaging character of an irritant, the earliest stage being red macules or patches that very soon are surmounted by vesicles, bullae, or both.

All of the morphologic expressions of allergic contact dermatitis and of irritant contact dermatitis are a consequence of a basic pathologic process, to wit, delayed hypersensitivity for the former and nonhypersensitivity, often with necrotizing effects, for the latter. In short, papules, vesicles, and bullae that develop in response to contact allergens and contact irritants are a reflection of an inflammatory process that involves the dermis and epidermis. Spongiosis with little if any ballooning or necrosis is present in the case of allergic contact dermatitis, and ballooning accompanied by necrosis and little if any spongiosis is manifest in the case of irritant contact dermatitis.

THERAPY The patient must scrupulously avoid the suspected causative agent. Cold wet compresses and topical corticosteroids in a lotion or cream are beneficial for acute lesions, whereas a corticosteroid-containing ointment is helpful for chronic ones. A short-term course of oral corticosteroids is advisable in severe cases. Antihistamines taken orally usually are effective against severe pruritus that may interfere with sleep.

DEFINITION A systemic inflammatory process involving venules by deposits of fibrin within their wall in conjunction with neutrophils and nuclear "dust" of neutrophils. The clinical manifestations are urticarial papules, purpuric macules, papules, pustules, vesicles, and bullae, ulcers, and scars. The effects of the vasculitis in other organs are expressed variously, e.g., by gastrointestinal pain, hematuria, and arthritis.

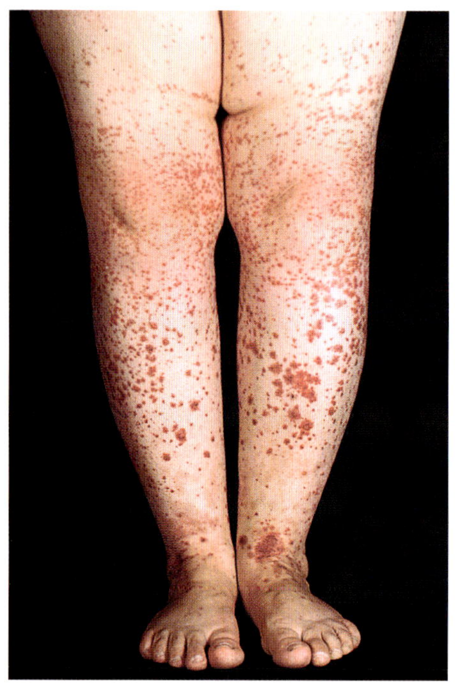

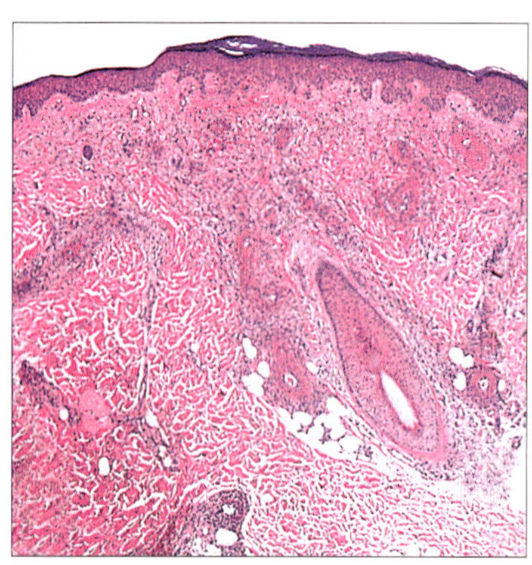

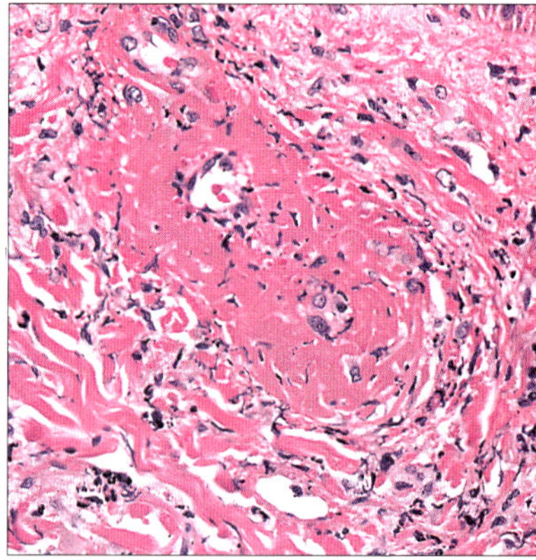

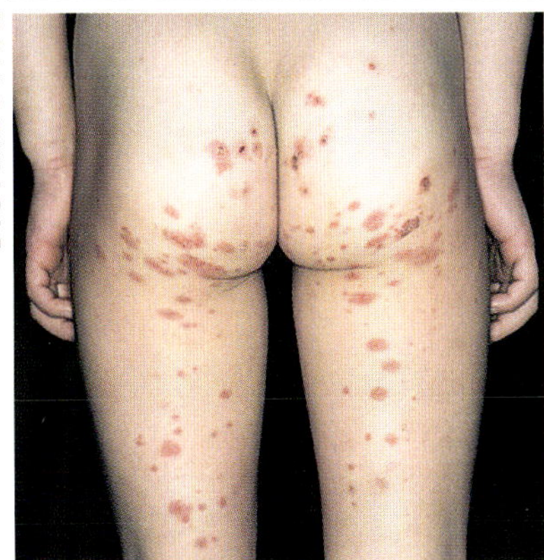

FIG. 4-1 *Purpuric macules, papules, and plaques in a patient with Schönlein-Henoch purpura.*

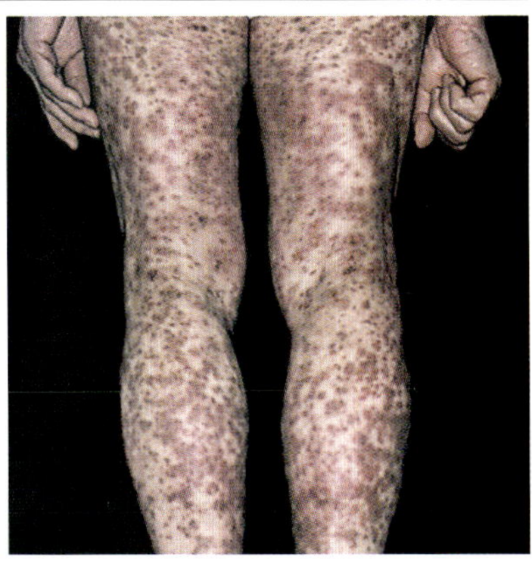

FIG. 4-2 *Purpuric macules, papules, and plaques, many of which have become confluent.*

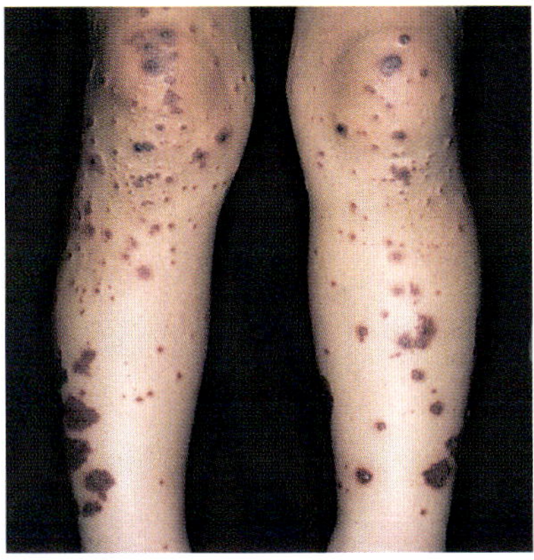

FIG. 4-3 *Purpuric macules, papules, and hemorrhagic bullae in a child with Schönlein-Henoch purpura.*

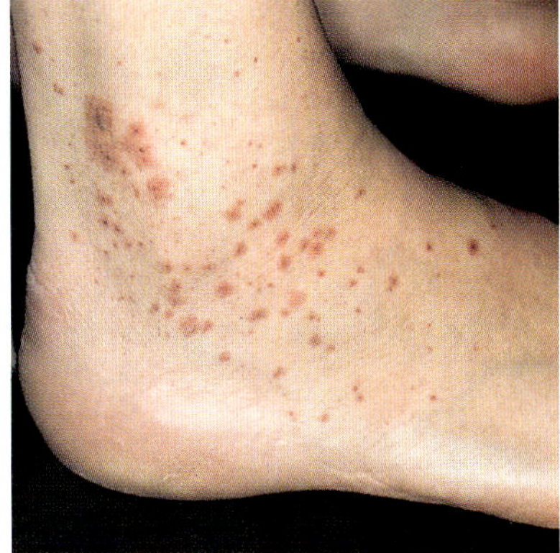

FIG. 4-4 *Purpuric papules, some of them agminated.*

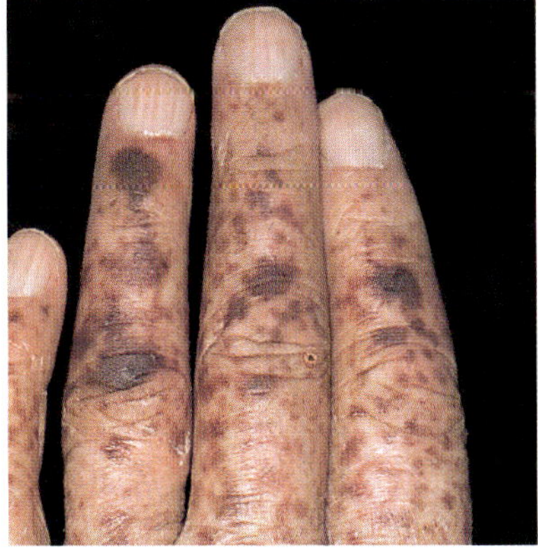

FIG. 4-5 *Purpuric macules, patches, and papules.*

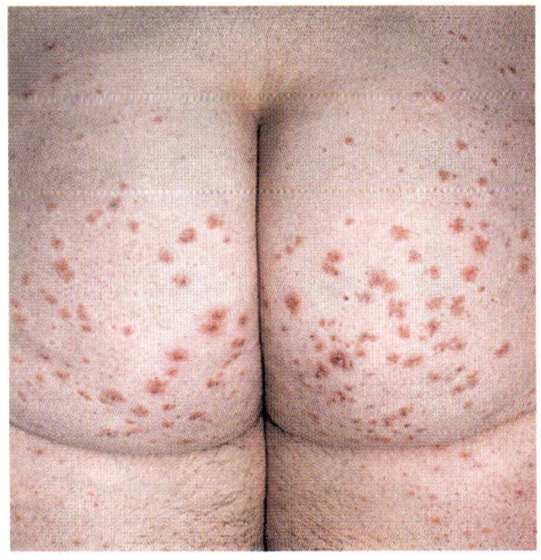

FIG. 4-6 *Purpuric macules and papules.*

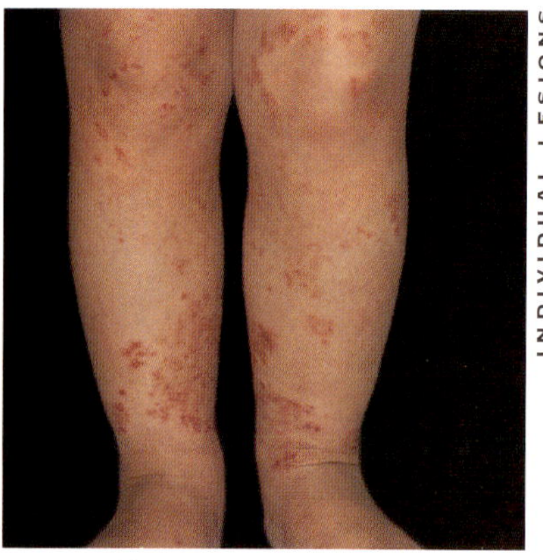

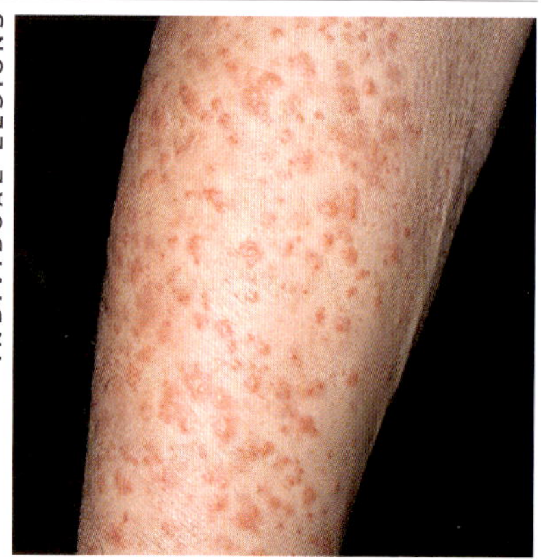

FIG. 4-7 *Purpuric macules and papules in a child.*

FIG. 4-8 *Urticarial papules.*

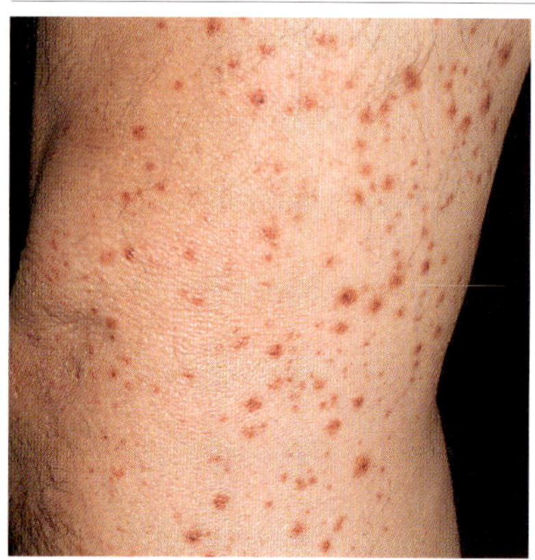

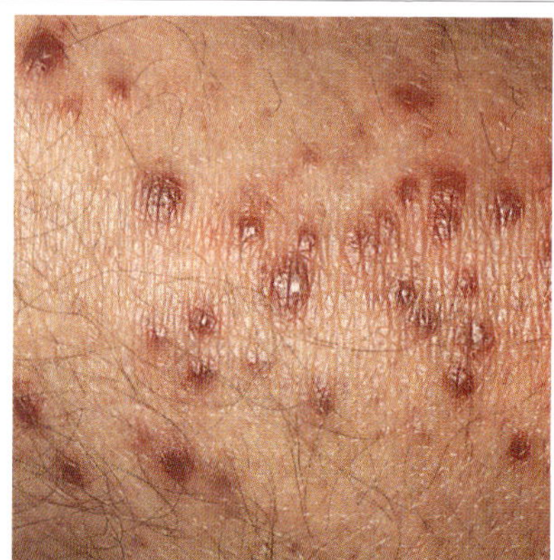

FIG. 4-9 *Purpuric macules and papules.*

FIG. 4-10 *Purpuric papules.*

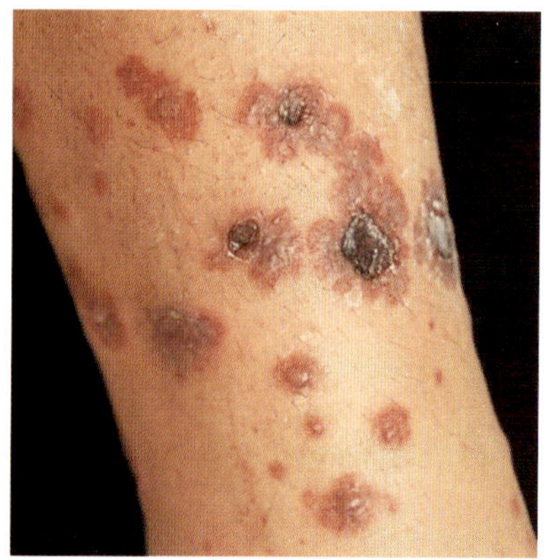

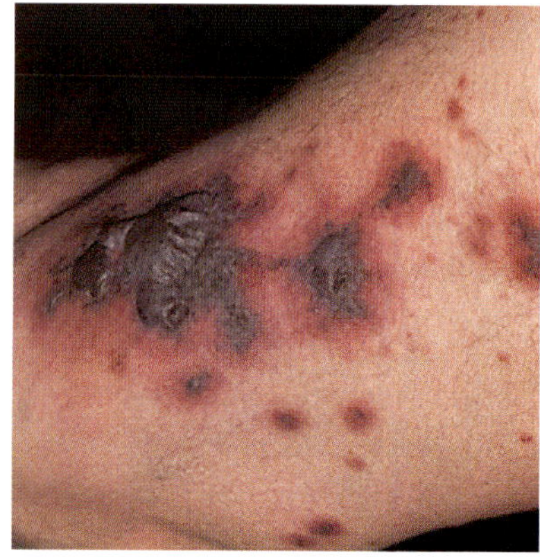

FIG. 4-11 *Purpuric macules, papules, and plaques, vesicles on a purpuric base, and ulcers covered by an eschar.*

FIG. 4-12 *Purpuric macules and papules, as well as hemorrhagic bullae.*

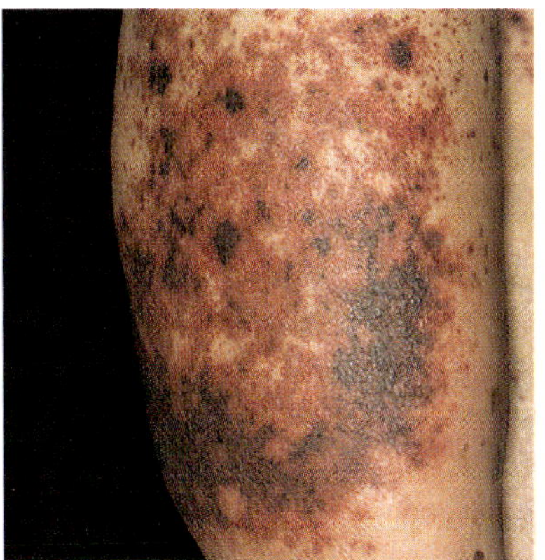

FIG. 4-13 *Purpuric macules, patches, and papules.*

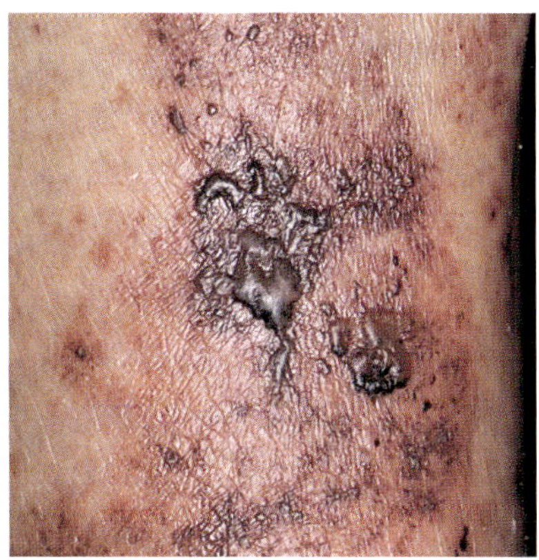

FIG. 4-14 *Hemorrhagic vesicles and bullae in company with purpuric macules and patches.*

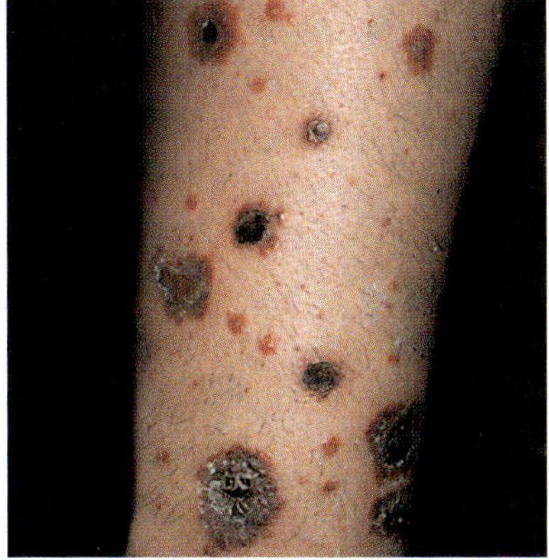

FIG. 4-15 *Purpuric papules and plaques, the latter covered by a hemorrhagic crust.*

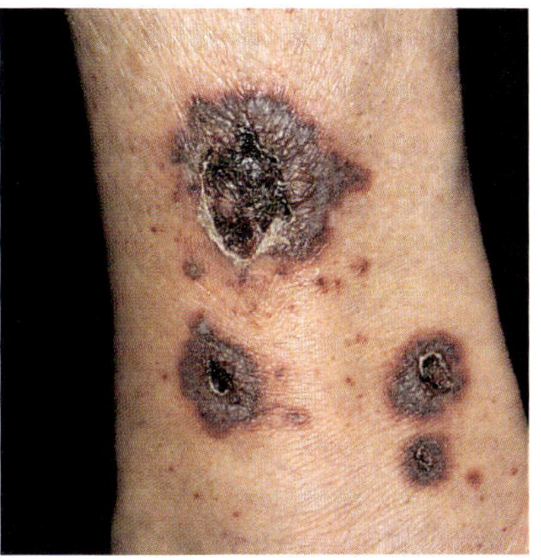

FIG. 4-16 *Purpuric macules and papules, and hemorrhagic bullae with a gray roof.*

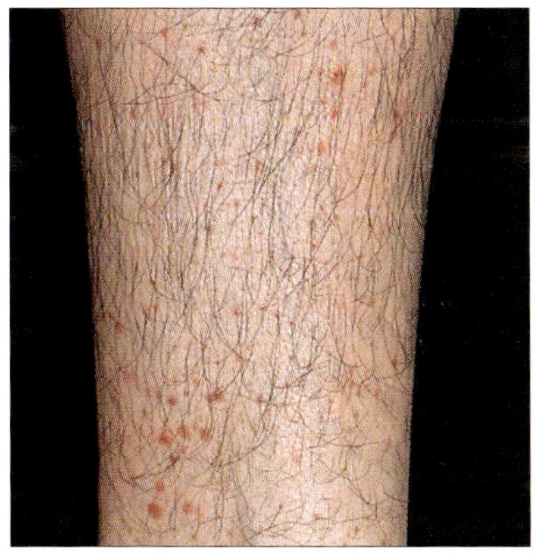

FIG. 4-17 *Punctate purpuric macules and subtle papules.*

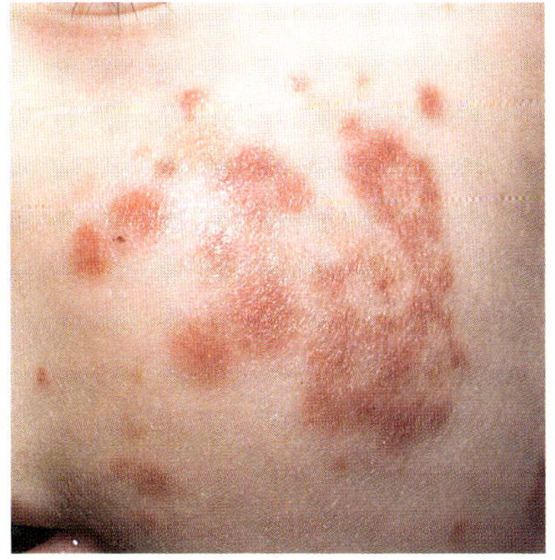

FIG. 4-18 *Edematous purpuric papules and plaques of Finkelstein's disease.*

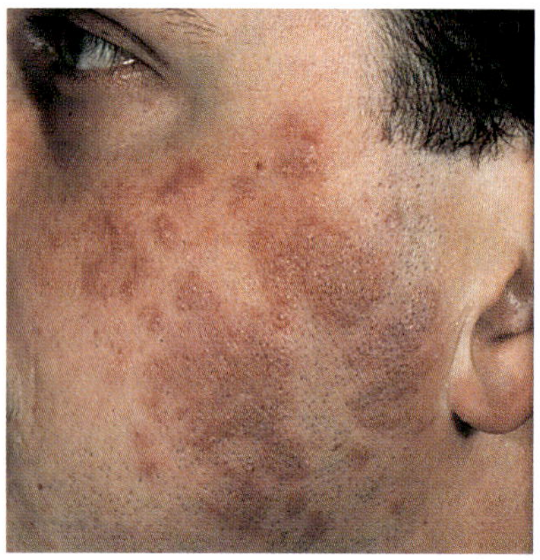

FIG. 4-19 *Papules and plaques of granuloma faciale.*

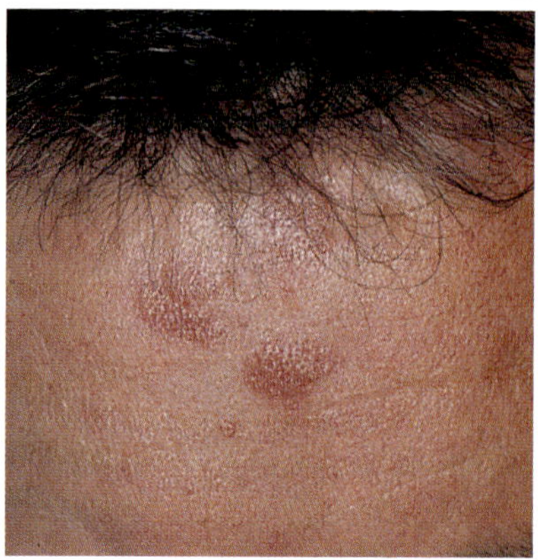

FIG. 4-20 *Plaques with patulous follicular ostia of granuloma faciale.*

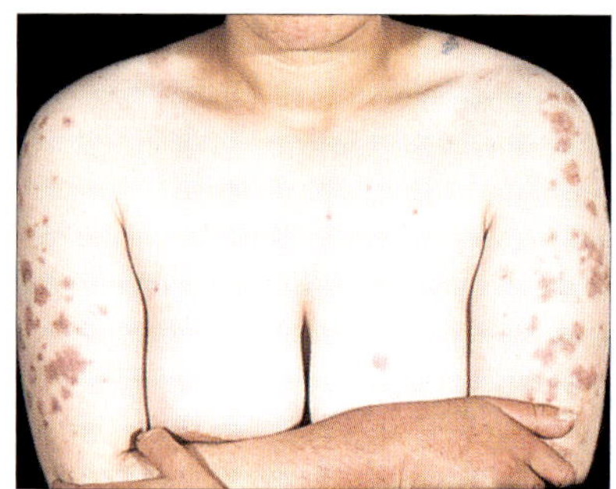

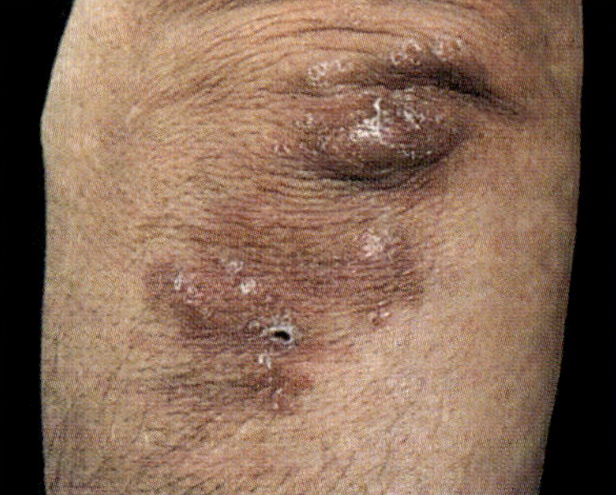

FIG. 4-21 (A, B) *Macules, papules, and plaques on the arms, including the vicinity of an elbow, in a patient with erythema elevatum diutinum, an expression of allergic vasculitis.*

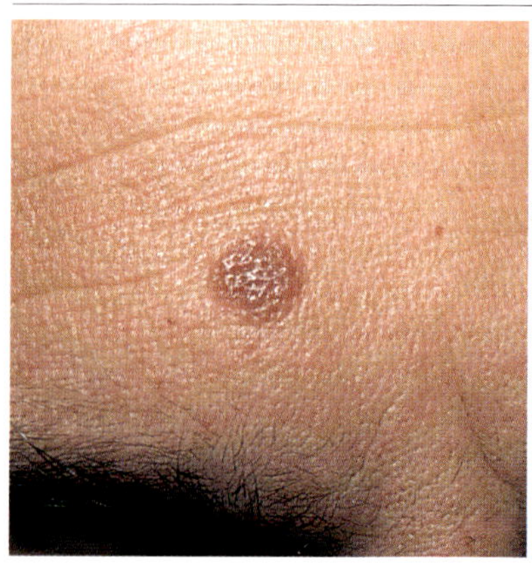

FIG. 4-22 *Plaque with markedly dilated ostia of follicles of granuloma faciale.*

ADJUNCTIVE DIAGNOSTIC TEST By application of the direct immuno-fluorescence technique, fibrin, immunoglobulins, and complement can be detected in the wall of venules.

COURSE Urticarial papules are an uncommon expression of allergic vasculitis and they tend to become purpuric quickly. Purpuric papules, the most common presentation of allergic vasculitis, often remain just that, progressing neither to vesicles or pustules nor to ulcers. Purpuric pustules resolve as hemorrhagic crusts. Purpuric vesicles and bullae often develop a gray roof, a sign of complete epidermal necrosis.

As a rule, papules and blisters of allergic vasculitis continue to form, as others resolve, over time. In the case of Schönlein-Henoch purpura, for example, the process usually comes to a halt in weeks. In the case of allergic vasculitis that results from administration of a drug, the lesions persist as long as the drug is given; when the drug is withdrawn, new lesions cease to appear and established lesions soon disappear. A peculiar presentation of allergic vasculitis is the papules and nodules that accompany granuloma faciale/erythema elevatum diutinum. That slowly evolving, long-lasting process persists for years, devolution of it also being slow and long. In time, fibroplasia supervenes, but the lesions regress only slightly, changing in color (becoming less red or orange) more than they do in size.

In sum, depending on a variety of factors such as cause and anatomic site, and on others not yet known, allergic vasculitis may last for weeks, months, or years. Allergic vasculitis induced by a drug, such as penicillin or sulfonamide, may be relatively short lived, lasting weeks, whereas Finkelstein's disease and Schönlein-Henoch purpura may persist for months, and granuloma faciale/erythema elevatum diutinum for years.

INTEGRATION: UNIFYING CONCEPT Allergic vasculitis, known by histopathologists as leukocytoclastic vasculitis, is a distinctive form of vasculitis that affects venules in a particular way. They have fibrin in their wall in the context of neutrophils and nuclear "dust" of neutrophils within the dermis. The histopathologic findings are the same at the outset of all expressions of allergic vasculitis, including granuloma faciale/erythema elevatum diutinum. Only after many weeks can lesions of granuloma faciale/erythema elevatum diutinum be identified with specificity for what they are by histopathologists, and then on the basis of nodular infiltrates in the reticular dermis made up of a mixture of inflammatory cells, namely, eosinophils, lymphocytes, and plasma cells in addition to neutrophils and nuclear "dust" of neutrophils.

Despite the fact that allergic vasculitis is fundamentally a single pathologic process, its clinical manifestations vary remarkably and range from the discrete papules of Schönlein-Henoch purpura, to papules arranged in the cocarde pattern of Finkelstein's disease, to purpuric pustules, vesicles, and bullae induced by some drugs, to nodules and even tumors of granuloma faciale/erythema elevatum diutinum.

The mechanism whereby immune complexes come to be formed is responsible for allergic vasculitis.

THERAPY Management must be directed first to the inciting agent, e.g., infection in the case of Schönlein-Henoch purpura or a particular chemical in the case of a drug. When a drug is responsible, it must be interdicted. Oral administration of corticosteroids in sufficient dose is the most effective way to interrupt the immunologic process and stop the appearance of new lesions in the skin and other organs. In severe cases, cyclophosphamide may be extraordinarily helpful.

DEFINITION Loss of hair attributable either to the effects of inflammatory cells on follicles or to physiological or mechanical factors in which inflammatory cells play no role. Although the scalp is the site most often affected, any region of the skin that bears hair follicles may be involved by certain types of alopecia.

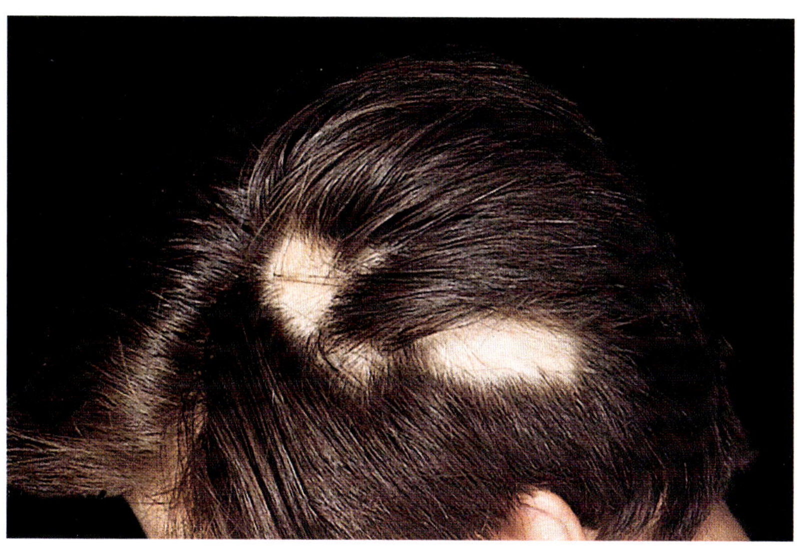

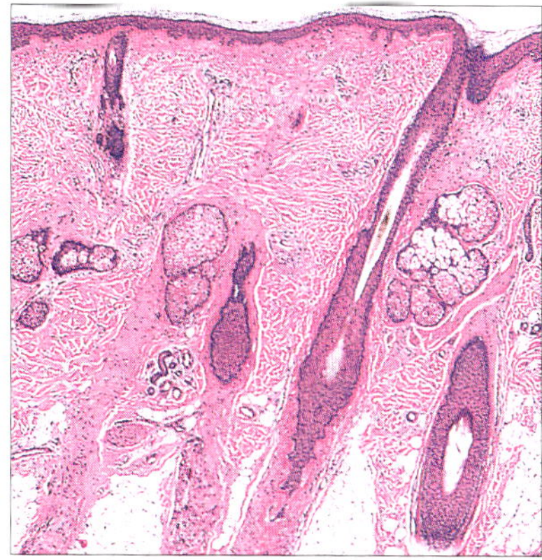

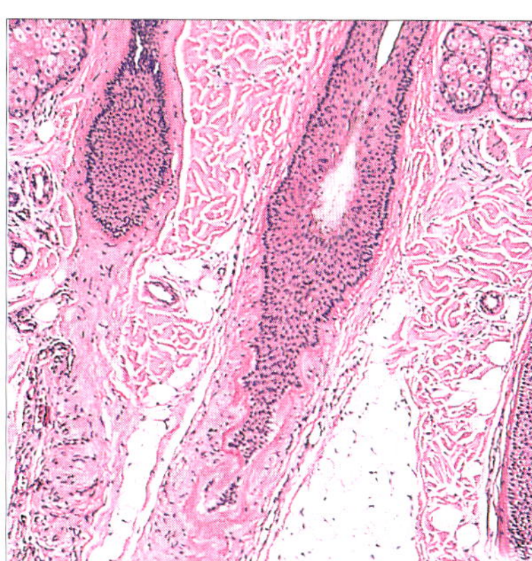

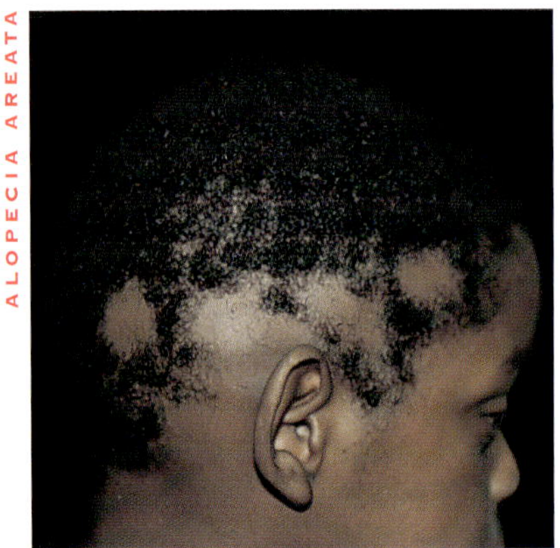

FIG. 5-1 *Lesions of alopecia areata.*

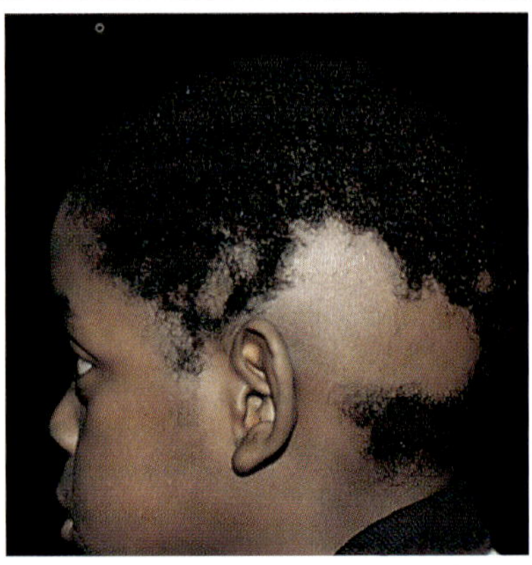

FIG. 5-2 *Small and large lesions of alopecia areata.*

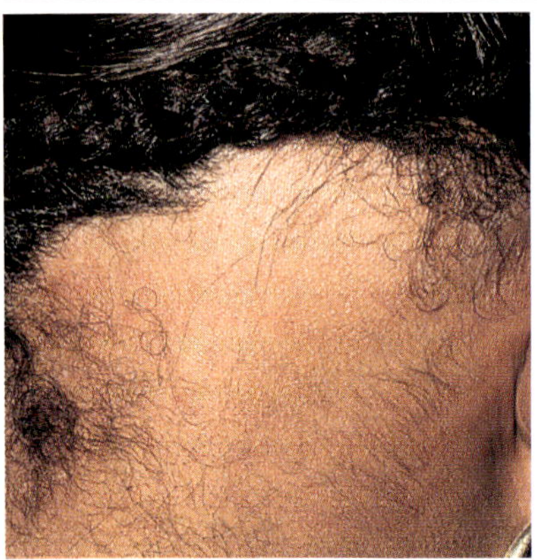

FIG. 5-3 *Large lesion of alopecia areata on the occipital region (ophiasis).*

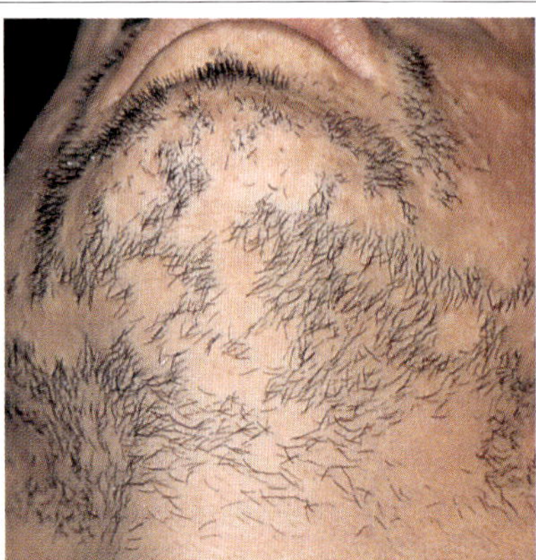

FIG. 5-4 *Many lesions of alopecia areata in the region of the beard.*

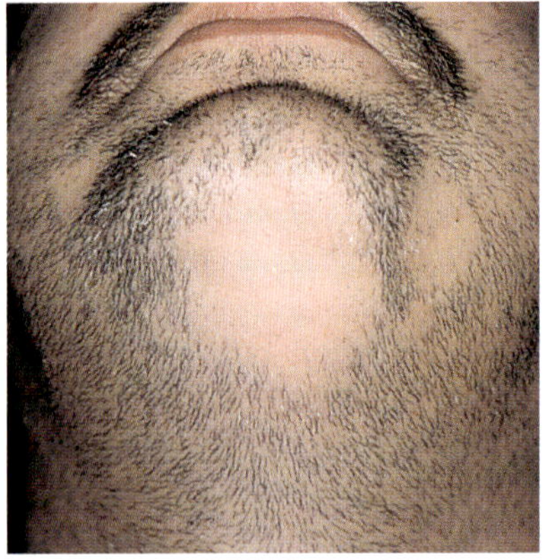

FIG. 5-5 *Lesions of alopecia areata of the beard.*

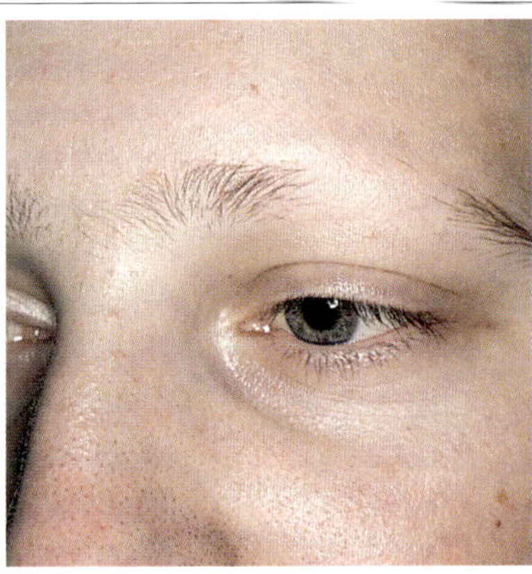

FIG. 5-6 *Discrete lesion of alopecia areata on the eyebrow.*

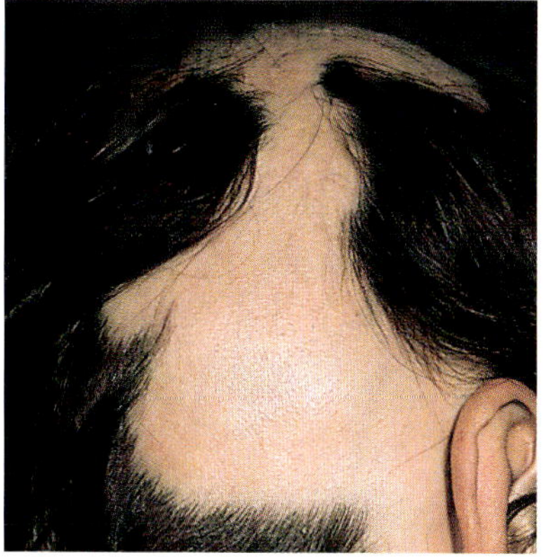

FIG. 5-7 *Lesions of alopecia areata that have become confluent.*

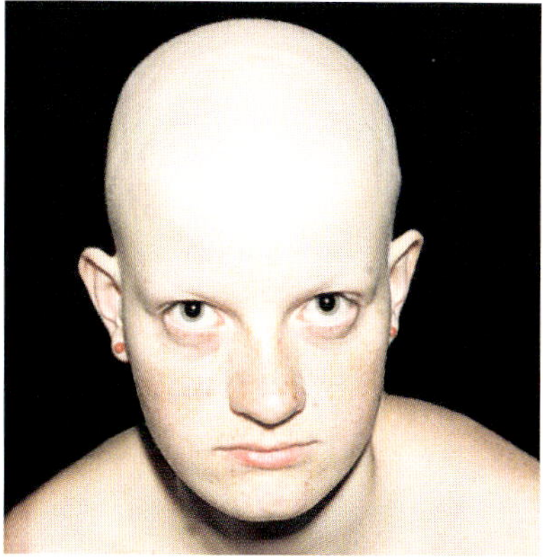

FIG. 5-8 *Alopecia universalis with absence of eyebrows and eyelashes.*

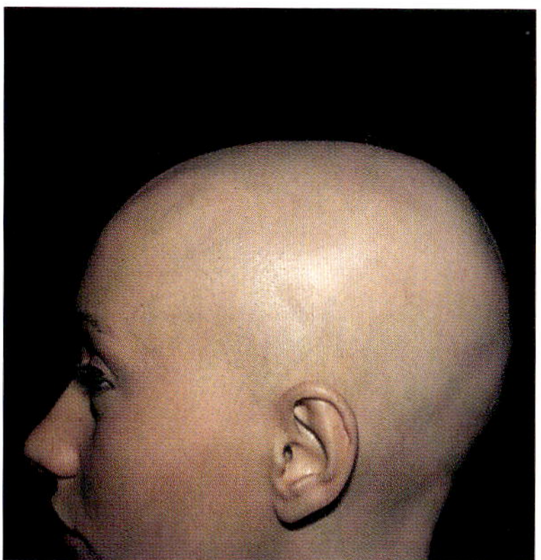

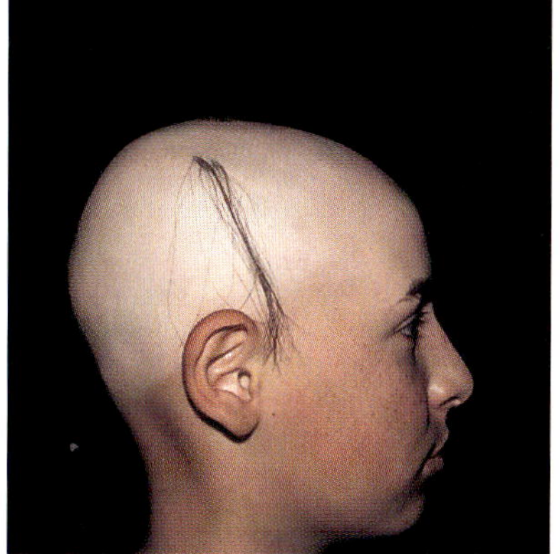

FIG. 5-9 (A, B) *Alopecia "universalis," i.e., nearly entire.*

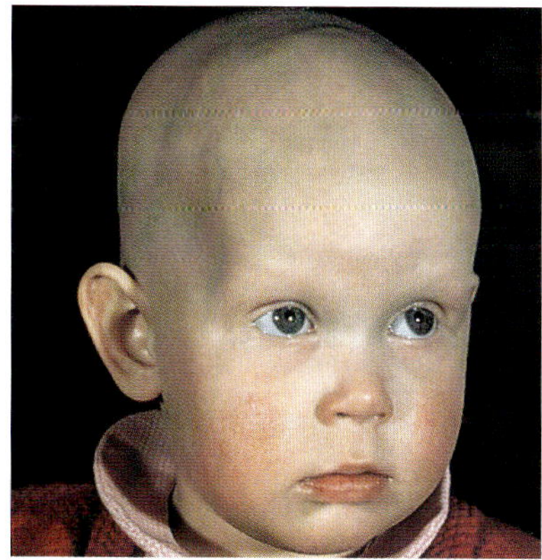

FIG. 5-10 *Alopecia universalis with complete absence of hair.*

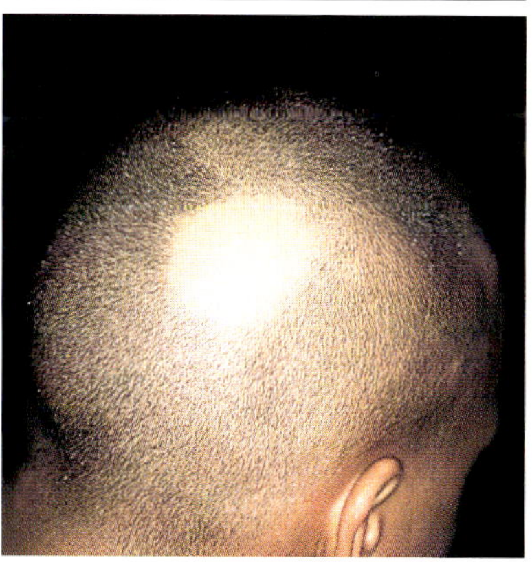

FIG. 5-11 *A single lesion of alopecia areata.*

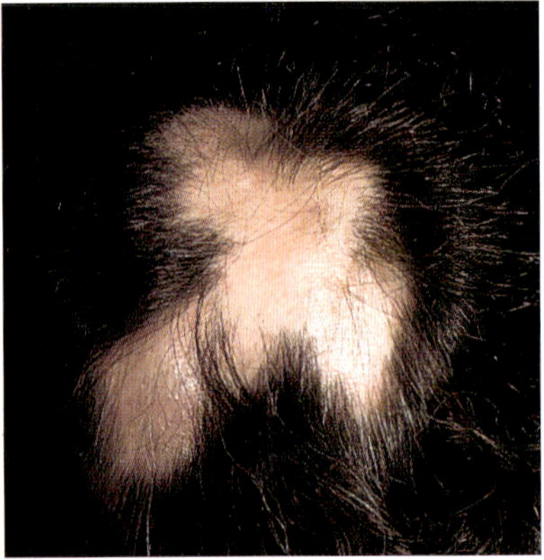 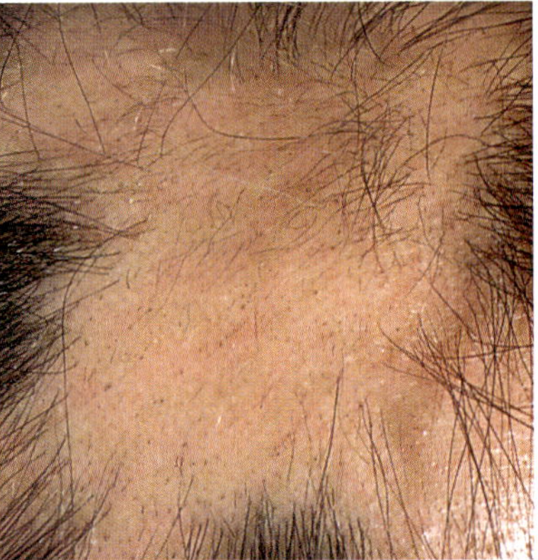

FIG. 5-12 (A, B) *"Exclamation point hairs" represent residual stubs of hair following breakage of shafts in alopecia areata.*

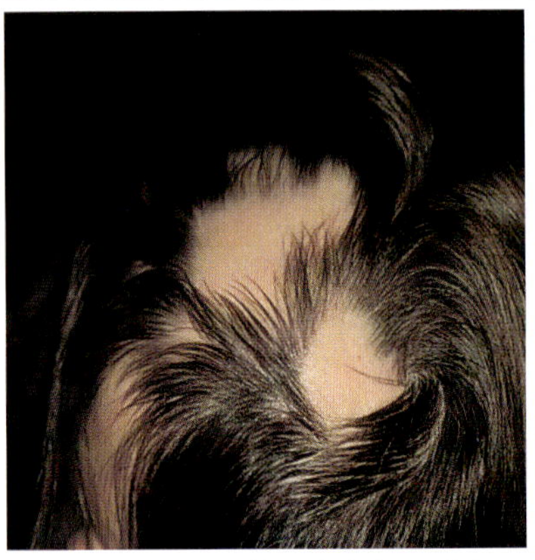 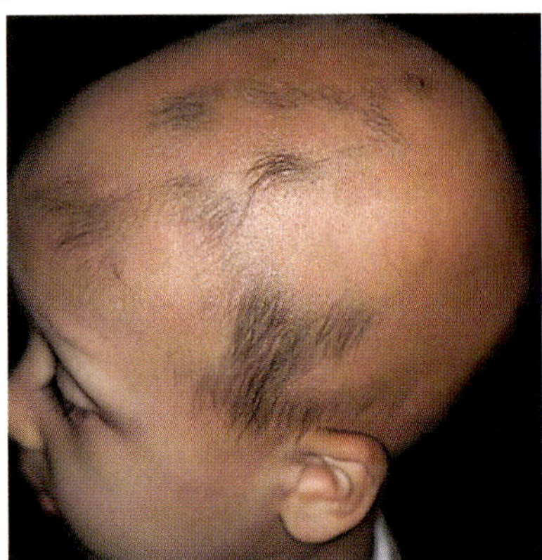

FIG. 5-13 *Absence of hair in lesions of alopecia areata.*

FIG. 5-14 *Extensive lesions of alopecia areata.*

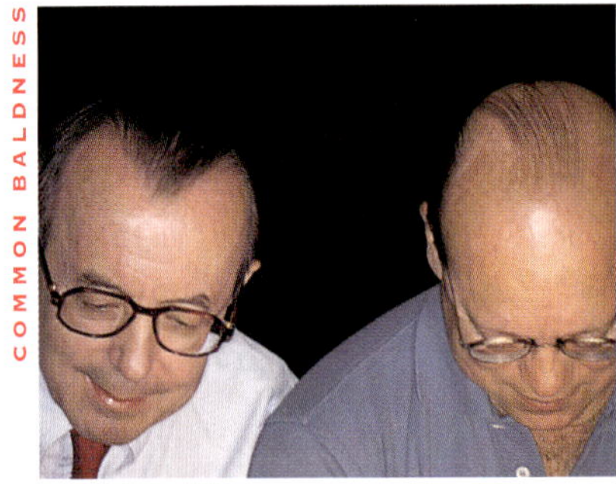 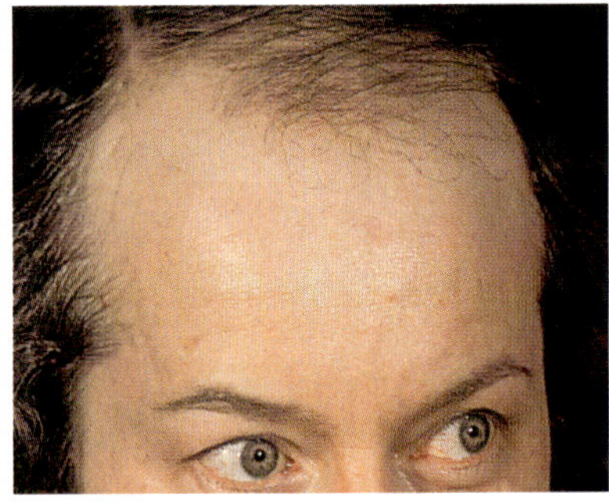

FIG. 5-15 *Different stages in progression of common baldness in two authors of this atlas.*

FIG. 5-16 *"Male pattern" baldness in a woman.*

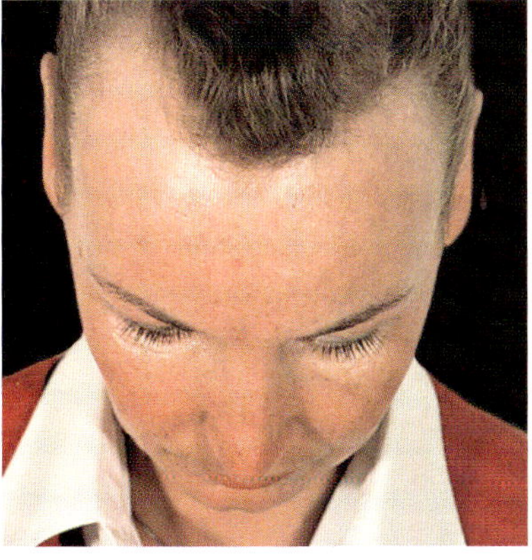

FIG. 5-17 *"Male pattern" baldness in a woman.*

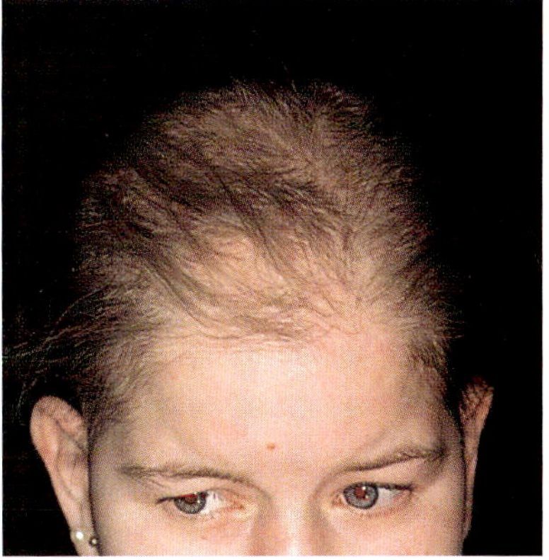

FIG. 5-18 *"Male pattern" baldness.*

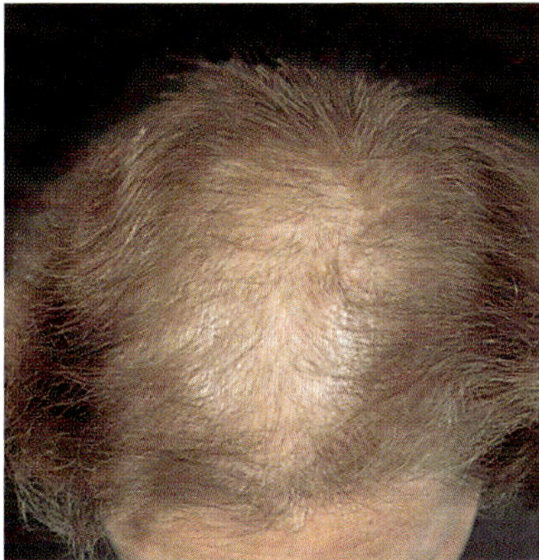

FIG. 5-19 *"Male pattern" baldness.*

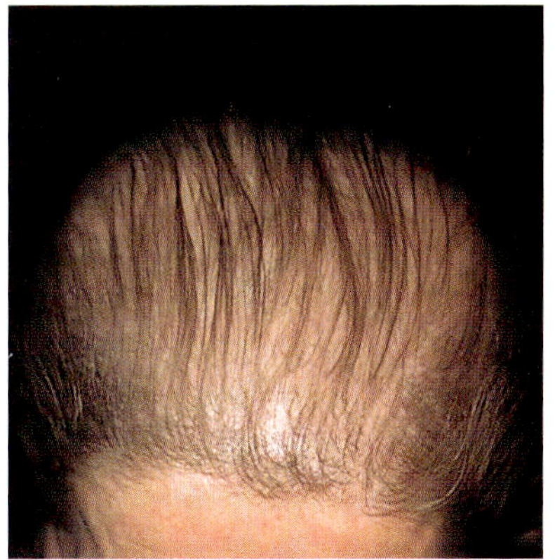

FIG. 5-20 *"Male pattern" baldness.*

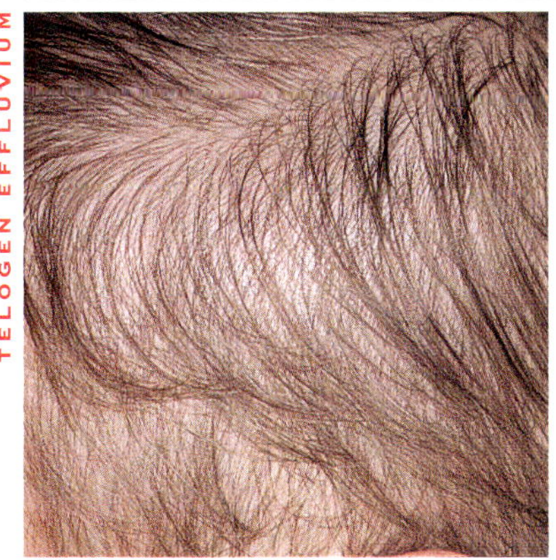

FIG. 5-21 *Diffuse loss of hair but with many normal hairs still in place.*

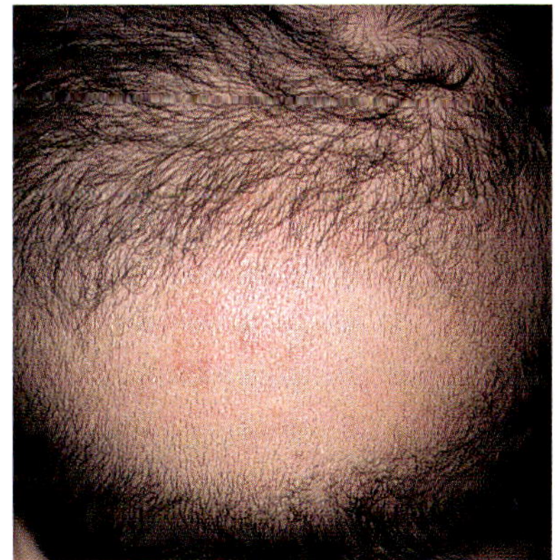

FIG. 5-22 *Alopecia confined to the occiput of an infant secondary to pressure and rubbing, a type of telogen effluvium.*

TELOGEN EFFLUVIUM

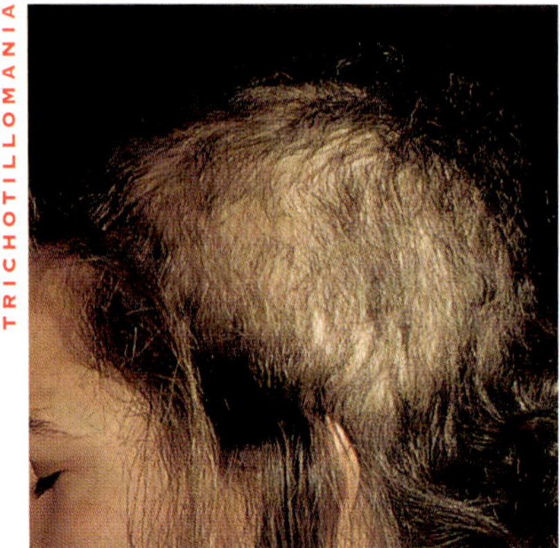

FIG. 5-23 *Shortened hairs of different lengths, the result of hairs having been twisted to and fro until they have fractured.*

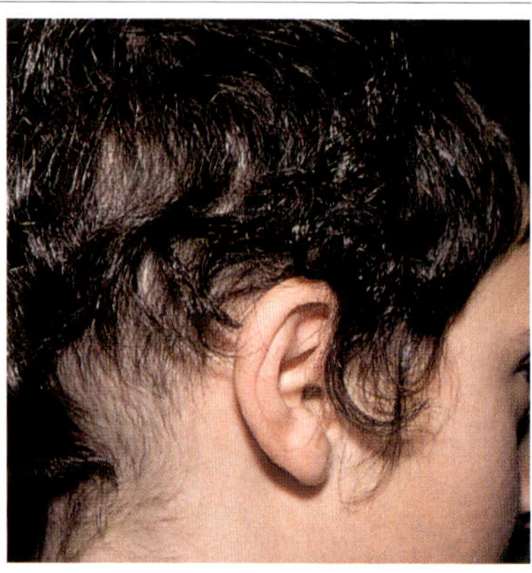

FIG. 5-24 *Diffuse alopecia with hairs of different lengths having broken secondary to their having been twisted back and forth.*

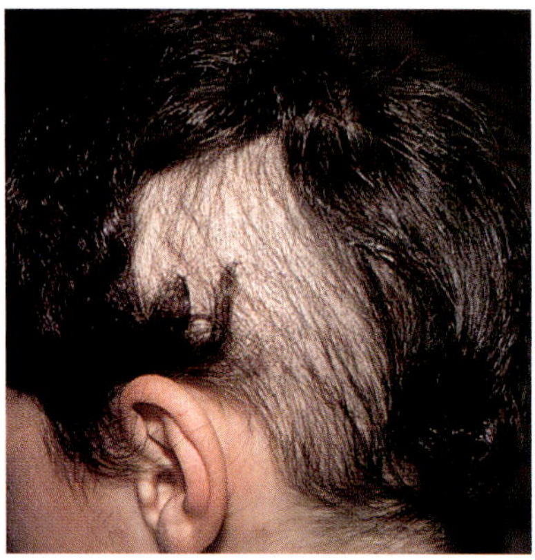

FIG. 5-25 *Patchy alopecia with hairs of different lengths.*

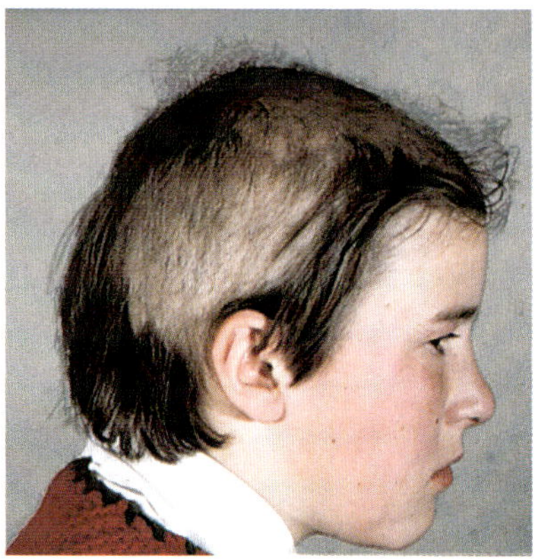

FIG. 5-26 *Diffuse alopecia with hairs of different lengths in a child who seems to be emotionally troubled.*

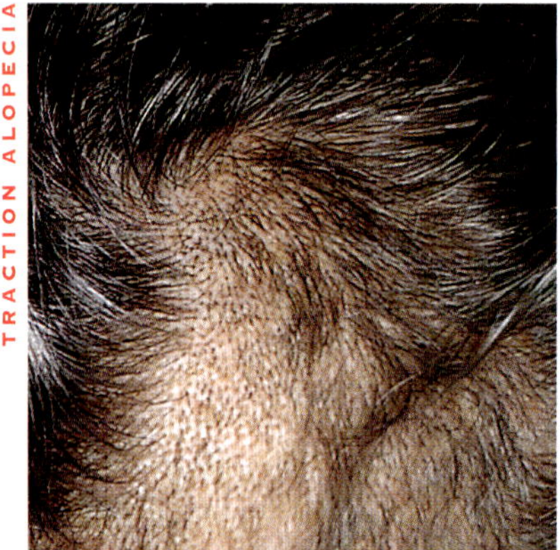

FIG. 5-27 *Loss of hairs in the frontotemporal region consequent to traction.*

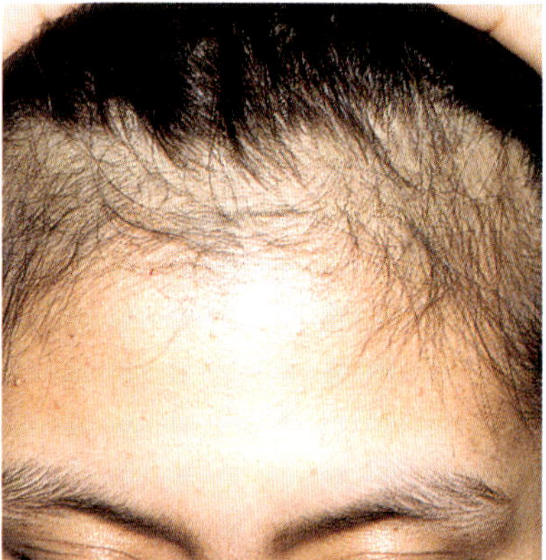

FIG. 5-28 *Loss of hairs in the frontal region as a result of traction for purpose of straightening hairs.*

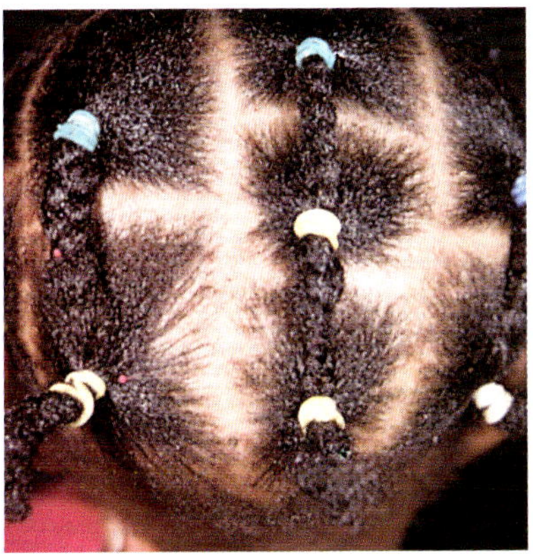
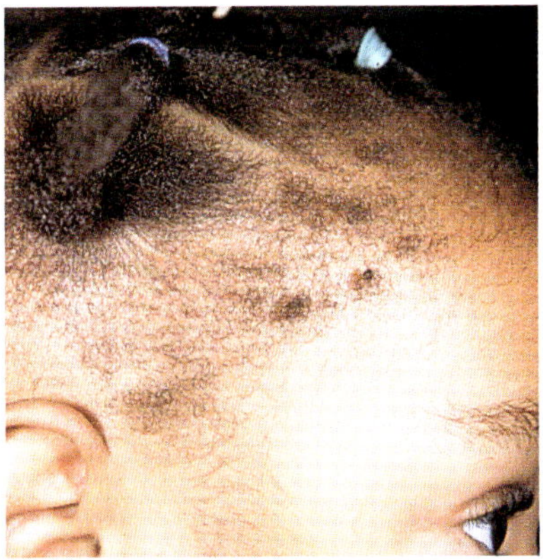

FIG. 5-29 (A, B) *Sharply circumscribed zones of alopecia over the temporoparietal region and vertex secondary to tight braiding of hair.*

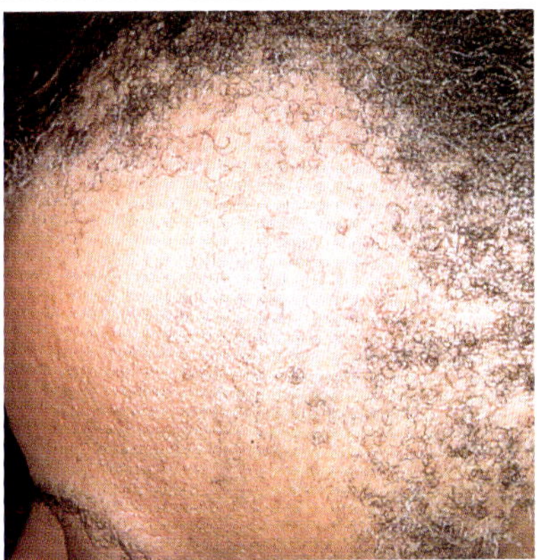

FIG. 5-30 *So-called follicular degeneration syndrome is really traction alopecia.*

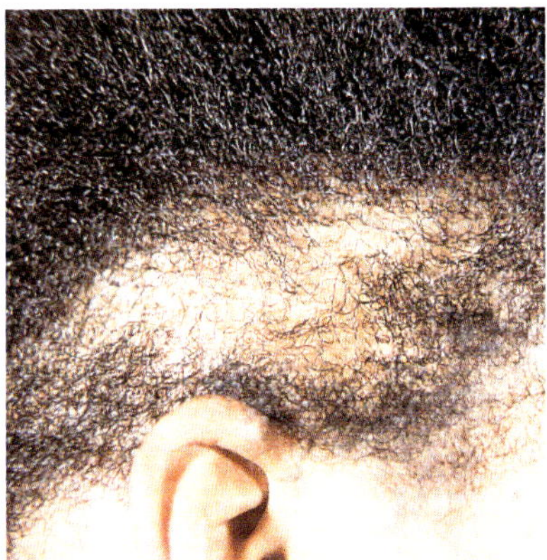

FIG. 5-31 *Loss of hair as a result of traction consequent to use of "rollers."*

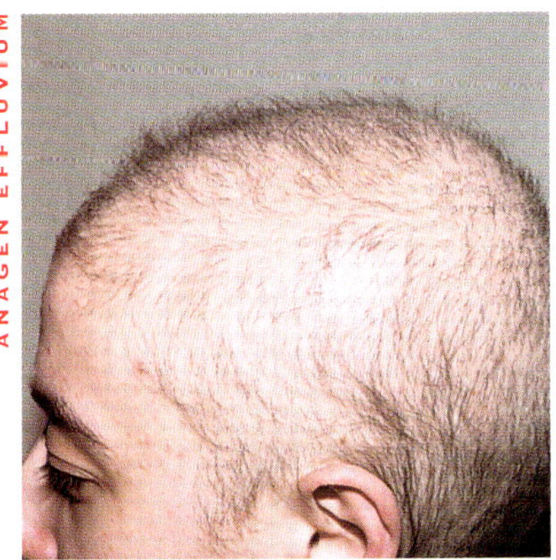

fig. 5-32 *Diffuse alopecia during chemotherapy for acute leukemia.*

ADJUNCTIVE DIAGNOSTIC TEST "Hair pull" to study by conventional microscopy the character of hair shafts and follicular bulbs. For example, the ratio of anagen to telogen hairs enables a physician to judge the nature of an alopecia, e.g., it is reversed in telogen effluvium, in a fashion analogous to inspection of gross morphologic attributes, e.g., "exclamation point hairs" in alopecia areata.

COURSE Both basic types of alopecia, namely, those unassociated with infiltrates of inflammatory cells (e.g., common baldness and telogen effluvium) and those associated with infiltrates of inflammatory cells (e.g., lichen planus and lupus erythematosus; see also the chapters on lichen planus and lupus erythematosus, respectively), display a characteristic sequence of clinical and histopathologic changes. In the case of common baldness, for example, the loss of hair at the outset is hardly noticeable, but after years a man may be nearly entirely bald. During this time, the follicular cycle (growing, involuting, and resting stages) shortens progressively so that each cycle becomes shorter than the last and each follicle becomes progressively thinner and situated higher in the subcutaneous fat and, in time, within the dermis. Eventually, the long terminal follicles with their long sturdy hairs are converted into short vellus follicles with their short wisp-like hairs.

In the case of lichen planus, for example, changes at the outset in the skin and in hairs are hardly noticeable clinically, but eventually reddish violet plaques become progressively alopecic and, still later, all that is left are white patches, some of them scarred, of alopecia. The dense lichenoid infiltrates of lymphocytes that surround follicles of lichen planopilaris at a relatively early stage of the process are responsible for destruction of follicular epithelium and for induction of alopecia by the effects of fibrotic tracks that eventually replace the follicles.

In common baldness and lichen planus, despite the fact that the former is a non-inflammatory process and the latter is an inflammatory one, the result is the same, namely, permanent loss of hair. In the case of common baldness, effete follicles are still present and there are no signs of scarring, either clinically or histopathologically. In lichen planus, however, no follicles remain at sites of alopecia; they have been destroyed, and there are signs of scarring at sites where formerly there were follicles.

A predictable sequence of events can be anticipated in non-inflammatory alopecias, like so-called telogen effluvium, and in inflammatory ones, like discoid lupus erythematosus. In the former, hairs always return, whereas in the latter, they do not.

It is impossible to predict accurately the course of alopecia areata, totalis, and universalis. As a rule, the longer the failure of hairs to regrow, the less likely will be their return, even should treatment eventually be instituted for that purpose. In the absence of any therapy, some patients with these three variants of a single distinctive type of inflammatory alopecia show signs of reappearance of hairs within weeks, others in months, and still others never. If therapy in alopecia areata and its more extensive equivalents is going to be effective, some evidence of regrowth of hair should become apparent in weeks. In many persons afflicted, however, therapy is ineffective.

INTEGRATION: UNIFYING CONCEPT Each specific type of alopecia—common baldness, telogen effluvium, trichotillomania, traction alopecia, alopecia areata, lichen planus, and discoid lupus erythematosus—represents a single specific process. Common baldness and telogen effluvium are physiologic processes, whereas trichotillomania, traction alopecia, lichen planus, discoid lupus erythematosus, and alopecia areata are pathologic ones. Lichen planus is a single process, whether it expresses itself as violaceous polygonal papules, dystrophic nails, or alopecia. So, too, is lupus dermatitis/panniculitis, whether its expression is evanescent pink patches (butterfly blush), subcutaneous nodules (lupus profundus), arcuate, annular, and serpiginous red scaly lesions (subacute cutaneous lupus erythematosus), bullae (bullous lupus erythematosus), or red plaques that sometimes involute as hypopigmented, alopecic, atrophic scars (discoid lupus erythematosus). Alopecia areata/totalis/universalis is an inflammatory disease of unknown cause in which the infiltrate of lymphocytes is centered around follicular bulbs.

Common baldness results from the effects of androgens on matrical cells in the bulb of follicles, telogen effluvium develops by virtue of interruption of anagen by a variety of factors, trichotillomania and traction alopecia are a consequence of mechanical influences, and alopecia areata and its variants are thought to be mediated by immunologic mechanisms. In trichotillomania, hairs are broken off by virtue of twisting them to and fro repeatedly; stopping the habit leads to return of normal pelage because the follicles themselves are undamaged. In contrast, in traction alopecia, a condition that occurs commonly in African-American women consequent to the effects of "rolling," "plaiting," and "cornrowing" (and wrongly termed "hot comb alopecia," "pseudopelade of black women," and "follicular degeneration syndrome"), hairs are lost by virtue of a lichenoid lymphocytic perifolliculitis that eventuates in perifollicular fibroplasia, a phenomenon that eventually "strangles" follicles and causes progressive permanent alopecia.

THERAPY

Alopecia areata: The inflammatory process tends to remit without treatment and in some patients hairs tend to regrow. Recurrences, however, are common. Systemic administration or intralesional injections of corticosteroids sometimes are helpful in interrupting the advance of lesions that are enlarging. Topical or oral methoxalen and ultraviolet A therapy sometimes are beneficial in severe cases. Induction of allergic contact hypersensitivity by application of diphencyprone at zones of alopecia may be effective.

Common baldness in men: Transplantation of hair certainly results in the appearance of pelage, but the cosmetic result varies from excellent to poor, the criterion being naturalness versus artificiality of appearance. In recent years, medications, such as minoxidil applied topically and finasteride (a 5 α-reductase inhibitor) given orally, have been introduced for the purpose of restoring growth of hair or slowing loss of it. Although the benefit for some men is undeniable, the result in general is not dramatic.

Male pattern baldness in women: Minoxidil applied topically may be of slight benefit.

Telogen effluvium: The process is self-limited and no treatment is either necessary or effective.

Trichotillomania: Psychotherapy is advisable if the underlying emotional disorder is deemed to be correctable. Psychopharmacologic agents may be instituted in lieu of psychotherapy or as an adjunct to it.

Traction alopecia: All manipulation of hairs must stop, especially the use of rollers and plaiting tightly in any manner.

DEFINITION A condition in which deposits of a fibrillary protein (amyloid) appear in the skin as macules, papules, and nodules consequent to the effects of local factors, or as patches (which may be purpuric), plaques, nodules, and tumors as a result of a systemic disease like myeloma.

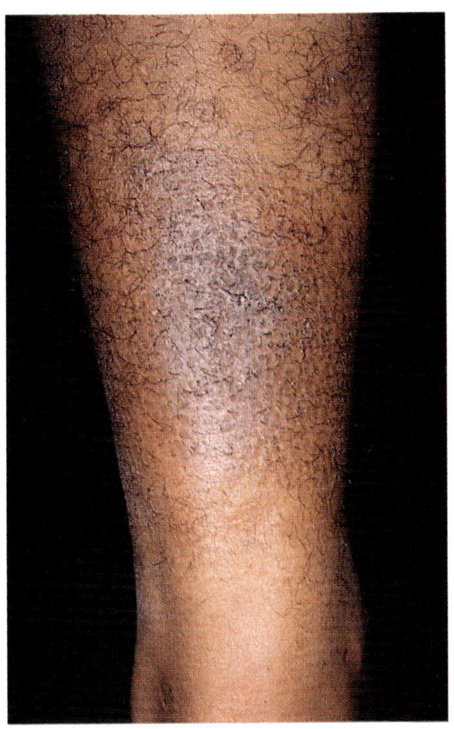

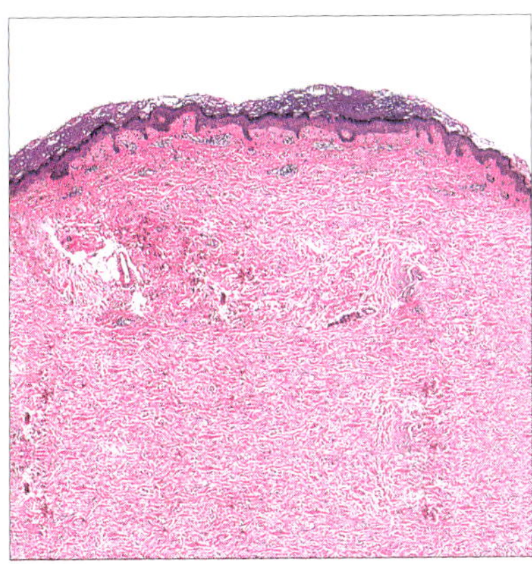

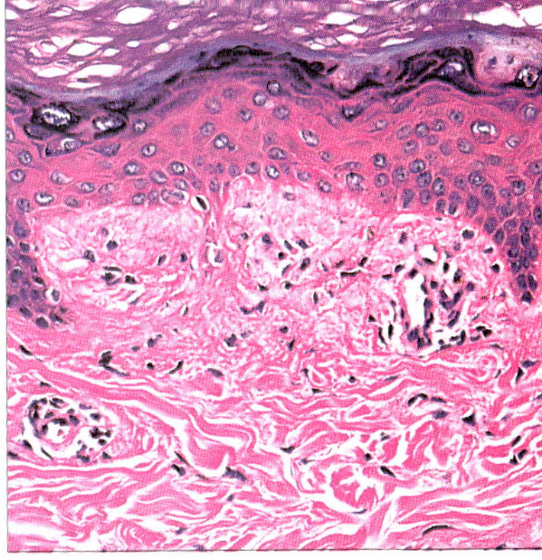

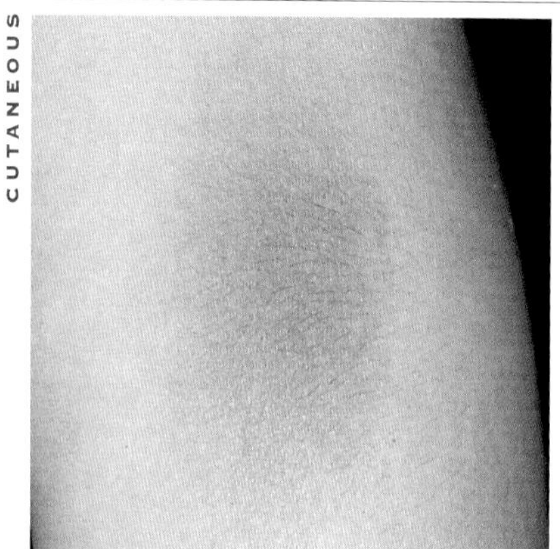

FIG. 6-1 *Macular amyloidosis. Pigmented macules remain flat if not rubbed persistently.*

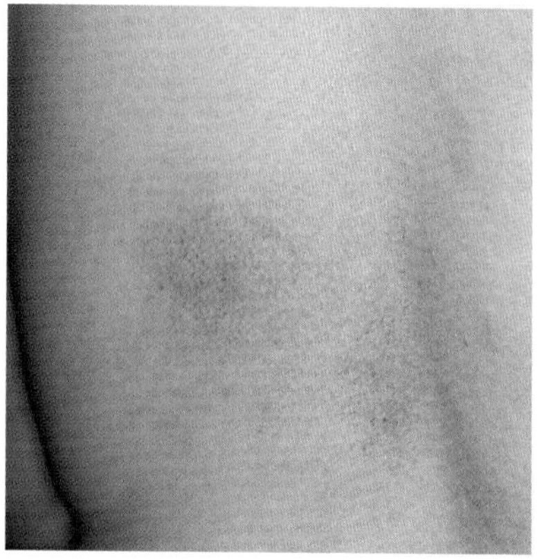

FIG. 6-2 *Macular/papular amyloidosis. The papules result from prolonged rubbing.*

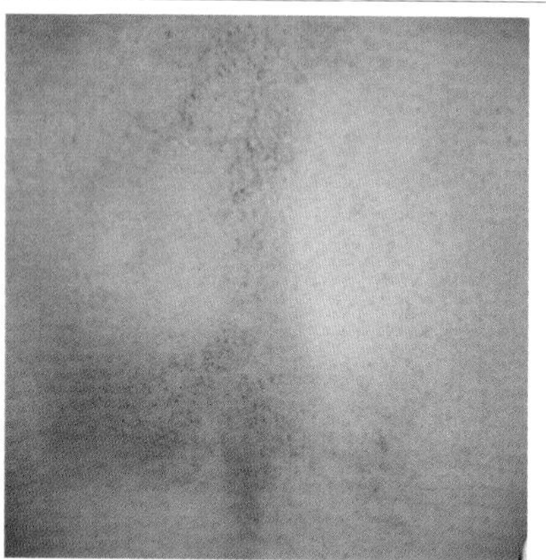

FIG. 6-3 *Reticulated pattern formed by pigmented macules.*

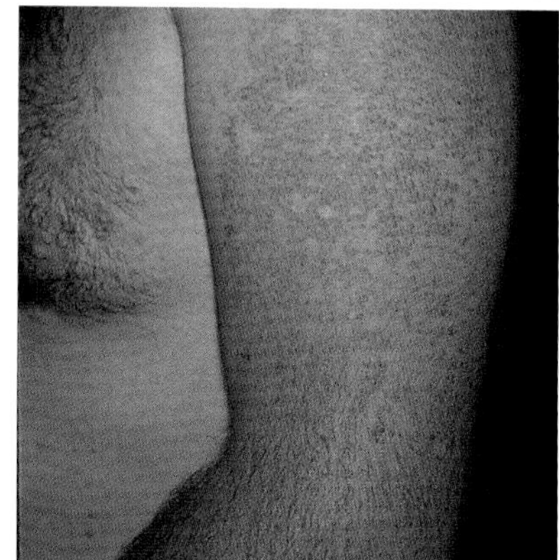

FIG. 6-4 *Widespread papules.*

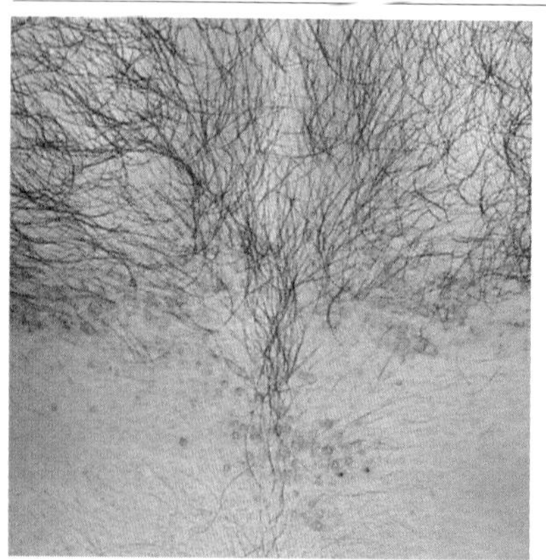

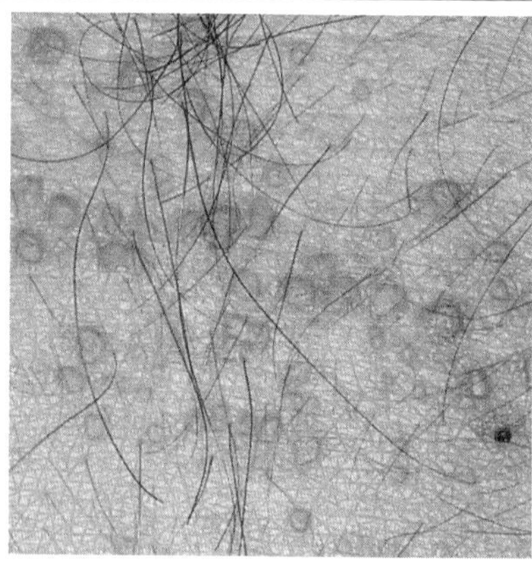

FIG. 6-5 (A, B) *Papules of amyloidosis.*

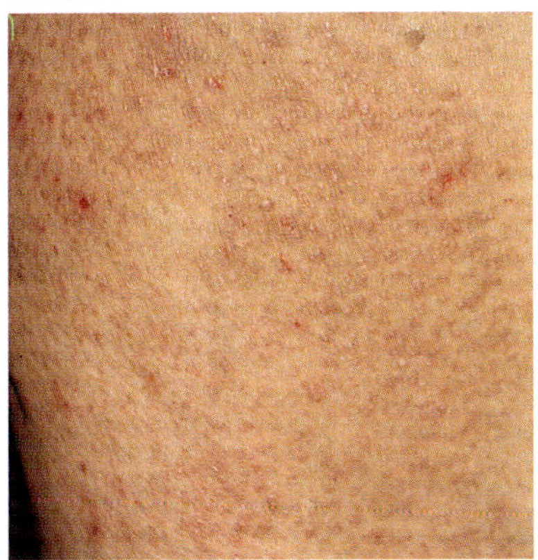

FIG. 6-6 *Papular (lichenoid) amyloidosis results from rubbing.*

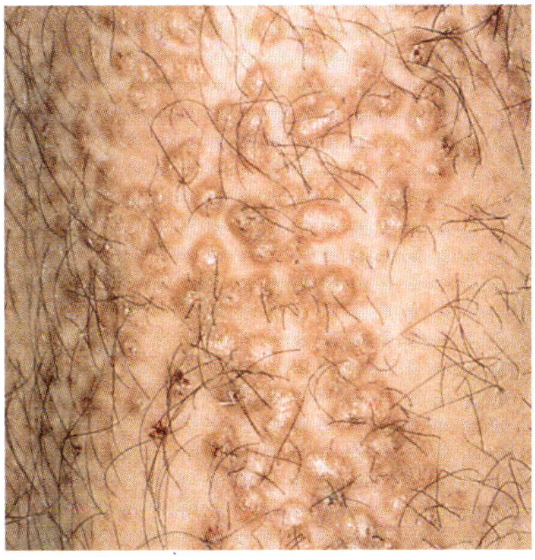

FIG. 6-7 *Discrete keratotic papules are like those of prurigo mitis.*

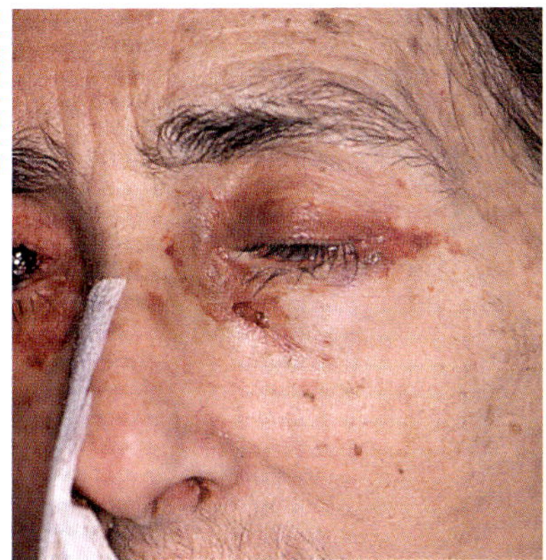

FIG. 6-8 *Periorbital purpura accompanied by hemorrhagic blisters.*

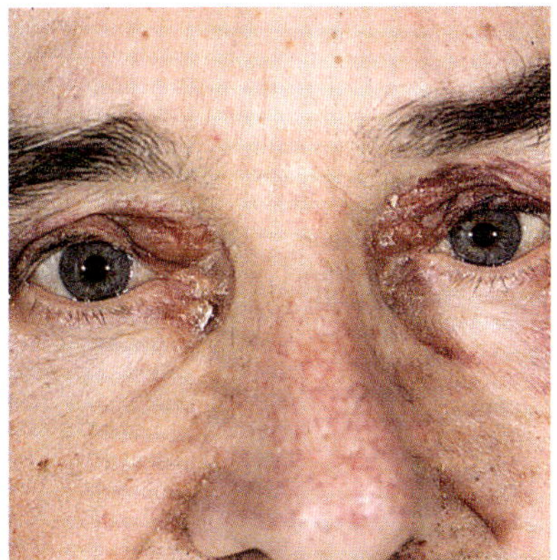

FIG. 6-9 *Purpuric macules, papules, and plaques.*

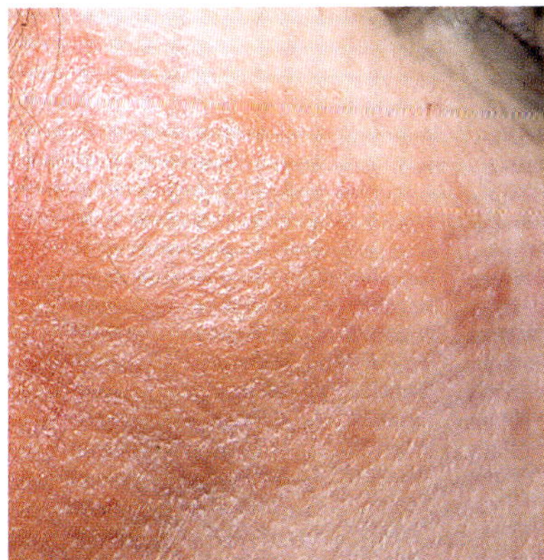

FIG. 6-10 *Confluent yellow-brown papules that have become plaques.*

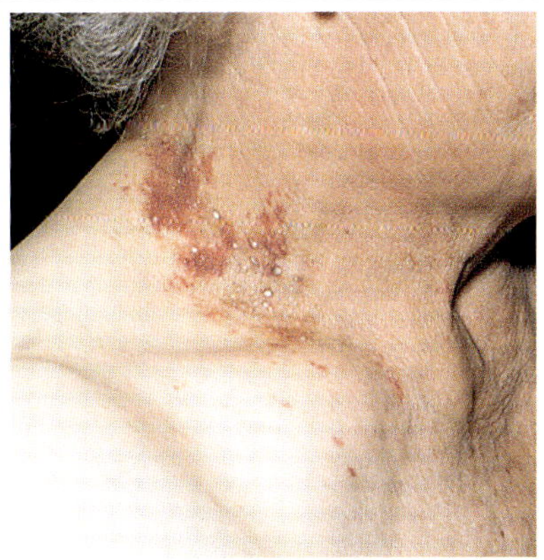

FIG. 6-11 *Ill-defined purpuric patches. The milia represent tiny infundibular cysts secondary to healing of subepidermal blisters.*

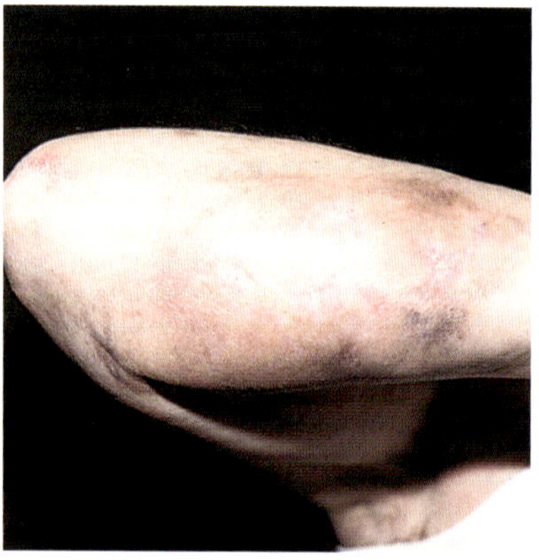

FIG. 6-12 *Plaque and tumor of amyloid that simulates panniculitis clinically.*

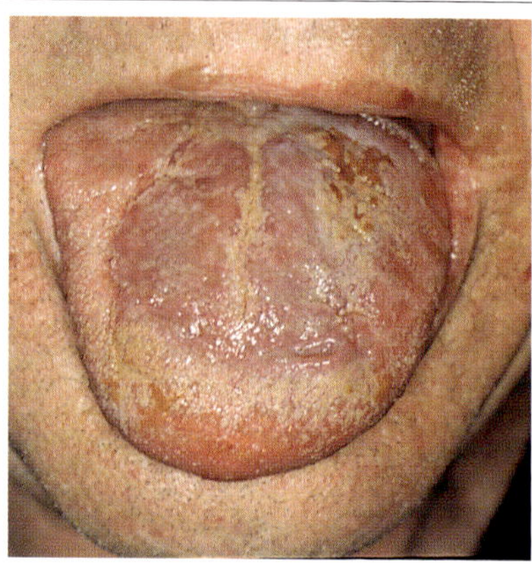

FIG. 6-13 *Macroglossia develops as a consequence of deposits of amyloid in the tongue.*

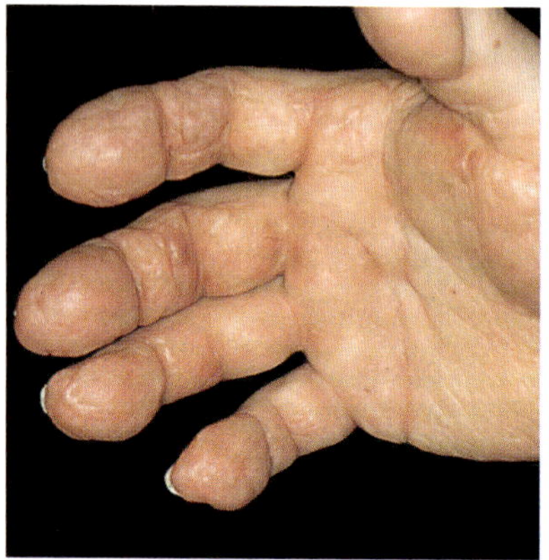

FIG. 6-14 *Acromegalic changes are a result of deposits of amyloid in skin and subcutaneous tissue.*

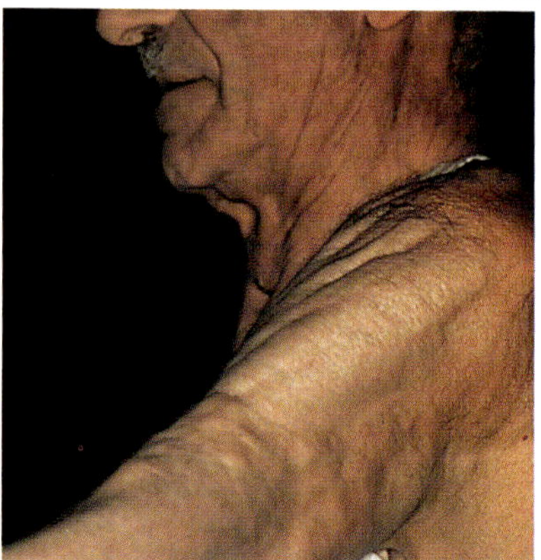

FIG. 6-15 *Cutaneous and subcutaneous nodules of amyloidosis.*

ADJUNCTIVE DIAGNOSTIC TESTS Specialized stains for amyloid include Congo red and thioflavin-T combined with fluorescence. Fine-needle biopsy of subcutaneous fat in clinically normal abdominal skin or biopsy of the mucosa of the rectum in systemic amyloidosis permits sampling of tissue that houses amyloid. Laboratory tests and special examinations are vehicles to demonstrate myeloma-associated systemic amyloidosis.

COURSE The course of cutaneous amyloidosis depends on the type of the disease. For example, the most common type of amyloidosis in the skin consists of pigmented macules that form a reticulated pattern on sites of predilection, namely, interscapular and pretibial areas. When the macules are rubbed firmly for years, they become keratotic papules. If macular and papular lesions of amyloidosis can be protected completely from being scratched and rubbed, the lesions slowly resolve and largely disappear, the only residuum being pigmentation.

A nodule of amyloidosis usually is a wholly cutaneous lesion unrelated to any systemic condition. It persists unless it is excised. The cause is not known.

Purpuric macules, patches, nodules, and blisters represent manifestations of systemic amyloidosis as occurs, for example, in paraproteinemia and myeloma. Those lesions come and go for as long as the systemic disease goes unchecked.

INTEGRATION: UNIFYING CONCEPT Amyloid in the skin, irrespective of type, has the same morphologic appearance when it is visualized through an electron microscope. When amyloid is viewed through a conventional microscope, however, macular and papular (lichenoid) lesions of a wholly cutaneous disease look very different from purpuric lesions of a systemic process. In macular and papular lesions, amyloid presents itself as homogeneous globules that when stained by hematoxylin and eosin may be slightly eosinophilic, amphophilic, or slightly basophilic. Those globules are situated mostly in dermal papillae.

When macular lesions of amyloidosis are rubbed vigorously and persistently, especially those situated over anterior tibiae, changes of lichen simplex chronicus are imposed on them. The combination of findings, to wit, macular amyloidosis plus lichen simplex chronicus, is known as lichenoid amyloidosis. If lesions of lichenoid amyloidosis can be occluded, such as by an Unna's boot, and thereby be protected from rubbing, the lesions in time become less and less papular and keratotic, and assume the appearance of reticulated patches of macular amyloidosis.

It is hypothesized that globules of amyloid in dermal papillae of macular and papular manifestations of amyloidosis represent keratinocytes that have become necrotic as a consequence of excited scratching and have "dropped off" into dermal papillae where they are coated by products of fibrocytes, the result being "amyloid." Lesions of macular and lichenoid amyloidosis occur on sites that are especially pruritic and that can be reached easily by fingernails, in particular, the interscapular and pretibial regions.

Amyloid in systemic expressions of amyloidosis does not present itself as homogeneous globules, but rather as deposits in confluence that can be recognized for what they are by their homogeneous amphophilic appearance. Those deposits are unrelated to necrotic keratinocytes, being either globulins or other serum proteins. The fibers of amyloid are composed of immunoglobulin light chain material.

THERAPY Amyloidosis confined to the skin must be managed by assisting the patient to avoid rubbing and scratching, and applying impediments, which include an Unna's boot on sites like the legs. Application of high-potency corticosteroids under occlusion seems to be beneficial. In some formidable lesions that are resistant to therapy, etretinate, laser surgery, and even dermabrasion have been effective.

Amyloidosis that is systemic must be treated systemically. Attention should be directed to the primary pathologic process; for example, use of chemotherapy for myeloma.

DEFINITION Papules, nodules, vesicles, and sometimes bullae that develop in response to "bites" of arthropods, among the most common offenders being mosquitoes, bedbugs, and mites of scabies.

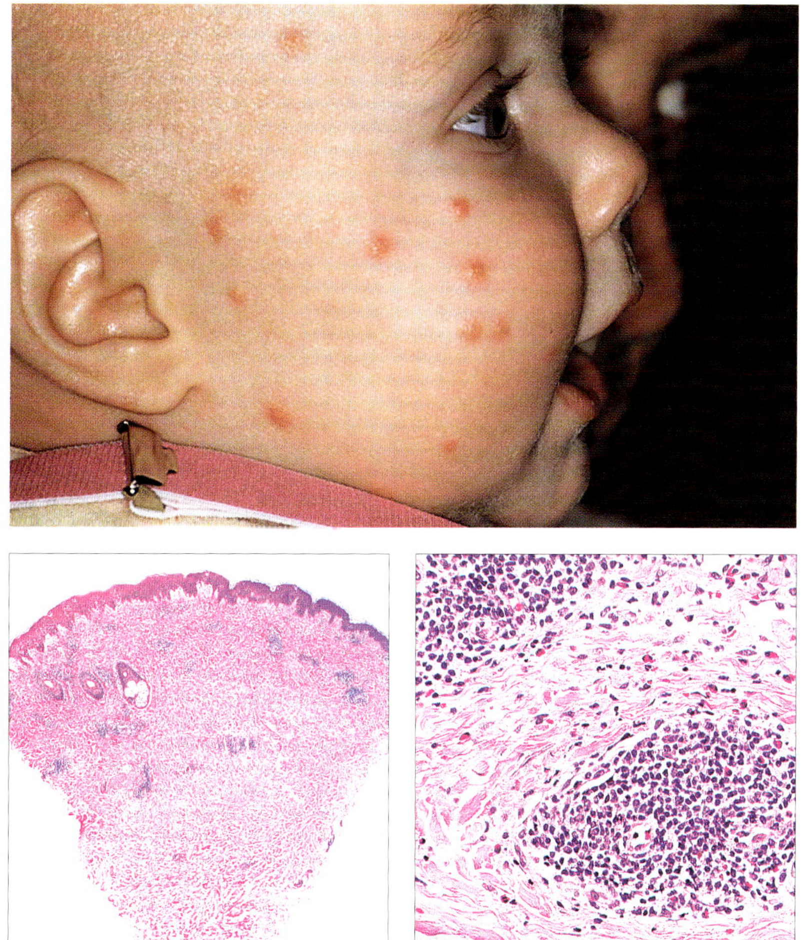

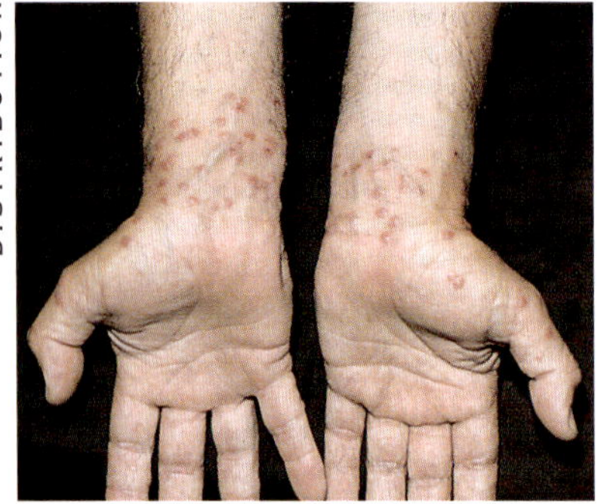

FIG. 7-1 *Discrete papules on the wrist and volar aspect of hands.*

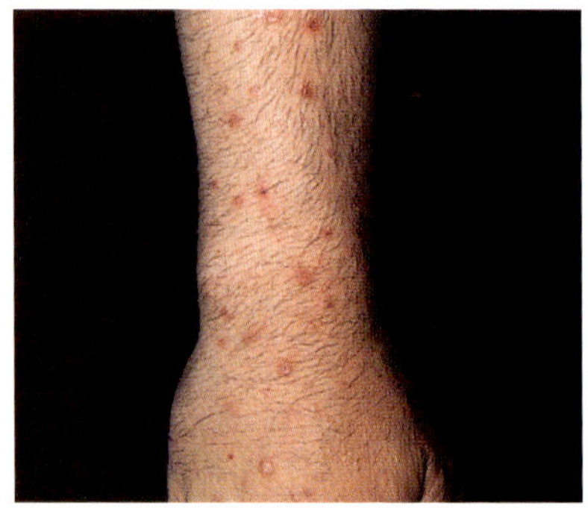

FIG. 7-2 *Excoriated papules.*

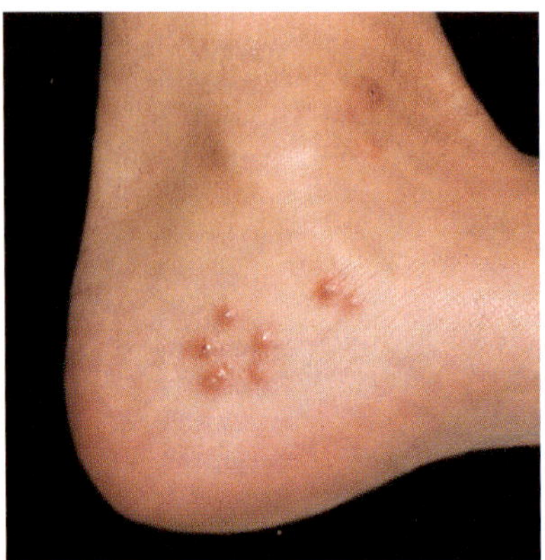

FIG. 7-3 *Discrete acuminate papules.*

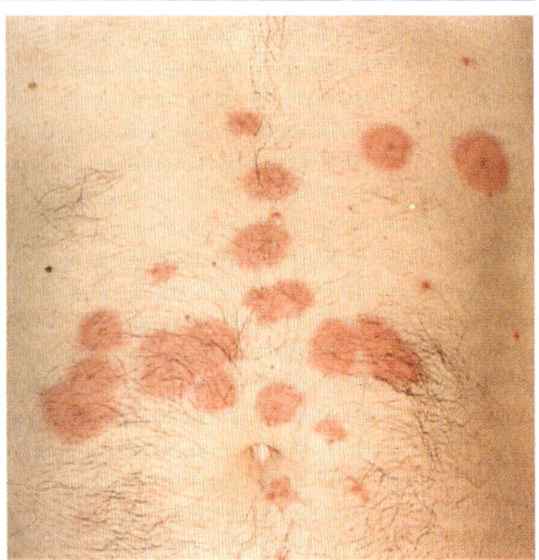

FIG. 7-4 *Many papules, each with a central purpuric punctum, on the abdomen.*

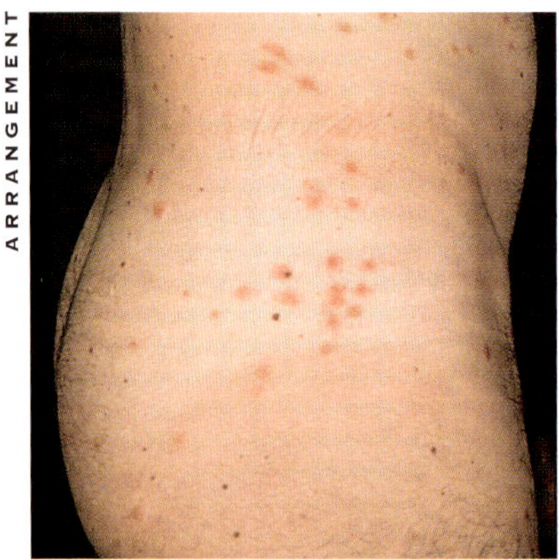

FIG. 7-5 *Numerous papules, some in clusters.*

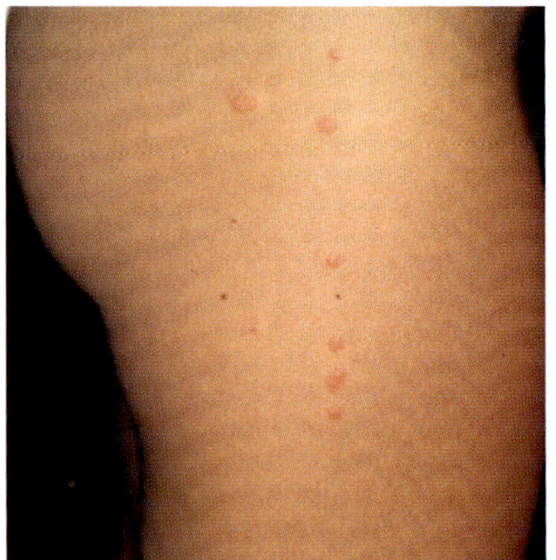

FIG. 7-6 *Papules in linear array, a common phenomenon consequent to fleabites.*

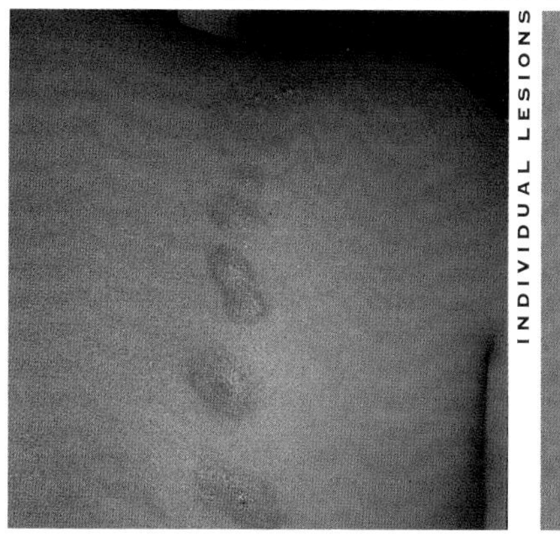

FIG. 7-7   *Papules and plaques in linear arrangement.*

FIG. 7-8 *A red macule.*

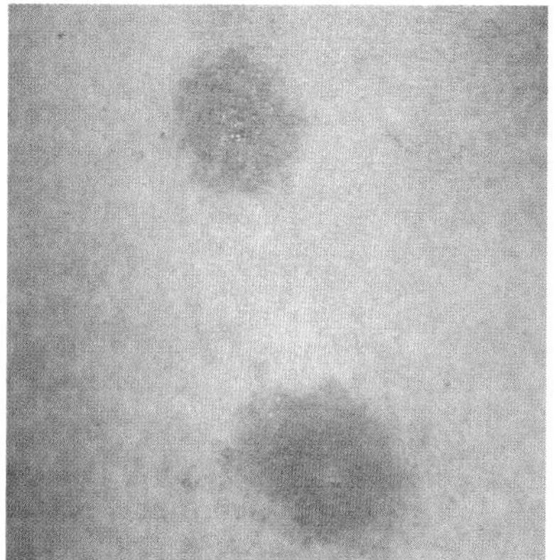
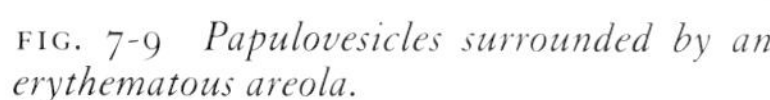

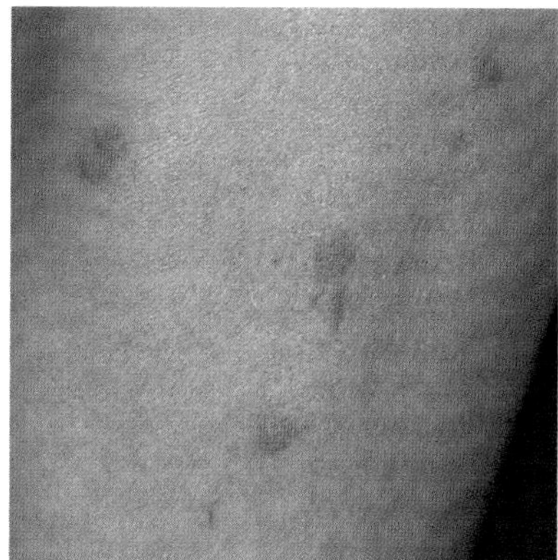

FIG. 7-9   *Papulovesicles surrounded by an erythematous areola.*

FIG. 7-10   *Discrete papules of different shapes.*

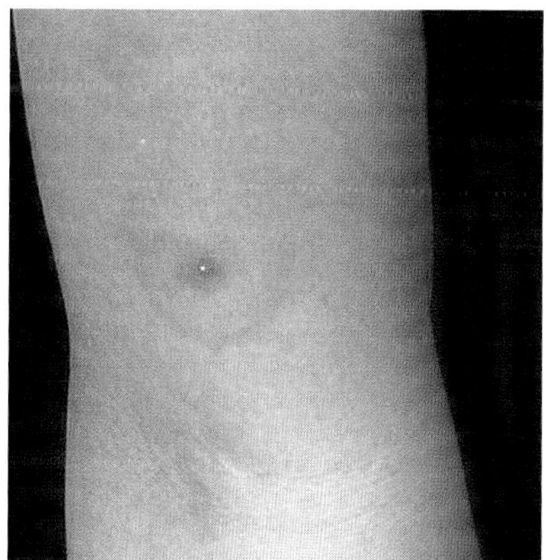

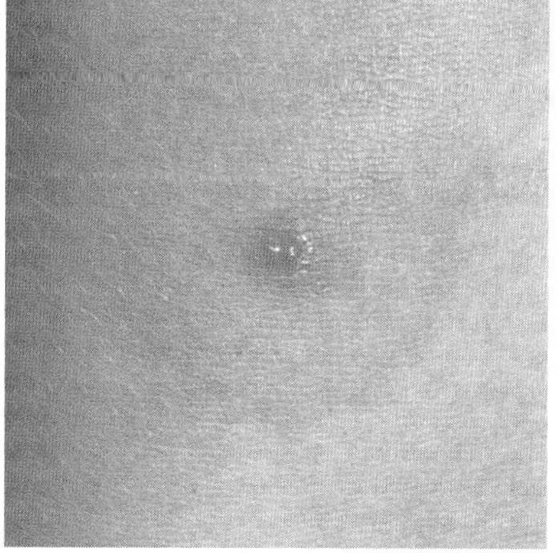

FIG. 7-11 (A, B) *A vesicle surrounded by a patch of erythema.*

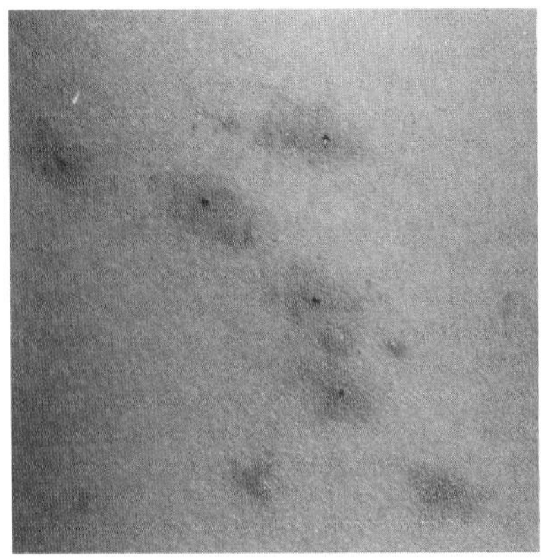

FIG. 7-12 *Papules punctuated in the center by an excoriation.*

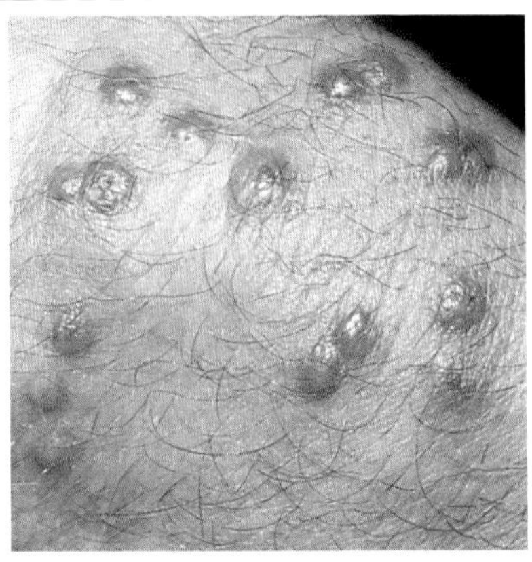

FIG. 7-13 *Papules, many excoriated, not equidistant from one another.*

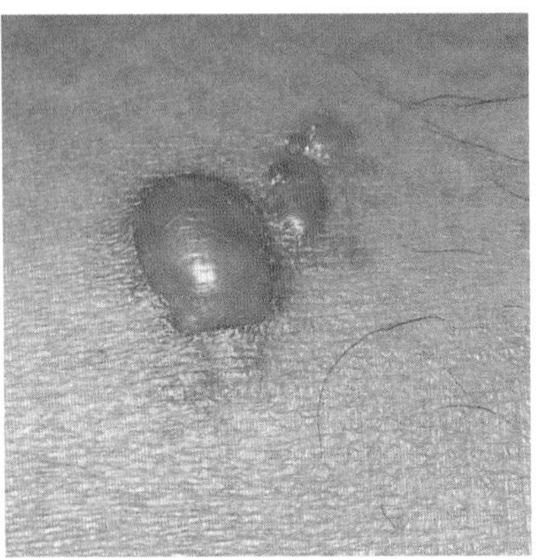

FIG. 7-14 *Vesicles and a bulla on an erythematous base.*

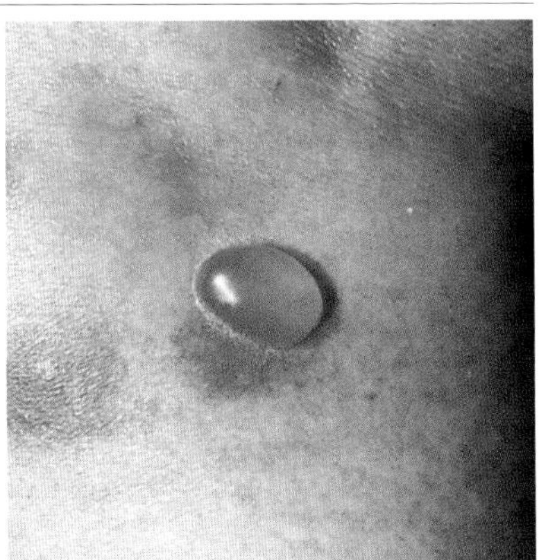

FIG. 7-15 *Tense bulla and erythematous patches and plaques.*

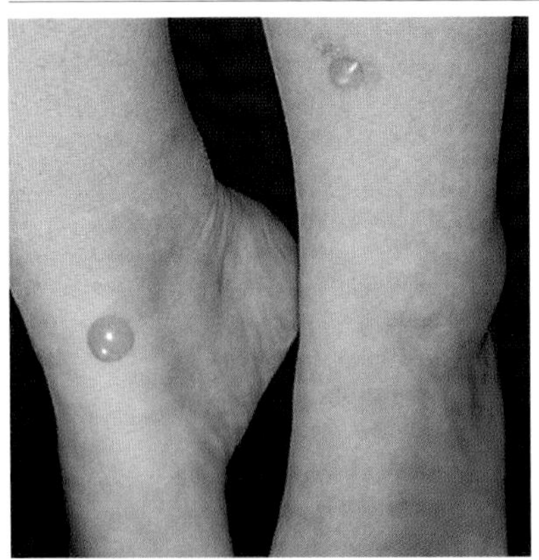

FIG. 7-16 *Bullae.*

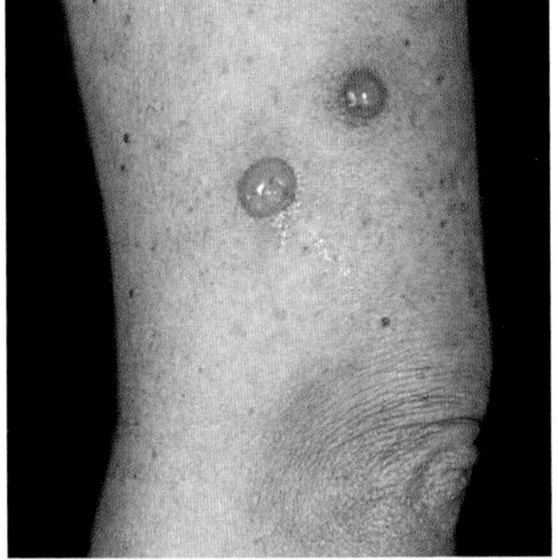

FIG. 7-17 *Bullae.*

VARIATIONS

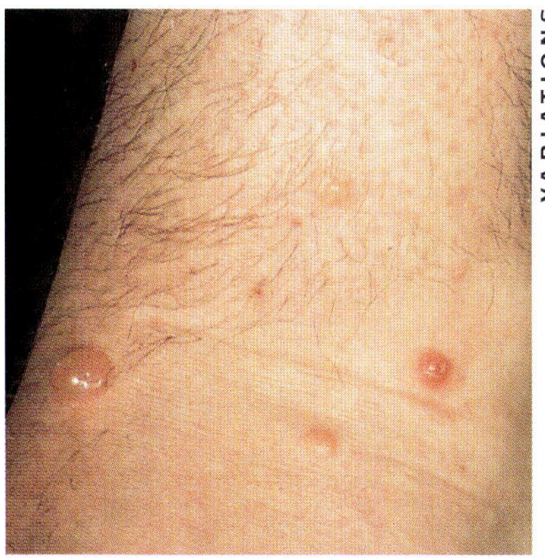

FIG. 7-18 *A papule, vesicle, and bulla.*

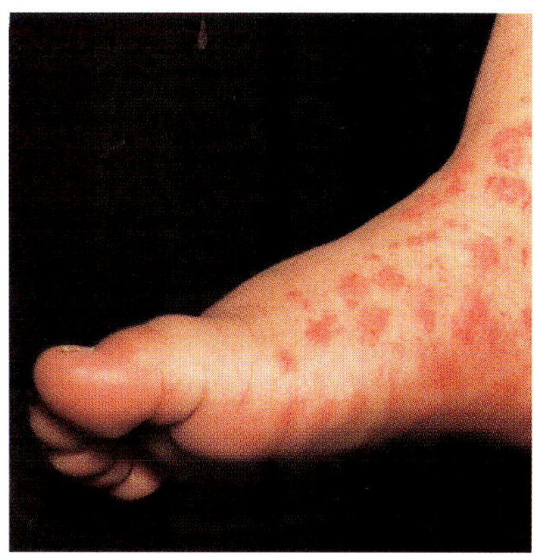

FIG. 7-19 *Papules, some excoriated, of what is called papular urticaria, strophulus, and lichen urticatus.*

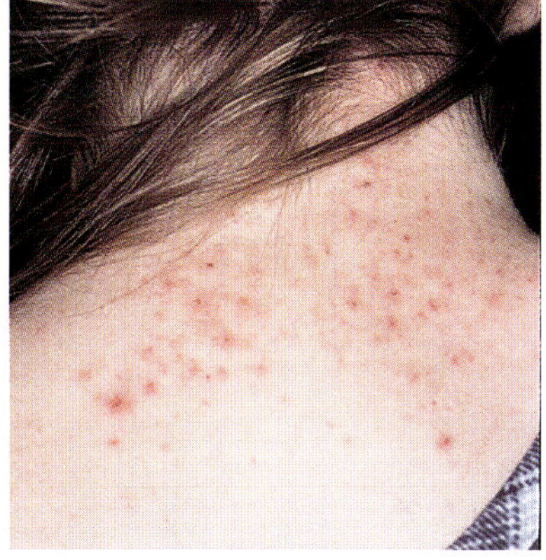

FIG. 7-20 *Macules and excoriated papules associated with nits of head lice.*

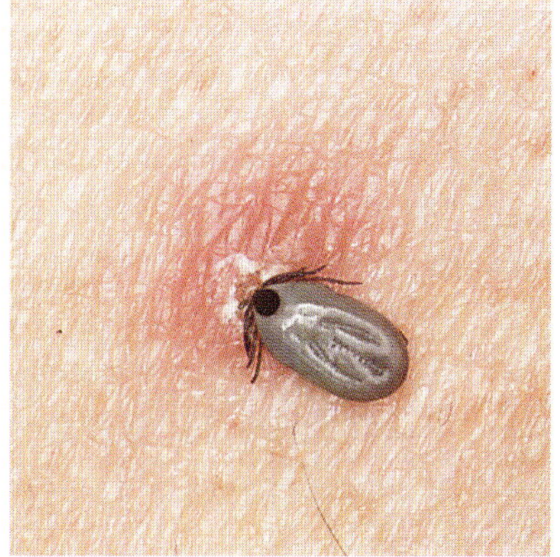

FIG. 7-21 *Tick whose head is buried in an erythematous papule.*

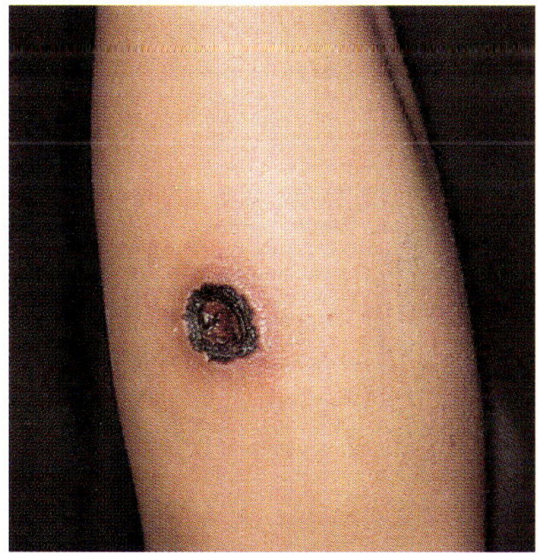

FIG. 7-22 *Eschar on an ulcer, a response to the bite of a spider.*

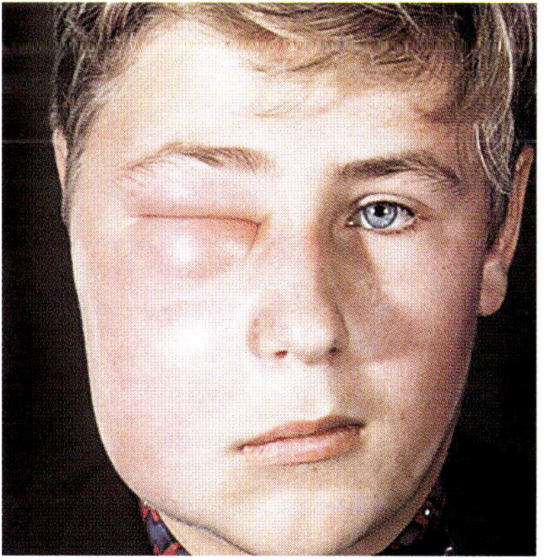

FIG. 7-23 *Extraordinary edema that developed within hours after a bee sting on one side of the face.*

COURSE Responses to insect "bites" vary enormously depending on the kind of insect and the particular sensitivity of the host. As a rule, most insects induce urticarial papules, in the center of which a tense vesicle may develop. Uncommonly, vesicles and bullae are the only manifestation of an insect "bite." Urticarial lesions resolve without residua in days or weeks, whereas vesicles and bullae involute more quickly as crusts that soon are shed. Almost always, urticarial responses to insect "bites" are accompanied by signs of excoriation. In time, persistent rubbing and scratching of lesions caused by bites may result in formation of picker's papules, lesions that may remain long after signs of bites themselves have disappeared.

INTEGRATION: UNIFYING CONCEPT Morphologically—that is, clinically and histopathologically—an individual lesion that results from the "bite" of an insect shows more or less the same features, whatever the offending agent, mosquito or bedbug. The urticarial component of those insect "bites" is characterized histopathologically by a wedge-shaped, superficial and deep, perivascular and interstitial mixed-cell infiltrate of lymphocytes and eosinophils around blood vessels and eosinophils scattered in the interstitium. Often the papillary dermis is edematous.

The vesicle that appears in the center of an urticarial lesion, which represents the actual site of the "bite," is at first intraepidermal and tense, resulting as it does from spongiosis and ballooning. Not uncommonly, the epidermis in the immediate vicinity of the vesicle is necrotic. If the vesicle becomes so distended that it can no longer be contained within the epidermis, it ruptures to become subepidermal. Such findings by conventional microscopy are specific for insect "bites" of various kinds, but the precise type of insect responsible for the "bite" cannot be inferred from histopathologic findings alone.

Clinical features related to distribution and arrangement of lesions are helpful in distinguishing among different types of insect bites. For example, mosquito "bites" are distributed randomly on sites not covered by clothing, whereas the lesions that develop in response to the "bites" of a bedbug usually are arranged in a line and are relatively equidistant from one another.

THERAPY Administration of a topical corticosteroid preparation, such as hydrocortisone lotion, and oral antihistamines in conjunction with application of cold compresses are sufficient for reactions to common insect "bites." Severe reactions may be managed by a short course of corticosteroids administered parenterally.

For pediculosis, permethrin or lindane are effective.

SCABIES

DEFINITION An inflammatory process caused by the acarus Sarcoptes scabiei and consisting of papules, papulovesicles, papulopustules, and vesicles, some arranged in linear or curvilinear tracks (burrows). Sometimes nodules are present, especially in the interdigital webs and on the genitalia, nipple and areola, chest, forearms, and wrists.

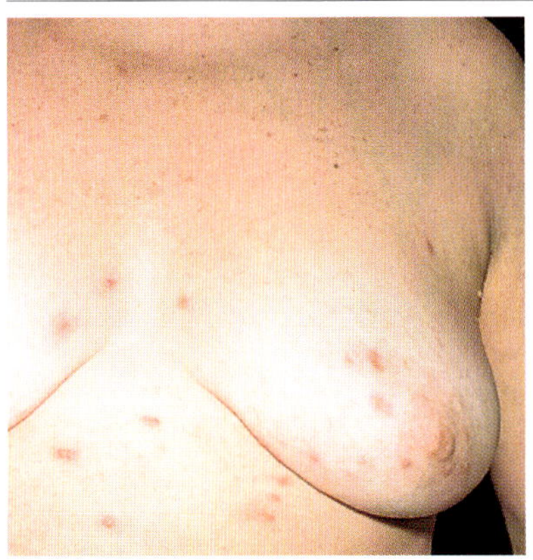
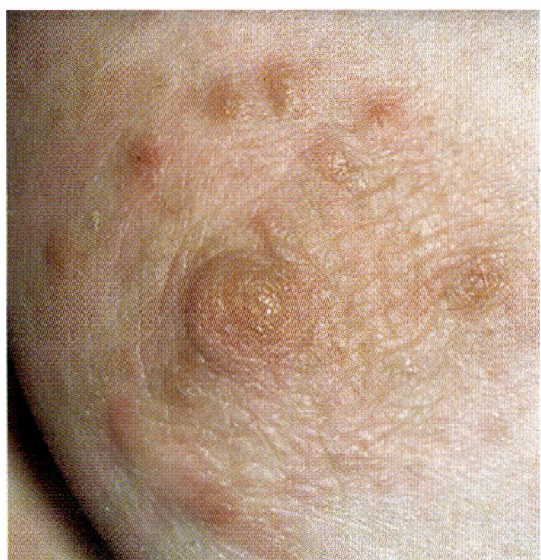

FIG. 7-24 (A, B) *Papules, some excoriated, on the breast and especially the areola, as well as on the trunk. The close-up (b) is of the nipple and areola of the right breast not shown in (a).*

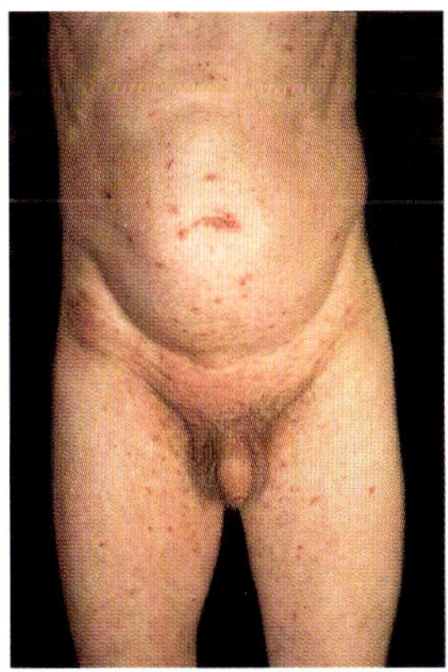
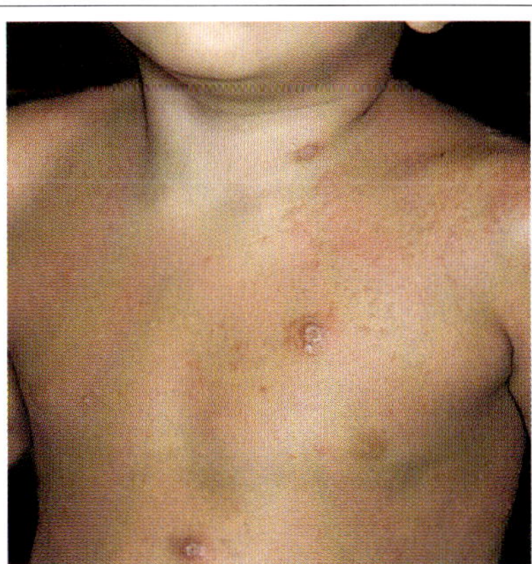

FIG. 7-25 *Widespread papules, many excoriated.*

FIG. 7-26 *Papules, some in clusters, and excoriated nodules on the trunk, and confluence of excoriated papules on the shoulder.*

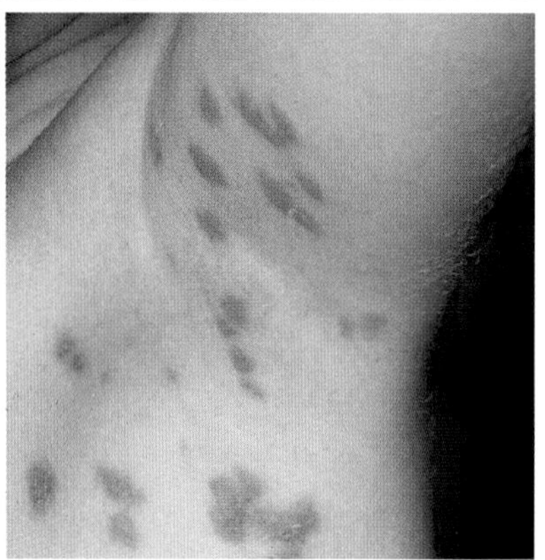

FIG. 7-27 *Papules, most of them discrete but some having become confluent.*

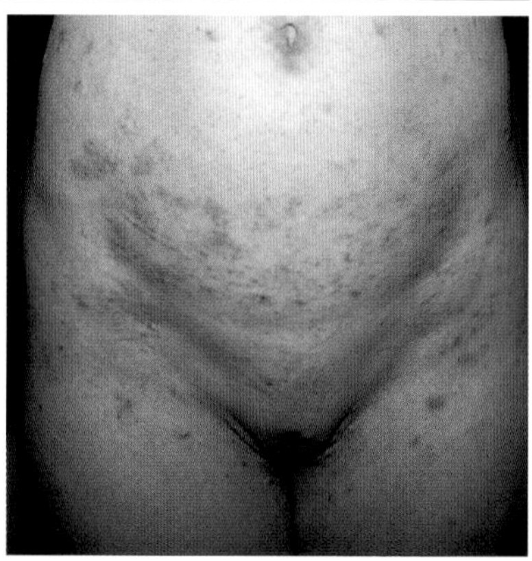

FIG. 7-28 *Papules, many of them excoriated, on the abdomen, genitalia, and thighs.*

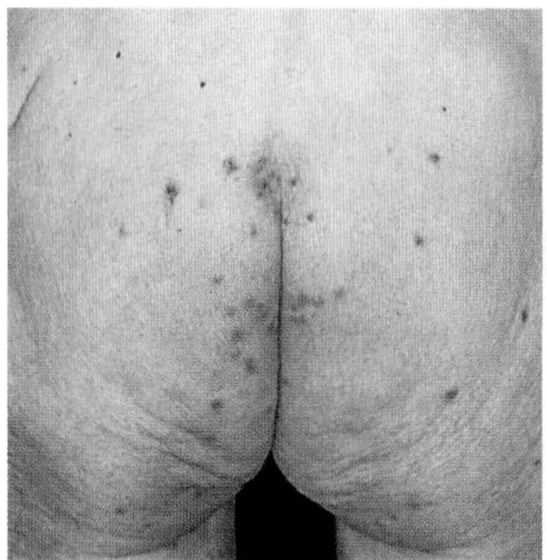

FIG. 7-29 *Excoriated papules in the inter-gluteal region, and on the buttocks and thighs.*

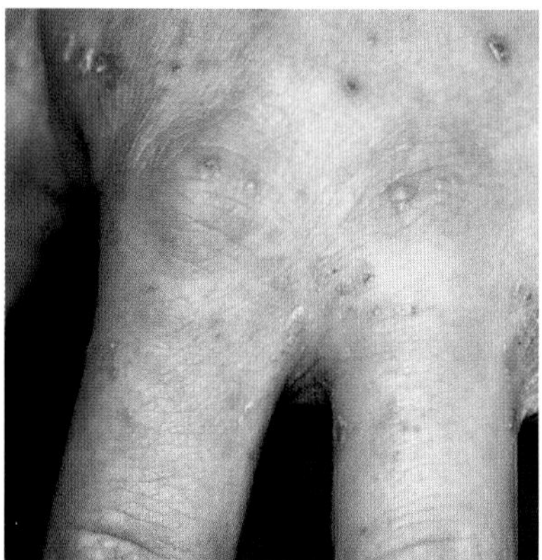

FIG. 7-30 *Macules, papules, some of them linear (burrows) and some of them excoriated, and papulovesicles.*

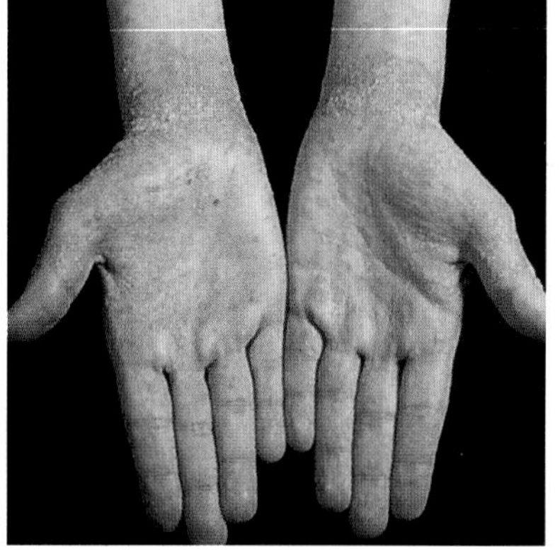

FIG. 7-31 *Scaly papules and collarettes of scale on the volar surface of the hands and fingers, and on the wrists.*

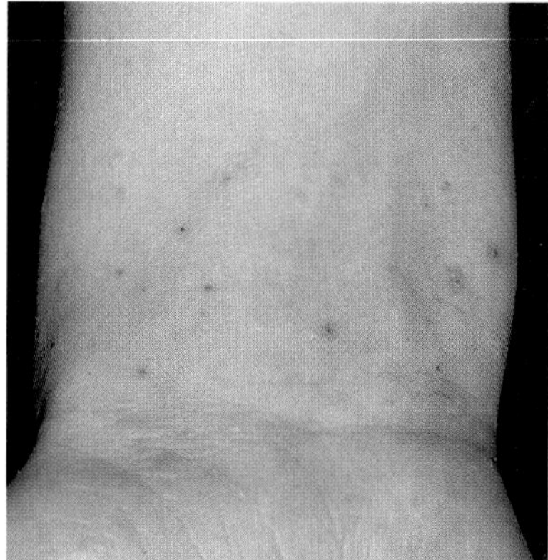

FIG. 7-32 *Excoriated papules on the wrist.*

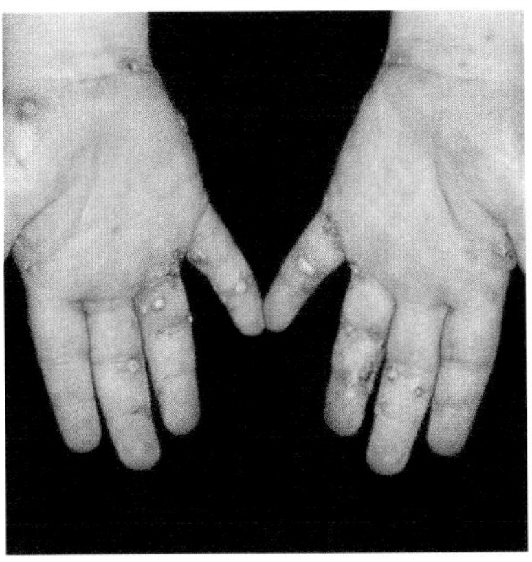

FIG. 7-33 *Pustules.*

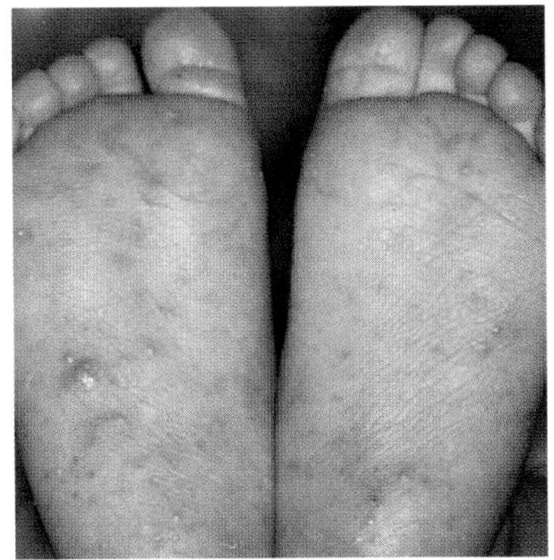

FIG. 7-34 *Papules, vesicles, and pustules.*

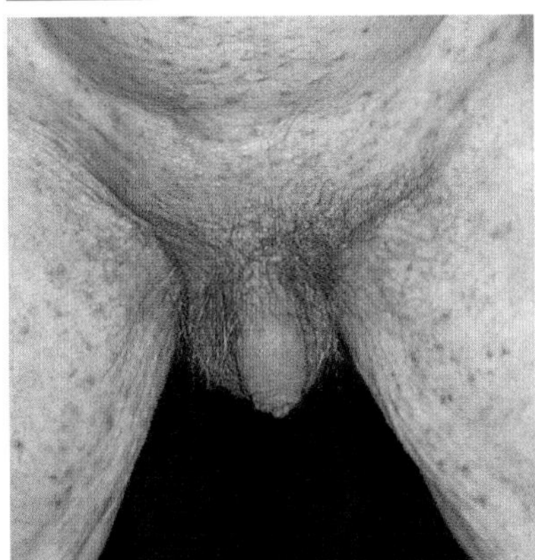

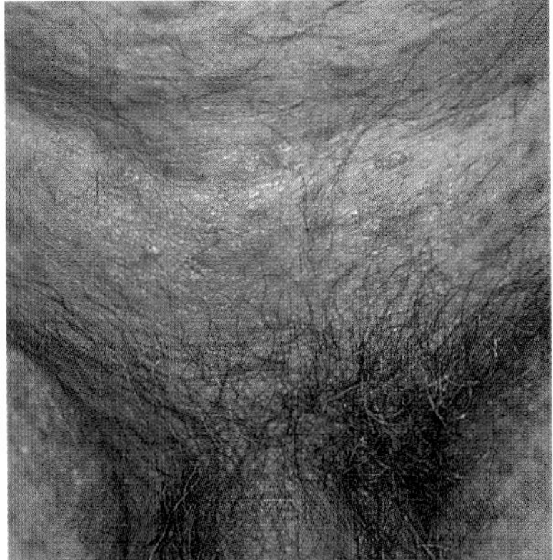

FIG. 7-35 (A, B) *Widespread papules, many excoriated, and vesicles.*

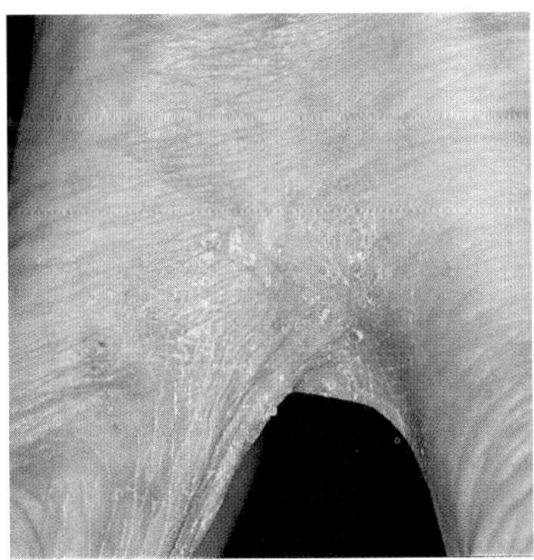

FIG. 7-36 *Collarettes of scales secondary to loss of central cap of parakeratosis.*

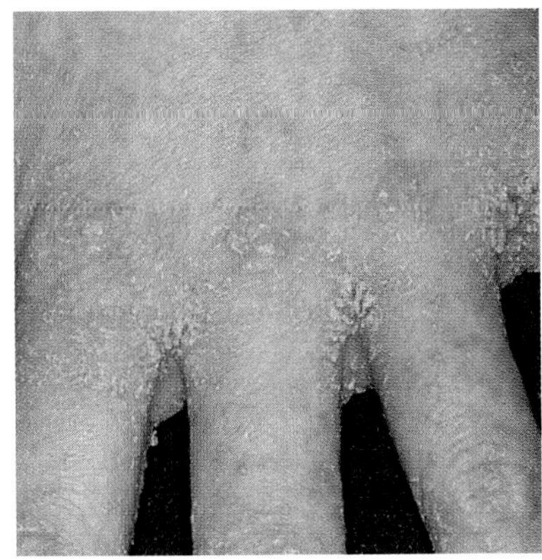

FIG. 7-37 (A) *Scaly papules, collarettes of scale-crusts, and fissures in interdigital webs and on the dorsal surface of the hand.*

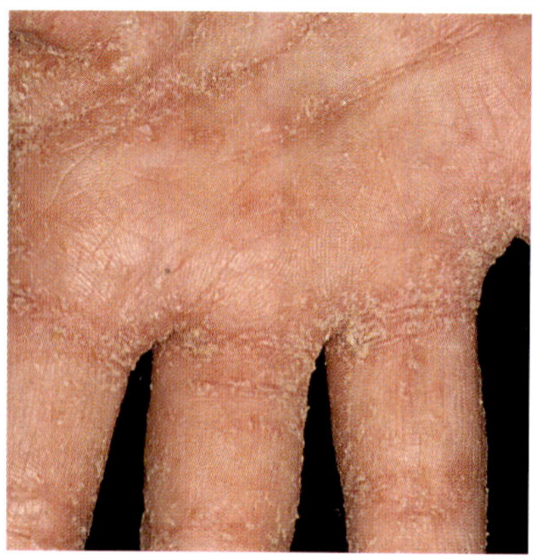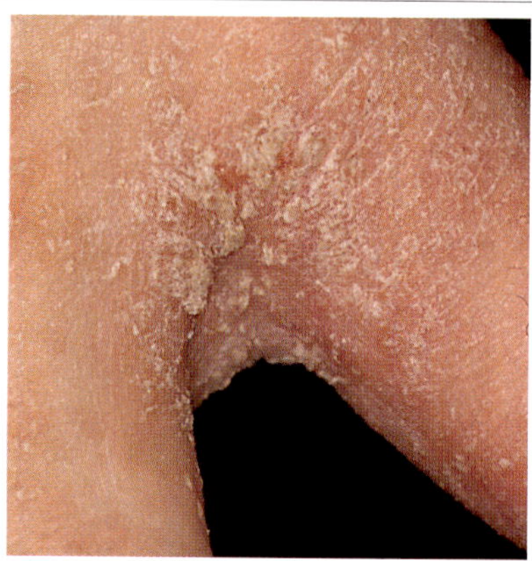

FIG. 7-37 (B, C) *Scaly papules, collarettes of scale-crusts, and fissures in interdigital webs and on the volar surface of the hand.*

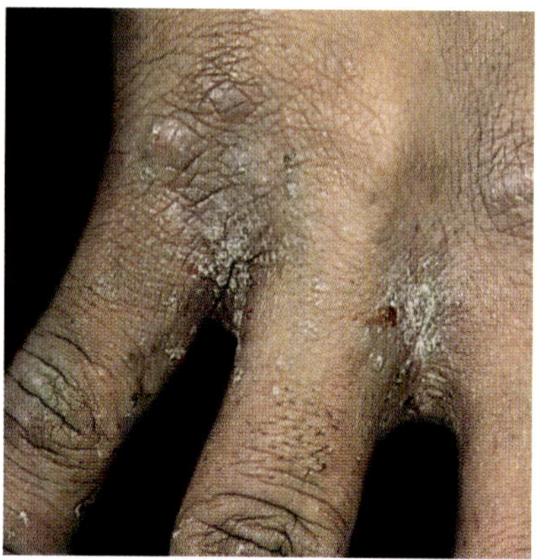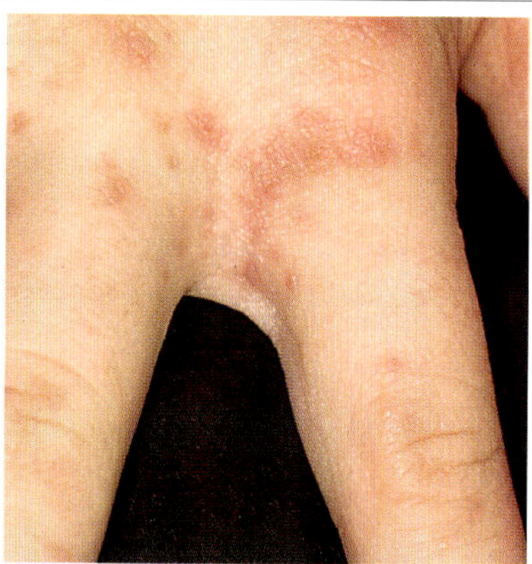

FIG. 7-38 *Scaly papules, some excoriated, especially in the interdigital webs.*

FIG. 7-39 *Papules, some excoriated, and burrows in curvilinear shape in an interdigital web and on the dorsum of the hand.*

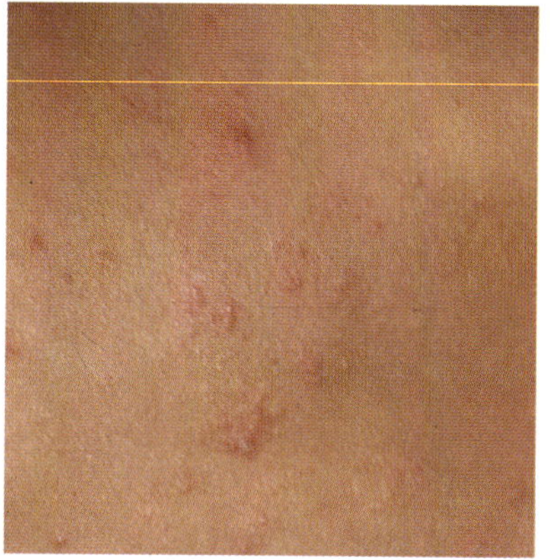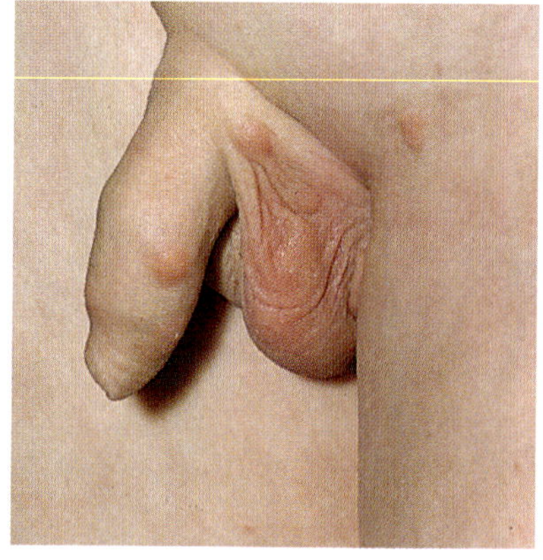

FIG. 7-40 *Pustules, papules, some of which are scaly, and burrows.*

FIG. 7-41 *Papules on the penis and scrotum, and in the groin ("nodular" scabies).*

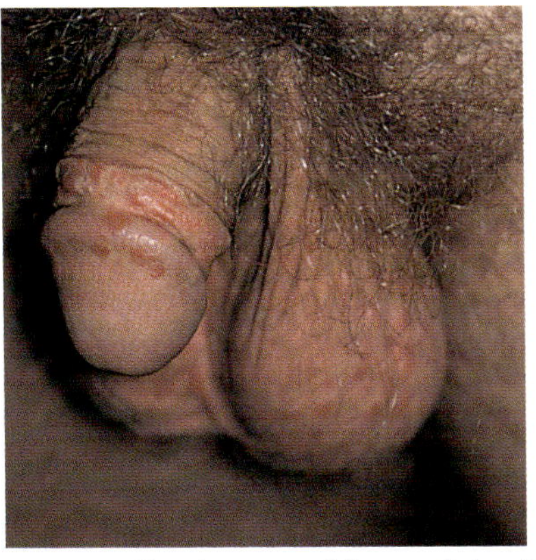

FIG. 7-42 *Papules, some of them eroded and crusted, on the penis, both glans and shaft.*

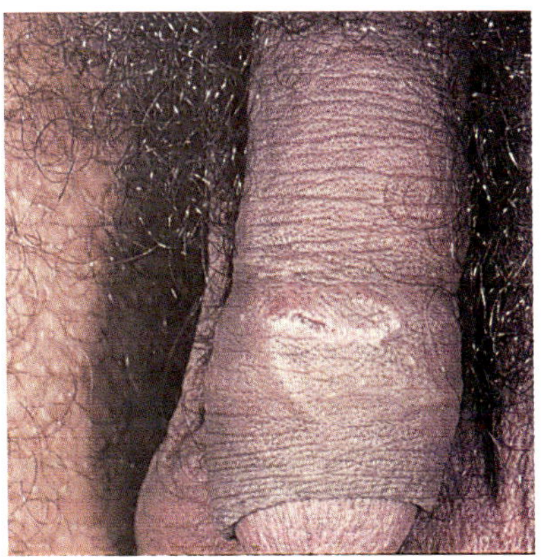

FIG. 7-43 *Burrow, scaly and crusted, on the foreskin.*

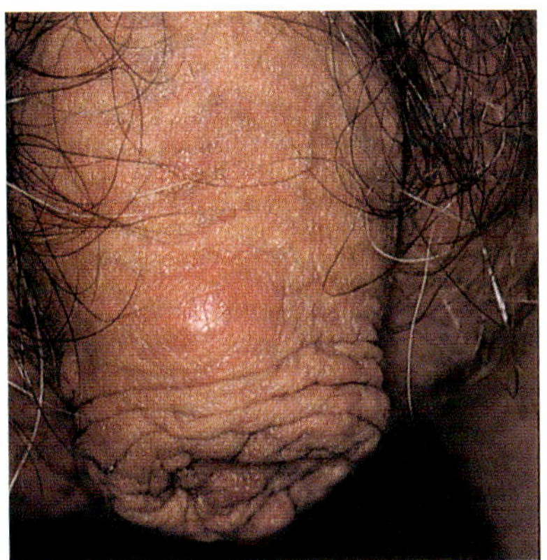

FIG. 7-44 *Papules of "nodular scabies."*

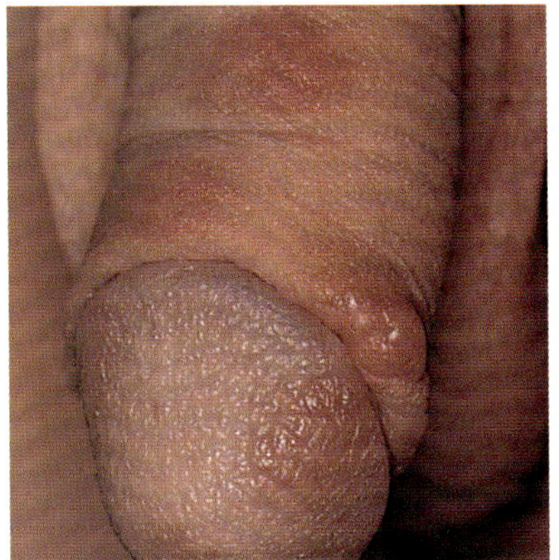

FIG. 7-45 *Papules of "nodular scabies."*

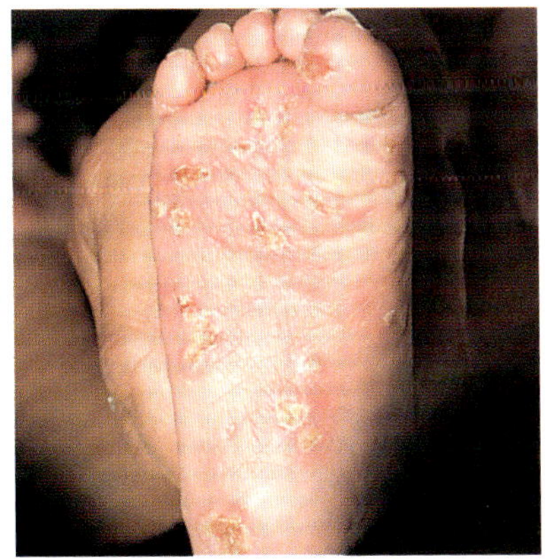

FIG. 7-46 *Vesicles, erosions, and crusts.*

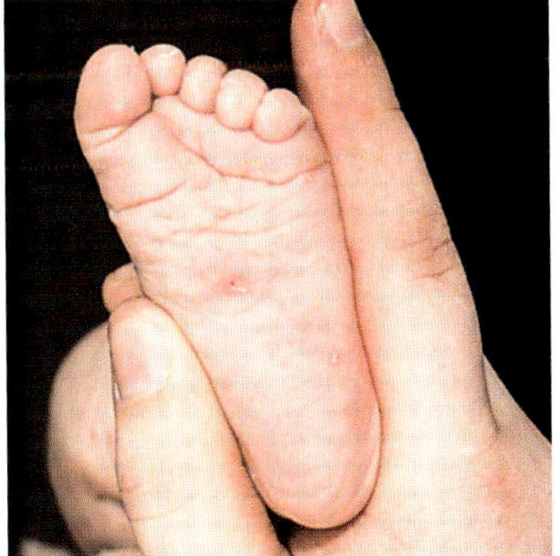

FIG. 7-47 *Papules, some of them scaly and others excoriated, on the foot and leg of a child and on the first finger of the mother.*

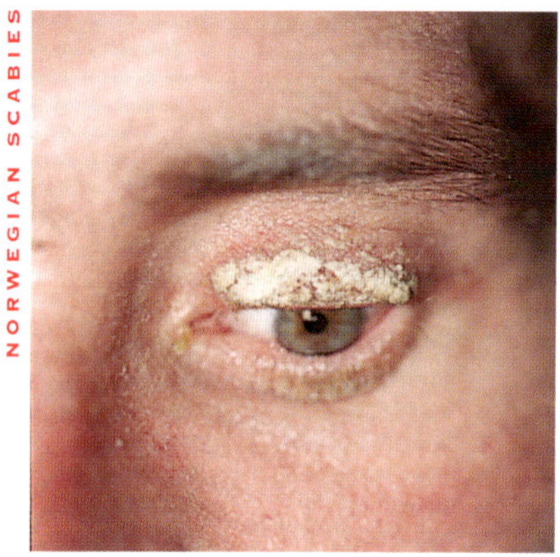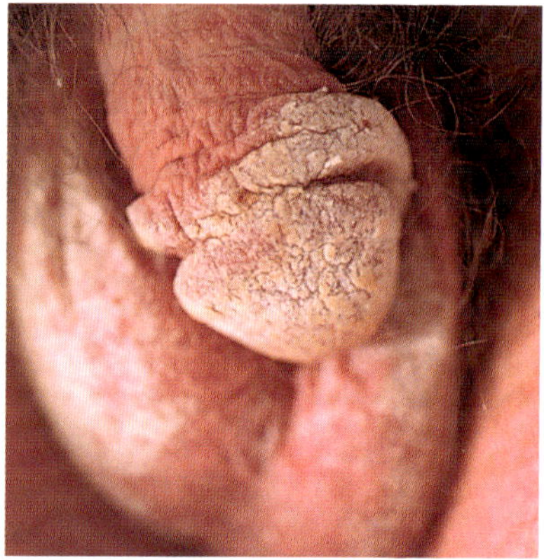

FIG. 7-48 (A, B) *Keratotic-crusted lesions on the eyelid, penis, and scrotum in an immuno-suppressed person.*

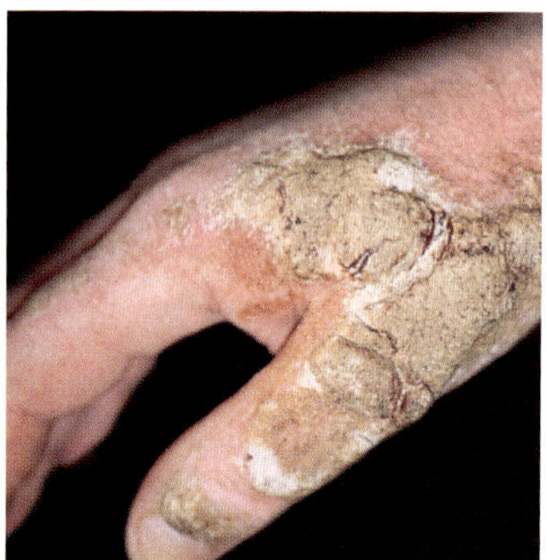

FIG. 7-48 (C) *Keratotic-crusted lesions on a hand in an immunosuppressed person.*

ADJUNCTIVE DIAGNOSTIC TEST Techniques include taking scrapings of skin lesions, especially burrows, or curetting them to prepare for search for the mite, her progeny, eggshells, or fecal nuggets by examination using conventional microscopy.

COURSE The papules, nodules, papulovesicles, and vesicles of scabies are a consequence of the effects of a female mite as she traverses the cornified layer of the epidermis, from which site she also takes her meals of nutrients provided by viable cells of the epidermis and juices from the papillary dermis.

The individual papules, papulovesicles, and vesicles of scabies usually wane in weeks. Nodules of scabies, however, may persist for months. The entire process of scabies usually ceases in months, presumably because the maddening pruritus induced by the effects of the female mite, her ova, her progeny, and her detritus leads to ferocious scratching, which serves to remove the mite and her train from their domicile in the stratum corneum ("post scabietic syndrome").

INTEGRATION: UNIFYING CONCEPT Scabies is diagnosable clinically by characteristic distribution of lesions and by types of lesions, especially burrows when they are present. Histopathologically, papules are made up of superficial and deep perivascular and interstitial infiltrates of lymphocytes and eosinophils. Those cells are present around venules, and eosinophils are scattered in the interstitium of the reticular dermis. Often the papillary dermis is edematous. That constellation of findings is not specific for scabies; it may be encountered in an assault by different types of arthropods.

Signs specific for scabies are found within the stratum corneum where it often is possible to detect the female mite, or parts of her, as well as ova, nymphs, larvae, and "fecal nuggets," excreta of the adult female. Nodular lesions of scabies are an exaggeration of changes seen within papules, to wit, rather discrete aggregations of lymphocytes, eosinophils, and sometimes plasma cells throughout the dermis. No edema is present in the upper part of the dermis, and there are no hints of the female mite or of her progeny in the stratum corneum. When a vesicle appears atop a papule of scabies or de novo, it can be seen to be intraepidermal as a consequence of prominent spongiosis and ballooning.

The widespread keratotic-crusted type of scabies that particularly affects immunosuppressed people, known as Norwegian scabies, is characterized by a moderately dense mixed infiltrate of inflammatory cells, above which there are uneven psoriasiform hyperplasia and a strikingly thickened cornified layer that houses countless adult mites, ova, nymphs, larvae, and "fecal nuggets."

Why scabies spares the face and scalp is not known.

THERAPY Application of permethrin, benzyl benzoate, lindane, or cro-tamiton topically is effective. Recently, ivermectin orally has been recommended.

ATOPIC DERMATITIS AND ITS ANALOGUES

*(lichen simplex chronicus, prurigo nodularis, picker's nodules,
and erosions and ulcerations secondary to excoriation)*

DEFINITION A condition of persons of any age, but particularly children with a genetic proclivity for allergic rhinitis and conjunctivitis, and allergic asthma. Intense pruritus induces patients to rub the skin intensely and to scratch furiously, the resultant factitious lesions being erythematous, often scaly, macules, patches, papules, and plaques that tend to become lichenified, eroded, ulcerated, and crusted.

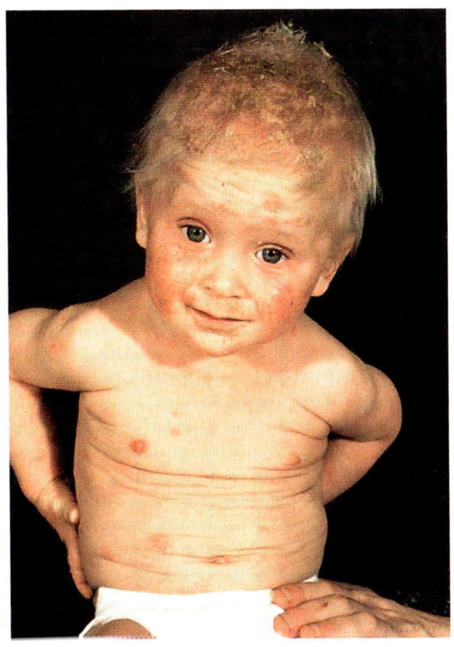

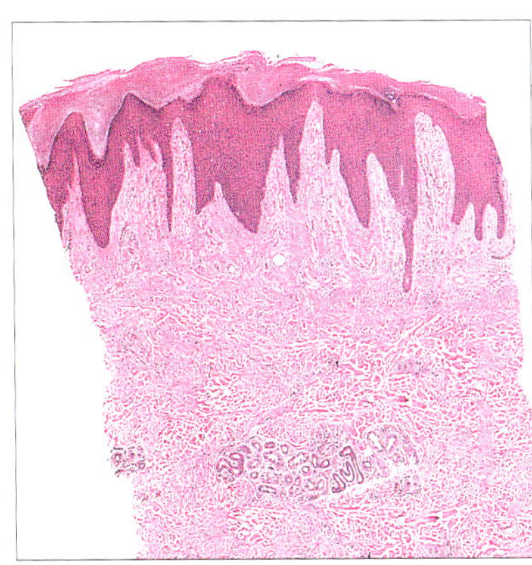

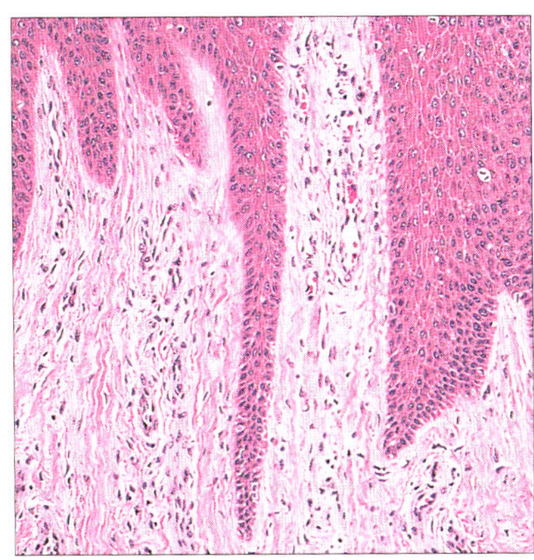

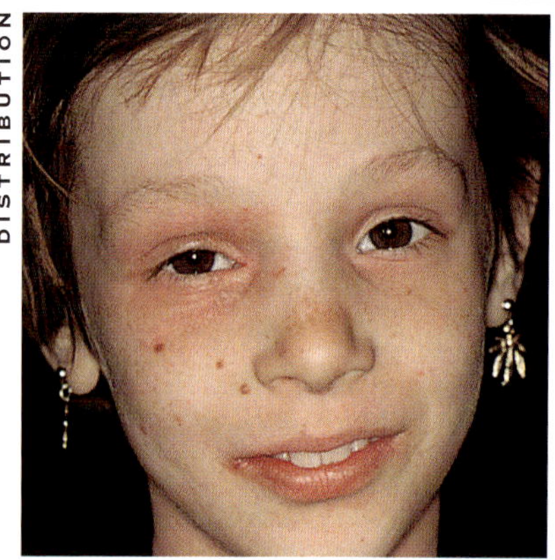

FIG. 8-1 *Periorbital erythematous, slightly scaly patches and plaques consequent to vigorous rubbing.*

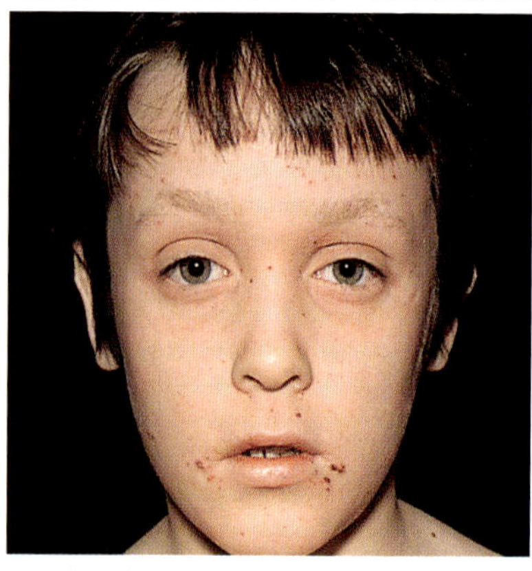

FIG. 8-2 *Hemorrhagic crusts atop excoriated papules, and periorbital dusky erythema ("allergic shiners").*

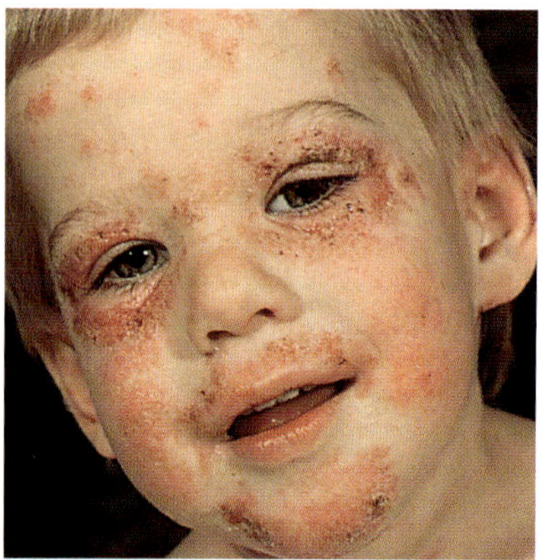

FIG. 8-3 *Red patches and plaques, erosions, hemorrhagic and yellow crusts, and scales. Note spared zones are untouched.*

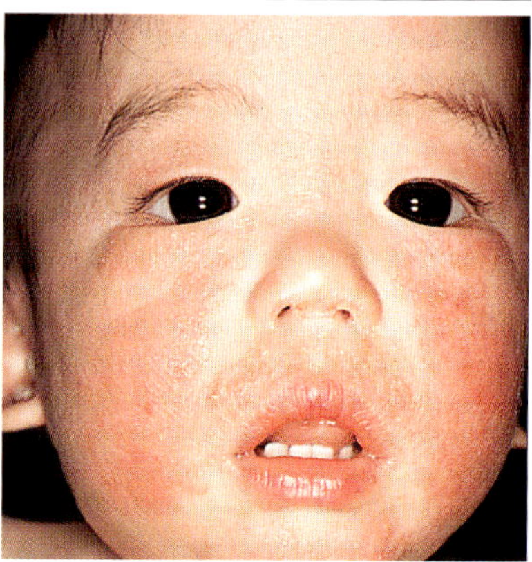

FIG. 8-4 *Erythematous scaly patches and plaques. Paranasal folds, tip of the nose, and skin below the lower lip are unaffected.*

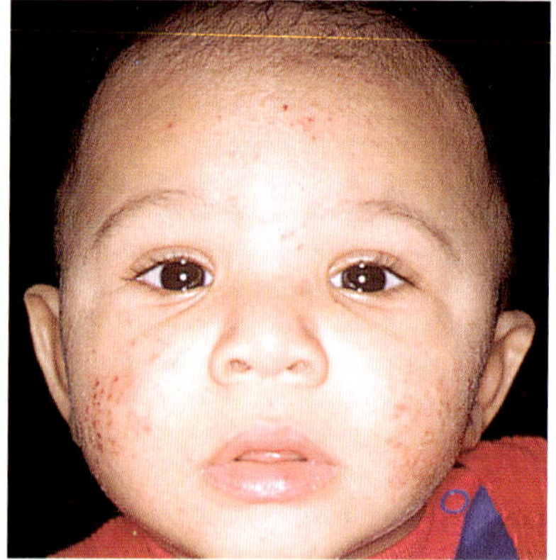

FIG. 8-5 *Erythematous papules, many excoriated.*

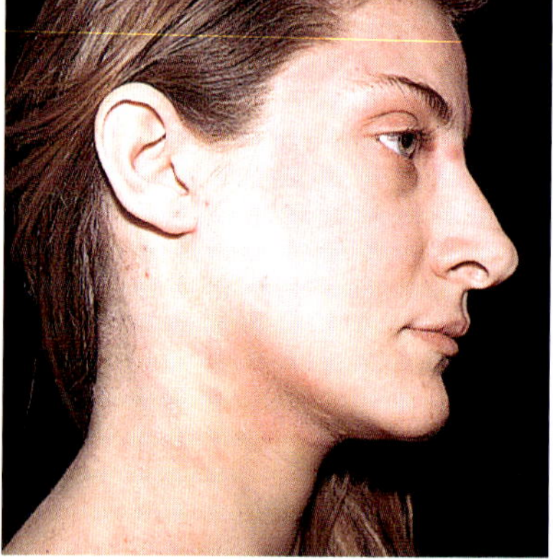

FIG. 8-6 *Erythematous, slightly scaly patches and plaques eroded secondary to excoriation.*

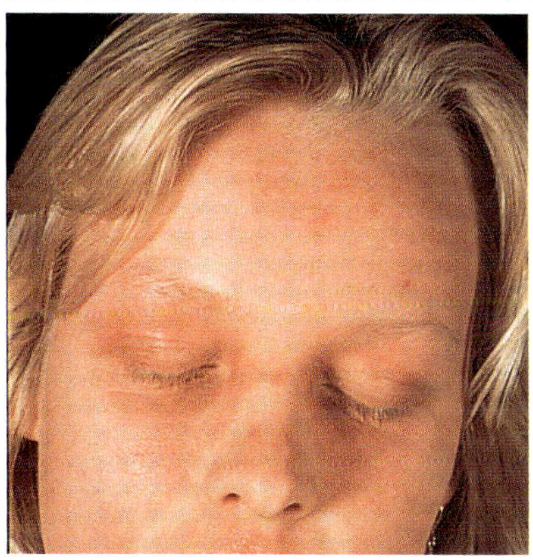

FIG. 8-7 *Erythematous scaly patches and plaques on cheeks. Sites spared are protected from rubbing and scratching.*

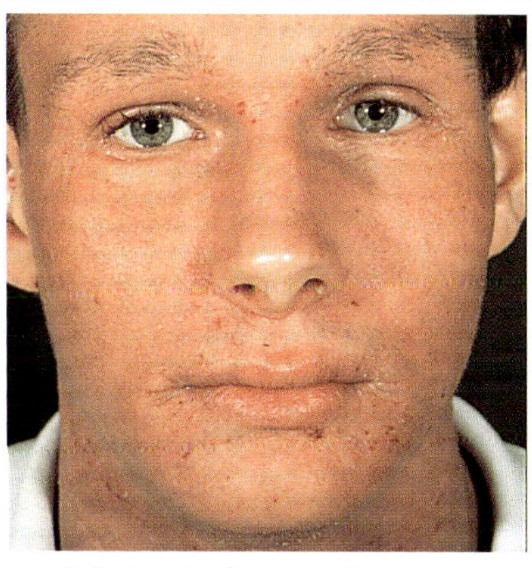

FIG. 8-8 *Erythroderma with erosions covered by hemorrhagic crusts.*

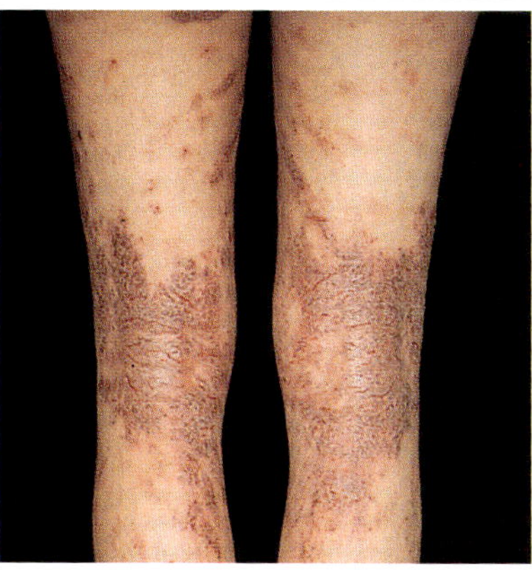

FIG. 8-9 *Lichenified dusky red plaques interrupted by fissures and covered by scales.*

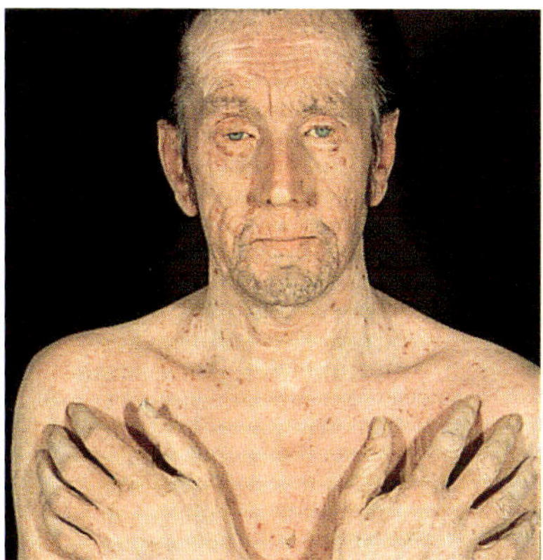

FIG. 8-10 *Erythematous patches, plaques, and papules, many eroded and covered by crust. Some plaques are lichenified.*

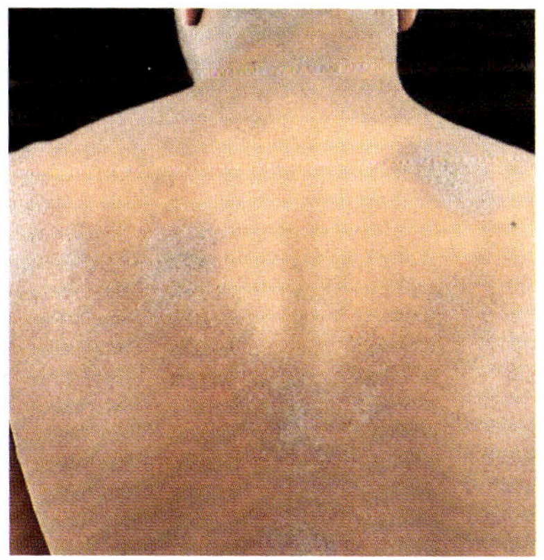

FIG. 8-11 *Keratotic papules and plaques.*

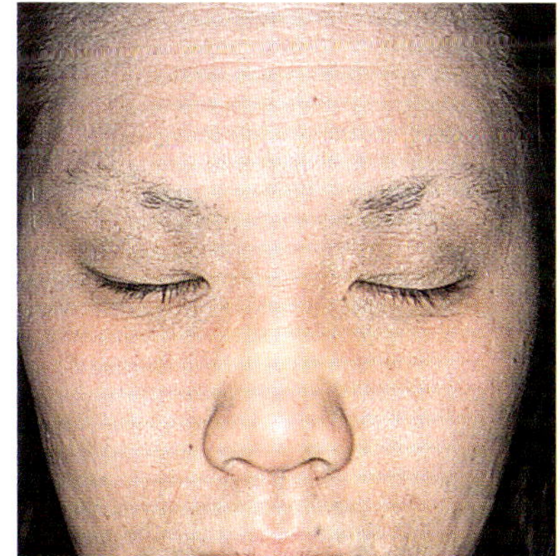

FIG. 8-12 *The lateral aspect of the eyebrows is missing as a consequence of prolonged rubbing ("Herthoge sign").*

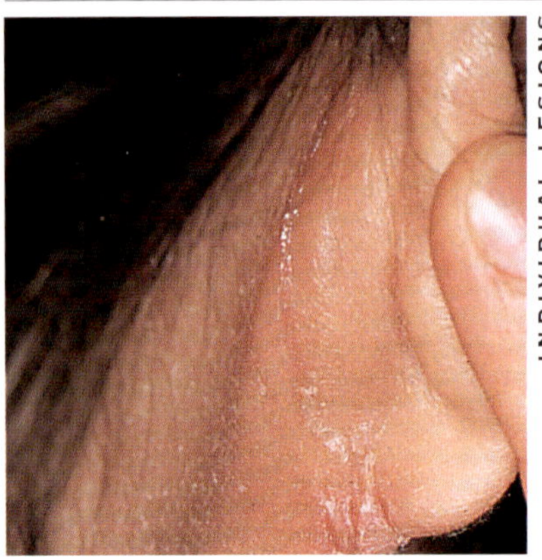

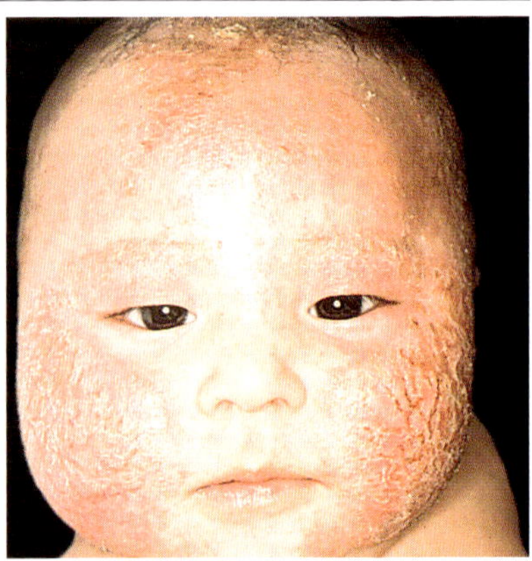

INDIVIDUAL LESIONS

FIG. 8-13 *Scales and fissures in the retroauricular region.*

FIG. 8-14 *Scale-crusts interrupted by fissures on cheeks ("eczema craquelé") and yellow crusts on scalp ("crusta lactea").*

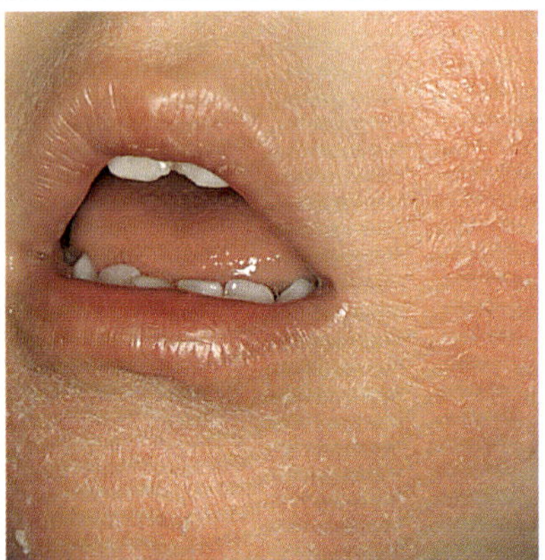

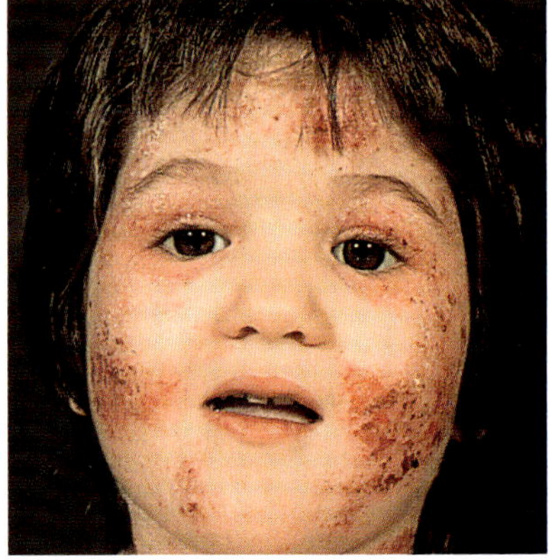

FIG. 8-15 *Excoriations covered by crusts in company with lichenification, erythema, and scaling.*

FIG. 8-16 *Erythematous scaly plaques. The paranasal folds are largely spared because they are indented.*

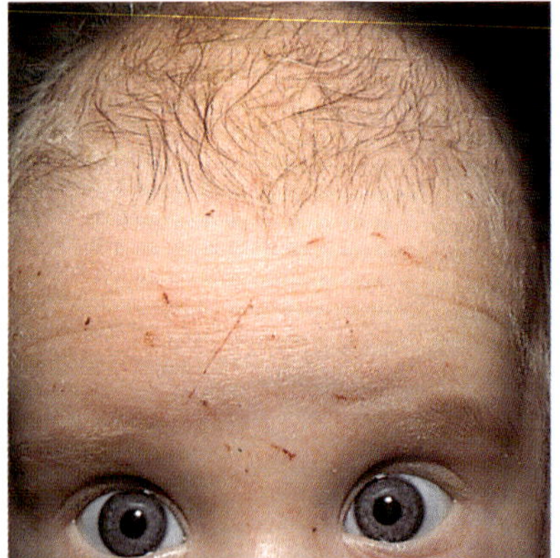

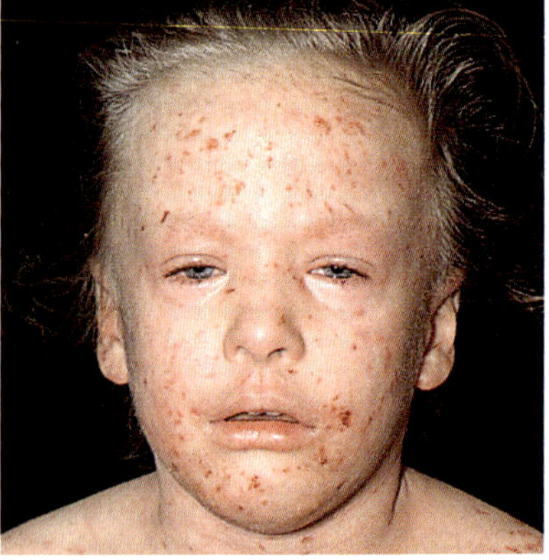

FIG. 8-17 *Erosions and hemorrhagic crusts atop lichenified plaques. Signs of scratching are the excoriations.*

FIG. 8-18 *Erythroderma, erosions covered by hemorrhagic crusts, and lichenification in an obviously atopic person.*

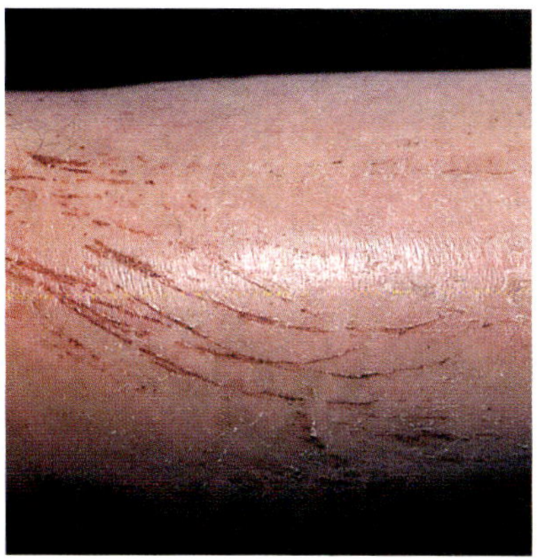

FIG. 8-19 *Diffuse erythema traversed by linear excoriations and covered by subtle scale-crusts.*

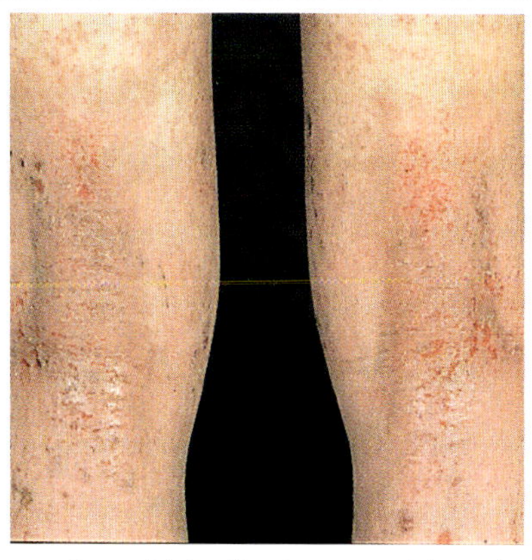

FIG. 8-20 *Lichenification covered by scales and associated with erosions and ulcerations.*

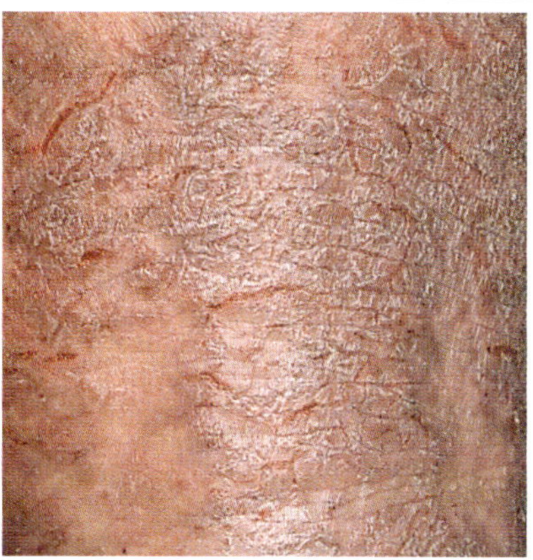

FIG. 8-21 *Lichenification surmounted by scales and traversed by fissures.*

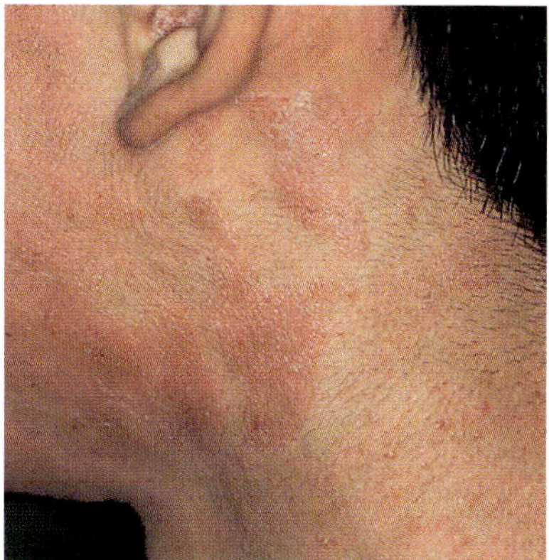

FIG. 8-22 *Erythematous scaly plaques with indistinct borders.*

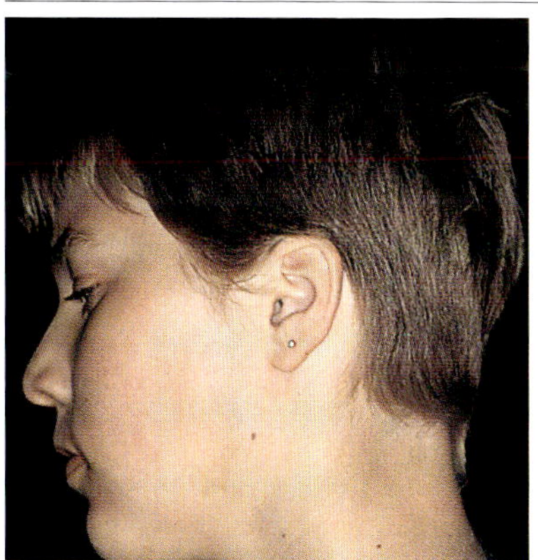

FIG. 8-23 *Reticulated hyperpigmentation and lichenification ("dirty neck").*

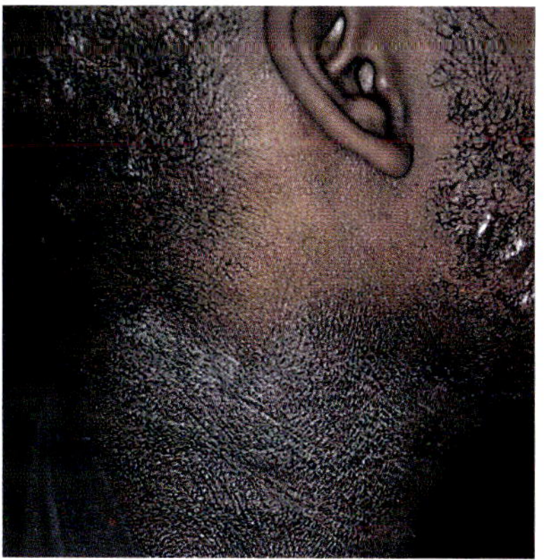

FIG. 8-24 *Hyperpigmentation and lichenification.*

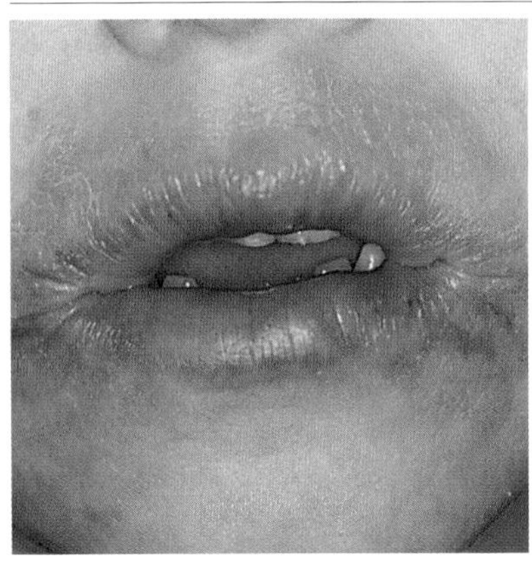

FIG. 8-25 *Lichenification and fissures at the angles of the mouth and lichenification of the upper lip.*

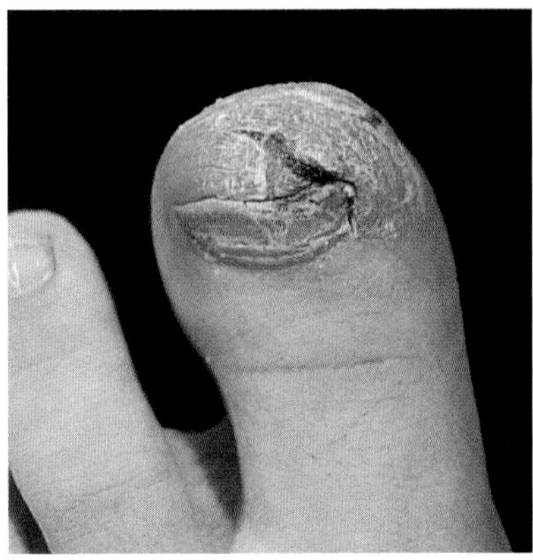

FIG. 8-26 *Erythema, scales, and a fissure of the tip of a toe whose nail is dystrophic.*

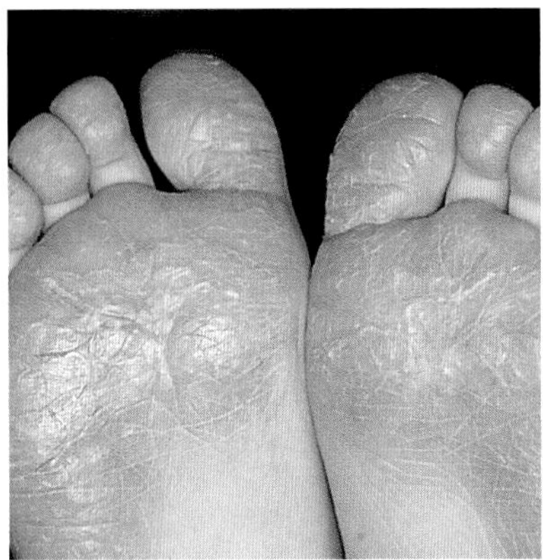

FIG. 8-27 *Dusky erythema, lichenification, and scales on wrinkled skin (juvenile plantar dermatosis). Arches are spared.*

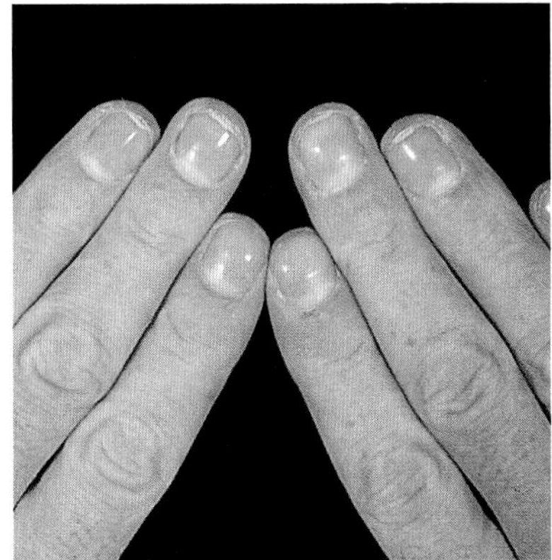

FIG. 8-28 *Shiny nails result from buffing them by longstanding intense rubbing.*

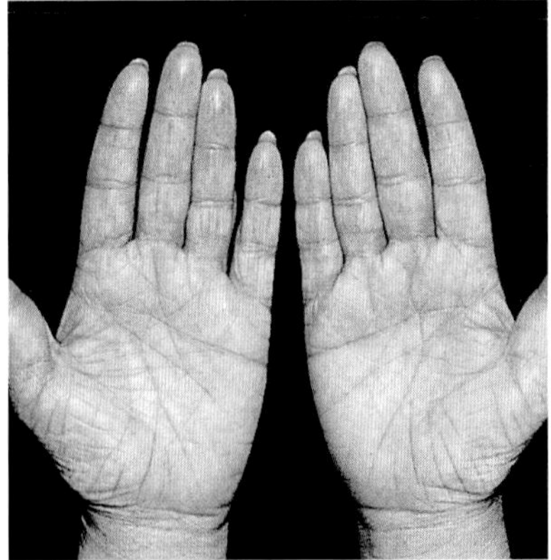

FIG. 8-29 *Accentuation of palmar creases (hyperlinearity of palms).*

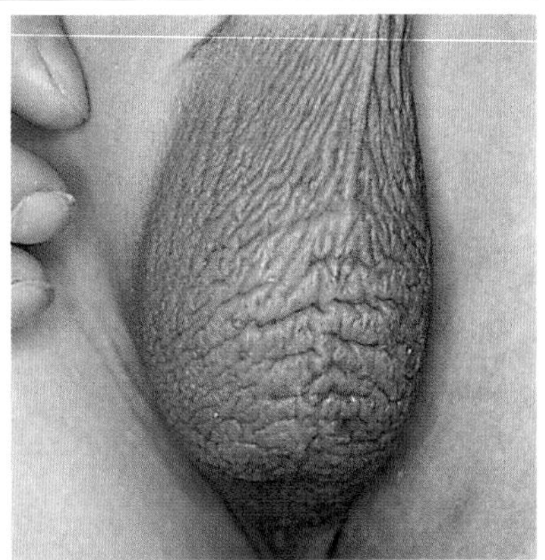

FIG. 8-30 *Lichenification of the scrotum.*

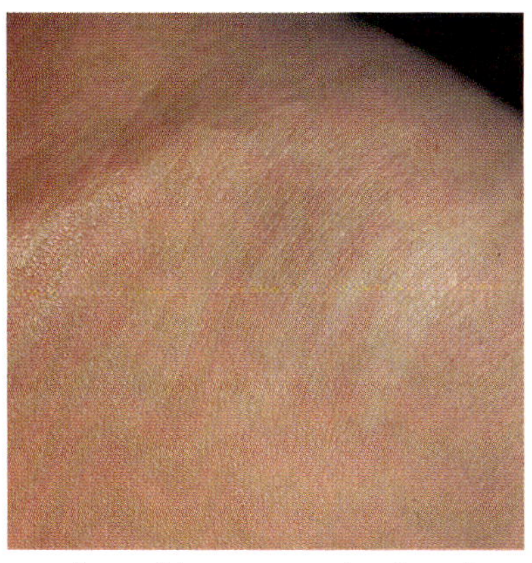

FIG. 8-31 *Linear zones of pallor after a recent scratch of erythematous skin ("white dermographism").*

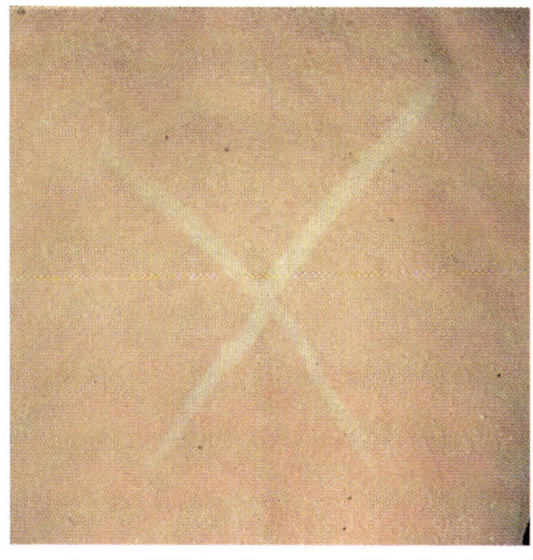

FIG. 8-32 *"White dermographism" induced artifactually by strokes of a blunt-tipped object against erythematous skin.*

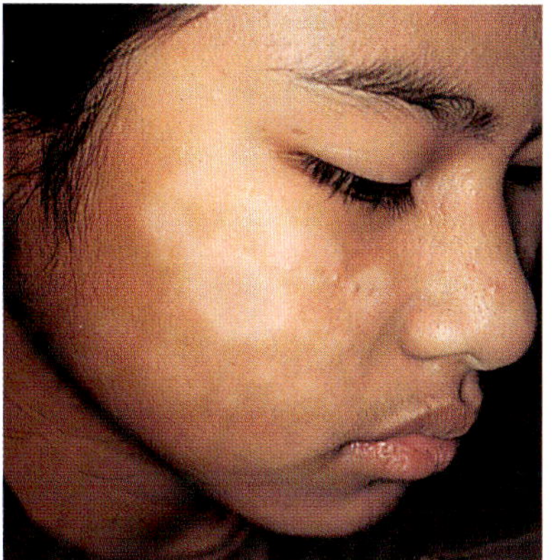

FIG. 8-33 *Hypopigmented scaly patches in an atopic child ("pityriasis alba").*

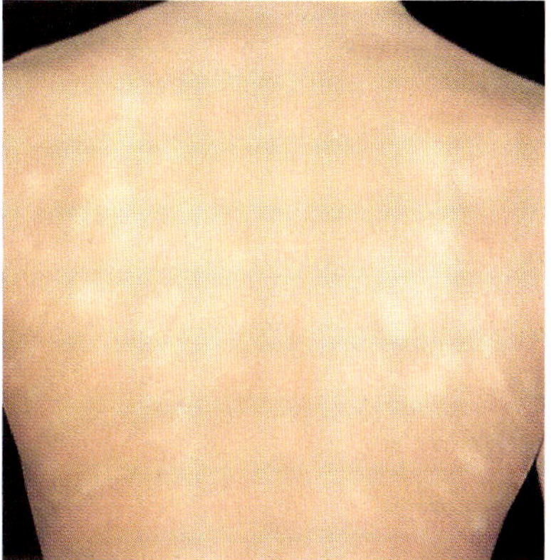

FIG. 8-34 *Hypopigmented scaly patches of pityriasis alba in an atopic child.*

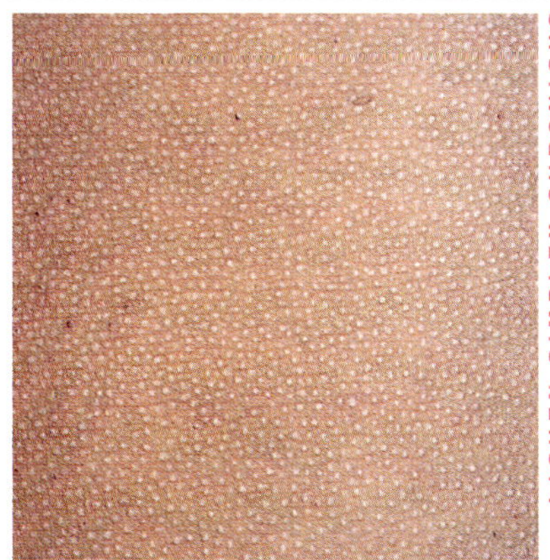

FIG. 8-35 *Monomorphous nonkeratotic follicular papules.*

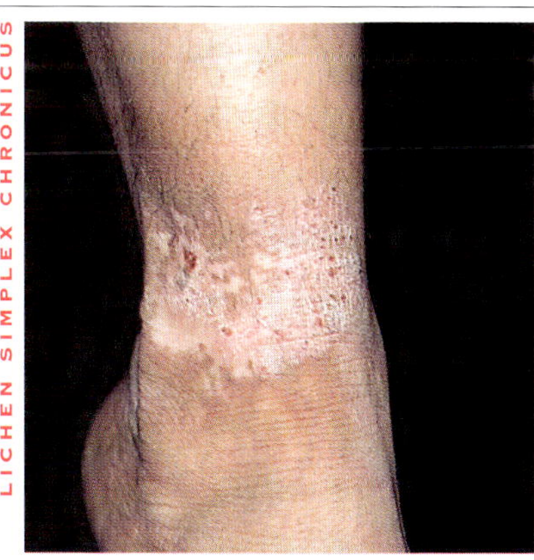

FIG. 8-36 *Ill-defined lichenified plaque.*

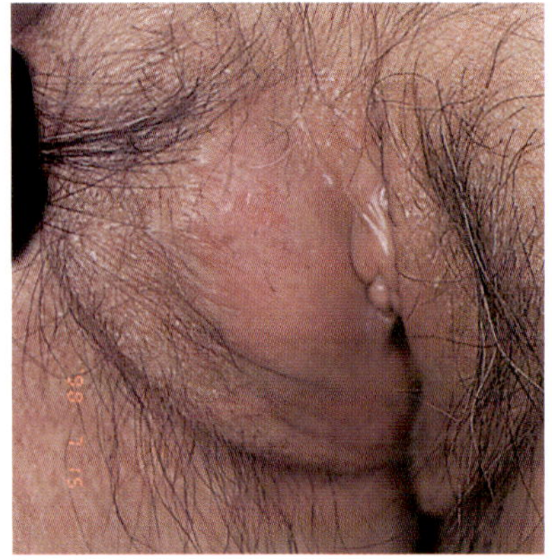

FIG. 8-37 *Zones of lichenification.*

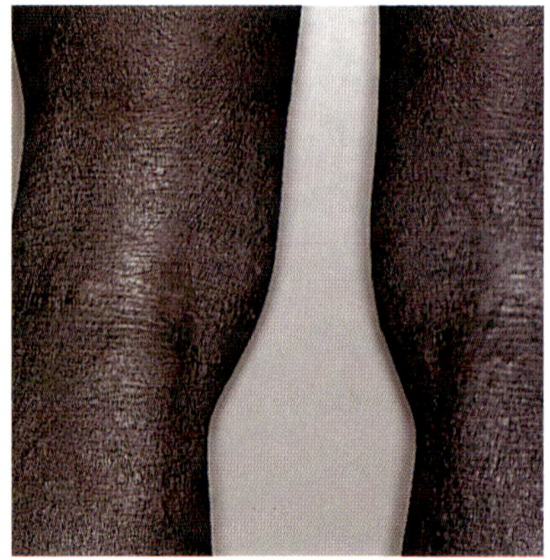

FIG. 8-38 *Lichenified hyperpigmented lesions secondary to rubbing.*

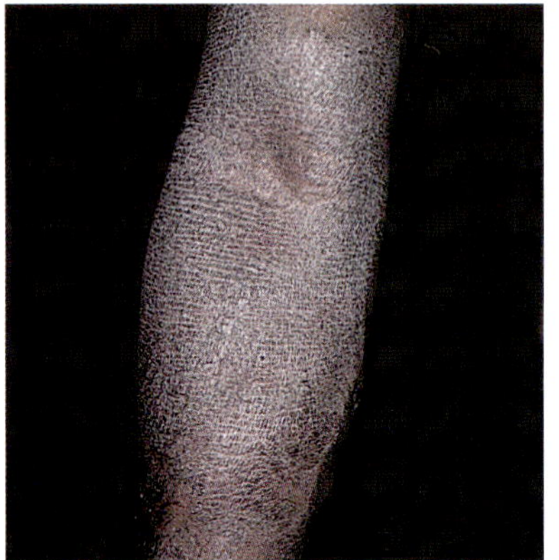

FIG. 8-39 *Lichenified plaque.*

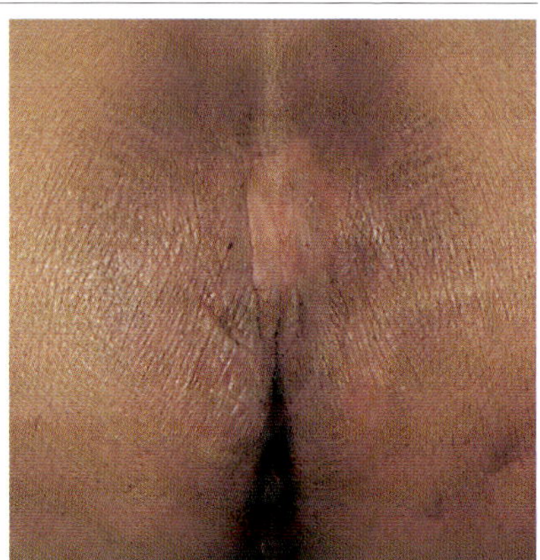

FIG. 8-40 *Lichenified plaque.*

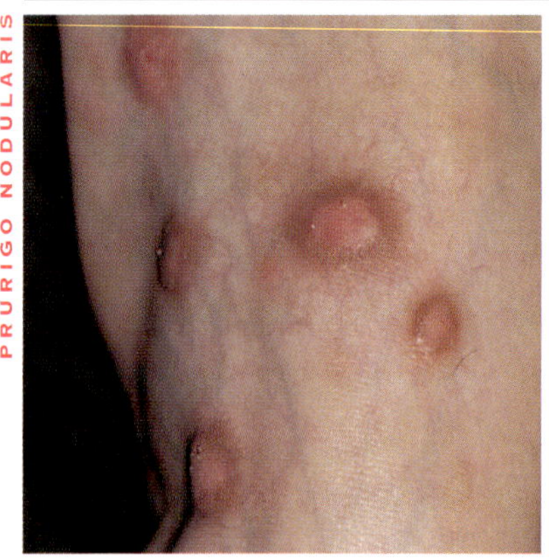

FIG. 8-41 *Papules consequent to persistent forceful rubbing of each discrete site.*

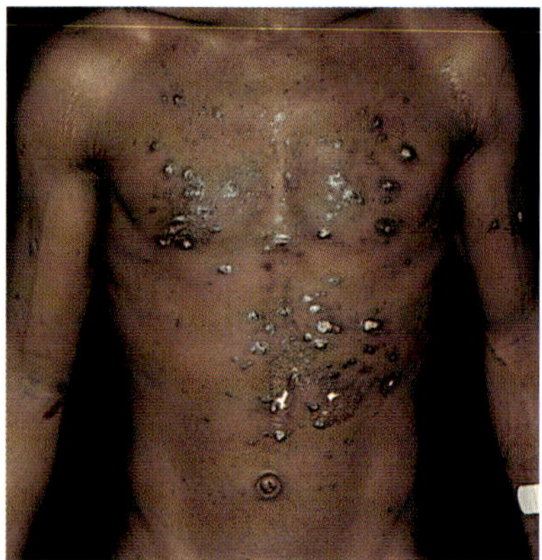

FIG. 8-42 *Hyperpigmented, hypopigmented, and depigmented papules have resulted from the effects of rubbing and scratching.*

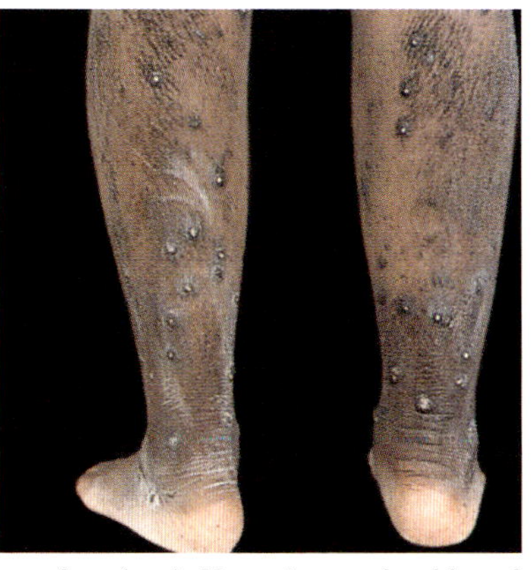 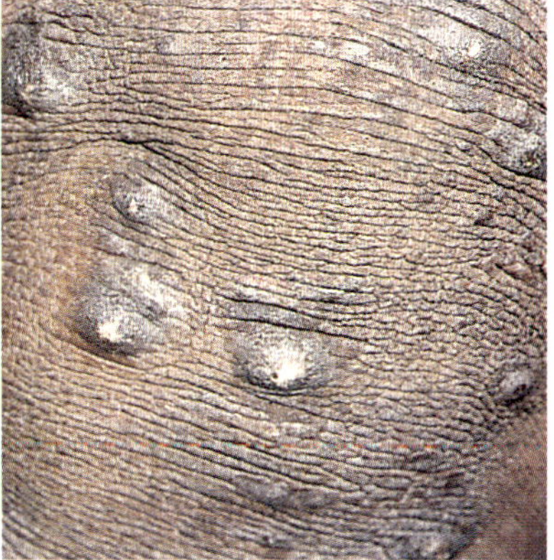

FIG. 8-43 (A, B) *Hyperpigmented and hyperkeratotic papules, and hyperpigmented lichenified plaques consequent to rubbing. The chalky appearance of linear lesions derives from scratching the keratotic surface of papules.*

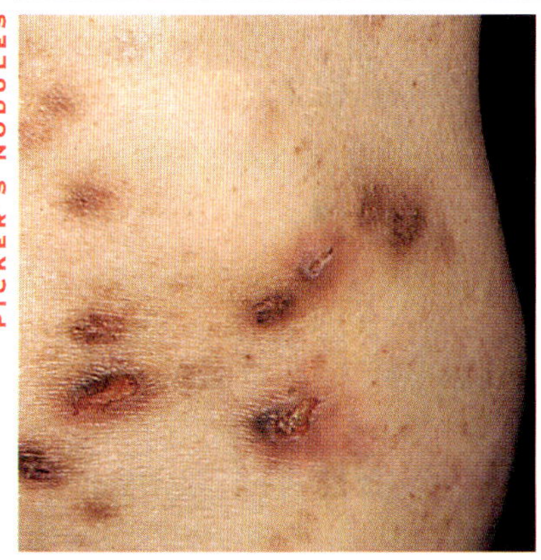 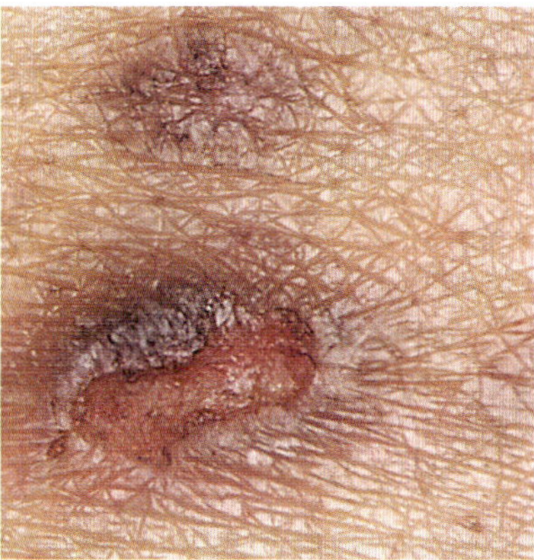

FIG. 8-44 (A, B) *Papules, many of which are ulcerated and hyperpigmented.*

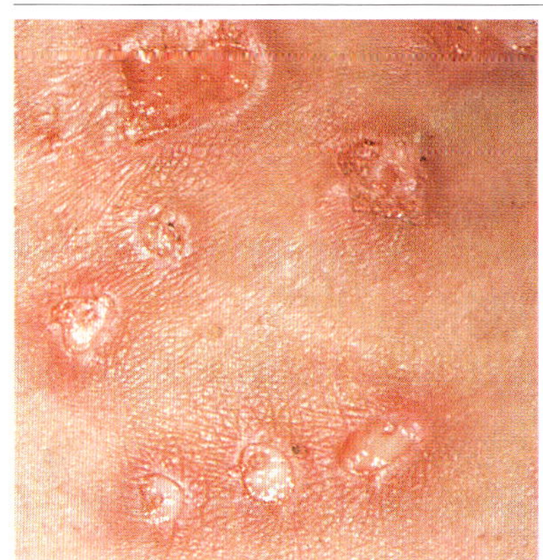 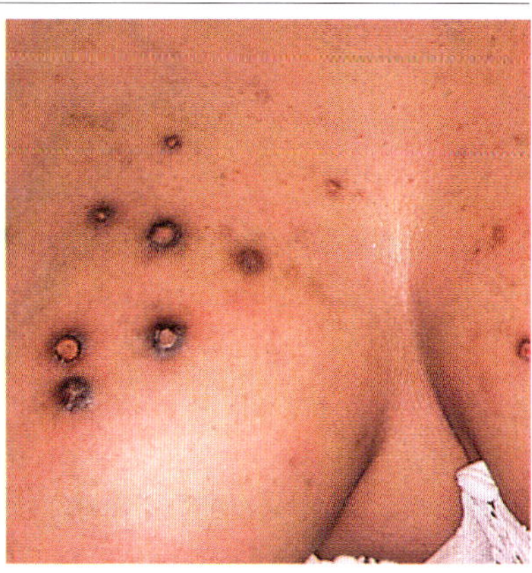

FIG. 8-45 *Ulcers covered by purulence and surrounded by redness and lichenification.*

FIG. 8-46 *Hyperpigmented ulcerated papules.*

ADJUNCTIVE DIAGNOSTIC TEST Detection of elevated serum IgE levels and serum IgE antibodies directed against various inhalant allergens can be accomplished by skin ("prick") tests.

COURSE Because in so-called atopic dermatitis none of the skin lesions are primary in the sense that they develop de novo, no statement can be made about chronological sequence, either of the lesions themselves or of the disease itself. For example, if a patient scratches lightly, only reddish discoloration may result, but if scratching is more animated, erosions may come into being. If scratching is furious, ulcerations may be produced. If rubbing is done very lightly, there may be no morphologic manifestations of it. If, however, rubbing is to and fro vigorously for a long period of time, a plaque of lichen simplex chronicus may be formed. If only a discrete site is rubbed persistently with the ball of a finger, a papule or nodule of prurigo nodularis may be brought into being. If a discrete focus is both rubbed and scratched, an eroded or ulcerated papule of picker's nodule may be brought forth.

Atopic dermatitis, because it results entirely from the effects of rubbing and scratching, may be reversed completely by cessation of external irritation. It may develop transiently if there are paroxysms of rubbing and scratching, and it may be sustained if there is nearly continuous rubbing and scratching.

In brief, lesions of what is called atopic dermatitis persist for as long as an atopic person rubs and scratches the skin. The skin of such a person surely may itch maddeningly, and the natural response to that sensation is forceful rubbing, which may result in lichenified papules and plaques, and furious scratching that may produce erosions, ulcerations, and crusts. All of the lesions of atopic dermatitis are induced by the patient; none "break out." If persons with atopic dermatitis can learn to stop rubbing and scratching, or if pruritus can be lessened markedly, the lesions disappear in time.

INTEGRATION: UNIFYING CONCEPT Atopic dermatitis is factitious dermatitis that occurs in persons who are atopic, to wit, those with a personal or family history of allergic rhinitis, allergic conjunctivitis, or allergic asthma. Such people also have a predilection for allergic urticaria. The state of atopy is determined genetically, and one of the cardinal symptoms of it is pruritus.

Persons who are atopic itch easily and in response to many causes. For example, a person who is not atopic has no difficulty wearing mohair, but on an atopic person a mohair sweater causes extraordinary pruritus, which is greeted by bouts of intense scratching. When an atopic person, whether child or adult, becomes unhinged emotionally at a particular moment, frenzied scratching of wildly pruritic skin may ensue, and, in minutes the entire integument may be transformed by the effects of fingernails. Those effects may range everywhere and into an erythroderma. If, however, the hands of an atopic could be shackled, the skin would be free of signs of rubbing and scratching that have come to be known, erroneously, as atopic dermatitis. This fact was demonstrated experimentally more than 100 years ago.

Lichen simplex chronicus appears in the skin of people who may or may not be atopic, and always as a consequence of mechanical trauma, such as in a variety of circumstances where trauma occurs expectedly. It might, for example, appear beneath the chin where a violin "rests" and on the elbows of a microscopist who "reads" sections of tissue for many hours daily. Lichen simplex chronicus, therefore, is not at all contingent on whether or not a person is atopic; vigorous rubbing of skin over the course of months or years is the common denominator.

The same principle applies to prurigo nodularis. When that condition occurs on the knees of surfers, it is called "surfers nodules," on the nose or behind the ear as a consequence of the pressure applied to the skin by parts of eyeglasses "granuloma fissuratum," and as a consequence of a prosthesis utilized because of amputation of a leg, "pressure papule." When pressure is applied to the helix or the antehelix of an ear damaged by the effects of ultraviolet light, the analogue of prurigo nodularis that develops is called "chondrodermatitis nodularis helicis," a misnomer. It is not truly a chondrodermatitis, but rather a papule that results from pressure against the cartilage, even pressure as light as is caused by sleeping on an ear.

THERAPY Reassurance, emotional support, and, depending on the debility caused by the skin disease, psychotherapy. Emollients, topical corticosteroids, and anti-histamines used to suppress pruritus are helpful but only palliative. Antibiotics are indicated for secondary bacterial infection. Phototherapy (UVA and UVB), cyclosporin, oral corticosteroids, and topical tacrolimus (FK506, a member of the immunosuppressive makrolide family) may be utilized in severe cases. In the ultimate analysis, a person with "atopic dermatitis" must be taught that the disease that goes by that name is entirely self-inflicted and that various strategies must be employed to lessen and control both the authentic pruritus and the legitimate tendency to obviate it by rubbing and scratching. Researchers engaged in study of atopic dermatitis would benefit, too, from learning this lesson.

CHONDRODERMATITIS NODULARIS HELICIS

DEFINITION A papule, sometimes eroded, ulcerated, crusted, or keratotic, on a helix or antehelix consequent to the effects of persistent trauma.

Because a lesion of chondrodermatitis nodularis helicis results from the effects of external trauma, analogous to picker's nodule but a consequence rather of pressure such as that imposed by an earphone, a wimple, or even that of a pillow while sleeping, it persists and often worsens for as long as the ear is offended by the object. When the cause of the compromising pressure is removed, the lesion slowly but surely wanes, and the ear returns mostly to normal.

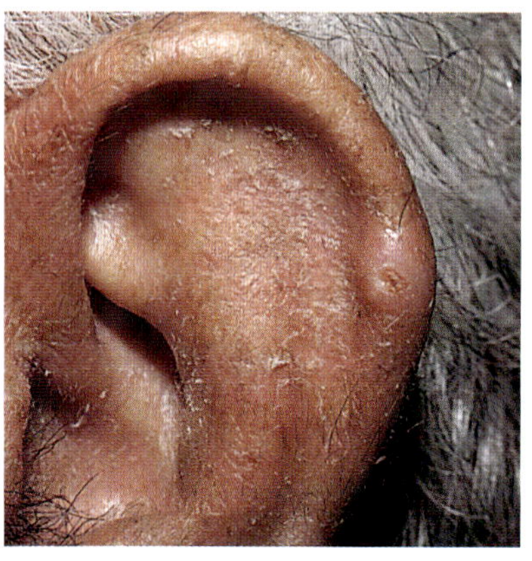

FIG. 8-47 *Eroded, crusted papule on a helix. A lesion such as this one is painful.*

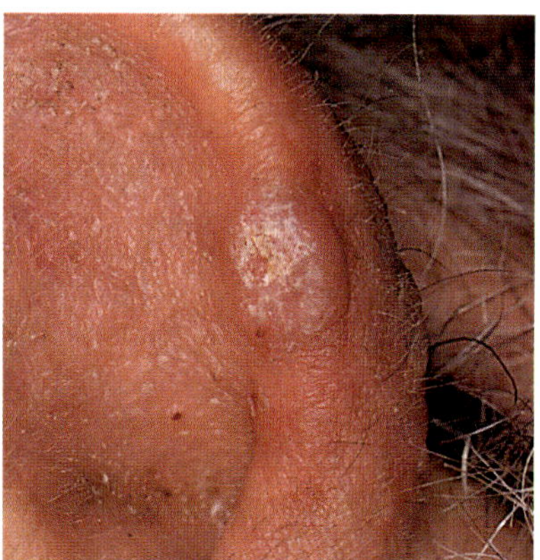

FIG. 8-48 *Keratotic papule on a helix.*

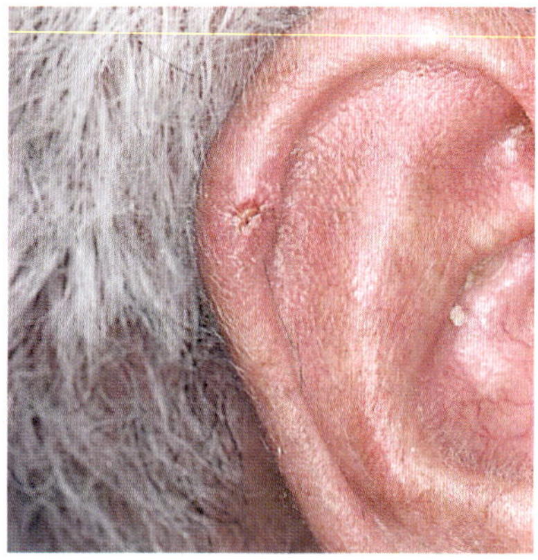

FIG. 8-49 *Keratotic papule.*

COURSE In time, the ulcer of chondrodermatitis nodularis helicis heals by re-epithelialization and by a distinctive kind of fibroplasia within the dermis in which a number of chondrocytoid fibrocytes are present in conjunction with altered bundles of collagen.

INTEGRATION: UNIFYING CONCEPT As has already been implied, chondrodermatitis nodularis helicis is not an inflammatory process of the cartilage, as its name denotes, but a response of sun-damaged skin of a helix or antehelix to the effects of sustained pressure. In this sense it is analogous to "granuloma fissuratum" and "pressure papule."

THERAPY The source of pressure to the ear must be mitigated. If the lesion is merely eroded or but slightly ulcerated, it may be injected with corticosteroid. If, however, the ulcer in a papule is deeper, intractable, and painful, excision of the lesion may be necessary.

DEFINITION Infection of skin and subcutaneous tissue by atypical mycobacteria, that is, mycobacteria other than those responsible for tuberculosis and leprosy, expressed clinically as keratotic and crusted papules, plaques, nodules, and tumors that may be punctuated by draining sinuses and by ulcers.

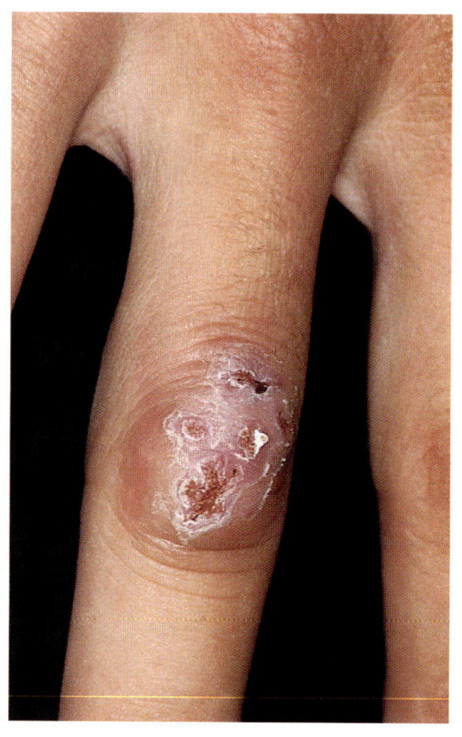

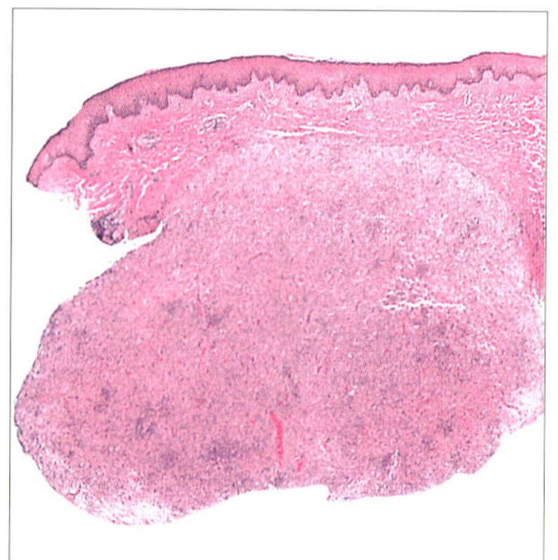

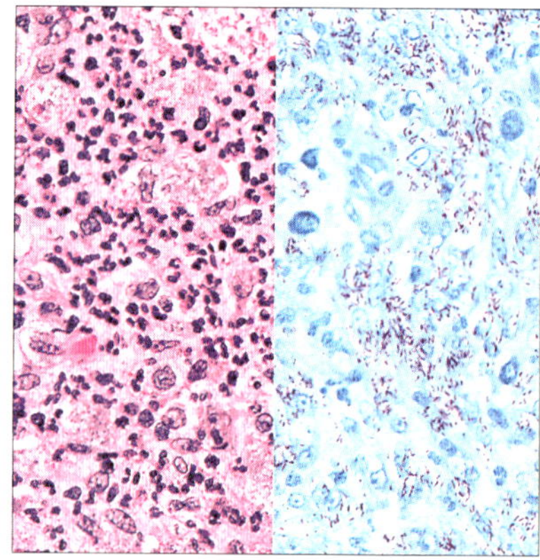

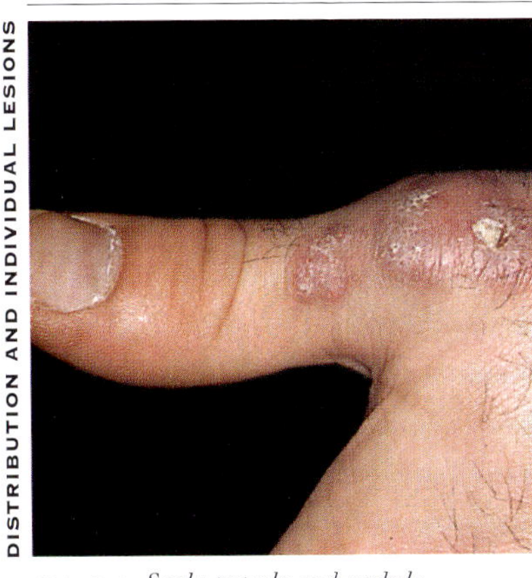

FIG. 9-1 *Scaly papule and nodule.*

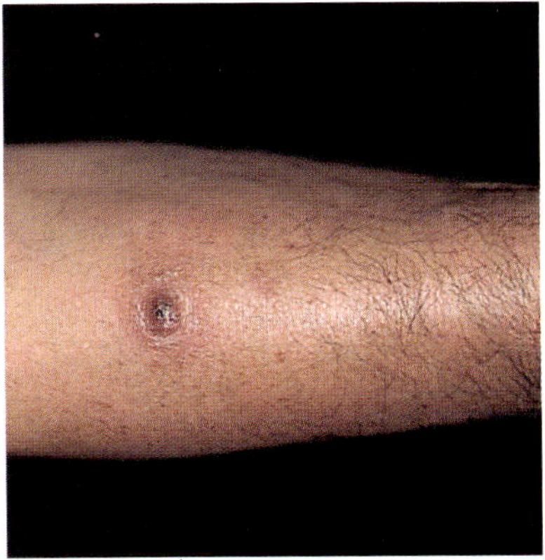

FIG. 9-2 *Crusted nodule on the forearm.*

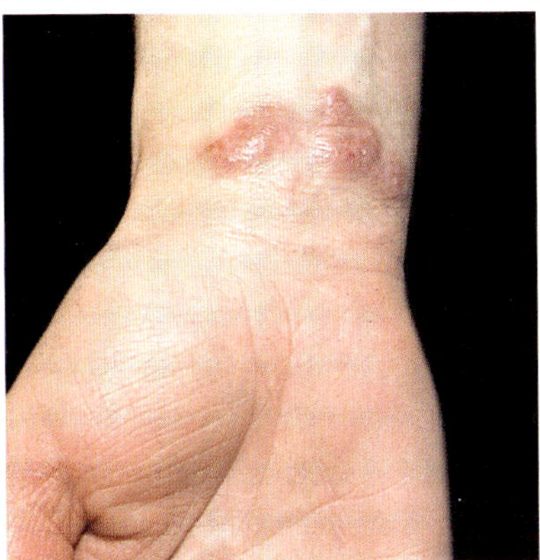

FIG. 9-3 *Nodules on the wrist.*

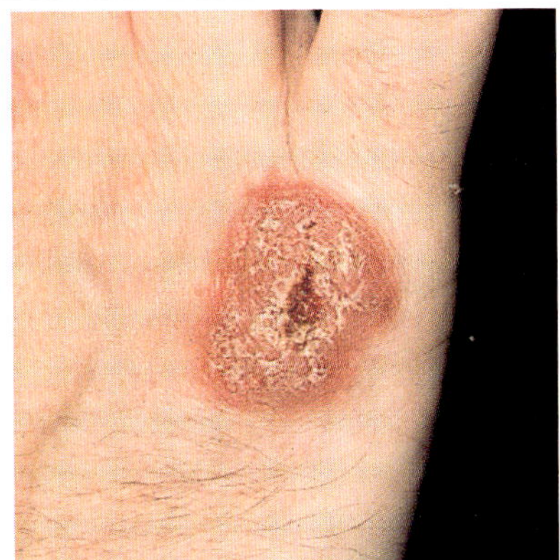

FIG. 9-4 *Nodule covered by scales and scale-crusts.*

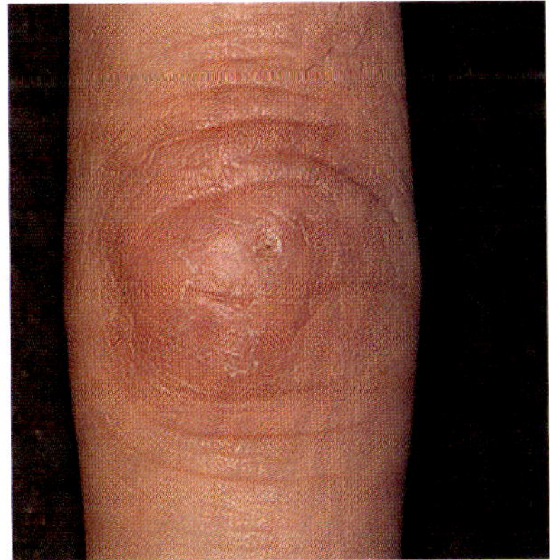

FIG. 9-5 *Nodule on the finger.*

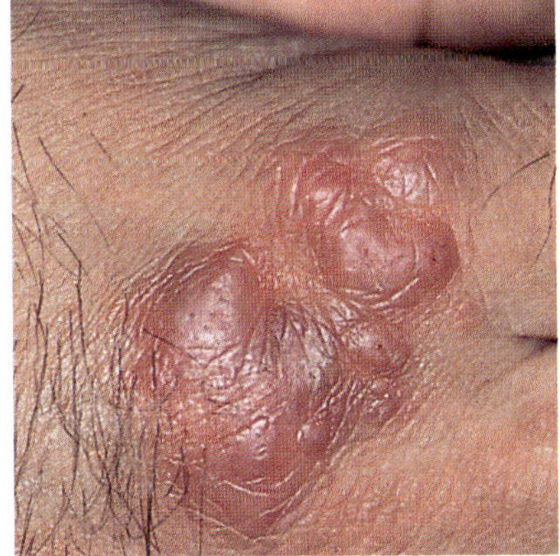

FIG. 9-6 *Papules and nodules in a cluster on the dorsum of the hand.*

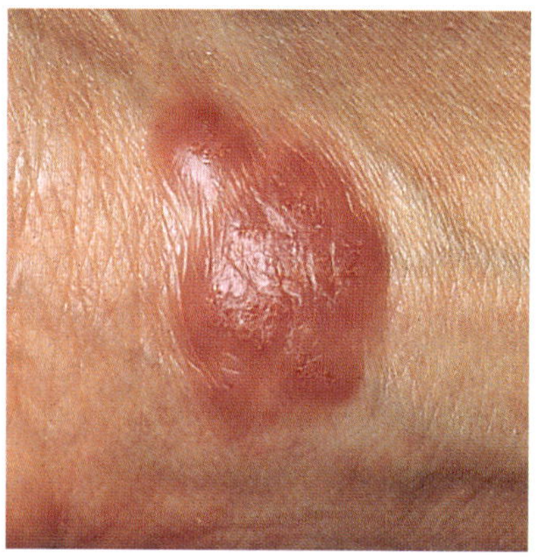

FIG. 9-7 *Smooth-surfaced papules that have become confluent to form a plaque on the wrist.*

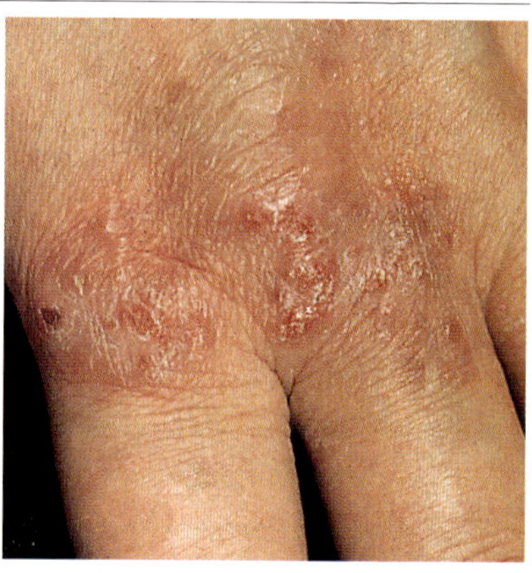

FIG. 9-8 *Confluence of crusted papules with formation of a plaque.*

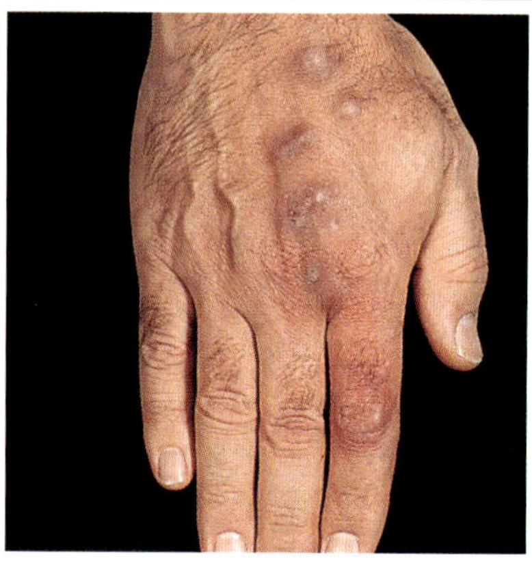

FIG. 9-9 *Papules in linear array.*

ADJUNCTIVE DIAGNOSTIC TESTS Ziehl-Neelsen stain in sections of tissue for purposes of coloring acid-fast organisms, and culture of tissue on specialized media. Mycobacterial DNA can also be demonstrated in skin by the polymerase chain reaction.

COURSE As a rule, lesions that represent infection by an atypical mycobacterium tend to persist and enlarge, although some actually undergo involution slowly over a period of many years, the result in the end being a scar.

INTEGRATION: UNIFYING CONCEPT All of the clinical/histopathological expressions of atypical mycobacterial infections, at every stage of their chronological course, are a consequence of the interplay between the bacilli on one hand and the host on the other. The bacilli induce, in sequence, suppuration, granulomatous inflammation, and fibrosis, and, as the process both evolves and resolves concurrently, all three may be present in a single section of tissue.

Nearly invariable in fully-formed lesions is the association of pseudocarcinomatous hyperplasia, which represents hyperplasia of epithelial structures of adnexa, especially of infundibula and eccrine ducts. That finding, coupled with scale-crusts that house neutrophils, often imparts the appearance of vegetations to the lesions clinically. In time, marked hyperkeratosis of the epidermis causes a lesion to appear keratotic. Later still, when all that is left of the process is extensive fibrosis, what may remain as residuum clinically is a scar associated with pigmentary abnormalities.

Atypical mycobacteria can be seen easily in sections that show suppurative and suppurative granulomatous, inflammation when tissue is stained by Ziehl-Neelsen's method. As the process becomes progressively granulomatous and increasingly fibrotic, no bacteria can be detected by any method.

On the basis of histopathologic findings alone, an accurate judgment cannot be made of the particular variant of atypical mycobacterium (e.g., marinum, fortuitum, or kansasii) that is responsible for the infectious process.

THERAPY Surgical excision is effective in removing disease localized to a single site. If a lesion is too large to be excised or if there is more than one lesion, minocycline or rifampicin and ethambutol are drugs of choice. Cryotherapy also has been claimed to be effective.

DEFINITION A malignant neoplasm made up of abnormal germinative cells analogous to those that compose the folliculosebaceous-apocrine germ in an embryo and that usually manifests clinically as a papule or nodule which may become ulcerated. On the basis of clinico-pathologic correlation, five distinctive types of basal-cell carcinoma have been identified, namely, nodular, superficial, morpheiform, fibroepithelial, and infundibulocystic.

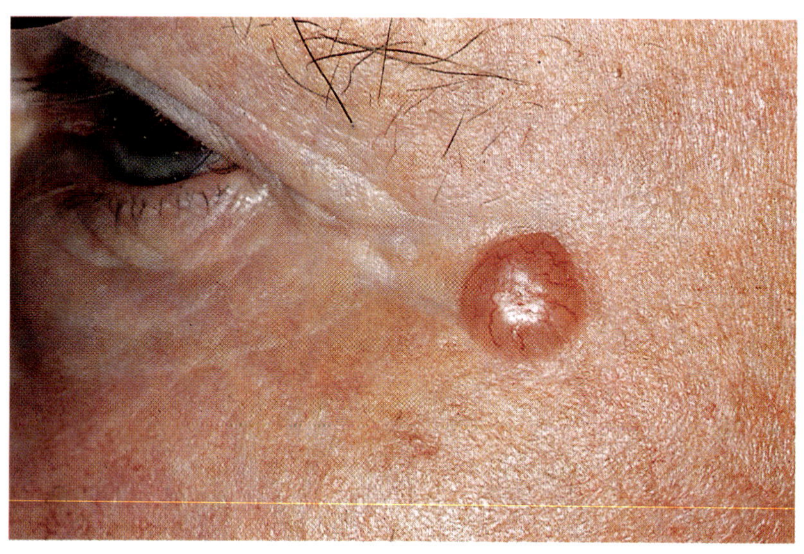

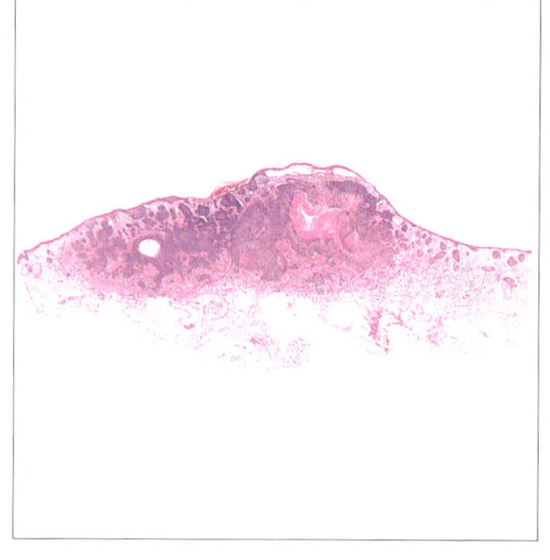

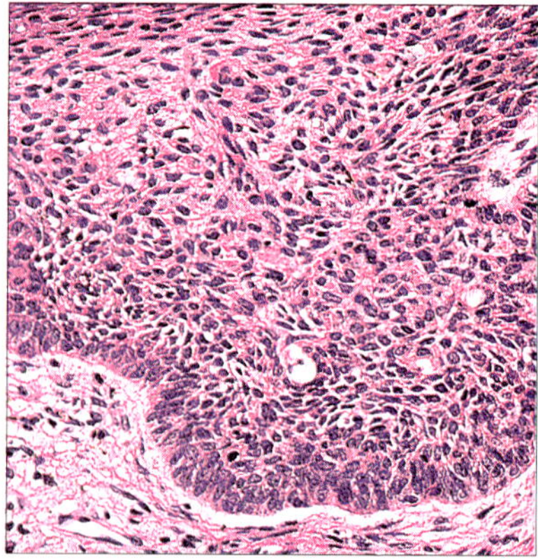

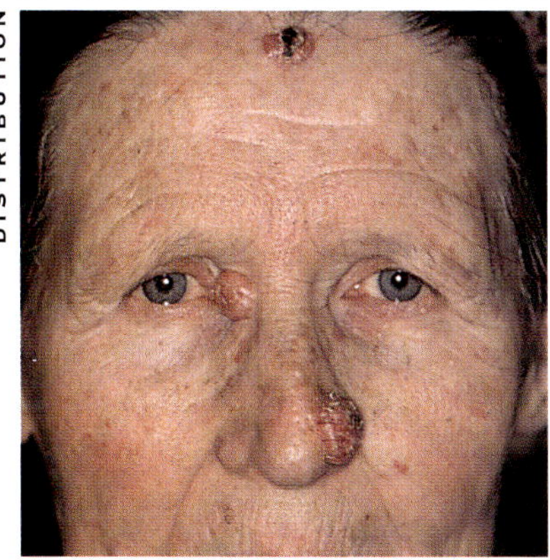

FIG. 10-1 *Numerous nodular basal-cell carcinomas.*

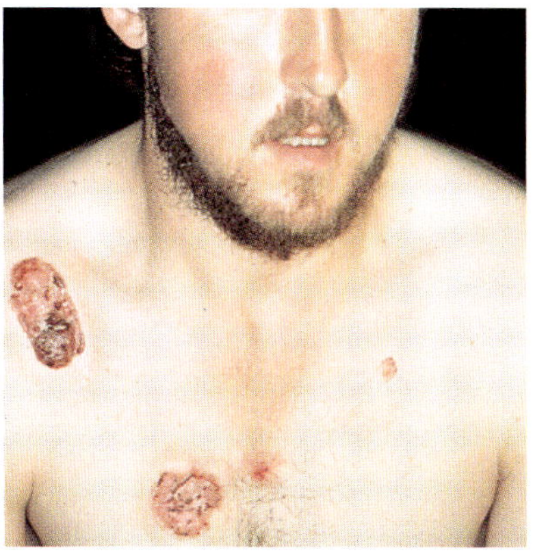

FIG. 10-2 *Superficial and nodular types of basal-cell carcinoma.*

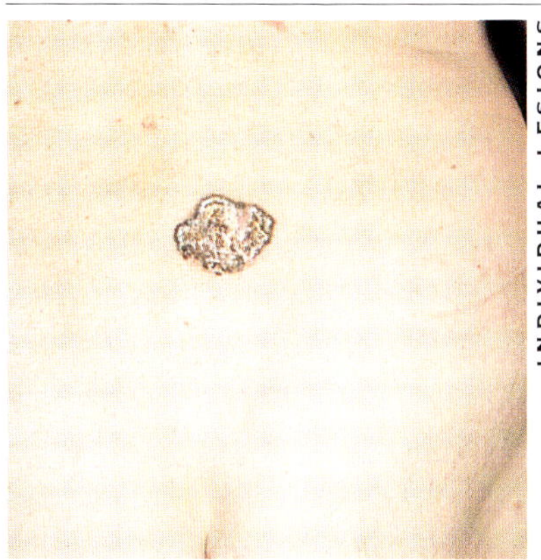

FIG. 10-3 *Pigmented superficial type of basal-cell carcinoma on the sacral region.*

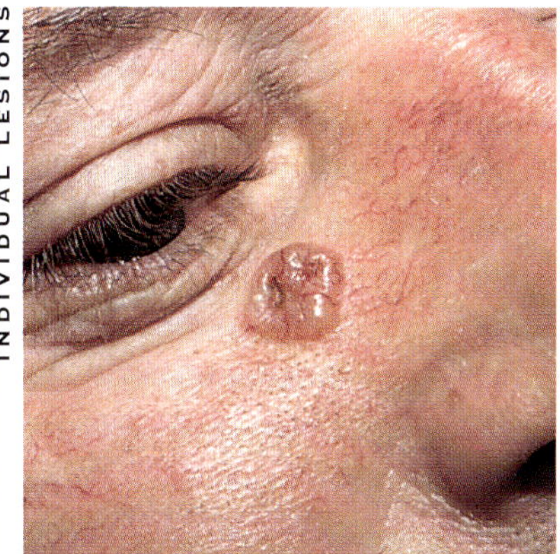

FIG. 10-4 *Basal-cell carcinoma in the form of agminated papules with telangiectases.*

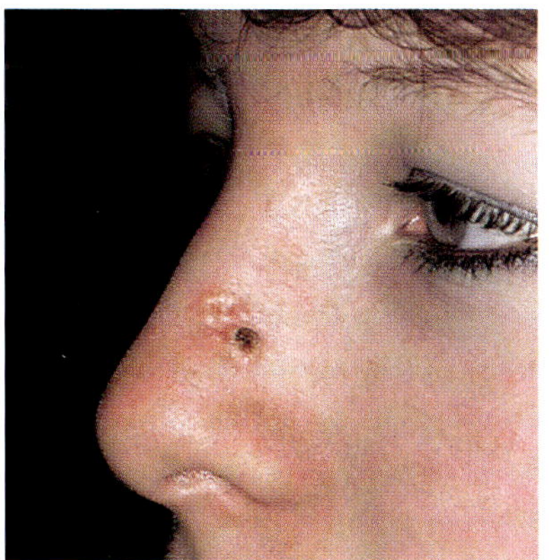

FIG. 10-5 *Nodular basal-cell carcinoma, ulcerated, with hemorrhagic crust.*

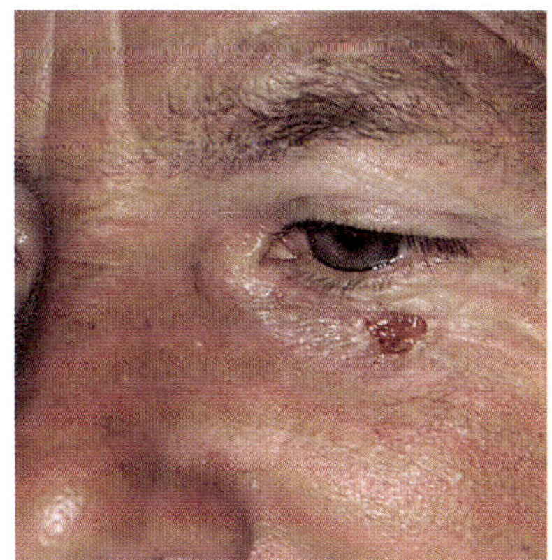

FIG. 10-6 *Noduloulcerative basal-cell carcinoma.*

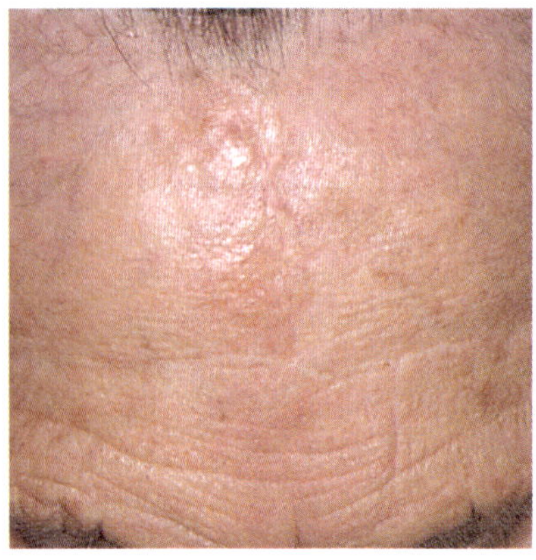

FIG. 10-7 *Papules that have become confluent to form a plaque.*

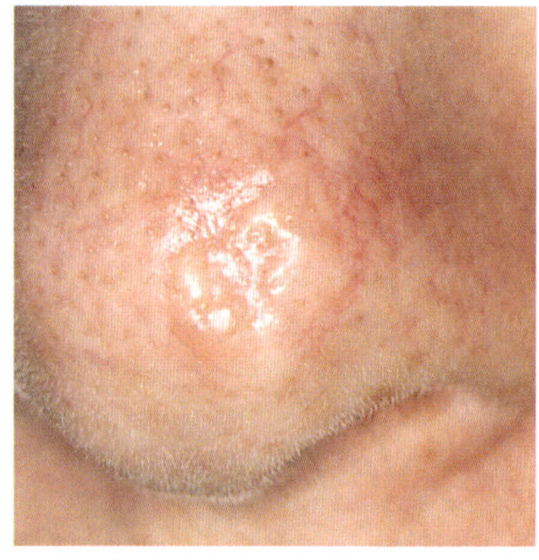

FIG. 10-8 *Nodular basal-cell carcinoma with central depression of morpheiform nature.*

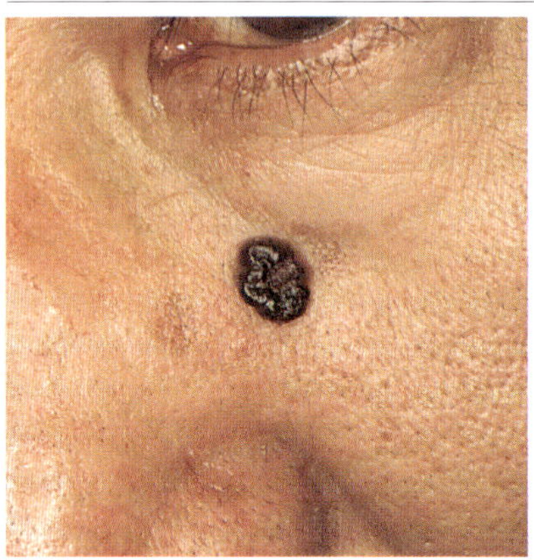

FIG. 10-9 *Nodular basal-cell carcinoma, pigmented.*

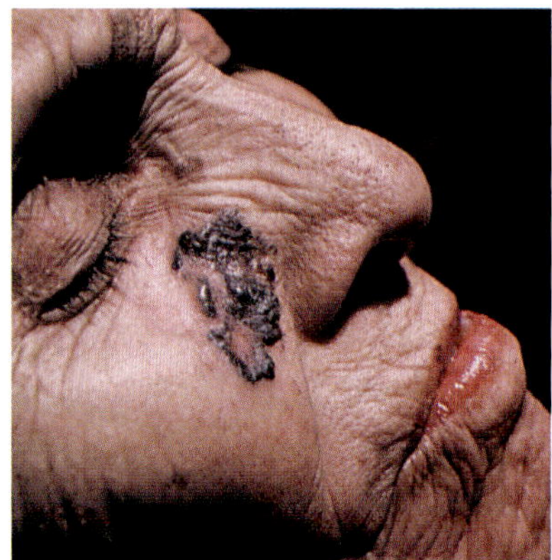

FIG. 10-10 *"Nodular" basal-cell carcinoma, plaque-like.*

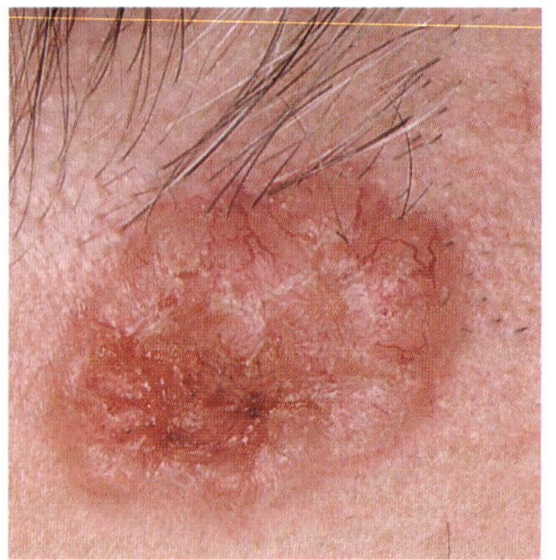

FIG. 10-11 *Nodular basal-cell carcinoma covered by telangiectases.*

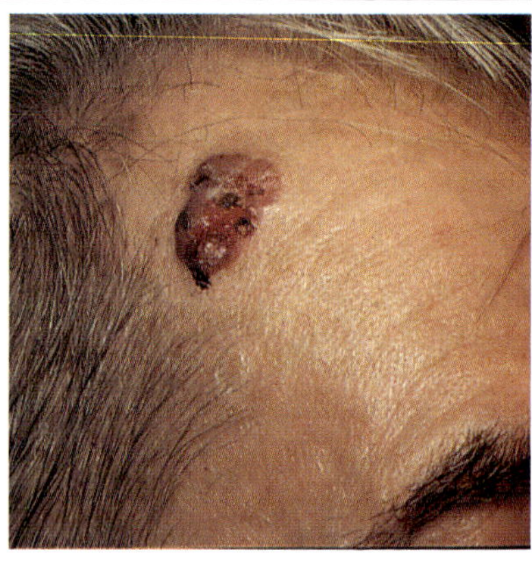

FIG. 10-12 *Noduloulcerative basal-cell carcinoma.*

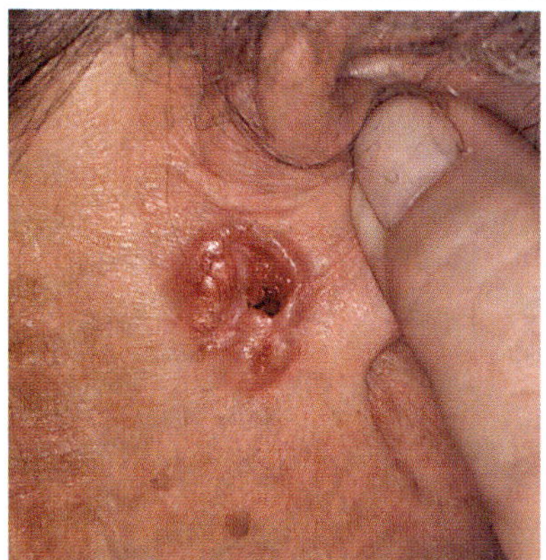

FIG. 10-13 *Noduloulcerative basal-cell carcinoma.*

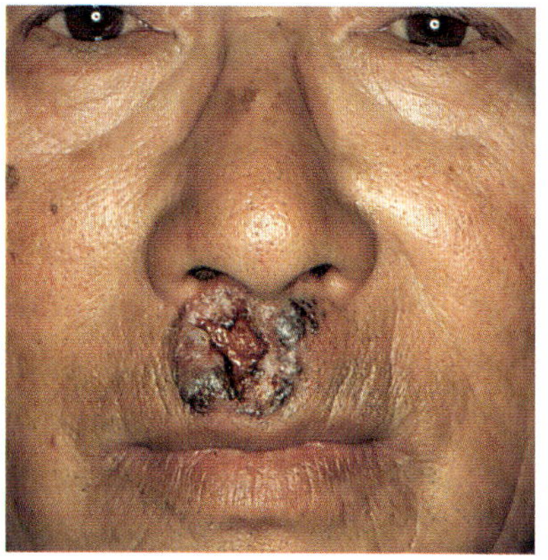

FIG. 10-14 *Noduloulcerative basal-cell carcinoma, pigmented.*

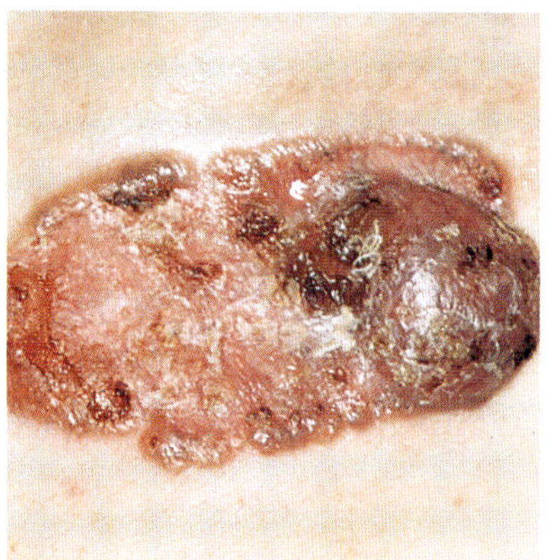

FIG. 10-15 *Superficial basal-cell carcinoma with a nodule.*

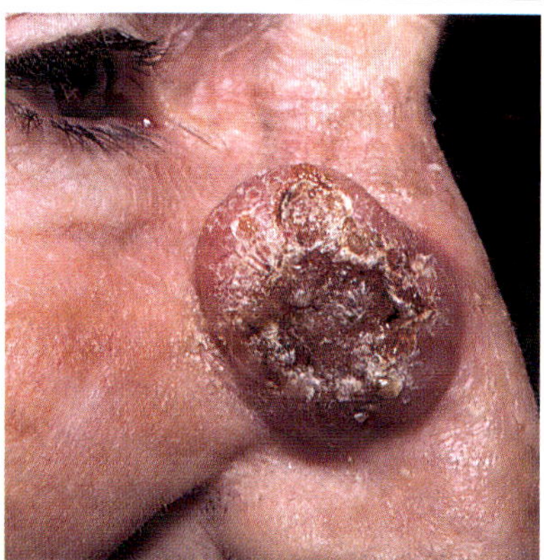

FIG. 10-16 *Noduloulcerative basal-cell carcinoma.*

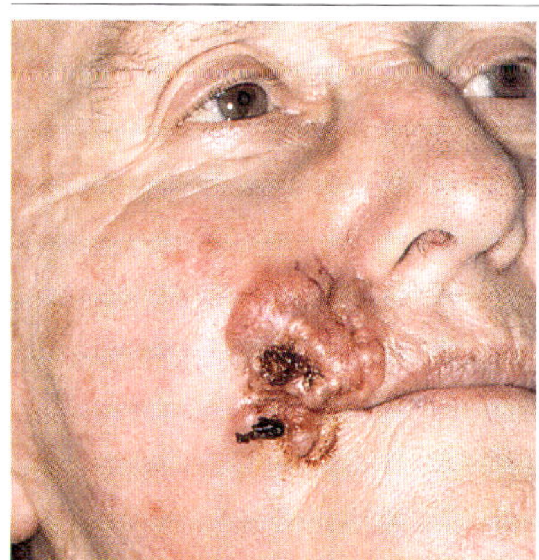

FIG. 10-17 *Noduloulcerative basal-cell carcinoma.*

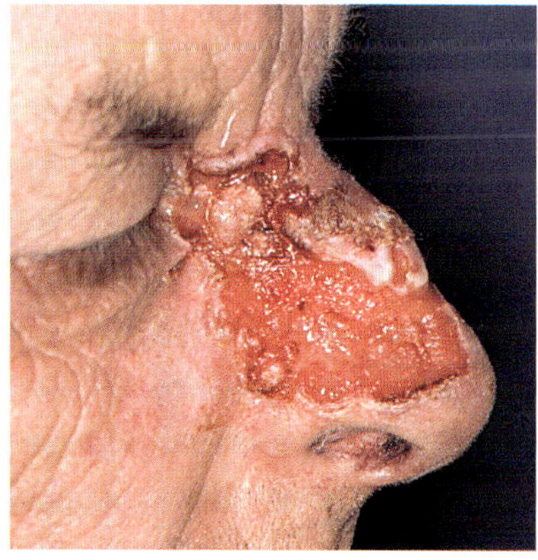

FIG. 10-18 *Noduloulcerative basal-cell carcinoma ("rodent ulcer").*

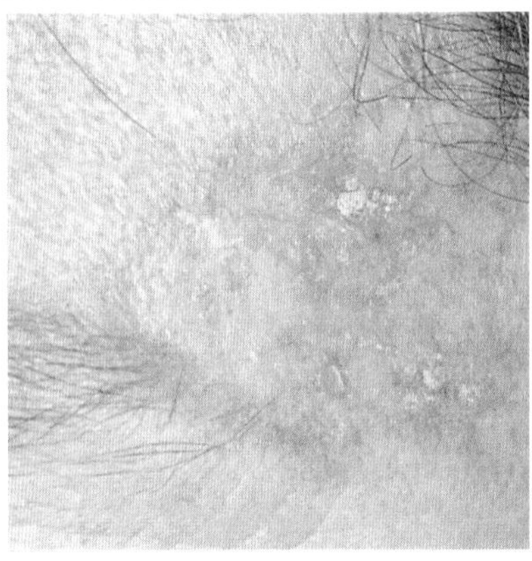

FIG. 10-19 *Morpheiform basal-cell carcinoma.*

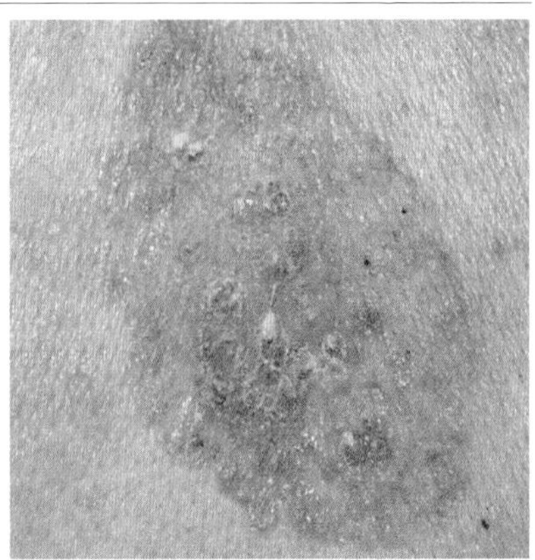

FIG. 10-20 *Superficial basal-cell carcinoma.*

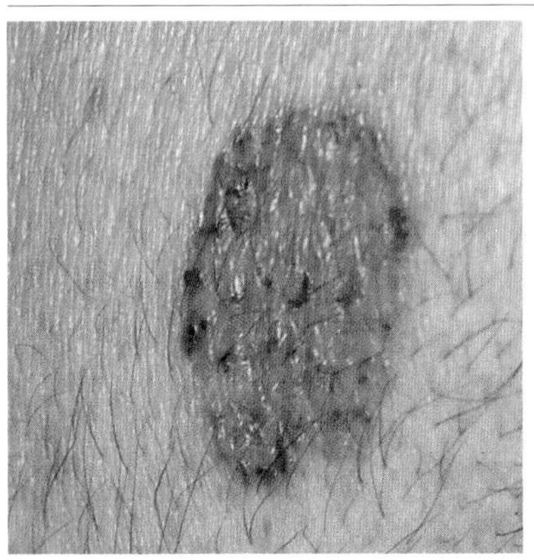

FIG. 10-21 *Superficial basal-cell carcinoma.*

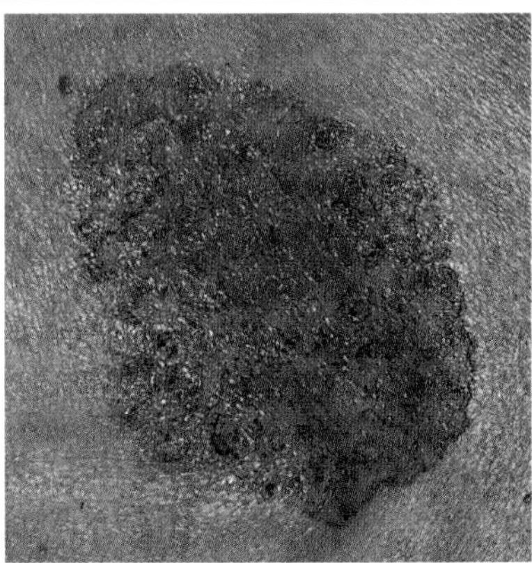

FIG. 10-22 *Superficial basal-cell carcinoma.*

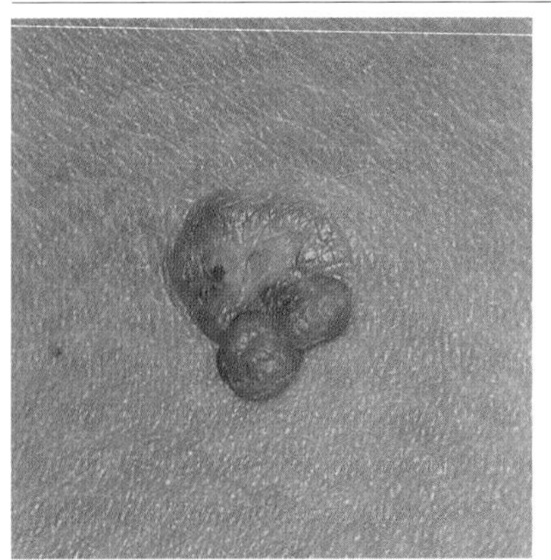

FIG. 10-23 *Fibroepithelial basal-cell carcinoma.*

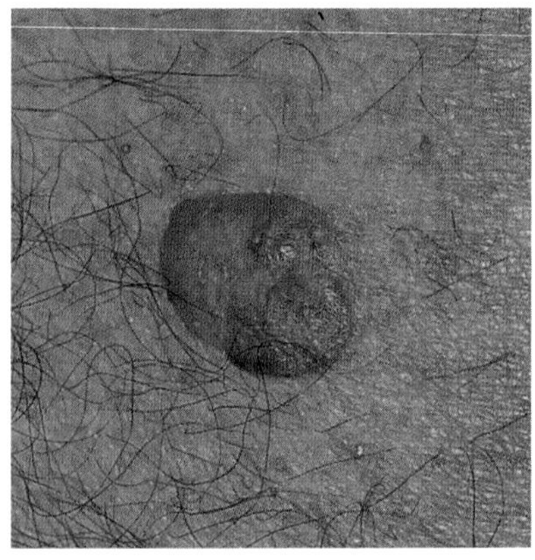

FIG. 10-24 *Fibroepithelial basal-cell carcinoma.*

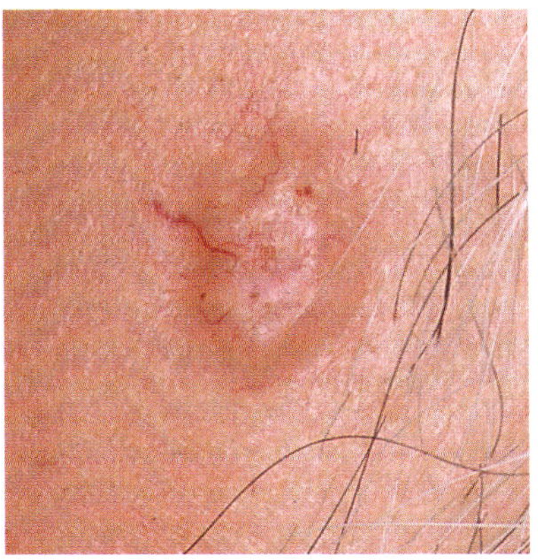

FIG. 10-25 *Nodular basal-cell carcinoma with a dell and telangiectases.*

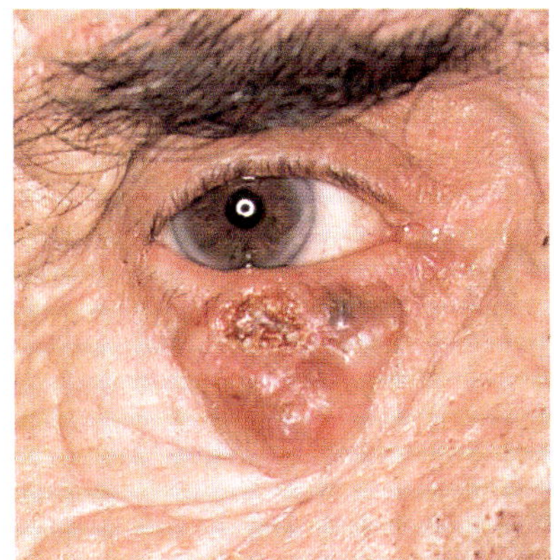

FIG. 10-26 *Noduloulcerative basal-cell carcinoma.*

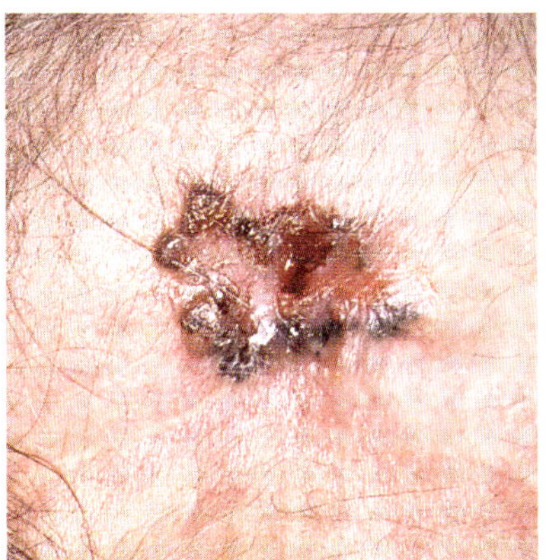

FIG. 10-27 *Noduloulcerative basal-cell carcinoma, pigmented, resembling melanoma.*

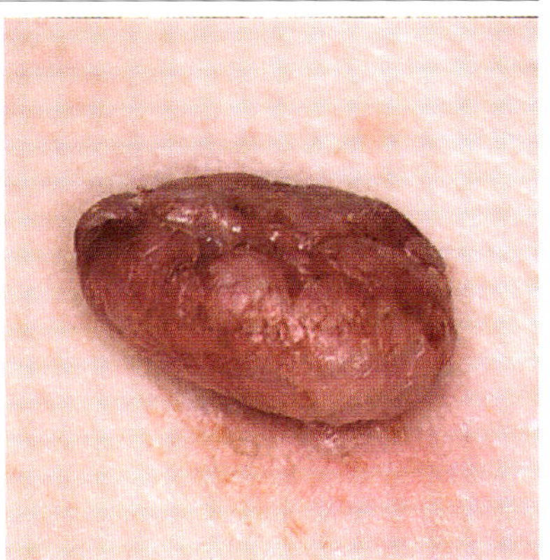

FIG. 10-28 *Fibroepithelial basal-cell carcinoma.*

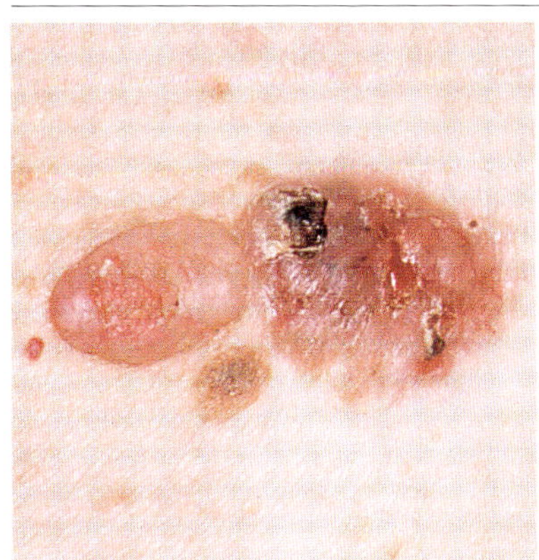

FIG. 10-29 *Noduloulcerative basal-cell carcinoma (right), fibroepithelial basal-cell carcinoma (left), and a seborrheic keratosis (between).*

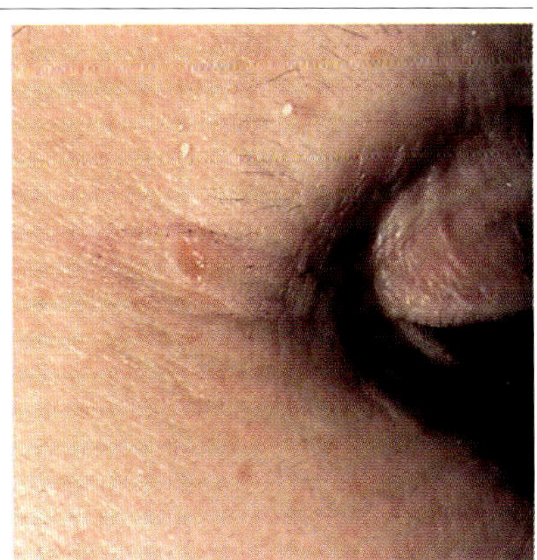

FIG. 10-30 *Infundibulocystic basal-cell carcinoma consisting of a papule with central depression.*

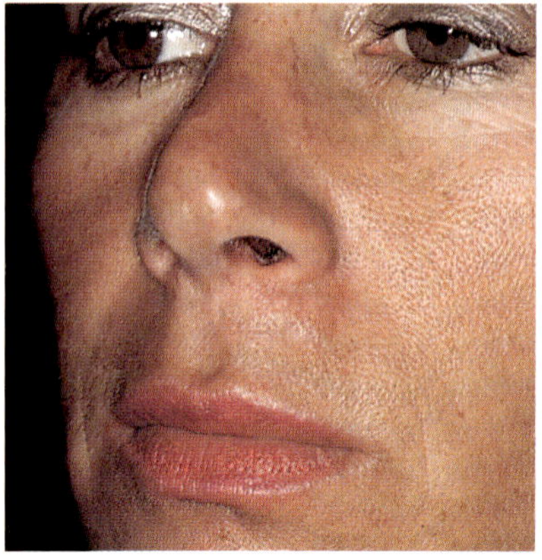
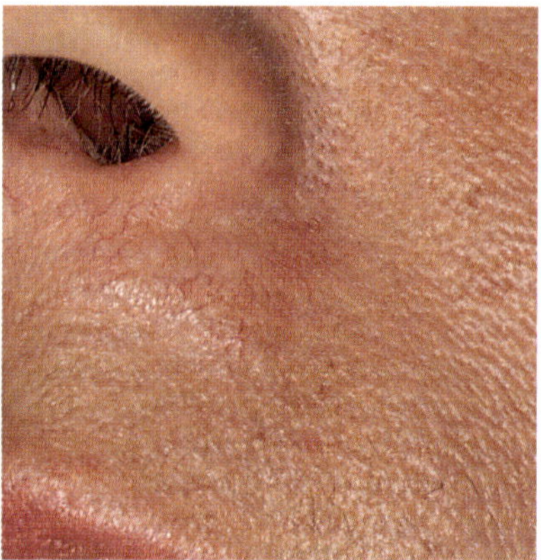

FIG. 10-31 (A, B) *Morpheiform basal-cell carcinoma in the form of a smooth-surfaced plaque.*

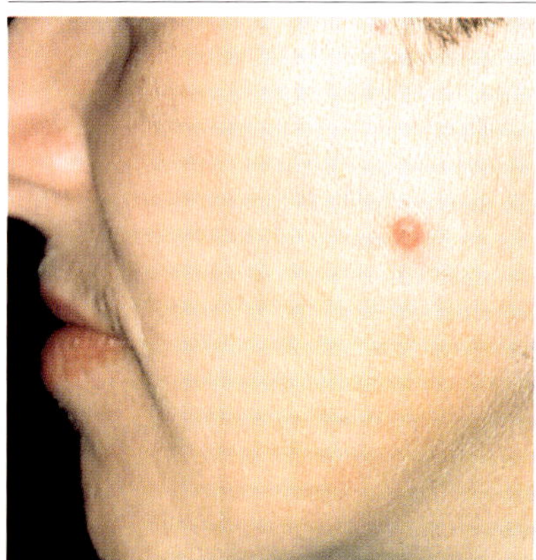

FIG. 10-32 *Basal-cell carcinomas, infundibulocystic type.*

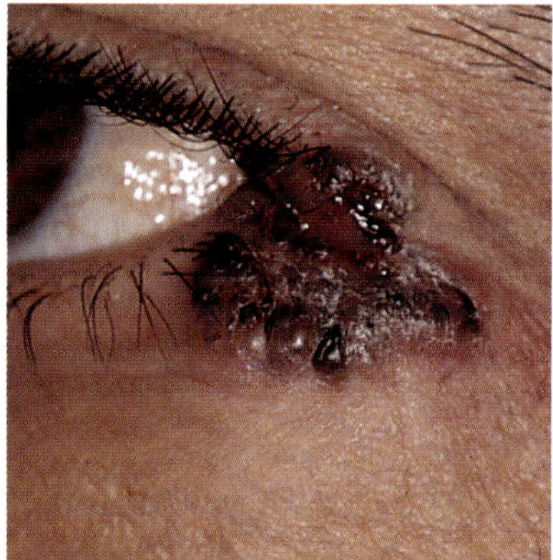

FIG. 10-33 *Noduloulcerative basal-cell carcinoma, pigmented.*

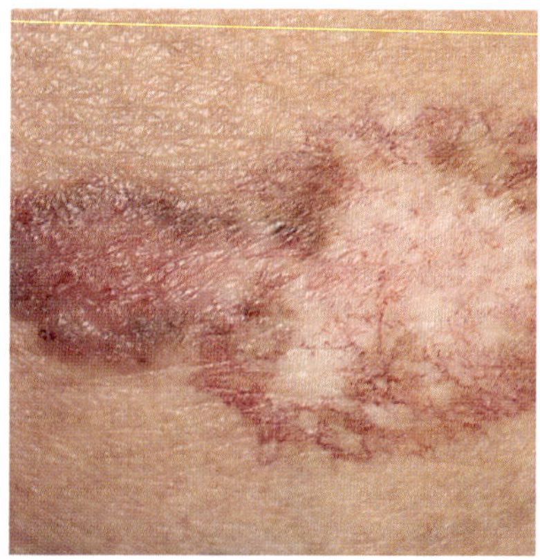

FIG. 10-34 *Superficial basal-cell carcinoma on left and depigmented telangiectatic patch of chronic radiodermatitis on right.*

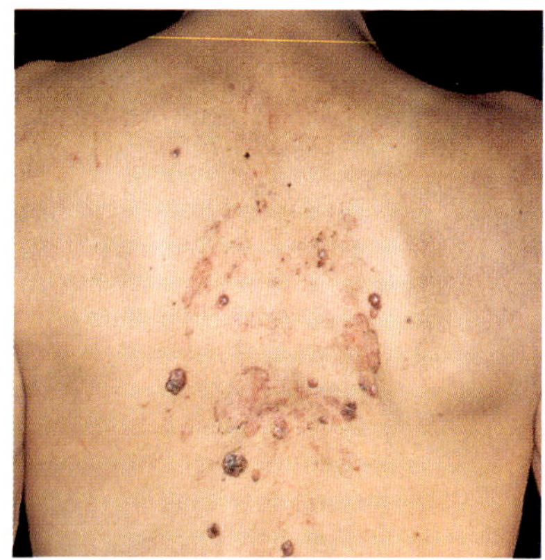

FIG. 10-35 *Nevoid basal-cell carcinoma syndrome with papules and nodules of basal-cell carcinoma.*

COURSE Five types of basal-cell carcinoma are recognizable on the basis of clinicopathologic correlation, namely, nodular, superficial, morpheiform, fibroepithelial, and infundibulocystic. As a rule, each of them grows slowly and does not do serious harm to a patient, but, episodically, a basal-cell carcinoma may kill by virtue of local destruction of tissue or, very rarely, of metastasis widely. It is the nodular type of basal-cell carcinoma, known also as noduloulcerative, that most often is responsible for extensive destruction of tissue locally and may even be associated with neurotropism. Most examples of so-called nodular basal-cell carcinoma remain papules, often ulcerated ones, for the lifetime of the person who bears them. In time, a papule may become a nodule and even a tumor. At times, a nodular basal-cell carcinoma can achieve gigantic proportions.

A superficial basal-cell carcinoma is usually flattish and, although it extends very slowly centrifugally, it usually remains flat or slightly elevated for a lifetime. Morpheiform basal-cell carcinoma, so named because it sometimes resembles morphea clinically, also grows slowly and rarely does serious damage. Because its borders are ill defined, however, this particular variant of basal-cell carcinoma tends to thwart excision completely and therefore is given to persist at the local site after incomplete excision of it. Fibroepithelial basal-cell carcinoma is a skin-colored indolent papule on a trunk that, for practical purposes, is innocuous. The same is true for the tiny papule on a face of infundibulocystic basal-cell carcinoma. That lesion rarely becomes larger than a tiny papule, growing extraordinarily slowly as it does for many years. It should be mentioned, parenthetically, that a nodular basal-cell carcinoma may develop in association with any of the other four types of basal-cell carcinoma, a fact that gives legitimacy to a unified concept of basal-cell carcinoma.

INTEGRATION: UNIFYING CONCEPT The neoplastic cells that compose basal-cell carcinoma are akin to the germinative cells in an embryo that give rise to the entire folliculosebaceous-apocrine unit. The benign analogue of basal-cell carcinoma is trichoblastoma, a neoplasm also made up of abnormal cells akin to the normal ones that constitute the folliculosebaceous-apocrine germ in an embryo. For this reason, a basal-cell carcinoma can rightfully be considered a trichoblastic carcinoma.

All five types of basal-cell carcinoma are related to one another because of a type of abnormal germinative cell that they possess in common. They are also related because of the concurrence of different types of basal-cell carcinoma in the same specimen, for example, fibroepithelial and nodular together, or infundibulocystic and nodular together. In short, basal-cell carcinoma is a distinctive pathologic process that expresses itself clinically and histopathologically as five morphologically distinct and distinctive variants. Although basal-cell carcinomas may be a consequence of a genetic disorder (nevoid basal-cell carcinoma syndrome), ingestion of a metal (arsenic), or x-rays (radiation dermatitis), the overwhelming majority of those neoplasms result from the deleterious effects of sunlight.

THERAPY Surgical excision, Mohs' micrographic surgery, cryosurgery, electrosurgery, photodynamic therapy, and radiotherapy are useful, depending on the general condition and the age of the patient, the size and location of the lesion, and the experience and ability of the treating physician.

DEFINITION An inflammatory disease caused by the spirochete Borrelia burgdorferi that manifests itself in the skin as figurate erythematous lesions (erythema chronicum migrans), pseudolymphomatous nodules (lymphadenosis benigna cutis), and acral patches and plaques that in time become atrophic (acrodermatitis chronica atrophicans). It may express itself in other organs as well, with cardiac, neurological, and arthritic symptoms and signs.

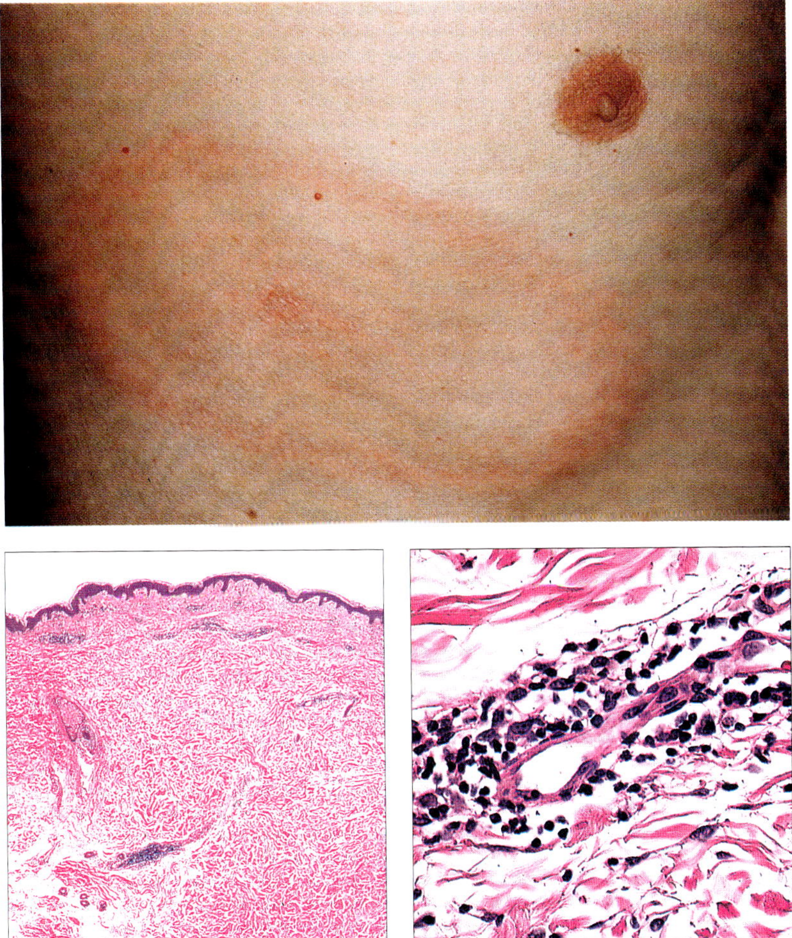

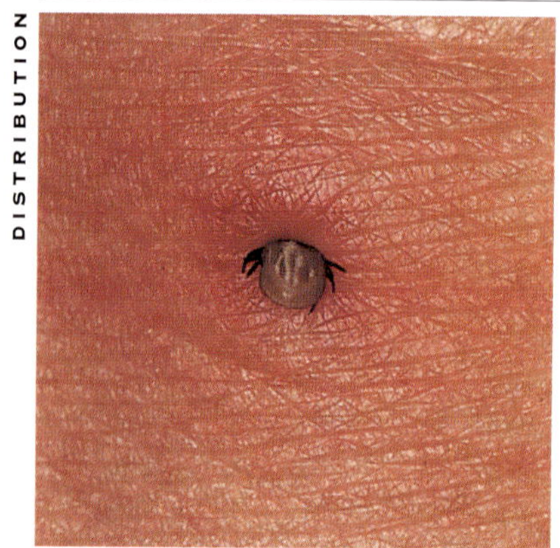

FIG. 11-1 *Tick dining on skin by sucking blood.*

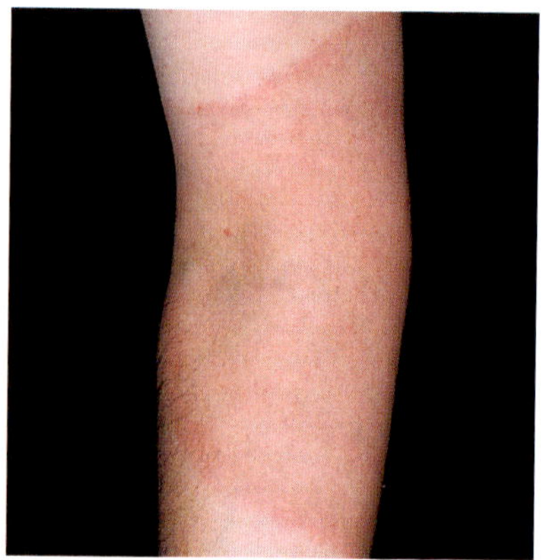

FIG. 11-2 *Plaque of erythema chronicum migrans.*

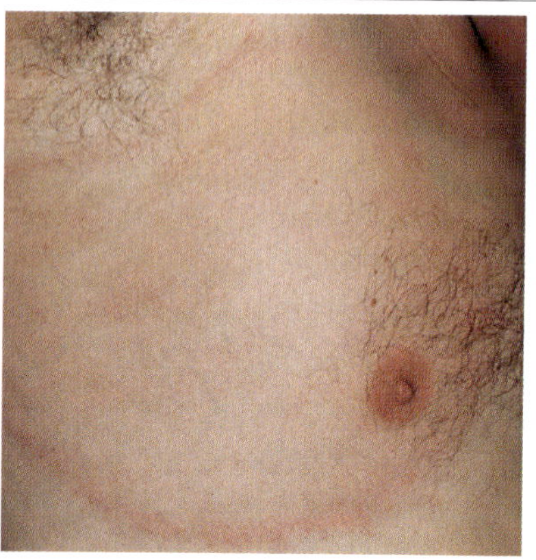

FIG. 11-3 *Erythema chronicum migrans.*

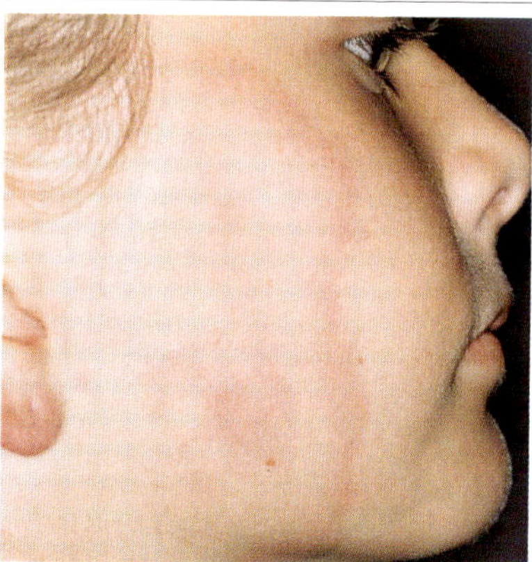

FIG. 11-4 *Erythema chronicum migrans.*

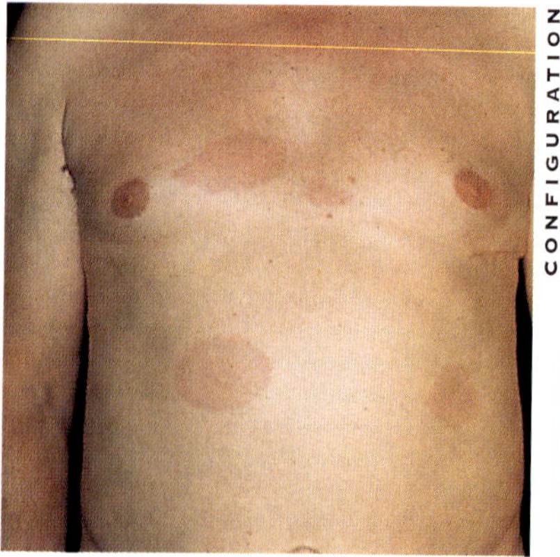

FIG. 11-5 *Widespread lesions of erythema chronicum migrans.*

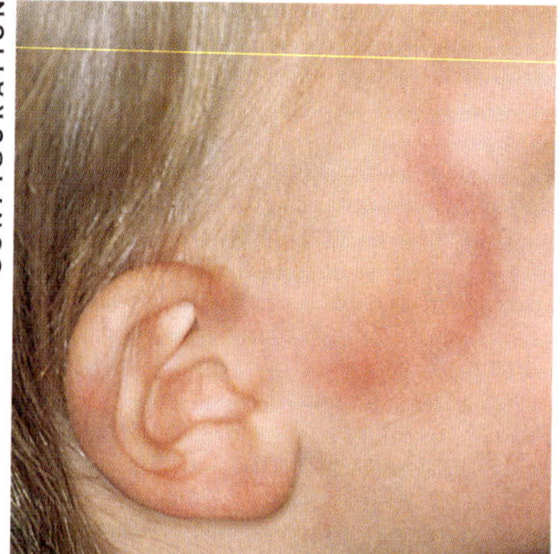

FIG. 11-6 *Arciform and serpiginous plaque of erythema chronicum migrans. The lesion extends across the ear.*

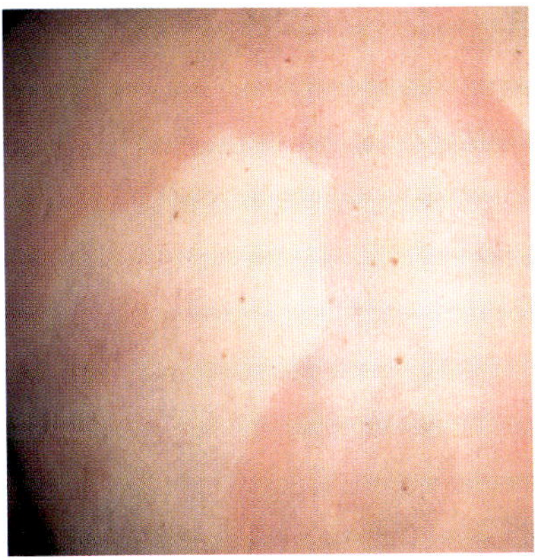

FIG. II-7 *Figurate outline of plaques of erythema chronicum migrans.*

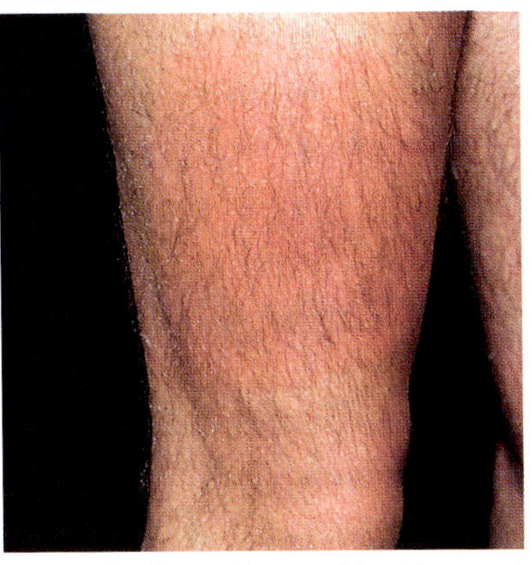

FIG. II-8 *Patch-plaque with collarette of scale in the center that represents the site of the "bite" of a tick.*

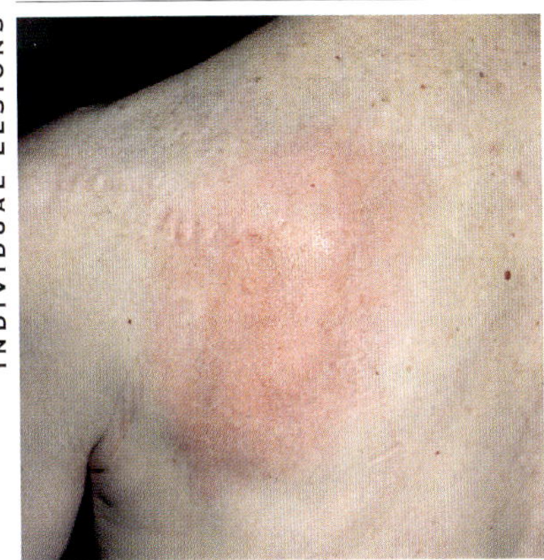

FIG. II-9 *Erythematous plaque of erythema chronicum migrans.*

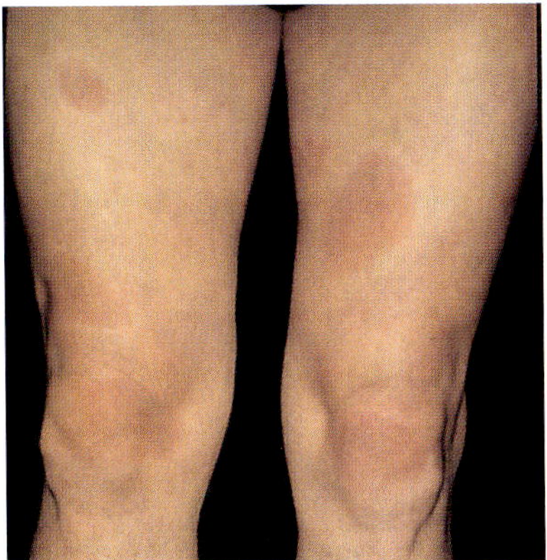

FIG. II-IO *Widespread erythematous circular patches of erythema chronicum migrans.*

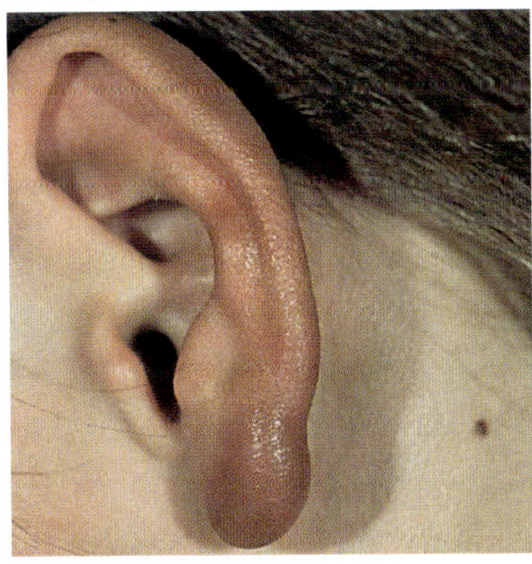

FIG. II-II *Dusky erythematous nodule of lymphadenosis benigna cutis.*

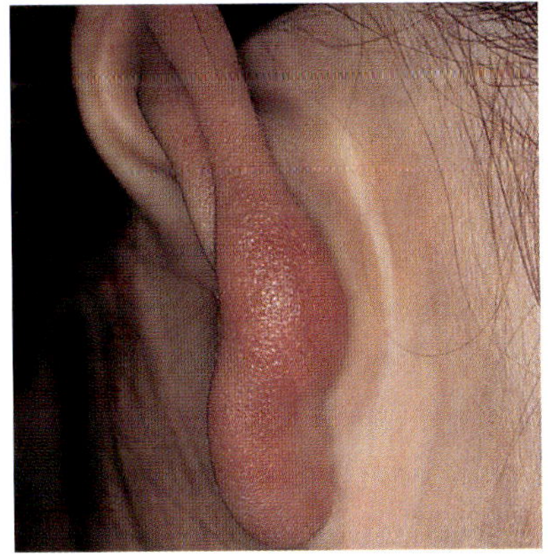

FIG. II-I2 *Erythematous nodule of lymphadenosis benigna cutis.*

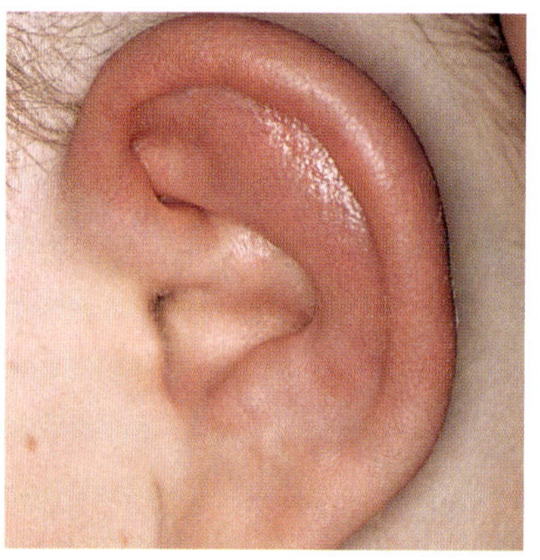

FIG. 11-13   *Erythematous plaque of lymphadenosis benigna cutis.*

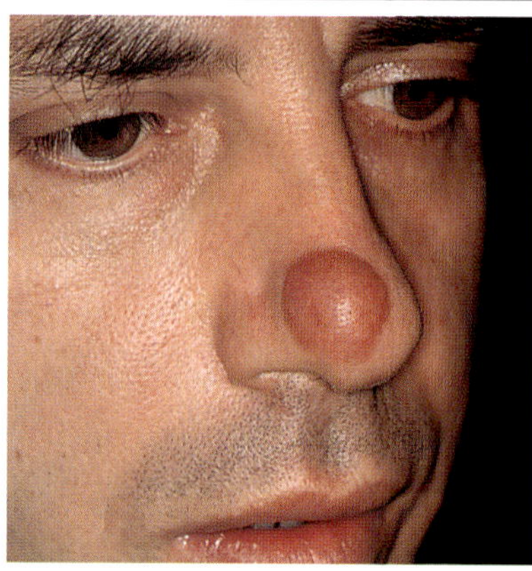

FIG. 11-14   *Dusky erythematous nodule of lymphadenosis benigna cutis.*

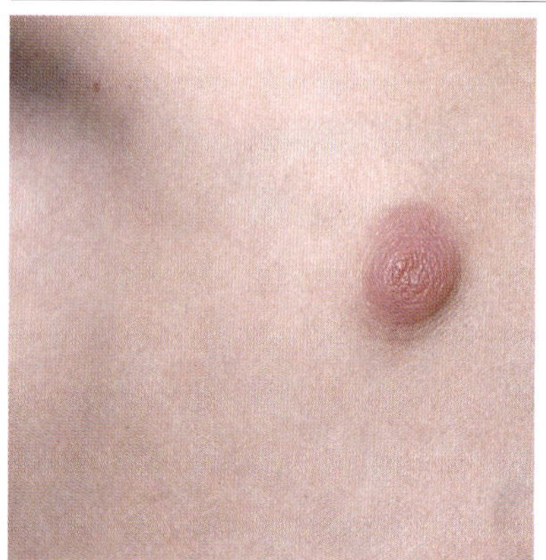

FIG. 11-15   *Erythematous nodule on the mammilla of lymphadenosis benigna cutis.*

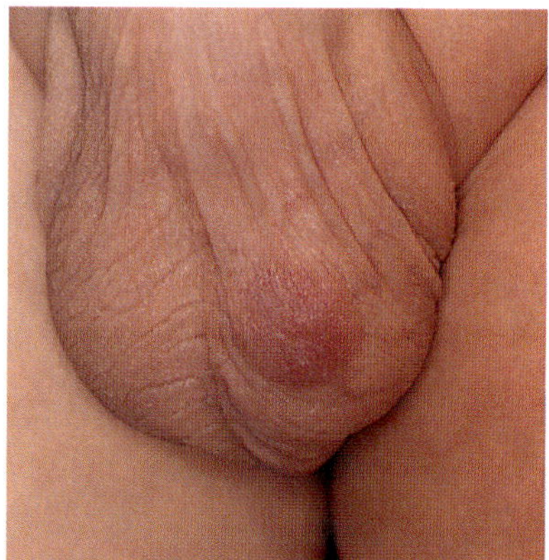

FIG. 11-16   *Erythematous nodule of lymphadenosis benigna cutis.*

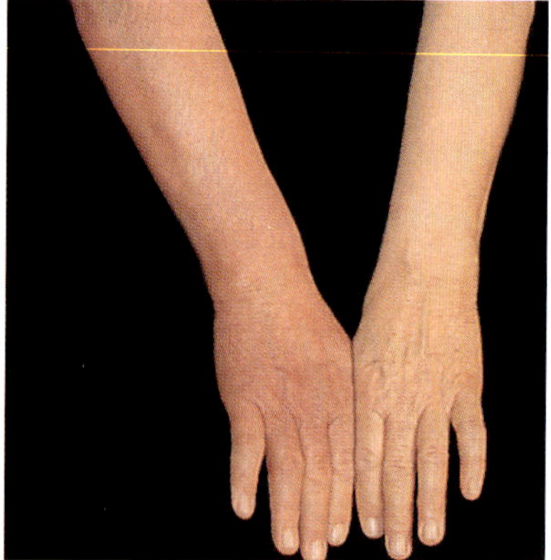

FIG. 11-17 *Acrodermatitis chronica atrophicans on an edematous right arm and hand.*

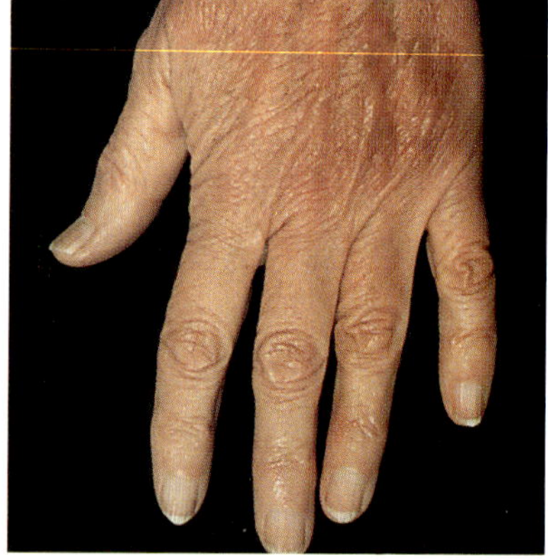

FIG. 11-18 *Atrophic hyperpigmented patch of acrodermatitis chronica atrophicans.*

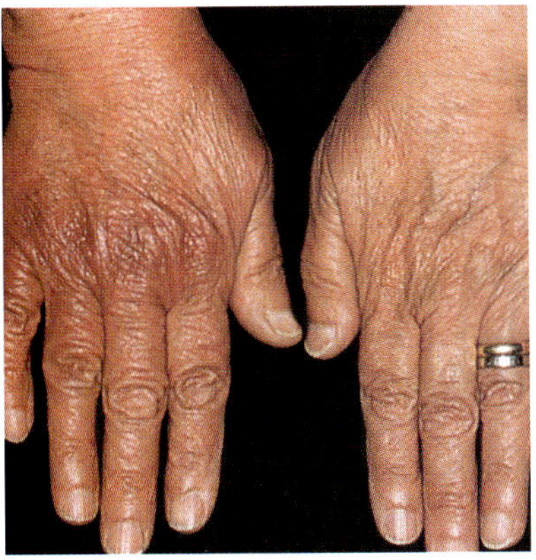

FIG. II-19 *Rust-colored atrophic patches of acrodermatitis chronica atrophicans.*

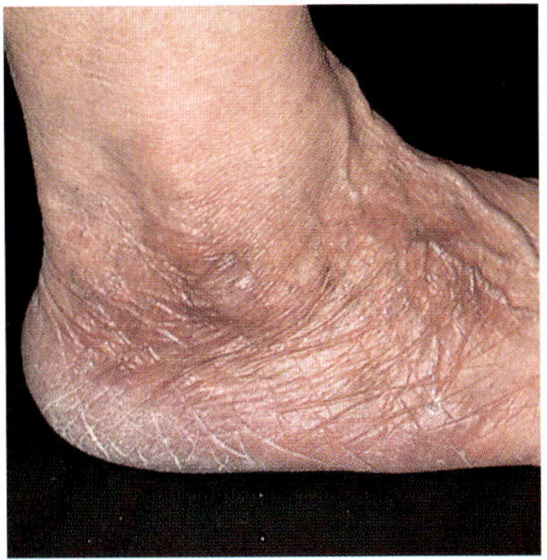

FIG. II-20 *Atrophic patch of acrodermatitis chronica atrophicans.*

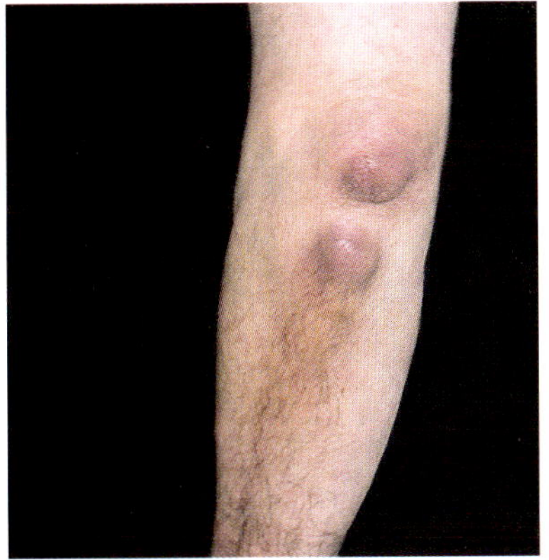

FIG. II-21 *Hyperpigmented plaque-like band ("ulnar band") beneath violaceous juxta-articular nodules (fibroid nodules).*

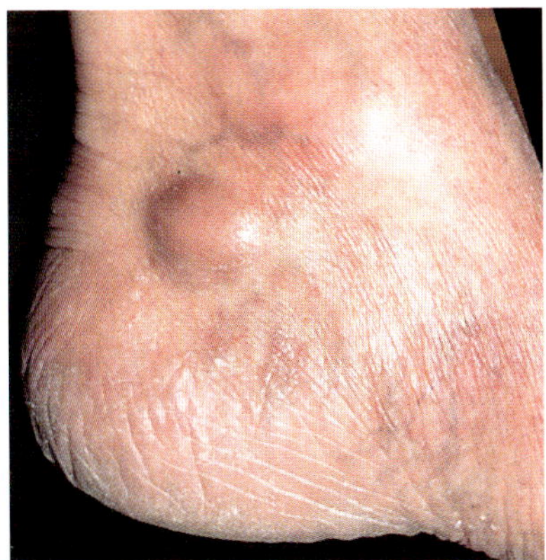

FIG. II-22 *Immunocytoma in a patch of acrodermatitis chronica atrophicans.*

ADJUNCTIVE DIAGNOSTIC TESTS Enzyme-linked immunosorbent assay (ELISA) and immunoblot techniques for measuring antibodies (IgM and IgG) to B. burgdorferi in serum. Detection by ELISA of immunoglobulins in serum specific for B. burgdorferi is confirmatory of infection by borrelia. Detection of borrelia DNA by polymerase chain reaction on tissue sections or in culture establishes the diagnosis.

COURSE As the name denotes, erythema chronicum migrans advances slowly but surely in centrifugal fashion for many weeks before eventually disappearing. The pseudolymphomatous nodules of lymphadenosis benigna cutis tend to persist for many months, and even years, before regressing slowly. The acral erythematous patches persist for years before ever so slowly involuting to become permanent atrophic patches of acrodermatitis chronica atrophicans.

INTEGRATION: UNIFYING CONCEPT The spirochete, B. burgdorferi, is responsible for all of the cutaneous manifestations of Lyme disease, to wit, erythema chronicum migrans, lymphadenosis benigna cutis, and acrodermatitis chronica atrophicans. The reasons, in terms of pathogenesis, for the different morphologic presentations of borreliosis are not known, but the basis for them seems to be immunologic. The situation is analogous, in some ways, to the different morphologic expressions of diseases caused by such disparate organisms as Mycobacterium tuberculosis, Mycobacterium leprae, and Treponema pallidum.

THERAPY Oral tetracyclines, penicillin, or cephalosporins (cefuroximaxetil) are effective in destroying B. burgdorferi.

BULLOUS PEMPHIGOID AND HERPES GESTATIONIS

BULLOUS PEMPHIGOID

DEFINITION An inflammatory disease of older people; signs include widespread erythematous macules and patches, urticarial papules and plaques, and vesicles and bullae, the blisters often arising on urticarial plaques. The cause is not known, but the mechanism is thought to be immunologic in response to antibodies to bullous pemphigoid antigens.

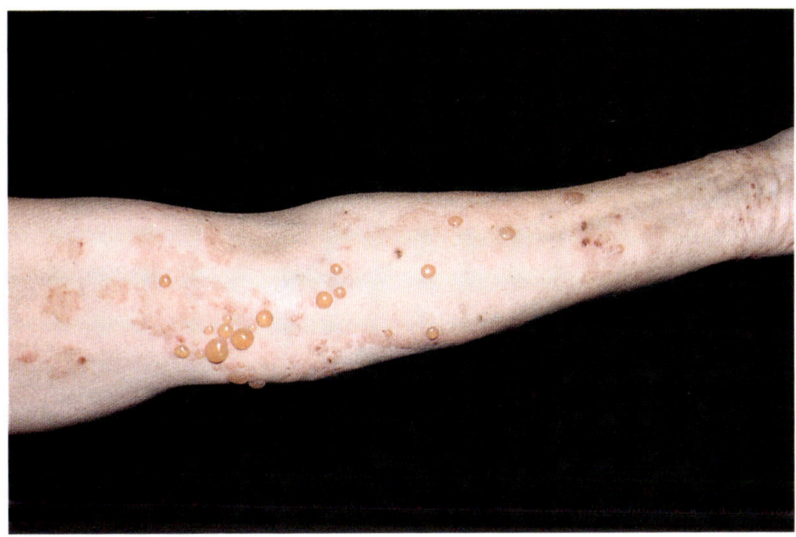

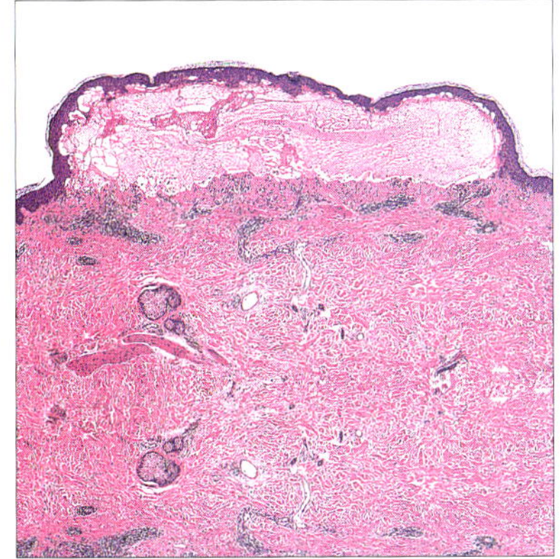

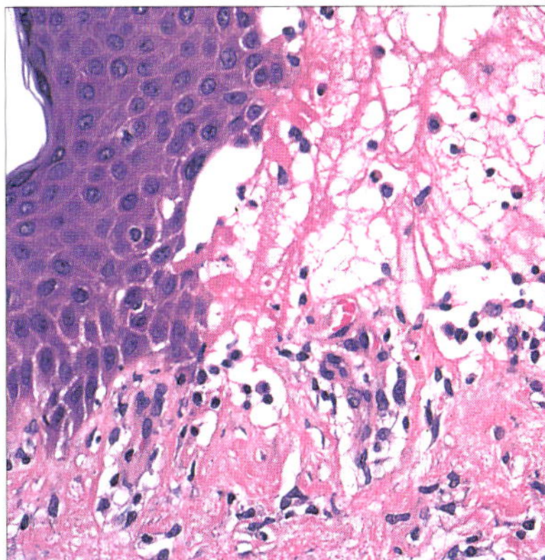

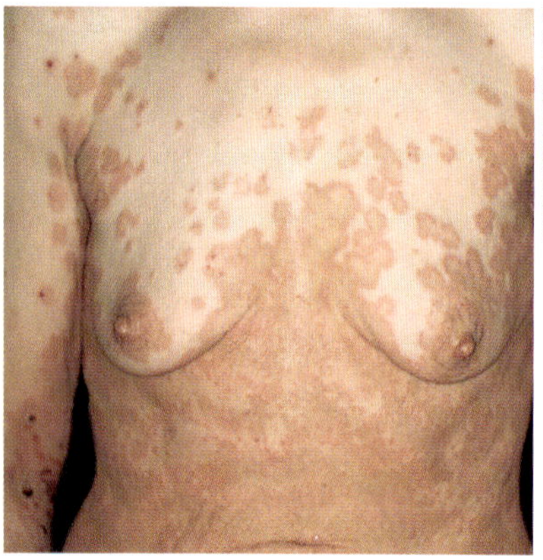

FIG. 12-1 *Urticarial papules, plaques with arcuate, annular, and polycyclic shapes, eroded vesicles, and hemorrhagic crusts.*

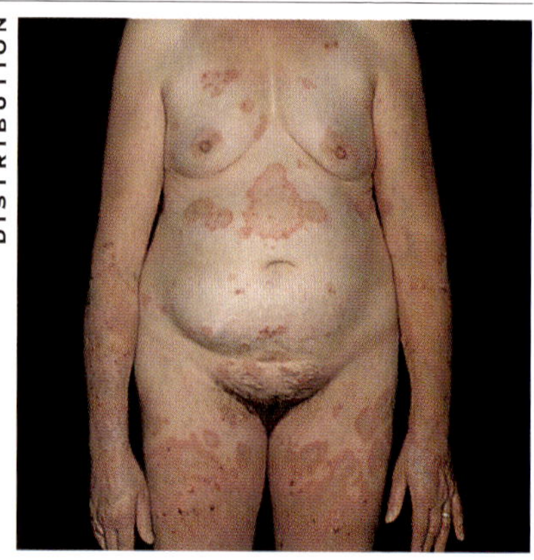

FIG. 12-2 *Urticarial papules and plaques with signs of excoriation.*

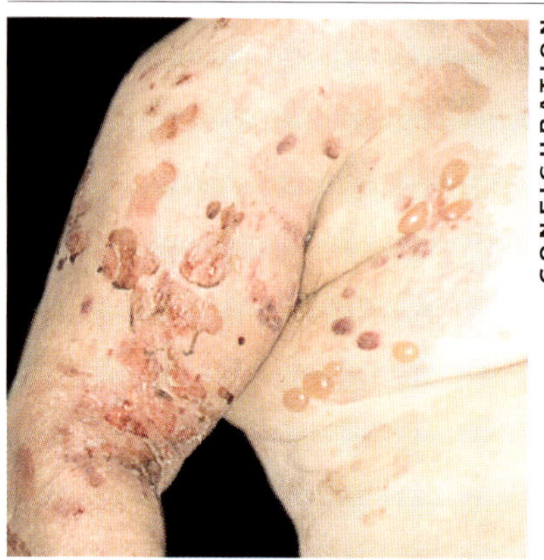

FIG. 12-3 *Urticarial papules and plaques with scalloped borders, vesicles, bullae, and erosions.*

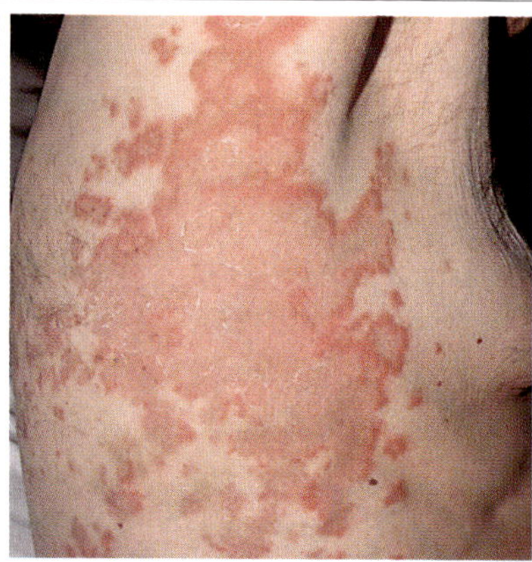

FIG. 12-4 *Urticarial plaques in arcuate, annular, and serpiginous patterns.*

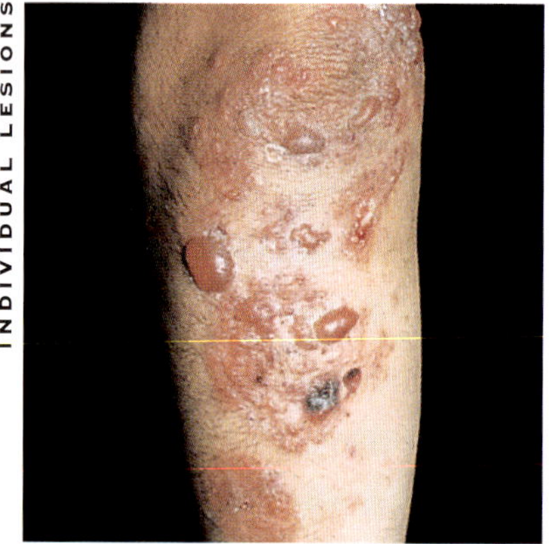

FIG. 12-5 *Urticarial papules and plaques, and bullae.*

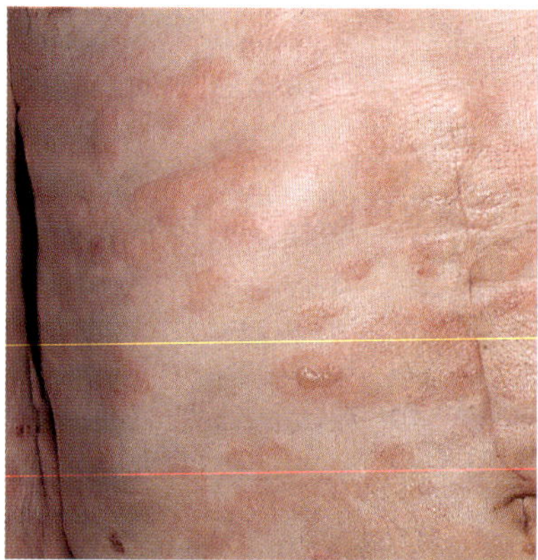

FIG. 12-6 *Urticarial plaques with round and polycyclic shapes, atop some of which are tense vesicles.*

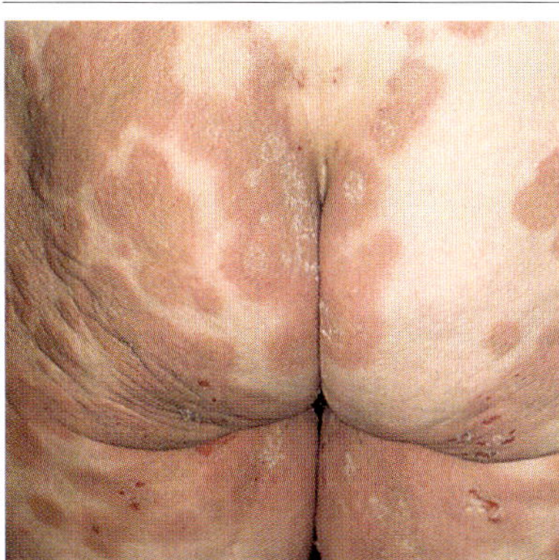

FIG. 12-7 *Urticarial papules and plaques, some of which are topped by tense vesicles and erosions.*

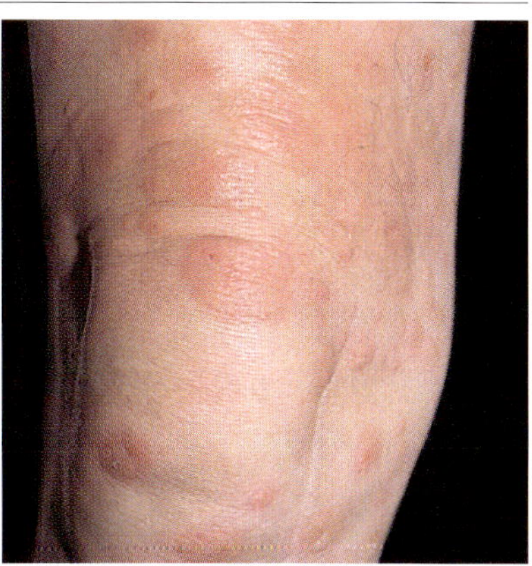

FIG. 12-8 *Urticarial papules and plaques with round and polycyclic shapes.*

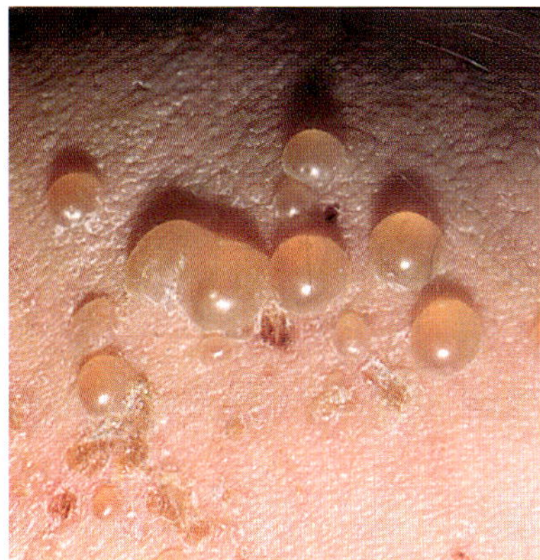

FIG. 12-9 *Tense vesicles and a bulla that resulted from confluence of vesicles, crusts, and scales.*

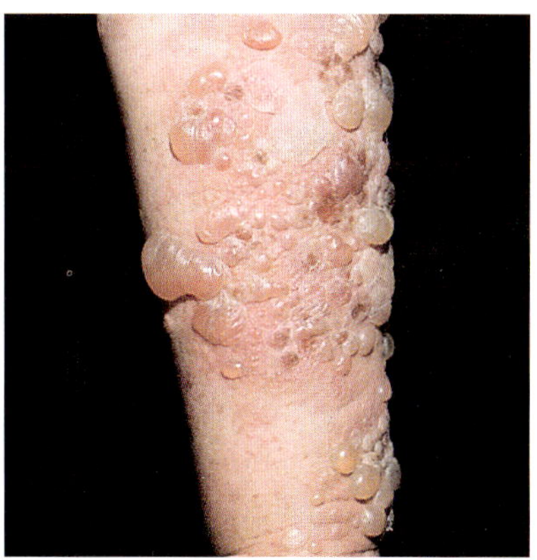

FIG. 12-10 *Vesicles and bullae on an erythematous urticarial base.*

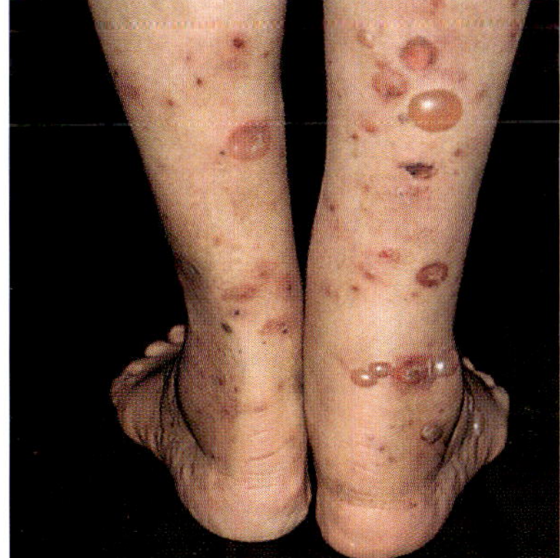

FIG. 12-11 *Vesicles, bullae, crusts, and postinflammatory hyperpigmentation.*

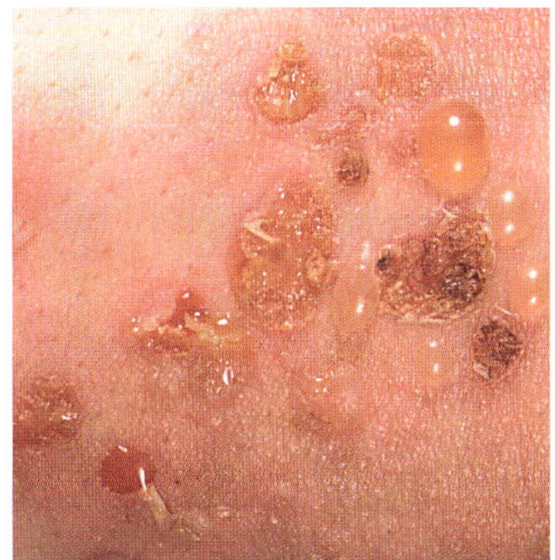

FIG. 12-12 *Tense vesicles, erosions, and crusts.*

ADJUNCTIVE DIAGNOSTIC TESTS Direct immunofluorescence of perilesional skin shows a linear band of IgG and C3 at the epidermal basement membrane. In 70 percent of patients with bullous pemphigoid, indirect immunofluorescence reveals circulating antibasement membrane IgG.

COURSE Some patients with bullous pemphigoid have urticarial papules and plaques for months before a single vesicle or bulla appears. Most patients, however, display both urticarial and blistering lesions from the outset. As a rule, the disease tends to become worse in time, i.e., the extent of distribution of lesions, the number of lesions, and the size of bullae increasing. Although the condition may wax and wane, it usually persists, if untreated, for the patient's lifetime.

INTEGRATION: UNIFYING CONCEPT Bullous pemphigoid is a single pathologic process that manifests itself as urticarial papules and plaques and as vesicles and bullae that are subepidermal and replete with eosinophils. Although the same fundamental lesions also are present in patients with herpes gestationis, the distribution and configuration of the lesions are different. So, too, is the age of the patients; bullous pemphigoid was known formerly as "bullous disease of the aged." The basis for bullous pemphigoid is immunologic, the disease presumably resulting from autoantibody-mediated disruption of adhesion between basal keratinocytes and basement membrane, a consequence of the binding by antibodies to antigens of bullous pemphigoid that are involved in attaching basal keratinocytes to the basement membrane. The antigens are bullous pemphigoid-antigen 1 (BPAG1; 230kD) which belongs to a family of genes that includes desmoplakin and bullous pemphigoid antigen 2 (BPAG2; 180kD; Type VII collagen).

THERAPY Oral corticosteroids in high dosage are tapered to a maintenance level. Immunosuppressants (azathioprine) are helpful adjuncts. For patients who do not respond to these measures, cyclophosphamide, dapsone, or tetracycline are worthy alternatives.

HERPES GESTATIONIS

DEFINITION An inflammatory disease of the second and third trimesters of pregnancy characterized by widespread urticarial papules and plaques accompanied by vesicles and bullae. Individual lesions are indistinguishable clinically and histopathologically from those of bullous pemphigoid. Although the cause is not known, the mechanism is thought to be immunologic in response to antibodies to an antigen peculiar to pregnancy.

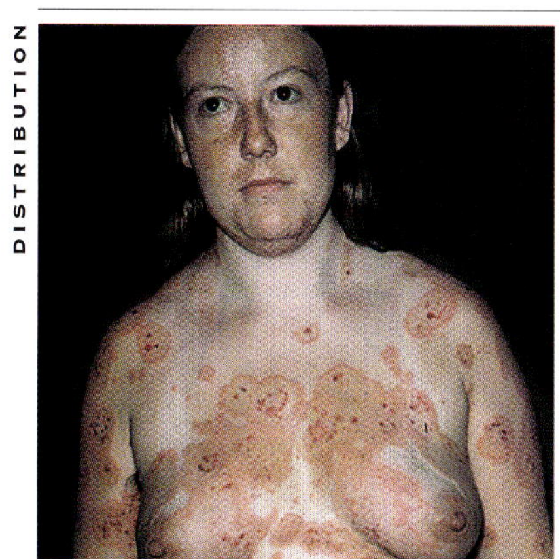

FIG. 12-13 *Widespread urticarial papules and plaques, vesicles, and bullae, some of them in cockade arrangement.*

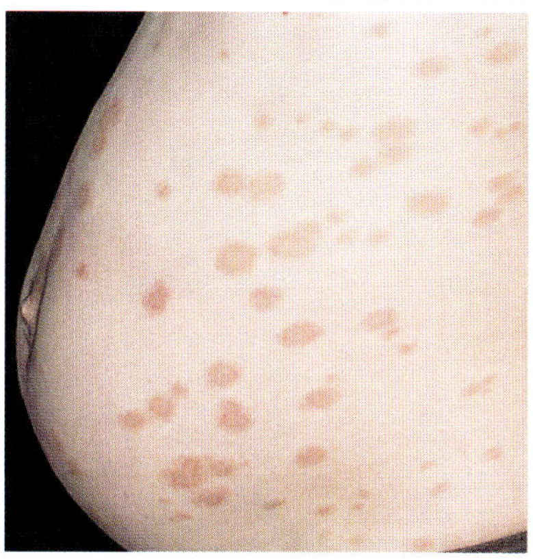

FIG. 12-14 *Urticarial papules and subtle nummular plaques in a woman in the third trimester of pregnancy.*

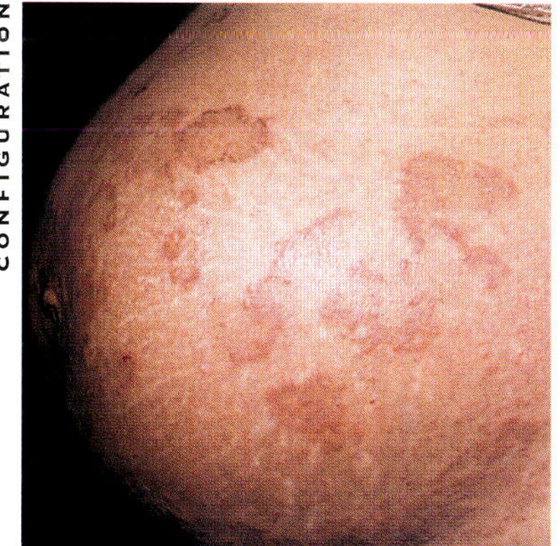

FIG. 12-15 *Widespread urticarial plaques characterized by round shape and by polycyclic outlines.*

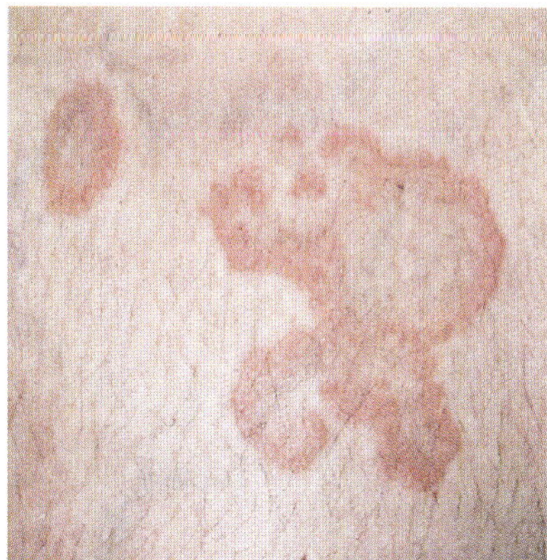

FIG. 12-16 *Urticarial papules and plaques have assumed round and polycyclic shapes.*

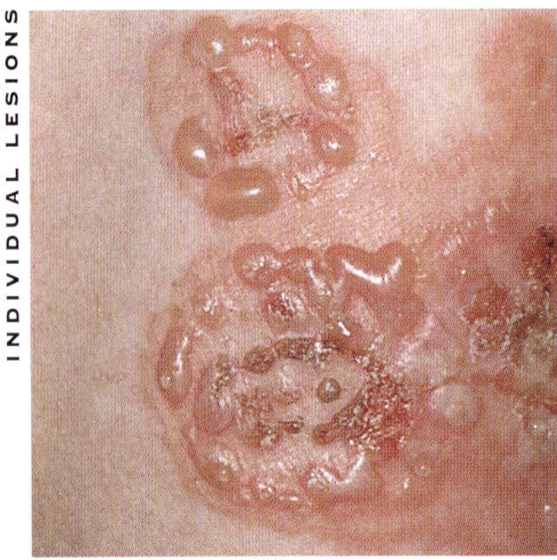

FIG. 12-17 *Tense vesicles in cockade pattern.*

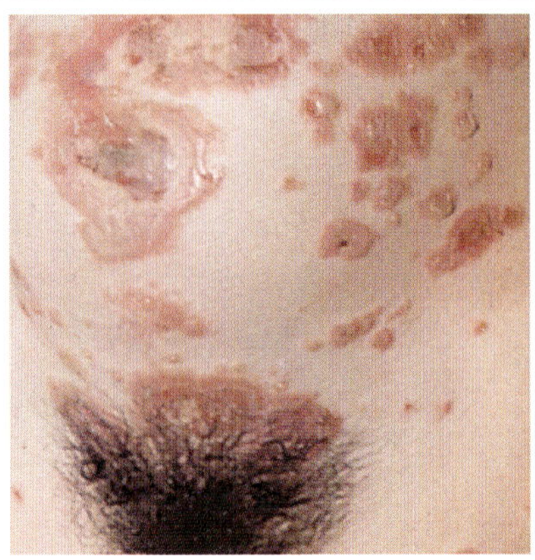

FIG. 12-18 *Urticarial papules and nummular plaques, the latter surmounted by vesicles.*

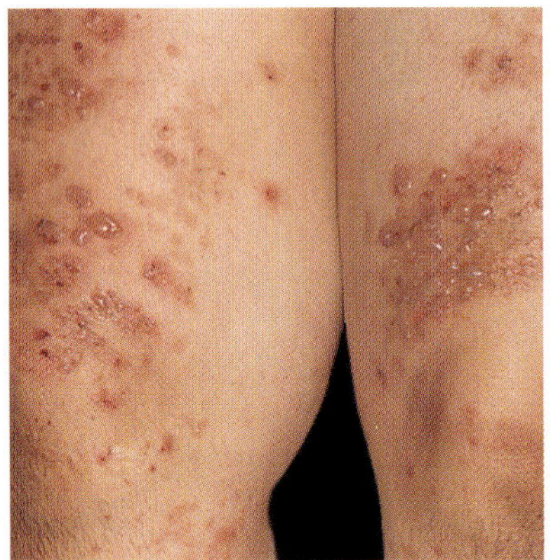

FIG. 12-19 *Vesicles atop urticarial plaques.*

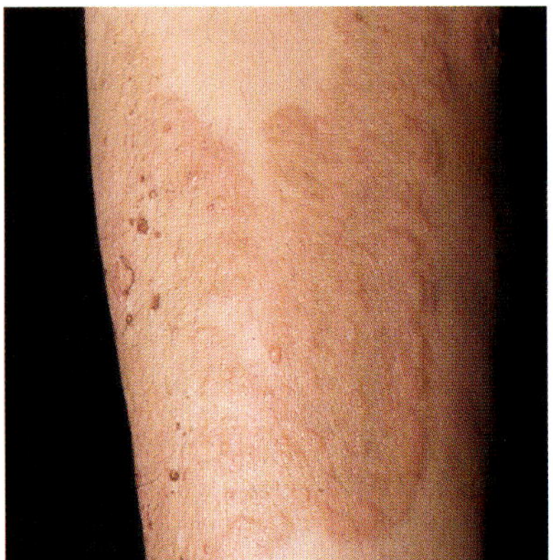

FIG. 12-20 *Urticarial plaques with scalloped outlines on which tiny vesicles and erosions reside.*

ADJUNCTIVE DIAGNOSTIC TEST Studies of peribullous and urticarial lesions by direct immunofluorescence reveal linear deposits of C3 and IgG (in about 30 percent of patients) along the basement membrane zone.

COURSE The disease does not begin in a first pregnancy, but in a subsequent one and then usually in each pregnancy thereafter. The urticarial and blistering lesions tend to erupt during the second trimester and then come and go until parturition, at which time they either cease altogether or sputter for a few more days before being extinguished (until the next pregnancy).

INTEGRATION: UNIFYING CONCEPT The urticarial papules, vesicles, and bullae of herpes gestationis are thought to be a consequence of an immune mechanism in which an antigenic stimulus peculiar to pregnancy causes a failure of adhesion between basal keratinocytes and basement membrane, in much the same way as happens in bullous pemphigoid. The blisters, like those of bullous pemphigoid, are subepidermal and abounding in eosinophils.

THERAPY Oral corticosteroids in high dosage are tapered during the postpartum period. Topical corticosteroids and emollients bring limited relief from itching, but are not efficacious in suppressing the eruption of urticarial and blistering lesions.

DEFINITION An inflammatory disease caused by the yeast Candida albi-cans and manifested clinically as erythematous papules and pustules that may become confluent to form plaques in the case of the former and erosions in the case of the latter. The nail unit may be affected by paronychia and the oral cavity by "thrush."

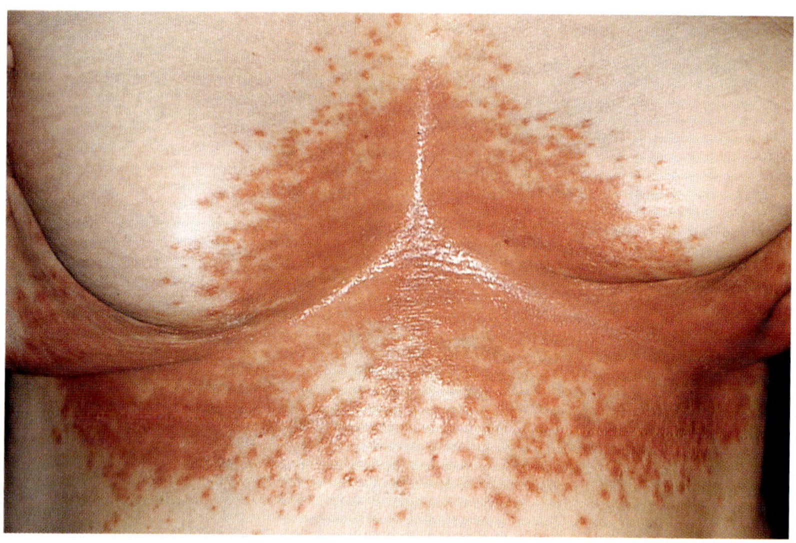

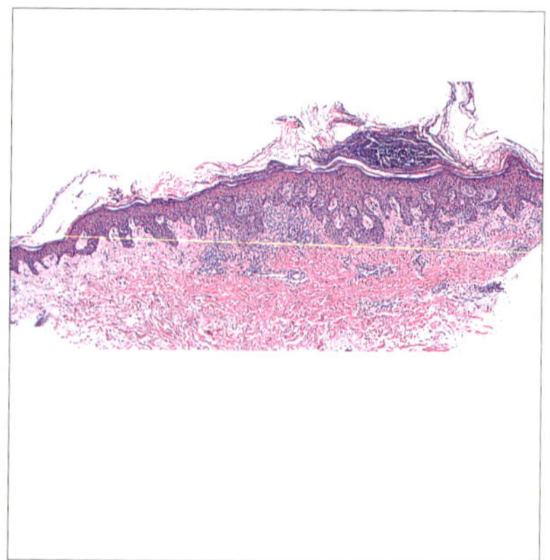

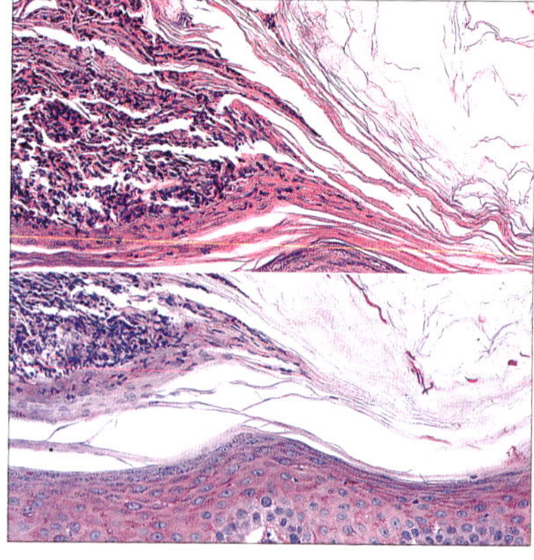

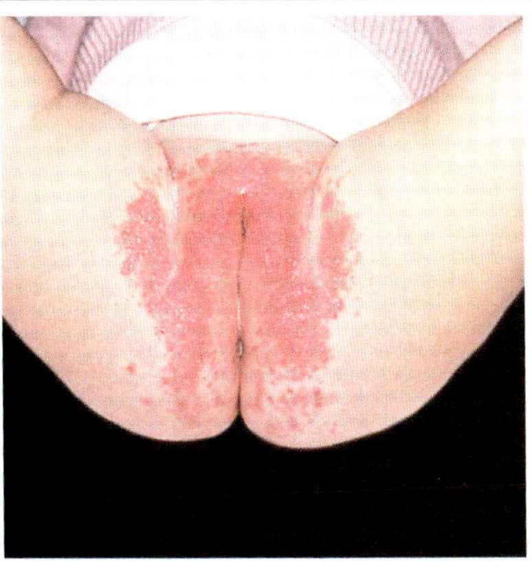

FIG. 13-1 *Dusky erythematous plaques, papules, pustules, and scales distributed symmetrically in the diaper region.*

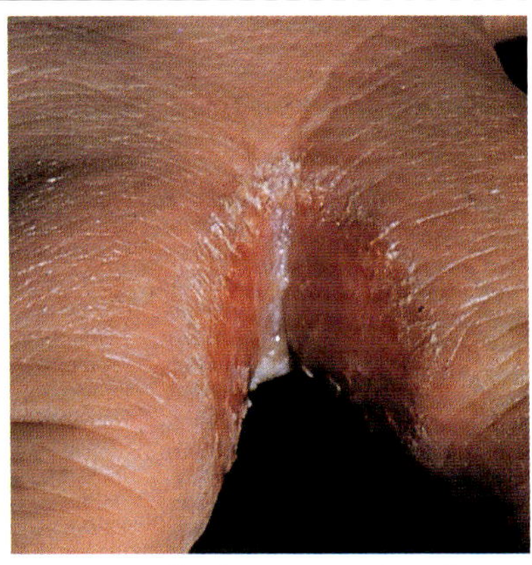

FIG. 13-2 *Erosions, maceration, fissures, and scales ("erosio interdigitalis candidomycetica").*

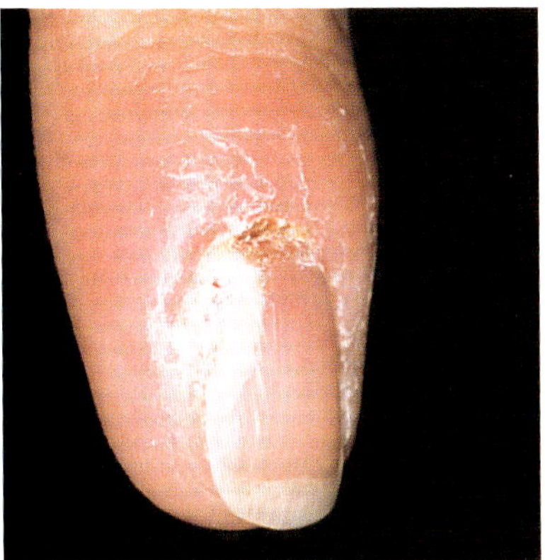

FIG. 13-3 *Paronychia.*

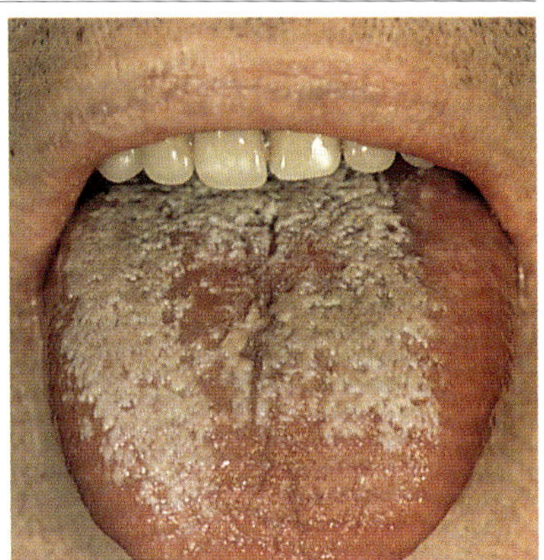

FIG. 13-4 *Colonies of Candida albicans make up the cheesy material that coats the tongue.*

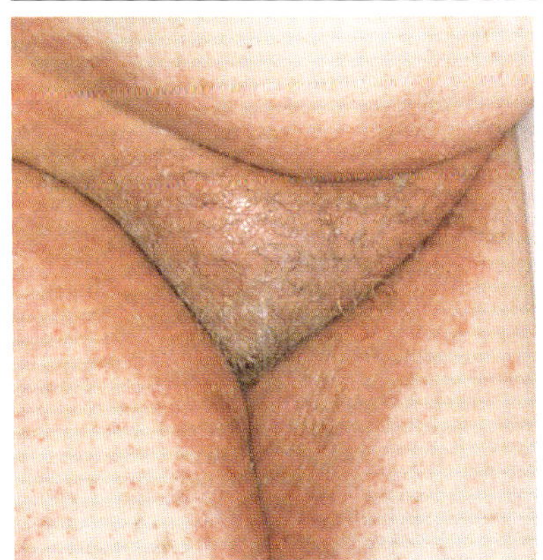

FIG. 13-5 *Papules and plaques in the crural region.*

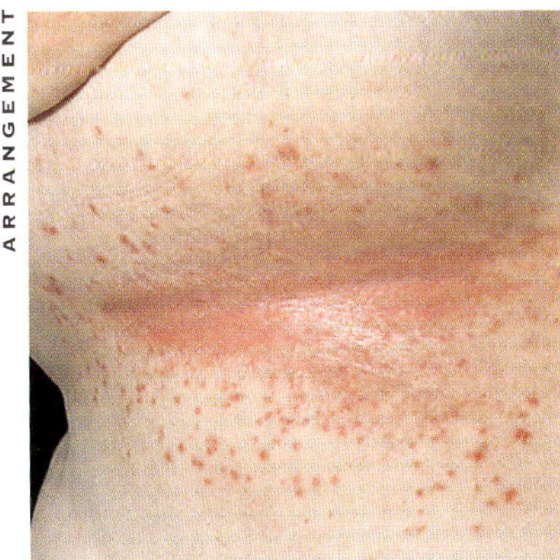

FIG. 13-6 *Papules in satellite array around an erythematous plaque at an intertriginous site.*

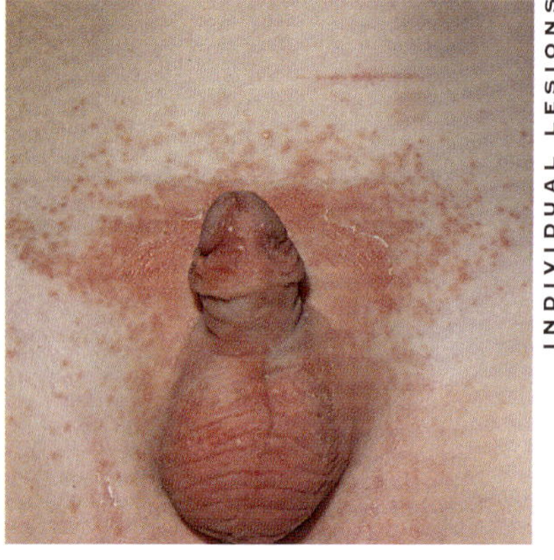

FIG. 13-7 *Erythematous plaques and papules, pustules, and collarettes of scale-crust.*

FIG. 13-8 *Erosions and ulcerations (balanoposthitis).*

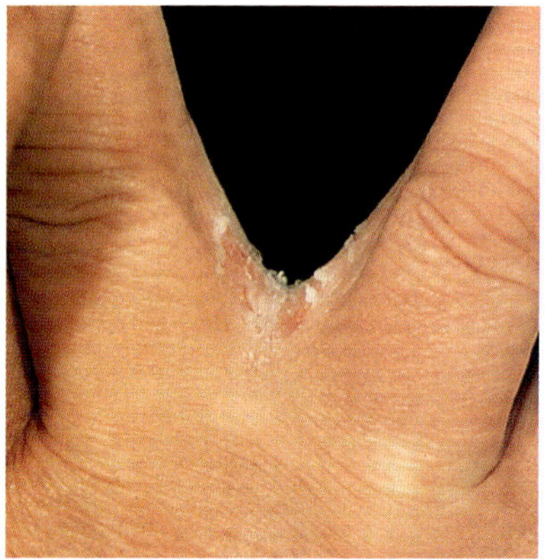

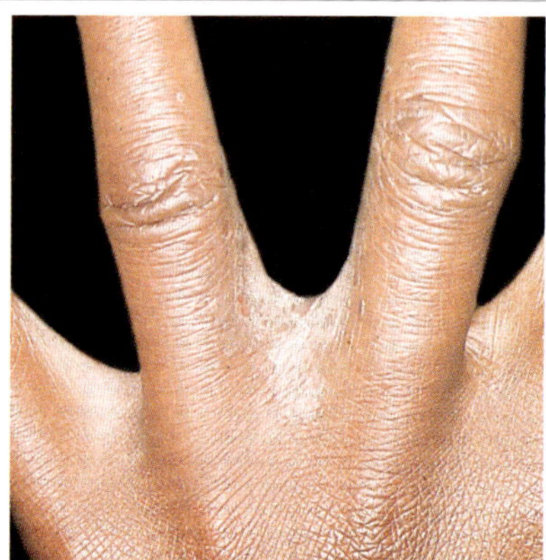

FIG. 13-9 *Erosion, maceration, and scale.*

FIG. 13-10 *Erosion and scale.*

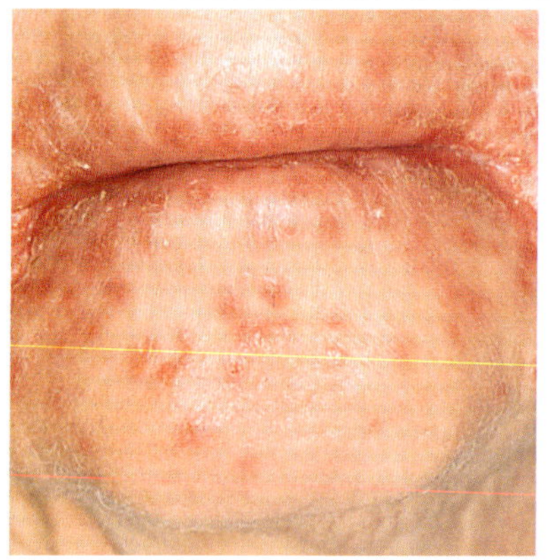

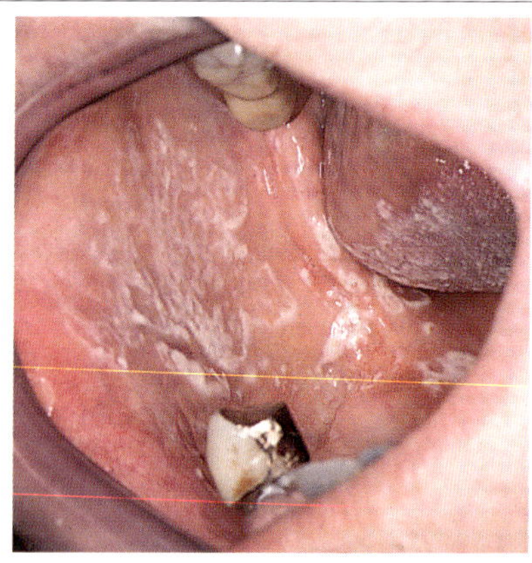

FIG. 13-11 *Erythematous papules, pustules, crusts, and scales (angular cheilitis).*

FIG. 13-12 *Creamy white "pseudomembrane" with scalloped borders.*

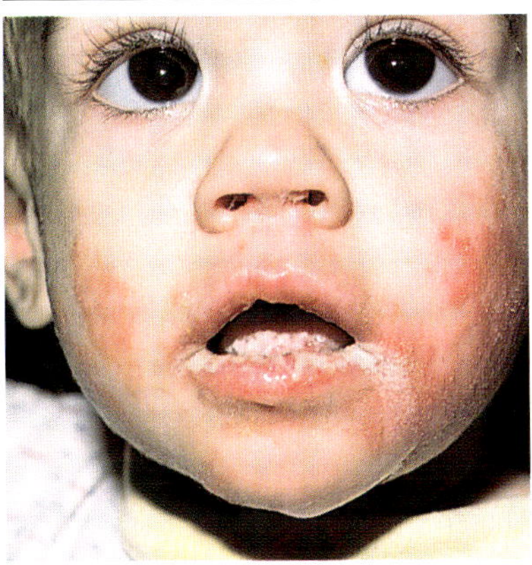

FIG. 13-13 *Chronic mucocutaneous candidiasis in an immunosuppressed child.*

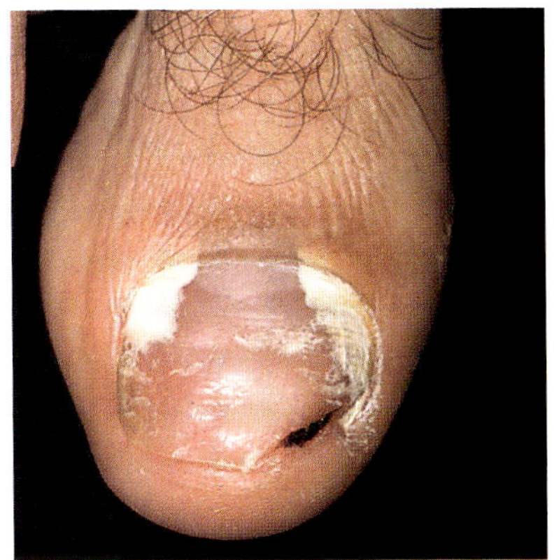

FIG. 13-14 *Paronychia with colonies of C. albicans as cheesy material emanating from beneath posterior nail fold.*

ADJUNCTIVE DIAGNOSTIC TESTS Examination of skin scrapings by conventional microscopy in order to demonstrate budding yeasts with hyphae or pseudohyphae. Culture of tissue on Sabouraud's agar enables colonies of yeast to grow.

COURSE Lesions of candidiasis may be self-limited if the factor(s) responsible for their development is eliminated. For example, housekeepers and bartenders who have candidal intertrigo should keep their hands out of water as much as possible. Lesions of candidiasis sometimes persist and even worsen, such as in a person immunosuppressed consequent to long-term, high-dose therapy with corticosteroids administered systemically or secondary to a systemic disease like leukemia or lymphoma.

INTEGRATION: UNIFYING CONCEPT All the cutaneous, ungual, and mucous membrane lesions of the disease are a direct result of the effects of the yeast C. albicans. That organism flourishes in corneocytes of the stratum corneum and, occasionally, in those of the nail plate, but not in those of the hair shaft or inner sheath. It also luxuriates in corneocytes whose nuclei are retained in mucous membranes, such as those of the oral cavity and vagina. In patients who are severely immunosuppressed, candida may be carried by blood vessels to tissues throughout the body; in the skin, the yeast may proliferate wildly in the dermis and sometimes within the epidermis and epithelial structures of adnexa.

THERAPY Topical antimycotics (azoles or nystatin) are effective for disease of the skin. Oral antimycotics reduce intestinal overgrowth of yeasts. Derivatives of azoles taken orally may be beneficial for infection of the gastrointestinal tract as well as for chronic mucocutaneous candidiasis. For vaginal candidiasis, topical and systemic antimycotics (azoles) are beneficial.

DEFINITION Papules, nodules, and tumors that, on gross examination, are usually skin colored and, on histopathologic examination, consist of an epithelium-lined sac that contains fluid, cells, or both in the case of true cysts and of cysts that are associated with other epithelial elements of adnexa in the case of cystic hamartomas.

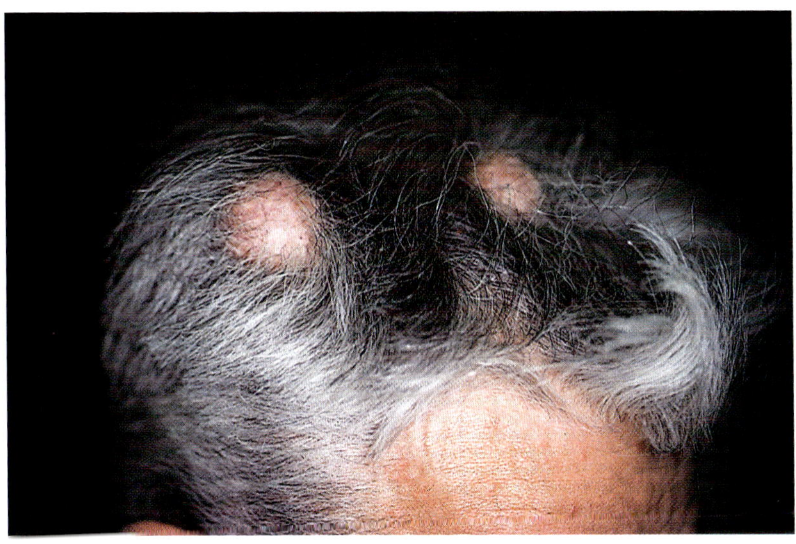

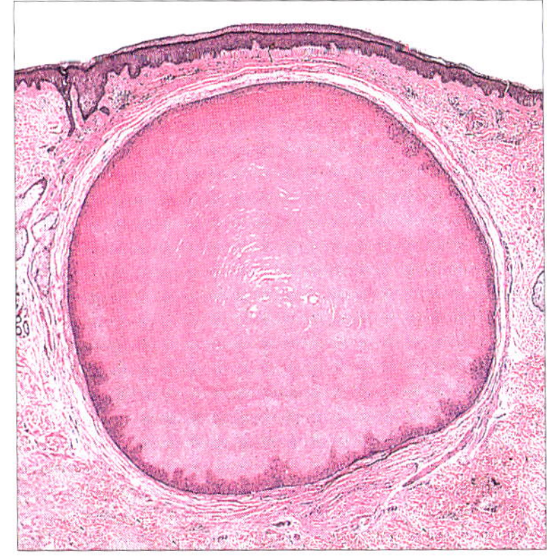

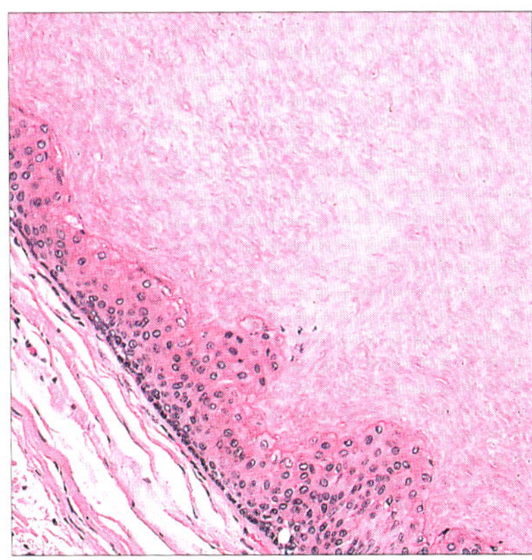

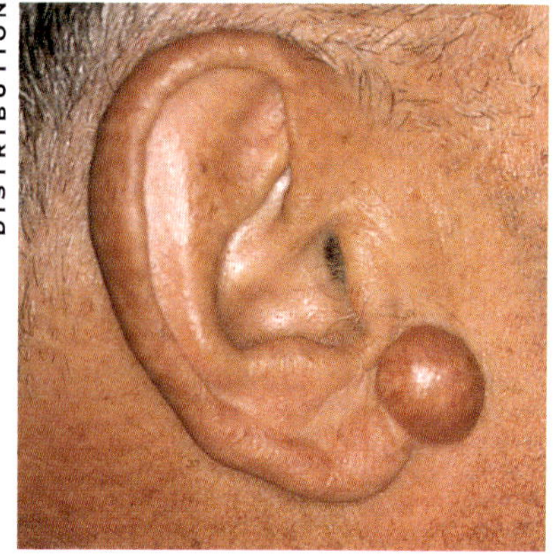

FIG. 14-1 *Dome-shaped, smooth-surfaced tumor of an infundibular cyst.*

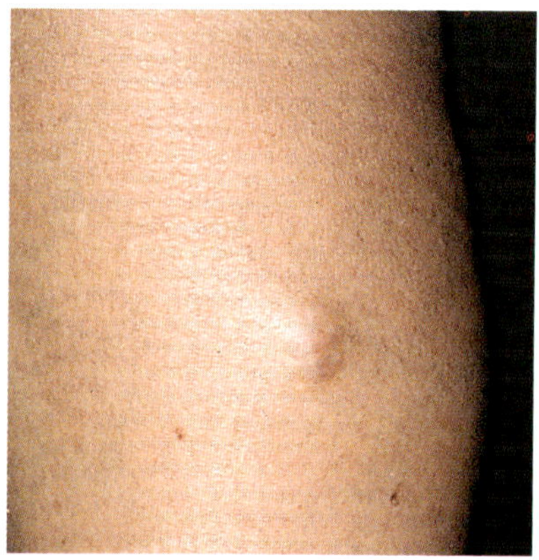

FIG. 14-2 *Skin-colored, smooth-surfaced nodule of an infundibular cyst.*

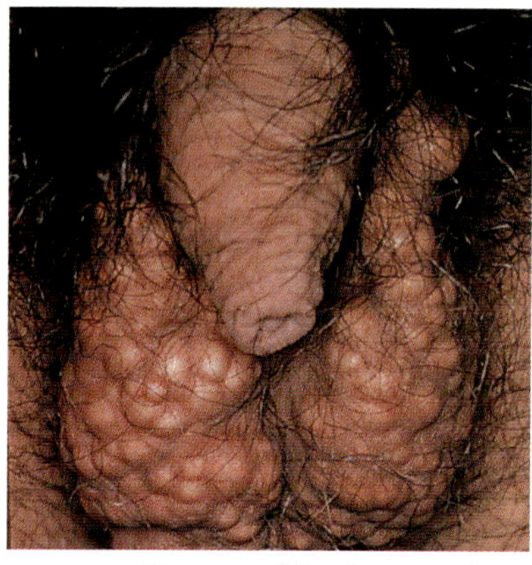

FIG. 14-3 *Numerous follicular cysts of near equal size on the scrotum (or the vulva) eventually calcify (idiopathic calcinosis).*

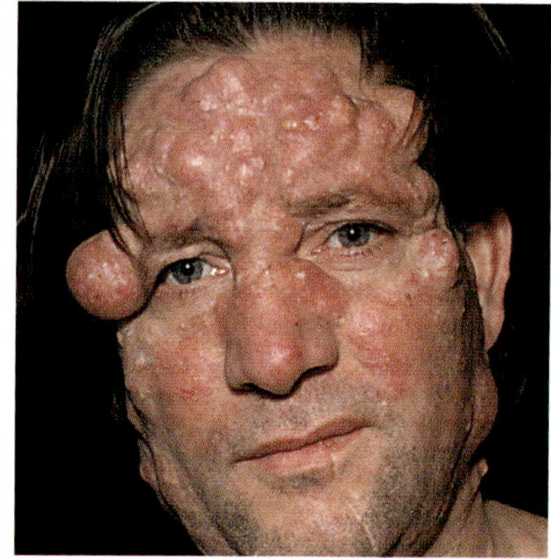

FIG. 14-4 *Dome-shaped, smooth-surfaced nodules of the infundibular type of follicular cyst.*

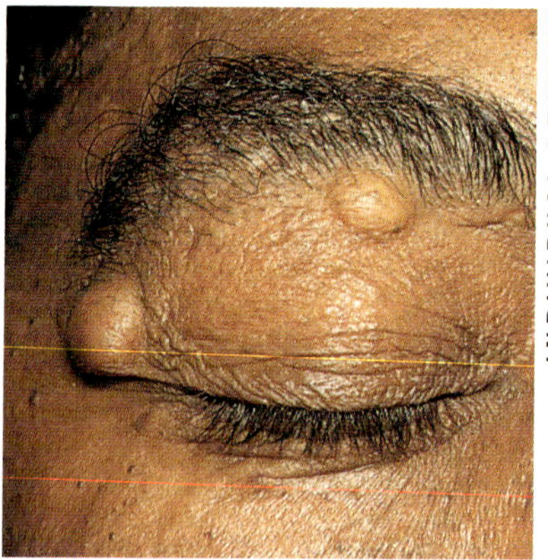

FIG. 14-5 *Dome-shaped papule and nodule of the infundibular type of follicular cyst.*

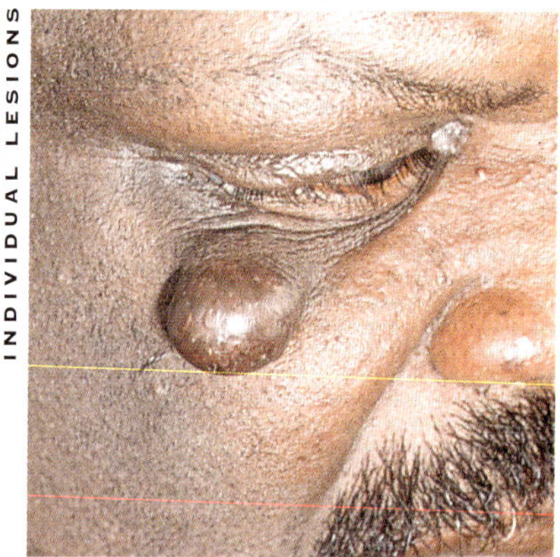

FIG. 14-6 *Dome-shaped nodule of an infundibular cyst and white papules of tiny infundibular cysts (milia).*

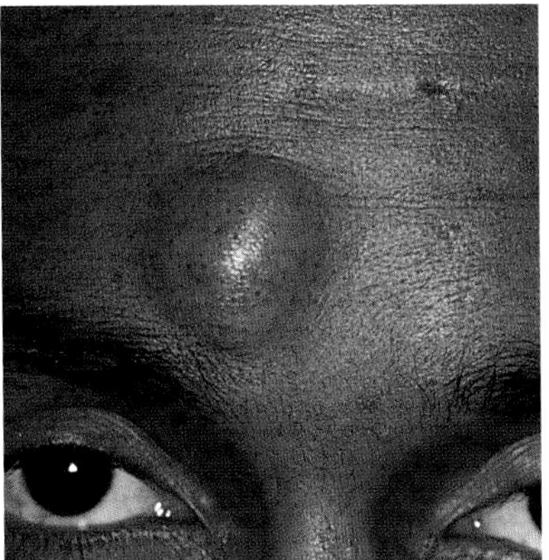

FIG. 14-7 *Dome-shaped tumor of an infundibular type of follicular cyst.*

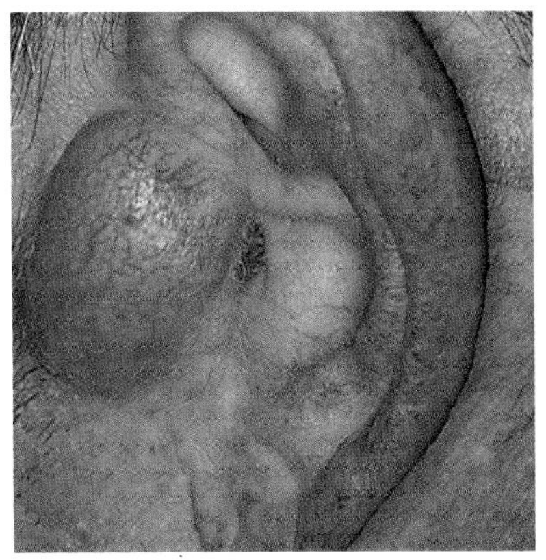

FIG. 14-8 *Tense, dome-shaped, smooth-surfaced tumor covered by telangiectases of an infundibular type of follicular cyst.*

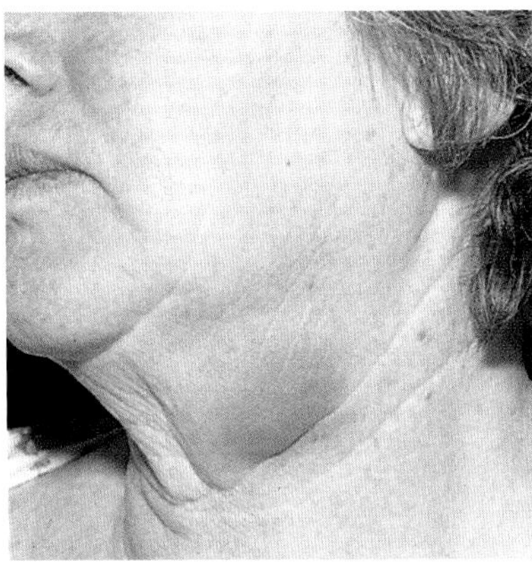

FIG. 14-9 *Red, slightly dome-shaped tumor of an infundibular cyst that has ruptured, inducing suppuration.*

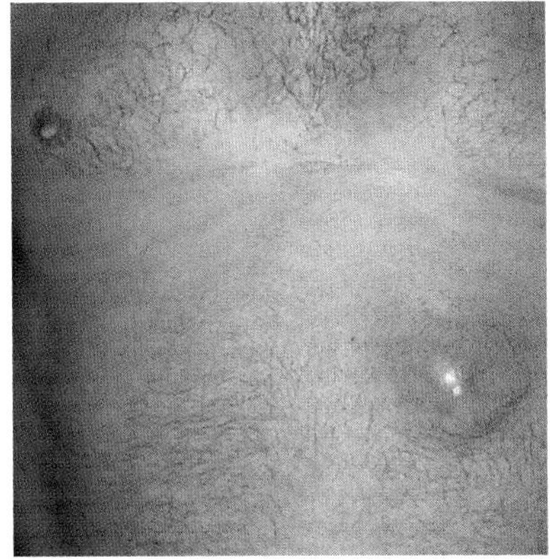

FIG. 14-10 *A tense, dome-shaped, smooth-surfaced shiny nodule that developed consequent to rupture of an infundibular cyst.*

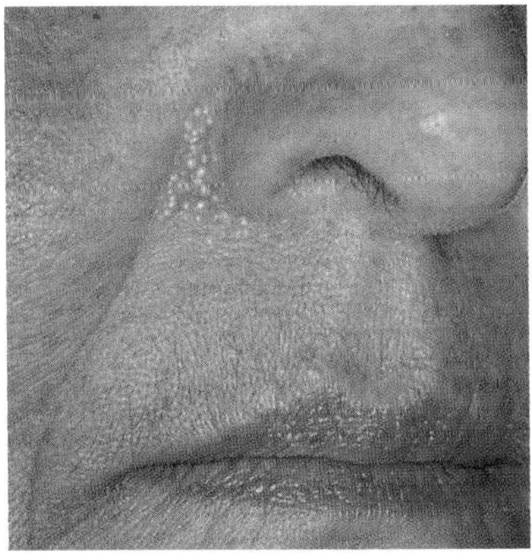

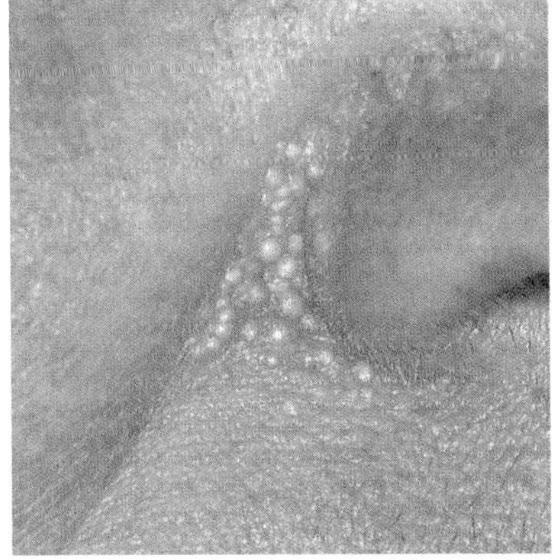

FIG. 14-11 (A, B) *Milia, some of the papules being in agminated arrangement, in the nasolabial fold.*

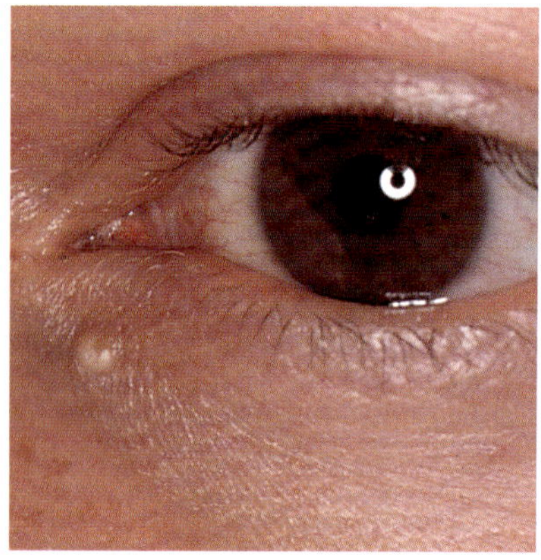

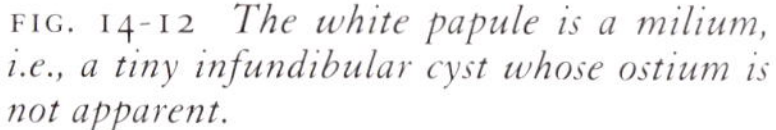

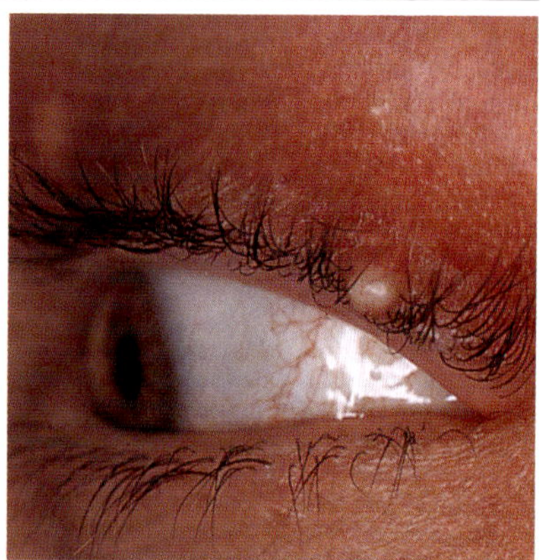

FIG. 14-12 *The white papule is a milium, i.e., a tiny infundibular cyst whose ostium is not apparent.*

FIG. 14-13 *White papule (milium).*

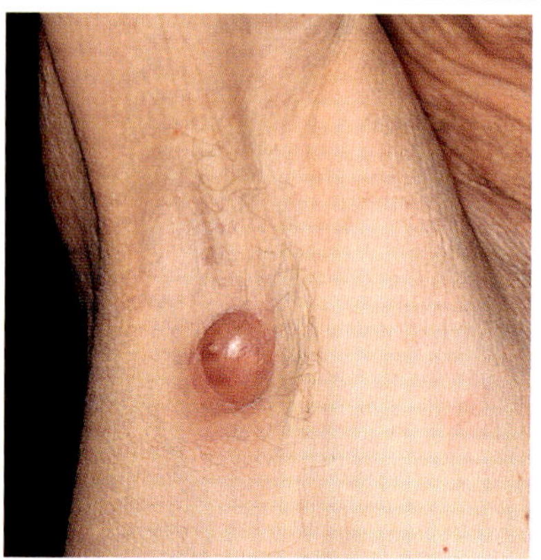

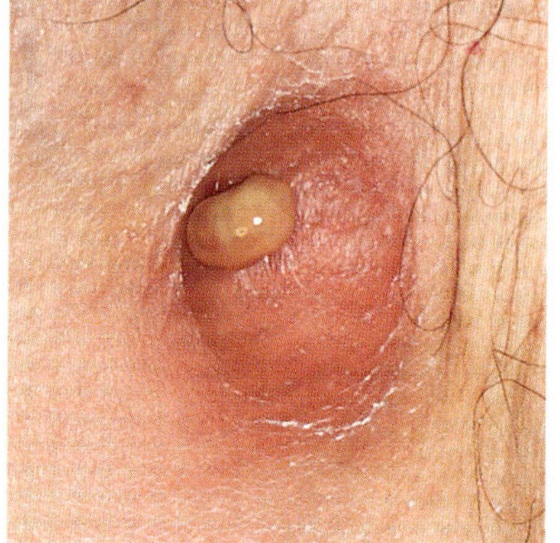

FIG. 14-14 (A, B) *Infundibular type of follicular cyst, ruptured, with extensive suppuration seen here as pus.*

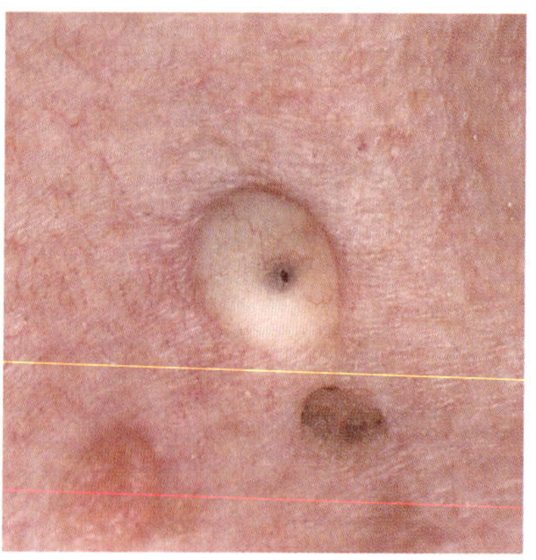

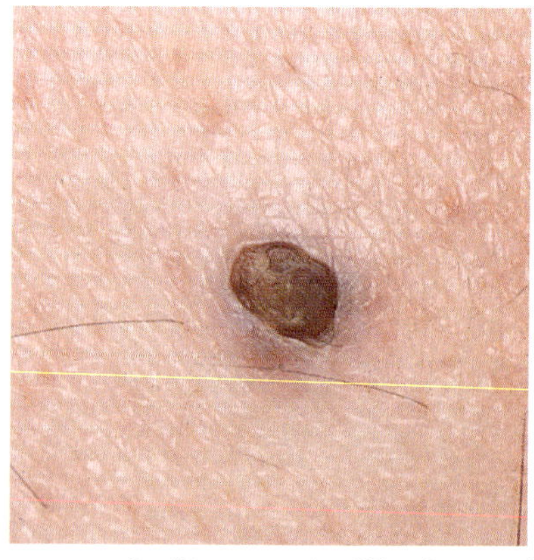

FIG. 14-15 *Dome-shaped, smooth-surfaced nodule with a central comedo of an infundibular type of follicular cyst.*

FIG. 14-16 *Giant comedo (dilated pore of Winer).*

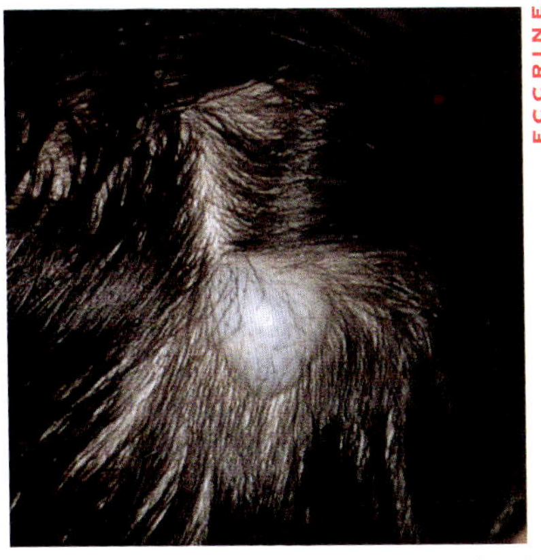

FIG. 14-17 *Dome-shaped, smooth-surfaced bluish nodule of an isthmic-catagen type of follicular cyst.*

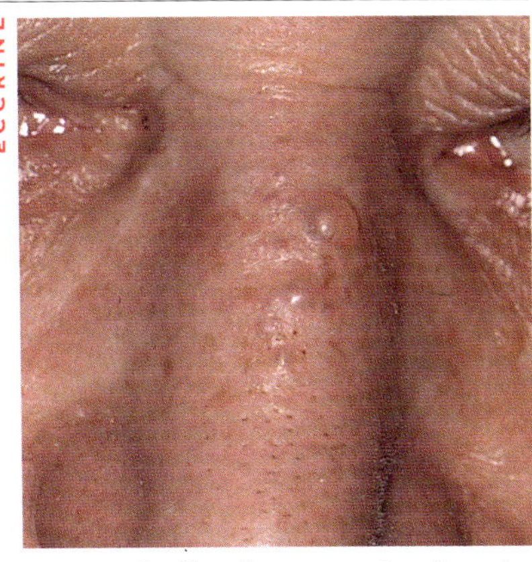

FIG. 14-18 *Translucent papules of eccrine hidrocystoma resemble vesicles arranged in a cluster.*

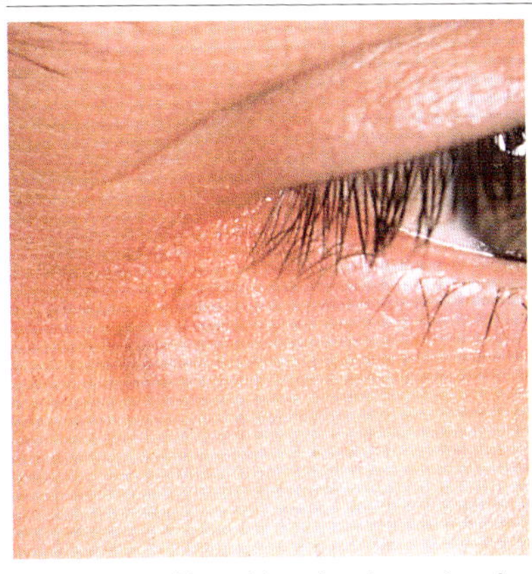

FIG. 14-19 *Two skin-colored papules that represent apocrine gland cysts (apocrine hidrocystomas).*

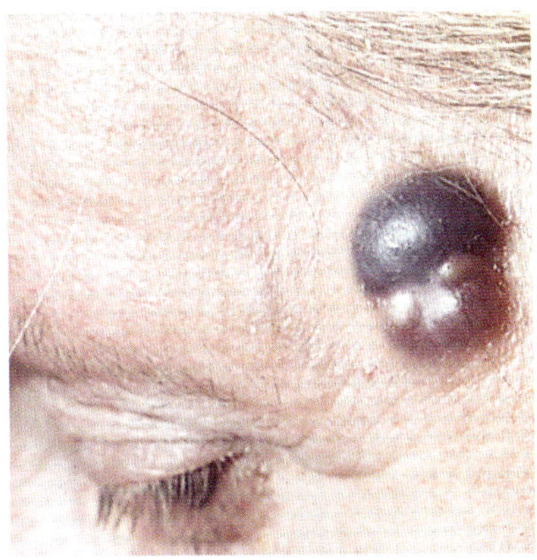

FIG. 14-20 *Blue-brown, multi-lobulated, smooth-surfaced nodule of an apocrine gland cyst ("blue-domed cyst").*

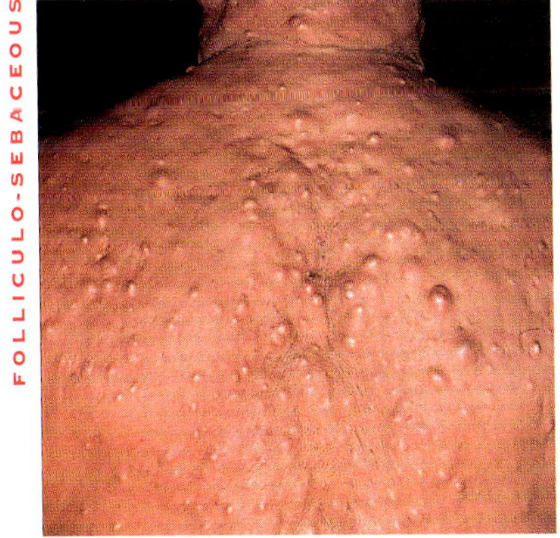

FIG. 14-21 *Numerous papules of steatocystoma, a cystic hamartoma.*

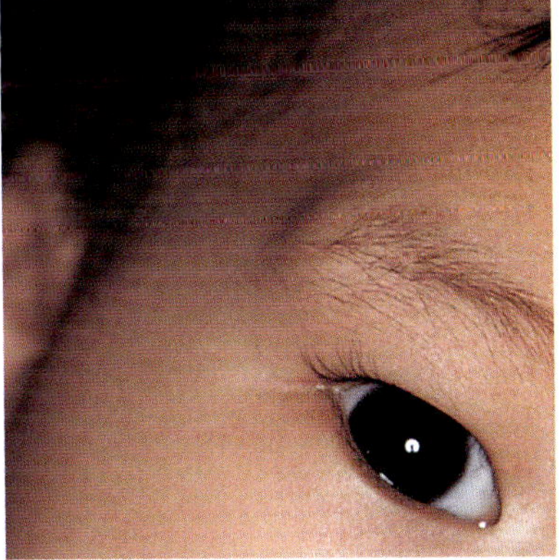

FIG. 14-22 *Dome-shaped, smooth-surfaced nodule of a dermoid cyst.*

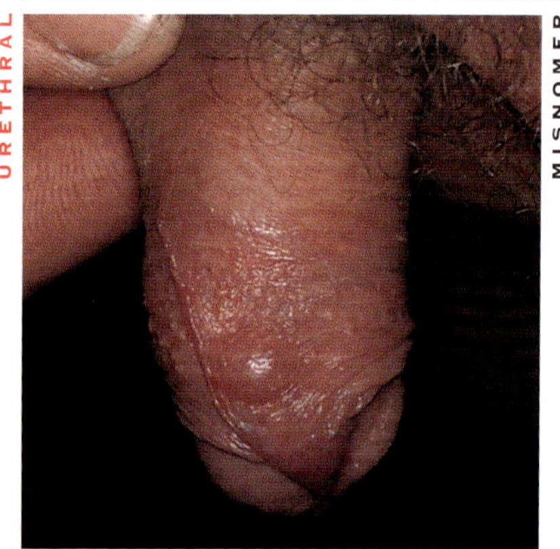
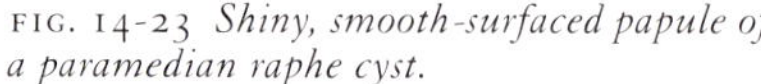

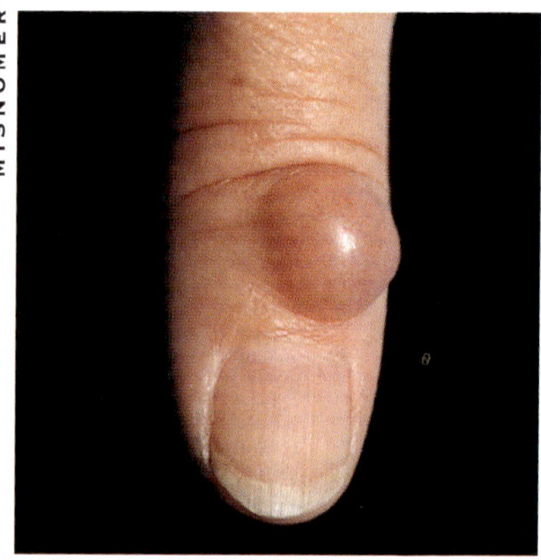

FIG. 14-23 *Shiny, smooth-surfaced papule of a paramedian raphe cyst.*

FIG. 14-24 *"Myxoid cyst" is not a true cyst but a deposit of mucin (focal mucinosis).*

COURSE Cysts of all kinds may remain intact for years, even decades, or they may rupture and heal eventually with scar. The common follicular cyst of the face and back is lined by epithelium like that of the infundibulum of a follicle (infundibular cyst) and often ruptures, inducing suppurative, then granulomatous, and finally fibrosing inflammation (as is the case in so-called cystic acne). The common follicular cyst on the scalp is lined by epithelium like the isthmus of a follicle and a follicle well advanced in catagen (isthmic-catagen cyst). It ruptures far less often than does an infundibular cyst and tends instead to proceed to calcification of its compactly-arranged cornified contents. A bluish cyst of the face known conventionally as hidrocystoma is lined by apocrine glandular epithelium (apocrine gland cyst) and it usually persists unchanged for a lifetime.

INTEGRATION: UNIFYING CONCEPT Each cyst and cystic hamartoma in the skin has its own distinctive character. Virtually every cyst is lined by epithelium that resembles that of adnexal epithelium of normal skin. For that reason, we name cysts according to the epithelial structure of adnexa that the lining of the cyst most closely resembles. With that system there are infundibular cysts (whose lining is like that of the normal infundibulum), isthmic-catagen cysts (whose lining is like that of the isthmus of a normal follicle or of a follicle well advanced in catagen), and apocrine gland cysts (whose lining is like that of an apocrine gland). An apocrine gland cyst usually presents itself as a solitary papule (or sometimes a very few papules) that does not enlarge when the person bearing it sweats; by contrast, eccrine gland cysts occur in large numbers and tend to enlarge when the person who displays them perspires profusely. As the name denotes, eccrine gland cysts are lined by epithelium like that of a normal eccrine gland.

Each cystic hamartoma in the skin and subcutaneous fat is composed of elements that develop during embryogenesis and that are present normally in human skin. For example, the cystic component of steatocystoma is lined by epithelium like that of a sebaceous duct. Continuous with that cystic structure are sebaceous lobules, vellus follicles, and, sometimes, apocrine glands and ducts. Fascicles of smooth muscle of hair erection sometimes accompany the epithelial elements of the hamartoma.

By contrast, folliculosebaceous cystic hamartoma is centered around an infundibular cyst to which sebaceous lobules and ducts are connected. The cyst is surrounded by mesenchyme that resembles that of embryonal skin, being replete with primitive fibrocytes, mucin, and, in foci, adipocytes. Changes identical to those of fibrous papule of the face—one of several types of cutaneous hamartomas of mostly follicular nature—are present, episodically, within the substance of a folliculosebaceous cystic hamartoma.

In short, each cyst and cystic hamartoma in the skin has a distinctive character. Some, such as infundibular cysts, seem to be a consequence of dilation of a pre-existing normal structure, whereas others, such as isthmic-catagen cysts, appear to result from a block in normal involution during the follicular cycle, i.e., from catagen to telogen, and still others, such as apocrine gland cysts, seem to be a developmental abnormality. Virtually all cystic hamartomas, as the name denotes, represent an aberration in embryogenesis.

THERAPY Removal of the cyst, including its epithelial lining and contents, by simple surgical excision is curative. A cystic hamartoma also can be excised, if the patient or physician so desires.

DEFINITION A genetically determined disorder in which numerous closely set keratotic papules are present on the skin, especially the trunk, in nail units, and on mucous membranes, particularly the palate, but also rarely in other parts of the gastrointestinal tract.

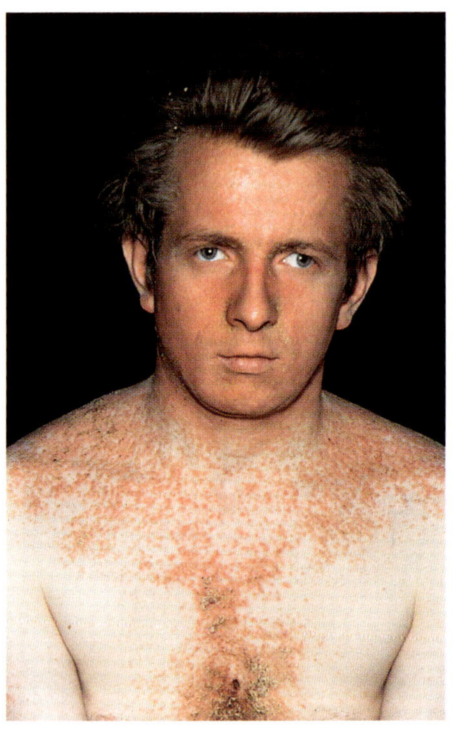

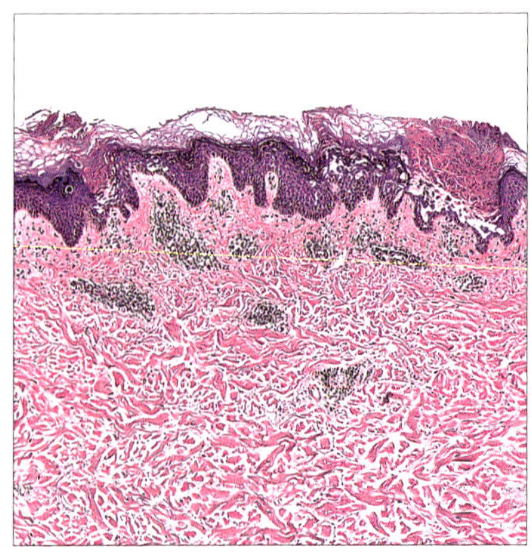

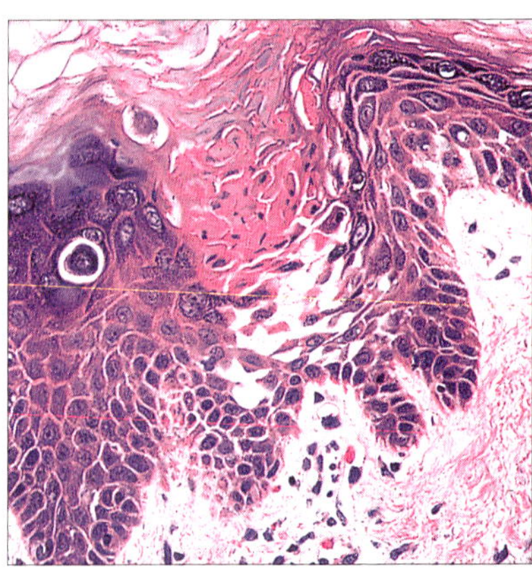

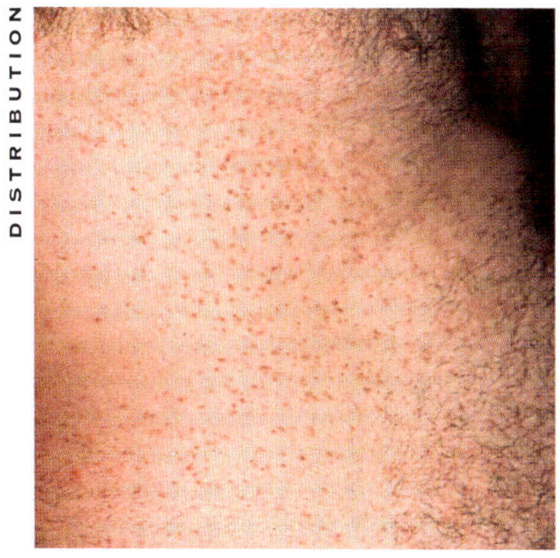

FIG. 15-1 *Widespread keratotic papules.*

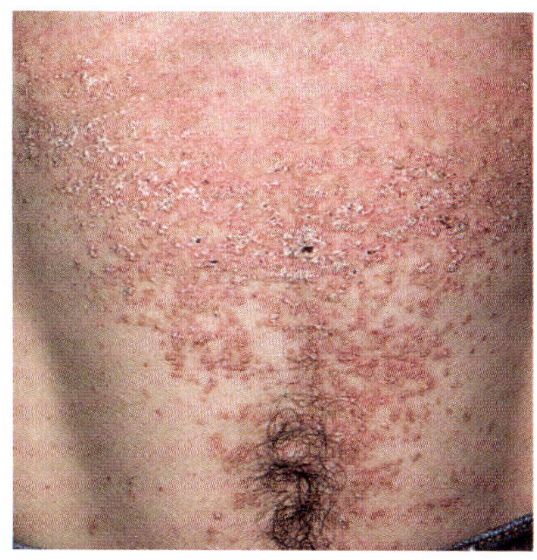

FIG. 15-2 *Scaly papules, some discrete and crusted, and some confluent.*

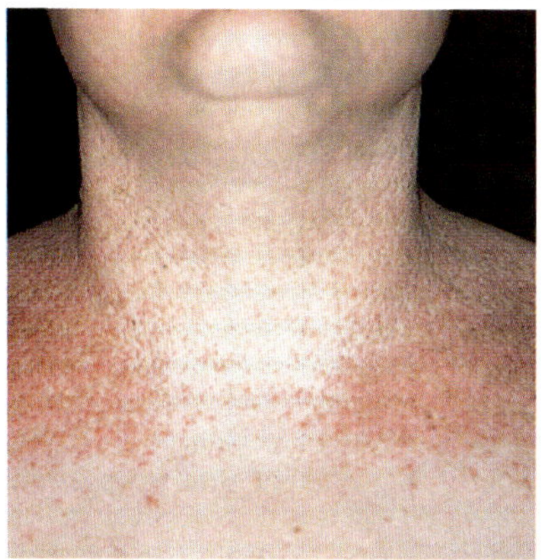

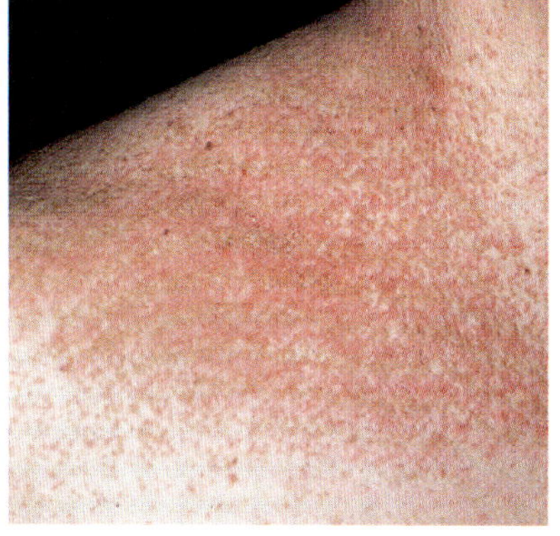

FIG. 15-3 (A, B) *Keratotic pigmented papules distributed symmetrically.*

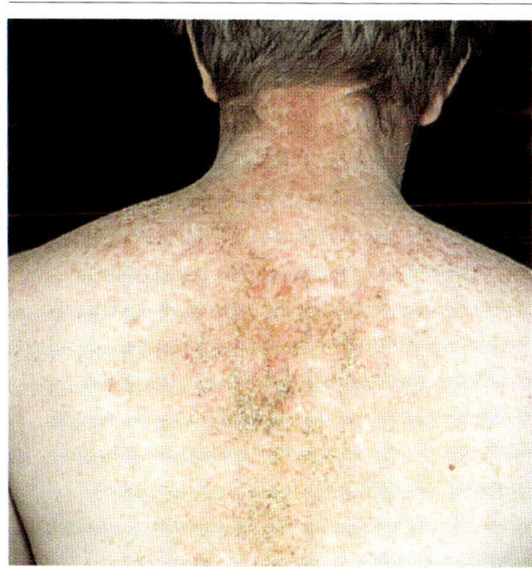

FIG. 15-4 *Keratotic papules in wedge-shaped pattern.*

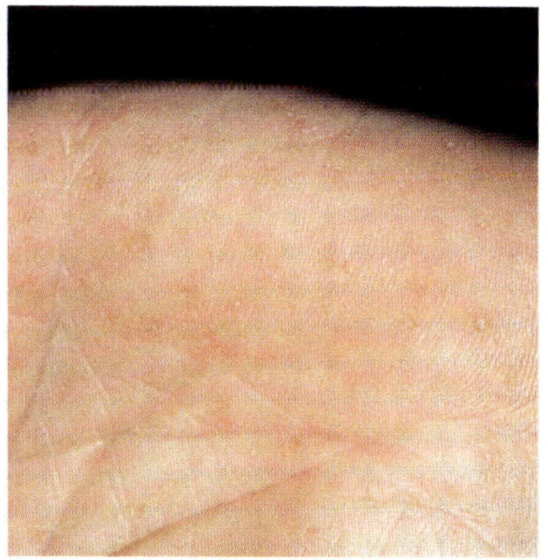

FIG. 15-5 *Keratotic papules.*

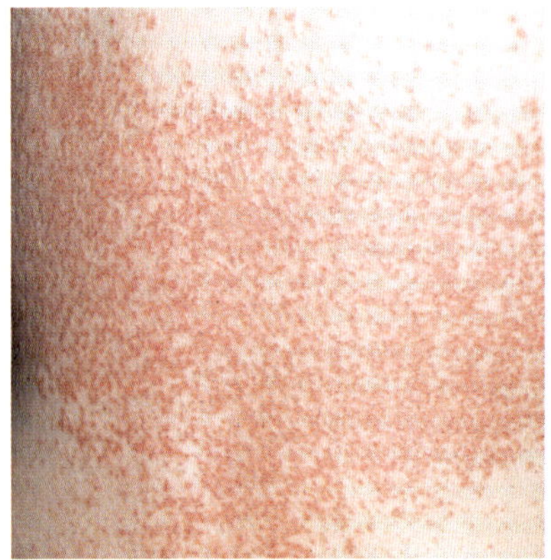

FIG. 15-6 *Keratotic papules.*

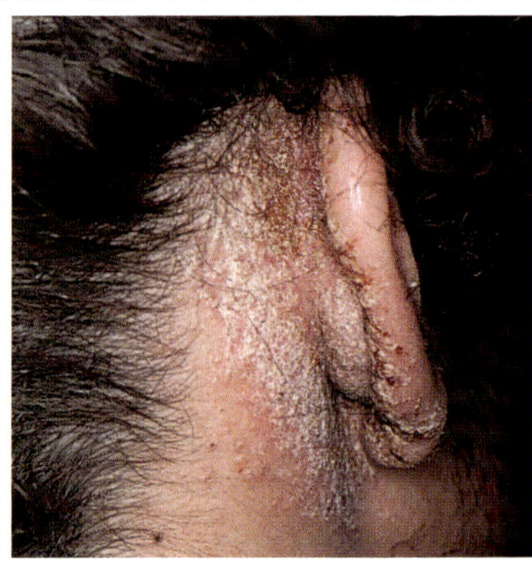

FIG. 15-7 *Keratotic crusted papules and plaques, the effects of impetiginization of lesions in the retroauricular region.*

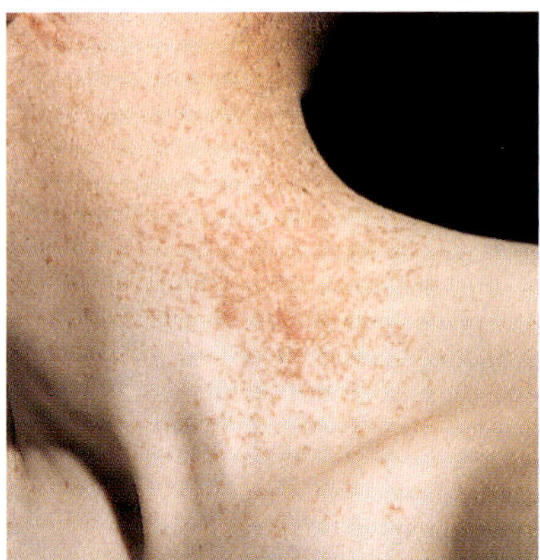

FIG. 15-8 *Keratotic papules on the neck and face.*

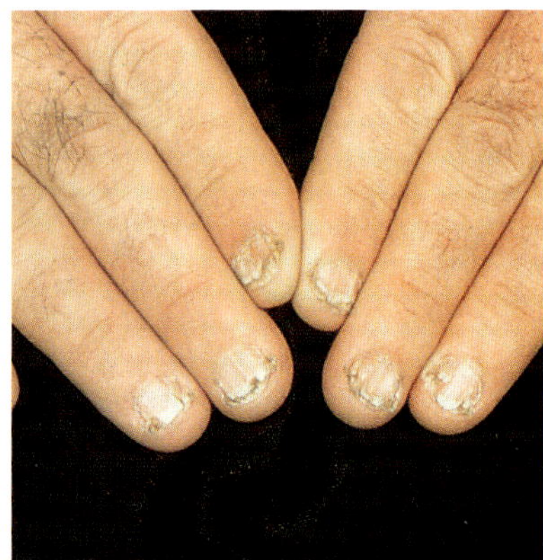

FIG. 15-9 *Each nail plate is involved, one by a pterygium, some by ridges, and some by distal onycholysis.*

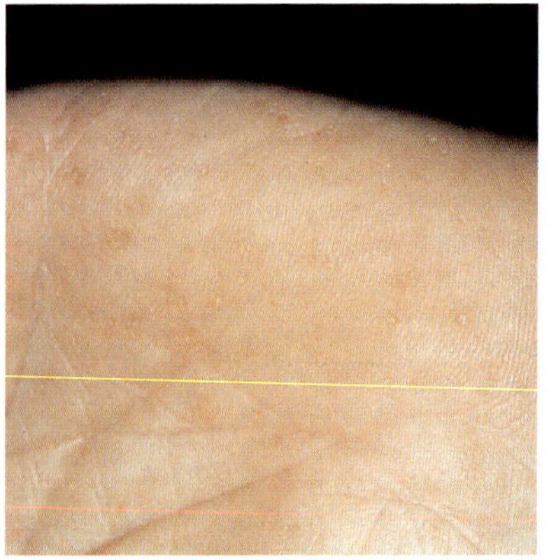

FIG. 15-10 *Palmar pits.*

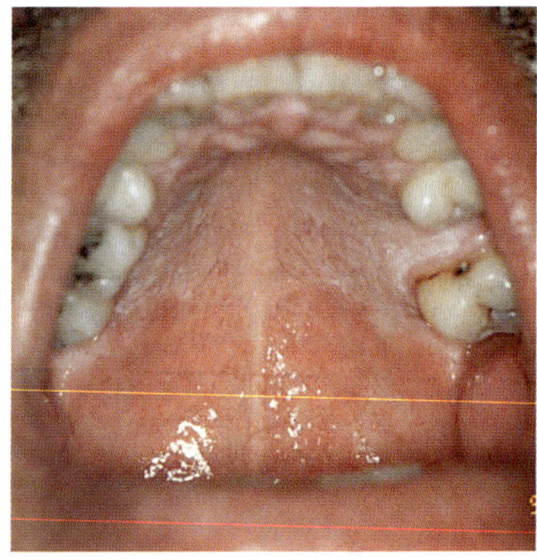

FIG. 15-11 *Cobblestone pattern formed by keratotic papules on the palate.*

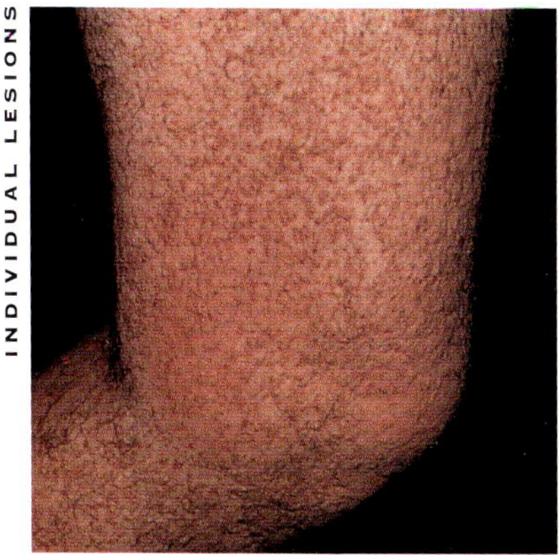

FIG. 15-12 *Keratotic papules are both discrete and confluent.*

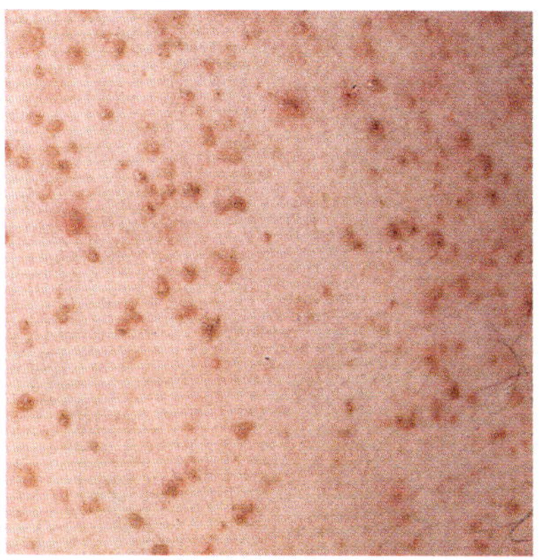

FIG. 15-13 *Keratotic papules are discrete.*

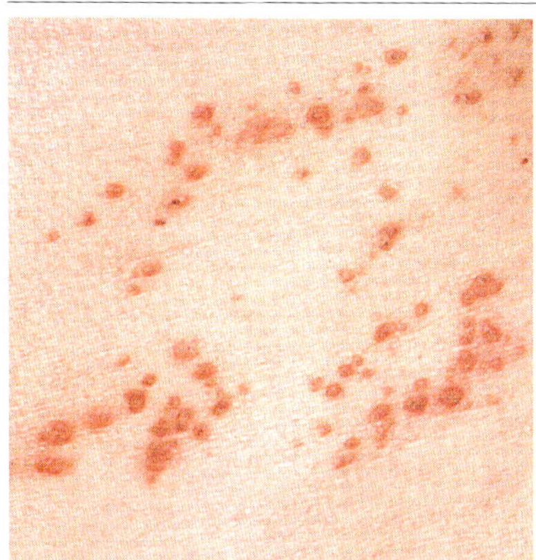

FIG. 15-14 *Keratotic papules in clusters.*

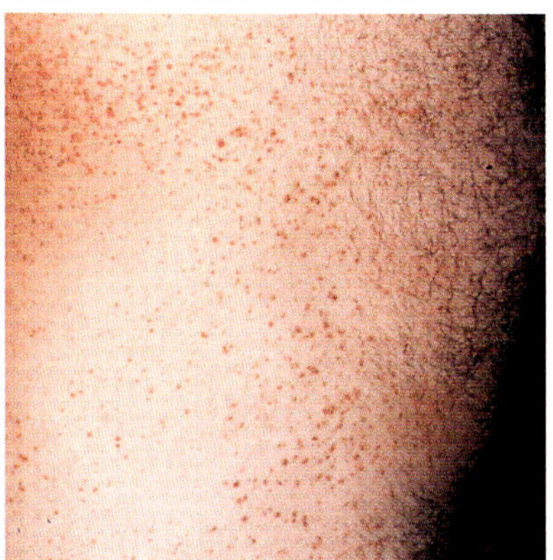

FIG. 15-15 *Keratotic papules.*

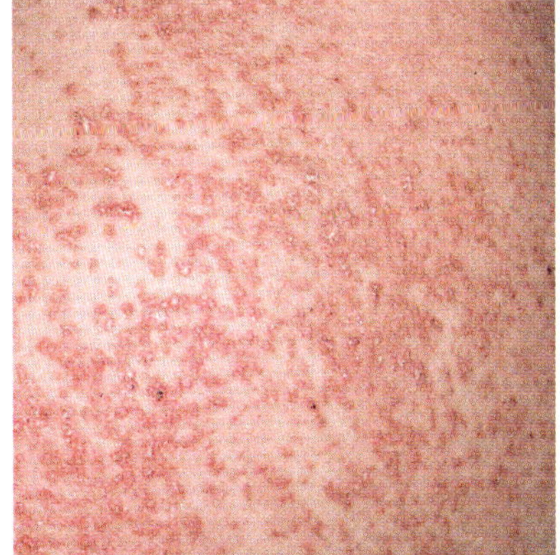

FIG. 15-16 *Confluence of keratotic papules with formation of ill-defined incipient plaques.*

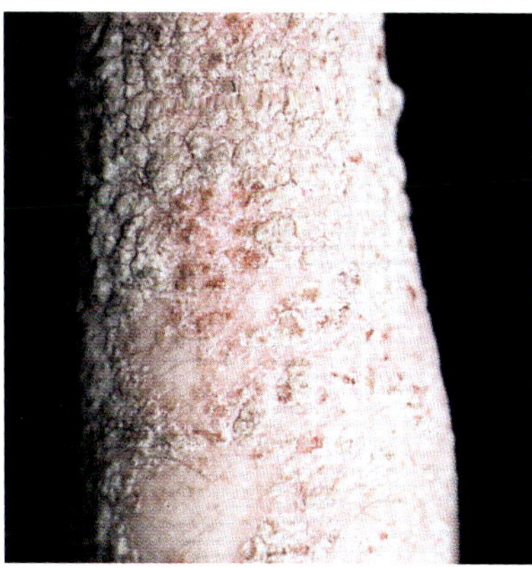

FIG. 15-17 *Keratotic papules in confluence have formed a plaque.*

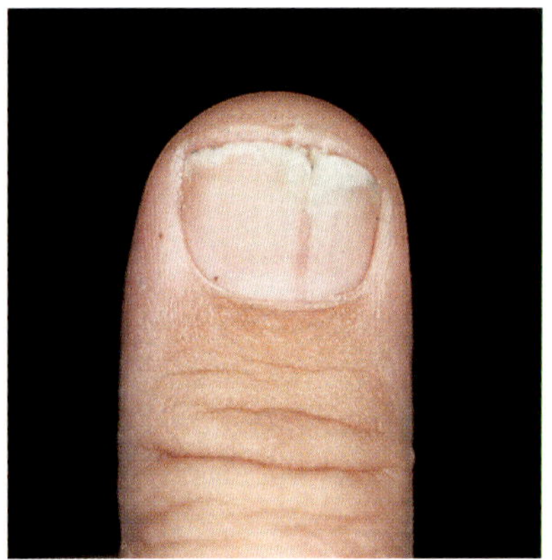

FIG. 15-18 *Wedge-shaped onycholysis.*

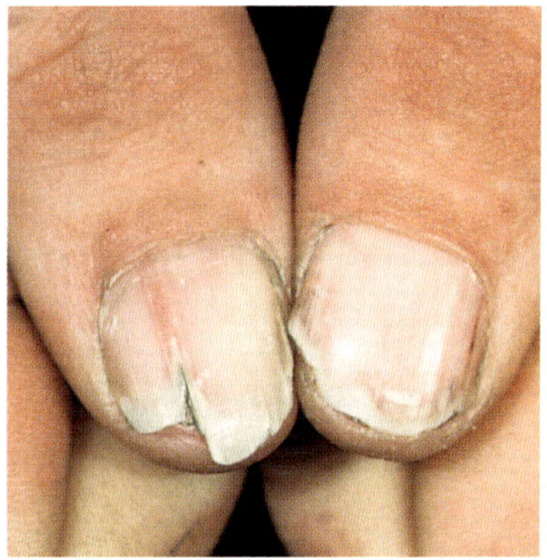

FIG. 15-19 *A dystrophic channel near the middle of one nail, and onycholysis and sub-ungual hyperkeratosis of both nails.*

COURSE Untreated lesions of Darier's disease persist and often worsen, i.e., they become more keratotic in time and are joined by new lesions in skin, nail units, and mucous membranes. Impetiginization secondary to animated scratching is common in patients with Darier's disease. Uncommon, but more serious, is secondary infection by herpesvirus (Kaposi's varicelliform eruption), a condition that tends to be widespread, i.e., wherever lesions of Darier's disease are present in the skin.

INTEGRATION: UNIFYING CONCEPT Darier's disease, known formerly and imprecisely as keratosis follicularis (it usually spares follicles and also involves sites devoid of follicles, such as nail units, the oral cavity, and even parts of the alimentary canal), is a distinctive genodermatosis that presents itself clinically as innumerable keratotic papules. Each papule consists of a focus of epidermal thickening typified by a suprabasal cleft, acantholytic dyskeratotic cells in the spinous and granular zones, and acantholytic parakeratotic cells at the base of a column of parakeratosis, a constellation of findings known descriptively as "focal acantholytic dyskeratosis." Even though those very histopathologic changes may be seen in other diseases, Darier's disease is distinctive clinically. Diseases characterized by focal acantholytic dyskeratosis include a variant of Grover's disease, a type of epidermal nevus that assumes linear, zosteriform, or systematized shapes, a condition that involves the palms and soles entirely in the manner of keratoderma palmaris et plantaris, and a solitary papule (acantholytic dyskeratotic acanthoma). The same histopathologic findings that typify Darier's disease in the skin are found, more or less, in nail units and on mucous membranes. Even when Darier's disease is complicated by impetiginization or by infection with herpesvirus, the underlying process is still identifiable, clinically and histopathologically.

Although Darier's disease usually is classified in textbooks of dermatology and dermatopathology as a type of intraepidermal vesicular dermatitis, it is not; it is a particular abnormality of keratinization, akin to other distinctive abnormalities of keratinization such as occur in bullous congenital ichthyosiform erythroderma (and its more circumscribed variants such as ichthyosis hystrix), and porokeratosis of Mibelli (and other variants of porokeratosis). The histopathologic findings in each of these keratotic conditions are unique, to wit, epidermolytic hyperkeratosis for bullous congenital ichthyosiform erythroderma and cornoid lamellation for porokeratosis of Mibelli.

THERAPY Retinoids (etretinate, acitretin) administered systemically are most effective in muting the process. Oral antibiotics are indicated for secondary infection by bacteria. Topical agents include "keratolytics" and retinoic acid gel. Dermabrasion has also been employed.

DEFINITION Cutaneous and subcutaneous lesions, usually nodules, that have become keratotic, crusted, and ulcerated as a consequence of infection by a variety of deep fungi, i.e., fungi situated in the dermis and subcutis, some of which may be disseminated to other organs.

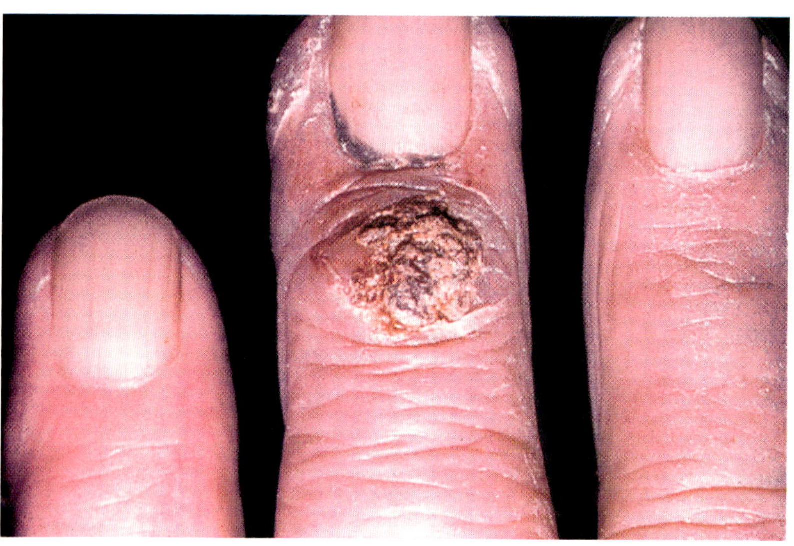

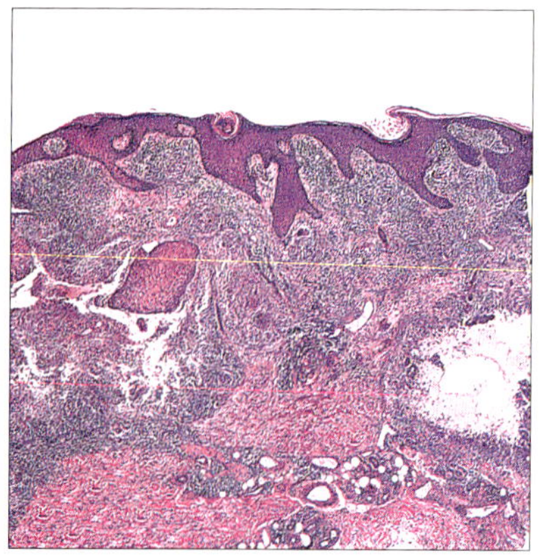

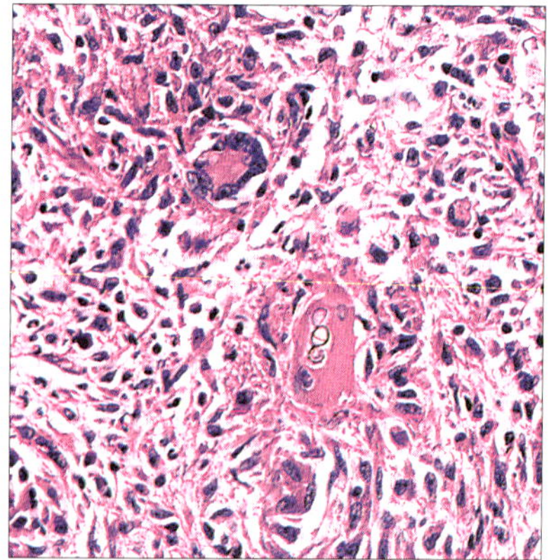

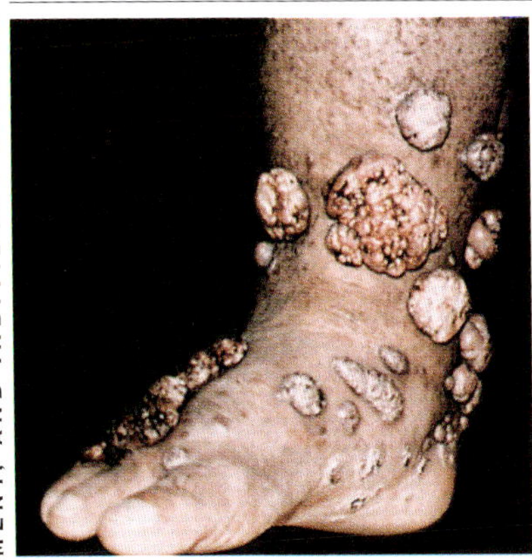

FIG. 16-1 *Papules, nodules, and tumors, one of them ulcerated, caused by a dermatiaceous fungus.*

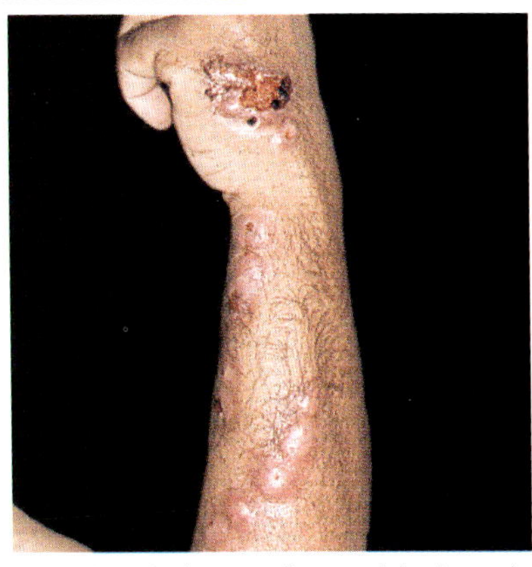

FIG. 16-2 *A chancre of sporotrichosis on the dorsum of the hand and nodules of the disease along lymphatics.*

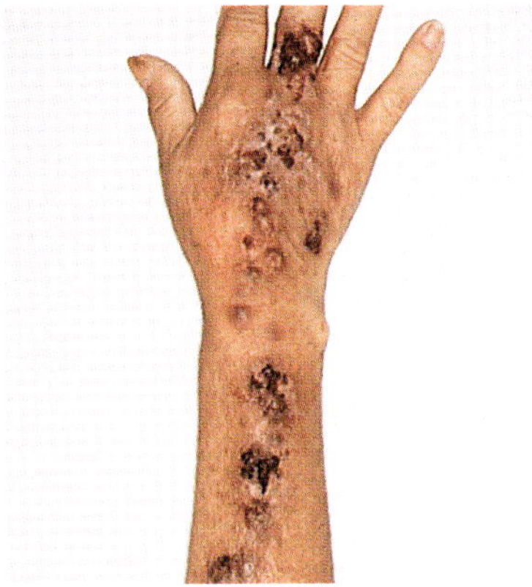

FIG. 16-3 *Crusted nodules in linear fashion along lymphatics in sporotrichosis.*

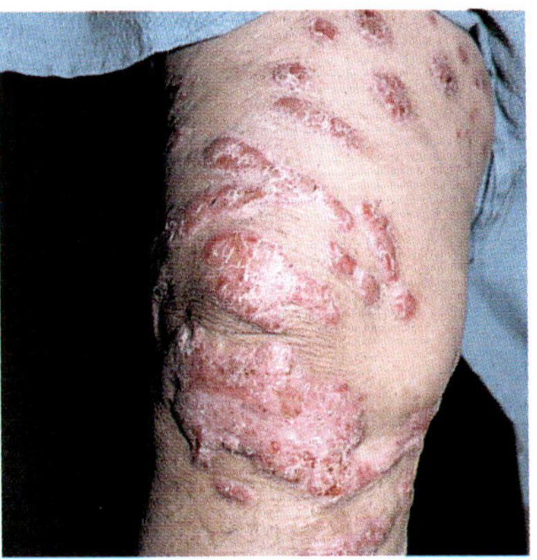

FIG. 16-4 *Crusted keratotic violaceous plaques of North American blastomycosis.*

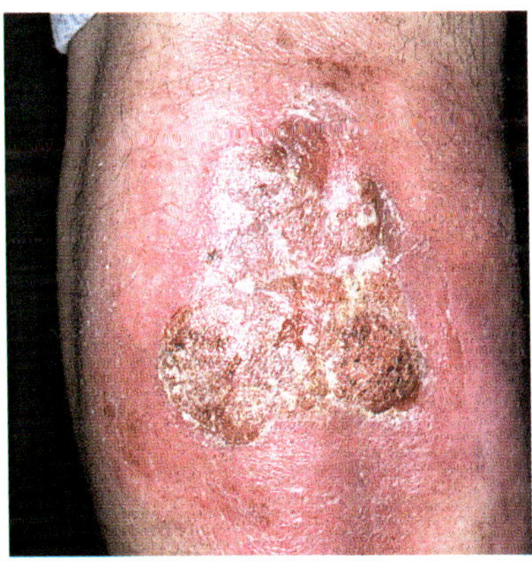

FIG. 16-5 *Plaques and nodules, some of them crusted and keratotic, surrounded by erythema of chromomycosis.*

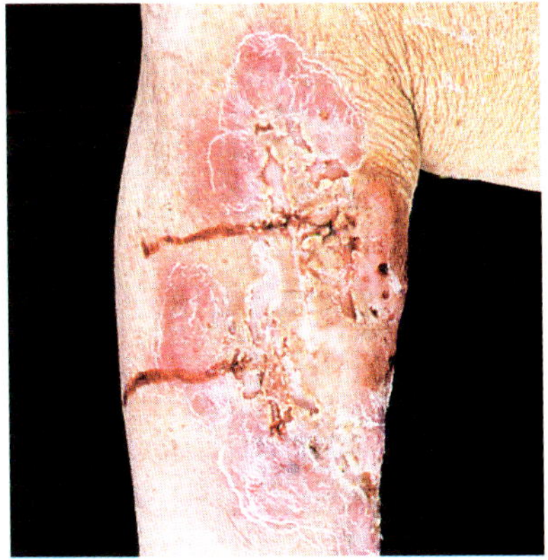

FIG. 16-6 *Large plaque with crusts and fissures of chromomycosis.*

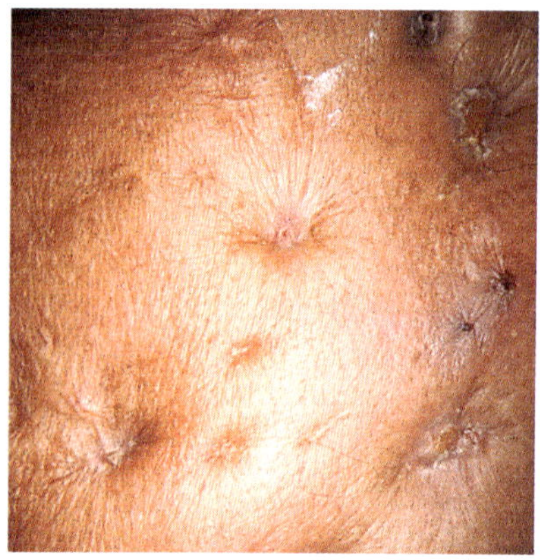

FIG. 16-7 *Dells that represent atrophic scars secondary to draining of sinuses of maduromycosis.*

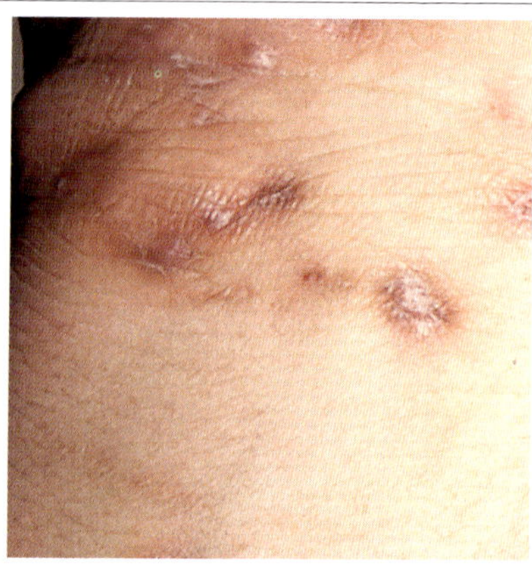

FIG. 16-8 *Atrophic scars at site of sinuses secondary to maduromycosis.*

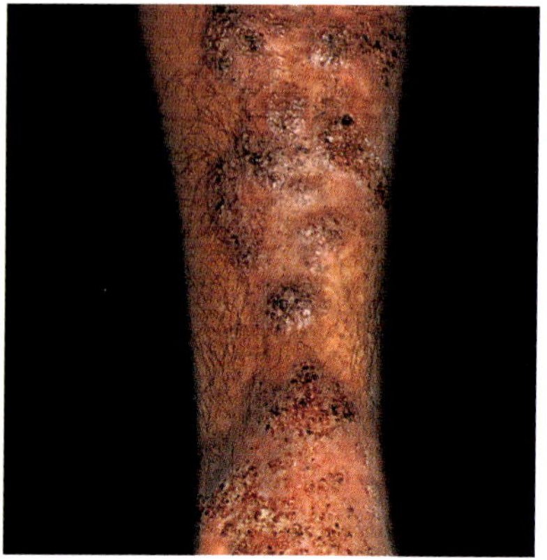

FIG. 16-9 *Crusted plaques of sporotrichosis.*

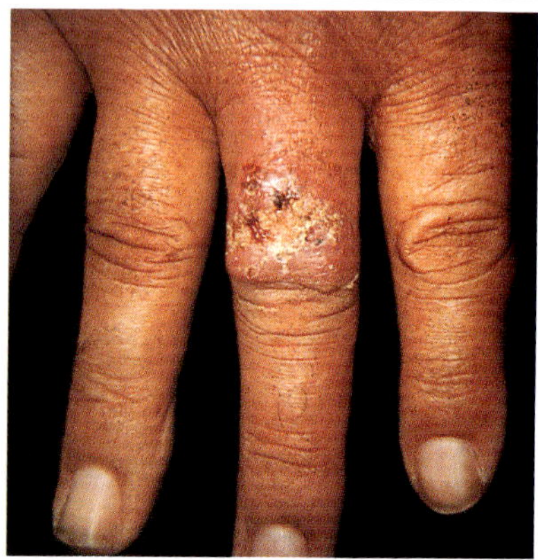

FIG. 16-10 *Crusted plaque with central ulcer of sporotrichosis.*

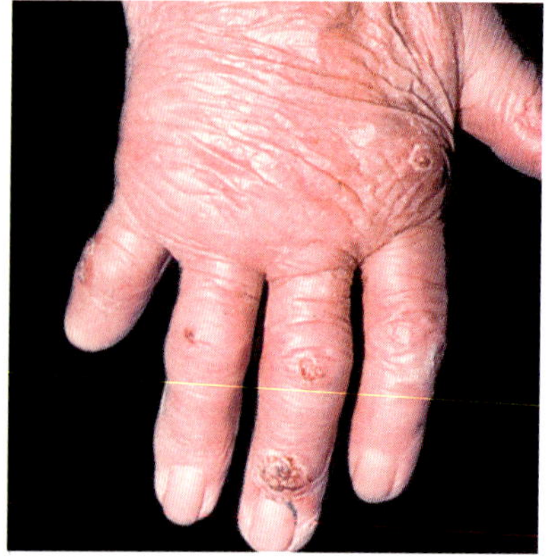

FIG. 16-11 *Crusted papules at sites of draining sinuses caused by maduromycosis, which has deformed the hand.*

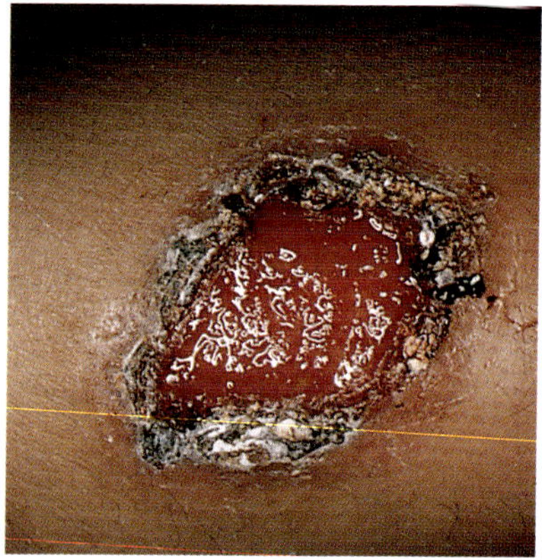

FIG. 16-12 *Plaque with central ulcer and peripheral crusts caused by* Sporotrichium schenckii.

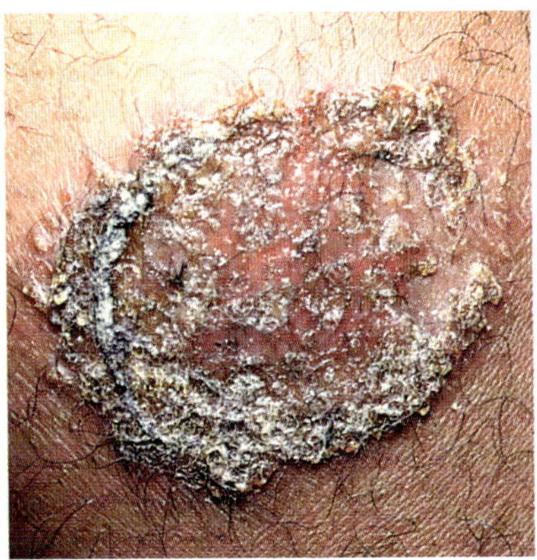

FIG. 16-13 *Plaque with verrucous papules and atrophic scars in the center of chromomycosis.*

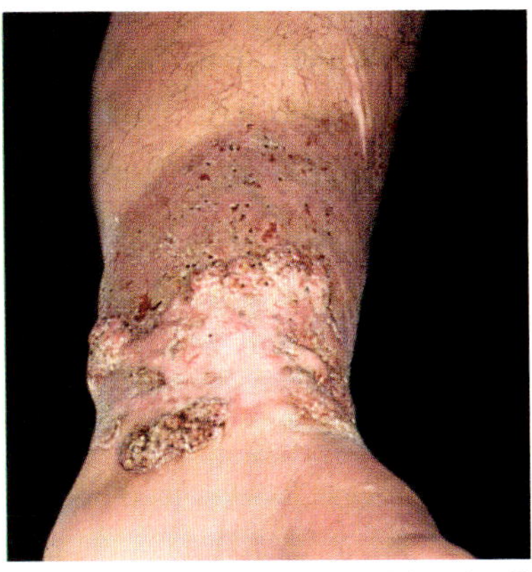

FIG. 16-14 *Scaly, crusted nodules, focally eroded plaque, and atrophic scar caused by a dermatiaceous fungus.*

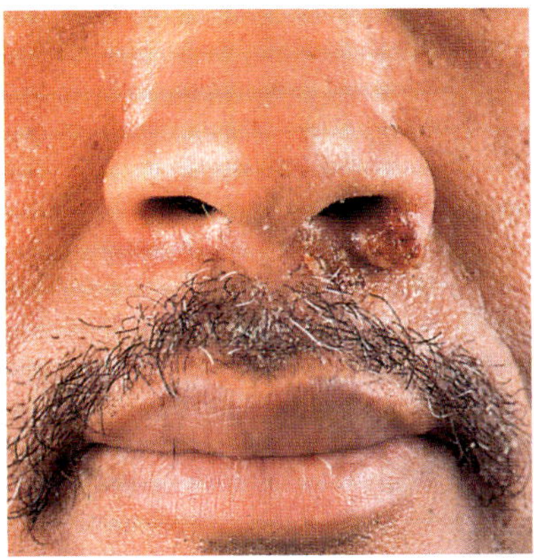

FIG. 16-15 *Ulcerated nodule of coccidioidomycosis on the nose.*

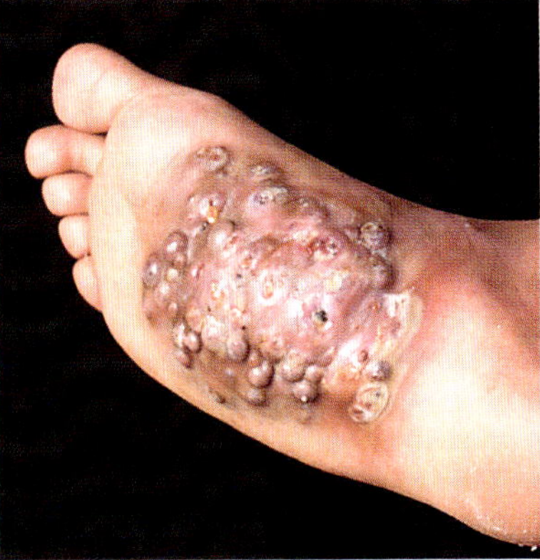

FIG. 16-16 *Verrucous plaque with draining sinuses of mycetoma.*

ADJUNCTIVE DIAGNOSTIC TESTS Specialized stains of sections of tissue for spores and sometimes hyphae, and culture.

COURSE Lesions that develop consequent to infection by deep fungi usually worsen steadily for years, only involuting rarely in the absence of specific therapy, and then often in parte rather than in toto. New lesions often appear, especially when the infectious agent is spread by lymphatics, as often is the case, for example, with sporotrichosis and chromomycosis.

INTEGRATION: UNIFYING CONCEPT What was written for "Integration: Unifying Concept" about atypical mycobacterial infections applies equally to deep fungal infections. The cause of each of the latter infections is a fungus, the types of which vary enormously and include, for example,

Sporotrichium schenckii, Histoplasma capsulatum, Blastomyces dermatitides, Coccidioides immitis, Paracoccidioides brasiliensis, and Loboa loboi. Although those organisms are very different from one another, they induce similar clinical features and histopathologic findings in the skin. The clinical ones are shown in photographs in this chapter. The histopathologic analogues of the clinical attributes, at different stages of the chronological course, are suppuration, granulomatous inflammation in conjunction often with pseudo-carcinomatous hyperplasia, and fibrosis. Those changes are responsible for fluctuance early, for vegetating and keratotic lesions later, and for scarring at the end.

As long as suppuration is present, organisms of deep fungal infections usually can be identified readily in sections stained only by hematoxylin and eosin, usually within zones of collections of neutrophils or in histiocytes, especially multinucleate ones. That is not the case in most instances, however, for sporotrichosis, which typically requires a specialized stain, such as periodic acid-Schiff with prior digestion by diastase, for identification of the organism responsible for it, namely, Sporotrichium schenckii. Once granulomatous dermatitis has replaced suppuration, and surely by the time there is fibrosis, organisms no longer are detectable in sections of tissue.

An exception to what has just been written about morphologic features of deep fungal infections is the manifestation in the skin of Cryptococcus neoformans. That organism does not induce suppuration, granulomatous inflammation, and fibrosis, but instead is made up of sheets of yeasts, many of them budding. Each of the yeasts displays a prominent gelatinous capsule. As a rule, because affected patients are so severely immunosuppressed, the yeasts do not induce any infiltrate of inflammatory cells; there are exceptions, however.

THERAPY Choice of agent depends on the specific causative organism. As a rule, oral itraconazole and ketoconazole, as well as intravenous amphotericin B, are likely to be curative.

Sporotrichosis: Oral treatment with saturated solution of potassium iodide or itraconazole, or terbinafine.

Mycetoma: When possible, small lesions can be removed surgically or treated with ketoconazole or miconazole. Actinomycotic mycetoma responds well to a combination of trimethoprim-sulfamethoxazole and dapsone.

Chromomycosis: Small lesions can be removed surgically or treated with itraconazole administered orally.

DEFINITION An inflammatory process characterized by symmetrical distribution, especially on the skin of the scalp, overlying the scapulae and the sacrum, on the buttocks, and on the extensor surface of the extremities, of clusters of urticarial papules, papulovesicles, and vesicles that are so intensely pruritic that they soon are scratched away, leaving in the wake erosions, ulcers, hemorrhagic crusts, and eventually pigmented macules and scars.

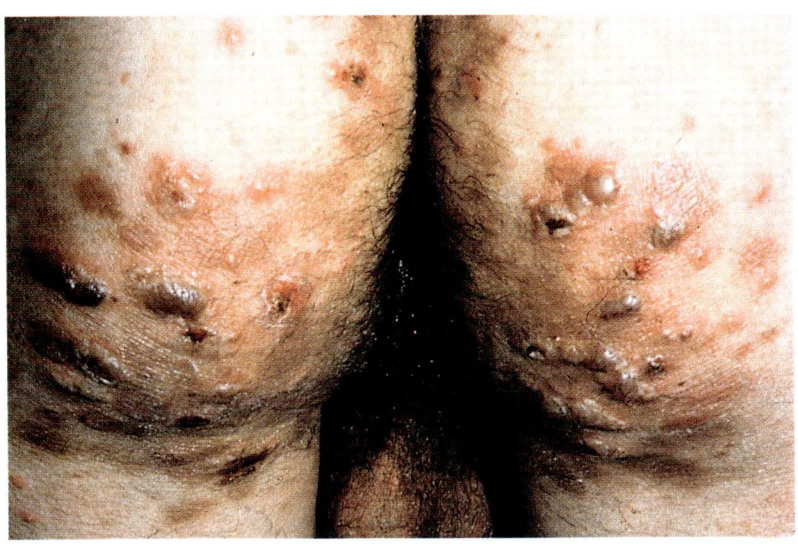

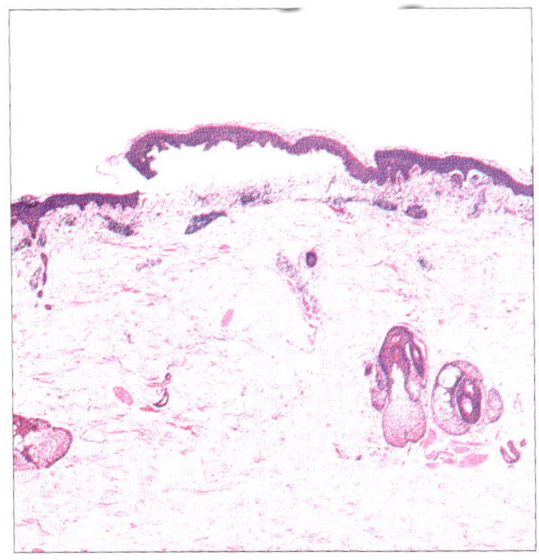

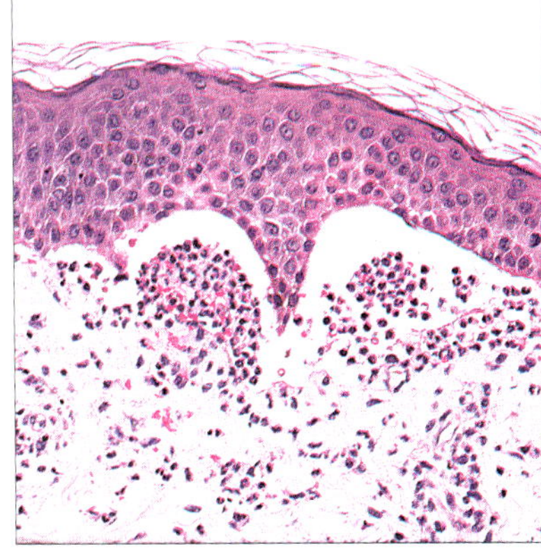

DISTRIBUTION

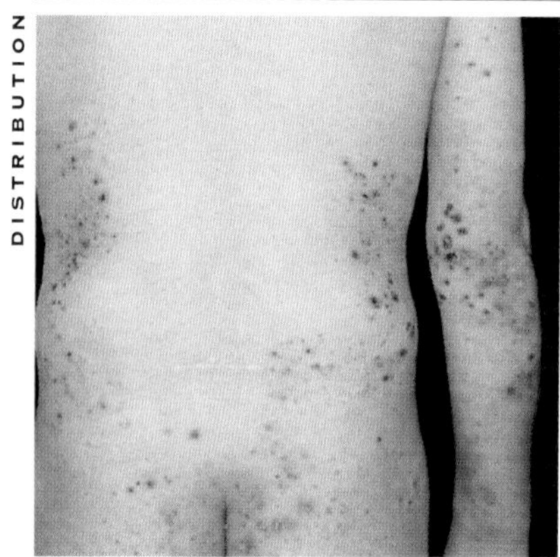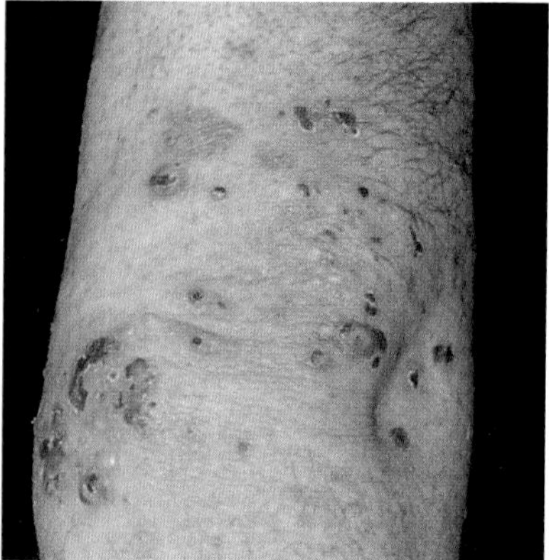

FIG. 17-1 (A, B) *Bilateral symmetrical distribution of urticarial papules, vesicles, erosions, and crusts.*

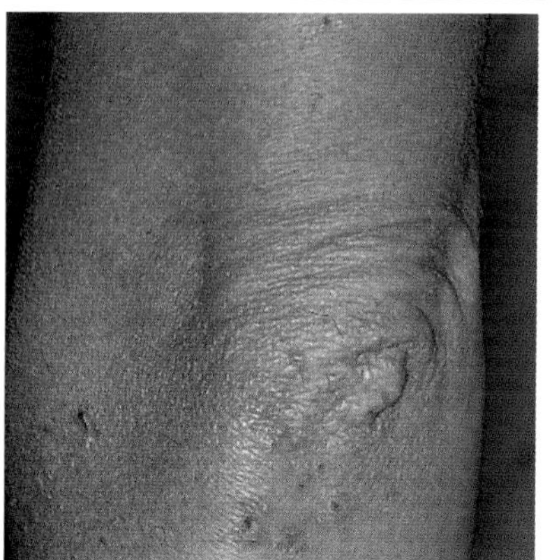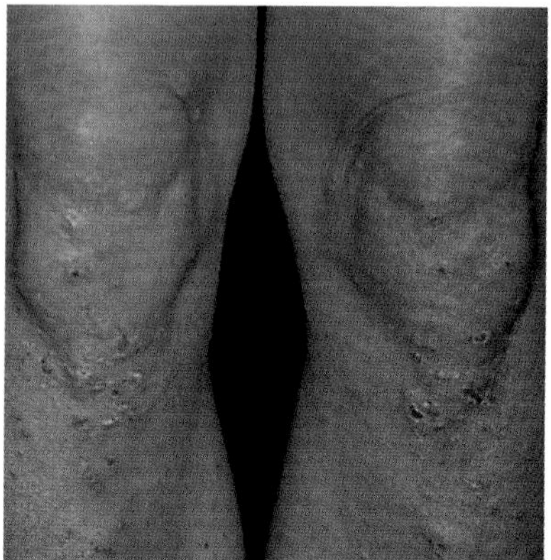

FIG. 17-2 *Cluster of papules, some of them excoriated and covered by hemorrhagic crusts.*

FIG. 17-3 *Scattered papules and vesicles.*

ARRANGEMENT

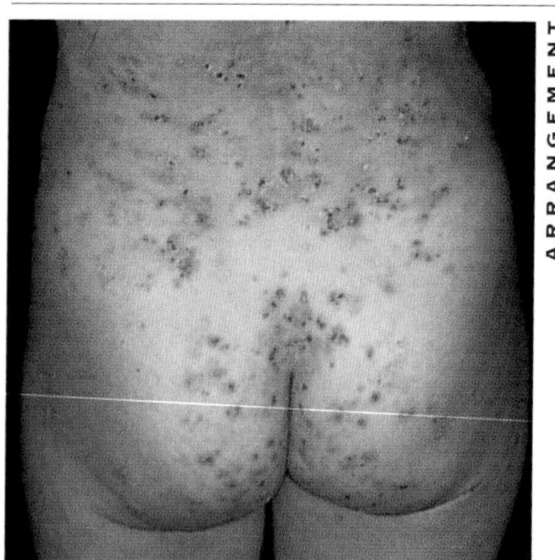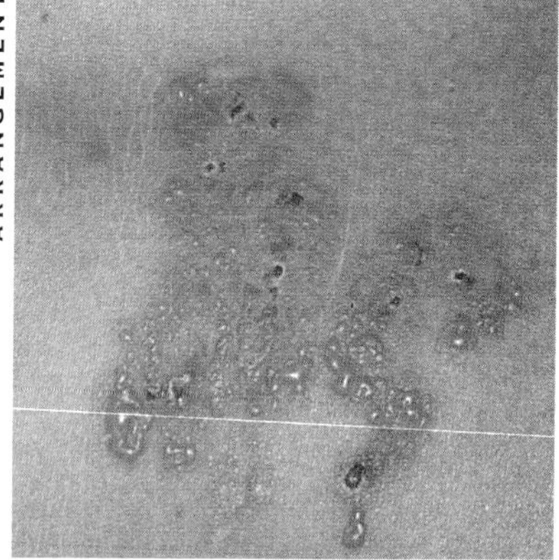

FIG. 17-4 *Clusters of papules, vesicles, hemorrhagic crusts, and scars, in bilateral symmetrical fashion.*

FIG. 17-5 *Grouped papules, vesicles, and hemorrhagic crusts, some of them on an erythematous base.*

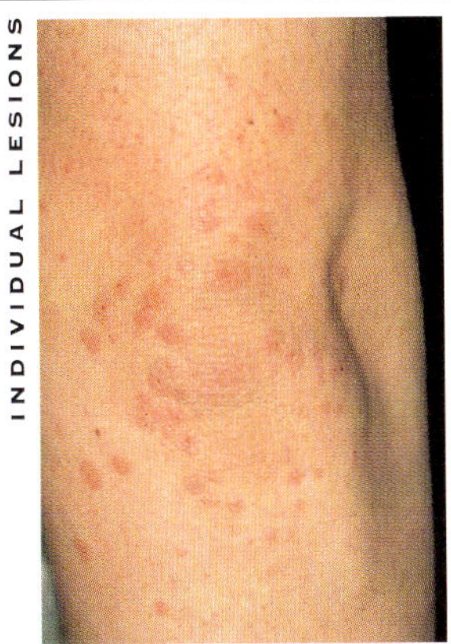

FIG. 17-6 *Urticarial papules, some excoriated.*

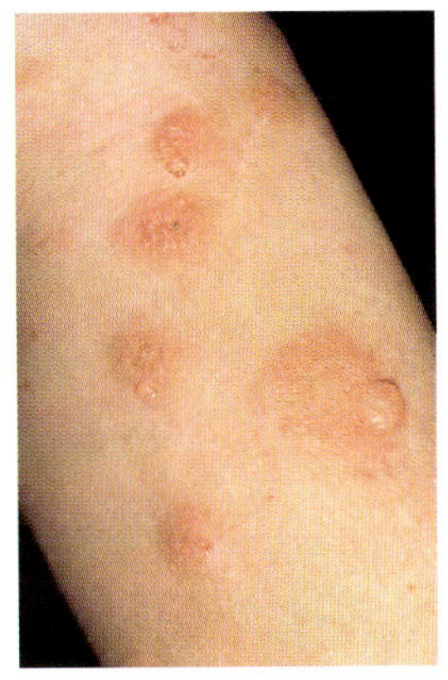

FIG. 17-7 *Groups of vesicles on an erythematous base.*

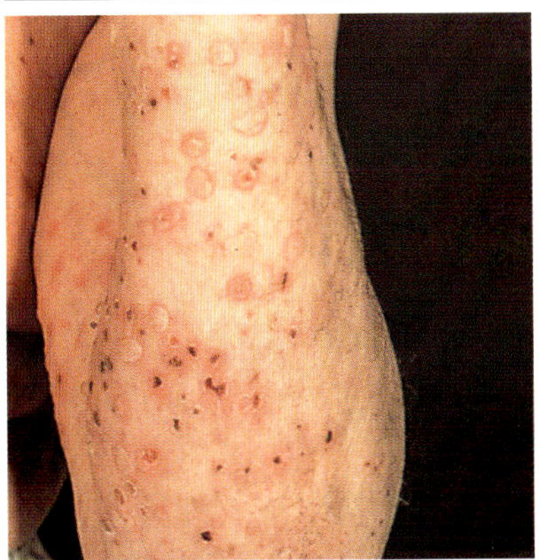

FIG. 17-8 *Vesicles, some of them in clusters, erosions, and hemorrhagic crusts.*

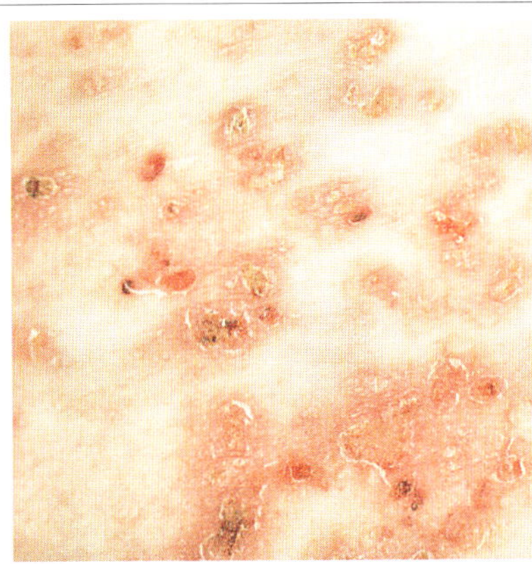

FIG. 17-9 *Erosions, hemorrhagic crusts, and collarettes of scale-crusts on an erythematous base.*

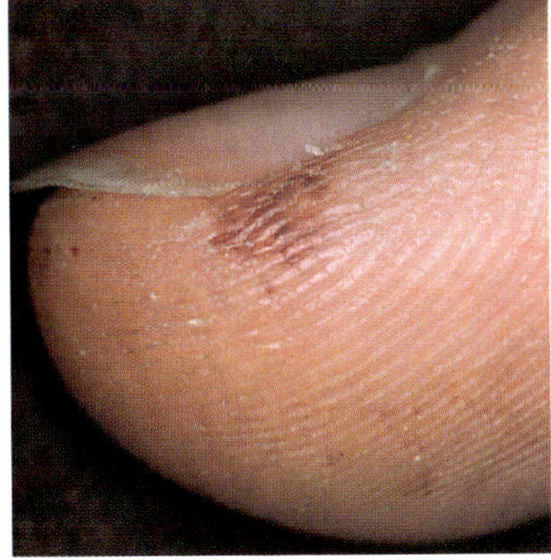

FIG. 17-10 *Purpuric macules on volar skin, a premonitory sign of fully expressed dermatitis herpetiformis.*

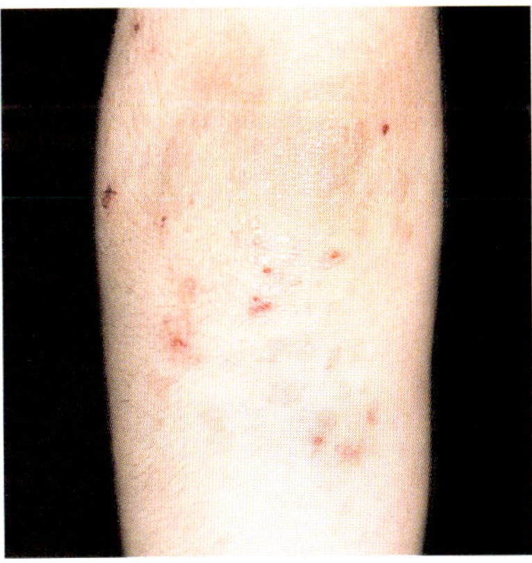

FIG. 17-11 *Papules, some of them excoriated.*

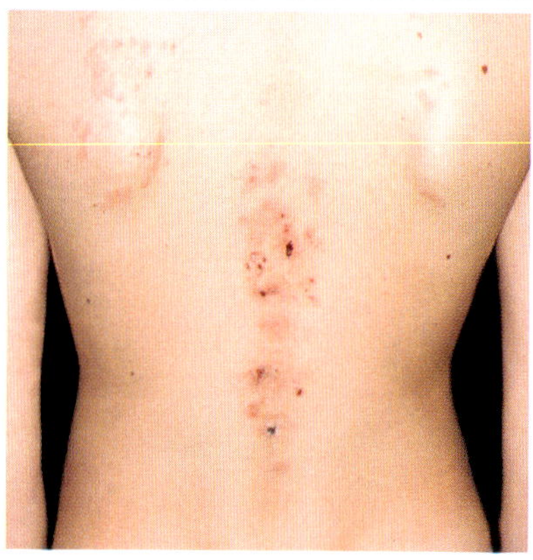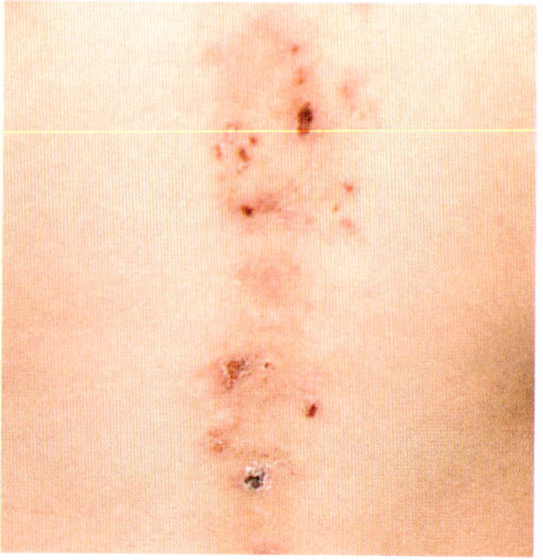

FIG. 17-12 (A, B) *Papules, some of them excoriated and covered by hemorrhagic crust.*

ADJUNCTIVE DIAGNOSTIC TESTS Demonstration of granular deposits of IgA situated at the tips of dermal papillae in both perilesional and normal-appearing skin. In severe cases, biopsy of the small intestine can be performed for the purpose of identifying celiac-like disease caused by sensitivity to gluten.

COURSE Dermatitis herpetiformis tends to appear in young adults, but it may develop in children and in the elderly, usually as urticarial papules and vesicles that are clustered in bilateral symmetrical fashion especially on the scalp, scapulae, extensor surface of arms and legs (in particular the region of the elbows and knees), sacrum, and buttocks. The lesions wax and wane, and in the absence of specific therapy, tend to come and go for a lifetime. Episodically, and exceptionally, the disease remits, not to reappear.

INTEGRATION: UNIFYING CONCEPT Dermatitis herpetiformis is a distinctive pathologic process that manifests itself as urticarial papules and vesicles; these lesions have a predilection for certain anatomic sites. Papules are made up mostly of neutrophils in edematous dermal papillae and in subepidermal clefts, and subepidermal vesicles also contain neutrophils. Neutrophils are joined by eosinophils within two or three days after a lesion first appears. The disease is thought to be autoimmune in nature, granular deposits of IgA alone or in combination with C3 being present at tips of dermal papillae.

Although the cause and mechanism of dermatitis herpetiformis are not known, it is thought currently that deposits of IgA in the papillary dermis are related to hypersensitivity to gluten. Ingestion of gluten is thought to initiate formation of IgA antibodies in the gastrointestinal tract, circulation of those antibodies, attachment of them to cutaneous structures, activation of complement, chemotaxis of neutrophils, and development of subepidermal blisters. The process is believed to be a consequence of the effects of products released by neutrophils on the attachment of the epidermis to the dermis. A gluten-sensitive enteropathy resembling celiac disease is commonly associated with dermatitis herpetiformis.

The histopathologic findings in linear IgA dermatosis are identical to those in dermatitis herpetiformis, but the clinical aspects and immunologic attributes of those diseases are different from one another.

THERAPY Dapsone is effective, presumably by suppressing neutrophils. An option therapeutically is sulfapyridine. A diet free of gluten may ameliorate the skin disease.

LINEAR IGA DERMATOSIS

DEFINITION An inflammatory disease characterized clinically by urticarial papules and vesicles, and sometimes by bullae on the trunk and flexural surfaces, that, by immunofluorescence, can be shown to exhibit deposits of IgA in linear array along the dermoepidermal junction.

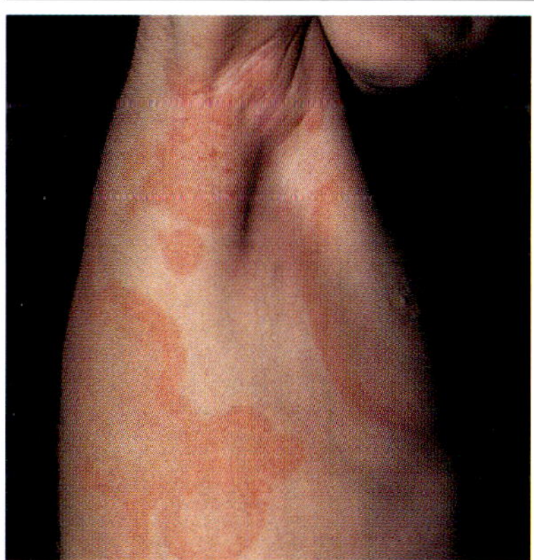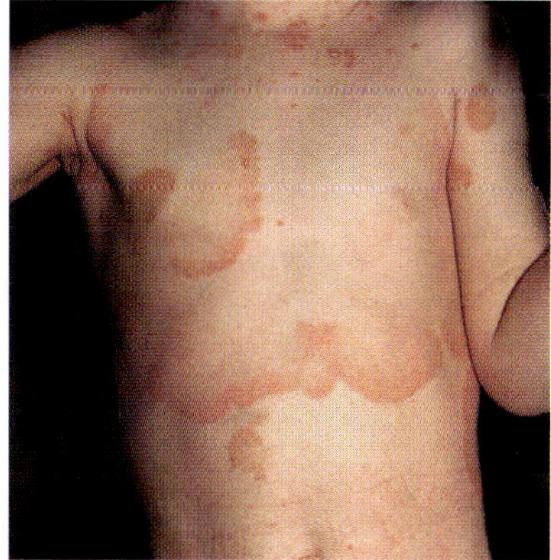

FIG. 17-13 (A, B) *Urticarial plaques in arcuate and annular configuration.*

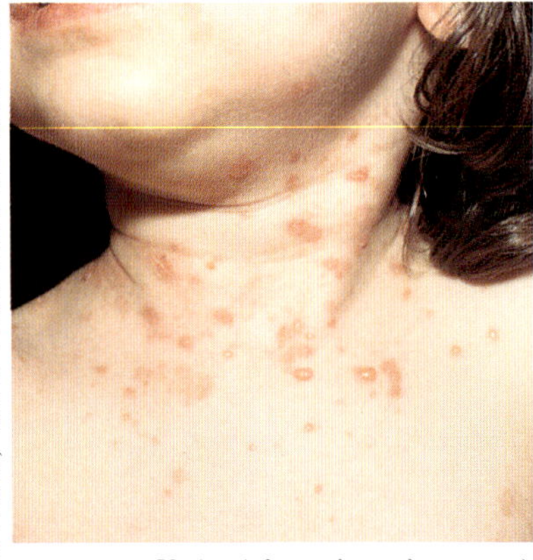

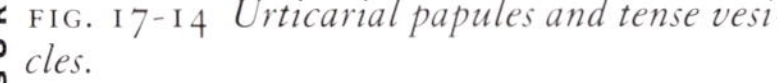

FIG. 17-14 *Urticarial papules and tense vesicles.*

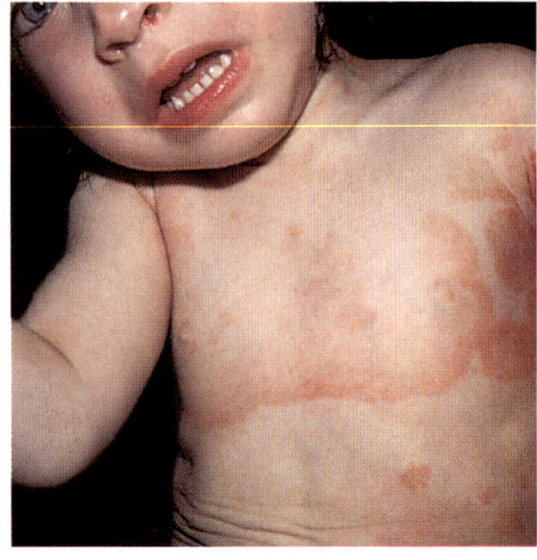

FIG. 17-15 *Urticarial plaques in annular configuration, as well as discrete papules and vesicles.*

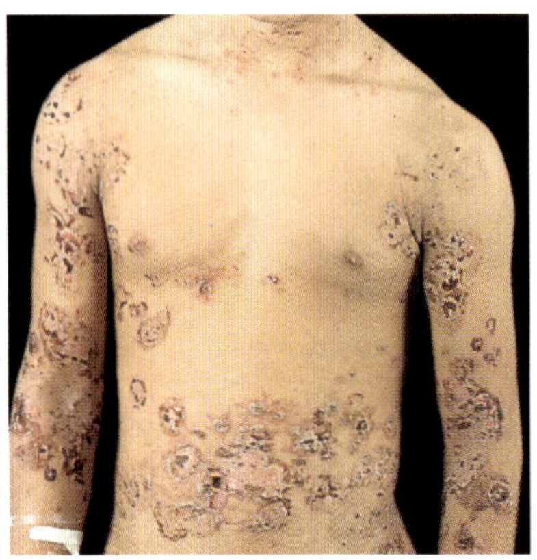

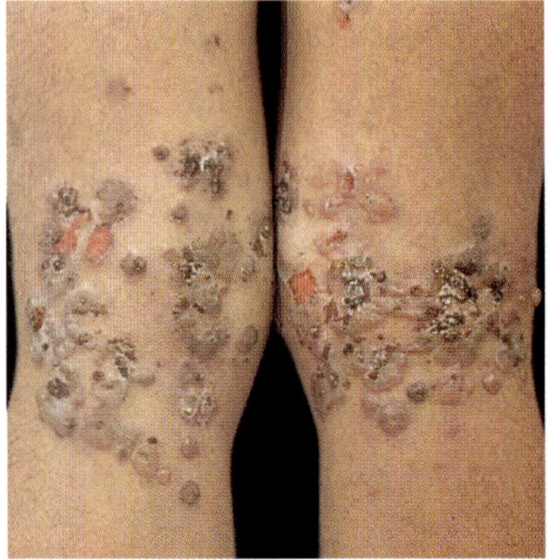

FIG. 17-16 (A, B) *Scale-crusts and hyperpigmentation in arcuate and annular configuration on the arms and trunk, and vesicles, crusts, and ulcers on the legs.*

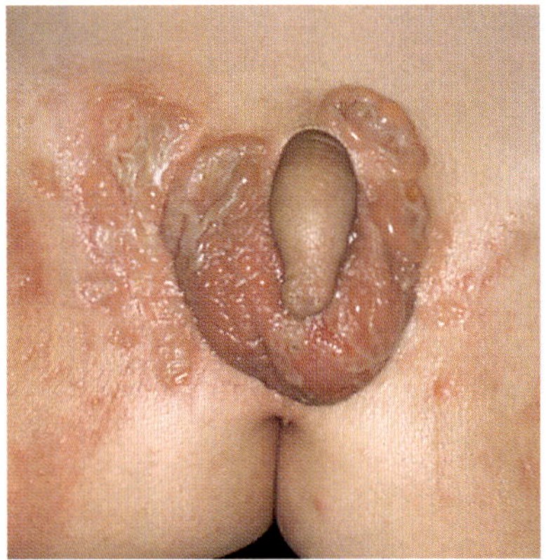

FIG. 17-17 *Vesicles, some of them in annular configuration, bullae, and erosions.*

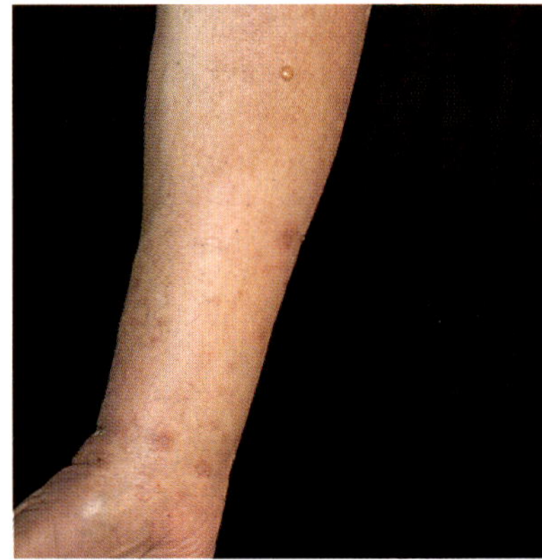

FIG. 17-18 *Papules, ill-defined plaques, and a tense vesicle.*

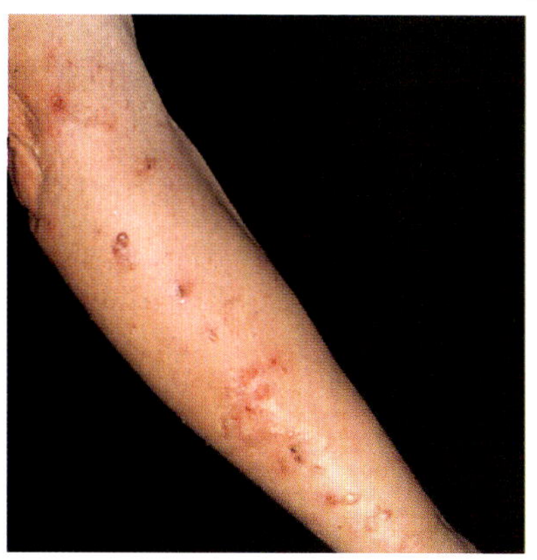

FIG. 17-19 *Papules, vesicles, erosions, and ulceration.*

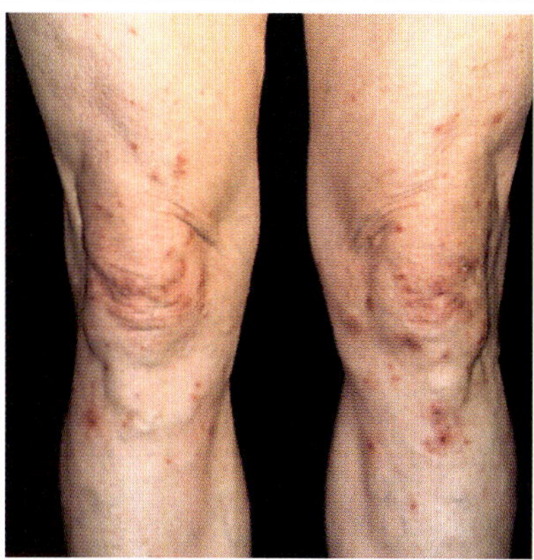

FIG. 17-20 *Papules, some of them excoriated, in clusters.*

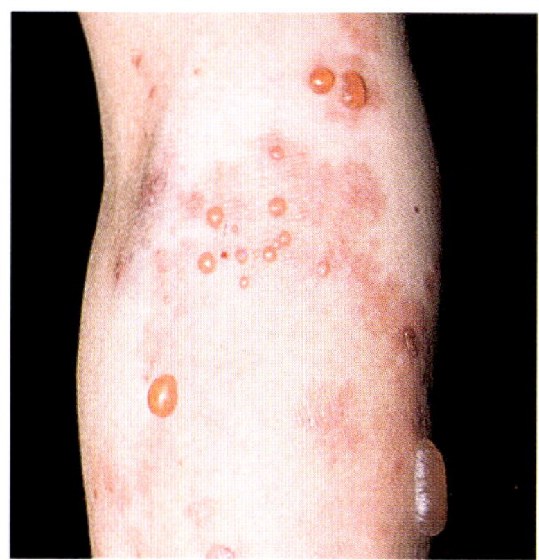

FIG. 17-21 *Vesicles and a bulla, most of them on an erythematous patch.*

ADJUNCTIVE DIAGNOSTIC TEST Direct immunofluorescence test to demonstrate linear deposits of IgA at the basement membrane.

COURSE The fundamental lesions of linear IgA dermatosis are urticarial papules, vesicles, and bullae, some of which may be large. The individual papules tend to last for no more than several weeks, and the vesicles and bullae even more briefly. Papules resolve without residua, whereas vesicles and bullae involute with crusts before healing as hyperpigmented or hypopigmented macules and patches. The disease itself is characterized by remissions and exacerbations, but may go on for years.

INTEGRATION: UNIFYING CONCEPT Histopathologic findings in papules and blisters of linear IgA dermatosis, in times past known as bullous dermatosis of childhood, are indistinguishable from those of dermatitis herpetiformis. Neutrophils are present in collections in dermal papillae and in subepidermal spaces, as well as in subepidermal blisters. Eosinophils follow neutrophils into the upper part of the dermis and into subepidermal blisters. Although linear deposits of IgA are discernible at the basement membrane zone of both dermatitis herpetiformis and linear IgA dermatosis, the deposits are granular in the former and linear in the latter. The cause of linear IgA dermatosis, like that of dermatitis herpetiformis, is not known.

THERAPY Dapsone is the treatment of choice. An alternative method is a combination of systemic corticosteroids and an immunosuppressant such as azathioprine.

DEFINITION An inflammatory process that develops secondary to trauma, usually in the form of a penetrating injury or rupture of a follicle, and that proceeds through stages of granulation tissue with numerous extravasated erythrocytes, granulomatous inflammation, and fibrosis. As is the case for other fibrosing dermatitides, such as scars and keloids, papules and nodules of dermatofibroma shrink in time and resolve as hyperpigmented macules, some of which even may be delled.

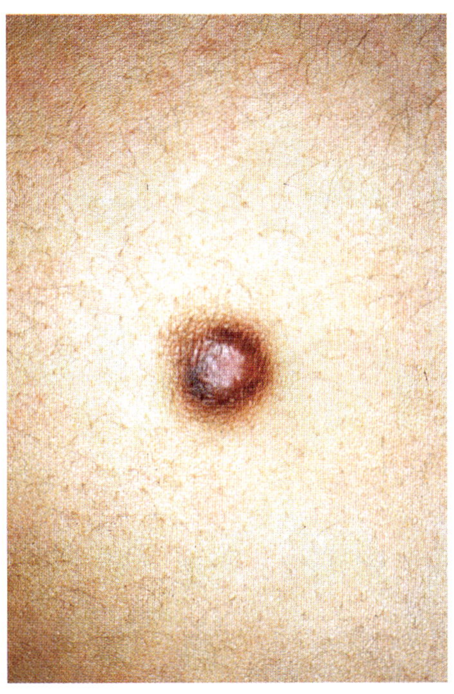

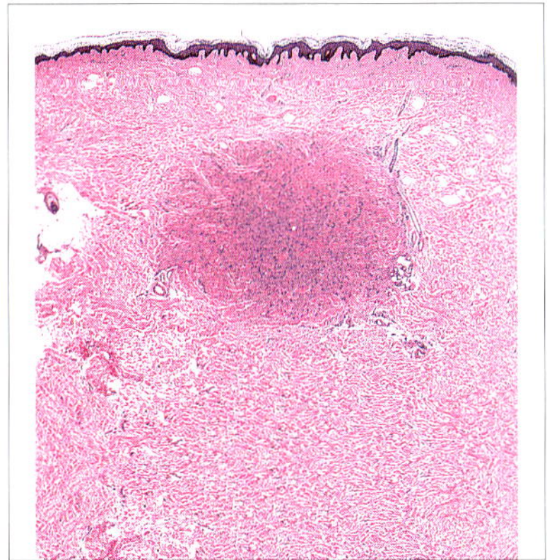

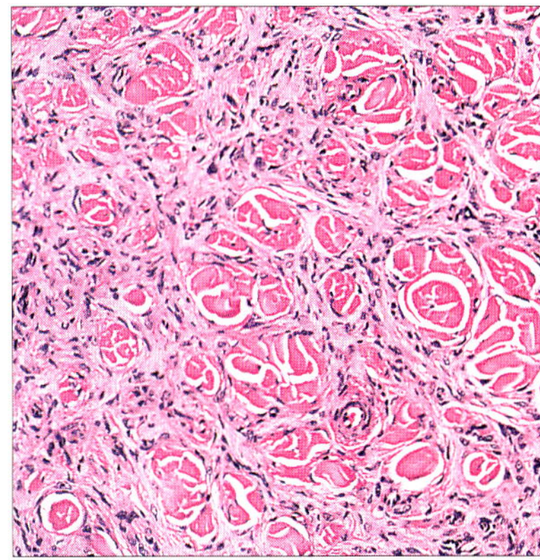

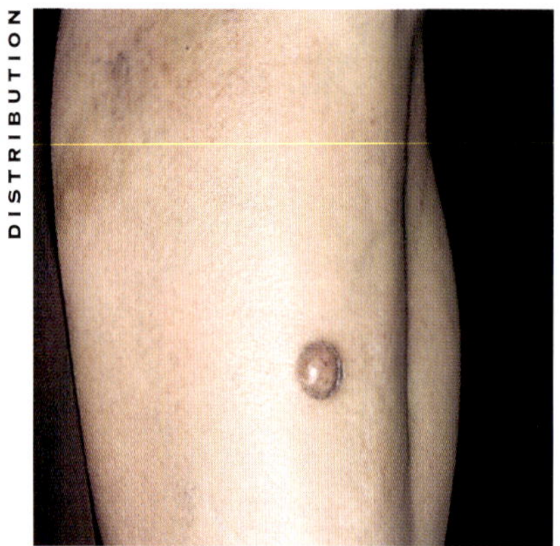

FIG. 18-1 *Dome-shaped pigmented nodule.*

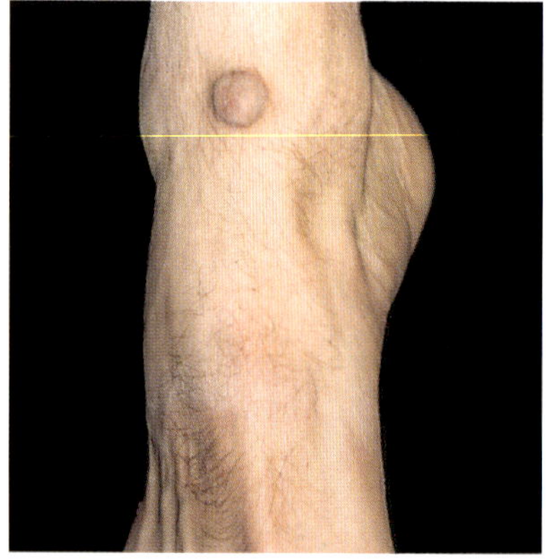

FIG. 18-2 *Dome-shaped pigmented nodule.*

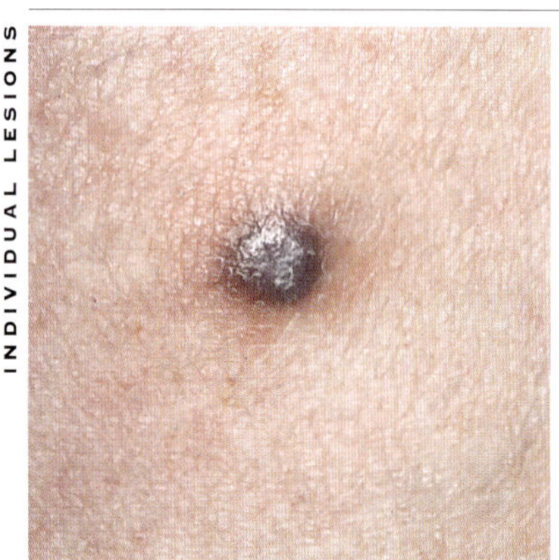

FIG. 18-3 *Hemorrhagic scaly papule.*

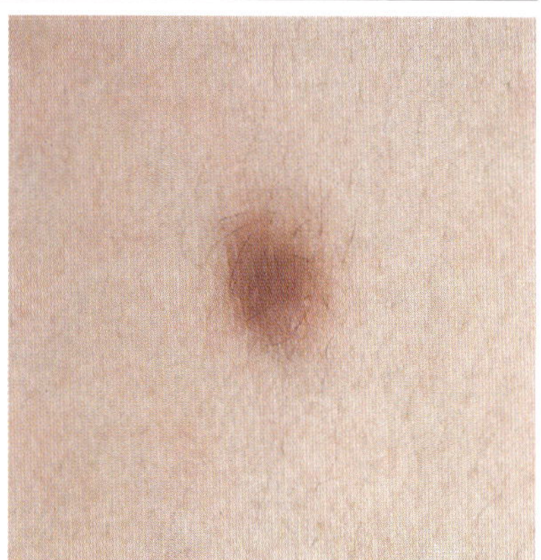

FIG. 18-4 *Rust-colored, smooth-surfaced papule.*

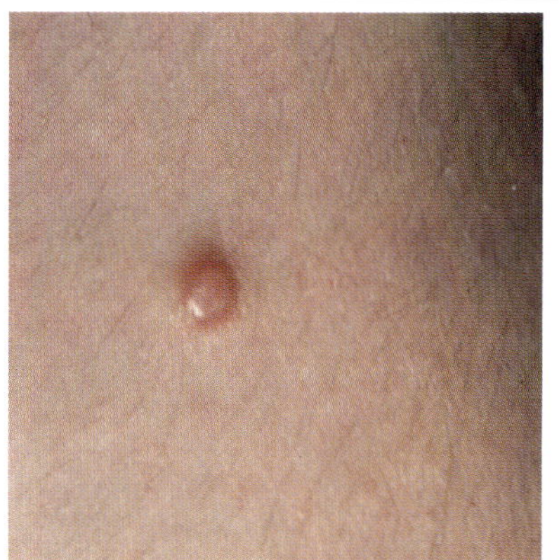

FIG. 18-5 *Gray, smooth-surfaced papule with a red-brown rim.*

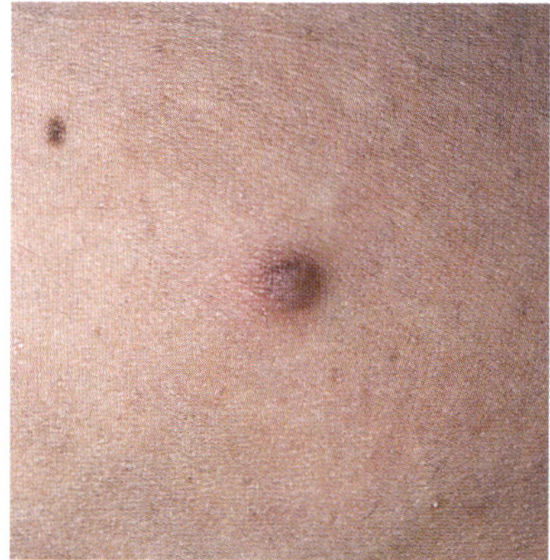

FIG. 18-6 *Dusky red, smooth-surfaced papule. A Clark's nevus is above and to the left of it.*

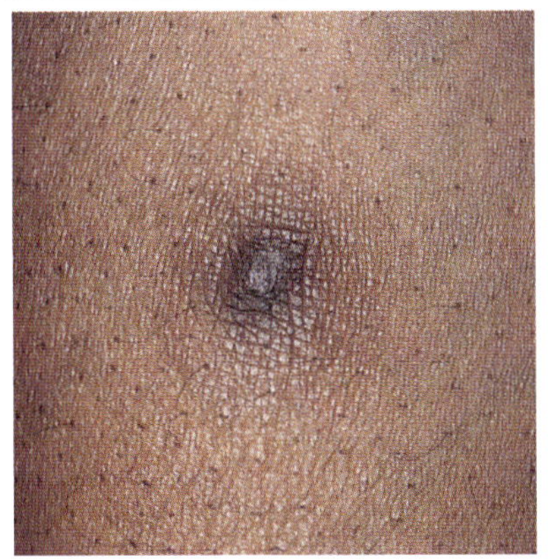

FIG. 18-7 *Dark brown papule.*

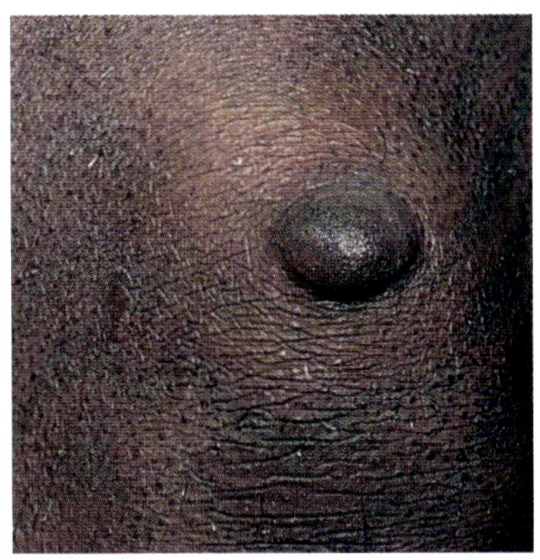

FIG. 18-8 *Dark brown, smooth-surfaced nodule.*

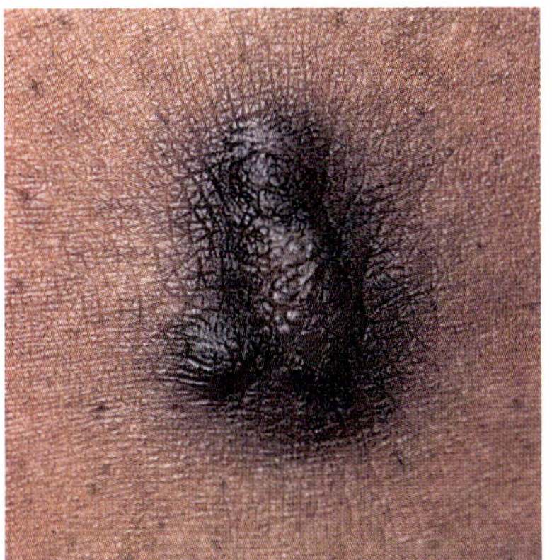

FIG. 18-9 *Black nodule upon which lichen simplex chronicus has been imposed.*

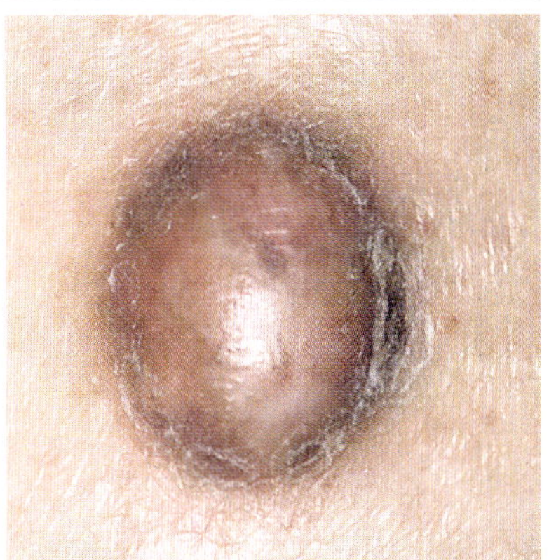

FIG. 18-10 *Chocolate brown, slightly scaly, dome-shaped nodule.*

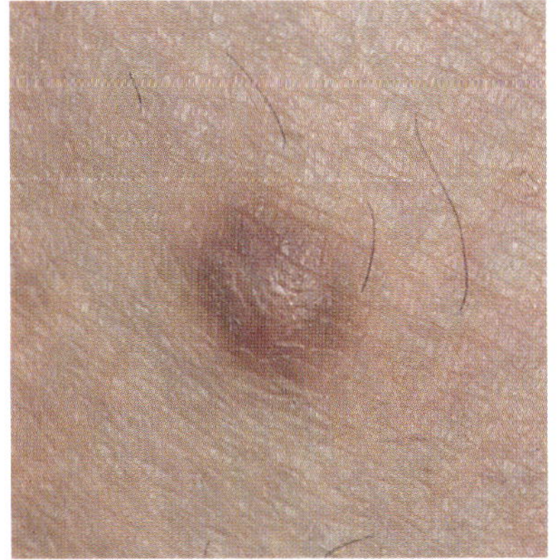

FIG. 18-11 *Reddish brown, slightly dome-shaped papule with accentuated skin markings.*

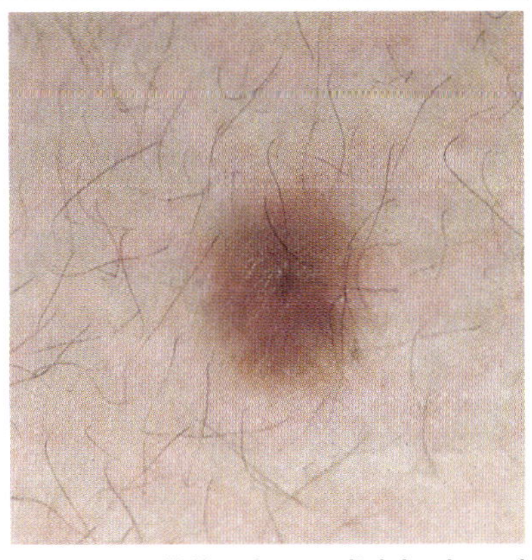

FIG. 18-12 *Yellow-brown slightly elevated papule.*

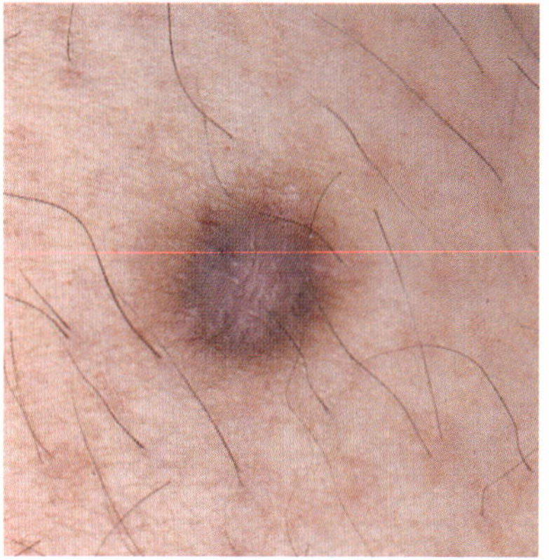

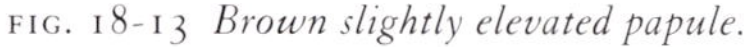

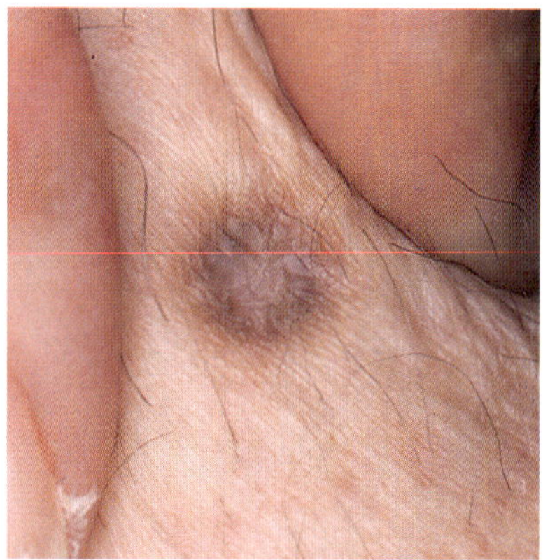

FIG. 18-13 *Brown slightly elevated papule.*　　FIG. 18-14 *Brown papule.*

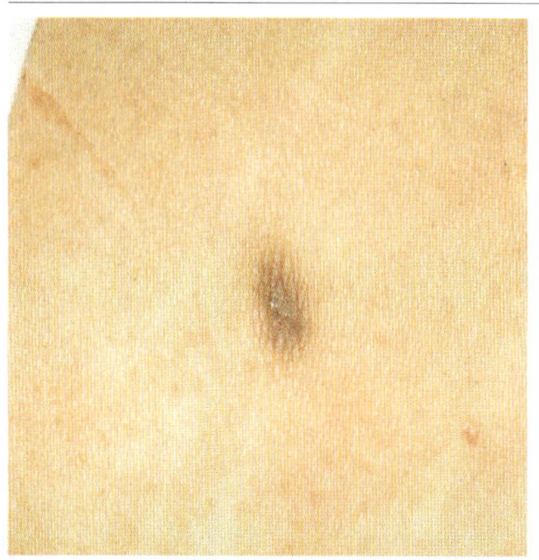

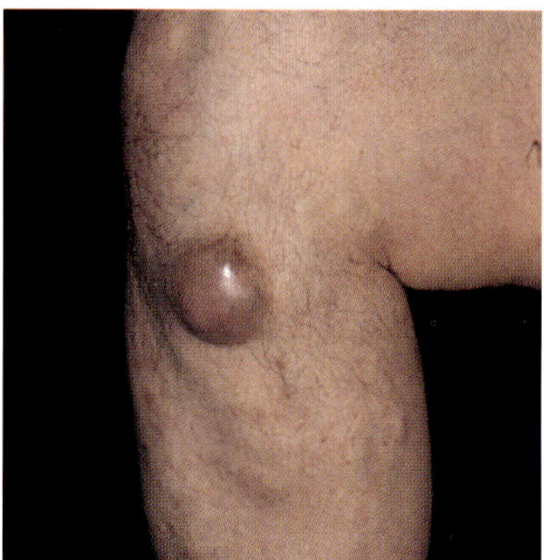

FIG. 18-15 *Brown delled macule ("dimple sign").*　　FIG. 18-16 *Reddish-brown nodule.*

COURSE Dermatofibroma begins as a dusky red macule that quickly becomes a papule composed mostly of granulation tissue in company with innumerable extravasated erythrocytes within the dermis. Soon macrophages appear in abundance, and by ingestion of components of blood acquire the attributes of siderophages and lipophages. The lesion may become nodular and even tumorous, and progressively more firm as a consequence of production of altered collagen by proliferating fibrocytes. In time, fibroplasia predominates over granulomatous inflammation, and as more melanin is formed within the epidermis, the hard, dome-shaped lesion becomes browner. In time, after many years, the lesion slowly flattens consequent to shrinkage by fibroplasia. Sometimes the shrinkage is so great that the lesion at last is a hyperpigmented dell.

INTEGRATION: UNIFYING CONCEPT Dermatofibroma is a distinctive type of granulomatous and fibrosing inflammation that results from trauma of some kind— a penetrating injury, for example, an insect "bite," or rupture of a follicle or a follicular cyst. Because the condition looks so different histopathologically (and also clinically) at different stages of its evolution and devolution, it has been given a variety of names, among them, sclerosing hemangioma (for the stage of granulation tissue), histiocytoma (for the stage of granulomatous inflammation with siderophages and lipophages), dermatofibroma (for the stage in which fibrosis is dominant), and subepidermal nodular sclerosis (for the end of the fibrotic stage). Dermatofibroma differs from other types of fibrosing inflammation that follow trauma, such as scar and keloid, by passing invariably through a stage of granulomatous inflammation. During that stage, histiocytes may sport strikingly abnormal nuclei, for which reason that expression of dermatofibroma is sometimes called "dermatofibroma with monster cells."

THERAPY None, unless a lesion grows to several centimeters in diameter, when simple surgical excision may be indicated.

DEFINITION A malignant nonepithelial neoplasm (a sarcoma) presumably of perineural fibrocytes that presents itself usually on the trunk, but sometimes elsewhere, such as the extremities, face, and scalp. A papule of it tends to become a plaque, a nodule, a tumor, or all of them concurrently. Sometimes a plaque is interspersed with many nodules and tumors in a cluster. The sarcoma is "low grade," i.e., it metastasizes only episodically and then rarely beyond lymph nodes, but it can also kill by destruction locally, e.g., by penetrating the calvarium and entering the brain.

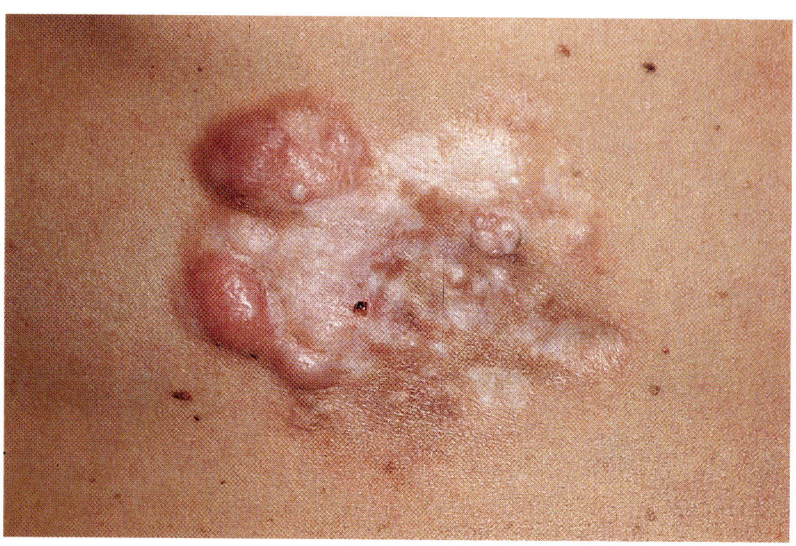

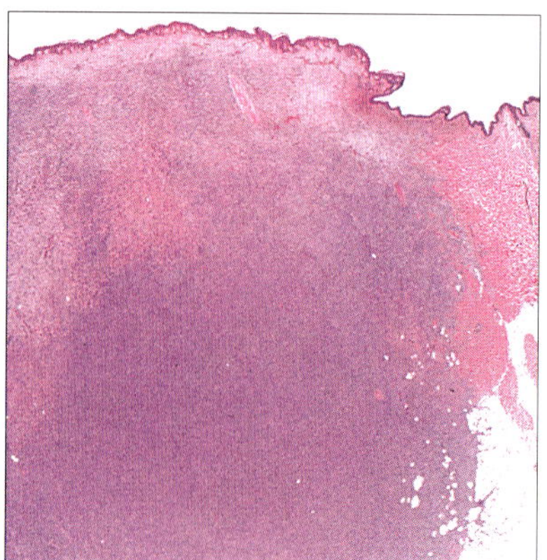

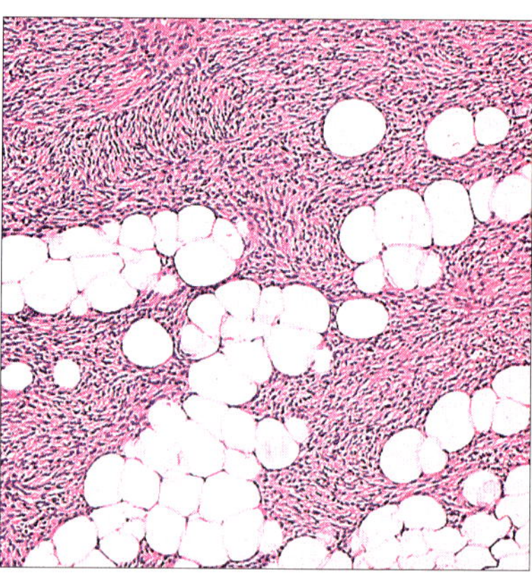

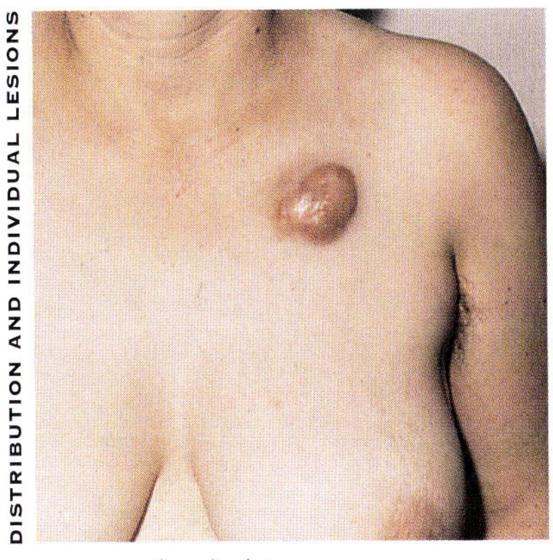

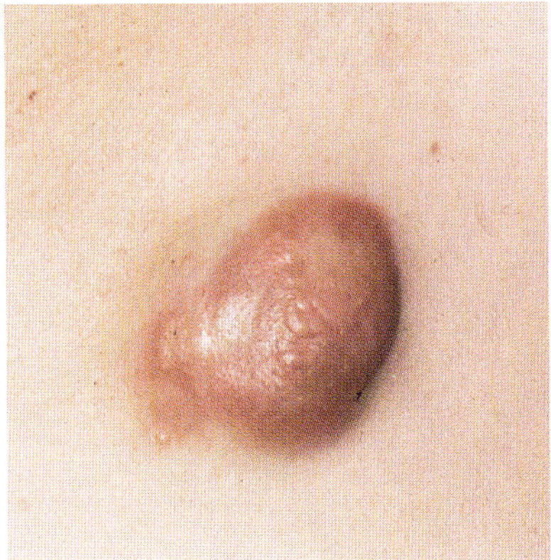

FIG. 19-1 (A, B) *A tumor.*

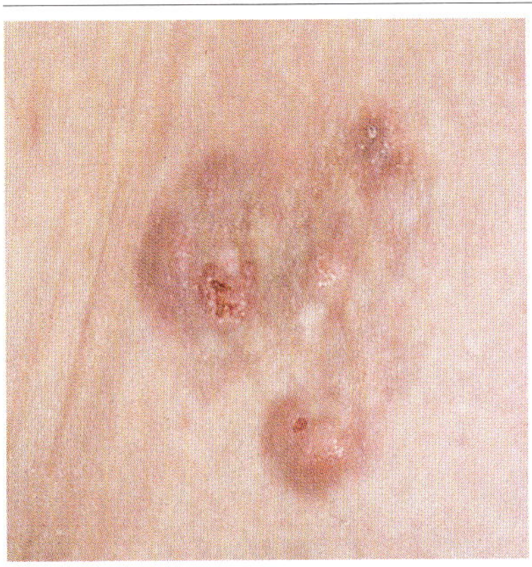

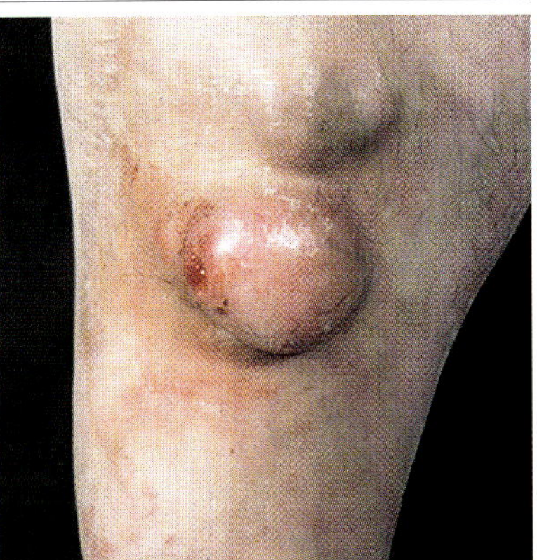

FIG. 19-2 *A patch atop which are papules and nodules, some of them ulcerated, on the abdomen.*

FIG. 19-3 *Tumors atop a plaque.*

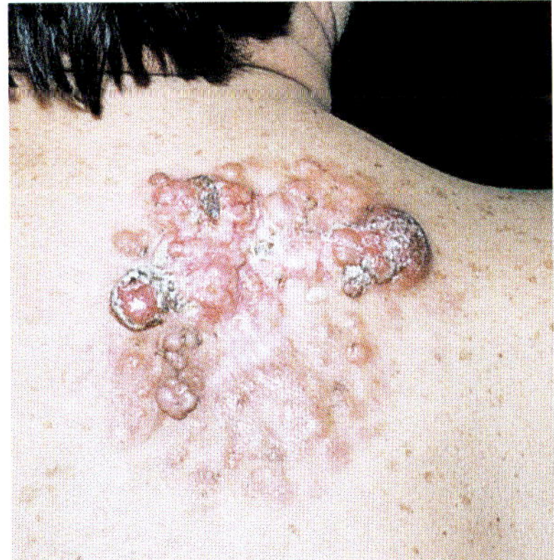

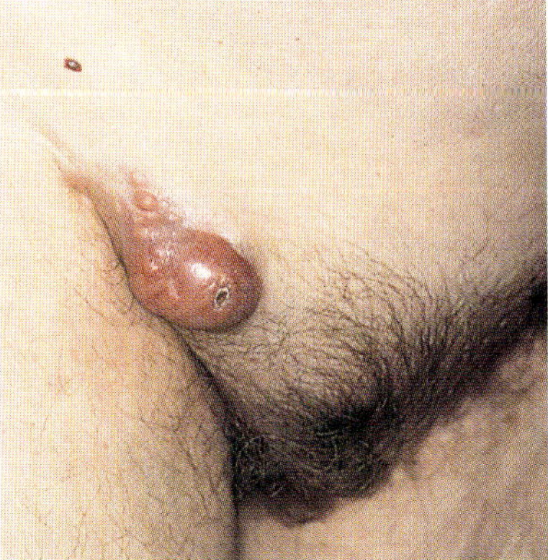

FIG. 19-4 *Agminated papules, nodules, and tumors. The scar in the center is from previous surgery.*

FIG. 19-5 *Tumor in continuity with a plaque and with papules.*

COURSE Dermatofibrosarcoma protuberans, because it is a malignant neoplasm, is relentless in its growth, although that advance tends to be slow. The neoplasm, like virtually all malignant neoplasms, begins as a macule that becomes a papule and, in time, a nodule and tumor. Often the neoplasm attains huge size, and nearly always is multinodular with a very uneven surface. As the neoplasm becomes increasingly exophytic, it also becomes progressively endophytic, extending from its site of origin in the dermis into the subcutaneous fat and into structures beneath it, such as fascia, skeletal muscle, and even bone itself. Once neoplastic cells of dermatofibrosarcoma protuberans have penetrated the bone of the skull, the patient affected is practically doomed. The brain becomes compromised progressively by virtue of the irrepressible assault upon it by neoplastic cells.

INTEGRATION: UNIFYING CONCEPT As the name denotes, dermatofibrosarcoma protuberans is a sarcoma, i.e., a nonepithelial malignant neoplasm. For reasons not understood, no matter how deep neoplastic cells extend, even into fascia, skeletal muscle, and bone, it does not usually metastasize. Nonetheless, in some instances, probably less than 5 percent of all examples, metastasis does occur, but then usually not beyond regional lymph nodes. Episodically, however, metastases may be widespread and death may ensue.

Clinically, dermatofibrosarcoma protuberans is hardly ever seen by a physician when it is still a papule. By the time patients present themselves to a physician, the lesion usually is nodular and sometimes tumorous. At times, the lesion is multilobate or a plaque upon which nodules and tumors have formed. Although the trunk is the site of predilection, any part of the skin, including the face, may be affected.

All of the clinical expressions of dermatofibrosarcoma protuberans show the same basic histopathologic changes, namely, short fascicles of nonepithelial cells that interweave in a storiform pattern. The cells themselves have thin nuclei that often are wavy. Hardly ever is there nuclear atypia and mitotic figures are few. Almost always, by the time a biopsy specimen has been obtained, the process involves the entire dermis diffusely, and usually much of the subcutaneous fat. In the fat, a characteristic fenestrated pattern is formed by struts made up of neoplastic tissue like that which has replaced much of the dermis, namely, wavy nuclei and scant cytoplasm of neoplastic cells and delicate fibrillary bundles of collagen.

There are many variants, histopathologically, of dermatofibrosarcoma protuberans, among them extensively mucinous and association with markedly pigmented bipolar dendritic melanocytes (Bednar's tumor). Other variants include zones in which there are numerous multinucleate cells that have been compared to the appearance of a flower, i.e., "floret cells" (giant-cell fibroblastoma). In short, all of these are merely morphologic variants of dermatofibrosarcoma protuberans.

In rare examples of dermatofibrosarcoma protuberans, another sarcoma may develop, to wit, malignant fibrous histiocytoma or fibrosarcoma. In that event, the prognosis changes from a relatively good one for dermatofibrosarcoma protuberans alone to a relatively bad one. We do not conceive of the phenomenon as either "conversion" or "transformation" of dermatofibrosarcoma protuberans, but simply as an expression of a particular pathologic process.

The essential cell in the sarcoma known as dermatofibrosarcoma protuberans has yet to be identified with precision. We infer on the basis of the wavy character of nuclei and the delicate fibrillary bundles of collagen, features seen often in neoplasms with neural differentiation, that it is a perineural fibrocyte. The presence of indubitable melanocytes within the substance of some examples of dermatofibrosarcoma protuberans gives further credence to this hypothesis. That dermatofibrosarcoma protuberans is not fundamentally a sarcoma with neural differentiation can be concluded from the fact that the neoplasm is negative for all immunoperoxidase stains said to be specific for neural differentiation.

Despite the similarities in appellation, dermatofibrosarcoma protuberans is completely unrelated to dermatofibroma. The former is a sarcoma, whereas the latter is an expression of granulomatous and fibrosing inflammation.

THERAPY Complete surgical excision is mandatory. Margins of excision must be scrutinized by a histopathologist in order to ensure that they are free of neoplastic cells. Not uncommonly, those cells extend to one or more margins of the specimen, which signifies inevitable persistence at the local site if additional curative surgery is not performed.

DEFINITION An inflammatory disease of children and adults that tends to involve skin and skeletal muscle mostly, the findings in the skin being patches with the color of heliotrope, especially in the periocular region. The disease manifests itself as poikiloderma on the extremities, as papules that tend to become atrophic on the dorsum of the joints of fingers, and in muscles as weakness, especially of shoulder and pelvic girdles. The disease seems to be immunologic in character and, in adults, is often a response to a malignant neoplasm situated in an internal organ.

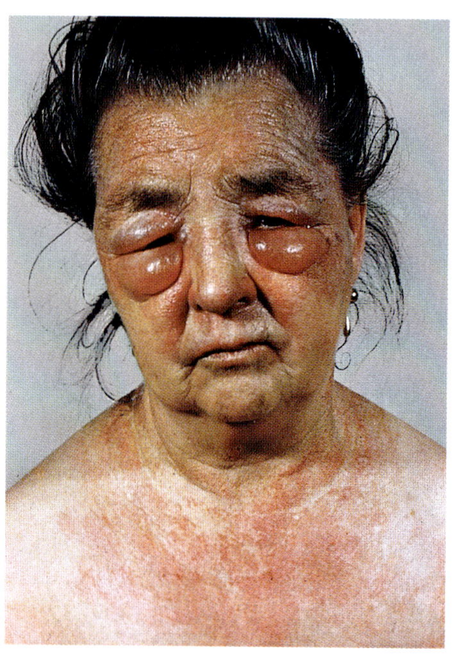

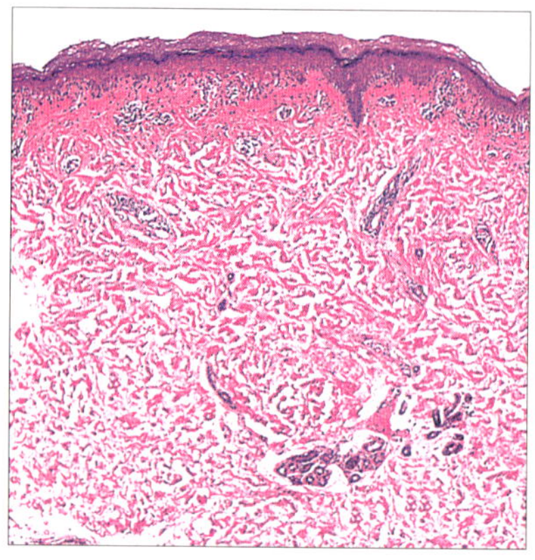

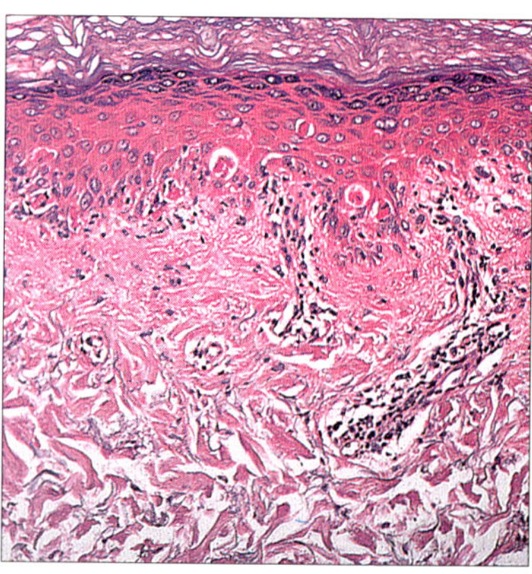

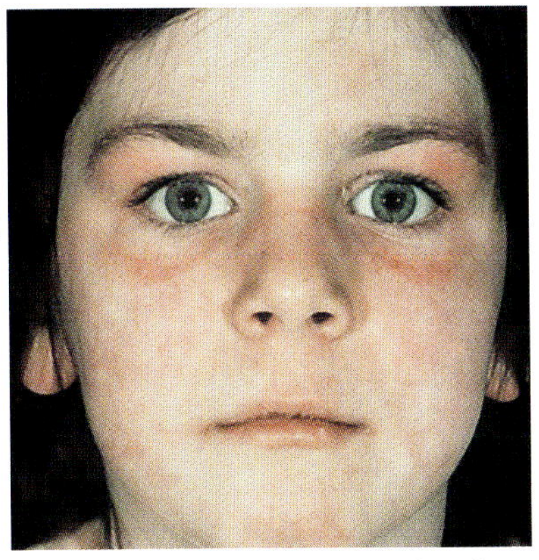

FIG. 20-1 *Symmetrical patches of erythema accompanied by slight periorbital swelling.*

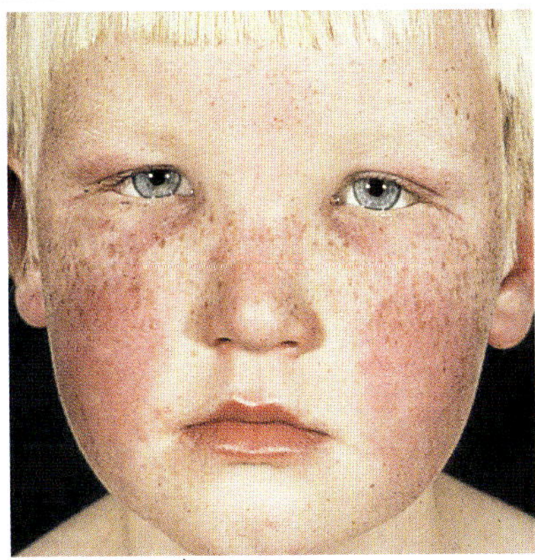

FIG. 20-2 *Symmetrical patches of erythema in periorbital distribution.*

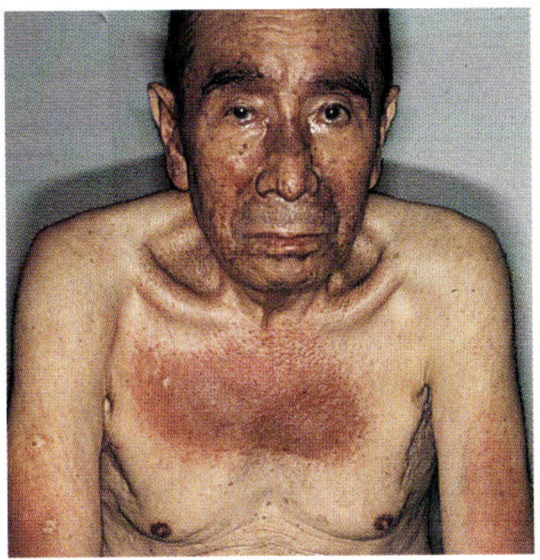

FIG. 20-3 *Patches of dusky erythema on the face, chest, and dorsal surface of the arms.*

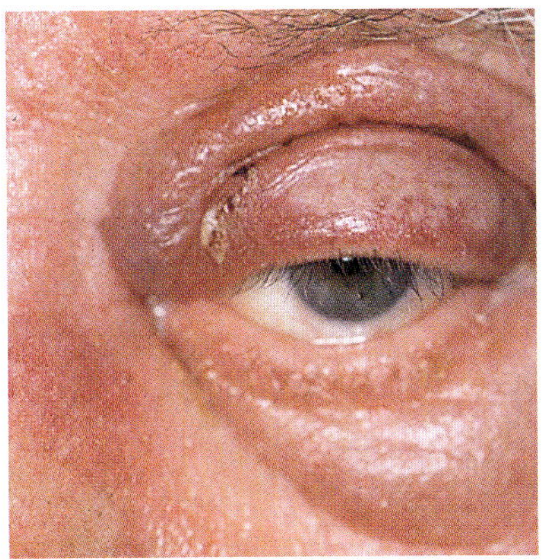

FIG. 20-4 *Erythema, telangiectases, and marked periorbital edema.*

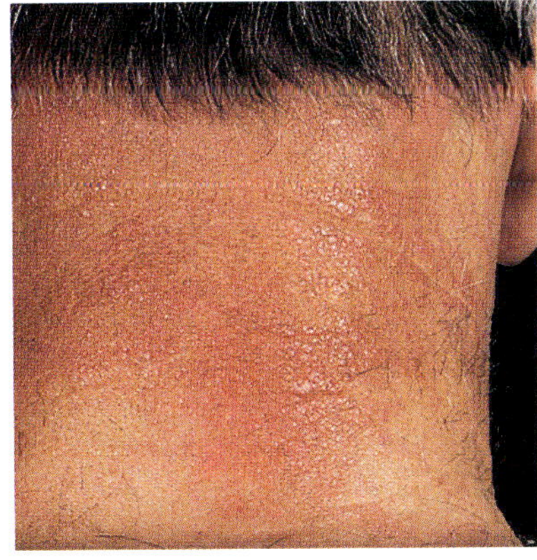

FIG. 20-5 *Dusky erythema.*

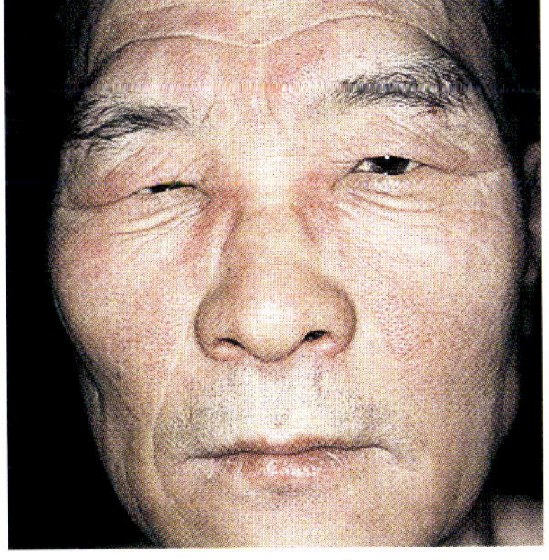

FIG. 20-6 *Patchy dusky erythema and periorbital swelling.*

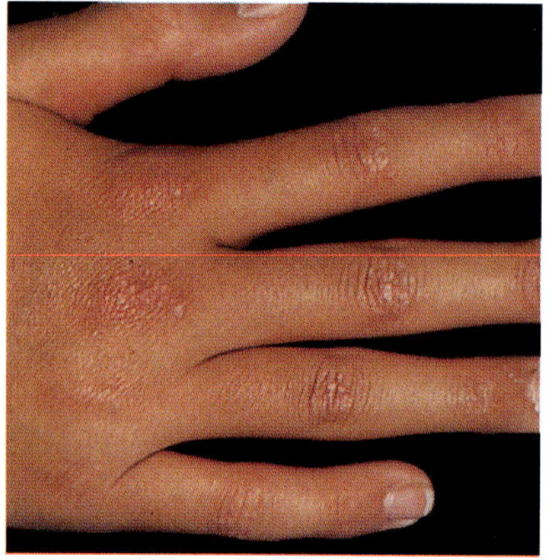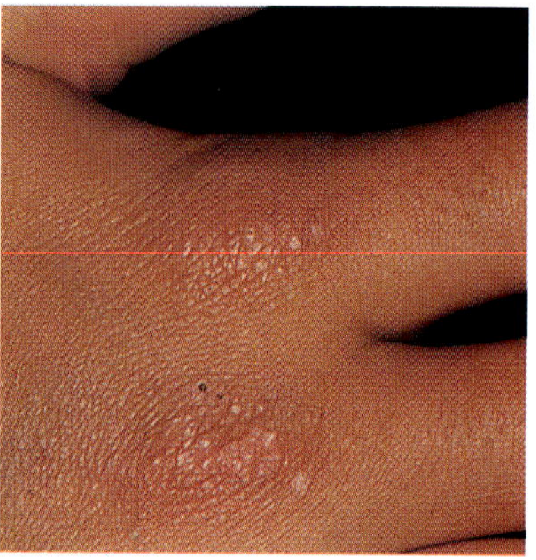

FIG. 20-7 (A, B) *White, flat-topped papules over the knuckles.*

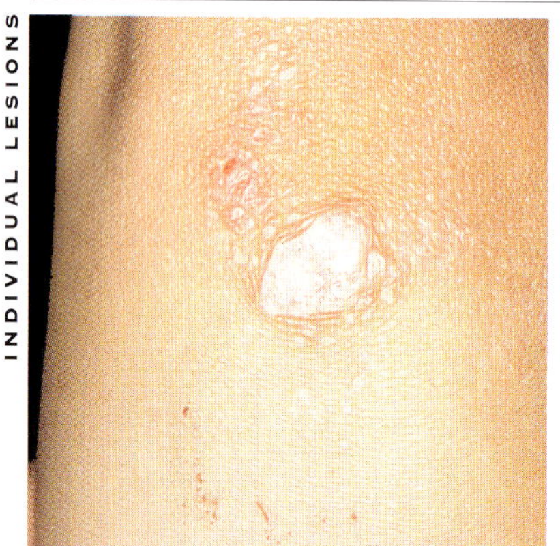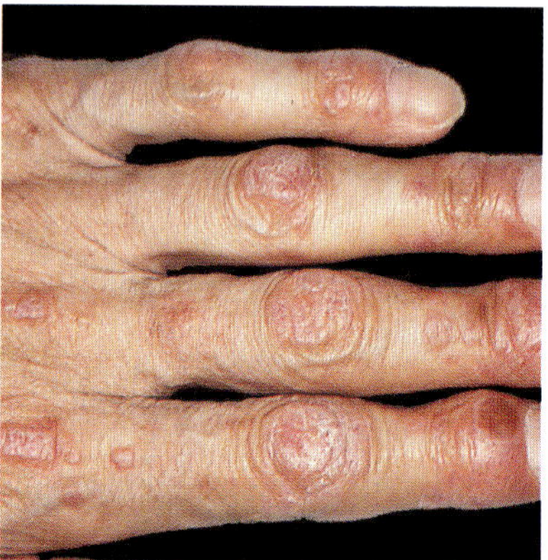

FIG. 20-8 *White, flat-topped papules and a white, flat-topped plaque.*

FIG. 20-9 *Scaly papules and plaques on the dorsa of the hands and fingers (Gottron's papules).*

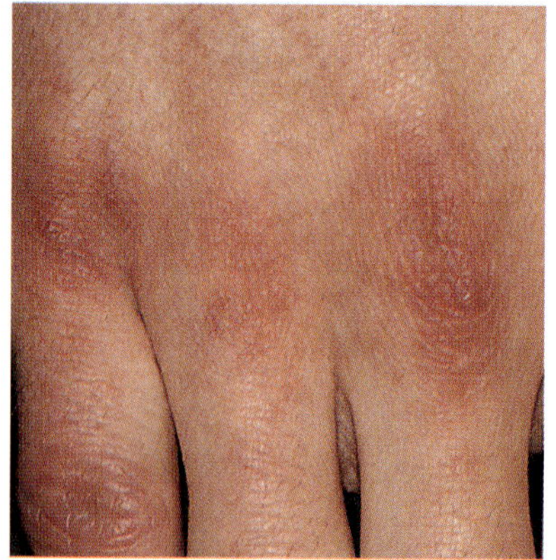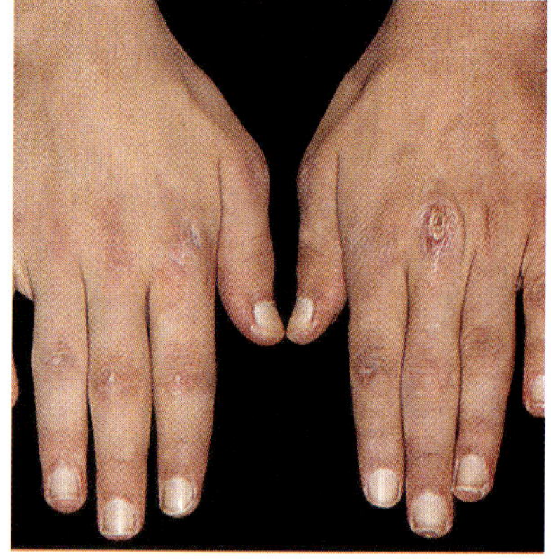

FIG. 20-10 *Erythematous macules and papules.*

FIG. 20-11 *Raynaud's phenomenon and foci of calcification.*

INDIVIDUAL LESIONS

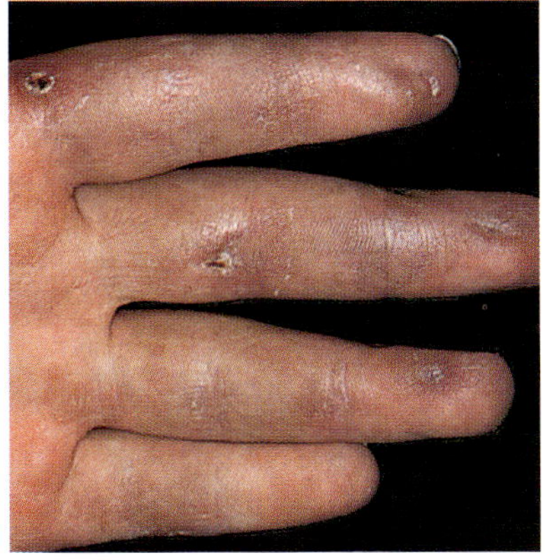

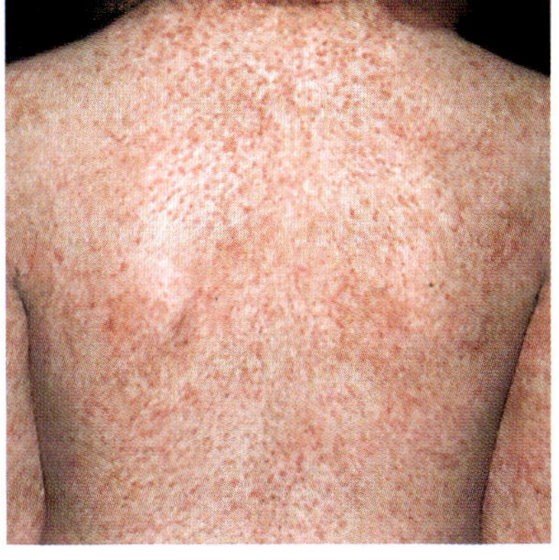

FIG. 20-12 *Raynaud's phenomenon, small depressed scars, and crusts. Beneath the crusts are deposits of calcium.*

FIG. 20-13 *Widespread poikiloderma.*

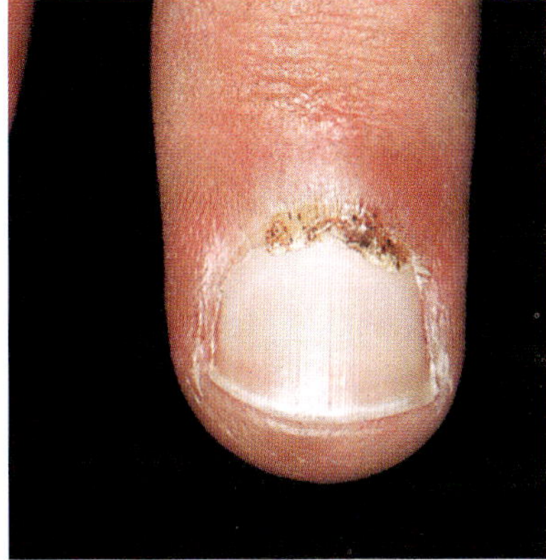

FIG. 20-14 *Petechiae and telangiectases in a thickened erythematous posterior nail fold and in lateral nail folds.*

ADJUNCTIVE DIAGNOSTIC TESTS Worthwhile are immunoserological assessment of levels of antinuclear antibodies (autoantibodies to Jo-1 and autoantibodies to Mi-2) and determination of levels of muscle enzymes (serum creatine kinase and serum aldolase). Electromyography and muscle biopsy are also valuable in establishing the diagnosis.

COURSE The lesions of dermatomyositis in children and adults are similar, namely, first redness and swelling, then the appearance of telangiectases, and later resolution, often with atrophy, hyperpigmentation and hypopigmentation, and telangiectases (poikiloderma). If lesions are treated early and effectively enough, they may completely regress when they are still red and edematous, and leave no residuum.

The course of dermatomyositis varies dramatically, from complete recovery, even without treatment, to rapid progression, in a matter of months, to death. Some patients neither recover rapidly nor die quickly; they have a long course marked by progressive disability in the form of profound weakness, deformities of extremities, and deposits of calcium in skin and muscle.

Rarely, skin lesions occur in the absence of muscle disease (amyopathic dermatomyositis).

INTEGRATION: UNIFYING CONCEPT The skin lesions of dermatomyositis are protean, ranging from discrete telangiectases, especially on the face but also in posterior nail folds, through innumerable closely approximated telangiectases on the eyelids that cause the skin to have a purplish ("heliotrope") hue, to poikiloderma and calcification. The eyelid changes almost always are accompanied, early in the course of the disease, by profound edema. When erythema, edema, and telangiectases of the skin of extremities and of the face especially persist for many months, the result is poikiloderma. Calcification is apparent readily as chalk-white material that extrudes from the skin.

Histopathologic findings in various clinical expressions of dermatomyositis, such as erythema, edema, and poikiloderma, are very similar to those in various lesions of lupus erythematosus. In both diseases, relatively early lesions are characterized by sparse infiltrates of lymphocytes around venules of the superficial plexus, a sprinkling of lymphocytes along the dermoepidermal junction in conjunction with vacuolar alteration there, a smudged appearance of the dermoepidermal junction, and a thinned epidermis devoid of discrete rete ridges. Later, lesions of both diseases are typified by a thickened basement membrane that is situated between epithelium (epidermal and adnexal) and dermis.

The epidermis, which may be extraordinarily thin in foci, exhibits variable amounts of compact orthokeratosis. At all stages of lesions of both dermatomyositis and lupus erythematosus, abundant mucin may be present in the reticular dermis. Unlike the situation in lupus erythematosus, however, the infiltrates of lymphocytes in dermatomyositis tend to be sparse and to involve only the venules of the superficial plexus, not the deep one.

The same histopathologic findings that typify lesions of dermatomyositis on eyelids and extremities, and that culminate in poikiloderma, also are seen in Gottron's papules and on posterior nail folds. The crucial findings for histopathologic diagnosis in each of those lesions are found at the dermoepidermal junction, especially a smudged appearance and a thickened basement membrane, and in the epidermis that is thinned focally.

Calcium is seen by conventional microscopy as chunks of purple material unassociated with infiltrates of inflammatory cells in a reticular dermis.

Skeletal muscle affected by dermatomyositis is characterized histopathologically by patchy infiltrates of lymphocytes that, in time, wane and are followed by permanent alteration of myofibrils.

The cause of dermatomyositis in more than 50 percent of adults over 40 years of age is an internal malignancy, usually a carcinoma, but sometimes a lymphoma. When the carcinoma is extirpated prior to development of metastases, or when a lymphoma is treated effectively, the signs of dermatomyositis in the skin and in muscle tend to disappear, except for those that are permanent, such as poikiloderma. The cause of dermatomyositis in adults who do not harbor a malignant neoplasm internally is not known. In them, as well as in children, an immunological mechanism or viral cause has been postulated.

THERAPY In adults it is necessary to search for an internal malignancy that may be causative. If one is found it should be treated expeditiously.

Systemic corticosteroids are the treatment of choice for dermatomyositis. Azathioprine may be an effective adjunct, as may be gamma globulin given intravenously at a high dosage.

DEFINITION An inflammatory process caused by superficial fungi, i.e., fungi situated superficially in the cornified layer and in other cornified structures, and expressed clinically as smooth-surfaced papules, scaly papules, scaly plaques, nodules, pustules, vesicles, and bullae. The papules, pustules, and nodules may be centered in follicles (Majocchi's granuloma). Lesions may occur on any anatomic site, but particularly on the scalp (tinea capitis), inguinal region (tinea cruris), hands (tinea manum), feet (tinea pedis), and nails (onychomycosis).

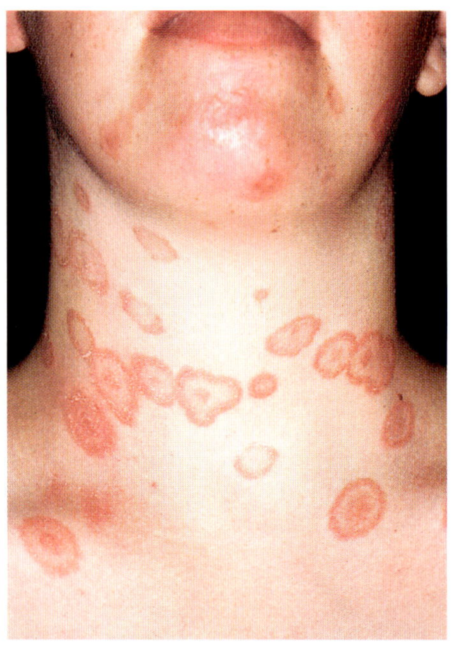

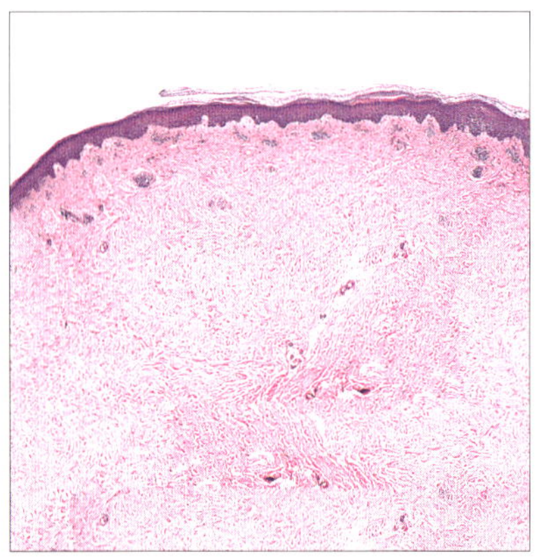

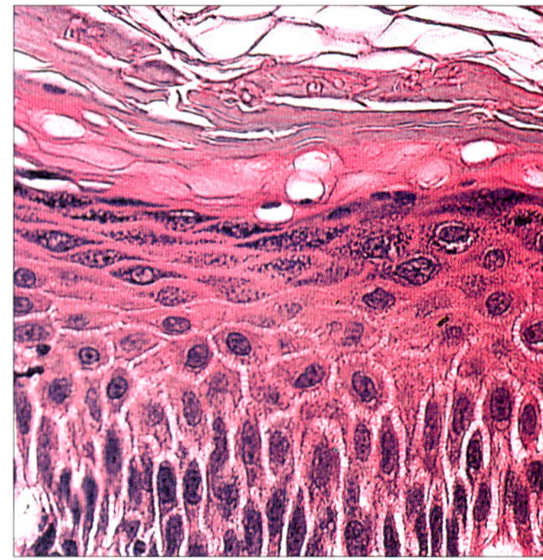

DISTRIBUTION

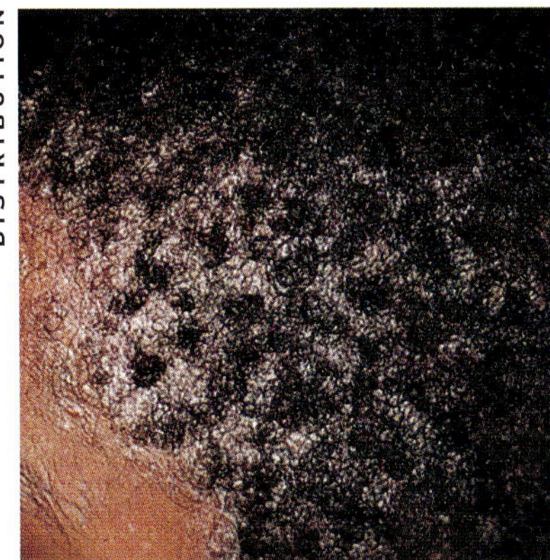

FIG. 21-1 *Scaly lesions of tinea capitis.*

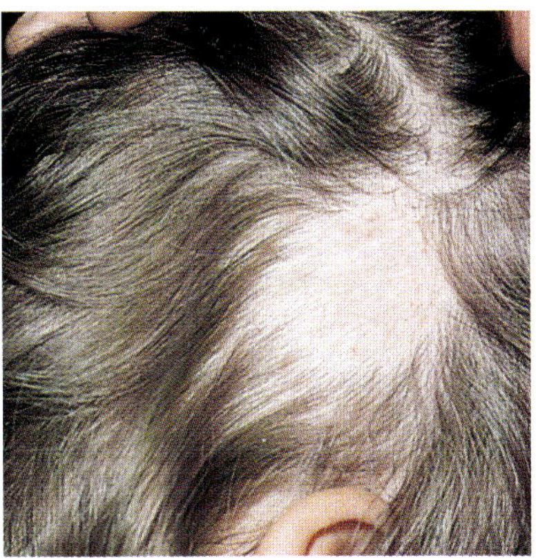

FIG. 21-2 *Alopecia with scales.*

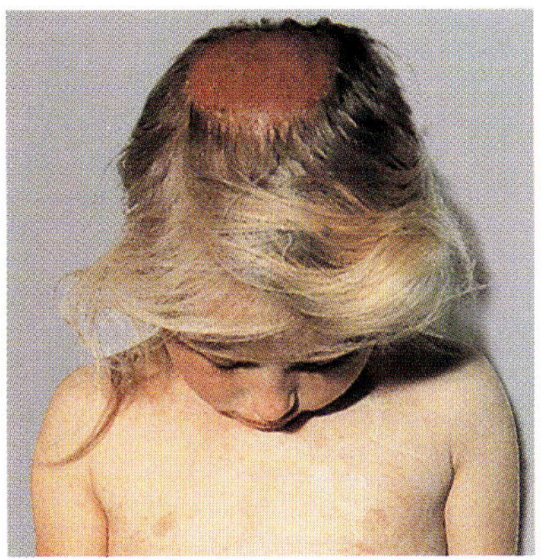

FIG. 21-3 *Alopecia with large erythematous plaque and widespread macules and papules (id reaction).*

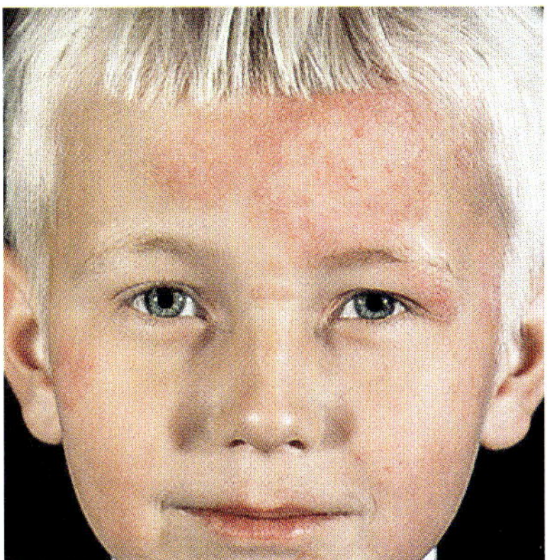

FIG. 21-4 *Papules and plaques in figurate arrangement.*

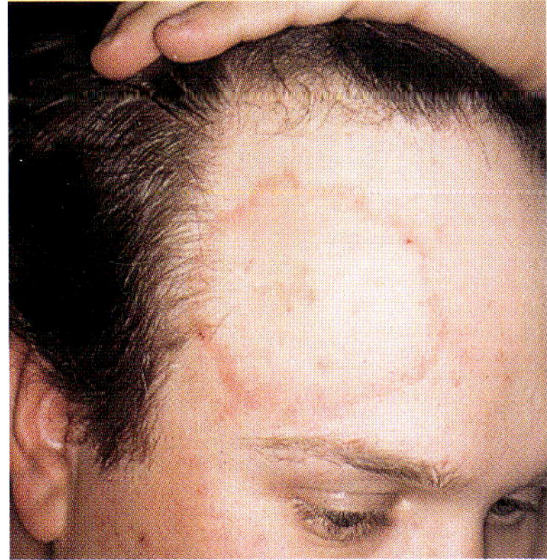

FIG. 21-5 *Plaque with annular border showing scales.*

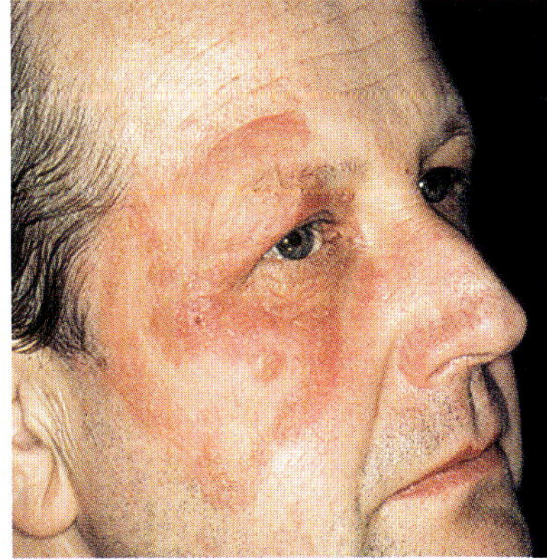

FIG. 21-6 *Papules and plaques with ill-defined borders on the forehead, nose, and cheeks.*

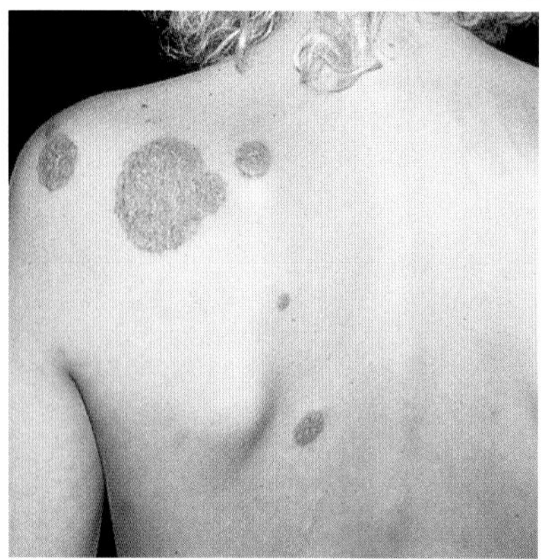

FIG. 21-7 *Erythematous scaly papules and nummular plaques.*

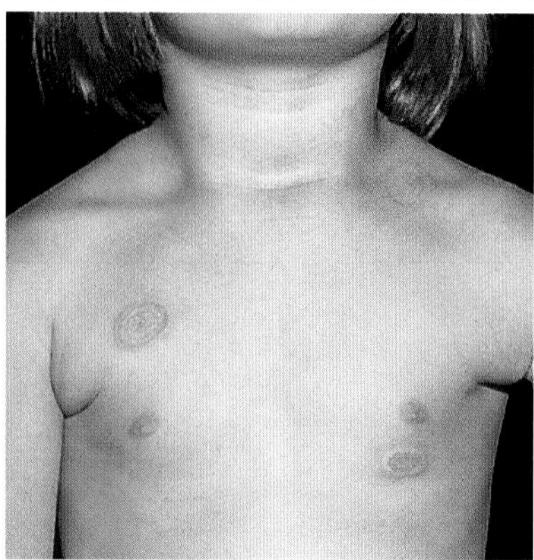

FIG. 21-8 *Erythematous scaly circinate plaques.*

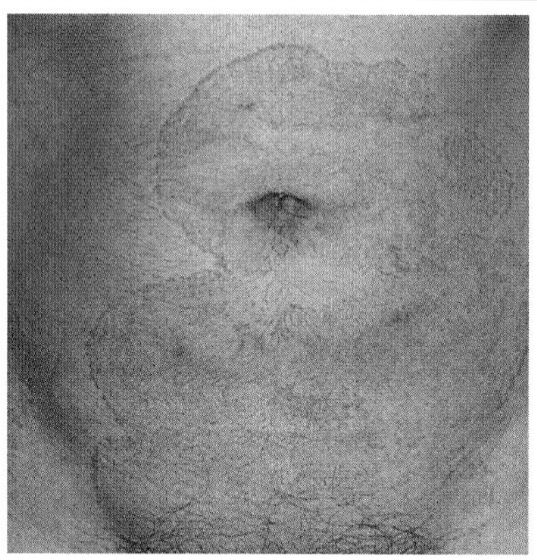

FIG. 21-9 *Arciform scaly plaques.*

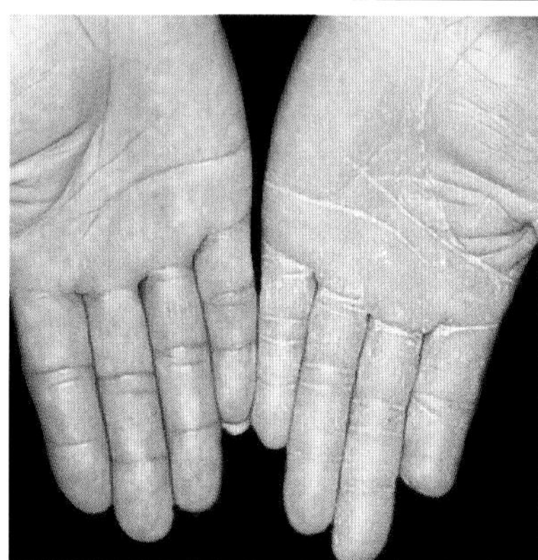

FIG. 21-10 *Scaly palms.*

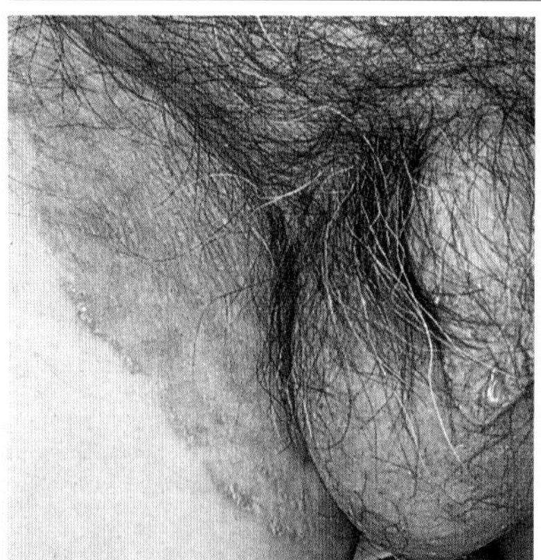

FIG. 21-11 *Erythematous scaly plaque with scalloped border.*

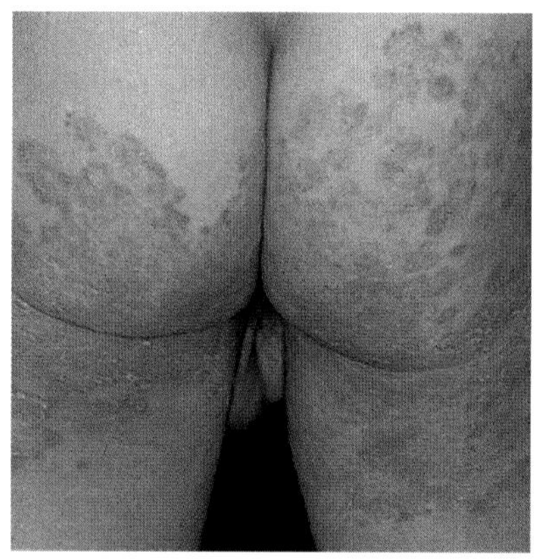

FIG. 21-12 *Erythematous scaly papules and plaques, some of them with arcuate and poly-cyclic outlines.*

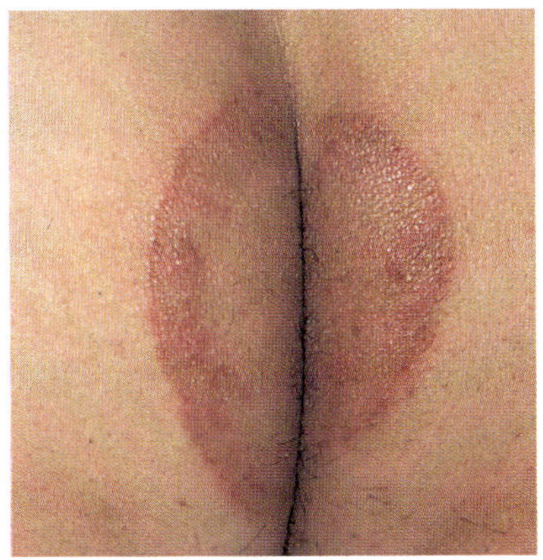

FIG. 21-13 *Patches with many papules near and at the border.*

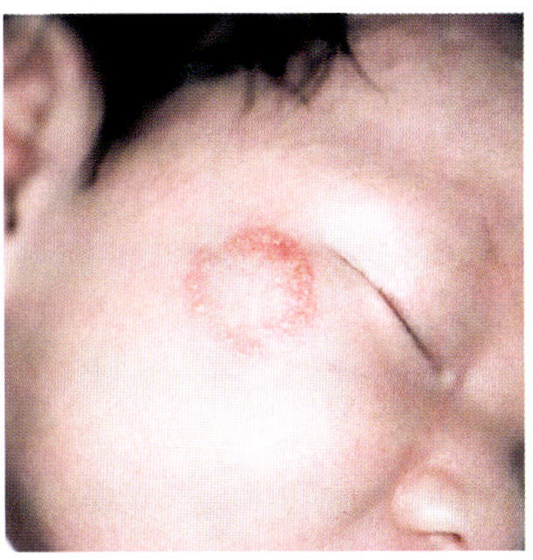

FIG. 21-14 *Annular scaly plaque.*

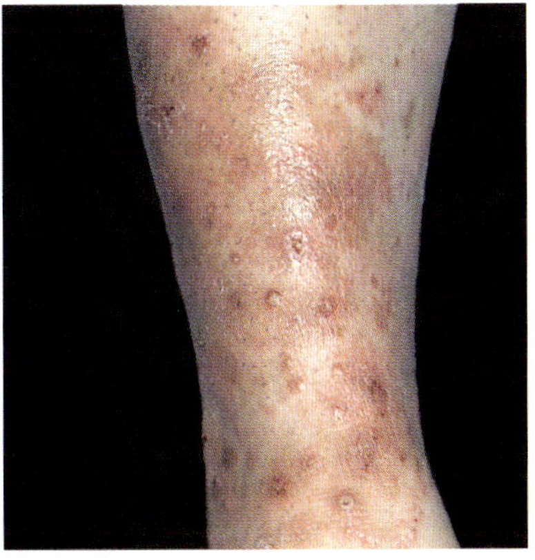

FIG. 21-15 *Follicular papules and pustules surrounded by erythema, the scaly periphery being scalloped (Majocchi's granuloma).*

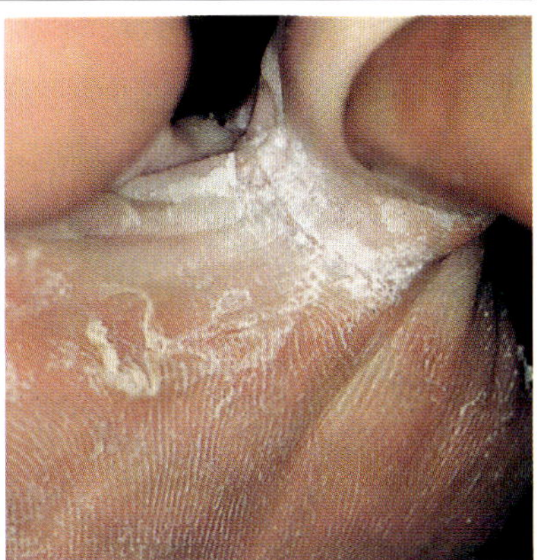

FIG. 21-16 *Maceration and scales, some of them in the form of a collarette.*

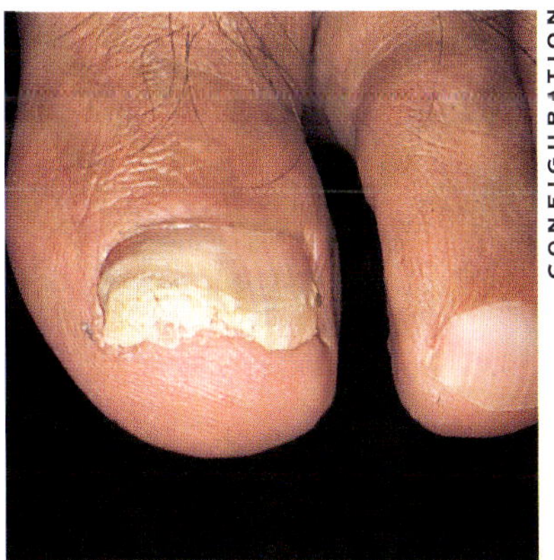

FIG. 21-17 *Thickened yellow nail plate with a ragged distal margin.*

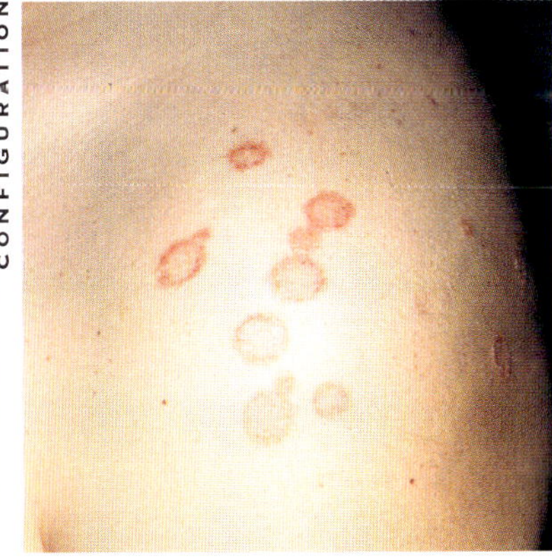

FIG. 21-18 *Erythematous scaly papules arranged in an annulus.*

CONFIGURATION

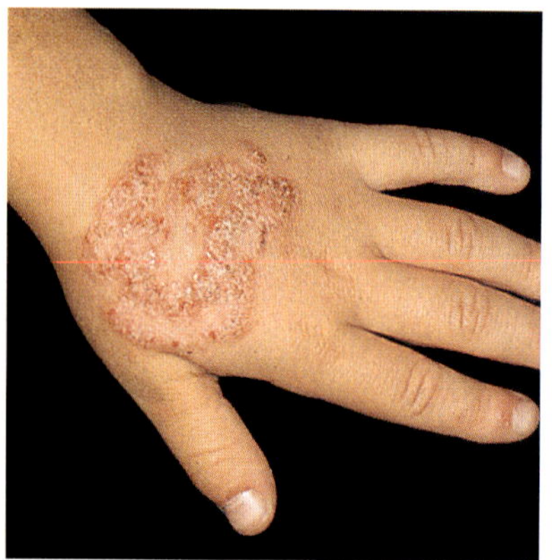

FIG. 21-19 *Papules and vesicles covered by scales and crusts, all of which combined have created a serpiginous outline.*

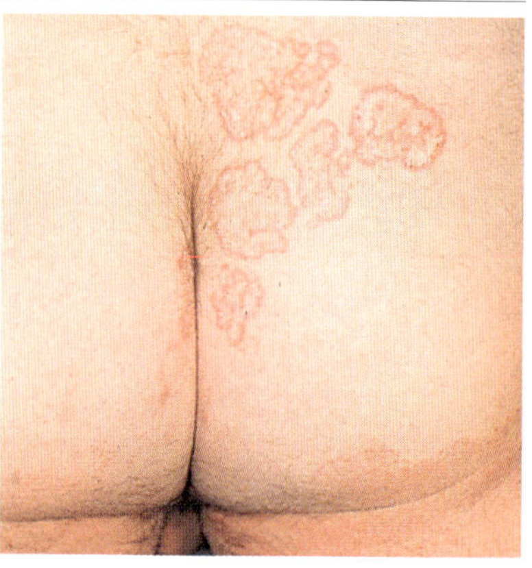

FIG. 21-20 *Labyrinthine arrangement of scaly papules.*

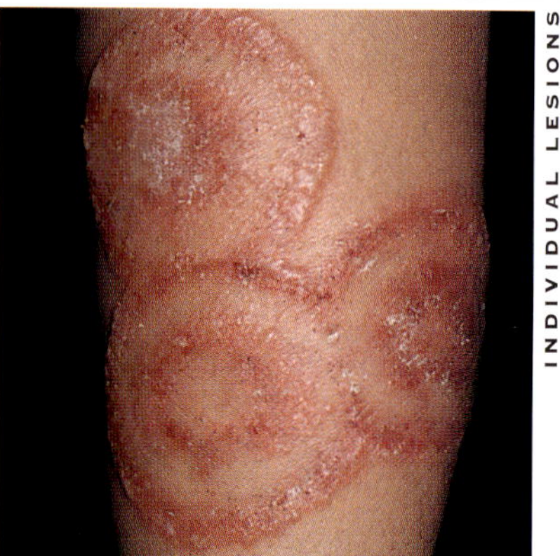

FIG. 21-21 *Scaly plaques in a pattern of concentric rings.*

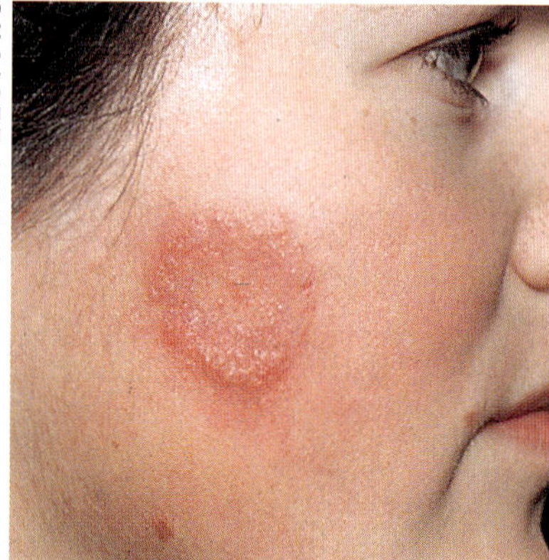

FIG. 21-22 *Erythematous plaque topped by pustules.*

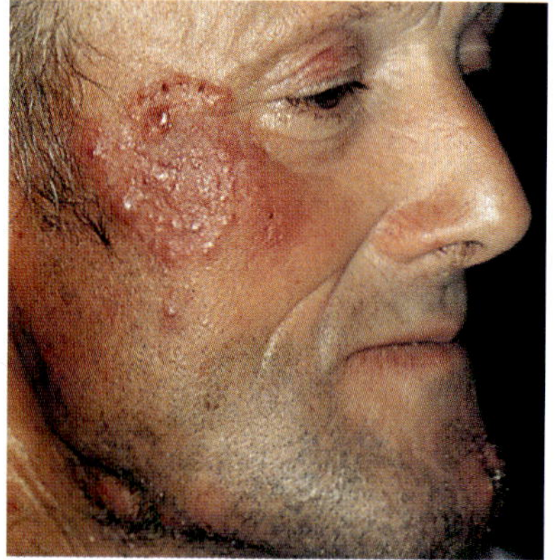

FIG. 21-23 *Crowded erythematous papules and pustules in nummular shape on the side of the face; nodules on the jawline and chin.*

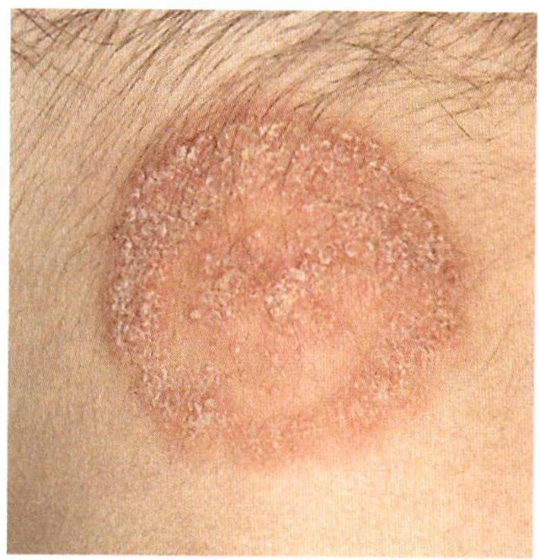

FIG. 21-24 *Large erythematous nummular plaque surmounted by innumerable pustules.*

INDIVIDUAL LESIONS

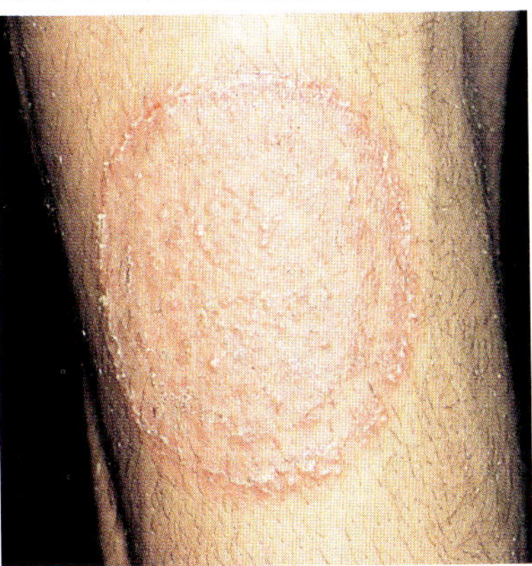

FIG. 21-25 *Papules and pustules on and within a circle.*

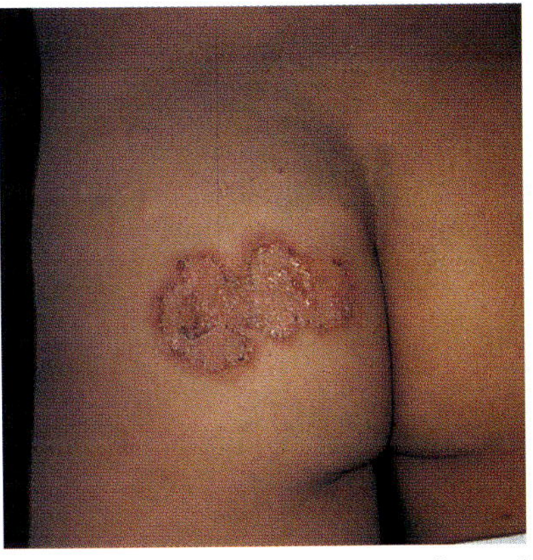

FIG. 21-26 *Plaque with figurate outline and an elevated border composed of papules, pustules, and crusts.*

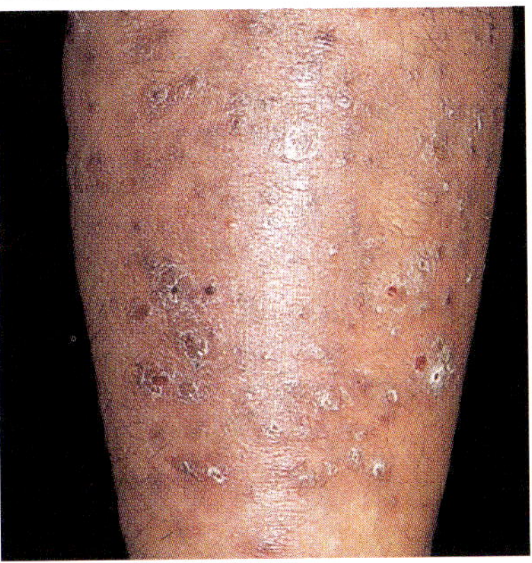

FIG. 21-27 *Follicular scaly papules, some of them eroded, with diffuse hyperpigmentation (Majocchi's granuloma).*

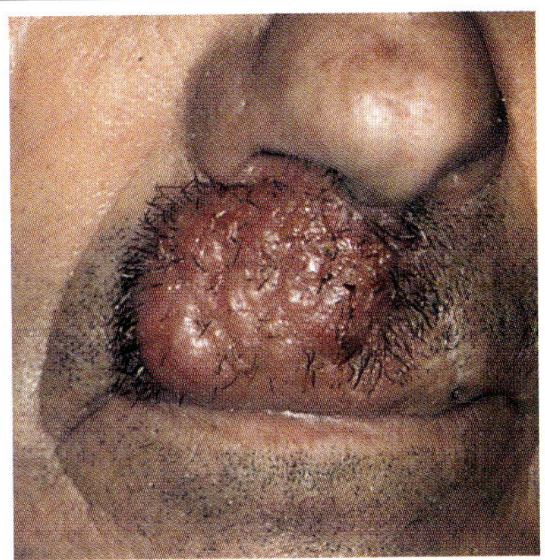

FIG. 21-28 *Partially alopecic erythematous tumor with a papillated surface (kerion).*

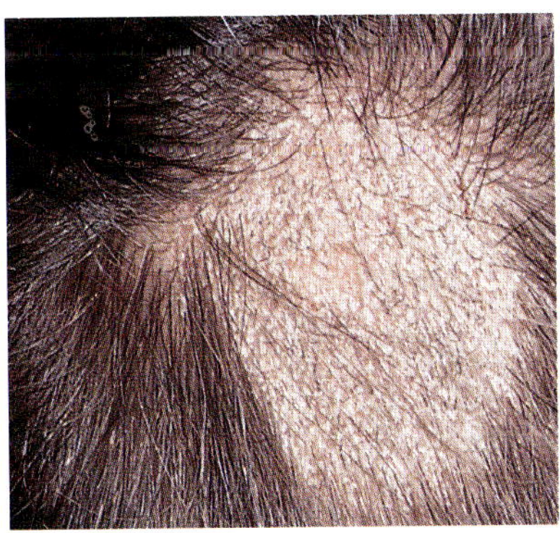

FIG. 21-29 *Patch of alopecia with scales.*

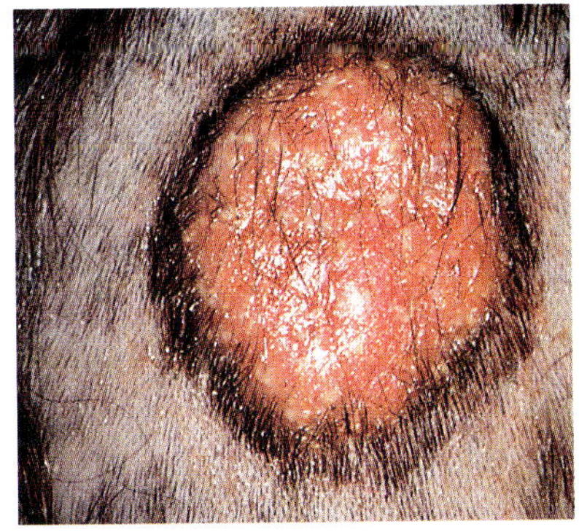

FIG. 21-30 *Plaque with draining sinuses and crusts (kerion).*

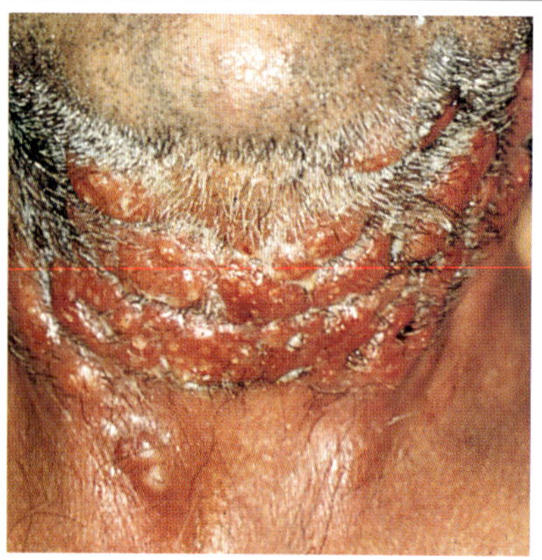

FIG. 21-31 *Closely-set nodules, pustules, and draining sinuses in a boggy mass (kerion).*

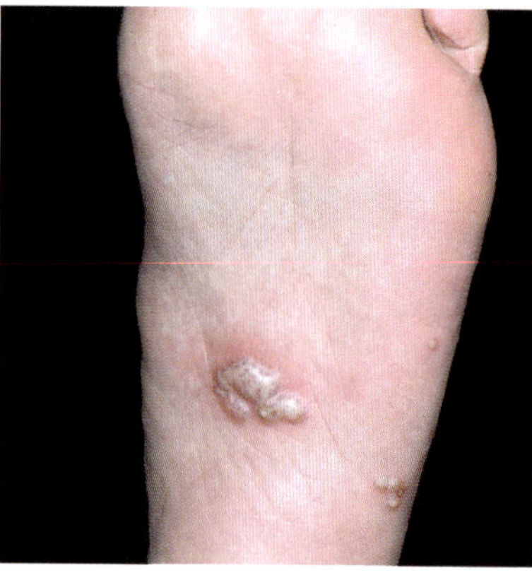

FIG. 21-32 *Tense vesicles and vesiculopustules, some of them grouped.*

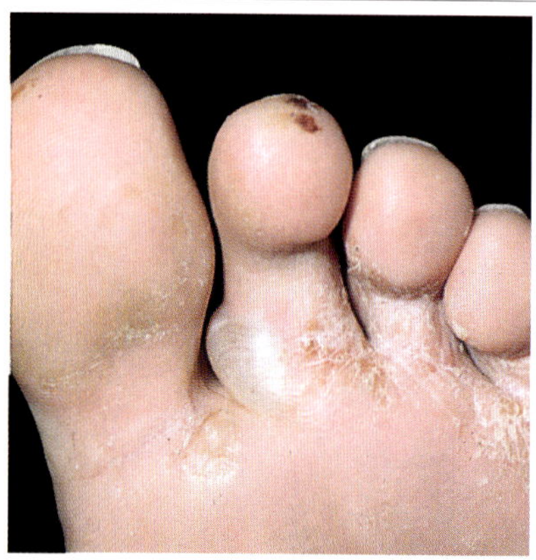

FIG. 21-33 *Vesicles, a tense bulla, and scale-crusts.*

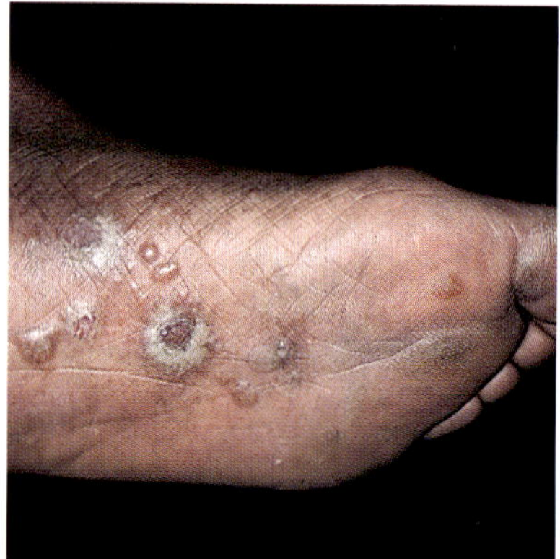

FIG. 21-34 *Vesicles and pustules.*

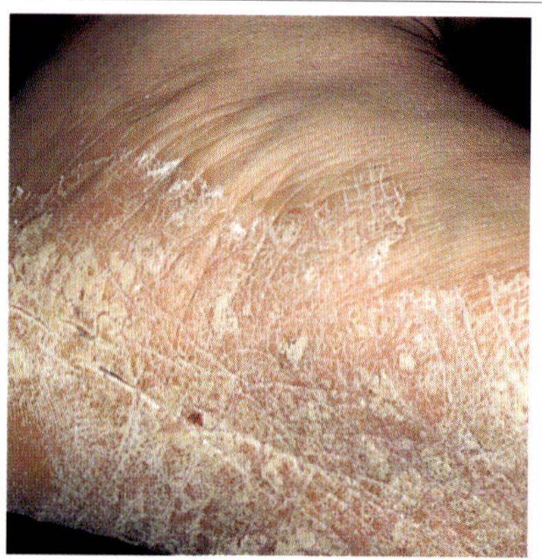

FIG. 21-35 *Scaly erythematous plaque with sharply defined scalloped borders (moccasin distribution).*

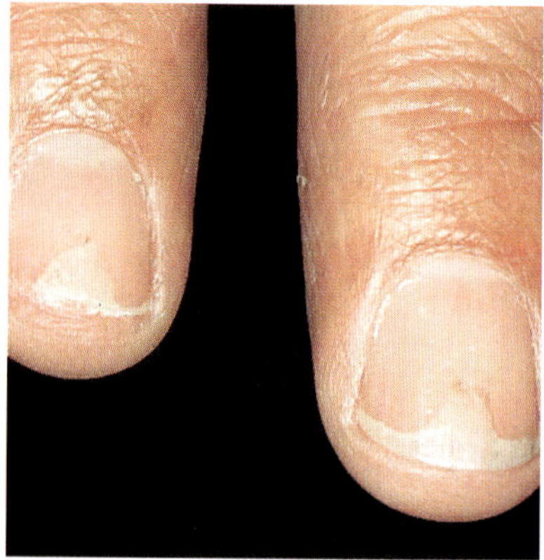

FIG. 21-36 *Wedge-shaped onycholysis and subungual hyperkeratosis (distal type of onychomycosis).*

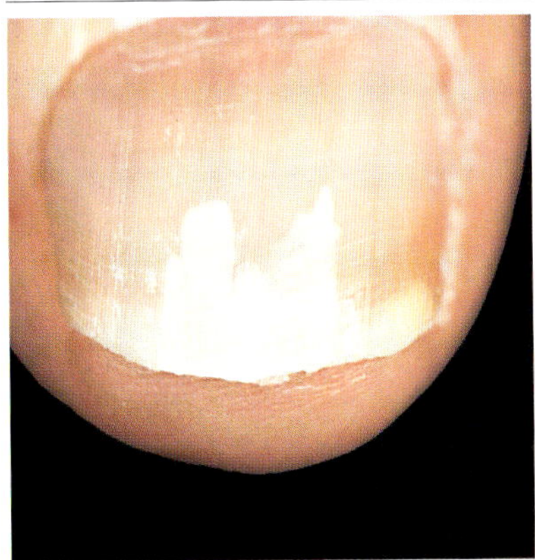

FIG. 21-37 *Chalky white discoloration of the distal nail plate.*

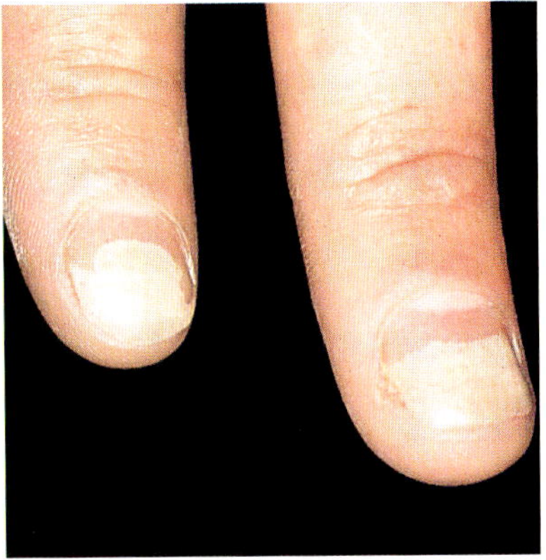

FIG. 21-38 *Yellow-white discoloration of the distal two-thirds of the nail plate and subungual hyperkeratosis.*

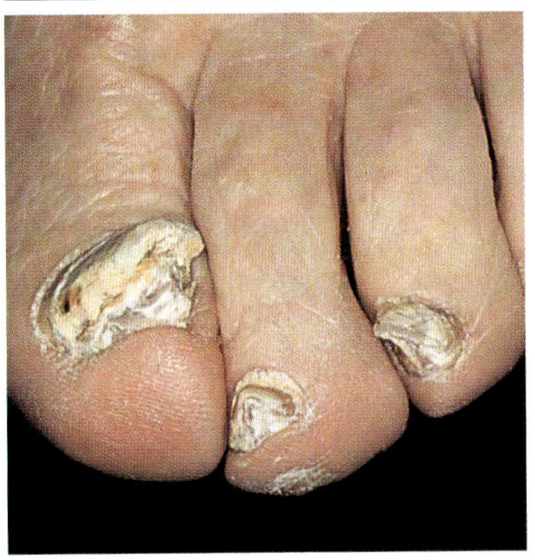

FIG. 21-39 *Severely dystrophic nails and scales in foci on volar skin.*

ADJUNCTIVE DIAGNOSTIC TESTS Wood's lamp examination enables infection by microsporum species to be confirmed. Examination by conventional microscopy of scrapings of skin and clippings of nails in KOH preparations reveals septate hyphae. Precise identification of the type of dermatophyte requires culture on Sabouraud's dextrose agar.

COURSE Dermatophytosis is common, especially the scaly papules, papulovesicles, and vesicles of "athlete's foot." As most people who have that condition know, in the absence of treatment, its lesions come and go for years. Some expressions of dermatophytosis are self-limited, such as the folliculocentric lesions of Majocchi's granuloma and, episodically, of kerion. Other manifestations, however, are tenaciously persistent, like onychomycosis and dermatophytosis in an immunosuppressed patient. In that latter circumstance, lesions of a superficial fungal infection may be widespread and chronic.

INTEGRATION: UNIFYING CONCEPT All of the morphologic features of dermatophytosis, among them, macules, papules, nodules, pustules, vesicles, and bullae, represent the effects of products of dermatophytes that reside in corneocytes within the skin, to wit, the stratum corneum, the cornified layer of the infundibulum, inner sheath, hair shaft, and nail plate. The range of histopathologic changes in dermatophytosis is great, among them spongiotic dermatitis, intraepidermal vesicular dermatitis, psoriasiform dermatitis, and suppurative folliculitis, the latter often expressing itself clinically as Majocchi's granuloma—a misnomer because the process is not fundamentally granulomatous, but suppurative folliculitic. Dermatophytic involvement of hair shafts leads to breakage of them, and involvement of nail plates to dystrophy of them.

THERAPY

Tinea pedis: Topical antimycotics.

Onychomycosis: Oral antimycotics (griseofulvin, triazoles, terbinafine).

Tinea capitis: Griseofulvin, oral azoles, or allylamine derivatives.

Tinea corporis: Topical antimycotics. If widespread, treatment with orally administered antimycotics.

DEFINITION An inflammatory process that results from the effects of a drug administered systemically, e.g., by ingestion, inhalation, injection, or application rectally, and manifested usually by lesions distributed widely and symmetrically. Any of the many clinical expressions of skin lesions may be induced by a drug, but the most common are macules and papules, the latter often being urticarial.

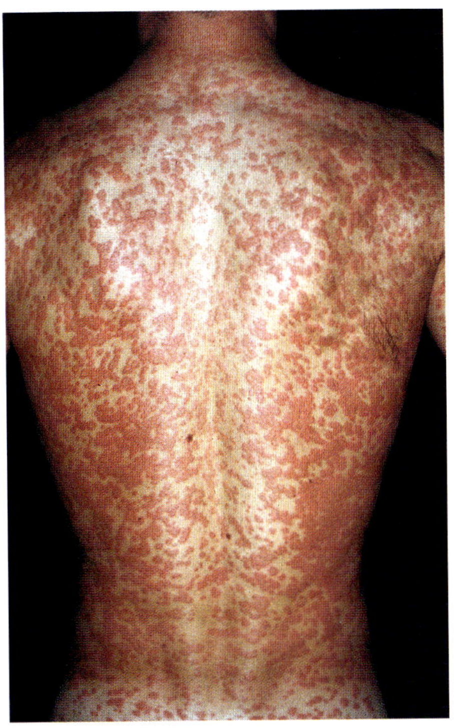

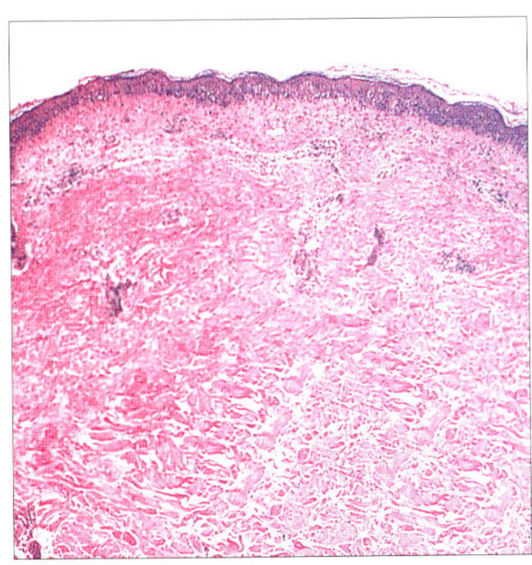

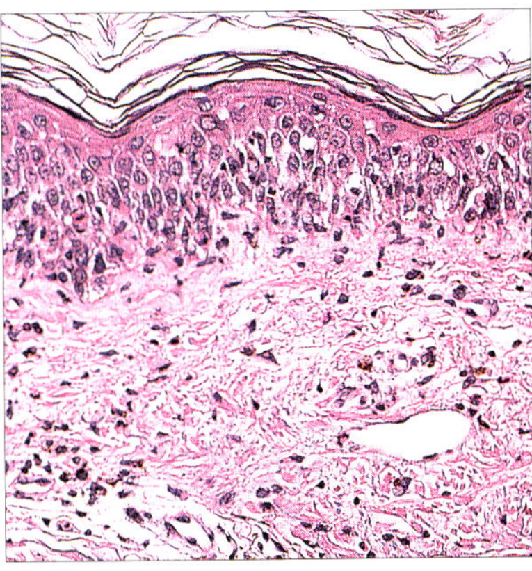

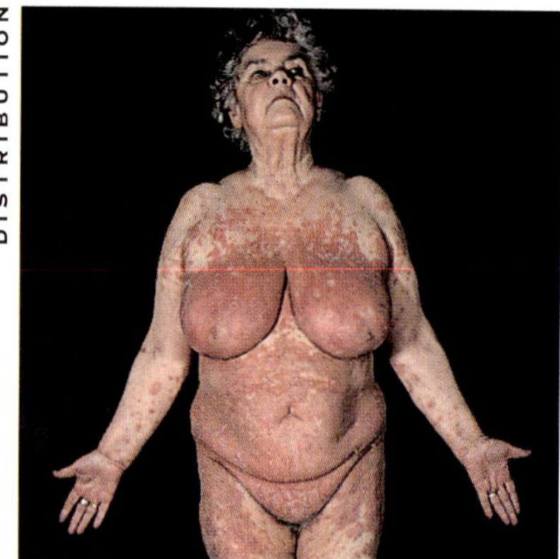

FIG. 22-1 *Widespread erythematous scaly macules and papules have become so confluent as to nearly create erythroderma.*

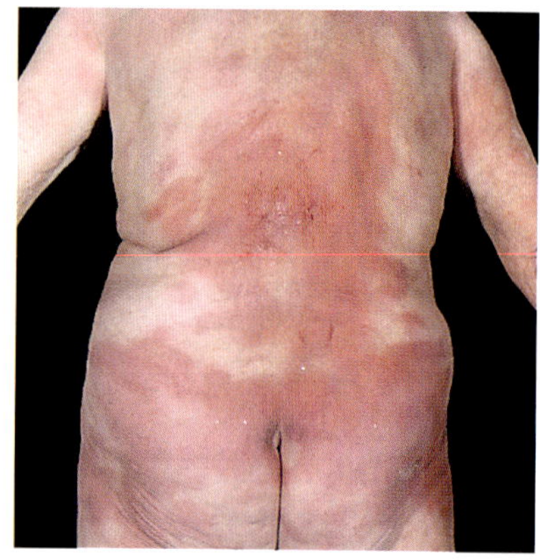

FIG. 22-2 *Widespread dusky, erythematous patches and urticarial plaques with erosions secondary to excoriation.*

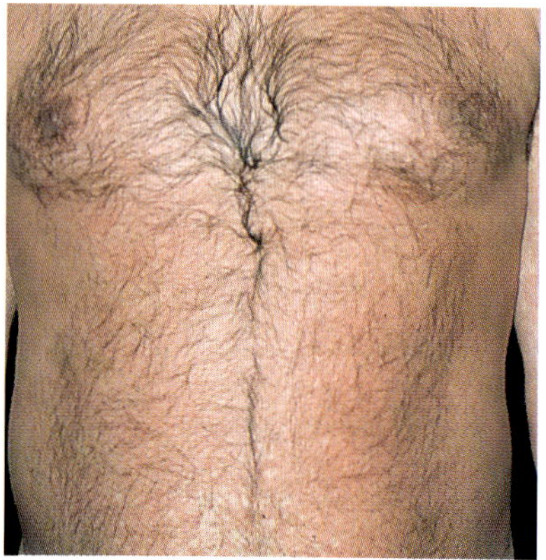

FIG. 22-3 *Widespread erythematous macules and papules in morbilliform pattern.*

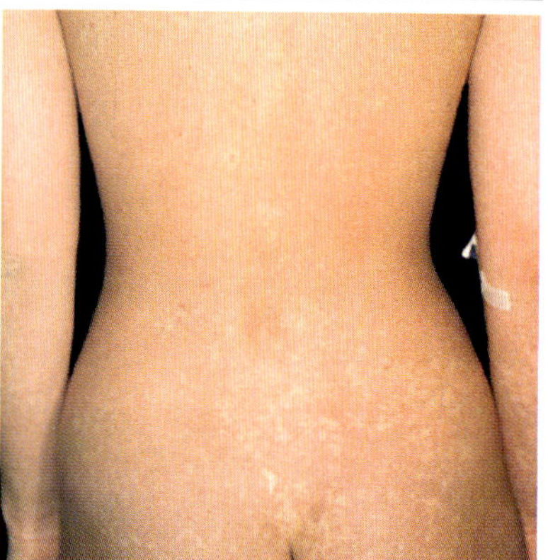

FIG. 22-4 *Widespread eruption of erythematous macules and papules in somewhat morbilliform pattern.*

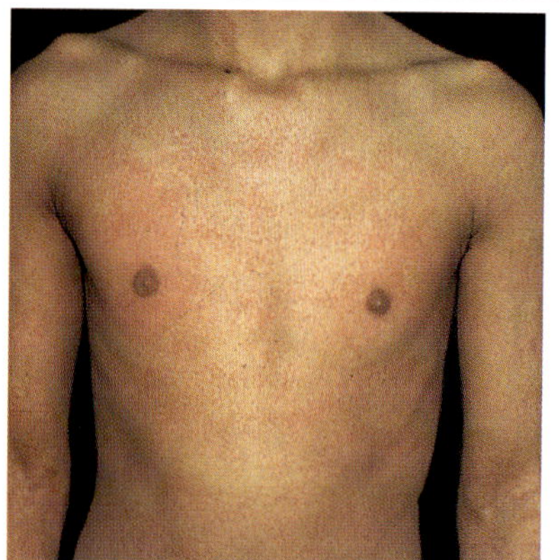

FIG. 22-5 *Widespread erythematous macules and papules that have become confluent.*

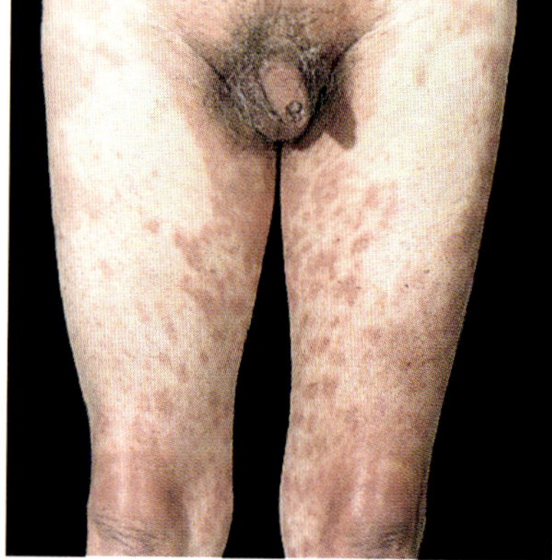

FIG. 22-6 *Erythematous macules, papules, patches, and plaques in bilateral, nearly symmetrical distribution.*

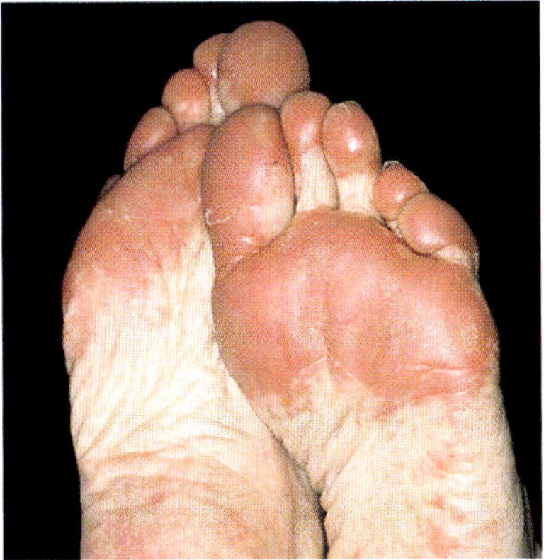

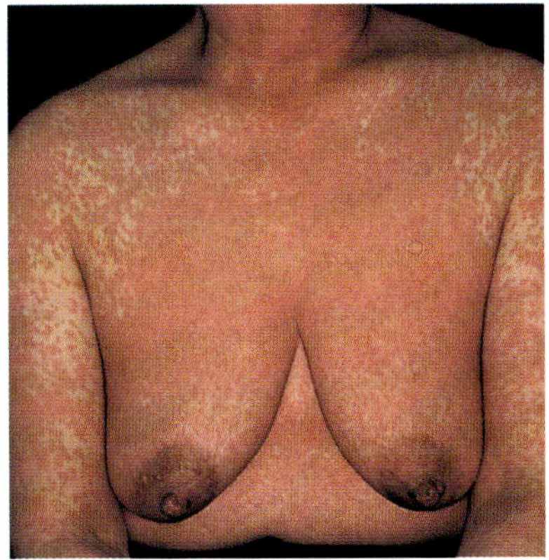

FIG. 22-7 *Erythematous macules and patches associated with edema in bilateral symmetrical distribution.*

FIG. 22-8 *Morbilliform erythematous eruption.*

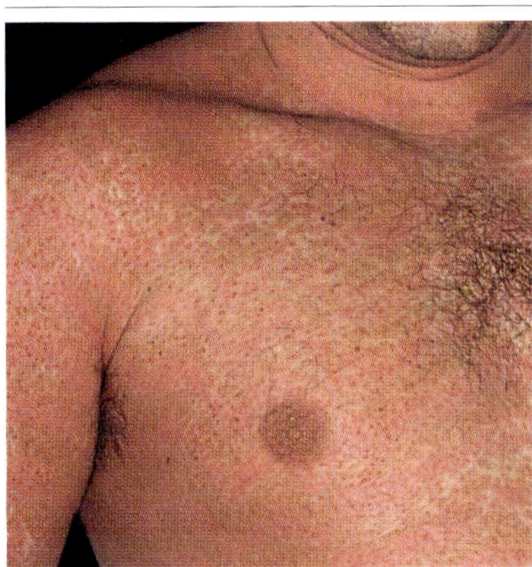

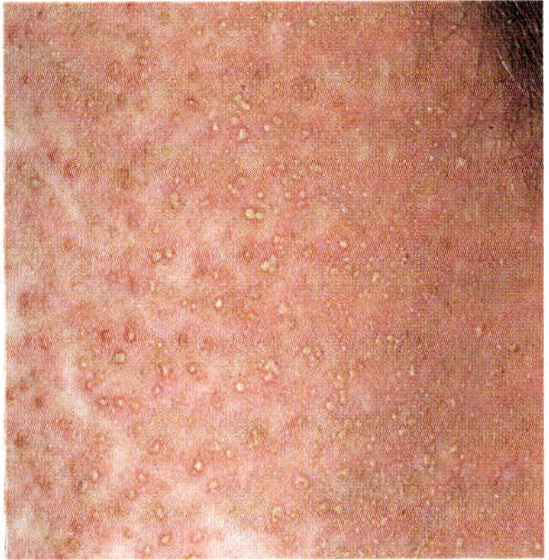

FIG. 22-9 (A, B) *Widespread erythematous papulopustular eruption.*

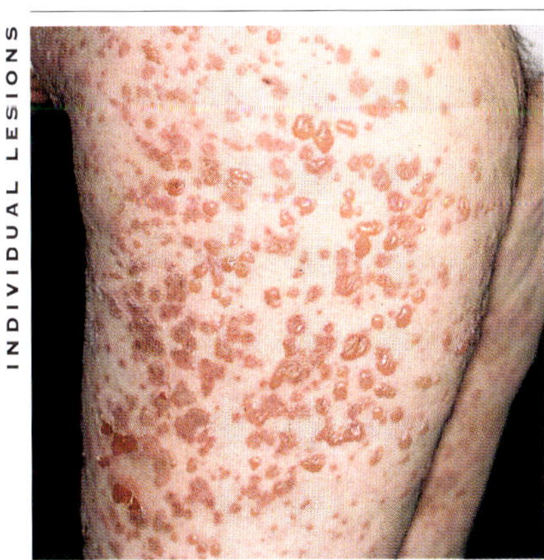

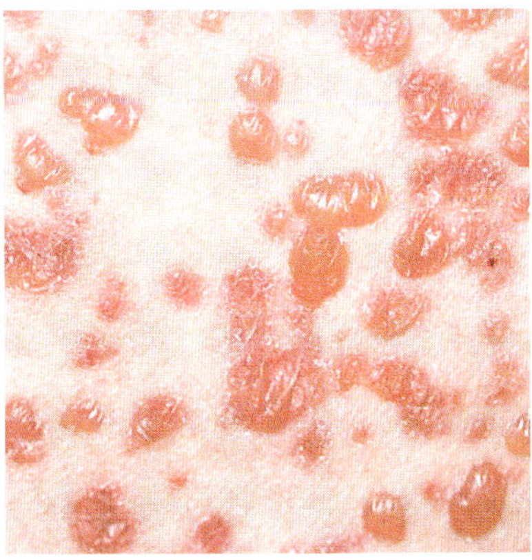

FIG. 22-10 (A, B) *Edematous papules and vesicles, some having become confluent, of a lymphomatoid drug eruption.*

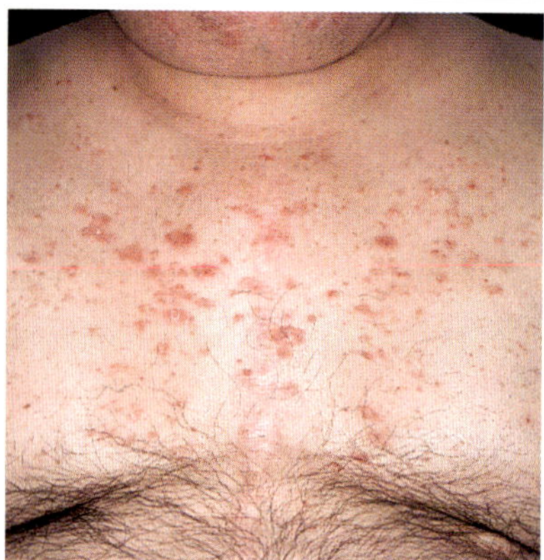

FIG. 22-11 *Erythematous lichenoid papules following injection of sulfonyl urea.*

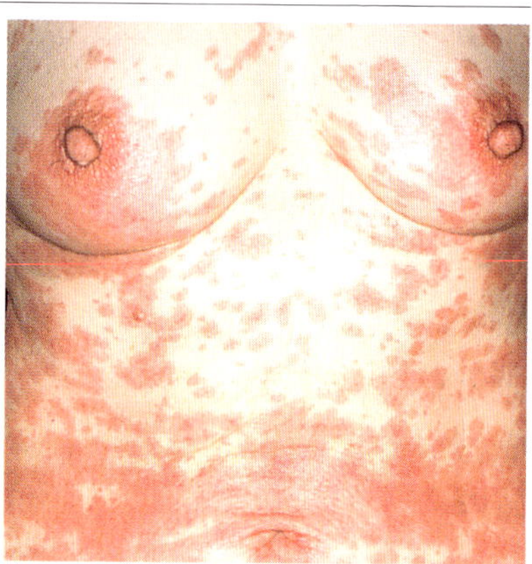

FIG. 22-12 *Erythematous macules and papules that have become confluent on the trunk.*

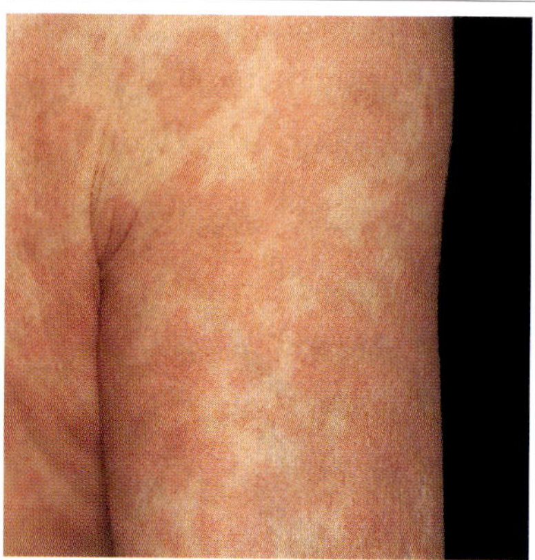

FIG. 22-13 *Erythematous macules and patches, and subtle papules and plaques.*

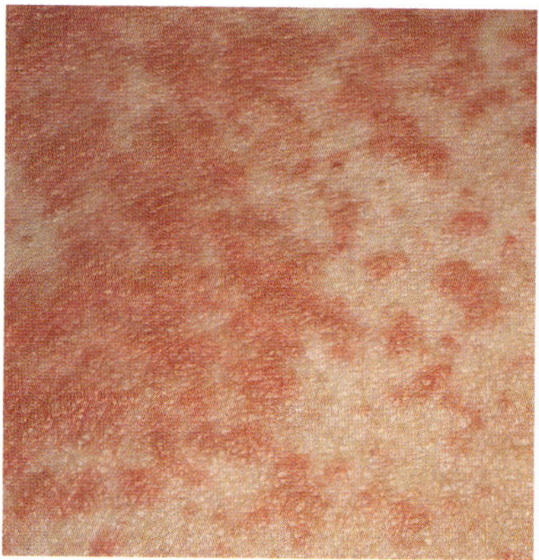

FIG. 22-14 *Erythematous macules and subtle papules that have become confluent to form a plaque.*

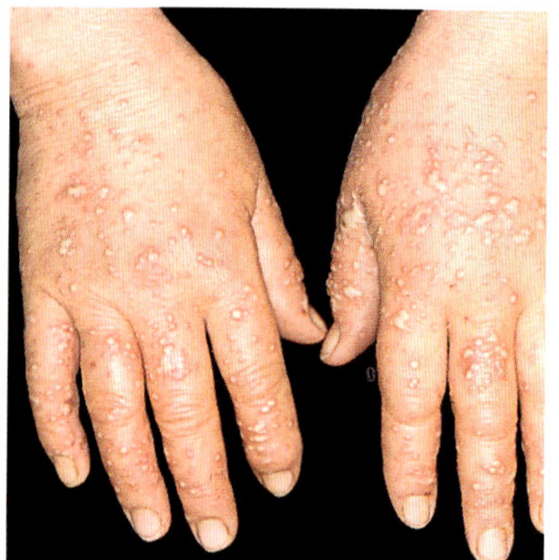

FIG. 22-15 *Pustules, some of which are grouped and distributed bilaterally.*

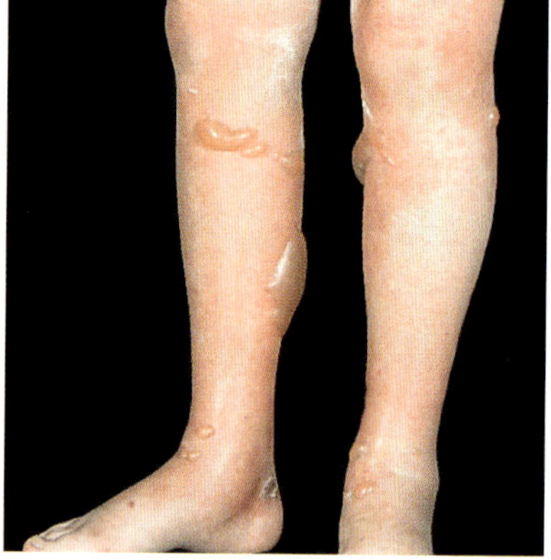

FIG. 22-16 *Erythematous macules, papules, patches, plaques, vesicles, and bullae distributed bilaterally.*

ADJUNCTIVE DIAGNOSTIC TESTS In vivo tests (intradermal and patch) and in vitro tests (RAST, i.e., radioallergosorbent or CAP-FEIA) may be advantageous for establishing the cause.

COURSE As a rule, an eruption caused by a drug given parenterally is sustained as long as the offending drug is administered. Individual lesions, of course, come and go, but the process itself often continues until a few days or weeks after use of the medication has ceased. If a drug responsible for an eruption, such as a morbilliform one, is not discontinued, an erythroderma may result.

INTEGRATION: UNIFYING CONCEPT The term "drug eruption" does not communicate how varied are the drugs that cause eruptions of the skin and how different are the morphologic expressions of those eruptions. Hundreds of drugs of different kinds are known to cause eruptions in skin. Some sense of how diverse are the manifestations of "drug eruption" can be gained from the contrast between a single patch or plaque of a fixed drug eruption and an erythroderma.

Virtually every pattern of inflammatory skin disease (superficial perivascular dermatitis, superficial and deep perivascular dermatitis, nodular and diffuse dermatitis, vasculitis, intraepidermal vesicular and pustular dermatitis, subepidermal vesicular dermatitis, folliculitis and perifolliculitis, fibrosing dermatitis, and panniculitis) may be induced by drugs. Each of those histopathologic patterns, as they are assessed by conventional microscopy at scanning magnification, has a corresponding clinical expression. Those manifestations include all the essential lesions of the skin, such as macules and patches (including a universal patch, which is erythroderma), papules and nodules, and vesicles and bullae. Some drug eruptions are utterly distinctive clinically and histopathologically, such as fixed drug eruption, whereas others simulate closely "authentic" diseases such as lichen planus, pityriasis rosea, and measles.

A clue to the clinical diagnosis of drug eruption is the appearance of widespread, bilateral lesions in symmetrical distribution of lesions that do not correspond exactly to any well-defined disease. The lack of precise histopathologic correspondence to a well-established condition is a clue to diagnosis of "drug eruption" by a microscopist. Although eosinophils are often present in drug eruptions, they are not invariably so, e.g., erythema multiforme usually is devoid of them. The most common of the histopathologic patterns of drug eruption (besides the perivascular and interstitial pattern seen in urticaria) is interface dermatitis. The mechanisms responsible for drug eruptions are varied and incompletely understood.

THERAPY Cessation of the offending drug. In severe examples, systemic administration of corticosteroids may be indicated. Antihistamines may alleviate pruritus.

FIXED DRUG ERUPTION

DEFINITION Circular orange-red-blue macule(s) or patch(es) that often becomes a papule(s) or plaque(s) and vesiculates, healing with hyperpigmentation, and that occurs repeatedly at the very same cutaneous and/or mucous membrane site(s), especially the genitalia, perioral region, and hands, in response to systemic administration of a particular drug or chemical, chief among them barbiturates and sulfonamides. It is the only type of drug eruption that can be diagnosed with surety histopathologically, the findings in it being entirely specific, unlike the situation in drug eruptions of all other kinds.

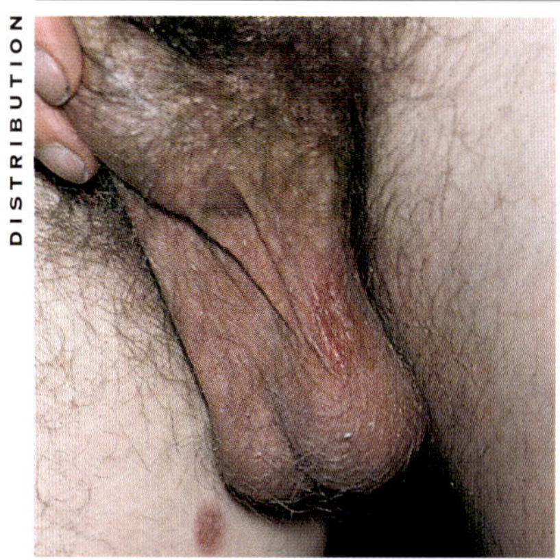

FIG. 22-17 *Circular, erythematous, eroded patch on the scrotum and circular red-blue plaque on the thigh.*

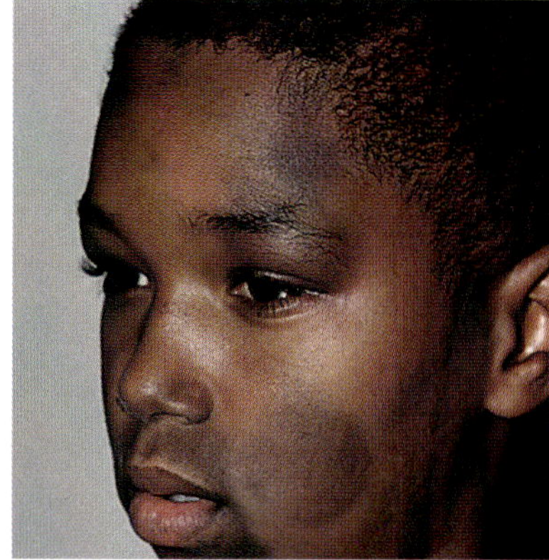

FIG. 22-18 *Circular hyperpigmented patches are signs of resolution of the process.*

INDIVIDUAL LESIONS

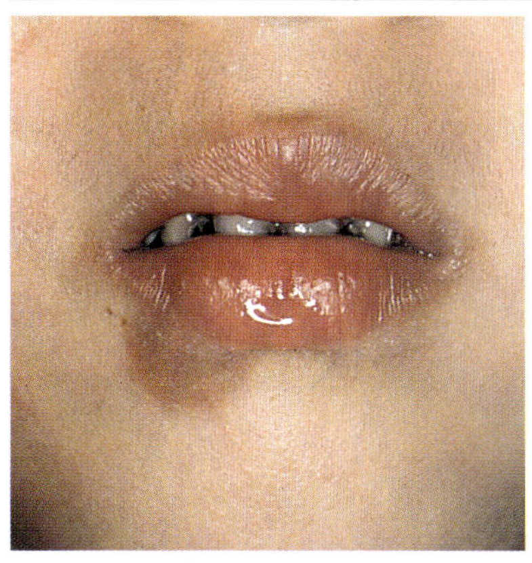

FIG. 22-19 *Semicircular hyperpigmented patch indicates a lesion has resolved.*

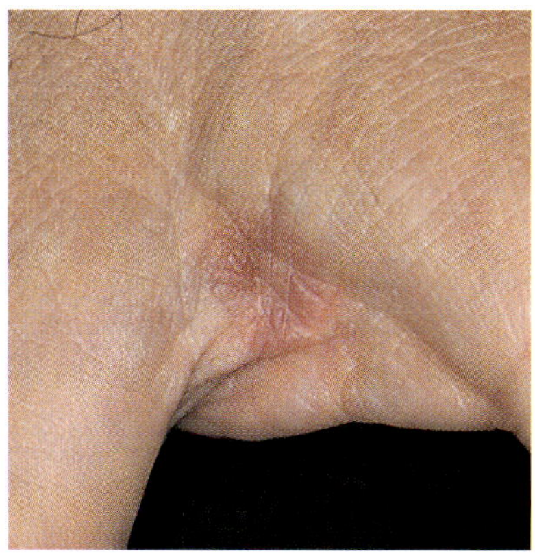

FIG. 22-20 *Interdigital, erythematous, rather well-circumscribed patch.*

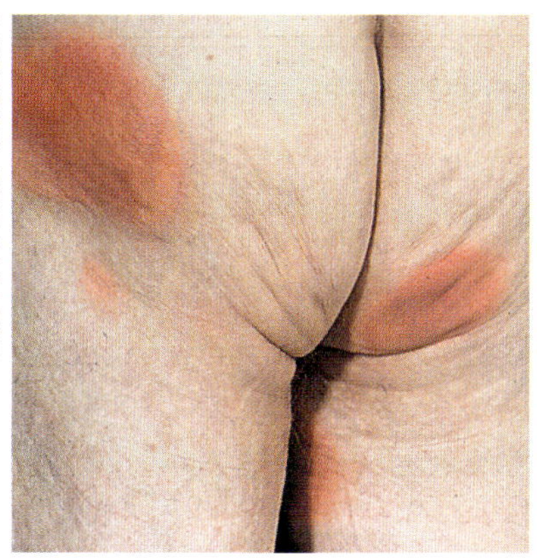

FIG. 22-21 *Circular orange-red macule and plaques.*

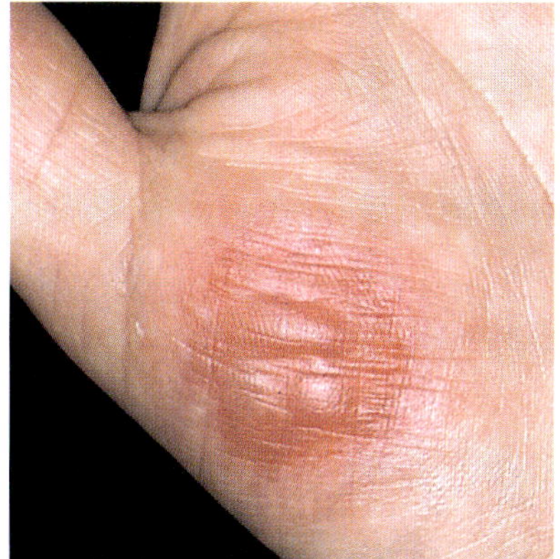

FIG. 22-22 *Vesicles atop an erythematous, edematous plaque.*

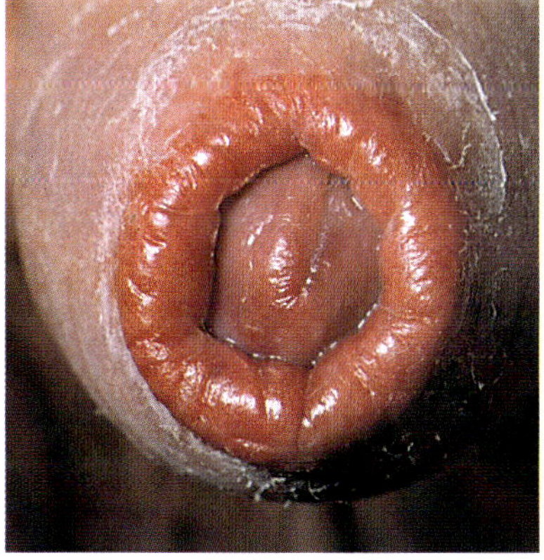

FIG. 22-23 *Phimosis with an annulus of edematous erythema covered by crusts.*

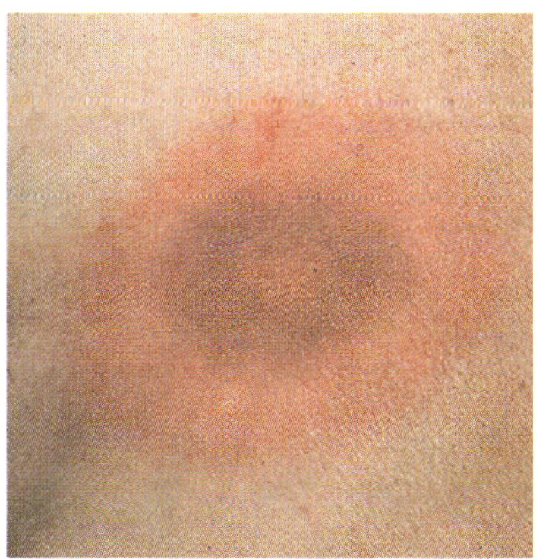

FIG. 22-24 *Circular patch with a salmon-colored rim and a dusky blue center.*

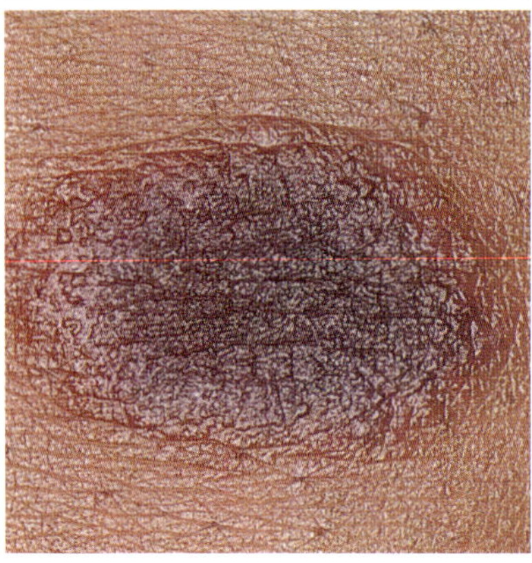

FIG. 22-25 *Nummular plaque with caramel-colored border and dark brown center.*

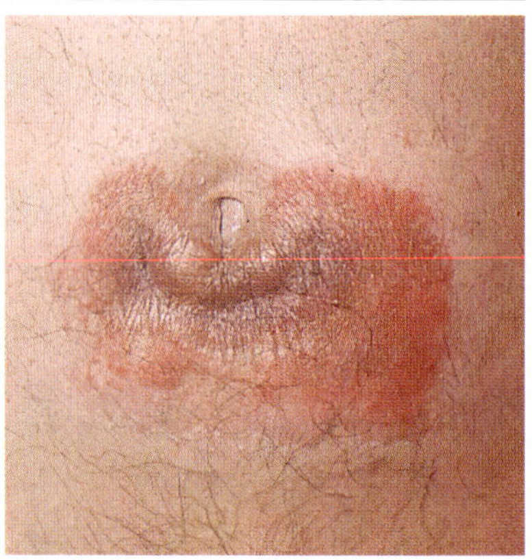

FIG. 22-26 *Somewhat rectangular perium-bilical erythematous plaque with a rust-colored periphery and dusky center.*

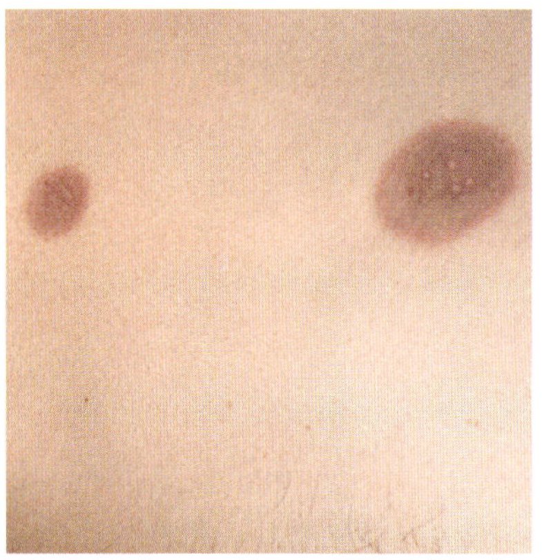

FIG. 22-27 *Two circular macules, both lesions showing a thin red rim and dusky center.*

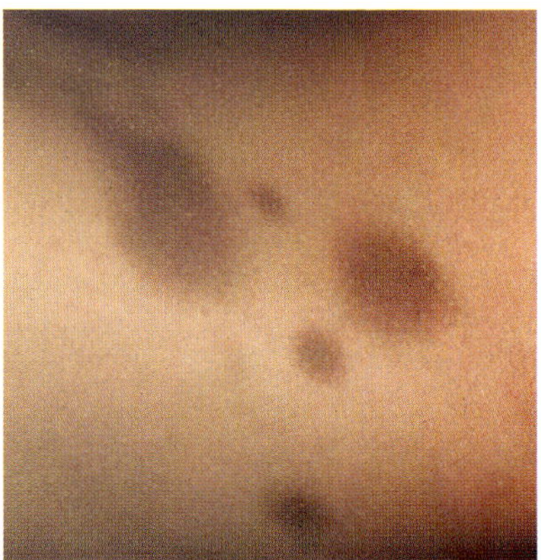

FIG. 22-28 *Circular hyperpigmented macules and patches, the end stage of the eruption.*

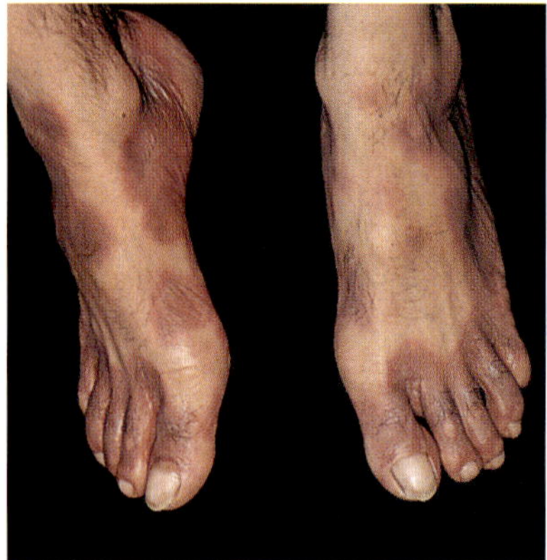

FIG. 22-29 *Hyperpigmented patches that represent the end of the eruption.*

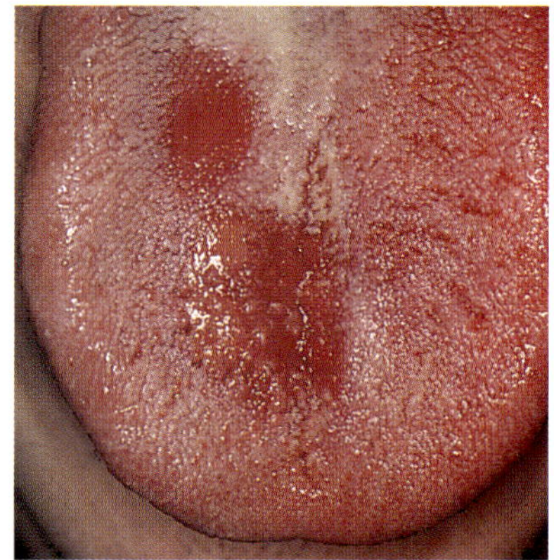

FIG. 22-30 *Circular erosions.*

ADJUNCTIVE DIAGNOSTIC TEST Epifocal patch test may be helpful.

COURSE Every time an offending drug or chemical responsible for a fixed drug eruption is ingested (or administered by another route), the lesion(s) reappears in the very same site(s).

INTEGRATION: UNIFYING CONCEPT Fixed drug eruption is the only drug eruption that can be diagnosed with confidence, clinically and histopathologically. The lesions are characteristic clinically, as is apparent in the pictures in this chapter, and they are characterized histopathologically by a superficial and deep perivascular mixed-cell infiltrate of lymphocytes, neutrophils, and eosinophils around venules, and neutrophils and eosinophils between collagen bundles in the upper part of the reticular dermis, in the papillary dermis, and along the dermoepidermal junction in conjunction there with vacuolar alteration and necrotic keratinocytes. Ballooning and spongiosis occur within the epidermis, changes that may eventuate in intraepidermal vesiculation. If the intraepidermal vesicles become sufficiently tense, they rupture, and the result is a subepidermal, as well as an intraepidermal, vesicle. In time, the entire epidermis becomes necrotic.

The major causes of fixed drug eruption are ingestion of barbiturates, analgesics, salicylates, tetracyclines, and sulfonamides. A common offender in times past was the chemical, phenolphthalein. The mechanism whereby fixed drug eruption develops is not known, but the name of the condition derives from its being fixed to the same site at each recurrence.

THERAPY The causative agent must be avoided. If only one or very few lesions are present, topical corticosteroids are indicated, but if there are many lesions, systemic administration of corticosteroids is necessary.

DEFINITION A pruritic papular and vesicular inflammatory process of unknown cause that tends to affect the sides of fingers and toes, as well as palms and soles. The name "dyshidrotic" is misleading; the condition has no relation whatever to eccrine glands or to sweating.

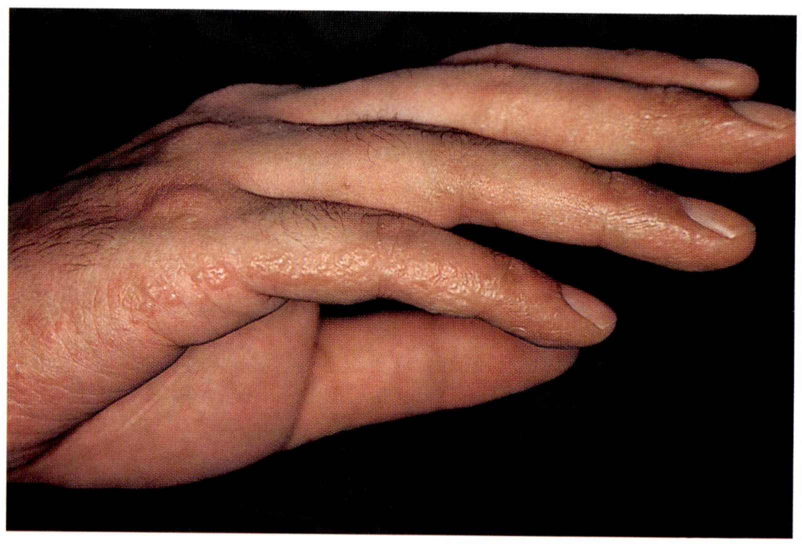

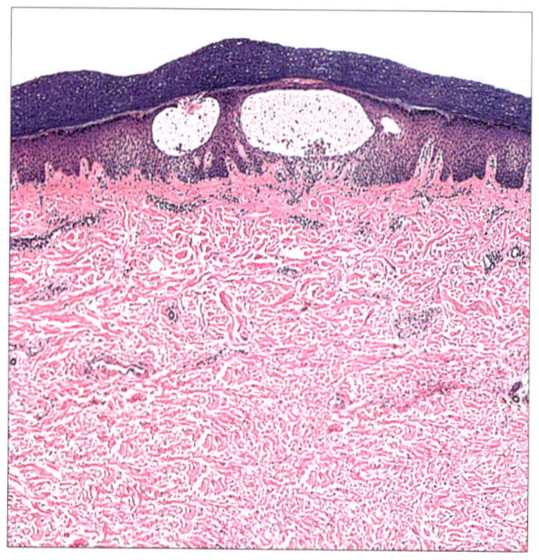

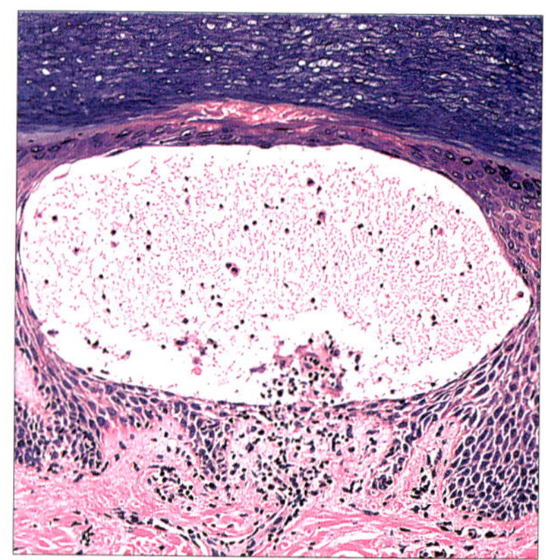

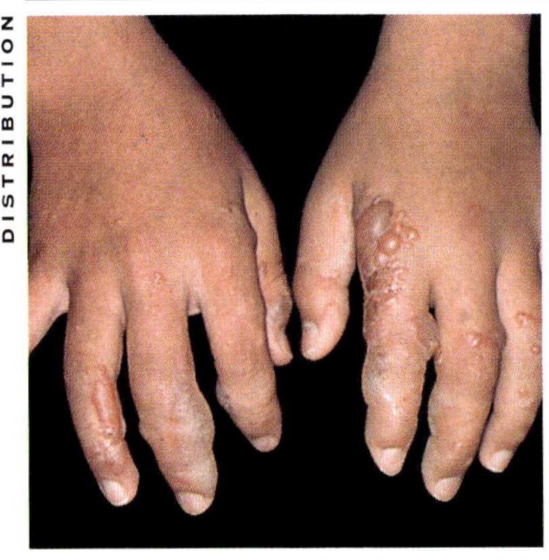

FIG. 23-1 *Vesicles and bullae, especially along the sides of fingers.*

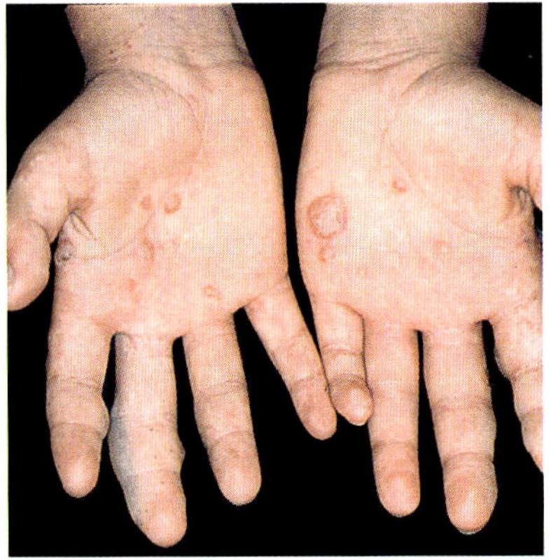

FIG. 23-2 *Vesicles have become confluent to form bullae along the sides of fingers and are present also on palms.*

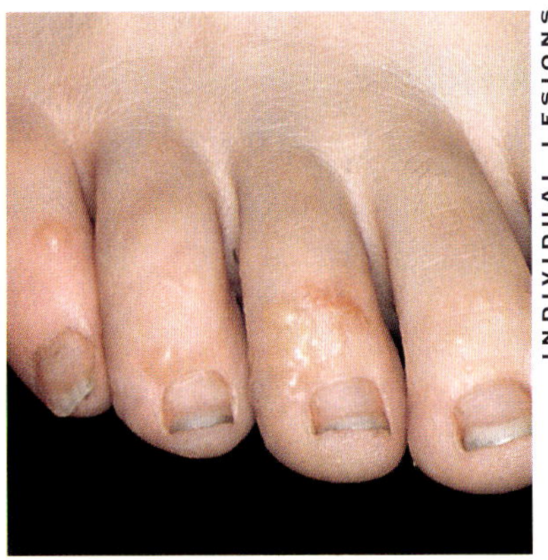

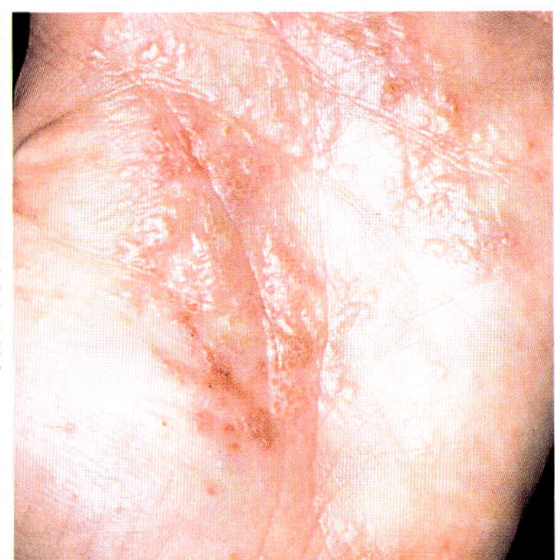

FIG. 23-3 *Tense vesicles along the sides of toes and on the dorsal surface of them.*

FIG. 23-4 *Confluence of vesicles.*

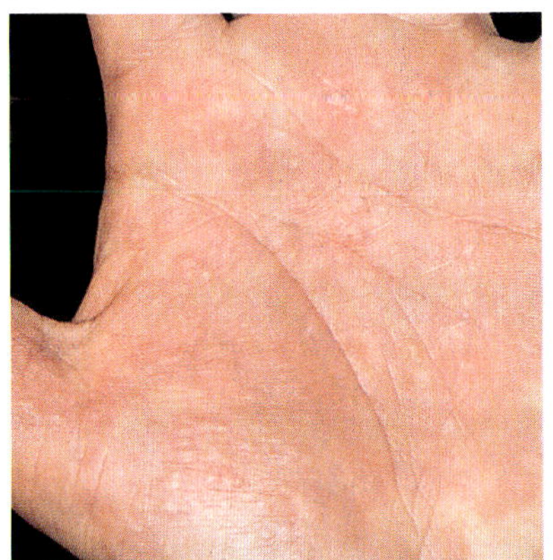

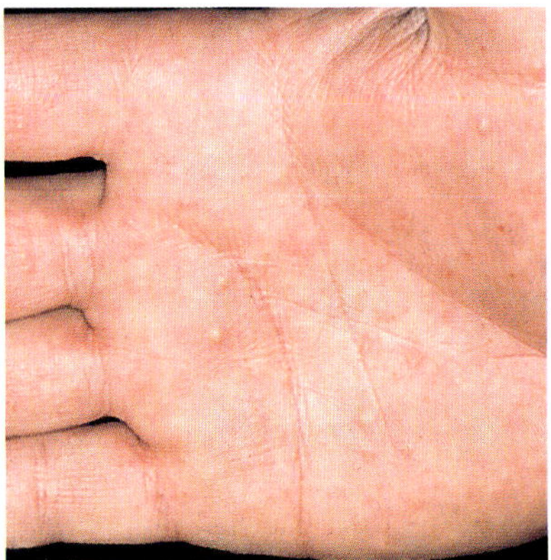

FIG. 23-5 *Erythematous patch on which are numerous papules and subtle papulovesicles.*

FIG. 23-6 *Tiny papules and vesicles on the fingers and palm.*

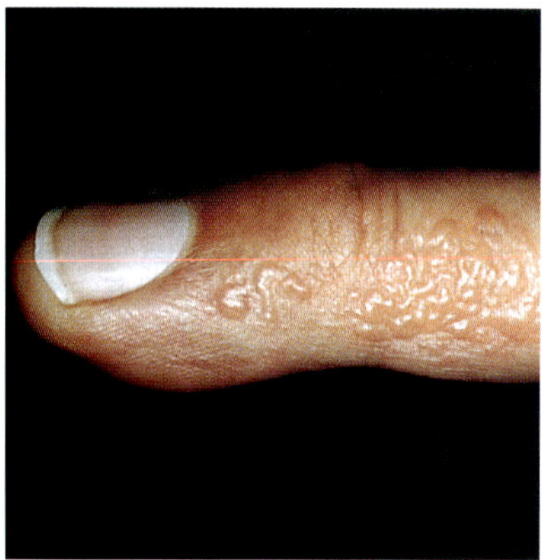

FIG. 23-7 *Vesicles along the side of a finger.*

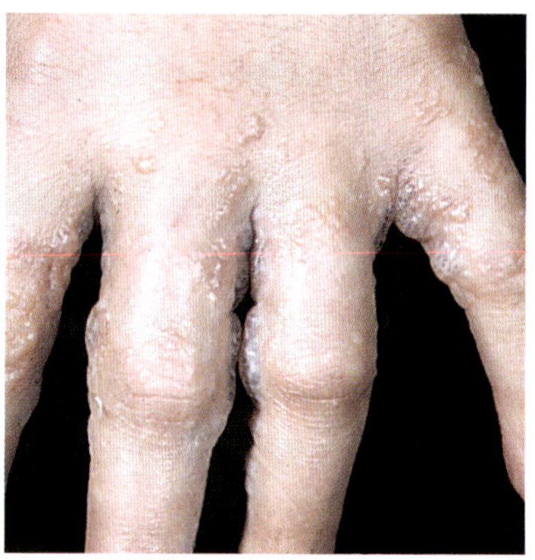

FIG. 23-8 *Tense vesicles, some of them in clusters and some in confluence forming small bullae.*

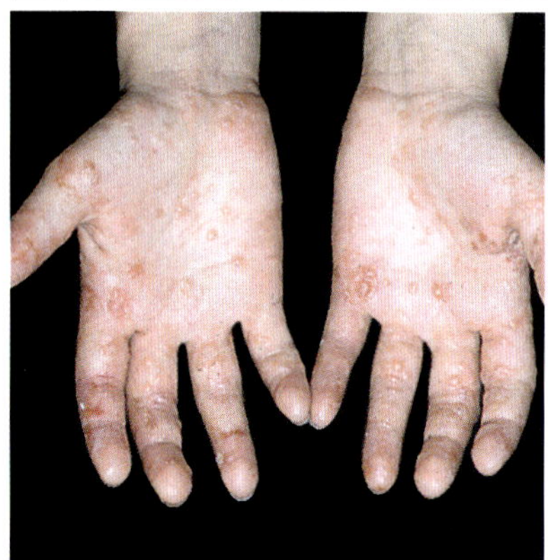
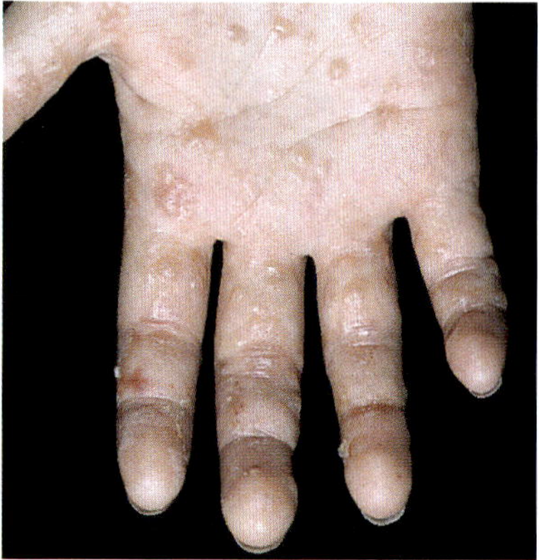

FIG. 23-9 (A, B) *Tense vesicles, some of them grouped, on the volar surface and sides of fingers, and on palms.*

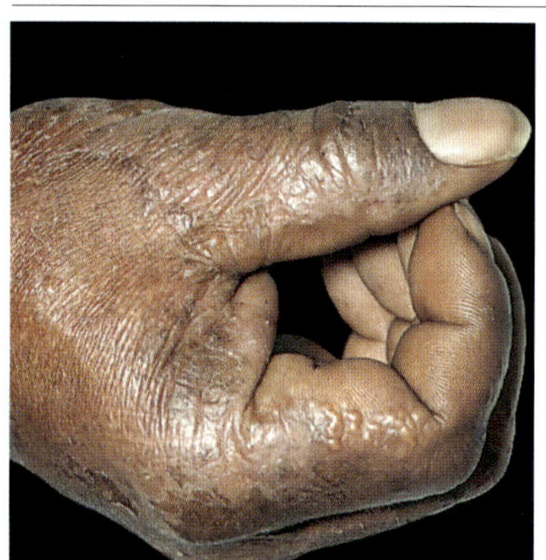

FIG. 23-10 *Tense vesicles along the sides of fingers and on their dorsal aspect.*

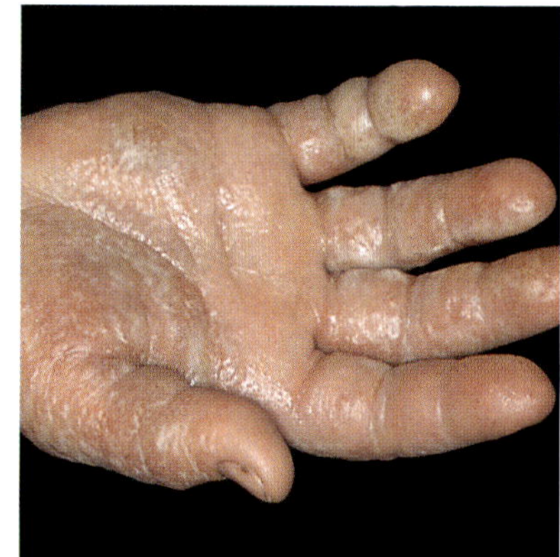

FIG. 23-11 *Diffuse involvement of edematous fingers and of the palm by vesicles, many of which have become confluent.*

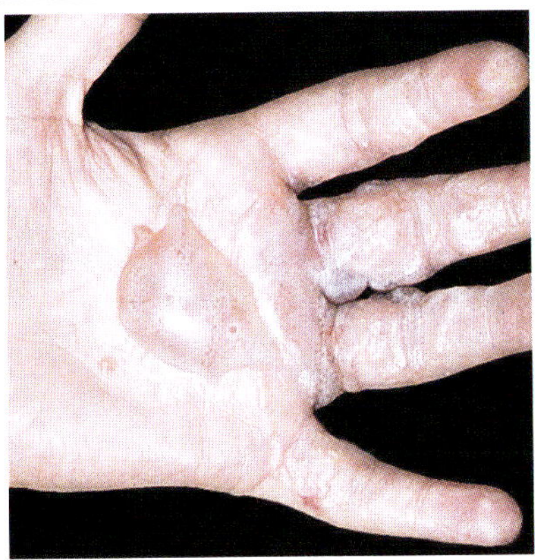

FIG. 23-12 *Tense vesicles and bullae.*

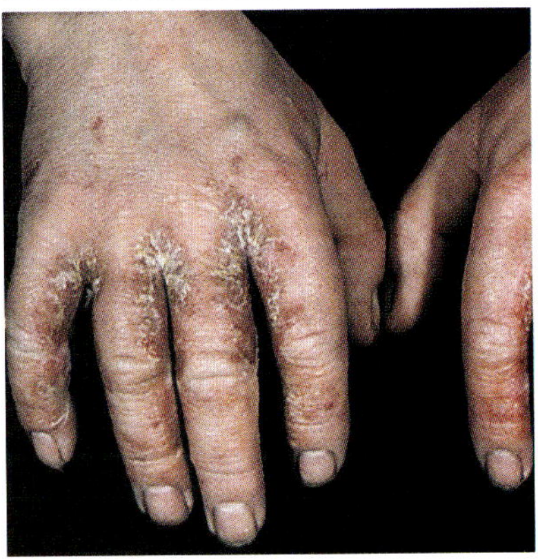

FIG. 23-13 *Erosions, scales, and scale-crusts at sites where previously there were tense blisters.*

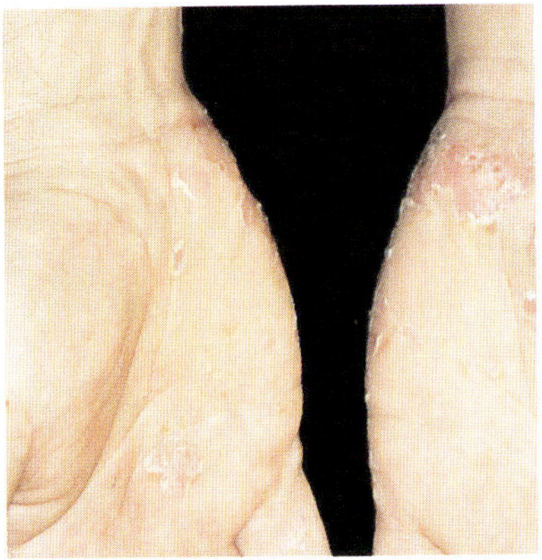

FIG. 23-14 *Collarettes of scale represent sites where vesicles were situated.*

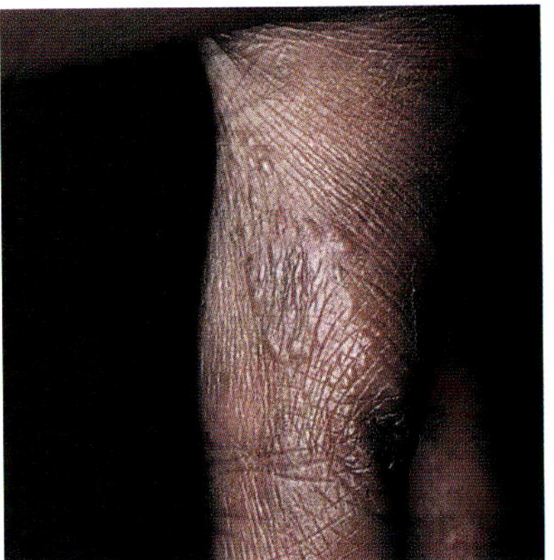

FIG. 23-15 *Papules and tiny vesicles.*

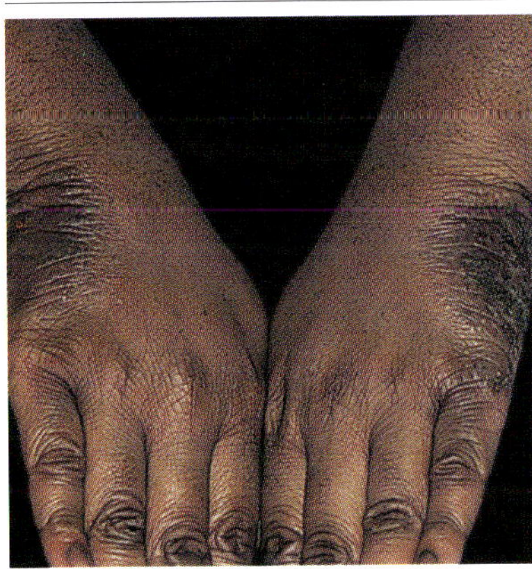

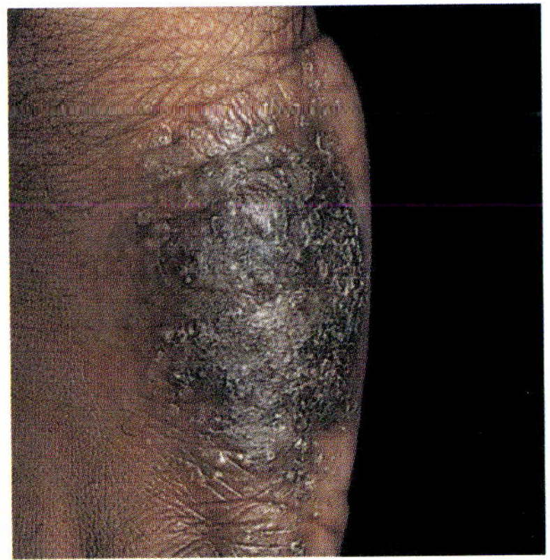

FIG. 23-16 (A, B) *Plaques with collarettes of scale, an evidence of resolution of spongiotic vesicles, and signs of lichen simplex chronicus.*

ADJUNCTIVE DIAGNOSTIC TEST Patch tests may be useful to rule out allergic contact dermatitis.

COURSE Dyshidrotic dermatitis has an unpredictable course. It may be remarkably evanescent, with vesicles appearing rapidly in hours and disappearing completely in days, or it may be intractable, e.g., vesicles coming and going for months or years with only short periods of remission. The vesicles are sometimes multilocular and resemble tapioca. The condition seems to flare when a susceptible person is under stress that is greater than can be handled with serenity.

INTEGRATION: UNIFYING CONCEPT The term "dyshidrotic dermatitis" is a misnomer; the spongiotic vesicular dermatitis has nothing to do with aberrations of sweating or with the eccrine unit. Vesicles in the condition, which tend to appear along the sides of fingers and sometimes of toes of persons who tend to be atopic, sometimes are present in conjunction with other clinical manifestations of spongiotic dermatitis, such as allergic contact dermatitis, nummular dermatitis, and id reaction. Even though these conditions are very different from one another clinically, they are indistinguishable from one another histopathologically. That fact, coupled episodically with the appearance of them concurrently in the same patient, leads us to the hypothesis that allergic contact dermatitis, nummular dermatitis, dyshidrotic dermatitis, and id reaction are very closely related to one another.

THERAPY Topical corticosteroid cream is palliative, but it does not seem to prevent new crops of vesicles from erupting. Flares of the disease may be suppressed by short-term oral administration of corticosteroids. PUVA bath therapy is claimed to be effective against active lesions.

DEFINITION Epidermal nevi are hamartomas in which the epidermis is abnormal, being hyperkeratotic, and in which lesions are aligned along Blaschko's lines.

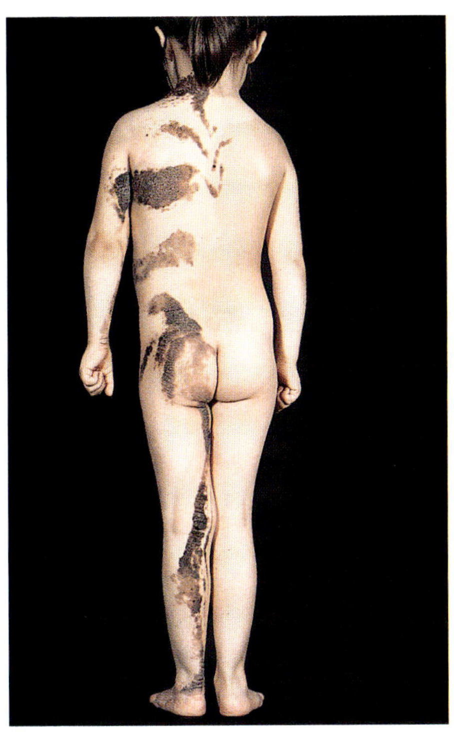

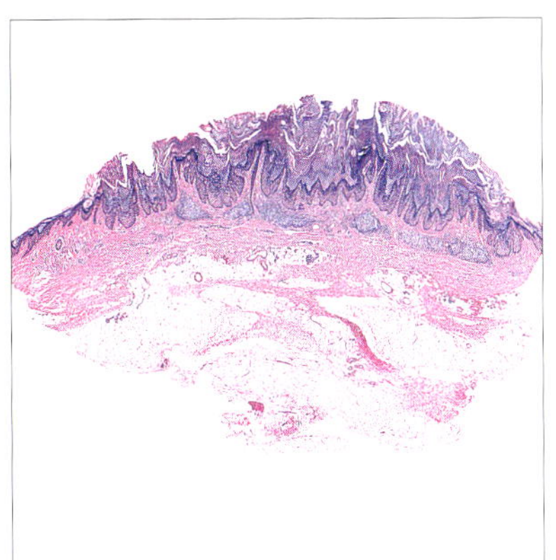

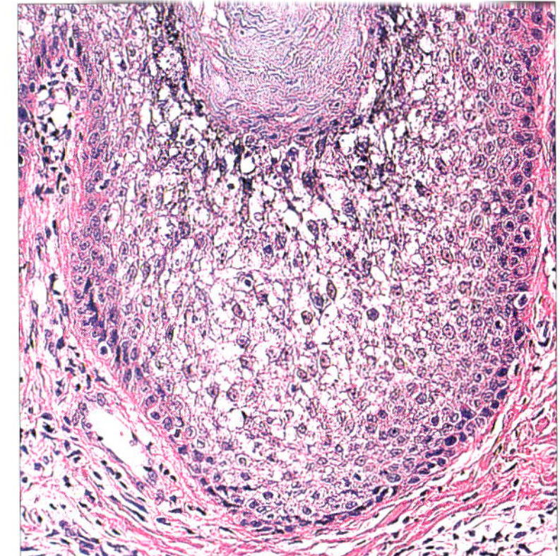

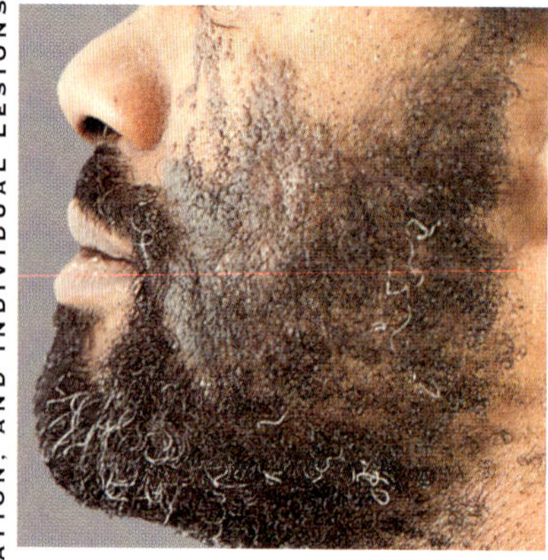

FIG. 24-1 *Pigmented papules that have become confluent to form plaques with a somewhat verrucous surface.*

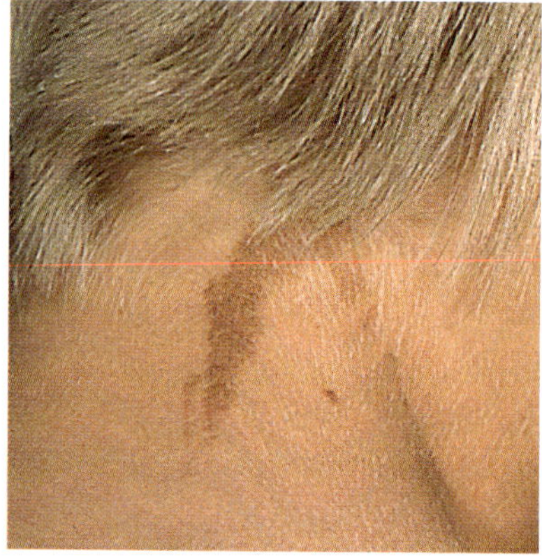

FIG. 24-2 *Pigmented curvilinear plaque on the nape.*

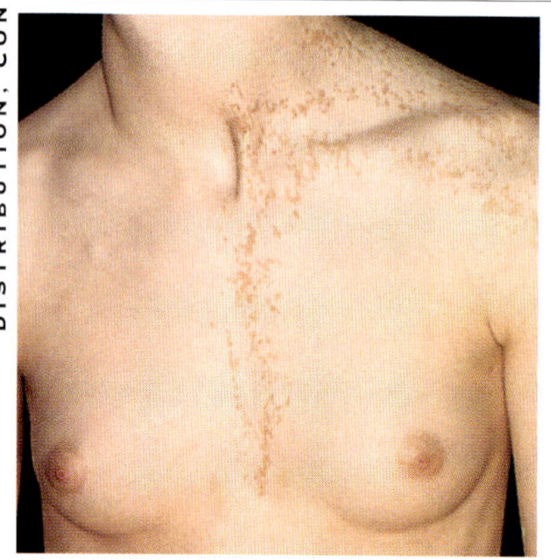
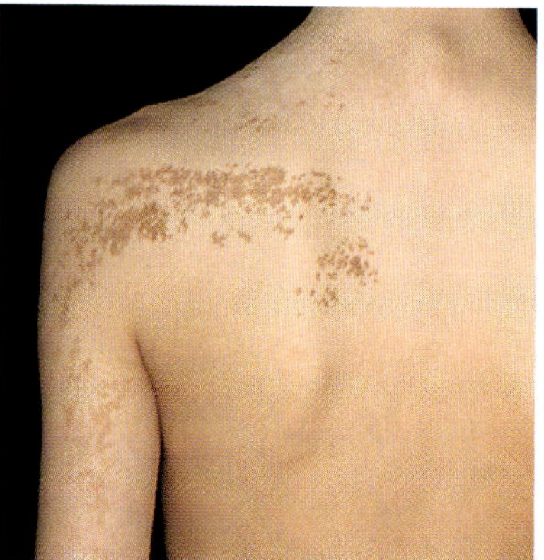

FIG. 24-3 (A, B) *Pigmented macules that have become confluent to form patches, and pigmented papules that have become confluent to form plaques.*

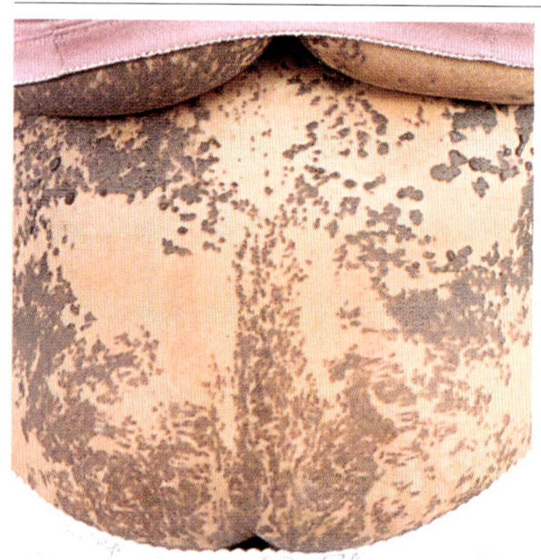
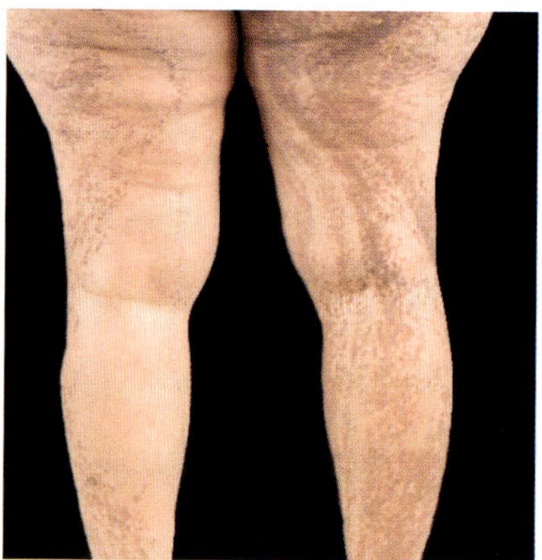

FIG. 24-4 (A, B) *Keratotic papules that have become confluent to form curvilinear plaques on the trunk and legs.*

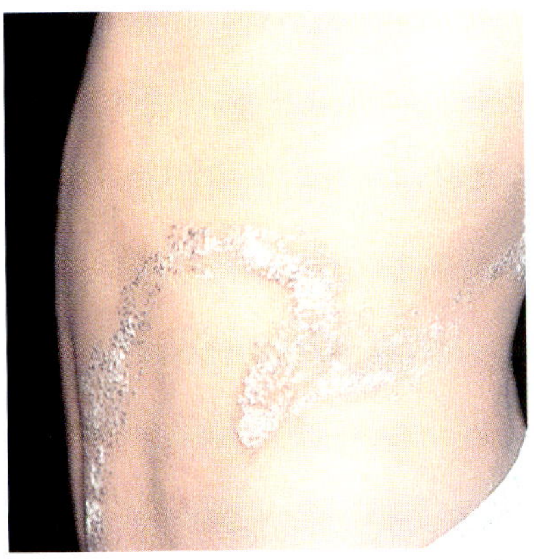

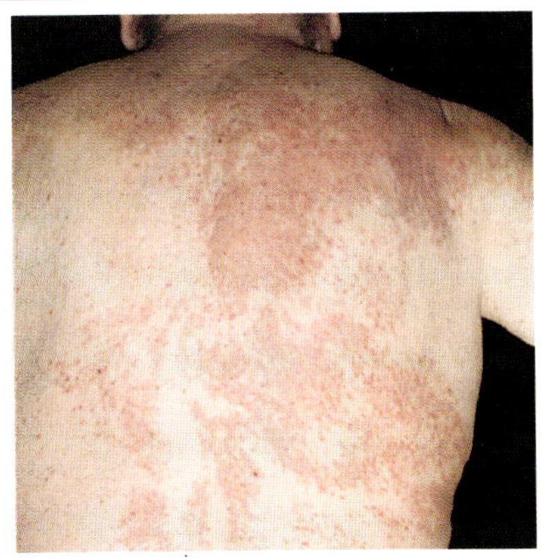

FIG. 24-5 *Pigmented macules, papules, patches, and plaques in a complex design.*

FIG. 24-6 (A) *Keratotic papules in mostly unilateral distribution and following Blaschko's lines (Systematized Darier-type nevus).*

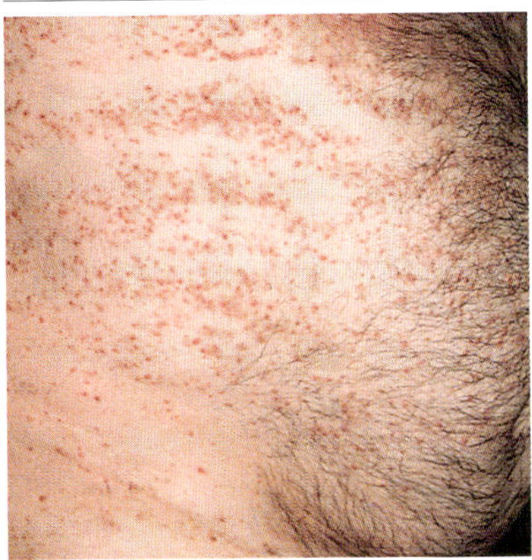

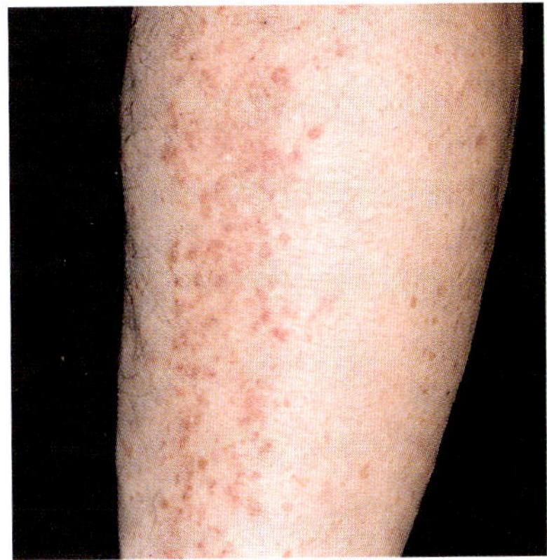

FIG. 24-6 (B, C) *Keratotic papules following Blaschko's lines.*

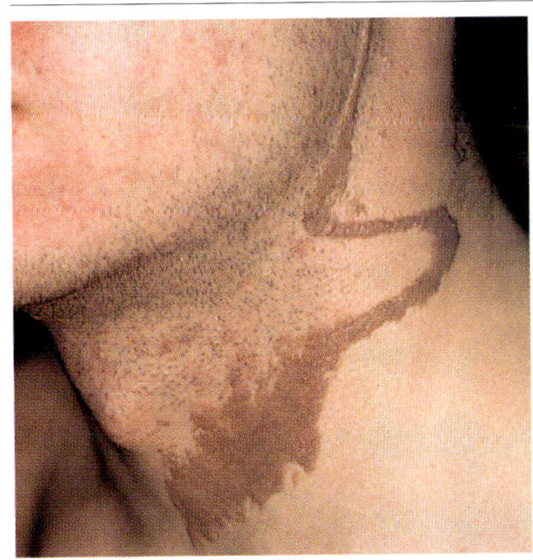

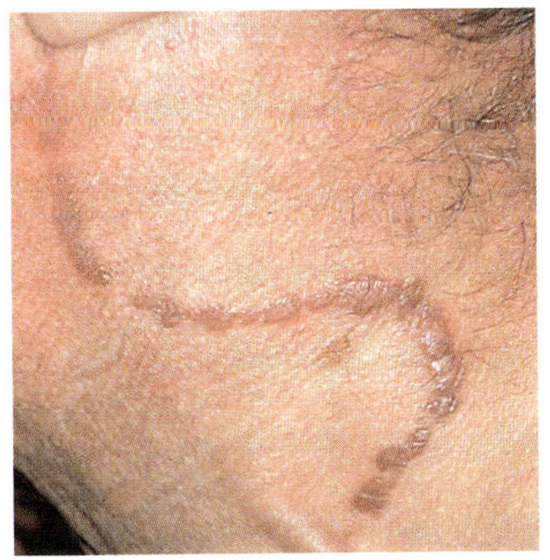

FIG. 24-7 *Pigmented keratotic plaque in serpiginous outline.*

FIG. 24-8 *Verrucous papules in serpentine array.*

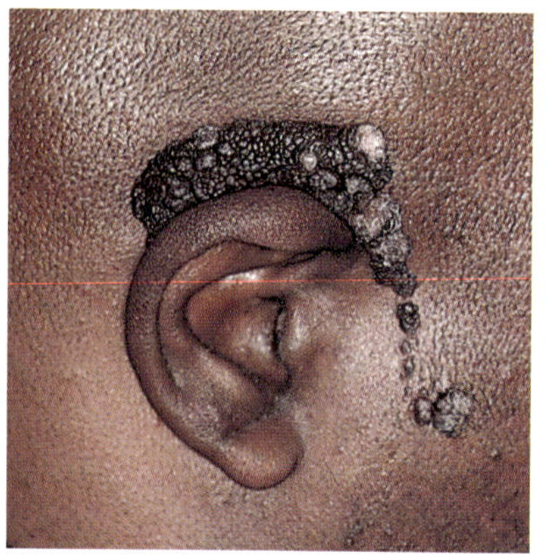

FIG. 24-9 *Keratotic papules and nodules in nearly arciform shape.*

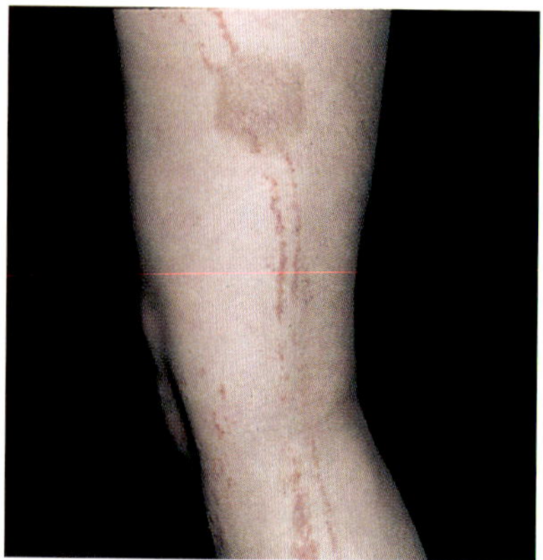

FIG. 24-10 *Verrucous papules with erythema in linear array.*

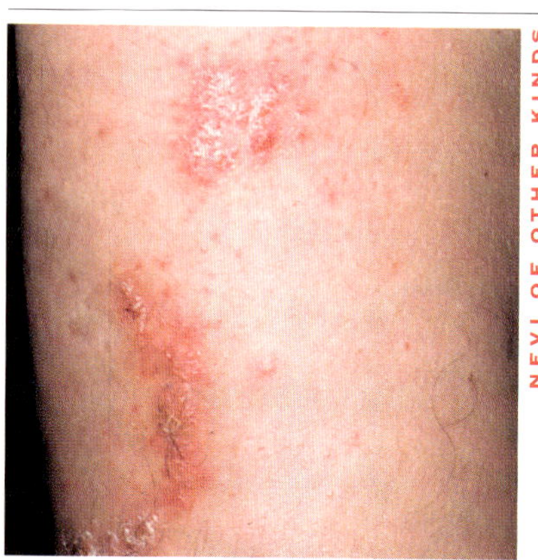

FIG. 24-11 *Keratotic papules on a red base and in linear array (inflammatory linear verrucous epidermal nevus).*

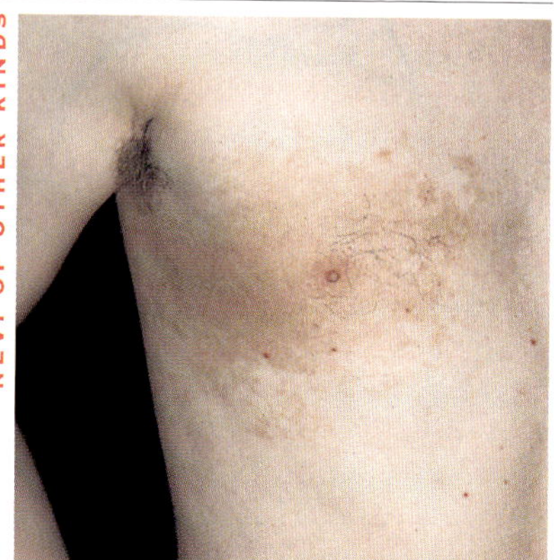

FIG. 24-12 *Becker's nevus, a type of organoid nevus.*

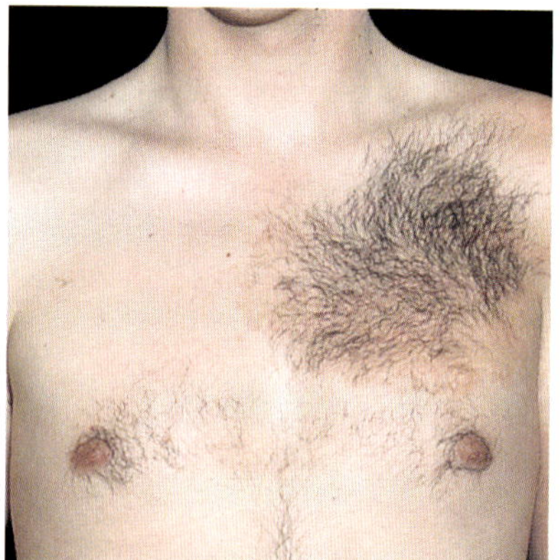

FIG. 24-13 *Pigmented patch with prominent hairs (Becker's nevus, which is a type of organoid nevus).*

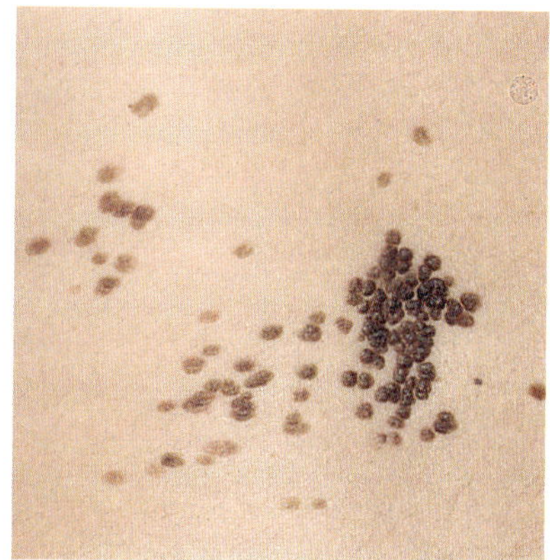

FIG. 24-14 *Connective tissue nevus with a smooth-surface and soft consistency.*

NEVI OF OTHER KINDS

COURSE Epidermal nevi and connective tissue nevi of all kinds often are visible at or soon after birth and persist for a lifetime. Those nevi, unlike neoplasms, do not grow more rapidly than the people who bear them, that is, they are in synchrony with a person's normal growth.

INTEGRATION: UNIFYING CONCEPT There are different types of epidermal nevi, many of them having a distinctive name, such as inflammatory linear verrucous epidermal nevus, ichthyosis hystrix, and so-called systematized Darier's disease. Some of those names telegraph a message of specific histopathologic findings. Such is the case with inflammatory linear verrucous epidermal nevus, which consists of stubby zones of parakeratosis that alternate with zones of orthokeratosis; with ichthyosis hystrix, which is characterized histopathologically by epidermolytic hyperkeratosis; and with "linear Darier's disease," which is typified histopathologically by numerous foci of acantholytic dyskeratosis. The designation ichthyosis hystrix, by the way, is a misnomer; it is not an ichthyosis of any kind but rather one expression of an epidermal nevus that when widespread is termed bullous congenital ichthyosiform erythroderma—also an incorrect designation, because it is not fundamentally an erythroderma.

The relationship between Darier's disease and "linear Darier's disease" is analogous to that between bullous congenital ichthyosiform erythroderma and ichthyosis hystrix; the first condition in each set is widespread, whereas the second is localized (systematized). All four are hamartomas, and the individual lesions of each set are identical morphologically. But Darier's disease is a specific malady that often involves nail units, mucous membranes, and the gastrointestinal tract, and "systematized Darier's disease" is unrelated to it.

Epidermal nevi assume a variety of patterns in terms of distribution, for example, linear, zosteriform, and systematized. Sometimes, as in the case with ichthyosis hystrix, the specific histopathologic findings may be inferred from the clinical appearance of the lesions. Linear epidermal nevi must be distinguished, clinically and histopathologically, from inflammatory diseases that present themselves in linear arrangement, such as linear lichen planus, linear psoriasis, and lichen striatus. The term nevus unius lateris is not specific for any particular condition, but signifies any epidermal (or connective tissue) nevus that is confined to one side of the body.

Distinction also must be made between epidermal nevi in which infundibula and acrosyringia also may be involved, such as systematized porokeratosis, and organoid nevi in which components of the skin besides the epidermis are represented, e.g., follicles, sebaceous glands, apocrine glands, and connective tissue elements, such as nevus sebaceus. Although Becker's nevus is invariably an abnormality of epidermis, it qualifies as an organoid nevus because aberrations of follicles (and consequently of hairs) and of smooth muscles of hair erection are common accompaniments. Epidermal nevi and some organoid nevi, especially those that are widespread, tend to be accompanied by developmental abnormalities, as in bones and in the central nervous system. Acronyms and eponyms given to some of those syndromes are CHILD, Proteus, and Schimmelpfennig.

What has just been written about epidermal nevi obtains also for nevi of connective tissue. Many different types of them exist, all of them are hamartomas made up of collagen, elastic tissue, or both together, and sometimes with acid mucosubstances, too. An example of those connective tissue nevi that involve collagen mostly is shagreen's plaque, of elastic tissue mostly, nevus elasticus, and of adipocytes mostly, nevus lipomatosus. The elastic tissue tends to be abnormal morphologically. Copious quantities of acid mucosubstances may accompany the fibrous and elastic tissue components of a connective tissue nevus.

Each of the different types of connective-tissue nevi has a characteristic clinical and histopathologic appearance. Just as certain types of epidermal nevi are associated with systemic abnormalities, so, too, it is for some kinds of connective tissue nevi. For example, a shagreen's patch signifies tuberous sclerosis, with all of its systemic implications. The connective tissue nevus known as dermatofibrosis lenticularis disseminata indicates Buschke-Ollendorff syndrome, and focal dermal hypoplasia, a so-called minus nevus because of the absence of some connective tissue elements, is a marker of Goltz syndrome.

THERAPY Complete excision when feasible, laser surgery, and dermabrasion are methods for removing epidermal nevi. Cryotherapy also has been advocated.

Only surgical excision is effective in removing nevi of connective tissue.

As a general principle, treatment of epidermal and connective tissue nevi should be predicated on cosmesis only and not on concerns about "malignant degeneration" of them.

DEFINITION A constellation of unrelated blistering diseases, many of them determined genetically but some of them not, that involve skin and sometimes mucous membranes, the blisters often developing after trauma and sometimes resulting in scarring and deformity. Longstanding atrophic scars are often the nidus for development of squamous-cell carcinoma that may prove to be fatal by virtue of metastasis.

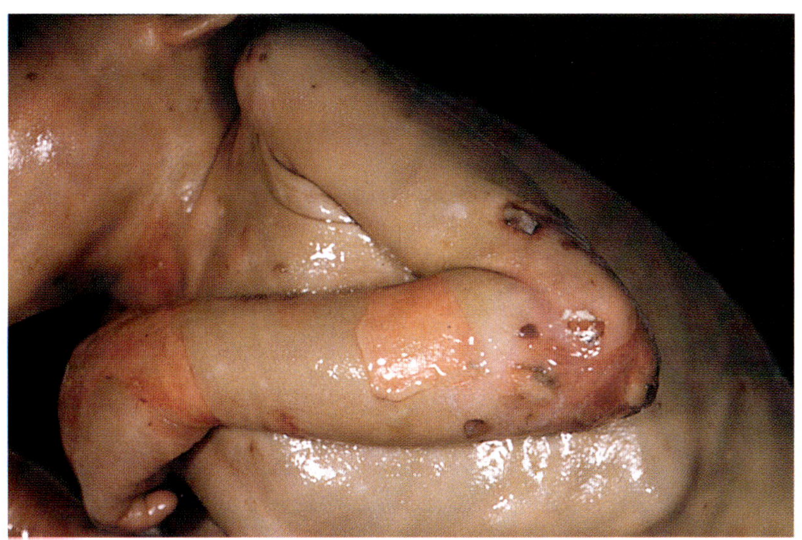

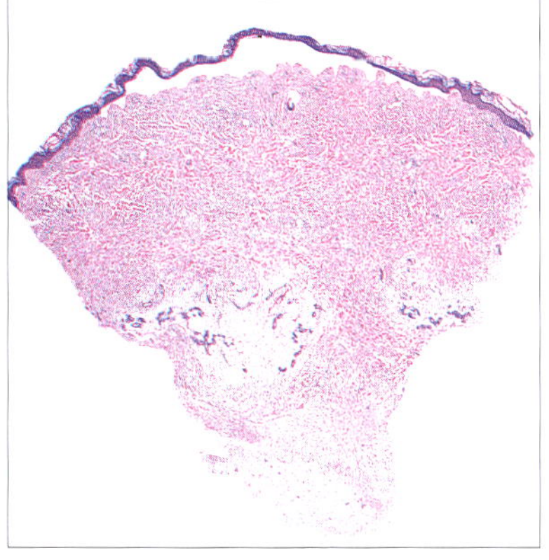

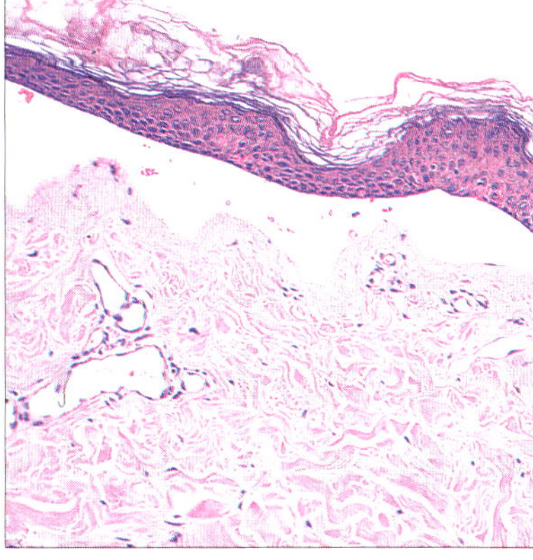

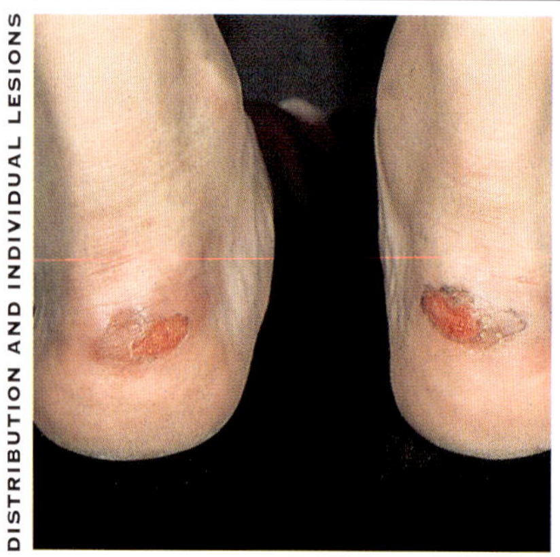

FIG. 25-1 *Bilateral erosions at sites of trauma in a patient with the Weber-Cockayne expression of epidermolysis bullosa.*

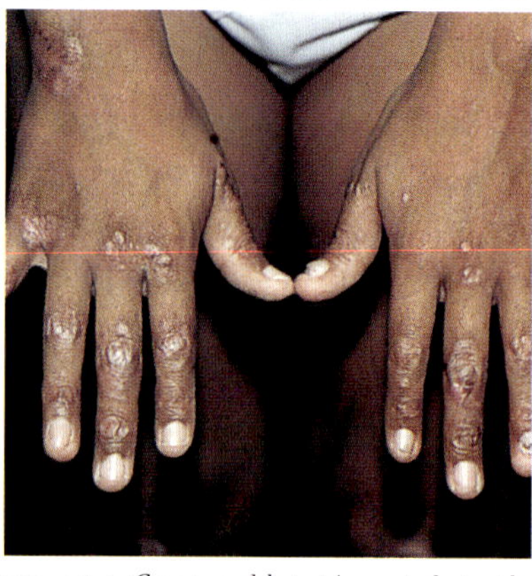

FIG. 25-2 *Crusts and hypopigmented atrophic scars of dominant dystrophic epidermolysis bullosa. Two nails are dystrophic.*

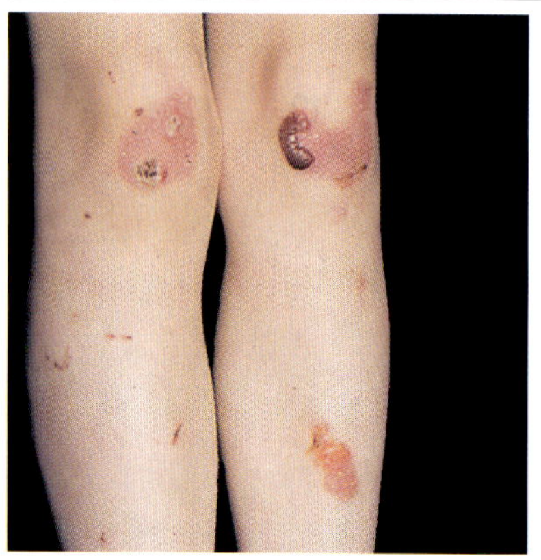

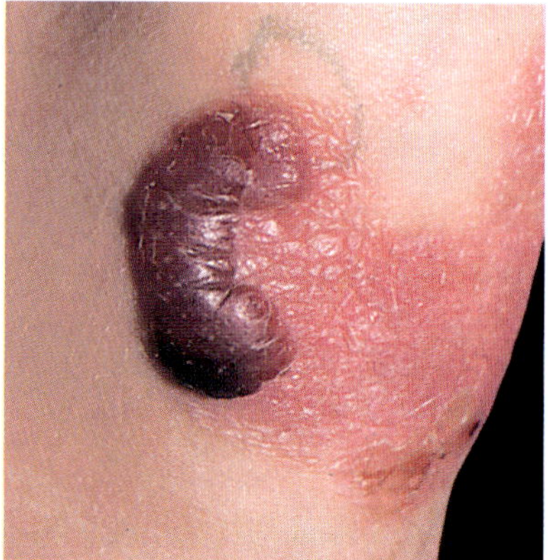

FIG. 25-3 (A, B) *Hemorrhagic blister with an arciform shape in company with crusts and scars of the dominant dystrophic type of epidermolysis bullosa.*

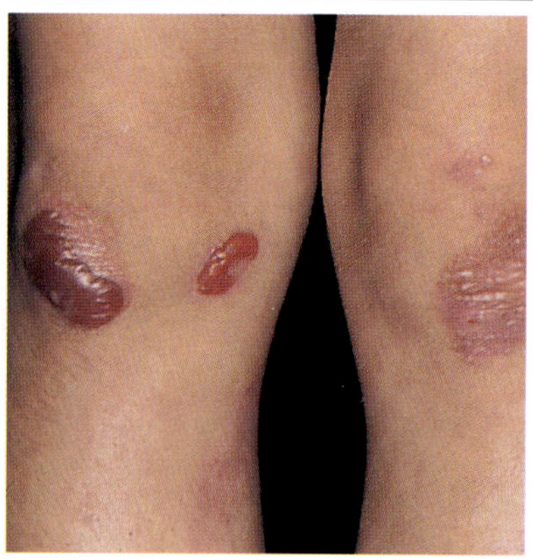

FIG. 25-4 *Blisters, scars, and milia of the dominant dystrophic expression of epidermolysis bullosa.*

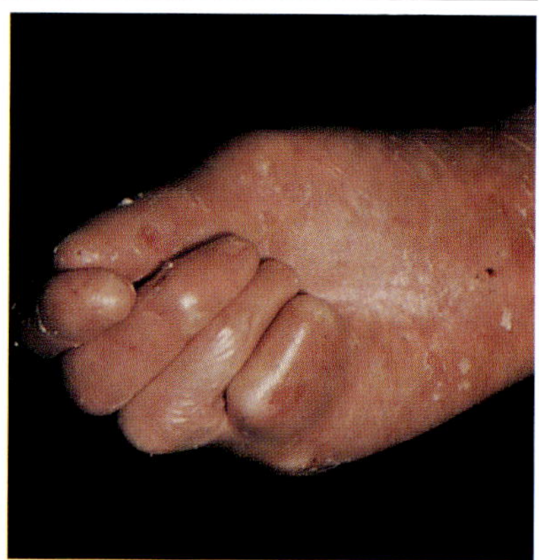

FIG. 25-5 *Atrophic scars that resulted in sclerodactyly and partial amputation of fingers in the recessive dystrophic type.*

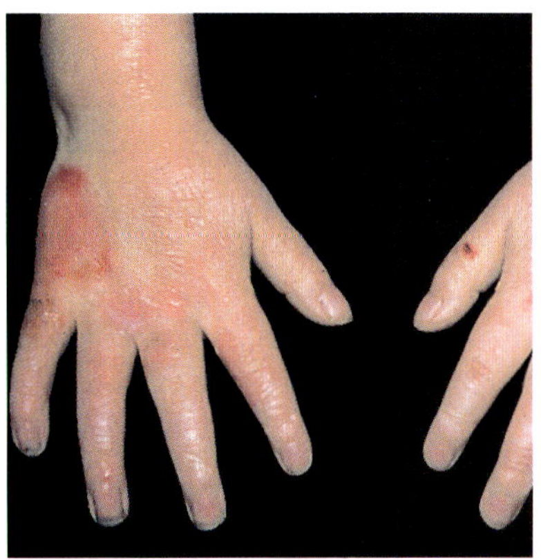

FIG. 25-6 *Blisters, erosions, and scars.*

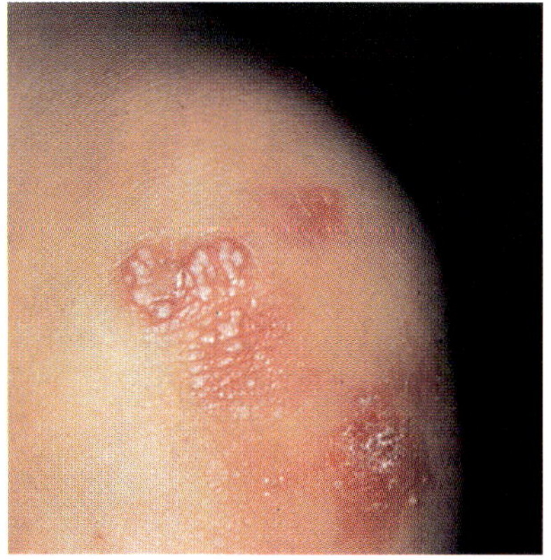

FIG. 25-7 *Milia secondary to the blisters of epidermolysis bullosa simplex.*

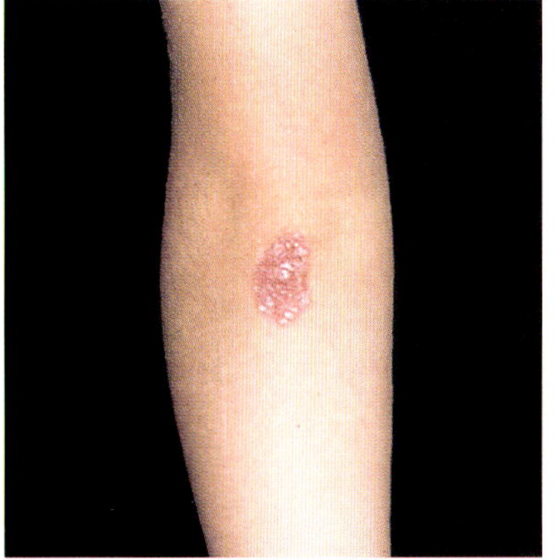

FIG. 25-8 *Clusters of milia secondary to subepidermal blisters of epidermolysis bullosa simplex.*

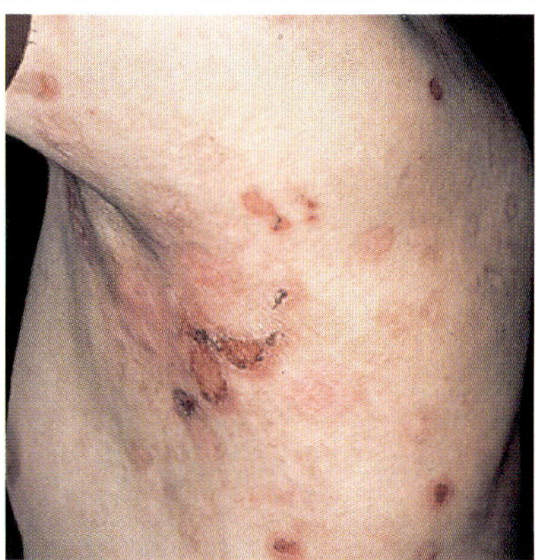

FIG. 25-9 *Vesicles, bullae, erosions, crusts, and pigmented patches of acquired epidermolysis bullosa.*

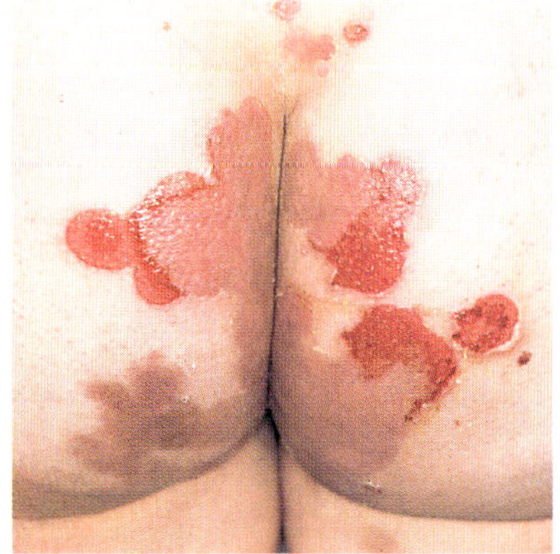

FIG. 25-10 *Erosions surrounded by collarettes of scale-crusts in the dominant dystrophic type of epidermolysis bullosa.*

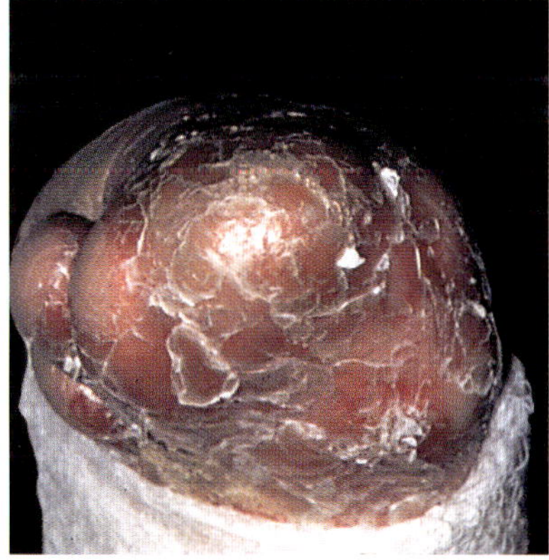

FIG. 25-11 *Stump of an extremity consequent to the destructive effects of repeated blisters of the recessive dystrophic type.*

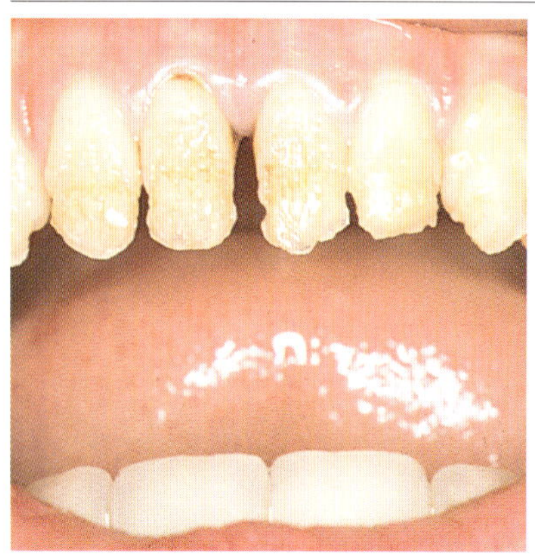

FIG. 25-12 *Deformities of teeth in a dystrophic type of epidermolysis bullosa.*

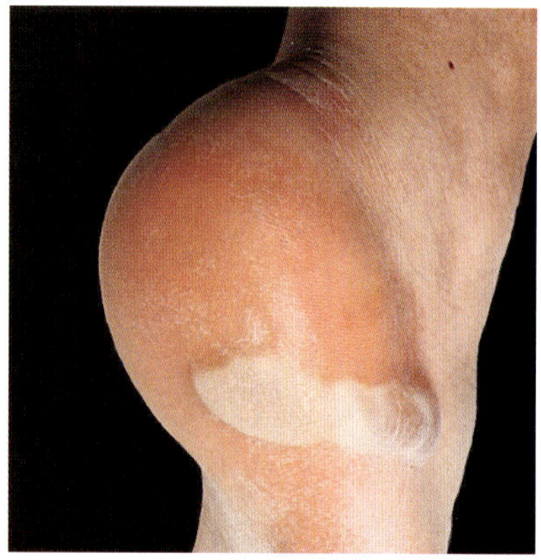

FIG. 25-13 *Tense bullae of epidermolysis bullosa simplex have become confluent.*

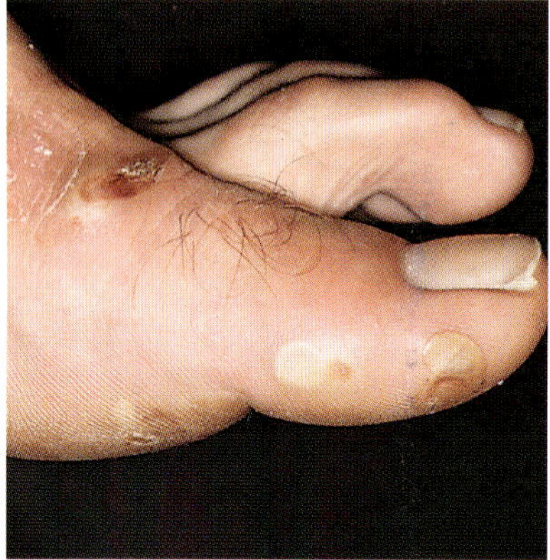

FIG. 25-14 *Vesicles, pustules, and crusted erosions of epidermolysis bullosa simplex.*

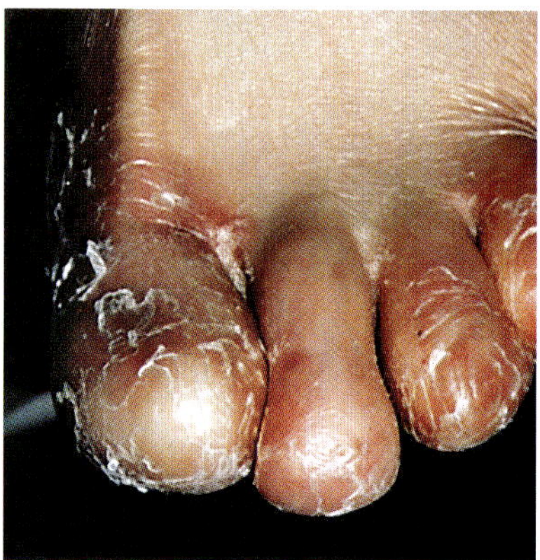

FIG. 25-15 *Atrophic scars and partial loss of toes in the recessive expression of dystrophic epidermolysis bullosa.*

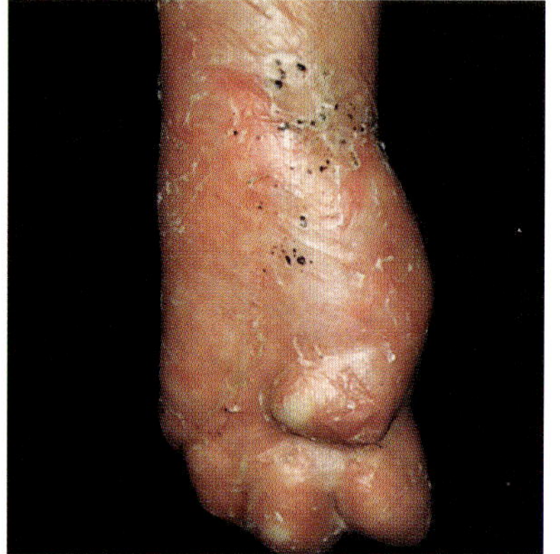

FIG. 25-16 *Stump of an extremity in a patient with the recessive expression of dystrophic epidermolysis bullosa.*

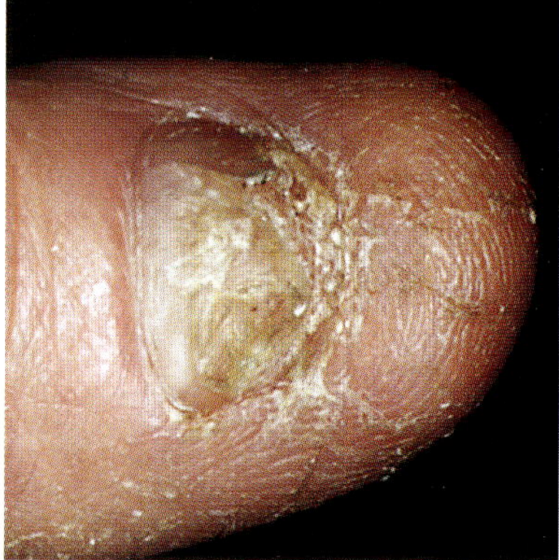

FIG. 25-17 *Partial loss of the nail and crusts in the Herlitz type of epidermolysis bullosa.*

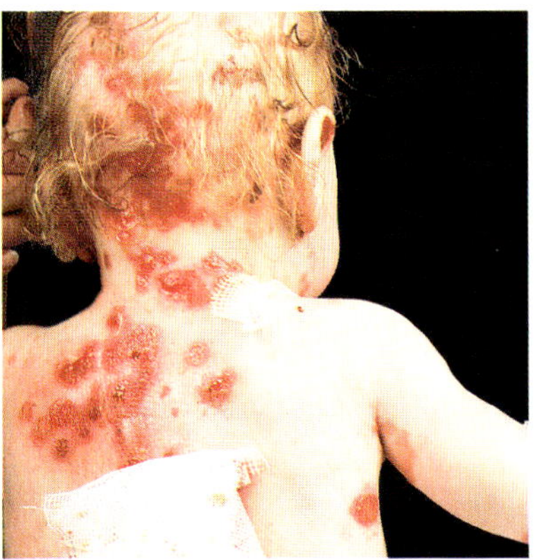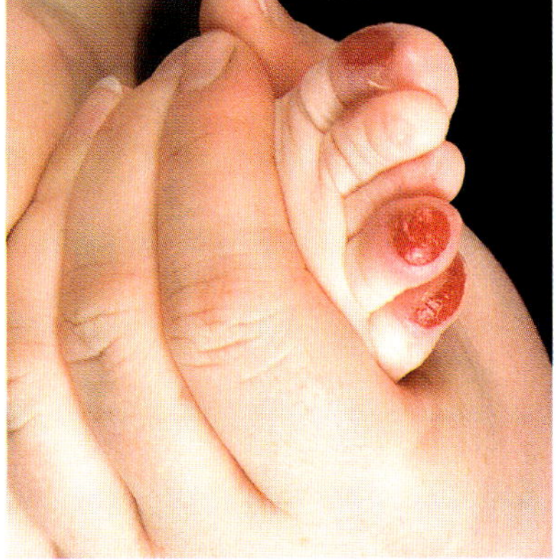

FIG. 25-18 (A, B) *Vesicles, erosions, and absence of nails in the Herlitz type of epidermolysis bullosa.*

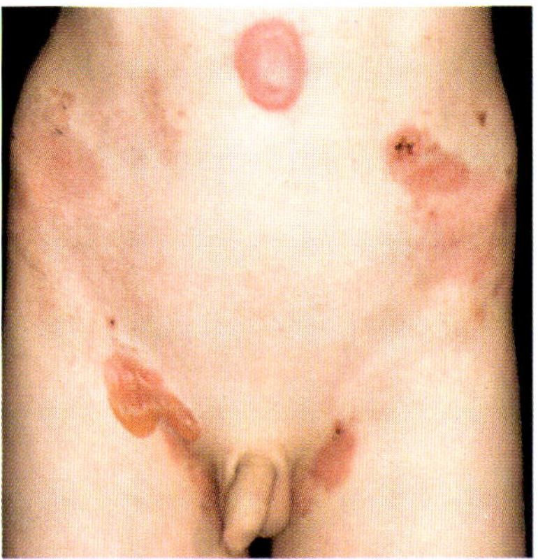

FIG. 25-19 *Erythematous patches and bulla of the dominant expression of dystrophic epidermolysis bullosa.*

ADJUNCTIVE DIAGNOSTIC TESTS Examination by electron microscopy permits identification of the precise site of cleavage and recognition of alterations of basal keratinocytes and anchoring complexes. Antigen mapping technique (immunofluorescence) with the use of immunodiagnostic reagents facilitates correlation of the site of cleavage with various antigens in the basement membrane zone.

COURSE Because all of the diseases called "epidermolysis bullosa" are different from one another, it is not surprising that the course of each of them is distinctive. Epidermolysis bullosa acquisita, for example, occurs in adults and in relatively untoward fashion, the blisters resolving only with scars that are not disfiguring. In contrast, epidermolysis bullosa letalis occurs in infants and, as its name denotes, progresses rapidly to death, usually in early childhood. Epidermolysis bullosa simplex is associated with blisters in children and the effects of it tend to lapse by puberty. The dominant dystrophic type of epidermolysis bullosa may be associated with blisters that come and go for a lifetime, but do not result in permanent severe injury to skin or structures that underlie it. Such is not the case for the recessive dystrophic type of epidermolysis bullosa. Its blisters develop on acral parts in response to only slight trauma and, in the course of years, lead to amputation of digits, synechia, and severely atrophic scars in which potentially metastasizing squamous-cell carcinomas often develop.

Individual blisters of epidermolysis bullosa acquisita and epidermolysis bullosa simplex break quickly and heal soon. By contrast, the blisters that develop in the recessive type of epidermolysis bullosa dystrophica heal with great difficulty over weeks and months. In a matter of years, nails no longer are present in patients with the recessive dystrophic type. The blisters also involve mucous membranes of the alimentary canal, sometimes eliciting subepithelial fibrosis that causes strictures and stenosis of the esophagus, a circumstance that results inevitably in death from inanition.

INTEGRATION: UNIFYING CONCEPT There is no way to synthesize all of the different diseases named "epidermolysis bullosa" because the only thing they have in common is blisters. Blisters of one manifestation of epidermolysis bullosa are intraepidermal (those of epidermolysis bullosa simplex occur within the basal layer of the epidermis), whereas those of the others are subepidermal. Subepidermal blisters form at different sites beneath the epidermis; for example, those of the letalis type form in the lamina lucida, and of the dominant dystrophic type beneath the lamina densa. Some do not heal with scars (e.g., epidermolysis bullosa simplex), whereas others, such as the recessive type of epidermolysis bullosa dystrophica, resolve with scars so deforming that stumps representing the residua are referred to as "mitten-like hands."

Some conditions titled epidermolysis bullosa involve the skin only—for example, epidermolysis bullosa simplex and epidermolysis bullosa acquisita—whereas other diseases termed epidermolysis bullosa involve the skin and other organs, especially mucous membranes, as in the dominant dystrophic and the recessive dystrophic types. Most of the conditions called epidermolysis bullosa are not associated with carcinomas, but in the recessive dystrophic type, squamous-cell carcinomas tend to appear in skin that has become extremely atrophic consequent to the effects of fibrosis. The fibrosis follows upon repeated blisters at a particular site, usually an extremity.

What is apparent, however, is that epidermolysis bullosa acquisita develops in adults presumably as a consequence of an immunologic reaction against constituents of the epidermal basement membrane. By contrast, all of the other diseases named "epidermolysis bullosa" appear in infancy or childhood, and result from genetic defects in the production of various proteins that are responsible for binding the epidermis to the dermis. The nature of some of those defects is now known precisely.

In sum, although the term "epidermolysis bullosa" is applied for historical reasons to a number of diseases, each is really different and distinctive, genetically, morphologically, and biologically. The same can be said of those different diseases classified indiscriminately as Ehlers-Danlos syndrome, the mucopolysaccharidoses, the ichthyoses, the sclerodermas, and the keratoacanthomas that were once thought to be manifestations of a single pathologic process but now are recognized to be unrelated.

THERAPY No effective treatment is available for preventing blisters of any expression of epidermolysis bullosa. Because trauma induces blisters, every effort must be made to minimize trauma to the skin. Systemically administered corticosteroids and immunosuppressive agents may be beneficial in the management of patients with epidermolysis bullosa acquisita. Antibiotics given topically or systemically are valuable in ridding bacteria responsible for impetiginization of blisters and of erosions that follow on breakage of them. Blisters and erosions may be managed with topical therapy such as ointments and special dressings. A new method for accelerating healing of erosions in patients with epidermolysis bullosa involves application of Apligraf, which also is being tested for replacing skin of those patients at sites subjected often to trauma. Patients with severe epidermolysis bullosa require much more than skin care; they need support in the form of nutritional supplements, physical therapy, and psychological counseling.

In patients with atrophic scars of the recessive dystrophic type, scrupulous attention must be paid to any sign of squamous-cell carcinoma in order to excise that neoplasm before it metastasizes.

DEFINITION An inflammatory process caused by one of several bacteria, especially Streptococcus pyogenes, and manifested clinically as erythematous patches and erythematous edematous plaques with scalloped outlines upon which vesicles and bullae, some of them hemorrhagic, may develop.

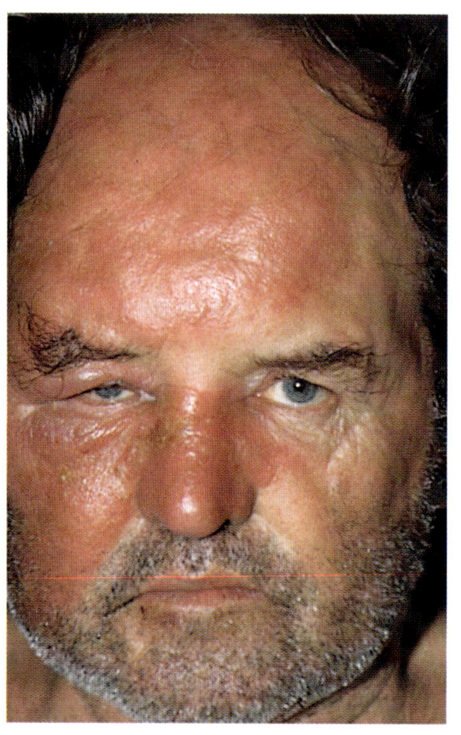

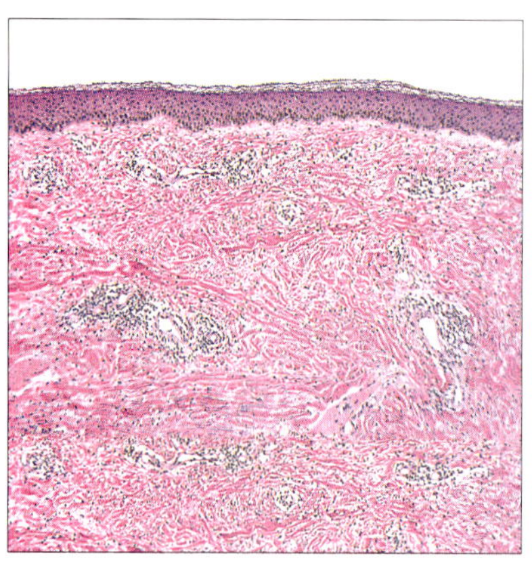

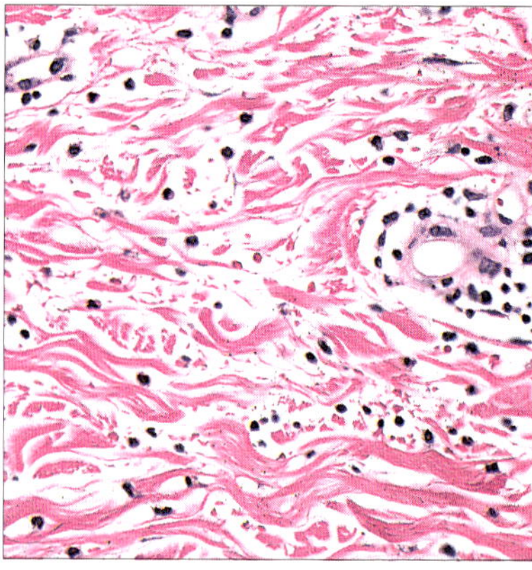

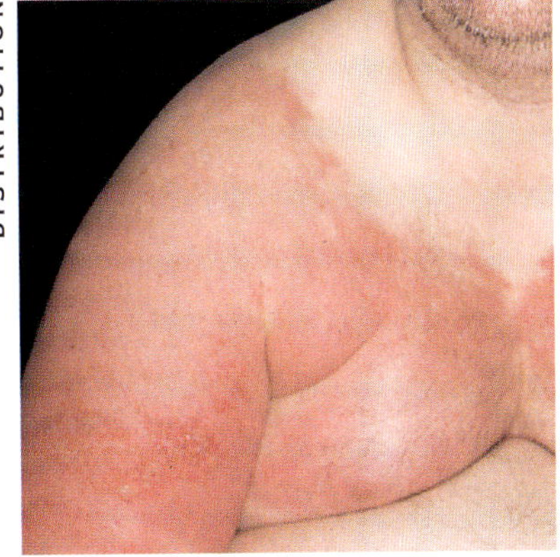

FIG. 26-1 *Broad erythematous plaque with scalloped margins, atop which are vesicles and erosions. Note signs of mastectomy.*

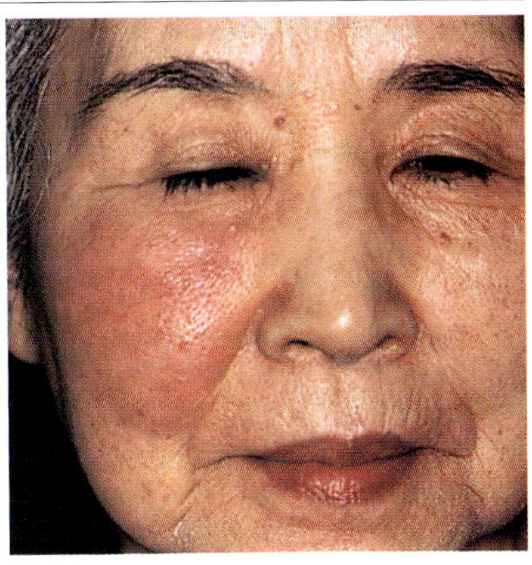

FIG. 26-2 *Erythematous edematous zone on one cheek.*

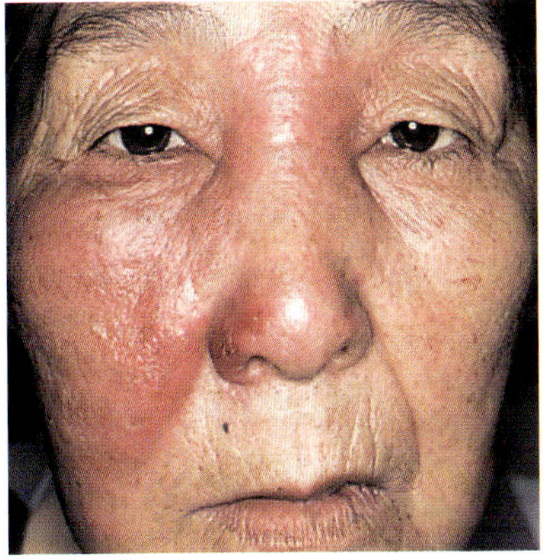

FIG. 26-3 *Edema, mostly unilateral, joined by erythema on the nose and cheek.*

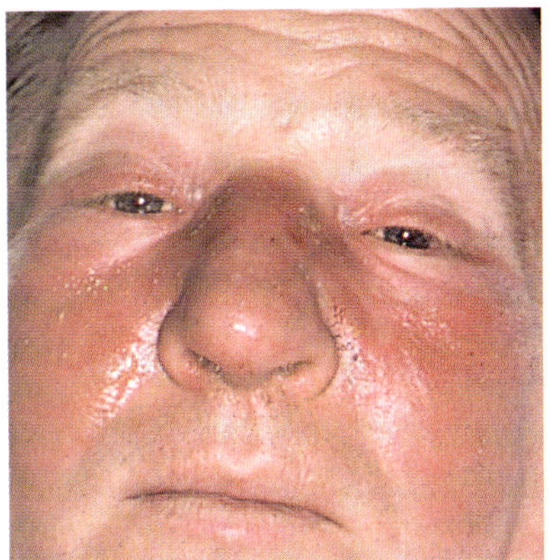

FIG. 26-4 *Erythema and swelling of the nose, eyelids, and cheeks associated with serous crusts.*

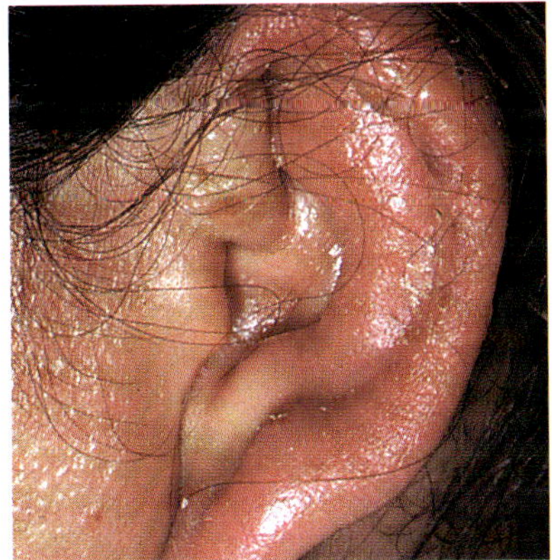

FIG. 26-5 *Erythema and swelling with blisters near the superior part of the pinna.*

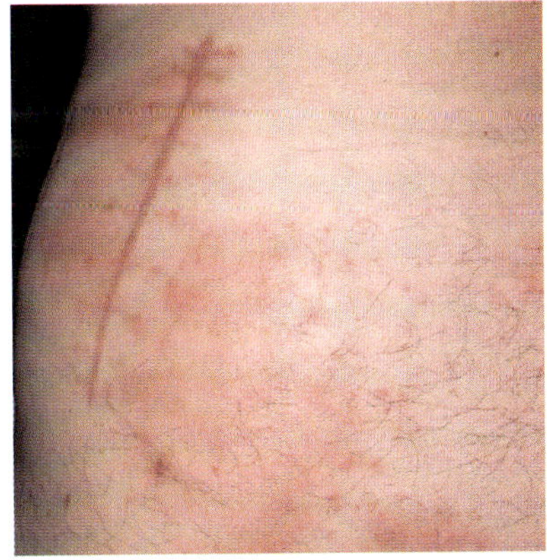

FIG. 26-6 *Erythema and edema following a surgical procedure.*

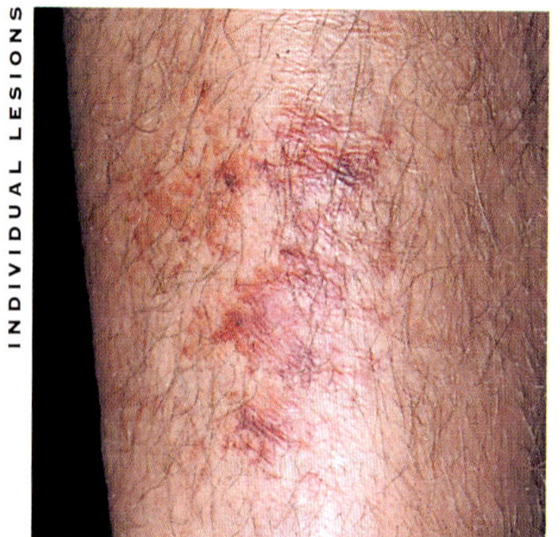

FIG. 26-7 *Erythematous and purpuric macules, hemorrhagic vesicles, and a plaque with a scalloped border.*

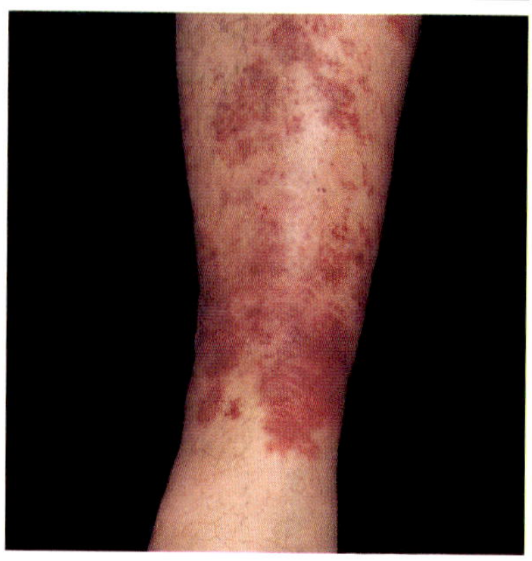

FIG. 26-8 *Purpuric macules, papules, and plaques, the latter with scalloped margins.*

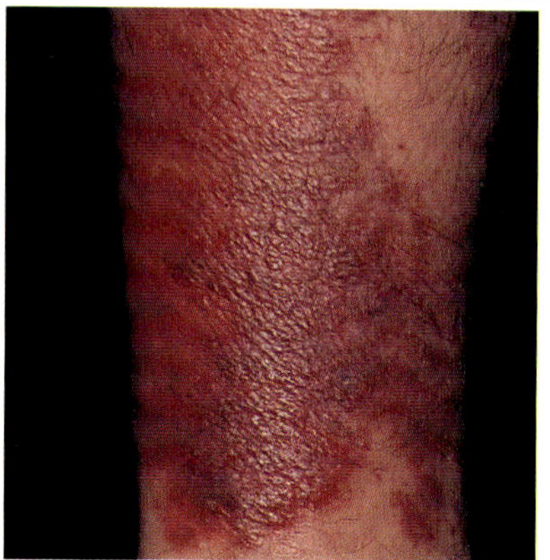

FIG. 26-9 *Purpuric plaque with scalloped borders and incipient hemorrhagic vesicles.*

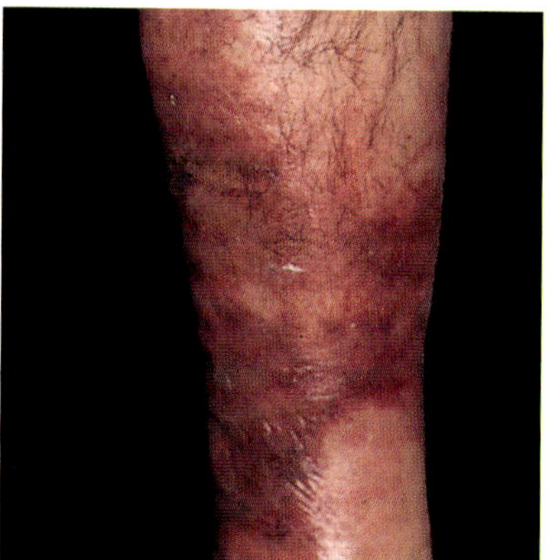

FIG. 26-10 *Purpuric plaque with hemorrhagic bullae.*

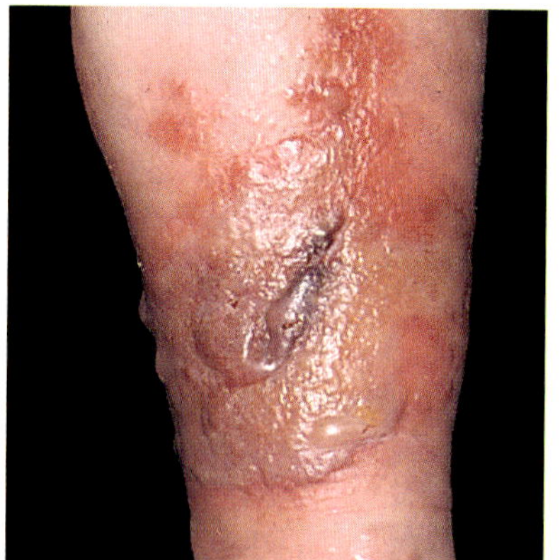

FIG. 26-11 *Vesicles and bullae on an erythematous base.*

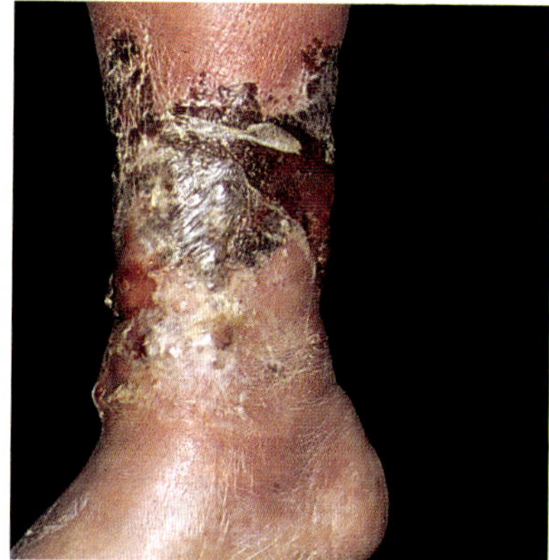

FIG. 26-12 *Crusted plaque with ulceration surrounded by erythema in a patient who is immunosuppressed.*

ADJUNCTIVE DIAGNOSTIC TEST Isolation of the causative organism by culture of the site of infection.

COURSE The most characteristic type of cellulitis is erysipelas, which is caused mostly by group A streptococci. The process evolves rapidly, and affected individuals display symptoms of systemic infection, among them fever and malaise. The condition, which often follows a penetrating wound of the skin, tends to heal without specific therapy and to disappear in about a week or two. The process sometimes recurs and, not uncommonly, at the same site, usually the face or leg. Numerous recurrences of cellulitis on a leg may result in unremitting brawny edema that ends as elephantiasis nostras.

INTEGRATION: UNIFYING CONCEPT Erysipelas in children and adults is caused by a bacterium. In children, the offending pathogens are mostly beta hemolytic streptococcus, Staphylococcus aureus, and Haemophilus influenzae, whereas in adults, the responsible organisms are mostly beta hemolytic streptococcus and Staphylococcus aureus. The mechanism whereby these organisms induce characteristic lesions—an erythematous patch or an erythematous edematous plaque that exhibits pseudopods and sometimes vesicles at its periphery—is not known.

THERAPY Antibiotics administered systemically, in particular, penicillin G delivered intramuscularly or intravenously, are curative. In severe infections, administration of penicillinase-resistant penicillins or broad coverage with other antibiotics is advisable.

DEFINITION An inflammatory disease characterized by lesions with arcuate, annular, and serpiginous outlines and by collarettes of scale on the inner margin of lesions that extend outward in centrifugal fashion, disappearing in months as a rule in the absence of treatment.

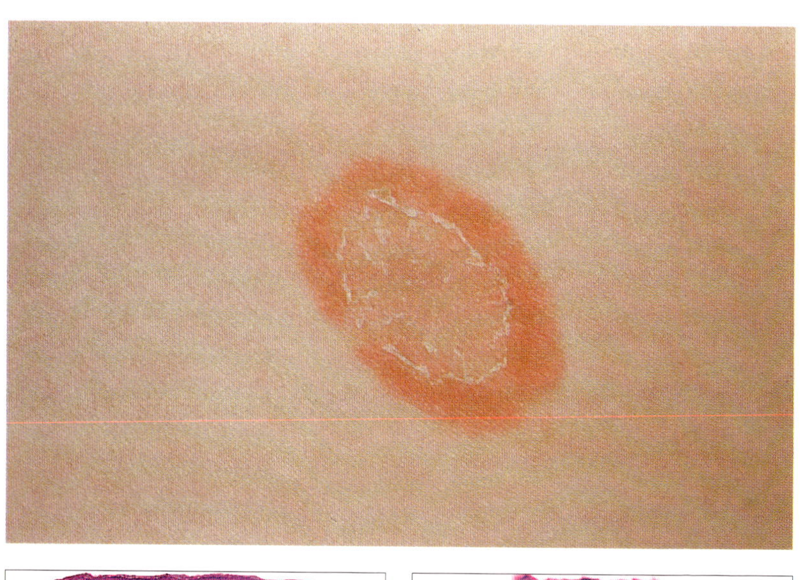

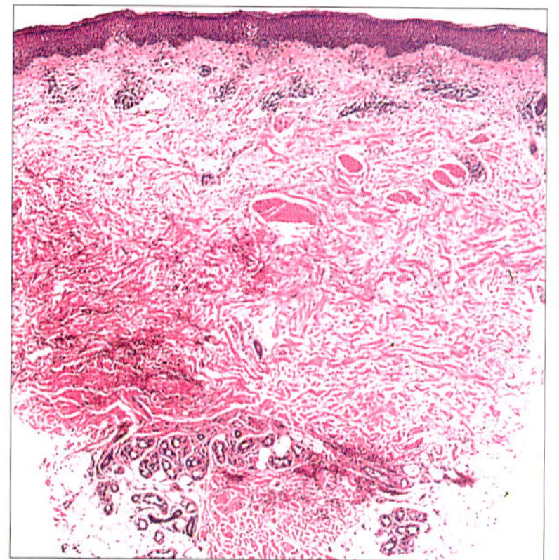

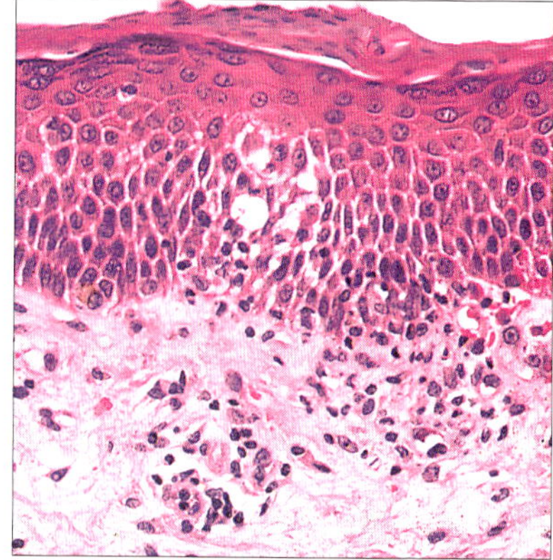

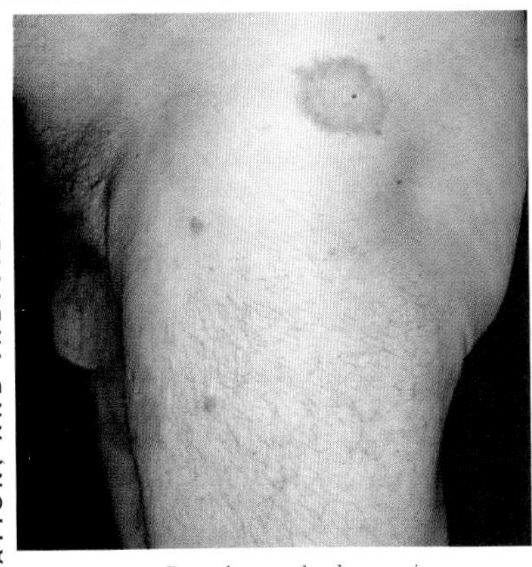

FIG. 27-1 *Papules and plaque in arcuate configuration, with thread-like scale along its inner margin.*

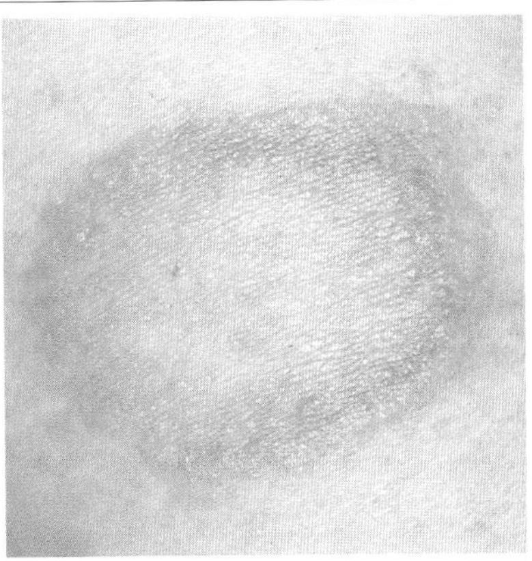

FIG. 27-2 *Plaque in arcuate shape with thread-like scale on its inner margin.*

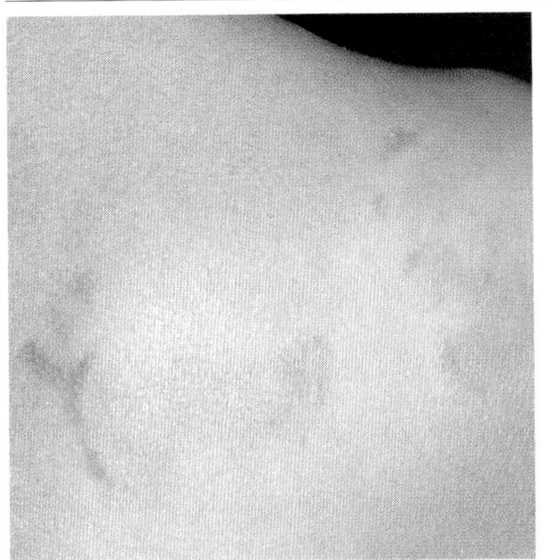

FIG. 27-3 *Plaques with annular shape and hyperpigmented patches.*

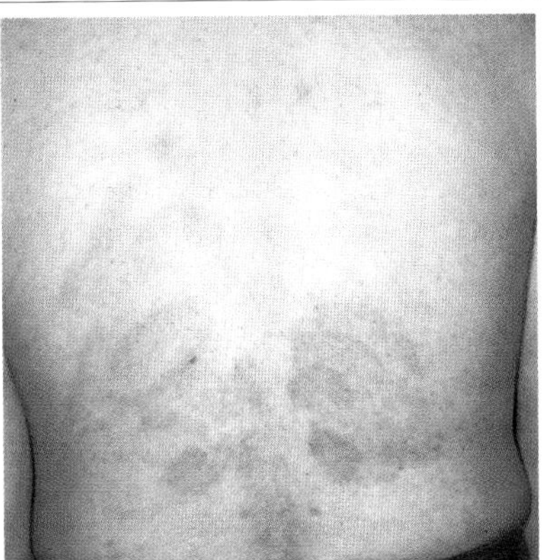

FIG. 27-4 *Arcuate lesions on the trunk have resolved with hyperpigmentation.*

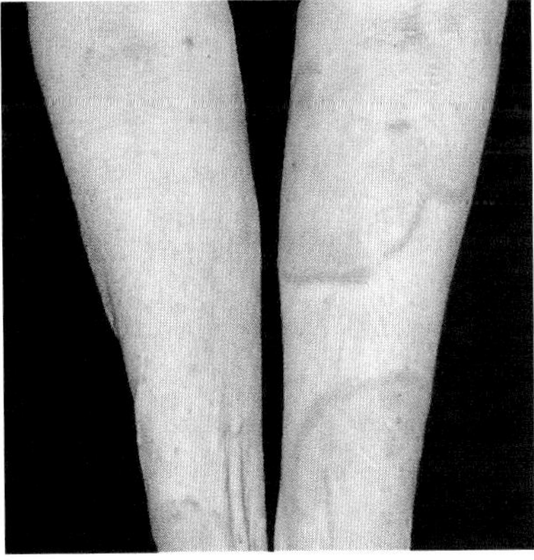

FIG. 27-5 *Arcuate lesions leave hyperpigmentation in their wake.*

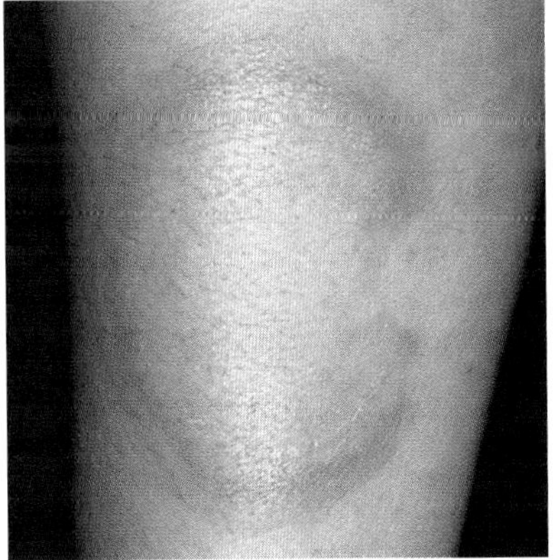

FIG. 27-6 *Plaque with arcuate shape and scale along the inner margin.*

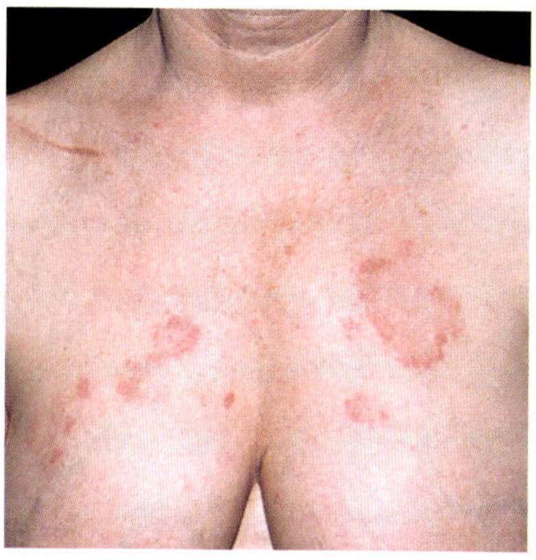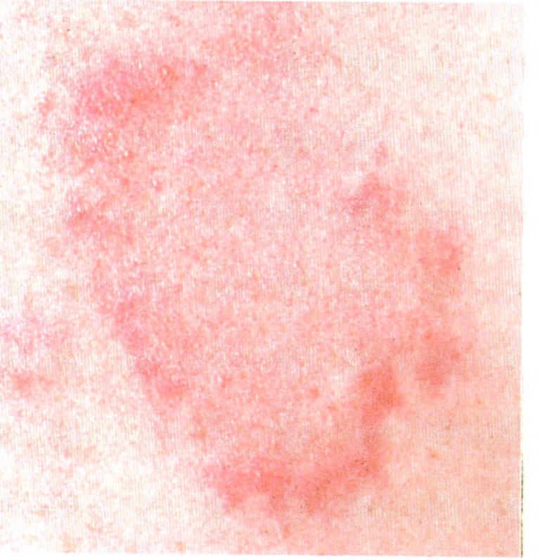

FIG. 27-7 (A, B) *Red papules in mostly arcuate and annular patterns.*

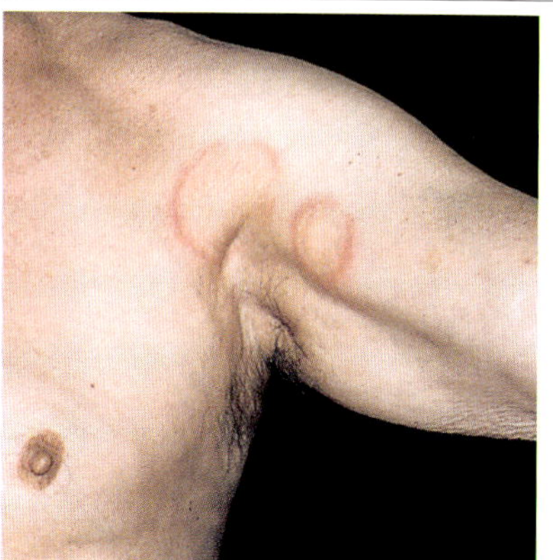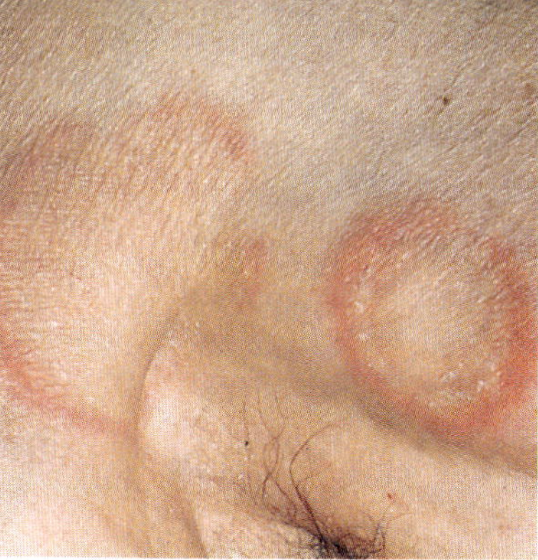

FIG. 27-8 (A, B) *Plaques in annular configuration, one of which has scale along its inner margin.*

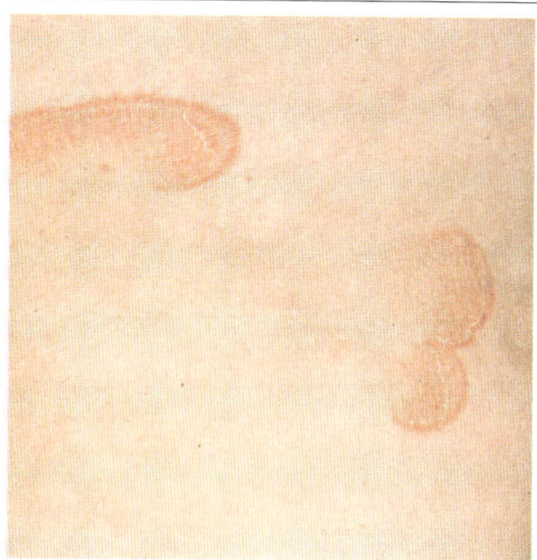

FIG. 27-9 *Patches of hyperpigmentation represent resolution of advancing arcuate plaques.*

COURSE Individual lesions of erythema annulare centrifugum usually expand centrifugally for weeks or months before disappearing. The condition may last for years.

INTEGRATION: UNIFYING CONCEPT Erythema annulare centrifugum is but one of many diseases characterized by spongiotic dermatitis. Histopathologically it is indistinguishable from pityriasis rosea. The scale of both conditions is made up of mounds of parakeratosis that sometimes house tiny globules of plasma. When a mound of parakeratosis is shed, the tiny residuum of parakeratosis at the very periphery forms what is seen clinically as a collarette of scale. The epidermis is slightly hyperplastic and punctuated by foci of spongiosis. The edematous papillary dermis harbors a few extravasated erythrocytes, and a rather sparse infiltrate of lymphocytes is present around venules of the superficial plexus. Rarely, and virtually only in black people, spongiosis in pityriasis rosea may eventuate in true vesicles. That is not the case, however, for erythema annulare centrifugum, in which vesicles never come into being.

The cause of erythema annulare centrifugum is not known, and neither are the mechanisms responsible for formation of its lesions.

THERAPY If a condition that underlies the development of the skin lesions can be identified, as is the case exceedingly rarely, it should be managed appropriately. Topical application of corticosteroids to the lesions themselves reduces redness, but does not alter the course of the process itself.

DEFINITION An inflammatory process that tends to involve mucous membranes, as well as skin, and of the latter the acra especially. The stereotypical presentation is lesions composed of concentric rings ("iris" and "target" type). The condition varies greatly in severity, the most extensive expressions of it going by names such as Stevens-Johnson syndrome and Lyell's syndrome (the adult type of toxic epidermal necrolysis).

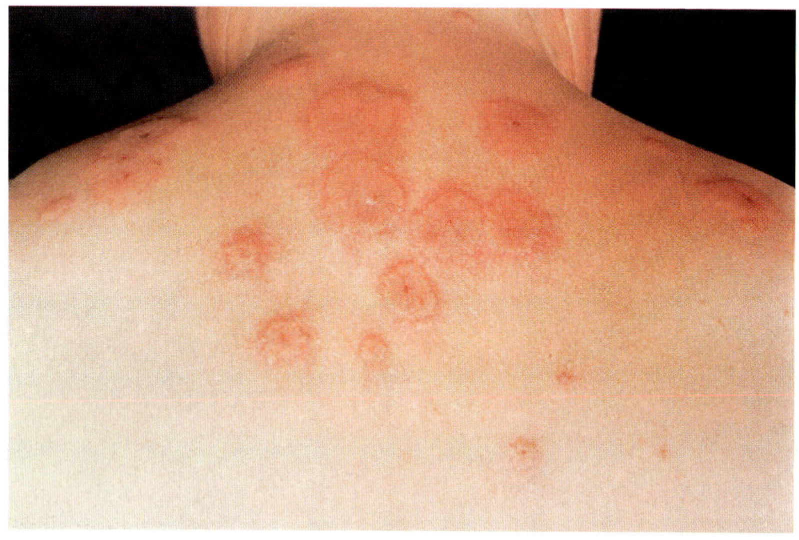

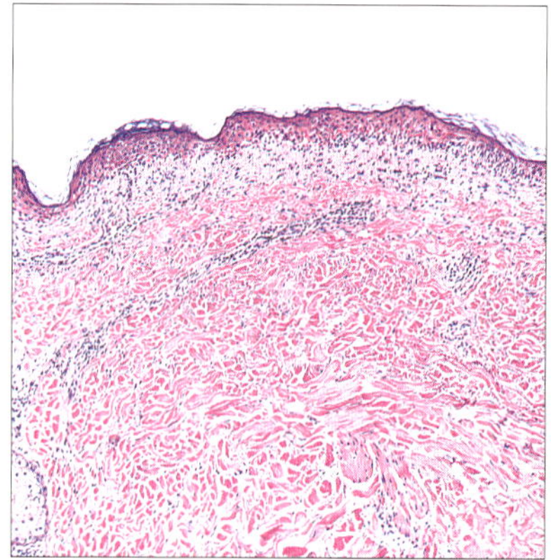

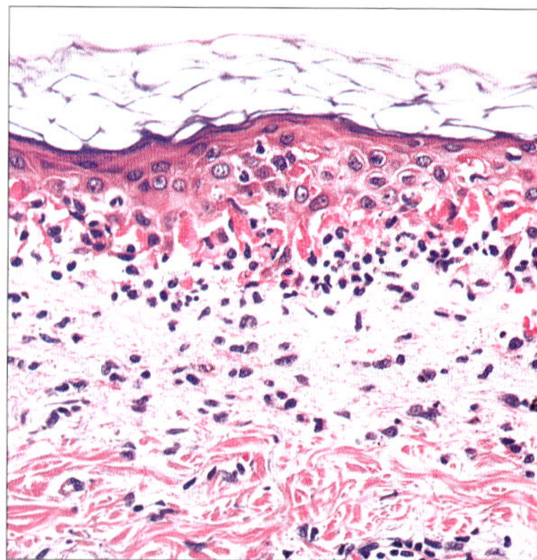

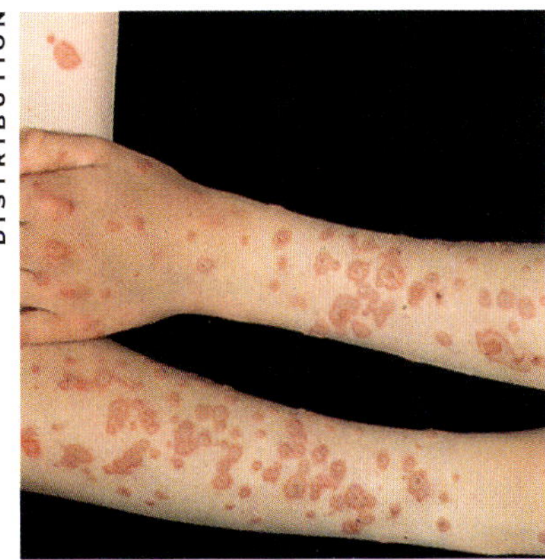

FIG. 28-1 *Erythematous papules, some with the appearance of an iris.*

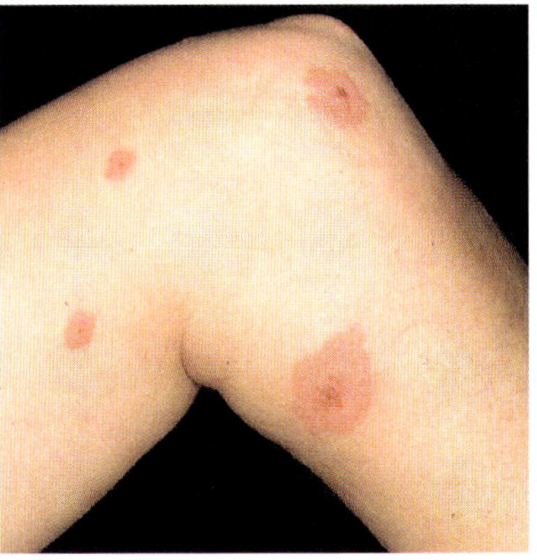

FIG. 28-2 *Erythematous papules and plaques with vesicles and crusts in the center.*

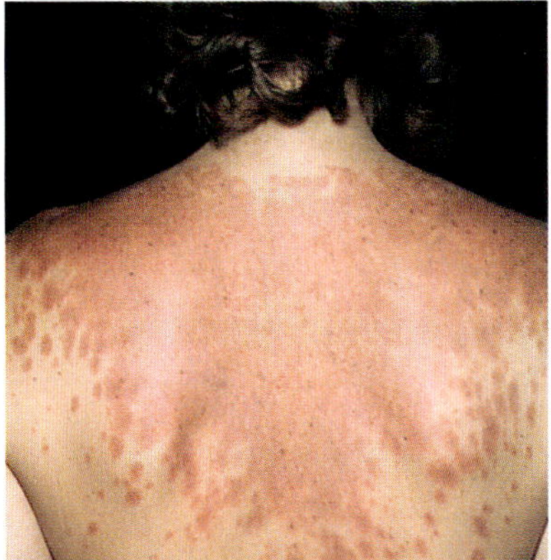

FIG. 28-3 *Round, dusky erythematous papules that have become confluent.*

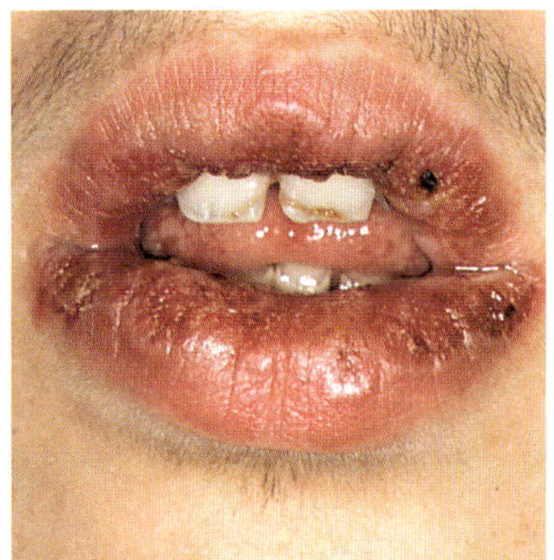

FIG. 28-4 *Erosions and hemorrhagic crusts, at the periphery of which are subtle blisters.*

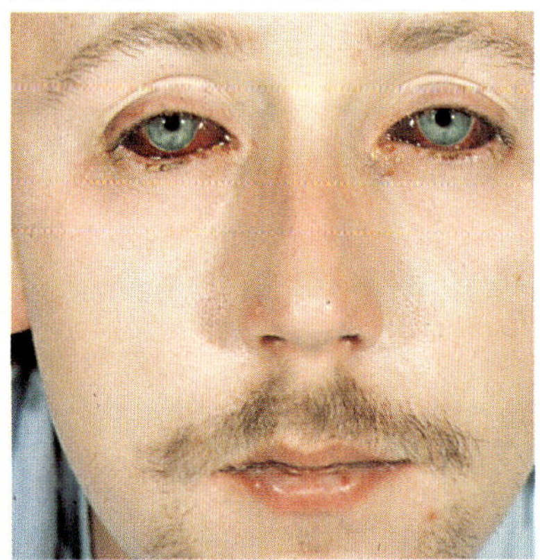

FIG. 28-5 *Involvement of the lower lip by crusts and scales, and of the sclerae by hemorrhage.*

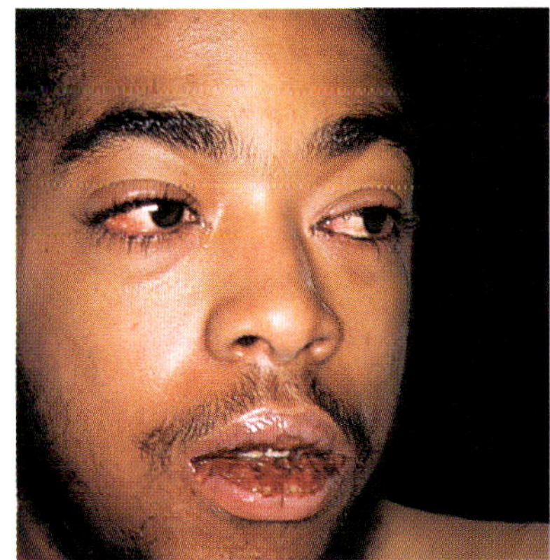

FIG. 28-6 *Erosions and hemorrhagic crusts of the lips, and erythema of the sclerae.*

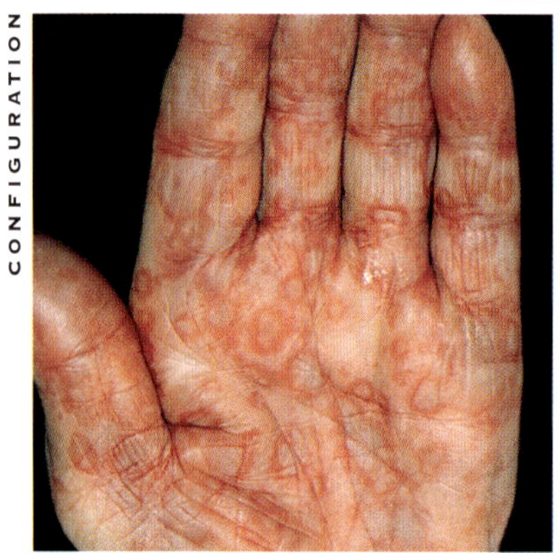

FIG. 28-7 *Annular lesions with a central gray-roofed blister and a red rim.*

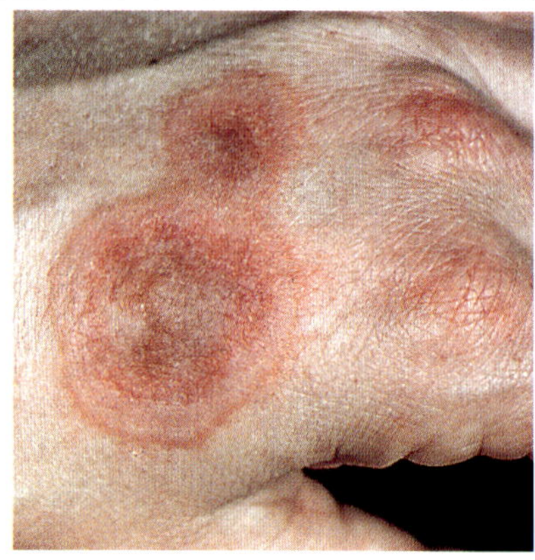

FIG. 28-8 *Plaques composed of concentric rings and a dusky erythematous center.*

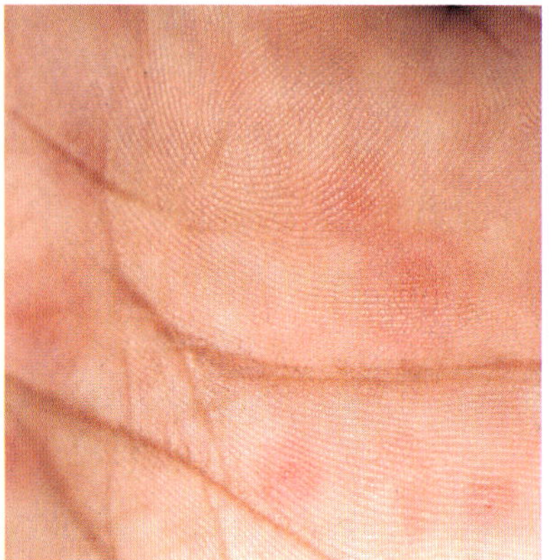

FIG. 28-9 *Round papules and plaques made up of a slightly darker zone in the center and a pale ring.*

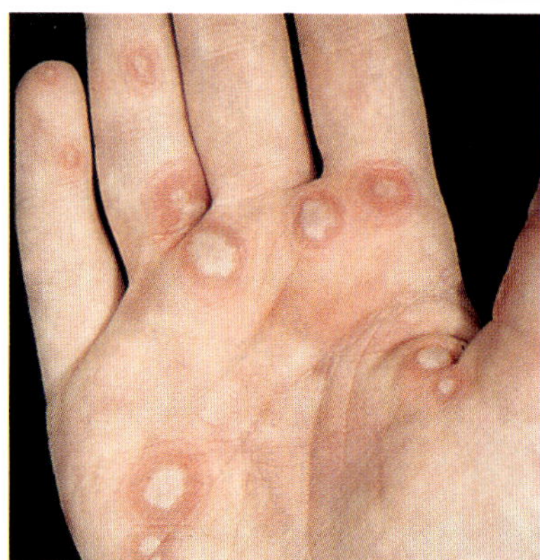

FIG. 28-10 *Some lesions made up of concentric rings that in their center display vesiculopustules.*

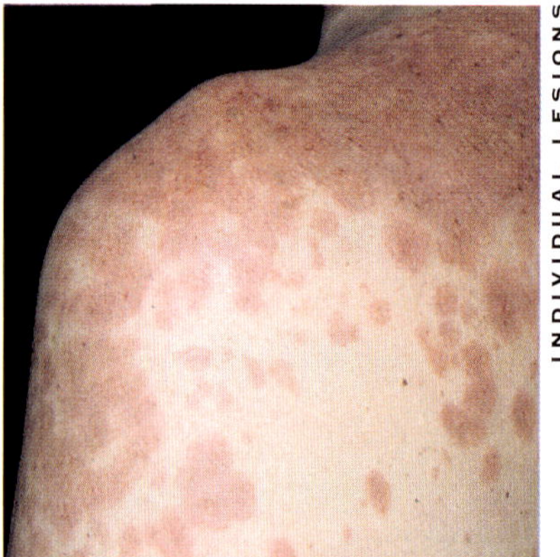

FIG. 28-11 *Dusky erythematous macules and papules, many of the latter having become confluent.*

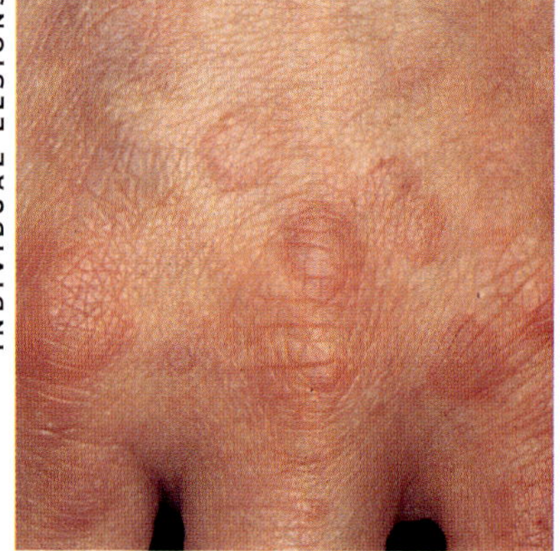

FIG. 28-12 *Erythematous edematous papules with a slightly darker rim.*

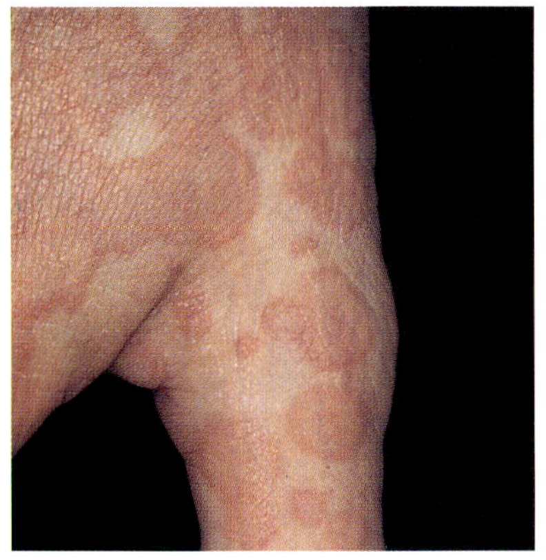

FIG. 28-13 *Papules, most of them round, with a dark center and dark rim. Some have become confluent to form plaques.*

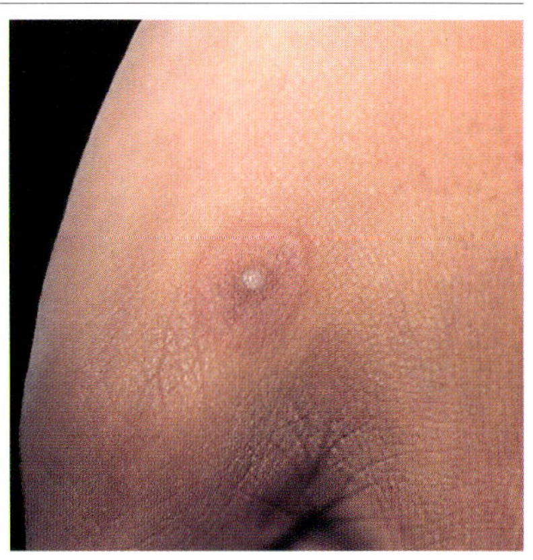

FIG. 28-14 *A pustule in the center of a papule that has a dark rim.*

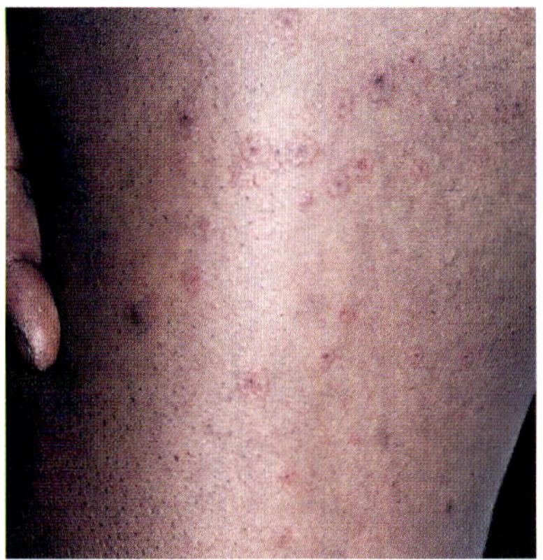

FIG. 28-15 *Small round papules with a dark punctate center and a dark rim.*

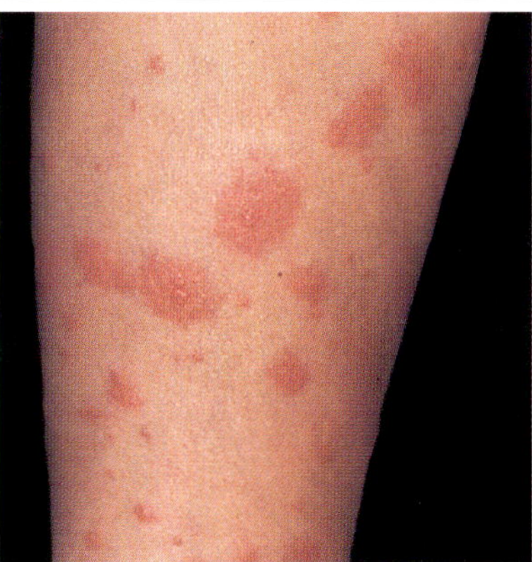

FIG. 28-16 *Erythematous papules with a central vesicle.*

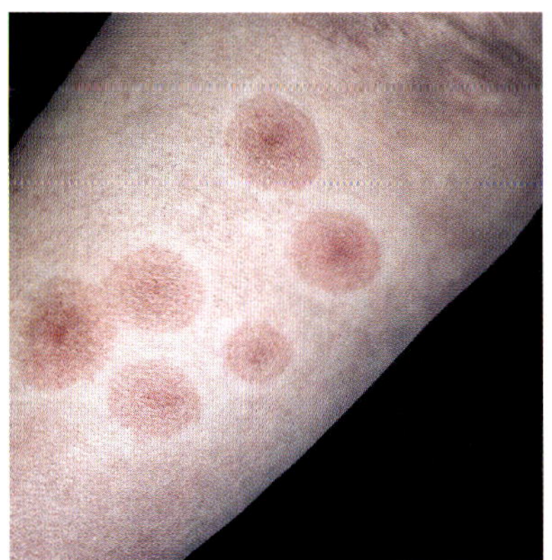

FIG. 28-17 *Dusky erythematous plaques in annular configuration.*

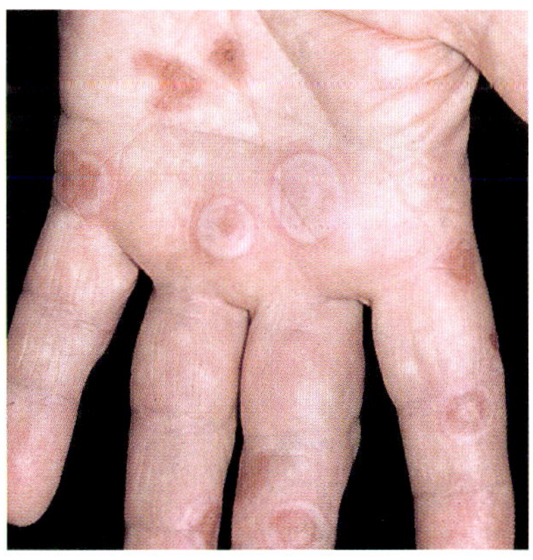

FIG. 28-18 *Vesicles with a gray roof and erosions.*

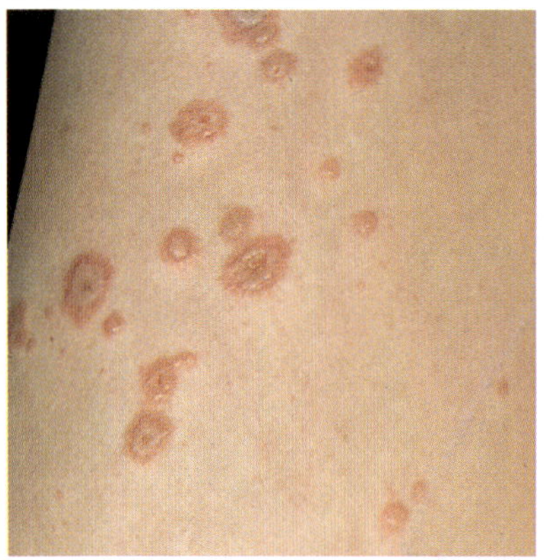

FIG. 28-19 *Erythematous papules surmounted by vesicles and vesiculopustules.*

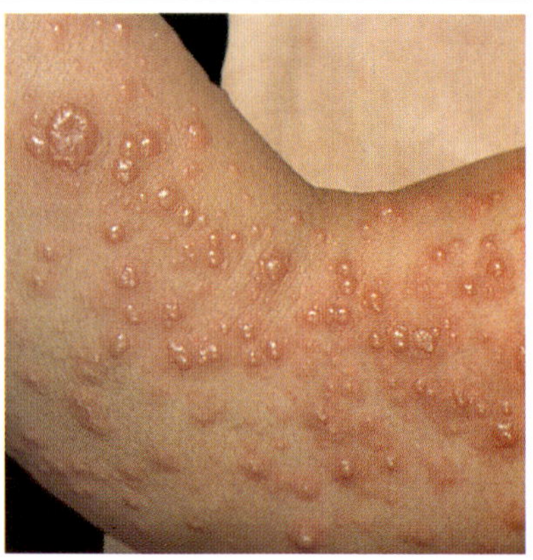

FIG. 28-20 *Numerous small erythematous papules, most of which are topped by a tense vesicle.*

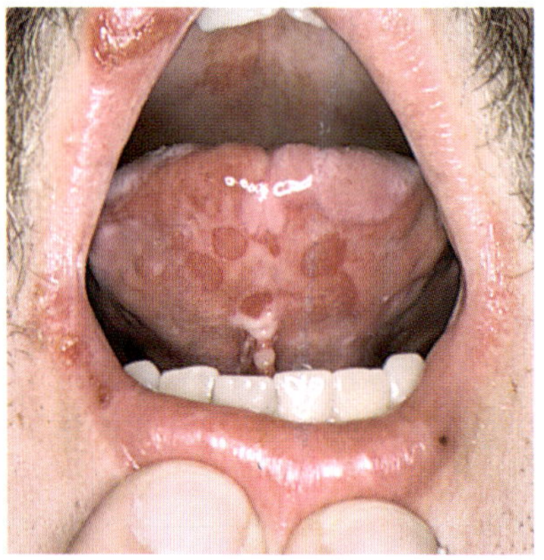

FIG. 28-21 *Round erosions on the lips, tongue, and floor of the mouth. Each erosion represents a site where a blister resided.*

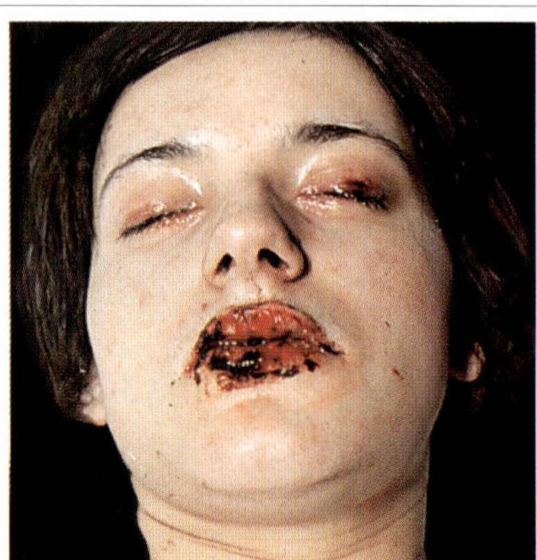

FIG. 28-22 *Erosions and hemorrhagic crusts on the lips and eyelids.*

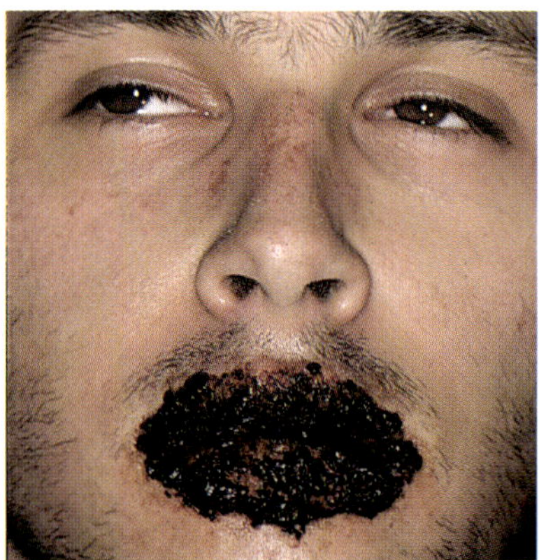

FIG. 28-23 *Extensive involvement of lips by hemorrhagic crusts.*

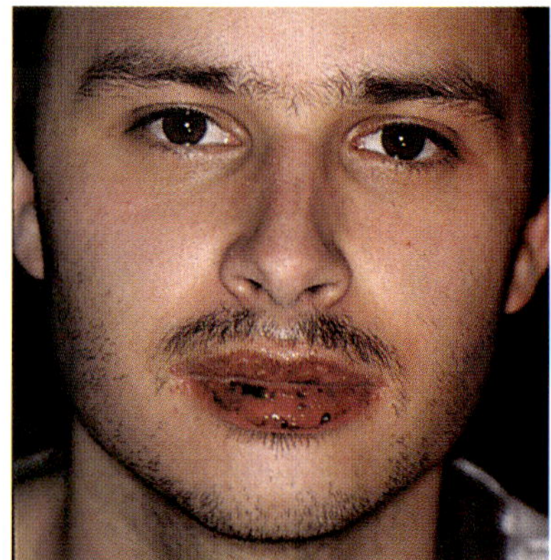

FIG. 28-24 *Extensive erosions, many covered by hemorrhagic crusts.*

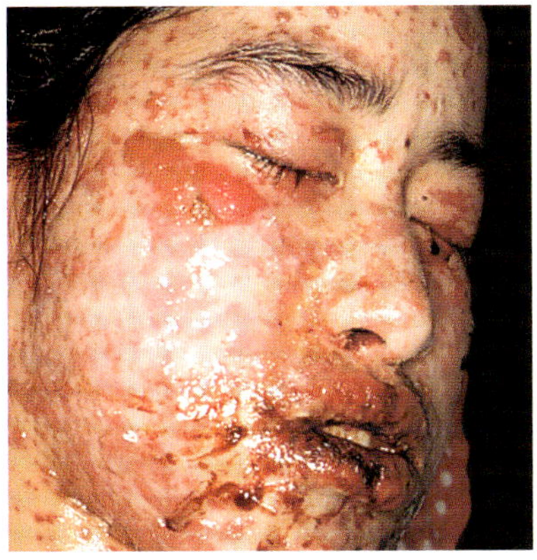

FIG. 28-25 *Blisters, erosions, and hemorrhagic crusts.*

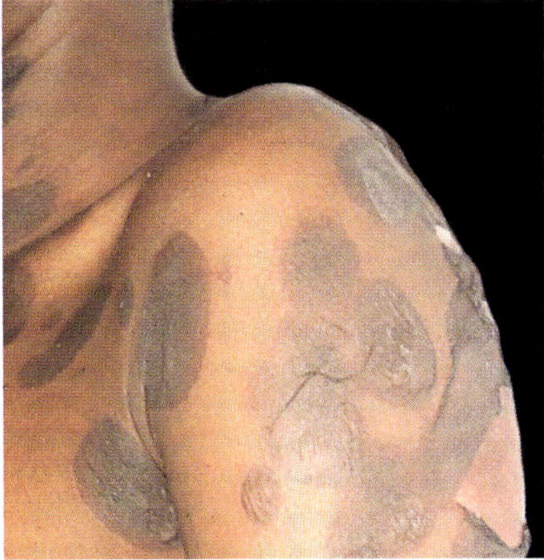

FIG. 28-26 *Dusky erythematous macules and patches that have become severely eroded secondary to blisters having broken.*

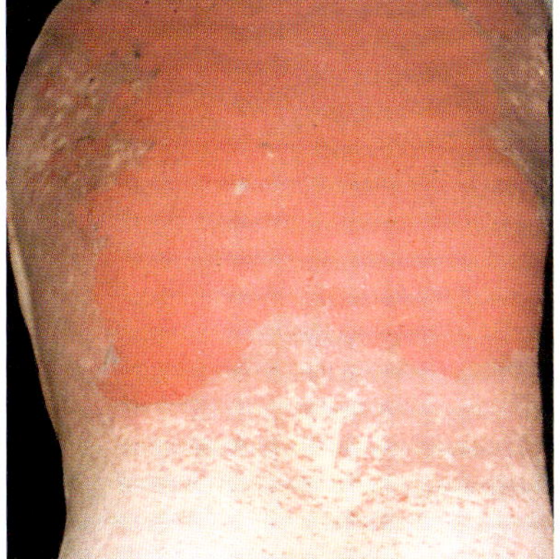

FIG. 28-27 *Dusky erythematous papules and plaques that have become severely eroded due to breakage of blisters.*

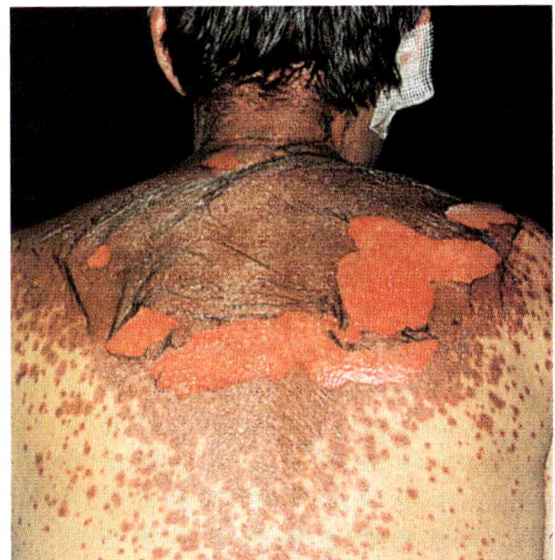

FIG. 28-28 *Purpuric macules and papules have become confluent and erosions have formed secondary to subepidermal blisters.*

COURSE Erythema multiforme manifests itself in widely divergent ways. It can appear as a few acral lesions that wane within a week or two, as often is the case with erythema multiforme precipitated by infection with herpesvirus, to a fulminant process that involves the skin universally and mucous membranes extensively. The virulent form may end fatally in only a few days, as in the expression of the disease in adults known popularly as toxic epidermal necrolysis, which commonly is induced by a drug. The usual presentation and course of erythema multiforme, however, is involvement of one or more mucous membranes, the oral and ocular, for example, with scores of skin lesions that favor acral sites. When a cause is identified, as it is in about half of the patients, and can be removed (in the case of a drug) or disappears on its own (in the instance of particular infections such as that caused by herpesvirus), the number of new lesions of erythema multiforme become fewer and fewer, and the condition remits completely in about two weeks.

INTEGRATION: UNIFYING CONCEPT Irrespective of cause, erythema multiforme exhibits a distinctive pattern whose morphologic expressions are diagnostic with specificity, clinically and histopathologically. The common denominators of erythema multiforme, when it is viewed in sections of tissue studied by conventional microscopy, are a superficial perivascular infiltrate of lymphocytes, obscuration of the dermoepidermal junction by lymphocytes in conjunction with vacuolar alteration and necrotic keratinocytes, and some lymphocytes in the spinous zone of the epidermis in company with ballooning, spongiosis, and individual necrotic keratinocytes. In time, intraepidermal vesiculation occurs as a consequence mostly of severe ballooning, and subepidermal vesiculation may result from progressive exaggeration of vacuolar alteration at the dermoepidermal junction. In time, the epidermis of erythema multiforme becomes completely necrotic.

Despite the fact that a diagnosis of erythema multiforme can be made clinically and histopathologically with confidence, no judgment can be made, on morphologic grounds alone, about the cause of it. Erythema multiforme induced by herpesvirus has the same morphologic features as erythema multiforme caused by a drug. The pathogenesis of erythema multiforme has yet to be elucidated, but it is thought to be a cell-mediated immune reaction. In the case of erythema multiforme secondary to infection by herpesvirus, the immune reaction is believed to be against keratinocytes that express antigens to herpesvirus.

THERAPY Specific treatment should be given for the condition that induced it, if known (e.g., antiviral for herpes simplex). Local application of soothing lotions and general supportive measures are indicated. If systemic corticosteroids are to be used in a patient with severe, widespread, life-threatening disease, they must be given in very large doses. Such a patient is managed best in a burn unit or in the equivalent of one. Parenthetically, intravenous administration of immunoglobulins is reputed to be beneficial in a circumstance of erythema multiforme that potentially is fatal.

DEFINITION An inflammatory process, i.e., a panniculitis, marked by tender erythematous plaques, nodules, or tumors (or combinations thereof) that usually affect the anterior aspect of the legs and, less often, the arms, and induced by processes, in an organ other than the skin, as dissimilar as sarcoidosis, Crohn's disease, and histoplasmosis.

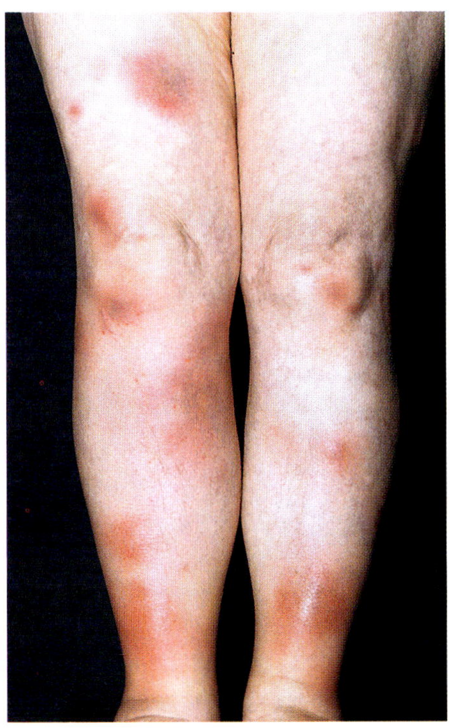

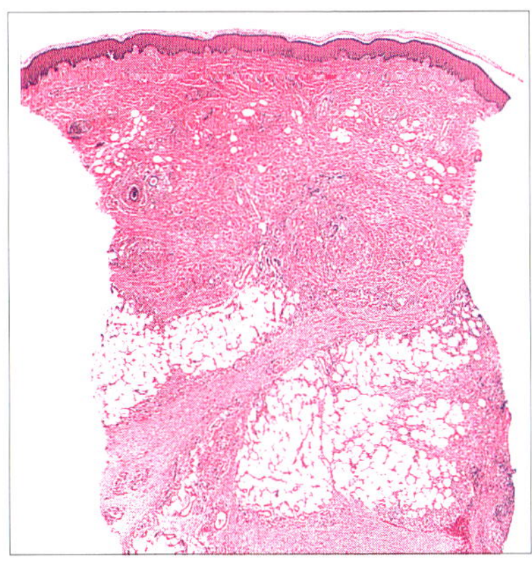

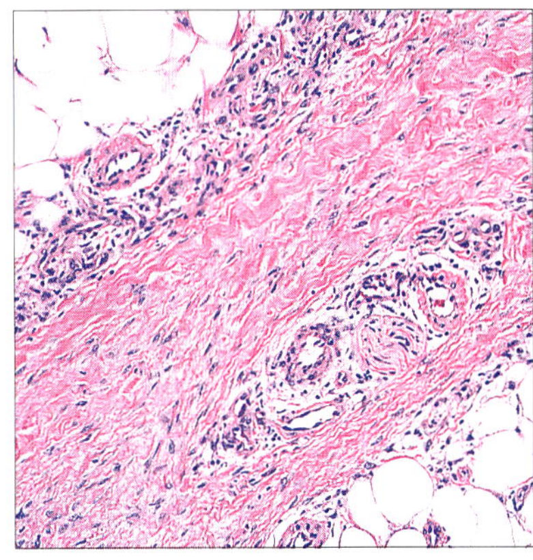

DISTRIBUTION

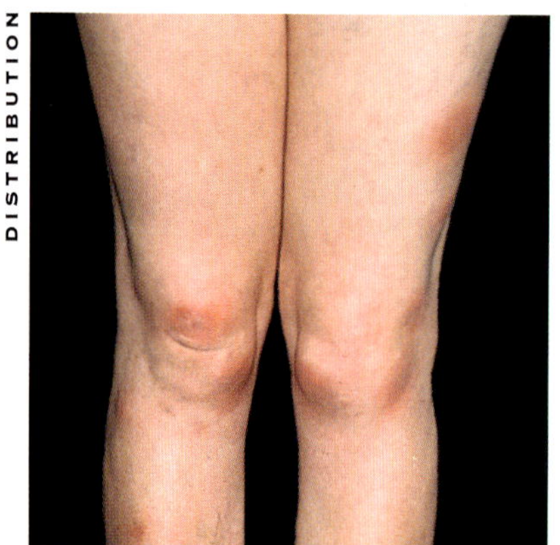

FIG. 29-1 *Dusky erythematous nodules.*

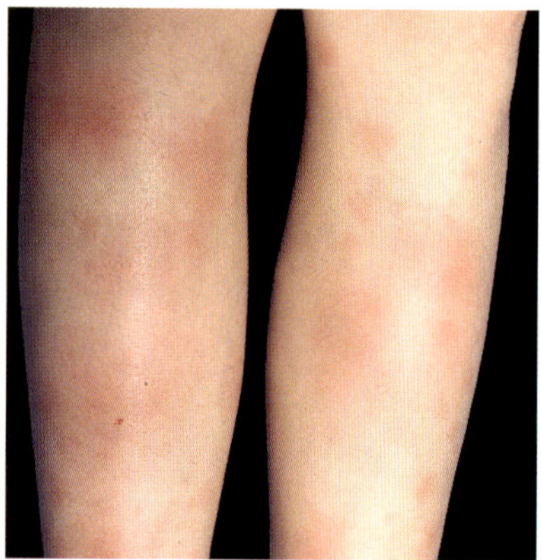

FIG. 29-2 *Slightly elevated dusky erythematous nodules, some of which have become confluent.*

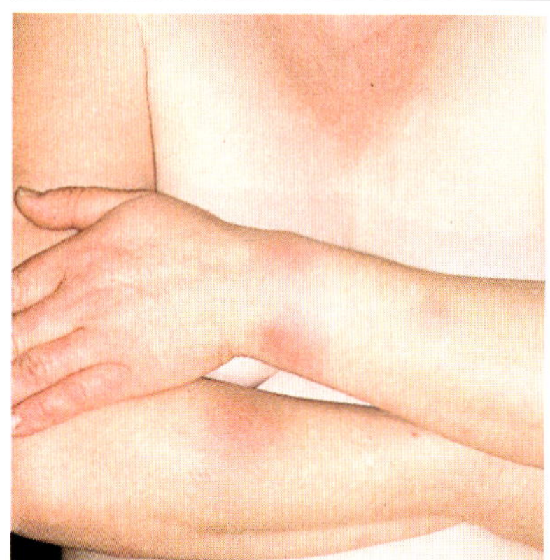

FIG. 29-3 *Dusky erythematous nodules.*

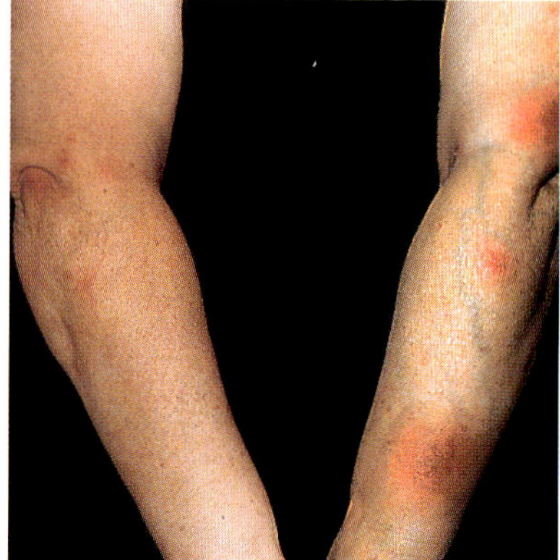

FIG. 29-4 *Dusky erythematous nodules and tumors.*

INDIVIDUAL LESIONS

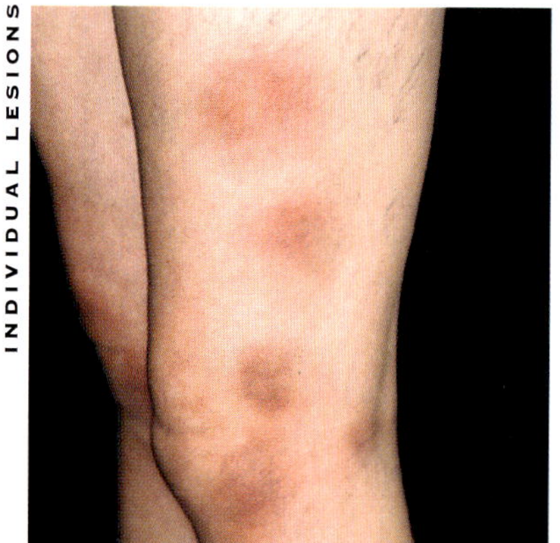

FIG. 29-5 *Discrete dusky nodules of various hues.*

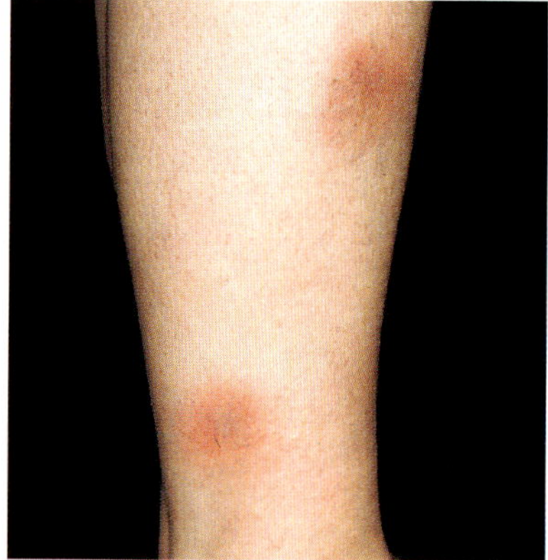

FIG. 29-6 *Slightly elevated erythematous nodules.*

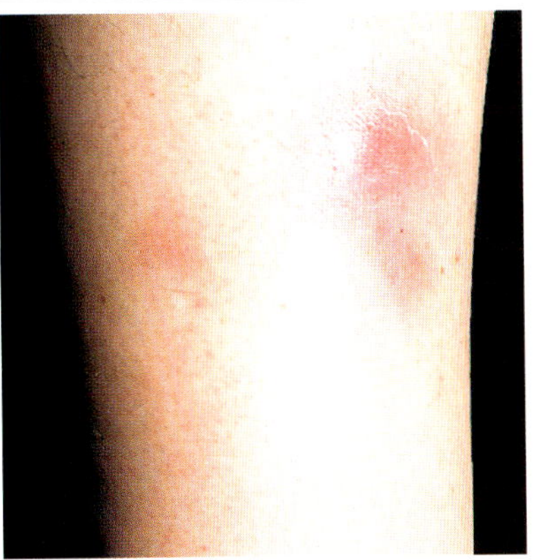

FIG. 29-7 *Shiny, dusky erythematous nodules.*

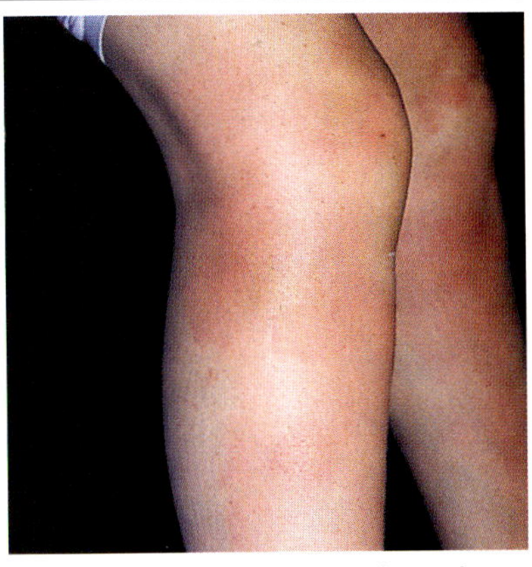

FIG. 29-8 *Slightly elevated, dusky erythematous nodules that have become confluent on edematous legs.*

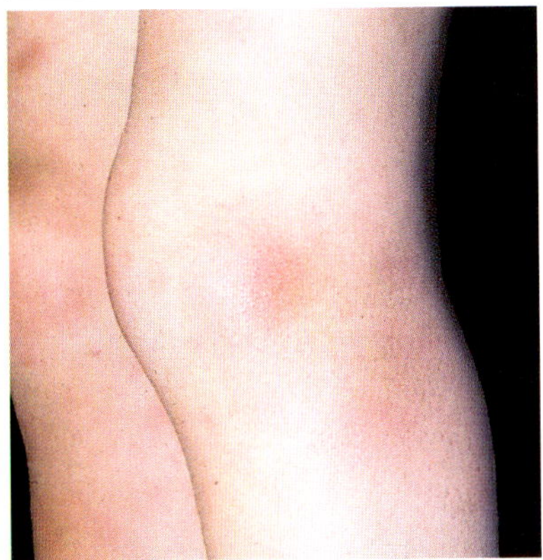

FIG. 29-9 *Slightly elevated, para-articular, dusky erythematous nodules whose border is indistinct.*

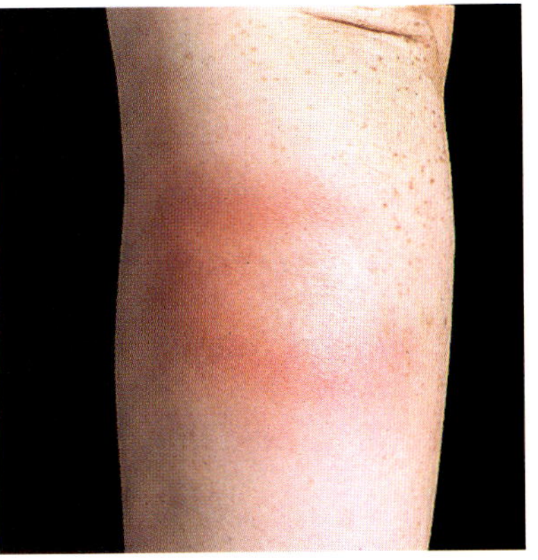

FIG. 29-10 *Arciform, dusky erythematous, poorly circumscribed nodule (subacute migratory panniculitis).*

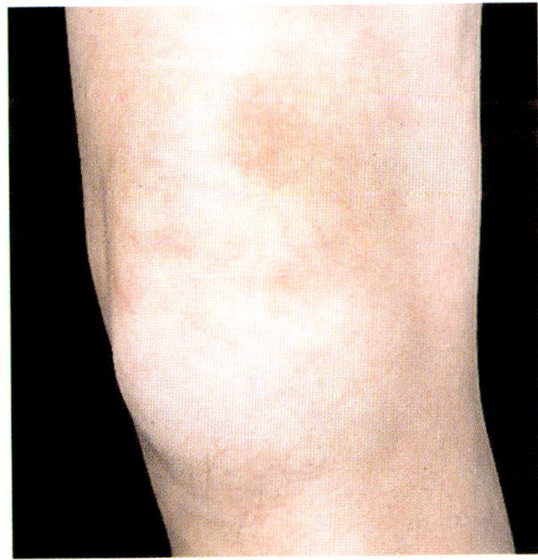

FIG. 29-11 *Plaques.*

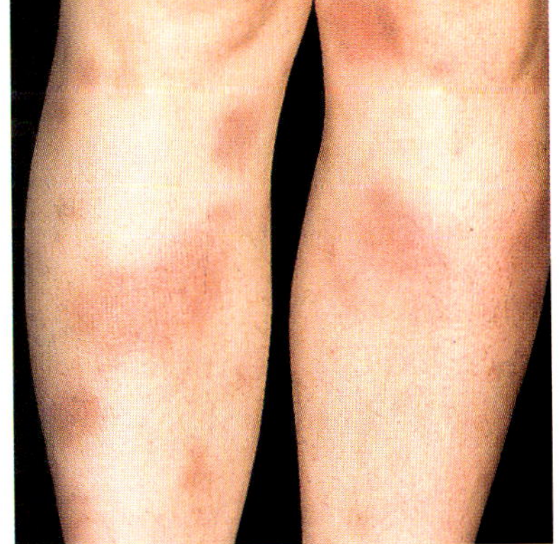

FIG. 29-12 *Patches and slightly elevated, dusky erythematous and hyperpigmented plaques.*

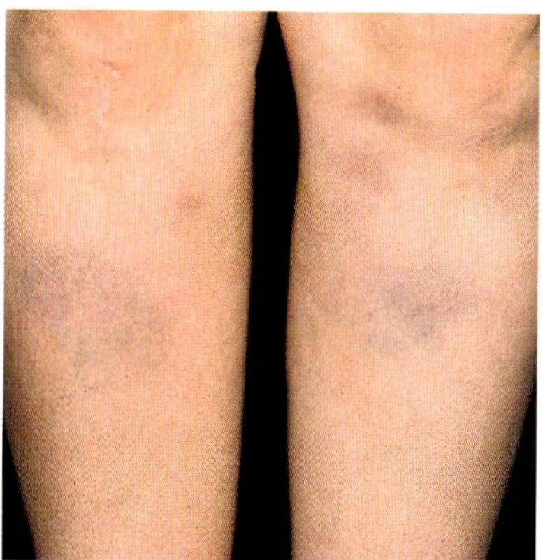
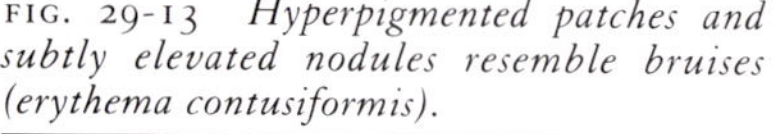

FIG. 29-13 *Hyperpigmented patches and subtly elevated nodules resemble bruises (erythema contusiformis).*

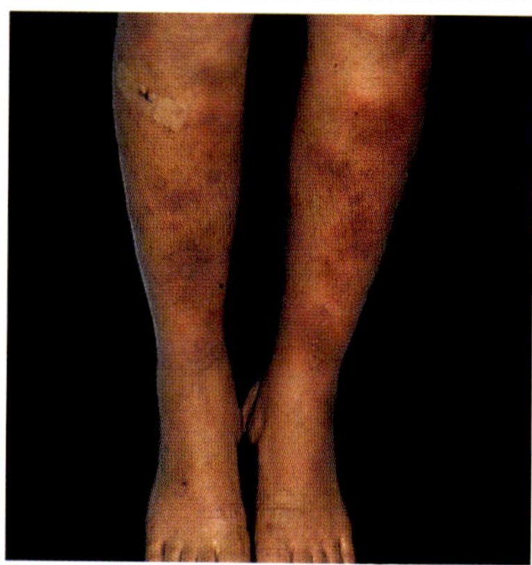

FIG. 29-14 *Plaques and nodules.*

ADJUNCTIVE DIAGNOSTIC TEST A chest x-ray is indicated in search for bilateral hilar adenopathy of sarcoidosis and signs of pulmonary infection, such as by a fungus.

COURSE The causes of erythema nodosum, which are many, influence the course of the panniculitic process. In about half the patients, no cause can be established. If lesions of erythema nodosum have been induced by a drug administered parenterally and use of that drug is stopped, very few or no new lesions of erythema nodosum will appear, and those already present will regress slowly in a matter of weeks. If, however, the precipitating cause of erythema nodosum is undetected, as may be the case for histoplasmosis or coccidioidomycosis, and therefore goes untreated, then new nodose lesions will appear as old ones slowly resolve.

INTEGRATION: UNIFYING CONCEPT Erythema nodosum, like erythema multiforme, leukocytoclastic vasculitis, Sweet's syndrome, and pyoderma gangrenosum, is a morphologic pattern that is easily recognizable clinically and histopathologically at every stage of its chronological course. When sections of tissue of a fully-developed lesion of erythema nodosum are studied by conventional microscopy, they show a granulomatous and fibrosing septal panniculitis.

The most common causes of erythema nodosum are infections of the upper respiratory tract, such as by Mycobacterium tuberculosis and Yersinia, drugs, including contraceptives, sarcoidosis, and inflammatory diseases of the gastrointestinal tract, such as Crohn's disease and ulcerative colitis. Those causes, however, cannot be determined by assessment of morphologic findings in the skin alone; other investigative methods are required. In sum, erythema nodosum is one of many morphologic patterns in the skin that are identifiable, clinically and histopathologically, by virtue of findings encountered repeatedly and that are of multiple causes.

THERAPY Treatment turns on determination of the primary condition responsible for erythema nodosum. Bed rest is advisable, as are nonsteroidal anti-inflammatory agents and, in the absence of any discernible infectious cause, oral corticosteroids if lesions are painful or incapacitating.

EXTRAMAMMARY PAGET'S DISEASE

DEFINITION Extramammary Paget's disease is an apocrine carcinoma that begins within the epidermis and presents itself clinically as a patch or a subtle plaque that extends centrifugally for many years before becoming a readily discernible thick plaque, a finding that signifies involvement by the carcinoma of the dermis, too.

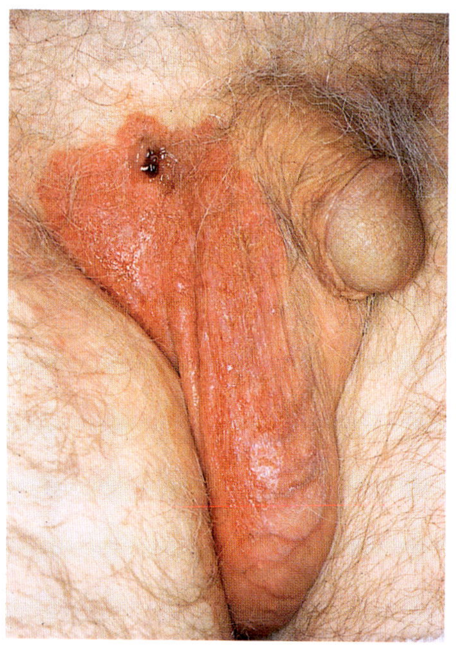

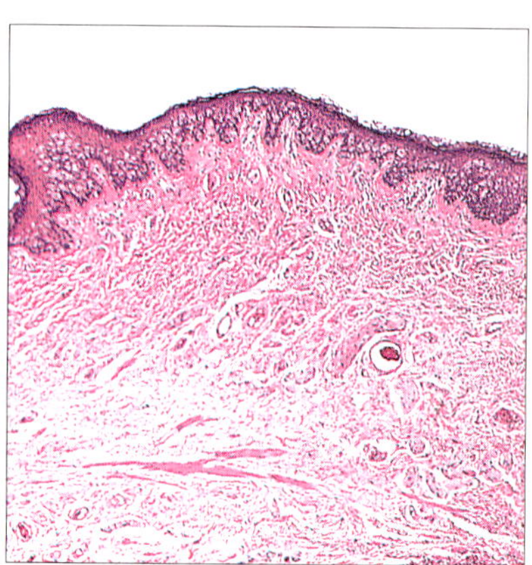

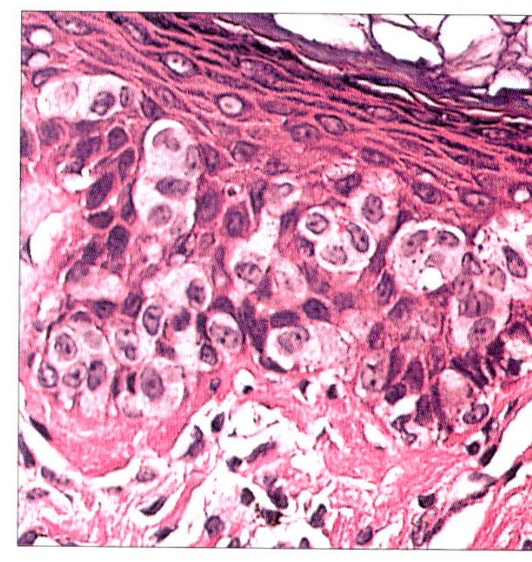

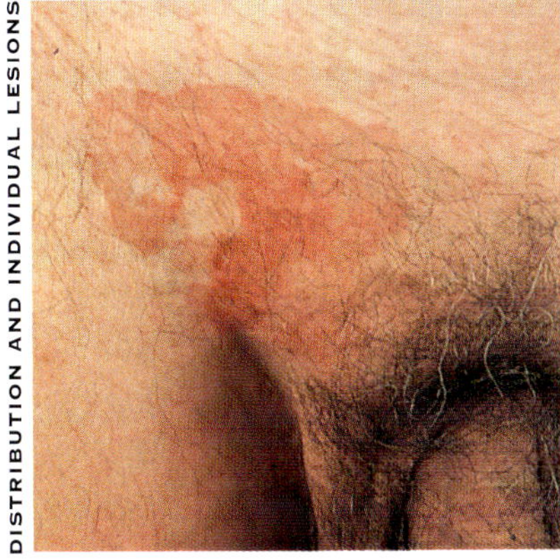

FIG. 30-1 *Focally eroded subtle plaque in figurate pattern in the suprapubic and inguinal regions.*

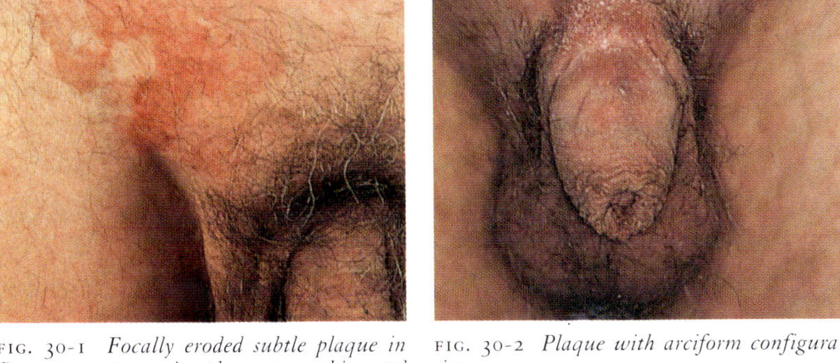

FIG. 30-2 *Plaque with arciform configuration.*

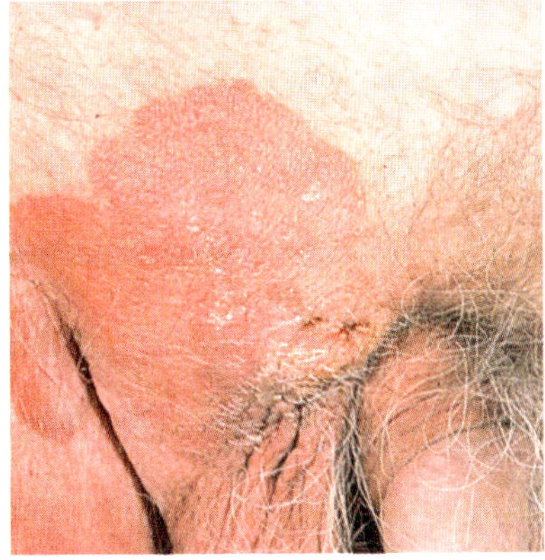

FIG. 30-3 *Plaque with focal erosions.*

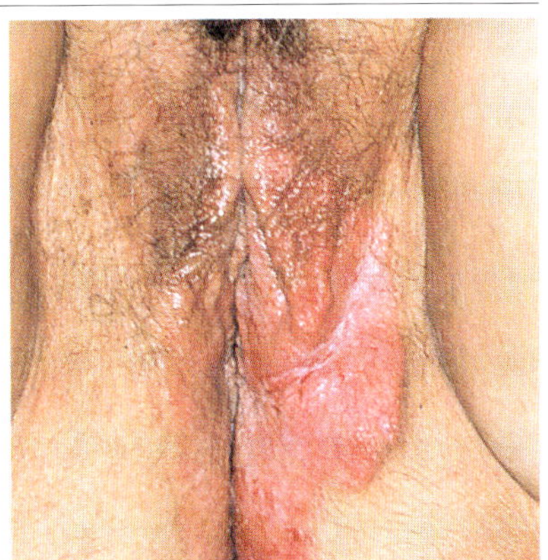

FIG. 30-4 *Plaque with erosions in foci.*

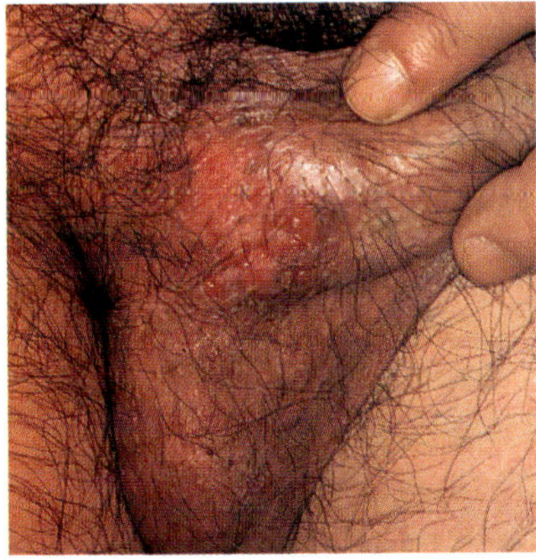

FIG. 30-5 *Partially-eroded, poorly-delimited plaque on the penis and scrotum.*

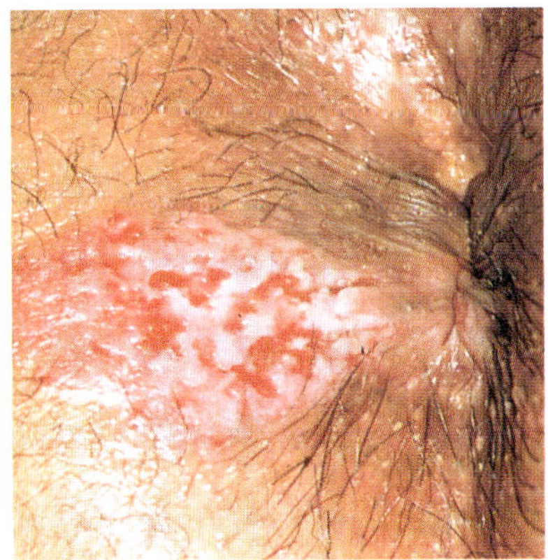

FIG. 30-6 *Focally ulcerated macerated plaque on the buttock and in the perianal region.*

COURSE Extramammary Paget's disease usually presents itself as a macule on genital skin and, less commonly, in the axilla. In time, the macule becomes slightly scaly and even crusted. Because extramammary Paget's disease is a malignant neoplasm, i.e., an apocrine carcinoma that begins with proliferation of individual neoplastic cells within the epidermis, it grows slowly, but irrepressibly. A scaly macule becomes a scaly patch and, in time, the epidermis thickens as a consequence of proliferation of Paget cells (cells of apocrine carcinoma). The patch may become a subtle plaque that then expands slowly to achieve a size of many centimeters.

As a rule, the neoplastic cells of extramammary Paget's disease remain in situ, i.e., confined to epidermal and adnexal (follicular, eccrine ductal, and apocrine ductal) epithelium for the lifetime of a person who has the disease. As long as the cells of the apocrine carcinoma remain confined to epidermal and adnexal epithelium, the neoplastic process is biologically benign. Only uncommonly do neoplastic cells of extramammary Paget's disease descend into the dermis, and then only after many years, where they also tend to grow slowly. Nonetheless, metastases from the primary apocrine carcinoma in the skin may appear in regional lymph nodes and beyond them. Patients have died from the effects of metastases of extramammary Paget's disease.

INTEGRATION: UNIFYING CONCEPT Extramammary Paget's disease is very different from mammary Paget's disease, although both of them are apocrine carcinomas. Paget's disease is a primary cutaneous apocrine carcinoma that begins within the epidermis and extends from it directly into epithelial structures of adnexa. Only uncommonly does it involve the dermis and rarely does it metastasize. In contrast, mammary Paget's disease is a primary apocrine carcinoma of the breast that begins in mammary glands, whence neoplastic cells ascend by way of lactiferous ducts to the epidermis. Not uncommonly, neoplastic cells of mammary Paget's disease extend from epidermal, mammary glandular, and lactiferous ductal epithelium into the dermis, from whence, not uncommonly, they metastasize. Like other forms of metastasizing breast carcinoma, the malignant neoplastic process of mammary Paget's disease all too often is fatal. Parenthetically, signet-ring cells replete with mucin are found often in extramammary Paget's disease, but not in mammary Paget's disease.

Despite the fact that the two conditions have in common the words "mammary" and "Paget's," extramammary Paget's disease and mammary Paget's disease, apocrine carcinomas both, are different neoplastic processes.

THERAPY Surgical excision with special attention being paid to margins at the periphery to ensure that the carcinoma has been removed completely.

MAMMARY PAGET'S DISEASE

DEFINITION Mammary Paget's disease is an apocrine carcinoma that begins in mammary glands and extends along lactiferous ducts to the epidermis where it is seen clinically as a scaly, crusted, or eroded plaque on the nipple or areola of women mostly, and uncommonly of men.

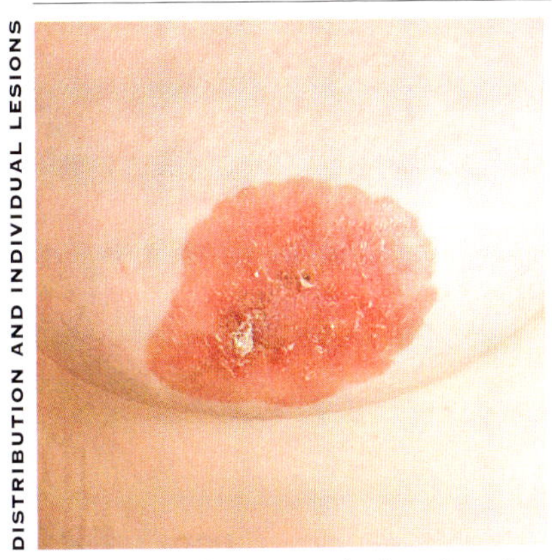

FIG. 30-7 *A plaque on a nipple and areola.*

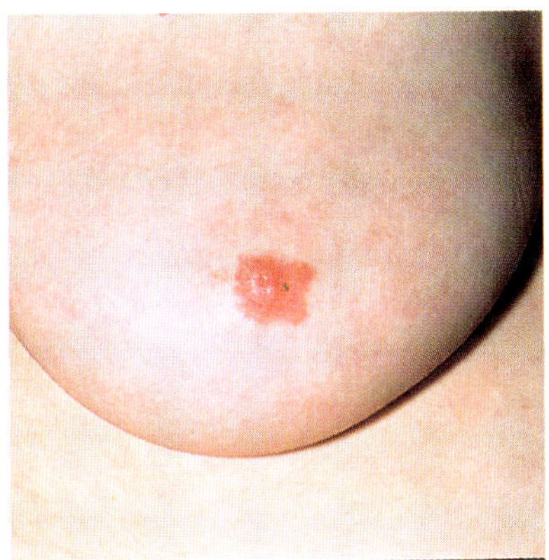

FIG. 30-8 *A plaque on a nipple and areola.*

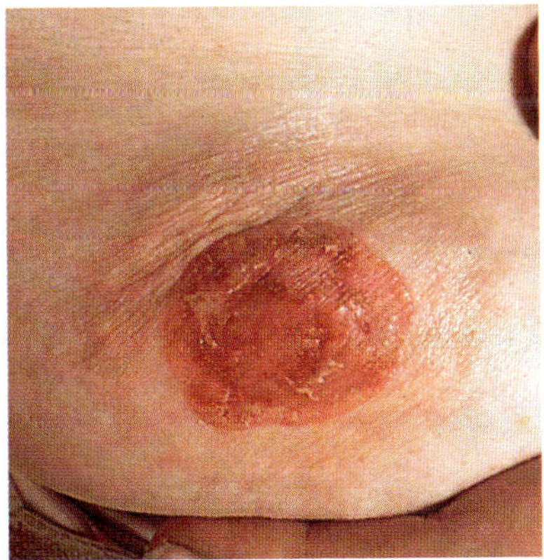

FIG. 30-9 *An eroded plaque on a nipple and areola.*

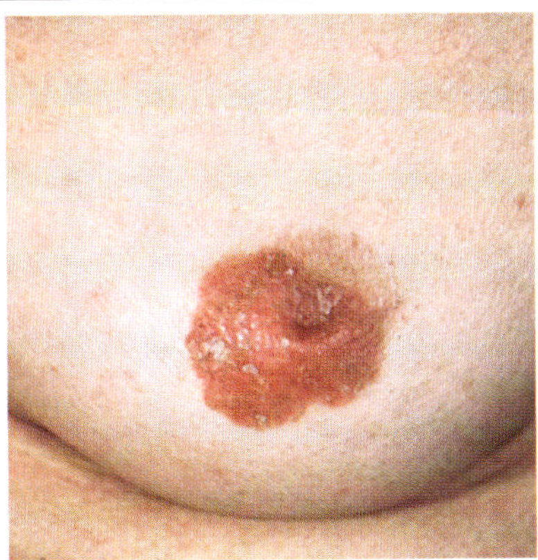

FIG. 30-10 *A scaly plaque on a nipple and areola extends onto adjacent skin.*

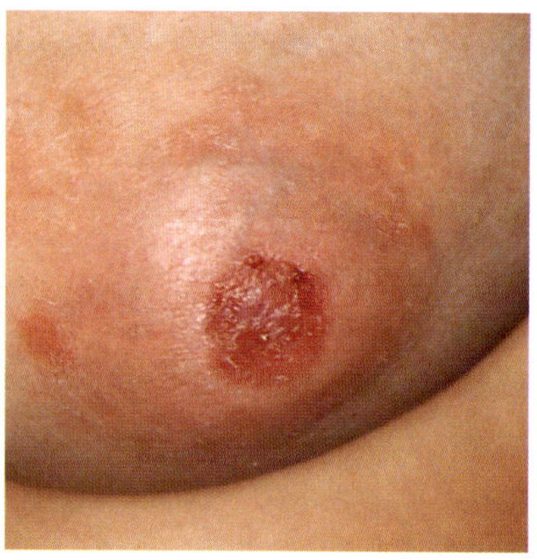

FIG. 30-11 *An eroded, scaly, crusted plaque of a nipple and areola above a tumor that represents the same carcinoma of the breast.*

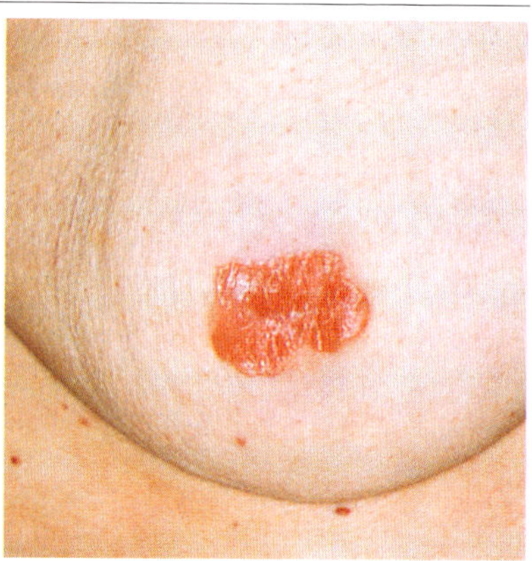

FIG. 30-12 *Scaly plaque.*

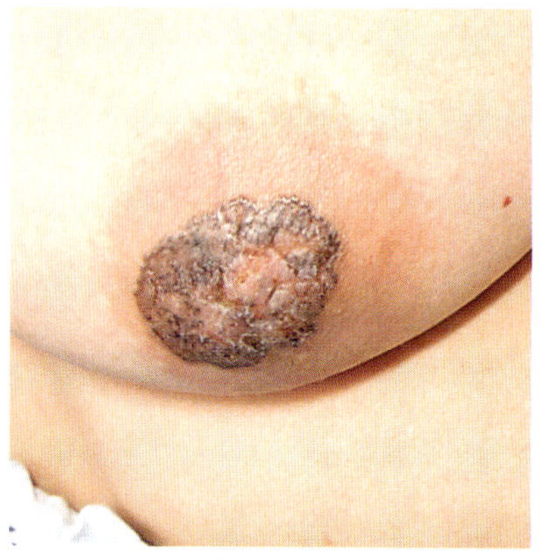

FIG. 30-13 *Scaly pigmented plaque with mammillated, focally eroded surface.*

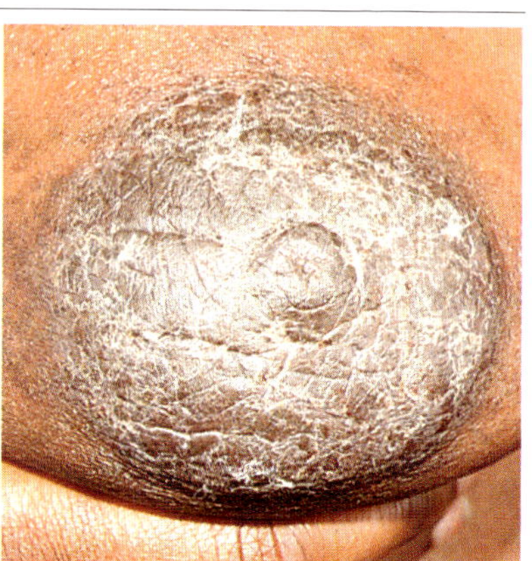

FIG. 30-14 *Scaly plaque.*

ADJUNCTIVE DIAGNOSTIC TEST Mammography in order to demonstrate a carcinoma of the breast.

COURSE Once a macule of mammary Paget's disease appears on a nipple or areola, it is destined to enlarge slowly there and to worsen, unless the carcinoma of the breast, of which it is the distal expression, is extirpated. In the absence of surgical intervention, the macule becomes a scaly, crusted plaque that, in the course of years, may become eroded or ulcerated. A plaque of mammary Paget's disease may extend far beyond the boundary of the areola to involve much of a breast.

INTEGRATION: UNIFYING CONCEPT The ostensible condition of the skin that appears on a nipple or areola and that is known as mammary Paget's disease is not a true primary cutaneous disease. The reason is not semantic; the nipple and areola are not true skin but represent a modification of it, and the basic pathologic process of mammary Paget's disease is a carcinoma of the breast itself. The neoplastic process begins, not on the nipple or areola, but in mammary glands. From there, the neoplastic epithelial cells ascend lactiferous ducts and eventually populate the surface epithelium of nipple and areola. A biopsy of those superficial sites produces a specimen from which sections of tissue, when studied by conventional microscopy, reveal a type of carcinoma, namely, apocrine. If the biopsy is performed by shave technique, the findings may only be those of apocrine carcinoma in situ.

Mammary glands are a type of apocrine gland, and the neoplastic cells that make up mammary Paget's disease are those of apocrine carcinoma. Within the surface epithelium, those Paget cells with their large roundish nuclei and abundant pale cytoplasm are present in Paget pattern, i.e., throughout the entire thickness of the surface epithelium, sometimes including the cornified layer. If tissue sections from the biopsy specimen house lactiferous ducts, the apocrine carcinoma also will be apparent within them. In short, mammary Paget's disease, which Paget himself thought to be a kind of "eczema," is simply the most superficial manifestation of a particular kind of apocrine carcinoma of the breast.

In contrast, extramammary Paget's disease is an apocrine carcinoma that begins within the epidermis and descends to epithelial structures of adnexa, namely, folliculosebaceous-apocrine units and eccrine units. The distribution of extramammary Paget's disease, unlike that of mammary Paget's disease, is skin of the genitalia and, sometimes, the axilla.

THERAPY Lumpectomy or modified radical mastectomy is the choice, and that decision can be made by a thoughtful surgeon who assesses the disease in the breast by observation and palpation.

DEFINITION Dermatitis (and/or panniculitis) induced artificially and deliberately by a patient and characterized clinically by findings unlike those of any "authentic" disease, for example, by lesions that have sharply angulated margins, lesions that are artificially linear, and ulcers that have a punched-out appearance, all of these changes occurring on sites that are within easy reach of manipulating hands.

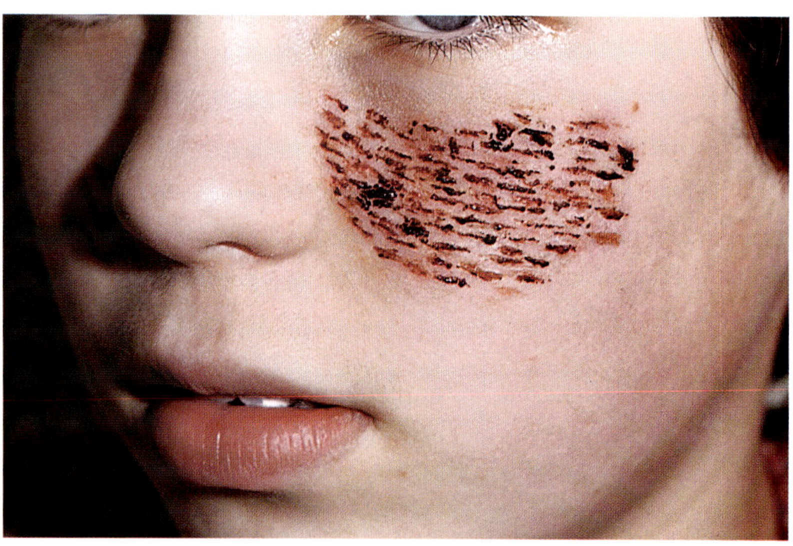

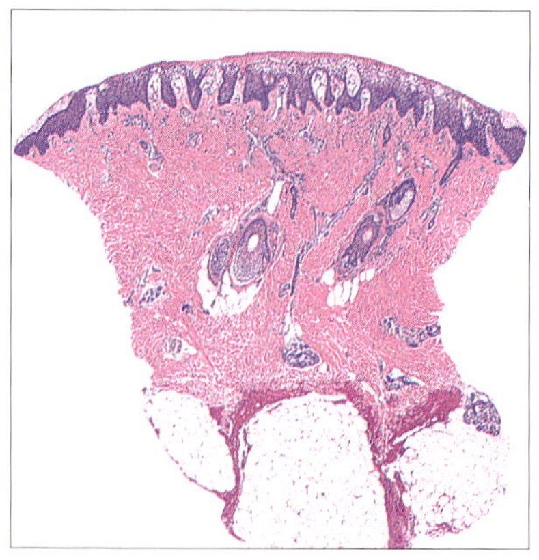

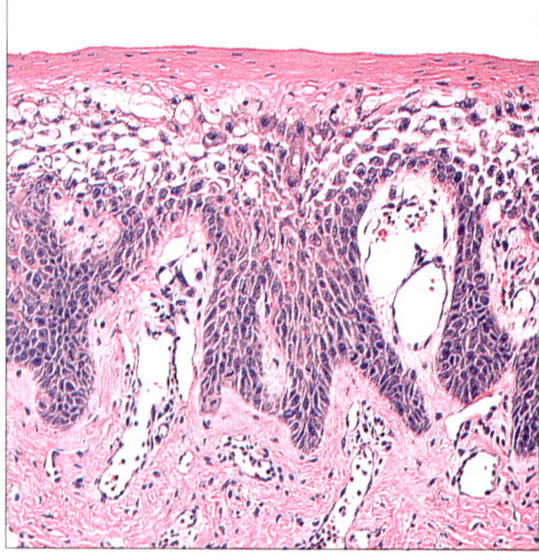

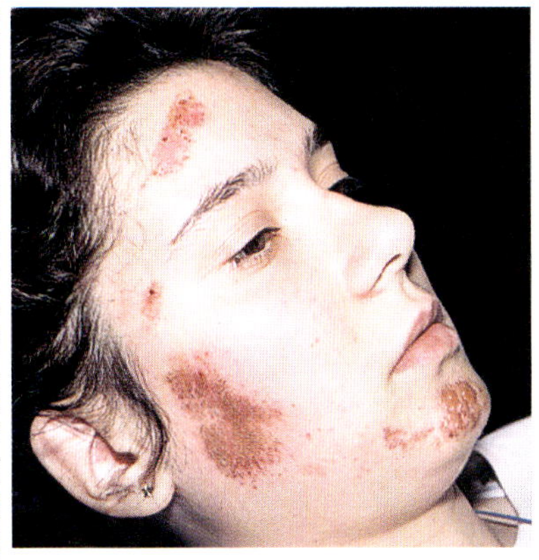

FIG. 31-1 *Abrasions and impetiginized crusts that do not conform to the effects of any accidental injury.*

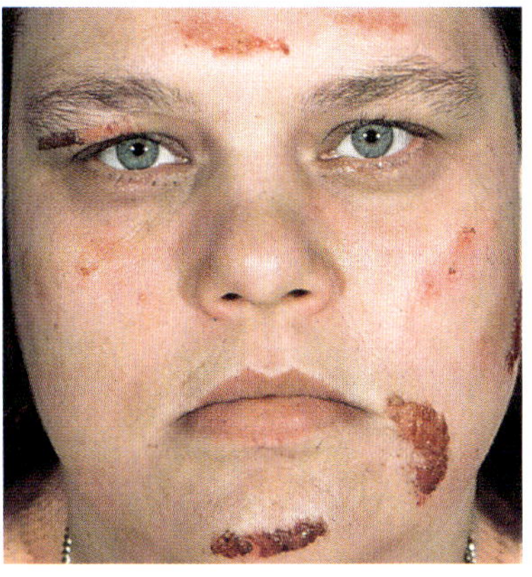

FIG. 31-2 *Abrasions and hemorrhagic crusts with bizarre, unnatural shapes.*

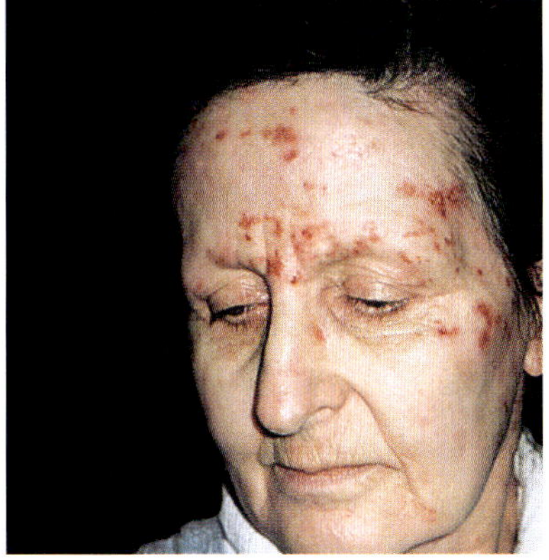

FIG. 31-3 *Erosions and ulcerations in artificial design.*

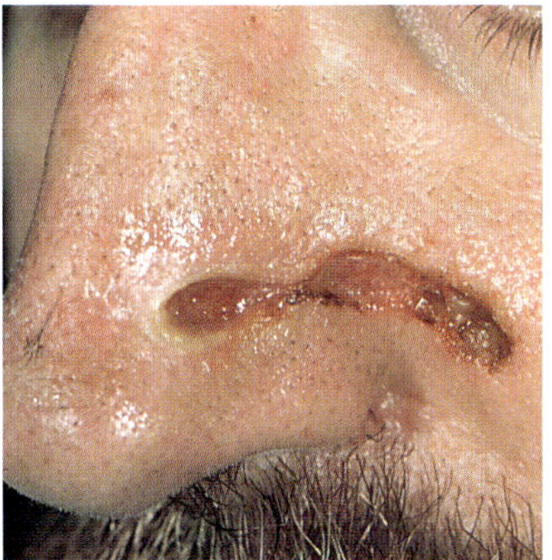

FIG. 31-4 *A deep, handmade ulcer in curvilinear shape.*

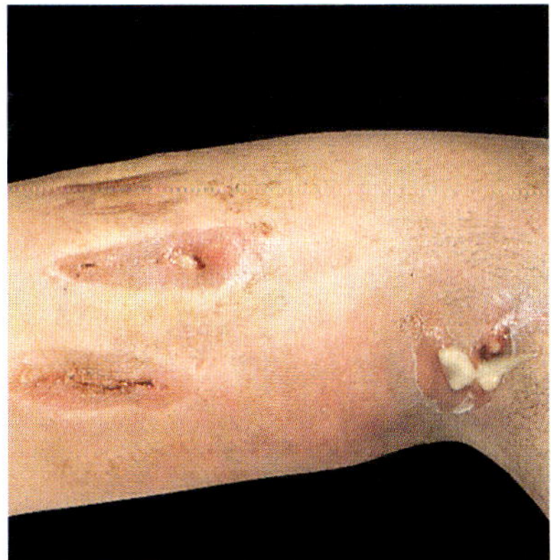

FIG. 31-5 *Atrophic linear scars and purulence emanating from a subcutaneous abscess.*

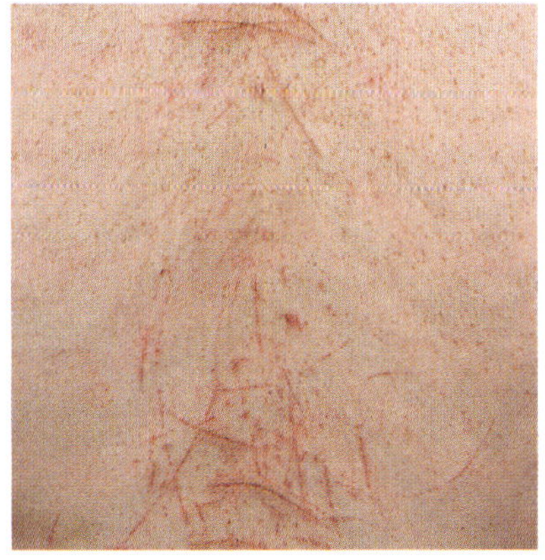

FIG. 31-6 *Superficial cuts in haphazard array.*

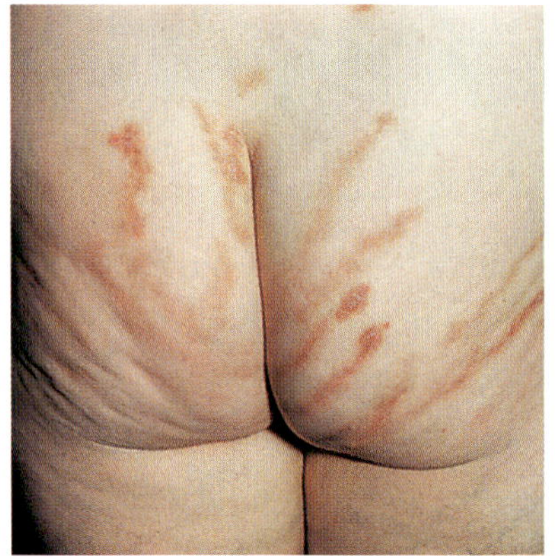

FIG. 31-7 *Artifactual lesions that have resulted from flagellation.*

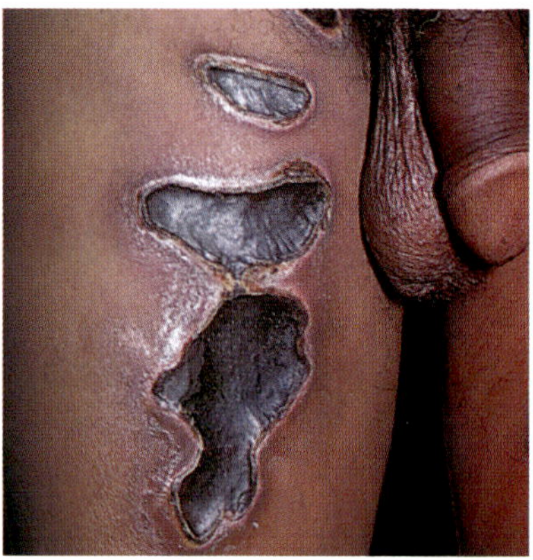

FIG. 31-8 *Deep ulcers with unnatural shapes, probably induced by application of acid.*

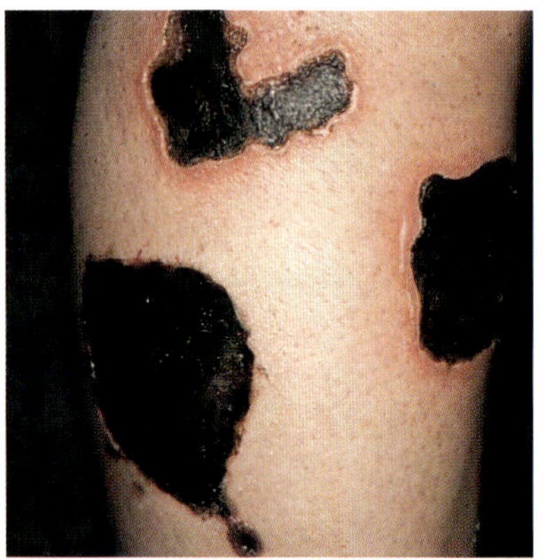

FIG. 31-9 *Eschars secondary to acid burns.*

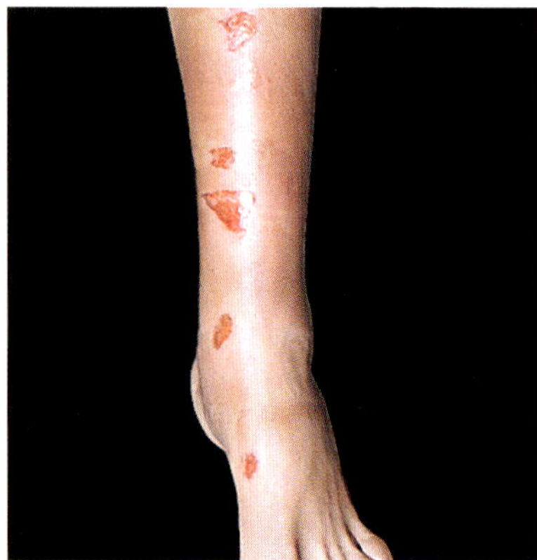

FIG. 31-10 *Erosions and ulcers with jagged outlines.*

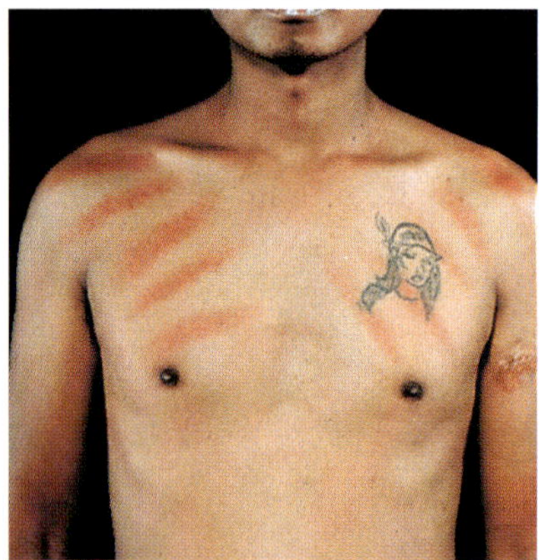

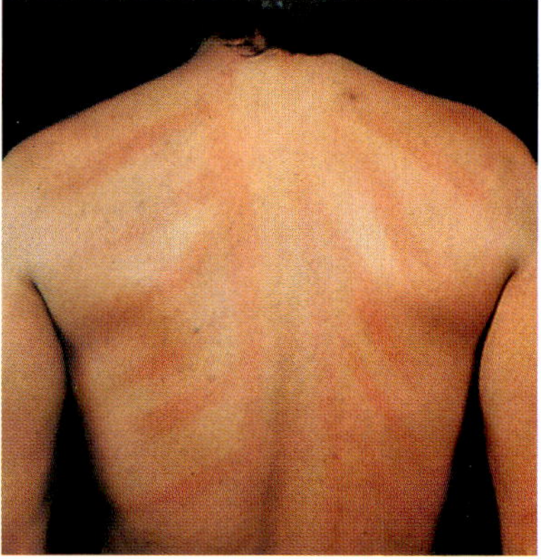

FIG. 31-11 (A, B) *Linear lesions distributed symmetrically consequent to rubbing a heated coin vigorously against the skin for purposes of mystical healing.*

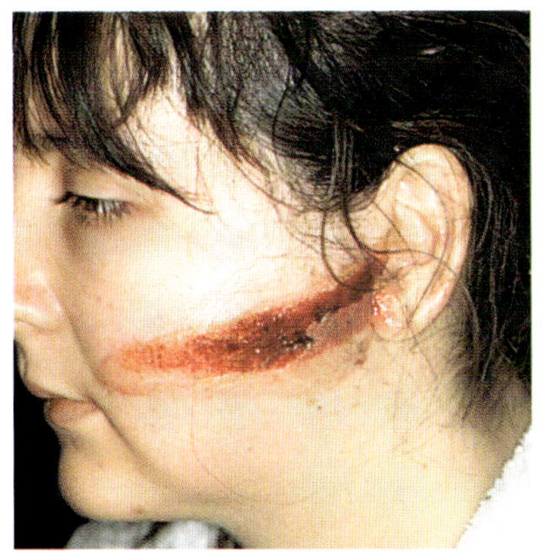

FIG. 31-12 *Erosion covered by hemorrhagic crusts in linear arrangement, secondary to a self-inflicted burn.*

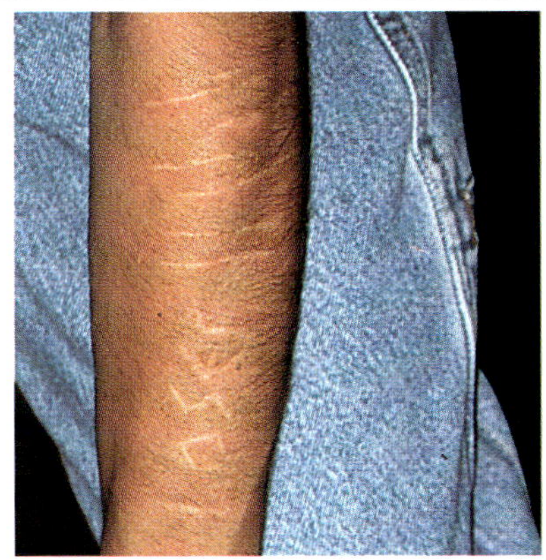

FIG. 31-13 *Scarification.*

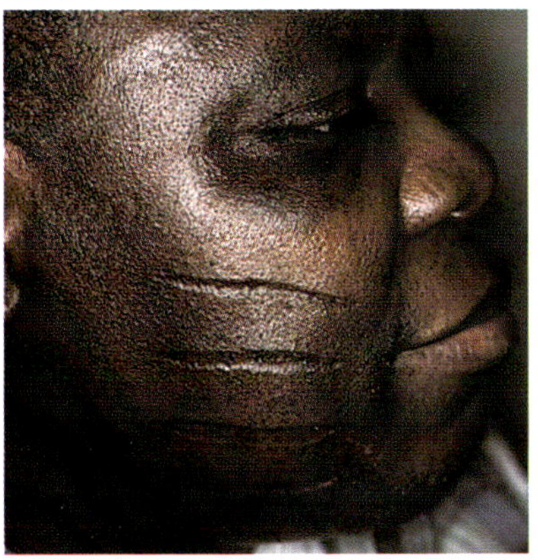

FIG. 31-14 *Scarification.*

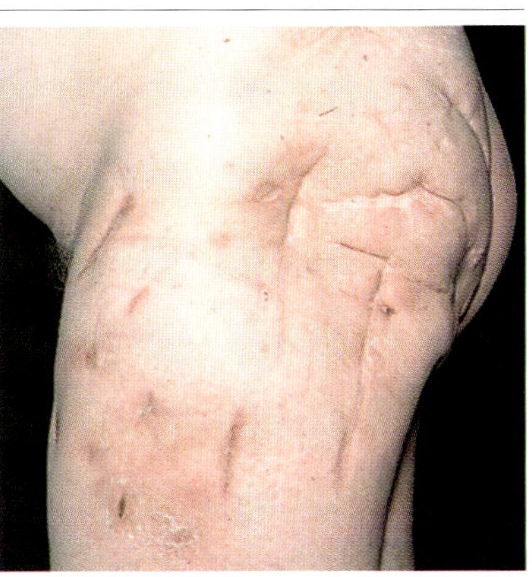

FIG. 31-15 *Linear scars after surgery for factitial panniculitis secondary to injections of milk.*

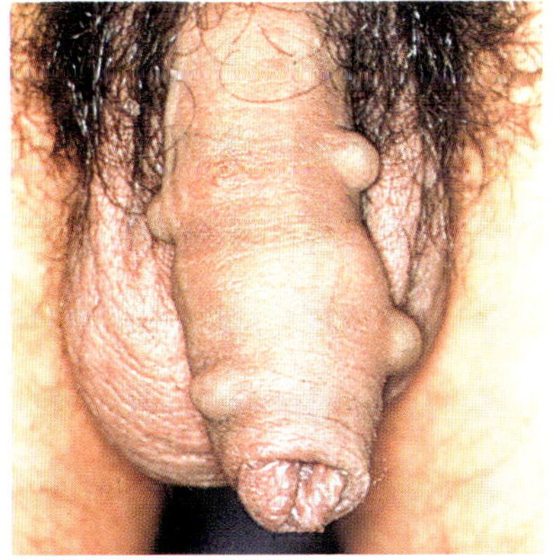

FIG. 31-16 *Nodules on the penis as a result of injection of plastic ("Tancho nodules").*

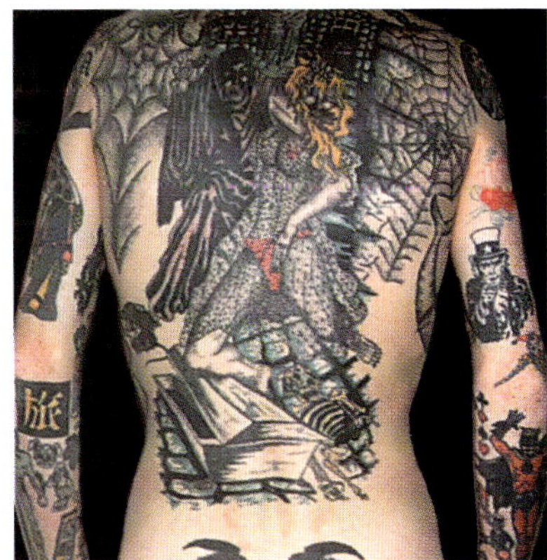

FIG. 31-17 *Extensive tattoo.*

COURSE Factitious dermatitis and panniculitis are caused entirely by a patient who presents herself (and less commonly himself) to a physician. The course of individual lesions depends on the method by which they were induced. If the lesions are abrasions, they heal quickly. If, however, the lesions are induced by application of acid or alkali to the skin, they may not heal for months, and then only with unsightly eschars and atrophic scars.

The course of the condition itself depends entirely on when, if ever, the person stops producing the lesions. For those neurotics who induce lesions factitially for purposes of secondary gain, there is every likelihood that they will become disenchanted with the exercise, realize that the gain is not being achieved, or improve with psychotherapy, and the activity will cease. For those persons who are psychotic, however, there may be no surcease from the demons driving the process and hence no end of it.

INTEGRATION: UNIFYING CONCEPT As a generalization, lesions are induced artifactually by persons who are either neurotic or psychotic. Those who are neurotic, in particular, hysteric, usually are women who seek to employ the skin lesions they have produced as a vehicle to ulterior gain. As a rule, such people do not cause serious injury to the skin or to themselves; almost always, the face is untouched. Often the women who induce lesions factitiously are nurses, physicians' assistants, healthcare workers of different types, or young daughters of persons employed in those vocations. It has been claimed that many neurotics with factitious disease were abused sexually in childhood.

In contrast to neurotics, psychotics produce lesions factitially because they cannot help themselves. They often do terrible damage to the skin and to themselves, producing lesions usually by using knives, acids and alkalis, and injections of material of all kinds, even feces.

A cliché heard often at conferences and meetings of dermatology is that "factitial dermatitis is a diagnosis of exclusion." Nothing could be further from the truth. The signs of factitious dermatitis and panniculitis, clinically and histopathologically, are just as specific as those of any so-called spontaneous disease. If the outlines of an ulcer are incredibly sharp, if lesions have a geometric pattern, such as near-perfect lines, circles, rectangles, or squares, or if bizarre lesions are present only on sites that are readily accessible, a diagnosis of factitious disease can be made with precision. It must be stressed further that no part of the skin is immune to factitious dermatitis/panniculitis. A person bent upon inducing lesions can do it in the mid-portion of the back by using implements such as knitting needles, hangers, and brushes. Never should it be averred that lesions are not factitious because they appear on a site that ordinarily would be difficult to reach.

The histopathologic findings in factitiously-produced dermatitis and panniculitis are as bizarre as the clinical lesions.

THERAPY Once a diagnosis of factitious skin disease has been established, psychotherapy is advisable for neurotics who produce those lesions and psychotherapeutic drugs for psychotics who cause them. Whatever the patient's psychologic profile, an attempt must be made to heal the skin lesions, and one method to enhance repair of ulcers is by occluding the site of them. In the ultimate analysis, however, it is the psyche of the person who produces lesions factitiously that must be healed. A physician managing such a patient should never be accusatory, but rather sympathetic; the patient is in pain emotionally.

DEFINITION Largely exophytic noninflammatory papules or nodules of various kinds made up mostly of collagen.

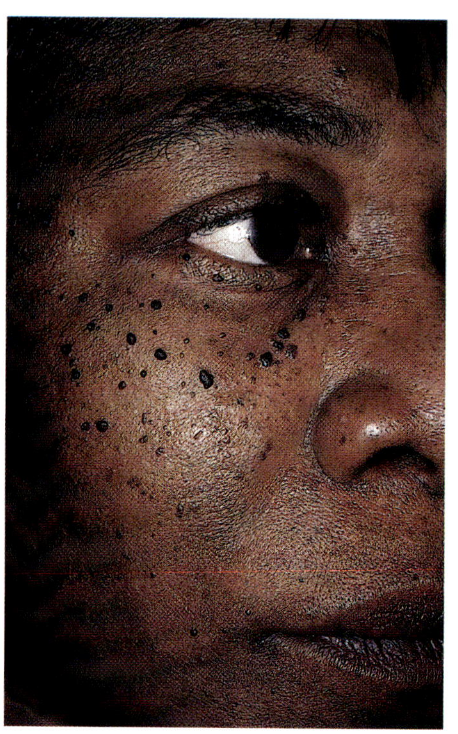

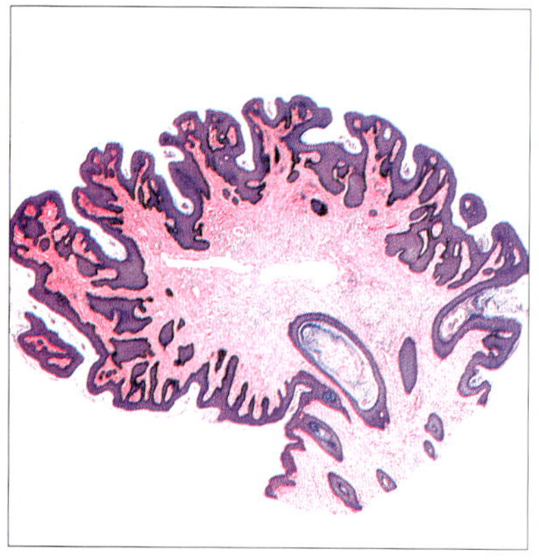

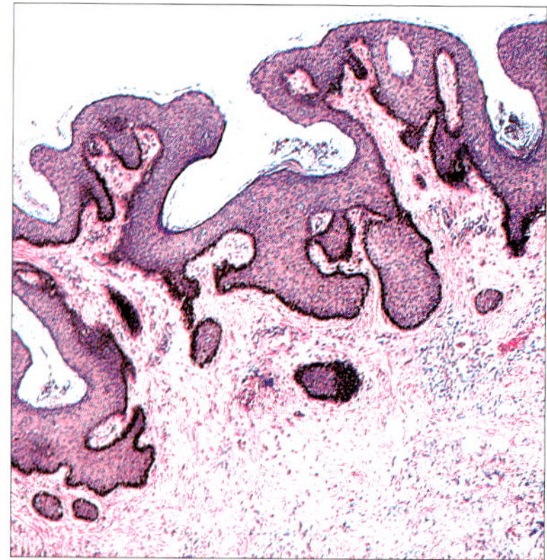

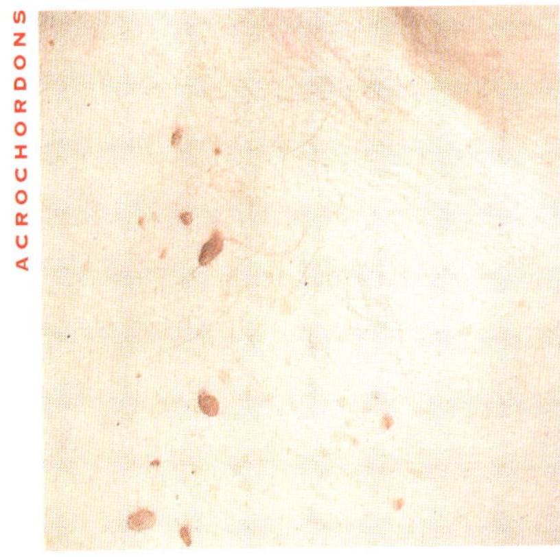

FIG. 32-1 *Pedunculated papules (skin tags).*

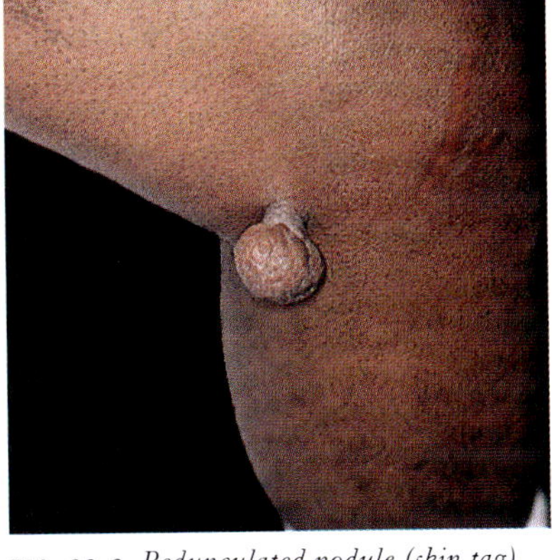

FIG. 32-2 *Pedunculated nodule (skin tag).*

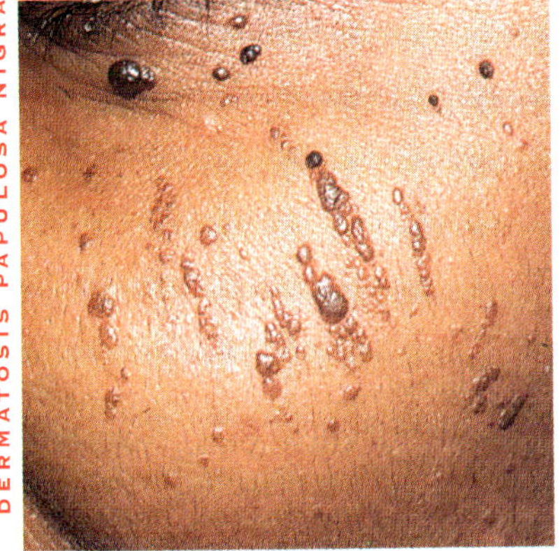

FIG. 32-3 *Pigmented papules, some in linear array (dermatosis papulosa nigra).*

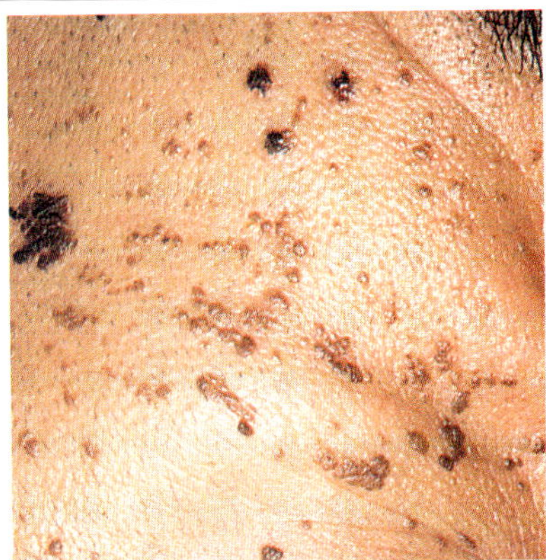

FIG. 32-4 *Pigmented papules of different sizes, shapes, and colors (dermatosis papulosa nigra).*

COURSE The fibromas under consideration in this chapter, namely, acrochordons and dermatosis papulosa nigra, usually appear after puberty and, once they have become manifest, remain the same, more or less, for a lifetime. Once these fibromas have become established, they usually neither grow perceptively nor do they involute. New lesions may continue to appear at any time during the life of the person.

INTEGRATION: UNIFYING CONCEPT The two types of fibromas pictured in this chapter, acrochordons and dermatosis papulosa nigra, are different from one another in terms of distribution, appearance of individual lesions, and histopathologic findings. They have in common, however, a polypoid shape and a core made up mostly of bundles of collagen. Acrochordons tend to involve intertriginous regions and the trunk, whereas dermatosis papulosa nigra is confined to a face. Histopathologically, although both have a core of fibrous tissue and a surface that may be papillated, the surface epithelium of dermatosis papulosa nigra vaguely resembles that of a seborrheic keratosis. The condition, however, is very different from seborrheic keratosis. The former is fundamentally fibrous, whereas the latter is basically epithelial.

It merits mention that there are fibromas in the skin besides acrochordons and dermatosis papulosa nigra. For example, subungual and periungual fibromas of tuberous sclerosis, and their lookalike, acquired digital fibroma, also are fibromas, but they, unlike acrochordons and dermatosis papulosa nigra, are not soft, but firm, and display entirely different histopathologic findings.

THERAPY Shave excision or electrocautery combined with curettage is an acceptable method of management, if the patient wishes treatment.

DEFINITION A hamartoma of mostly follicular elements that presents itself clinically as a firm, skin-colored papule. It usually occurs on the nose, but it can occur anywhere on the face. When solitary, or few, the lesion is termed "fibrous papule," but when innumerable on the face in the context of tuberous sclerosis it is designated "adenoma sebaceum."

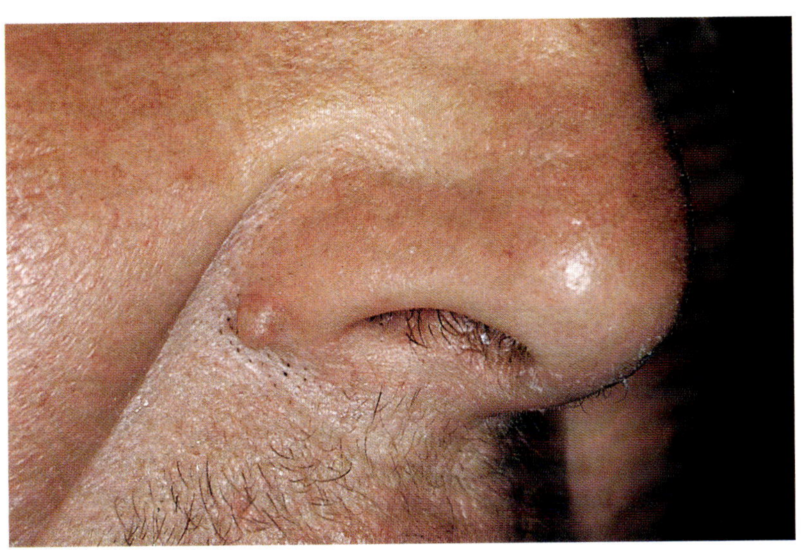

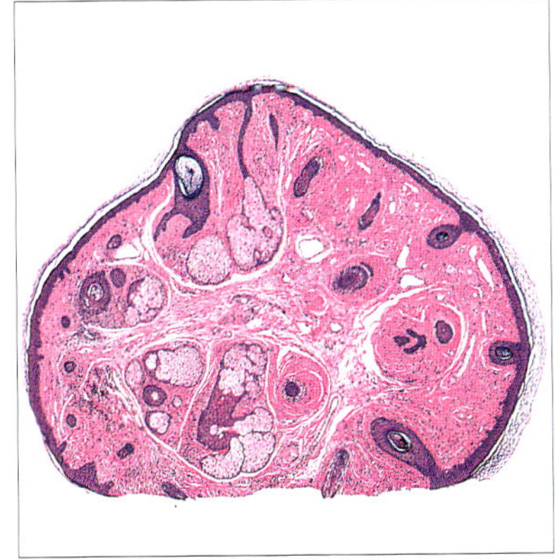

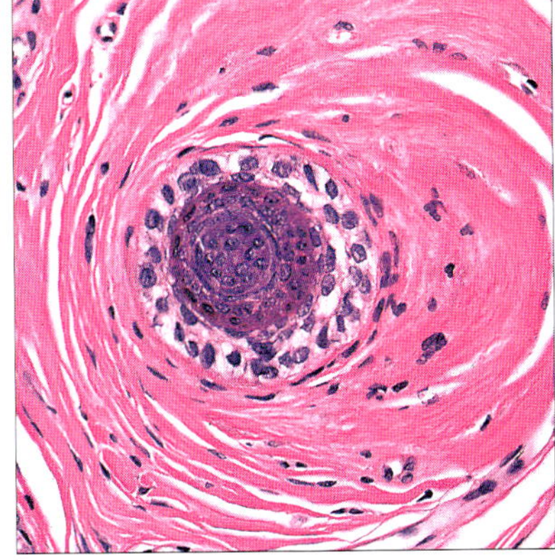

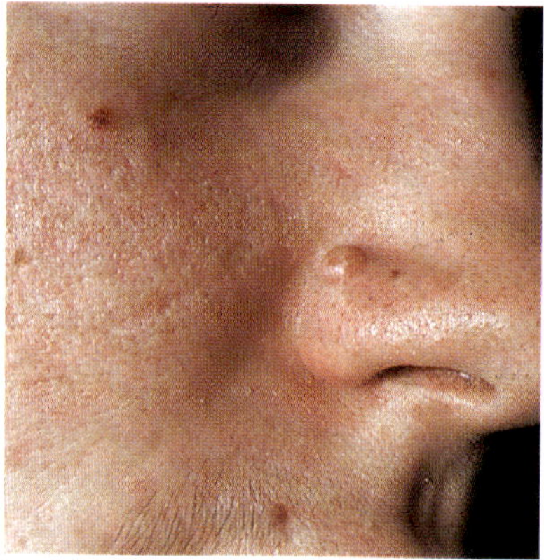

FIG. 33-1 *A smooth-surfaced, skin-colored, dome-shaped papule of fibrous papule on the ala.*

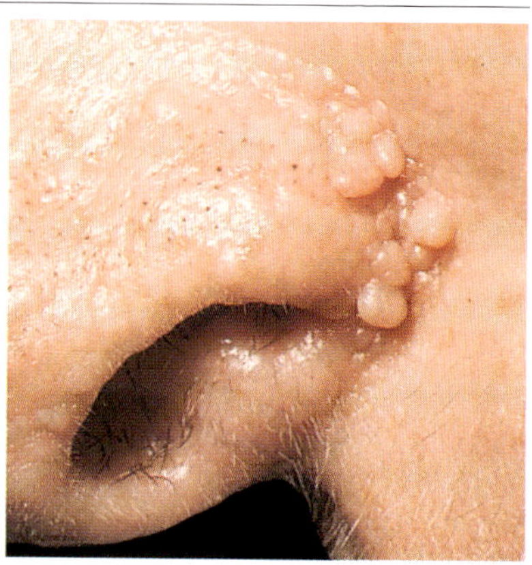

FIG. 33-2 *Smooth-surfaced agminated papules of adenoma sebaceum.*

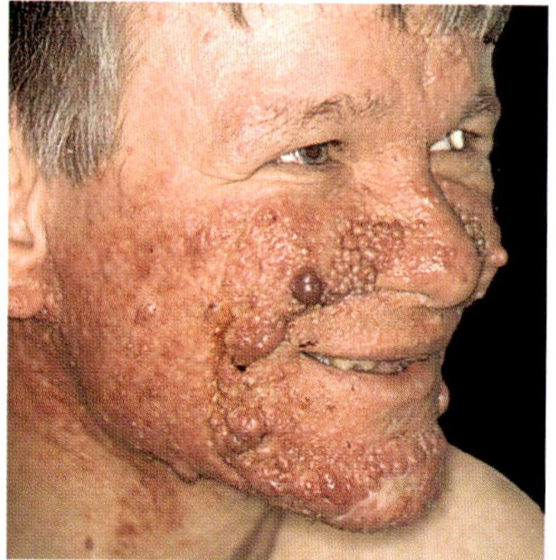

FIG. 33-3 *Innumerable smooth-surfaced papules of adenoma sebaceum.*

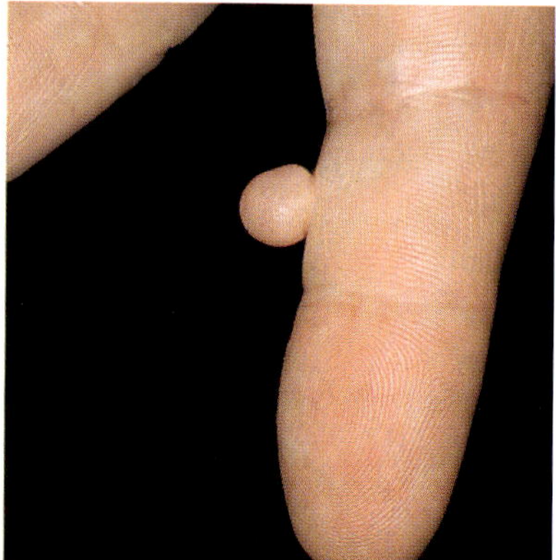

FIG. 33-4 *Papule on the finger (acquired digital fibroma).*

COURSE Once a fibrous papule (or papules) has appeared on the face, the lesion is destined to remain there for a person's lifetime. The same can be stated for hundreds, or even thousands, of fibrous papules in the condition known as adenoma sebaceum, which is one of the triad of epiloia, a mnemonic that stands for <u>epi</u>lepsy, <u>lo</u>w <u>i</u>ntelligence, and <u>a</u>denoma sebaceum.

INTEGRATION: UNIFYING CONCEPT Many myths surround the subject of fibrous papule of the face. When first described, it was said to be nothing more than a melanocytic nevus that had undergone regression. Although that point of view is still expressed by authors of some current textbooks, it has largely been discredited because it is wrong; there is no relationship of fibrous papule to a melanocytic nevus. Neither is fibrous papule of the face a mere "angiofibroma" as also has been proposed, nor is it a connective tissue nevus as some aver.

Fibrous papule is a hamartoma in which follicular elements are dominant. The papule is characterized by abnormal follicles; for example, instead of vellus follicles, which are typical of the face, the follicles are terminal ones. Instead of the follicles being oriented nearly vertical to the skin surface, which is the rule, they assume peculiar orientations, such as even being nearly parallel to the surface of the skin and, at times, even upside down. Sometimes, the follicles in a fibrous papule are bizarre, like having a huge bulb and a contiguous giant papilla. In addition to abnormalities of the follicles themselves, there usually is striking exaggeration of the perifollicular sheath, a phenomenon that prompted H. Pinkus to name it "perifollicular fibroma."

Much of the papule consists of altered bundles of collagen that are accompanied by an increased number of fibrocytes, many of them binucleate or multinucleate and associated with abundant stellate-shaped cytoplasm. Vessels are widely dilated. In the epidermis, there may be an increased number of melanocytes disposed as solitary units in the basal layer, but those melanocytes, even if large, are monomorphous and equidistant from one another. The very same findings that typify a single fibrous papule of the face are seen in the papules of adenoma sebaceum. Parenthetically, the term adenoma sebaceum is a misnomer; the condition, which is a follicular hamartoma, is neither adenomatous nor sebaceous.

THERAPY Shave excision or a combination of electrocautery and curettage is recommended for removal of one or a few fibrous papules, and laser surgery or dermabrasion for the lesions of adenoma sebaceum.

DEFINITION Folliculitis, usually a suppurative inflammatory process that involves infundibula, is either noninfectious, as in the case of pustules of acne vulgaris, or infectious, as in the case of pustules caused by Staphylococcus aureus. In contrast, pseudofolliculitis is a foreign-body type of inflammatory process that results from penetration of the dermis by an ingrown hair.

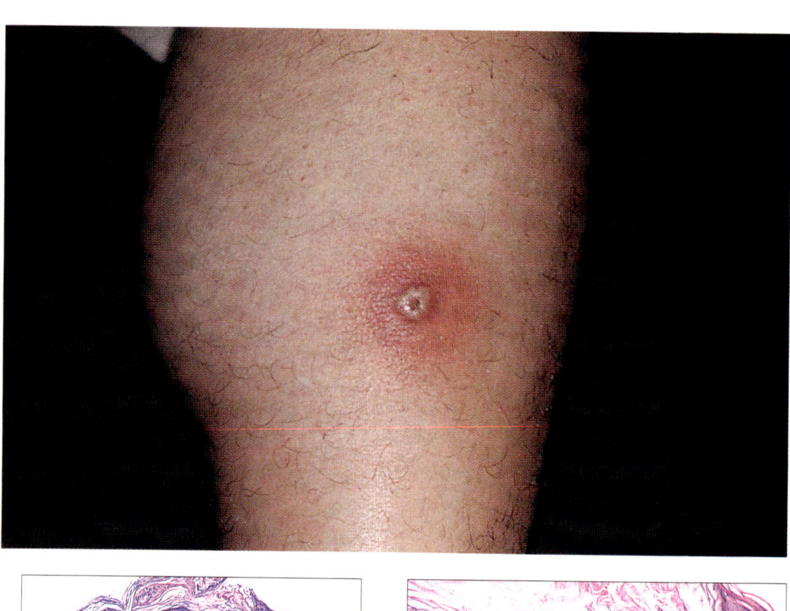

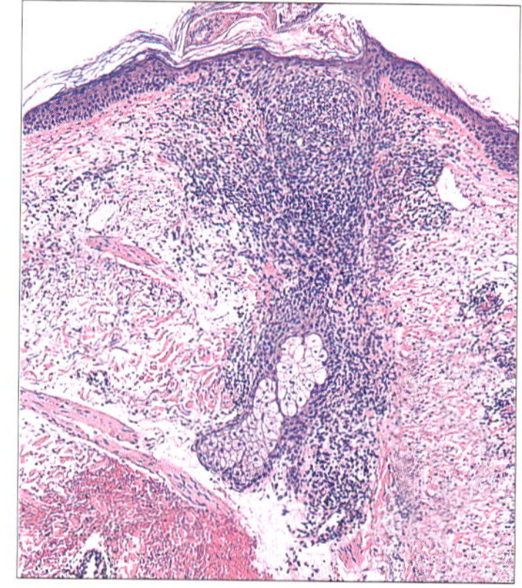

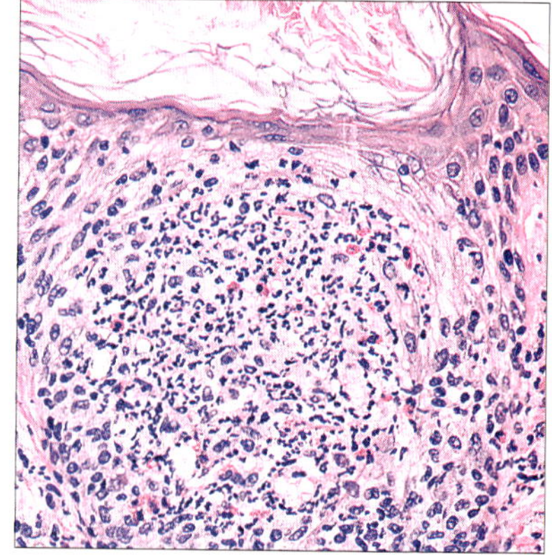

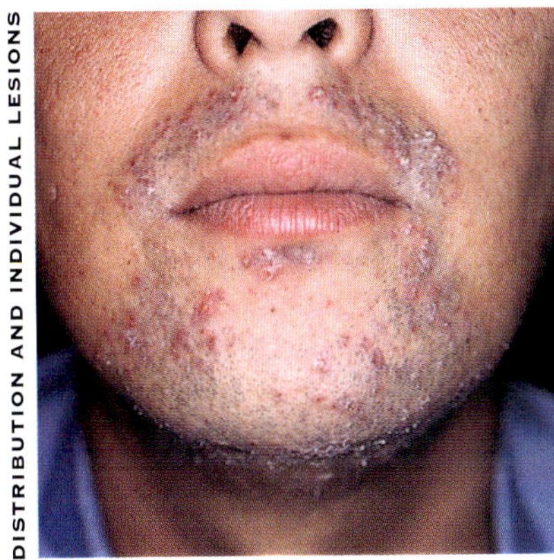

FIG. 34-1 *Papules of herpetic folliculitis.*

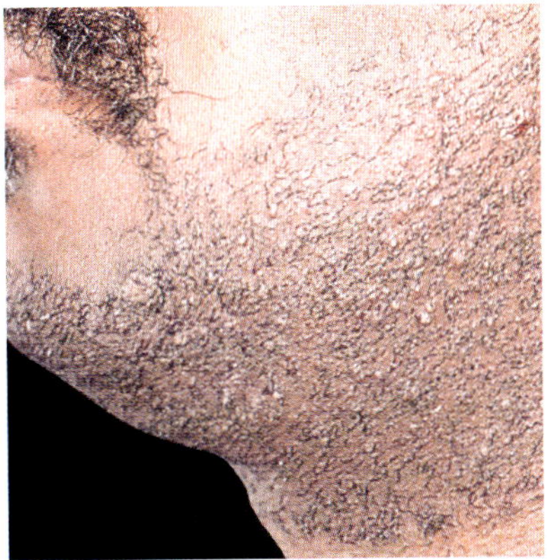

FIG. 34-2 *Innumerable discrete follicular papules of pseudofolliculitis barbae.*

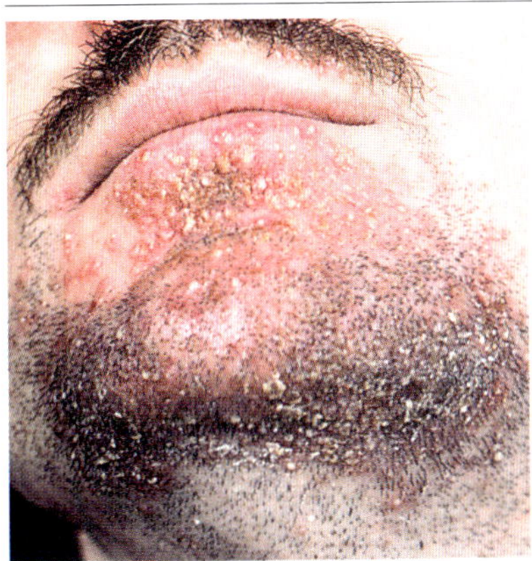

FIG. 34-3 *Crusts and pustules of staphylococcal folliculitis.*

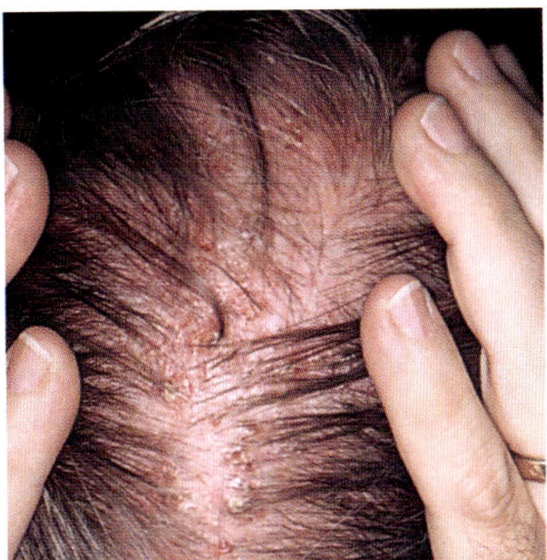

FIG. 34-4 *Pustules affiliated with tufts of hair ("tufted folliculitis").*

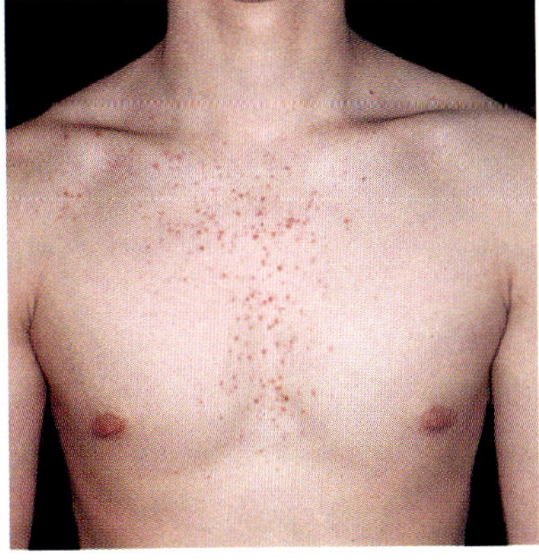

FIG. 34-5 *Monomorphous pustules of "pityrosporum folliculitis."*

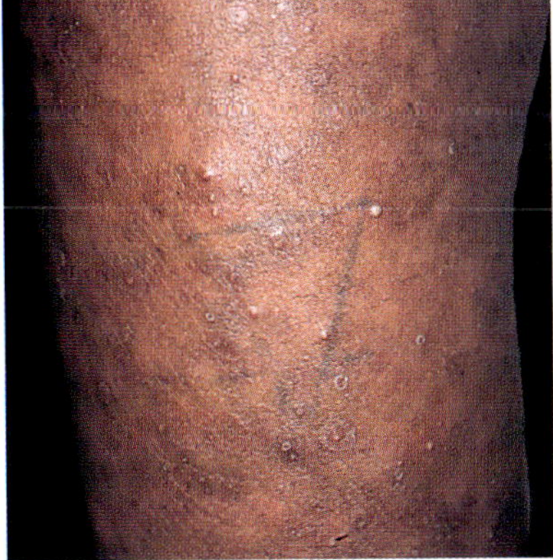

FIG. 34-6 *Eosinophilic folliculitis in an immunosuppressed patient.*

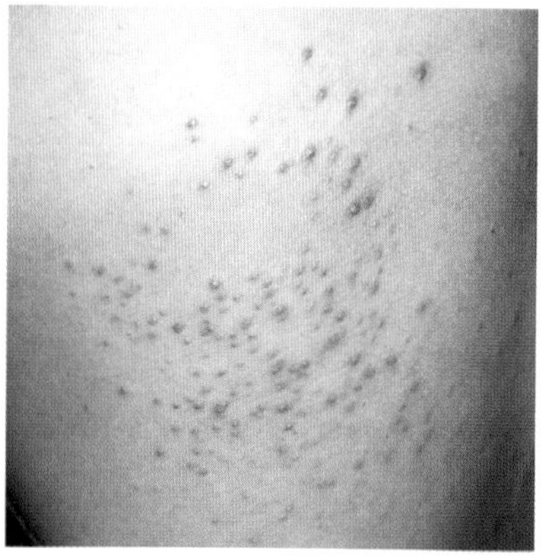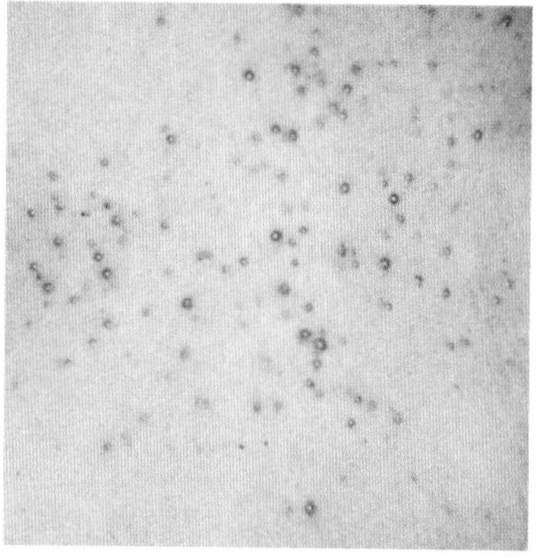

FIG. 34-7 (A, B) *Monomorphous follicular pustules of so-called pityrosporum folliculitis.*

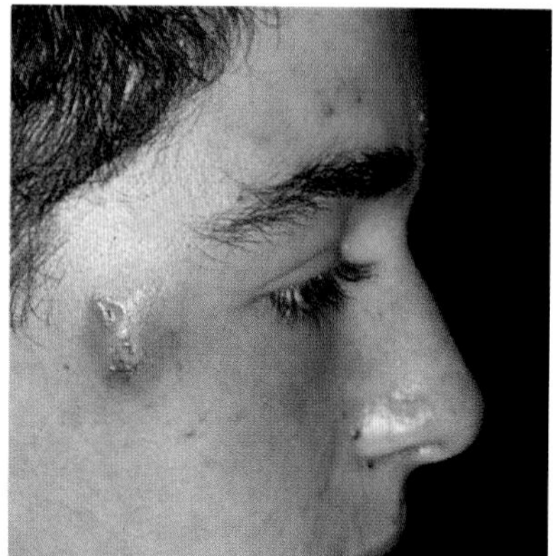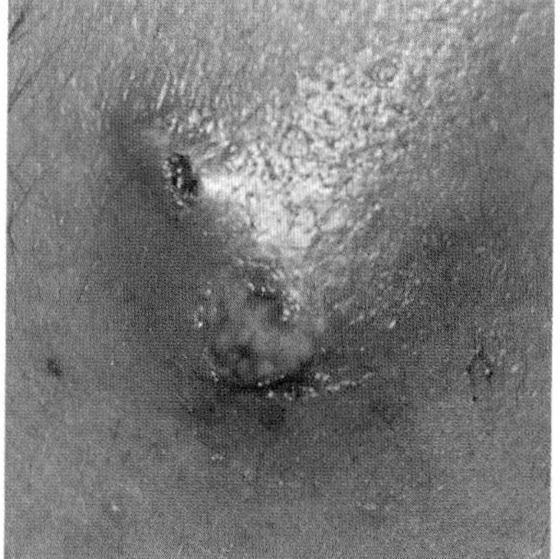

FIG. 34-8 (A, B) *Nodule with openings filled with purulent material (furuncle).*

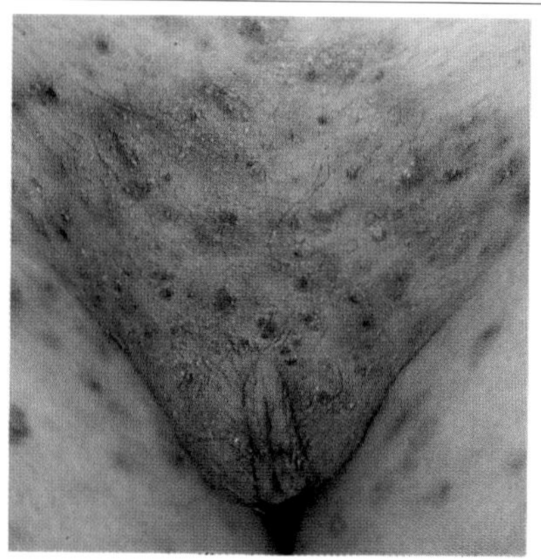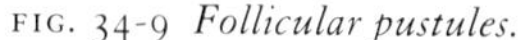

FIG. 34-9 *Follicular pustules.*

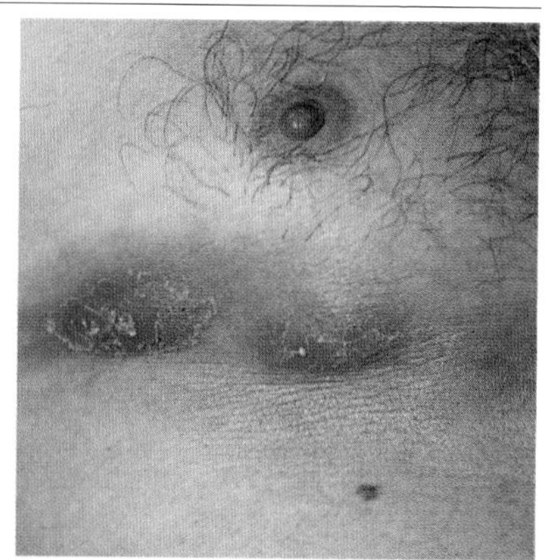

FIG. 34-10 *Erythematous nodules of furunculosis.*

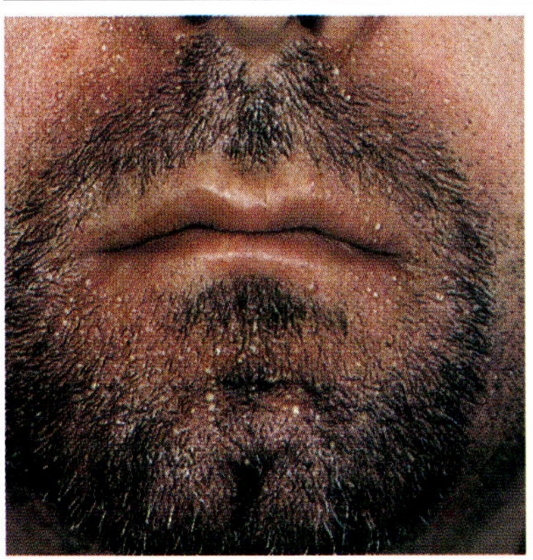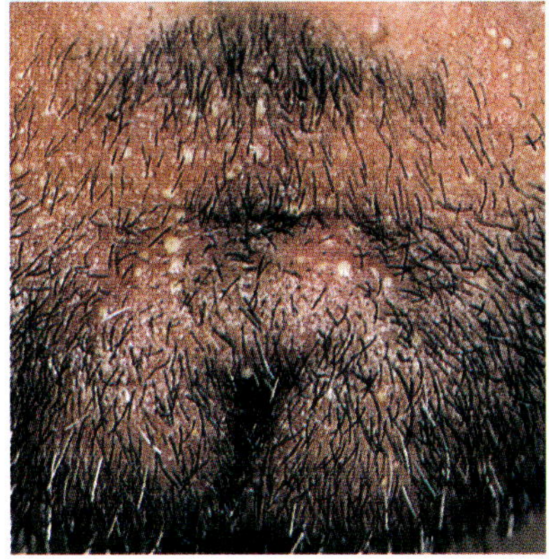

FIG. 34-11 (A, B) *Innumerable pustules in the beard and moustache region, each of them surrounding a hair.*

ADJUNCTIVE DIAGNOSTIC TEST Samples for culture may be taken and placed on specialized agar.

COURSE Folliculitis presents itself usually as pustules that appear quickly and disappear less quickly, first as crusts and then, at times, as hypopigmented or hyperpigmented macules. Often no residuum is left of the pustules of folliculitis. The course of folliculitis itself varies according to the cause of it. When pustules of folliculitis follow immersion in a whirlpool that has been contaminated by gram-negative bacteria, the pustules disappear in days if further exposure to those organisms is avoided. If, however, the cause of the folliculitis is machine oils to which a worker is exposed almost daily, the pustules will come and go for as long as there is occlusion of follicles by those oils.

Pseudofolliculitis is a consequence of "ingrown hairs," usually of persons who have hairs that coil. It tends to be more longer-lasting than folliculitis because the offending hairs penetrate the dermis where they act as foreign bodies.

INTEGRATION: UNIFYING CONCEPT Folliculitis can be divided generally into that which is infectious and that which is non-infectious. Infectious causes include bacteria, e.g., Staphylococci, superficial fungi, e.g., Trichophyton rubrum (Majocchi's granuloma), and viruses, e.g., herpesvirus. Those infectious agents also have capability to cause lesions in the skin that are not follicular. As a rule, the pustules of folliculitis may be identified for what they are by a hair that emanates from them, equidistance from one another, just as follicles themselves are, and appearance solely on hair-bearing sites.

Pustules of noninfectious folliculitis may be indistinguishable clinically from those of infectious folliculitis, but when they are studied through a conventional microscope, they are seen to lack telltale signs of an infectious process. No large clumps of bacteria, no hyphae in cornified cells of inner sheath, hair shaft, or infundibulum, and no nuclear and cytoplasmic changes typical of infection by herpesvirus are found. Often no cause can be determined for sterile pustules of folliculitis.

The most common folliculitis in skin is that of acne vulgaris, and that subject is addressed in the second chapter of this atlas. Acne vulgaris does not qualify as an infectious folliculitis, however, because the disease is not transferrable to either another person or to an experimental animal.

Pseudofolliculitis, as the name denotes, is not a true folliculitis, but results from hairs that, instead of growing straight out of follicles, coil, incurve, and penetrate the skin. In brief, pseudofolliculitis is a kind of "foreign body reaction" in which the "ingrown hair" acts as a foreign body that induces, in stages, suppurative, granulomatous, and fibrosing inflammation. When an abscess is present within the epidermis, it presents itself clinically as a pustule. Not surprisingly, the pustules of pseudofolliculitis are intraepidermal, in contrast to those of folliculitis which are intrainfundibular. When an abscess of pseudofolliculitis is present around a hair within the dermis, the lesion is seen clinically as an inflamed papule.

THERAPY Local cleaning and topical antibiotics are indicated for circumscribed disease caused by staphylococci, and oral antibiotics resistant to penicillinase are the preferred treatment for widespread bacterial disease. Systemically administered antifungal agents are effective in Majocchi's granuloma.

For noninfectious folliculitis, topical vitamin A acid is advisable.

DEFINITION An inflammatory, i.e., granulomatous, process that usually takes the form of papules which in constellation often assume annular, arcuate, and serpiginous shapes. Many variants exist, among them widespread papules, papules in photodistribution, papules marked by tiny crusts ("perforating" granuloma annulare), patches, plaques, and nodules (subcutaneous granuloma annulare).

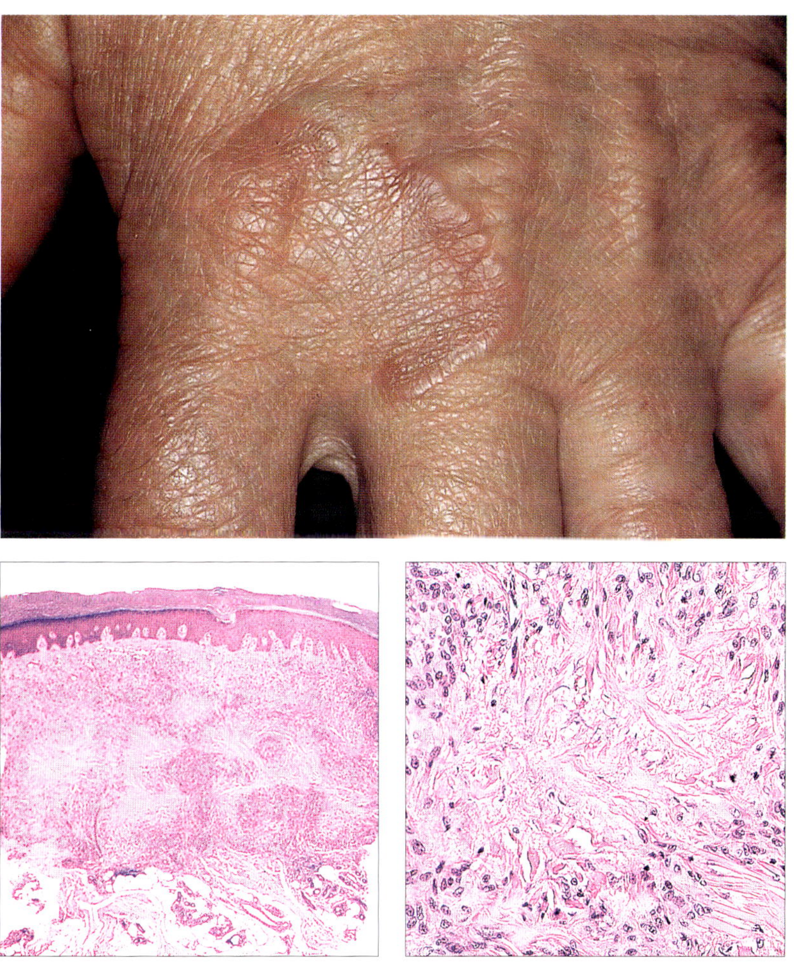

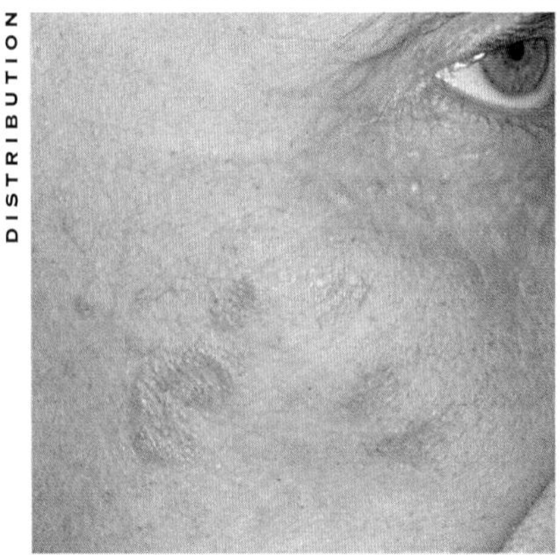

FIG. 35-1 *Annular papules and plaques.*

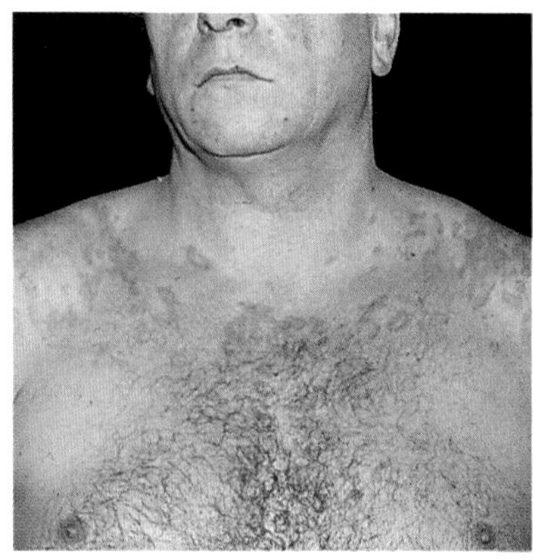

FIG. 35-2 *Macules and papules, some of them in annular configuration, as well as patches and plaques.*

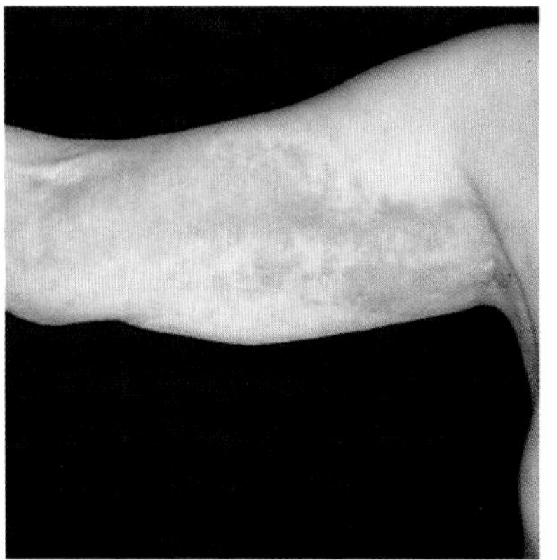

FIG. 35-3 *Macules and papules, some of them confluent forming patches and plaques.*

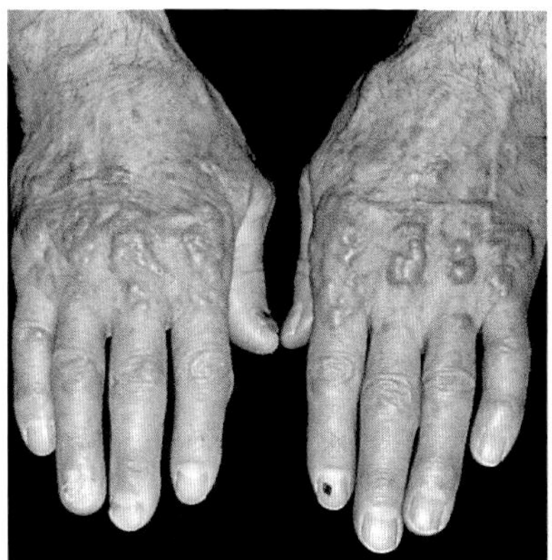

FIG. 35-4 *Papules and nodules.*

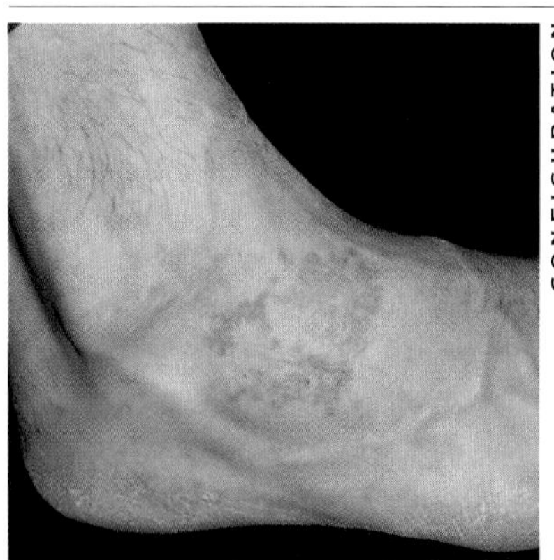

FIG. 35-5 *Papules, some having become confluent to form a plaque with scalloped outlines.*

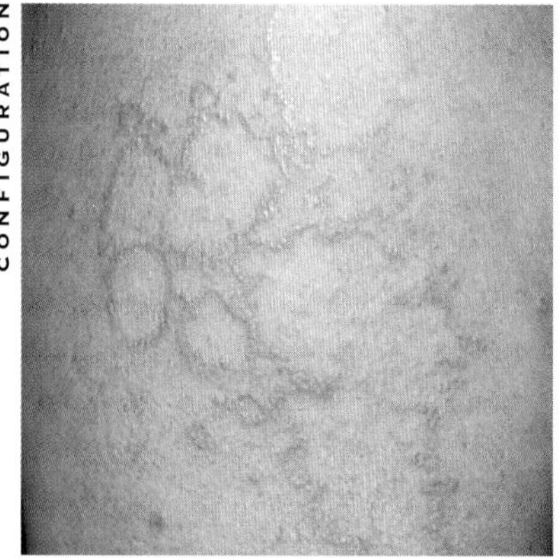

FIG. 35-6 *Papules in annular pattern secondary to confluence of them.*

INDIVIDUAL LESIONS

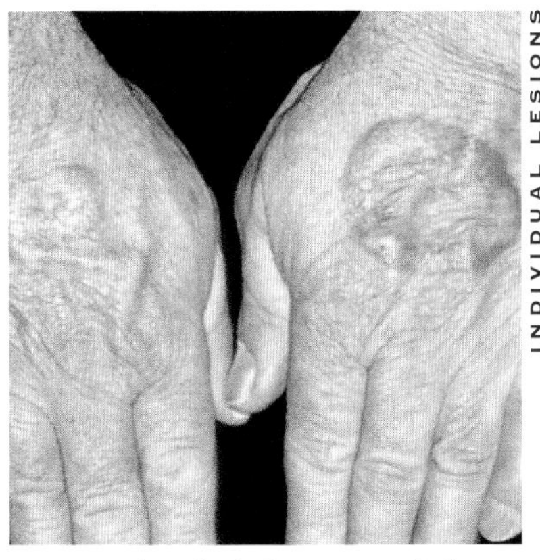

FIG. 35-7 *Annular lesions composed of many closely-set papules.*

FIG. 35-8 *Papules, some of them agminated.*

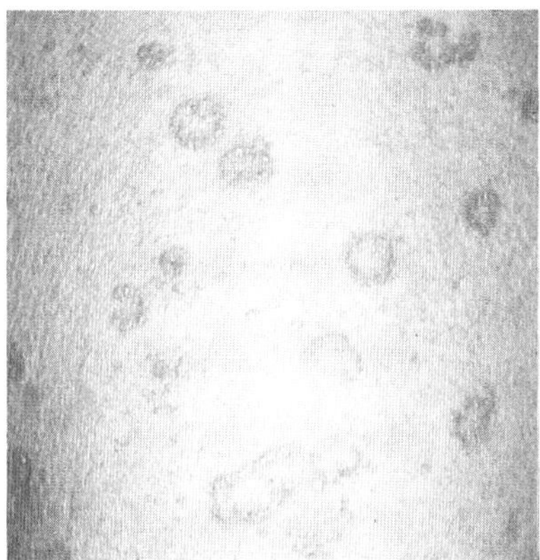

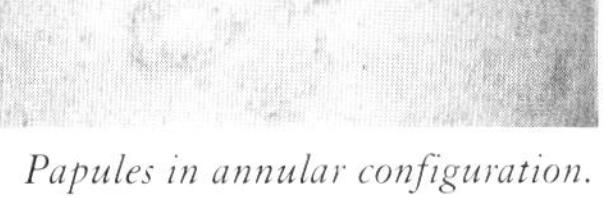

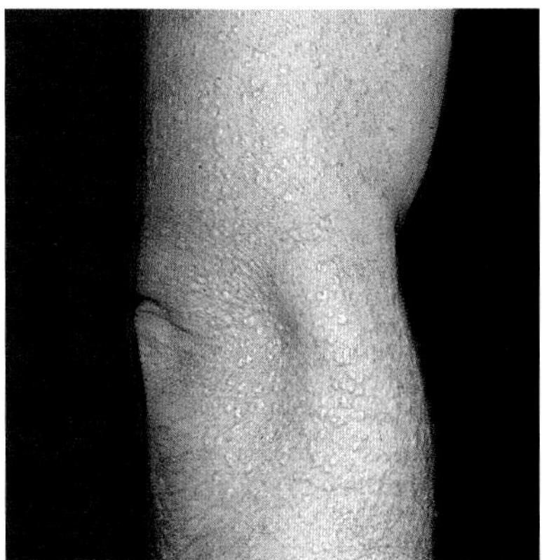

FIG. 35-9 *Papules in annular configuration.*

FIG. 35-10 *Widespread tiny papules.*

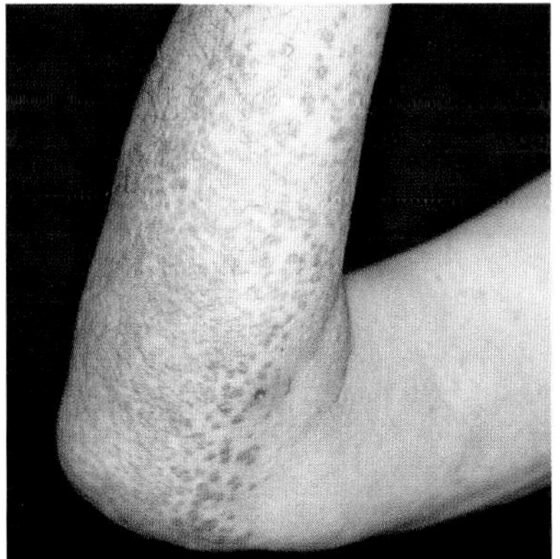

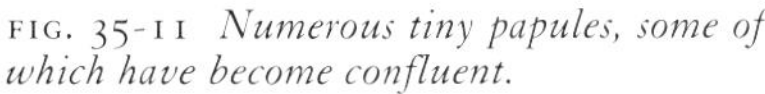

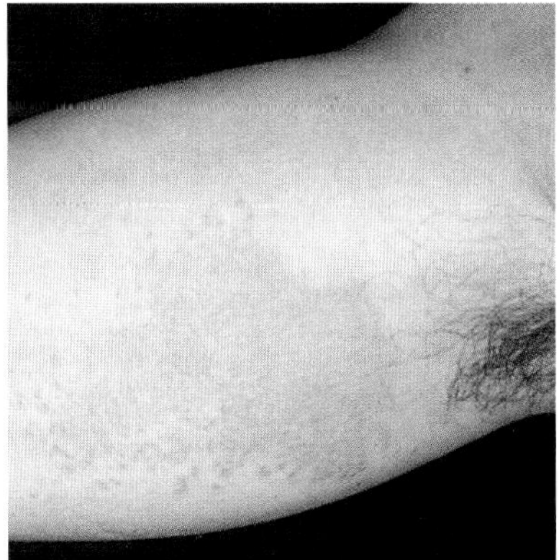

FIG. 35-11 *Numerous tiny papules, some of which have become confluent.*

FIG. 35-12 *Tiny papules that have become confluent to form a subtle plaque whose margin is scalloped.*

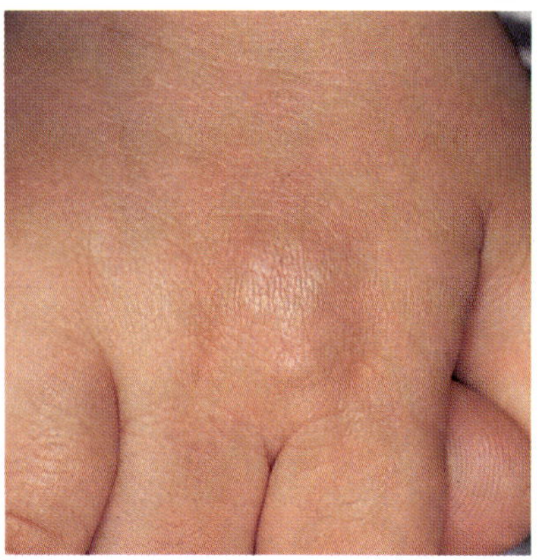

FIG. 35-13 *Plaque-like nodule on the dorsum of the hand of a child.*

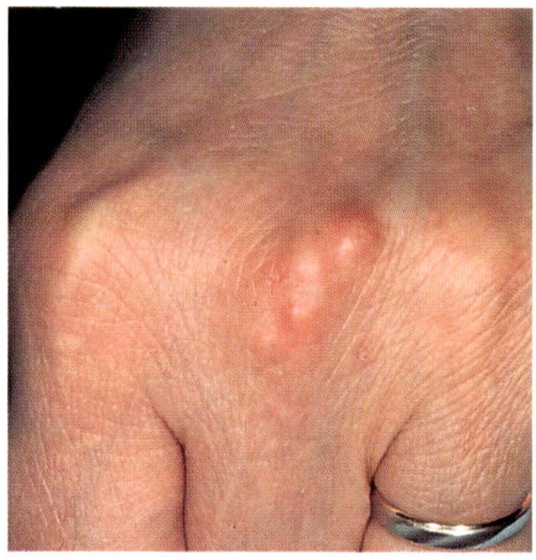

FIG. 35-14 *Cluster of papules forming a nodule of subcutaneous granuloma annulare.*

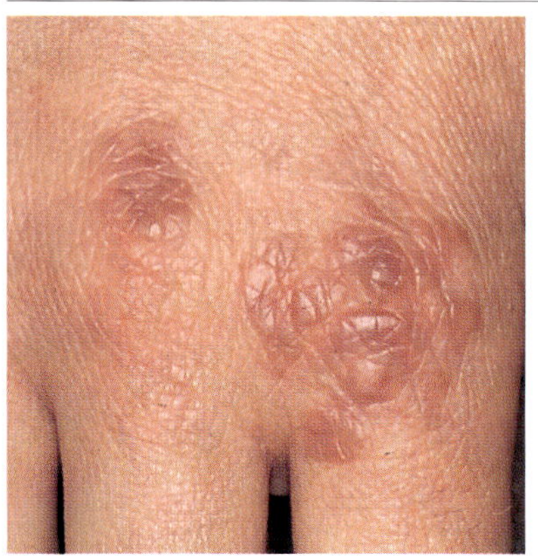

FIG. 35-15 *Papules in agminated and confluent array.*

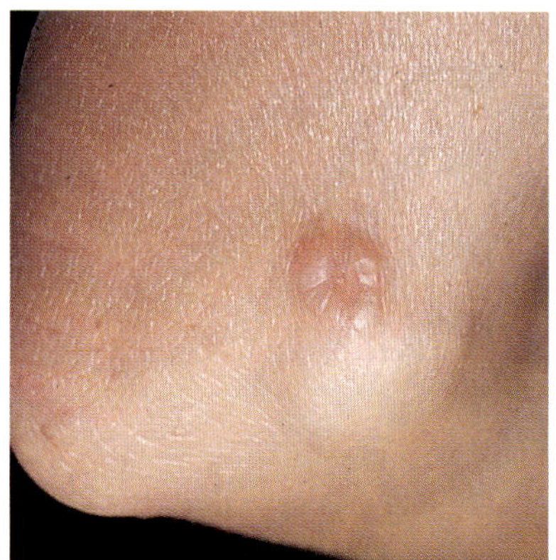

FIG. 35-16 *Papule with a central dell resulting in an annulus.*

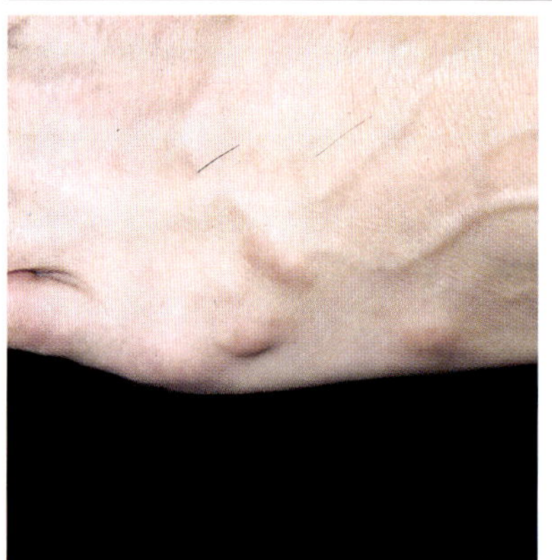

FIG. 35-17 *Papules and nodules of subcutaneous granuloma annulare.*

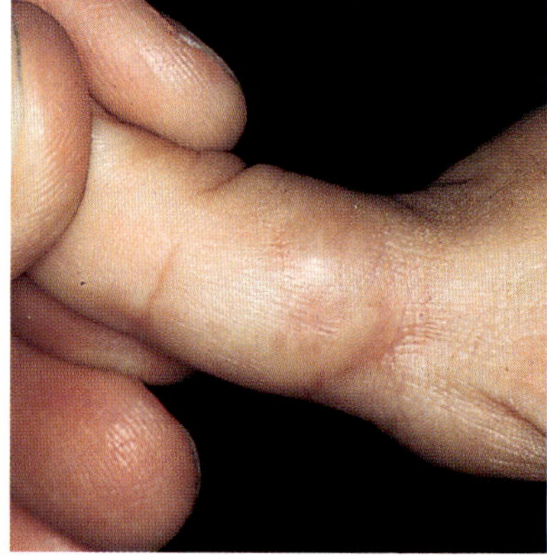

FIG. 35-18 *Nodule of subcutaneous granuloma annulare.*

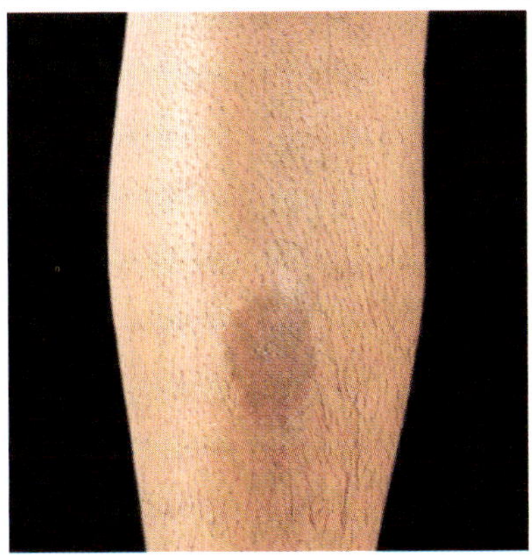

FIG. 35-19 *Plaque with slightly scalloped border.*

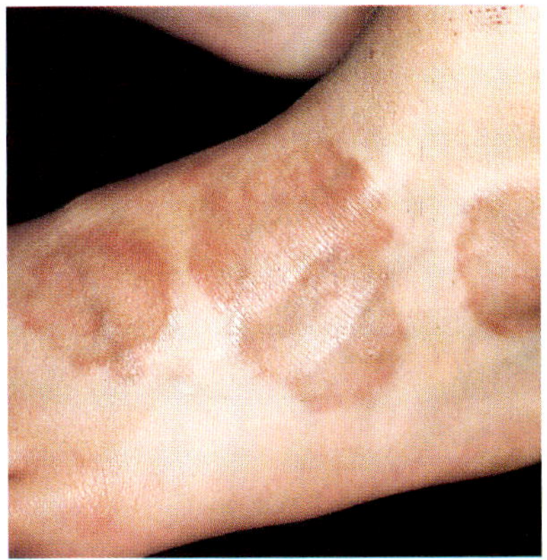

FIG. 35-20 *Papules in a scalloped pattern at the periphery of an atrophic patch.*

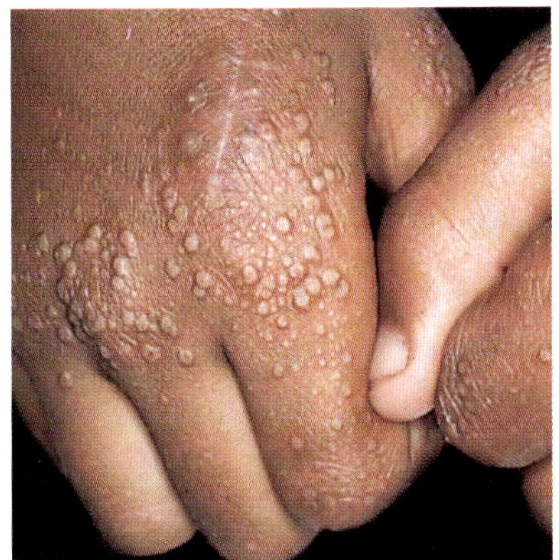

FIG. 35-21 *Numerous papules, some of them tiny and some of them marked by a central dell.*

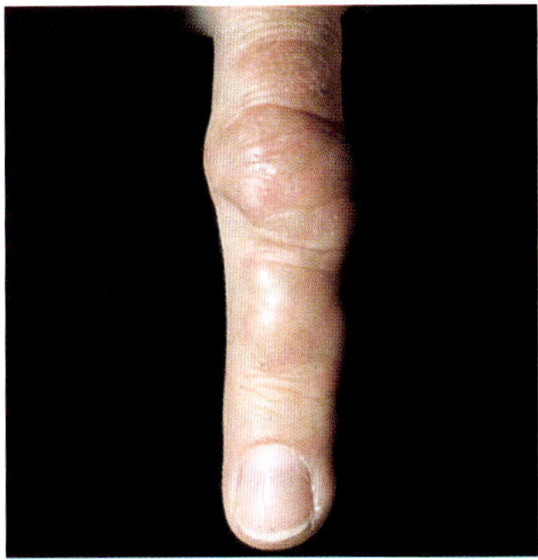

FIG. 35-22 *Nodules of subcutaneous granuloma annulare.*

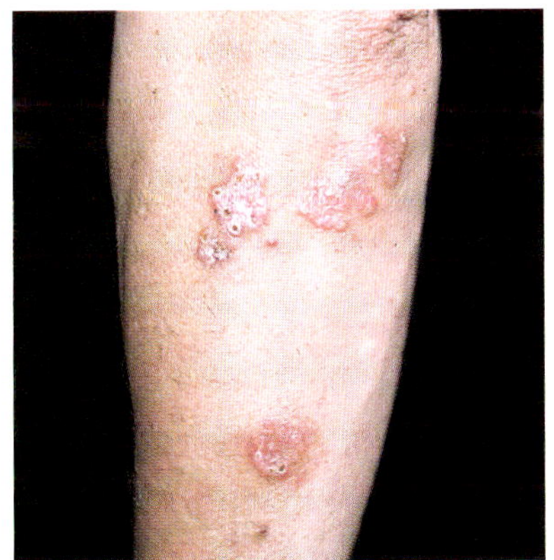

FIG. 35-23 *Papules clustered to form plaques punctuated by crusts (perforating granuloma annulare).*

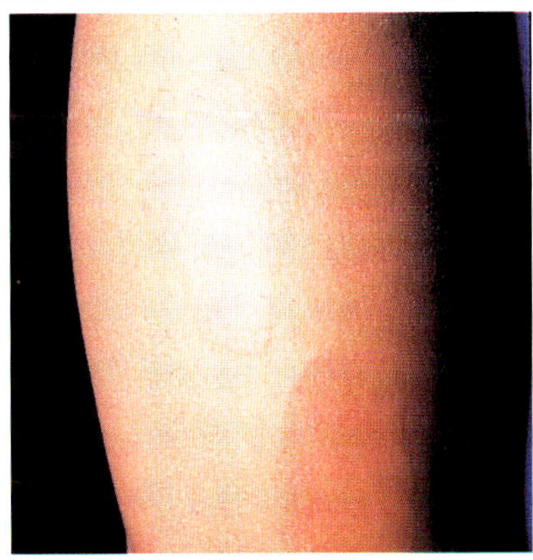

FIG. 35-24 *Patches rimmed by a border of tiny papules.*

COURSE Because lesions of granuloma annulare of all kinds, from tiny papules to subcutaneous nodules, are expressions of granulomatous inflammation, i.e., histiocytes predominate in foci, it follows that, in the absence of treatment, many months pass before they begin to regress. It also is apparent that, as a rule, except in children, nodules persist longer than papules. Curiously, a lesion of granuloma annulare in children often disappears after a biopsy is performed. The condition, however, is self-limited and in time it wanes and disappears.

INTEGRATION: UNIFYING CONCEPT Granuloma annulare presents itself clinically in many different guises, from the stereotypical annulus made up of small, smooth-surfaced papules to nodules that are subcutaneous; from widespread papules typified by central umbilication to tiny scale-crusts that represent sites of "perforation" through the epidermis of altered connective tissue in the upper part of the dermis; from patches rimmed by subtle papules on the legs to countless papules with a central dell on skin exposed to sunlight. What has been called actinic granuloma is simply granuloma annulare that expands centrifugally in skin damaged severely by sunlight, leaving in its wake an atrophic hypopigmented patch.

Although the histopathologic findings in each of these expressions of granuloma annulare reflect the findings seen clinically, the essential changes are typical and repeatable, namely, epithelioid histiocytes arranged in either a palisaded or interstitial pattern, or both together, in company with deposits of mucin. For example, in "subcutaneous" granuloma annulare, those changes are present as a rule in both the reticular dermis and the subcutaneous fat, in the latter first within septa from which the process extends progressively into lobules. In short, granuloma annulare, irrespective of clinical presentation, is diagnosable readily by conventional microscopy and all the manifestations of it have histopathologic findings in common. The cause of different expressions of granuloma annulare may be different, but the cause in none of them is yet known.

THERAPY There is no need for treatment because the lesions invariably involute and disappear. Intra-lesional injection of corticosteroids hastens the retreat of individual lesions. For widespread papules not induced by sunlight, either phototherapy (PUVA, UV-A-1) or dapsone may be effective.

DEFINITION An inflammatory process characterized by a pruritic, papular, and, uncommonly, papulovesicular eruption of unknown cause affecting persons over 40 years of age (and usually over 60), often in photodistribution, but sometimes widespread. Although named originally "transient acantholytic dermatosis" by Grover, the condition usually persists for many months and even for years.

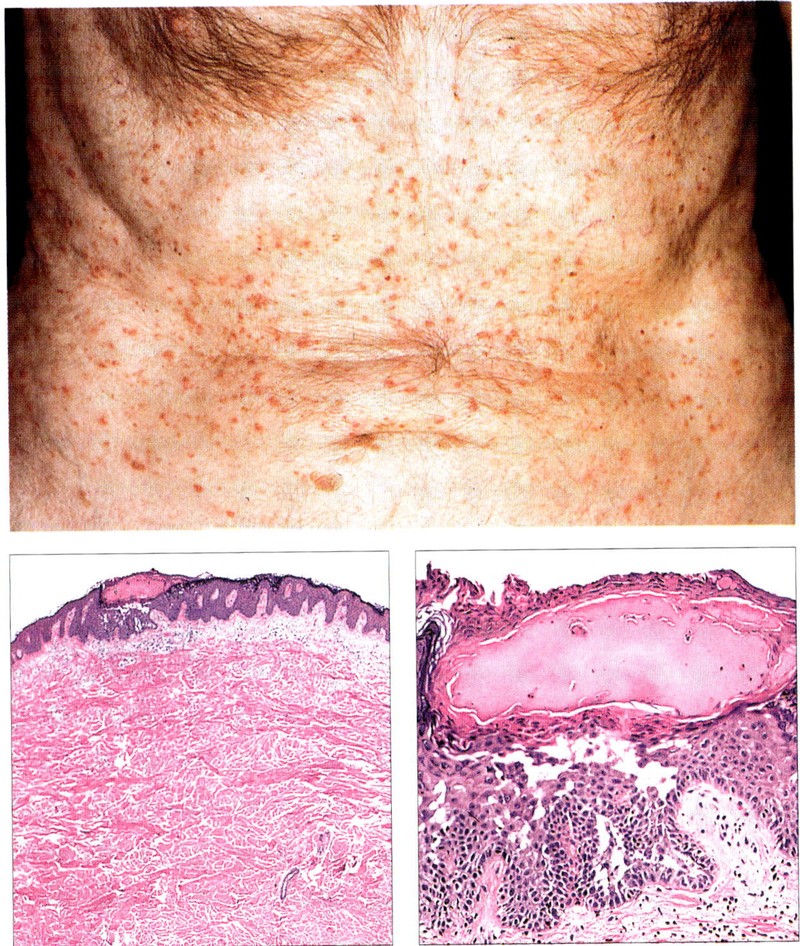

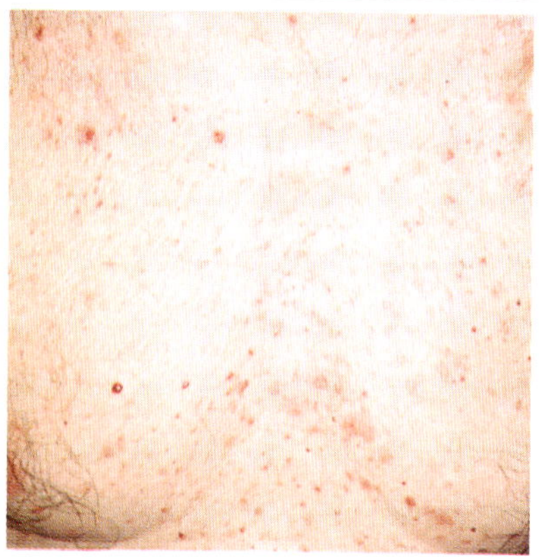

FIG. 36-1 *Papules, some of which are eroded secondary to excoriation.*

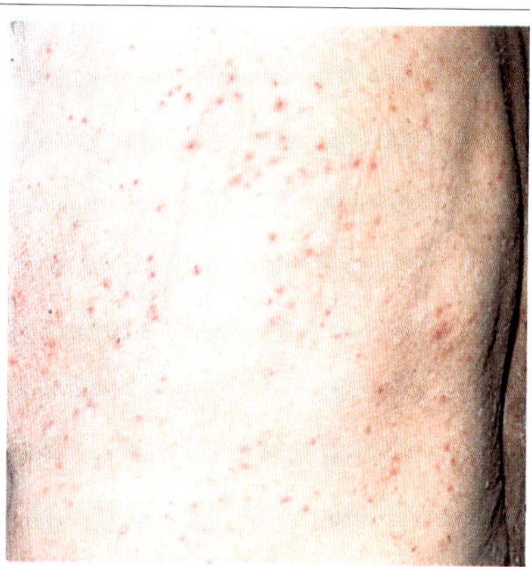

FIG. 36-2 *Discrete papules.*

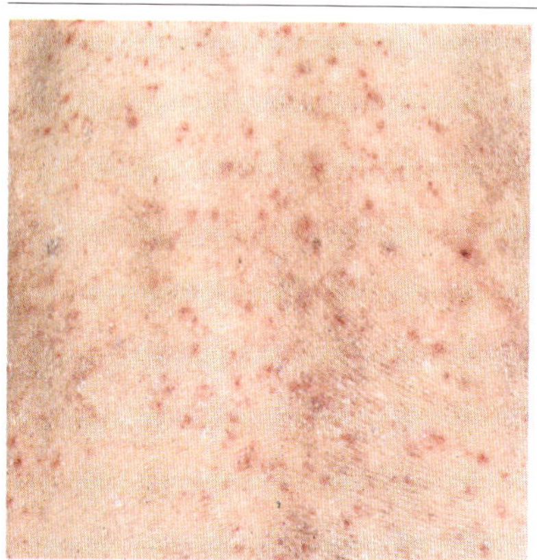

FIG. 36-3 *Discrete papules, some of which show signs of excoriation.*

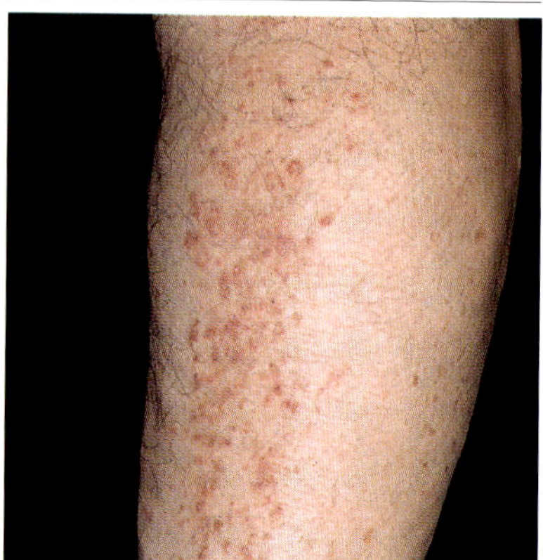

FIG. 36-4 *Discrete, slightly keratotic papules set close to one another.*

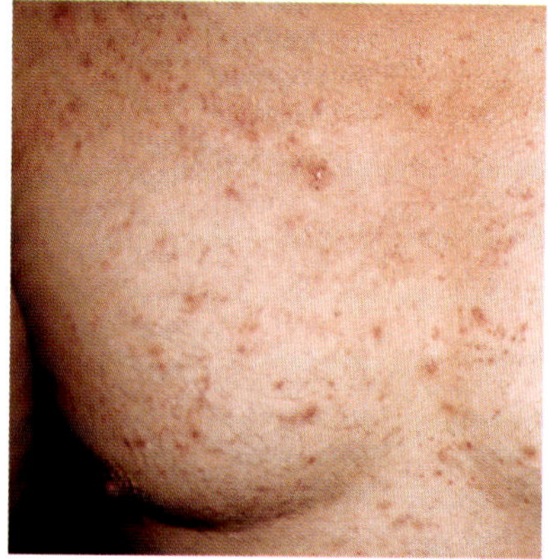

FIG. 36-5 *Discrete, scattered papules and hints of papulovesicles.*

COURSE Individual papules of Grover's disease may last for days (if they are smooth-surfaced) or weeks (if they are keratotic). As has already been stated, although the disease was first designated "transient acantholytic dermatosis" by Grover himself, it often lasts for months or years, rather than for weeks, as he originally thought. When, however, Grover's disease is induced by exposure to intense ultraviolet light, the lesions themselves, and the entire course of the disease, may last for little more than a week.

INTEGRATION: UNIFYING CONCEPT Clinically, papules are the common denominator of Grover's disease, and, histopathologically, the common denominator of individual lesions is the presence within the epidermis of some acantholytic cells. The papules have either a smooth or keratotic surface. Those with a smooth surface show acantholytic cells in a pattern that simulates those of pemphigus vulgaris, pemphigus foliaceus, or Hailey-Hailey disease. Keratotic papules show changes that closely resemble those of Darier's disease. Spongiosis may be an accompaniment of each of those histopathologic patterns. At times, more than one pattern may be seen in tissue sections of a single biopsy specimen of a lesion of Grover's disease.

The papules of Grover's disease are notoriously pruritic, and the most pruritic of all are those in which numerous eosinophils reside in the upper part of the dermis.

The cause of Grover's disease is not known.

THERAPY Topical corticosteroids, local antipruritics, and systemic antihistamines may be helpful in alleviating the intractable pruritus. Retinoids given systemically have sent the eruption into remission and caused lesions in some patients to involute.

DEFINITION A vesiculobullous disease in which blisters tend to be flaccid and localized to intertriginous regions, especially, the neck, axillary, infra-mammary, and inguinal ones. The disease is notoriously refractory to therapy. The name originally given to the condition by the brothers Hailey, familial benign chronic pemphigus, is misleading because the disease bears no relation to either pemphigus vulgaris or pemphigus foliaceus.

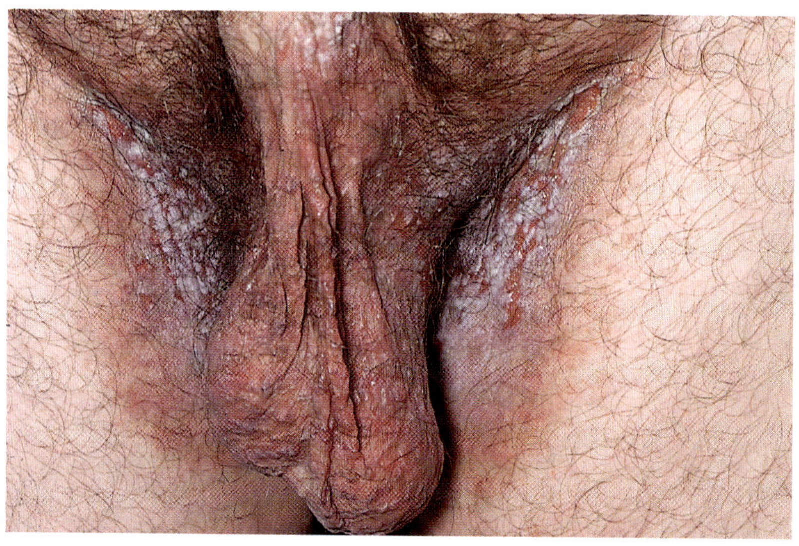

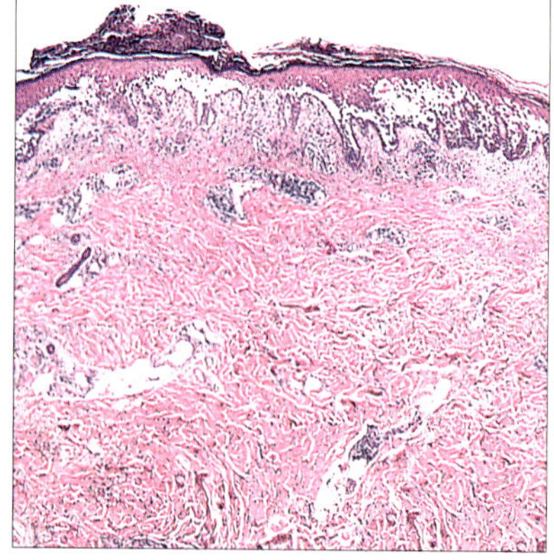

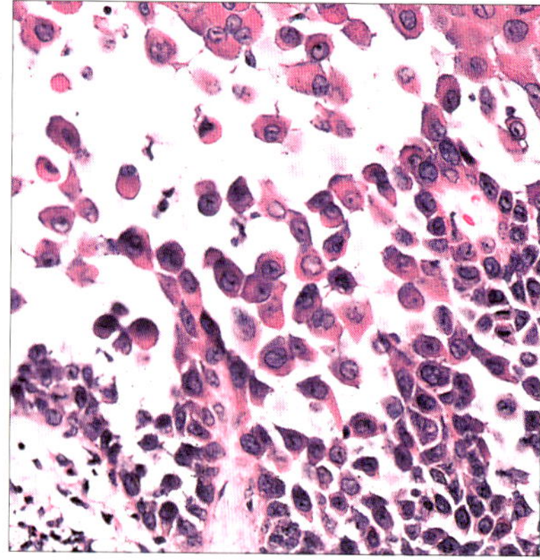

DISTRIBUTION

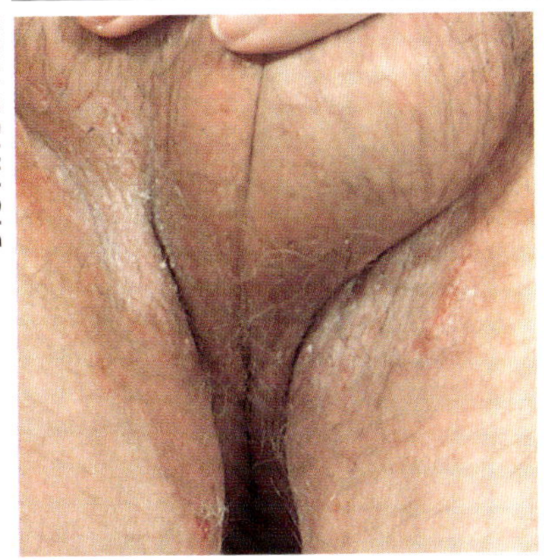

FIG. 37-1 *Vesiculopustules, maceration, erosions, scales, and hyperpigmentation in the groin.*

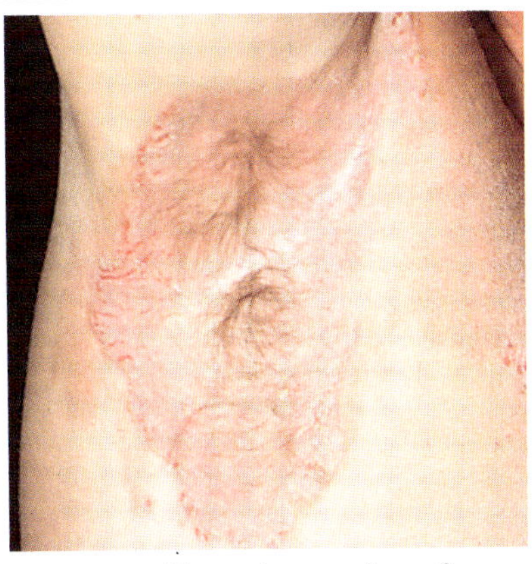

FIG. 37-2 *Maceration, erosions, fissures, scales, and scale-crusts in an axillary plaque whose periphery is hyperpigmented.*

INDIVIDUAL LESIONS

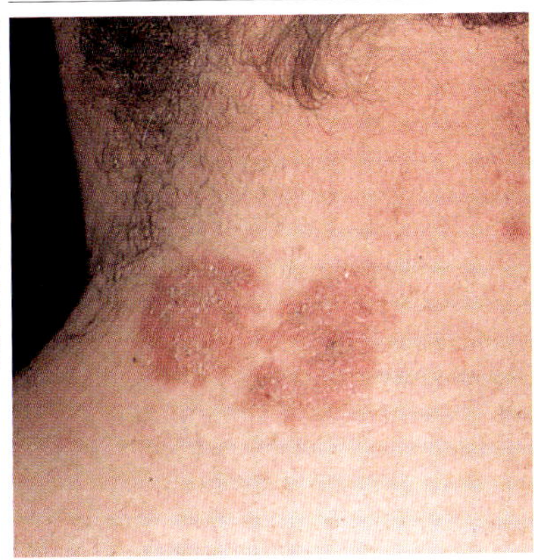

FIG. 37-3 *Papule and plaques covered by scale-crusts.*

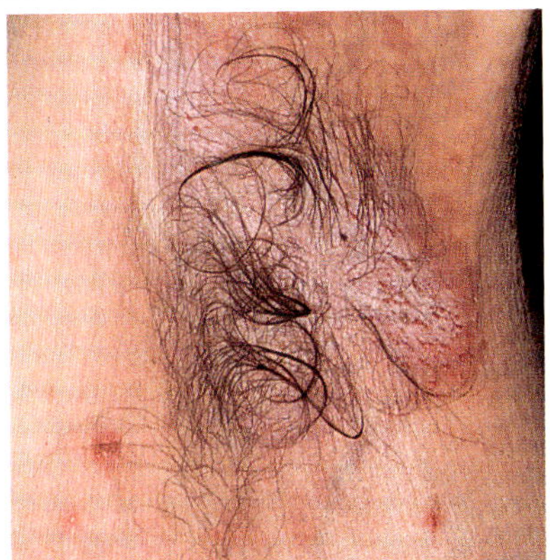

FIG. 37-4 *Plaque with signs of maceration and erosions.*

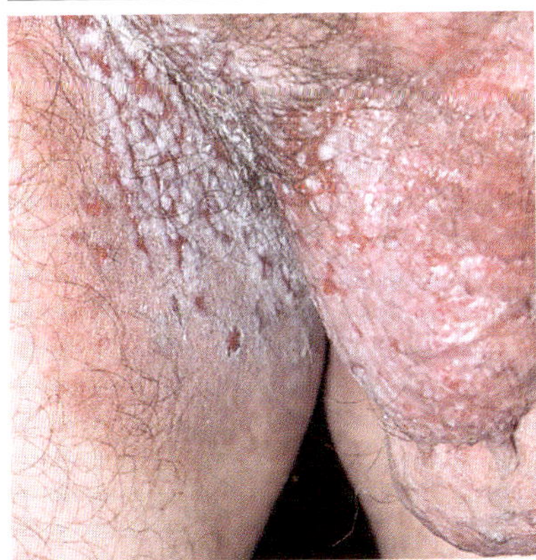

FIG. 37-5 *Extensive maceration, erosions, ulceration, and, at the periphery, a patch.*

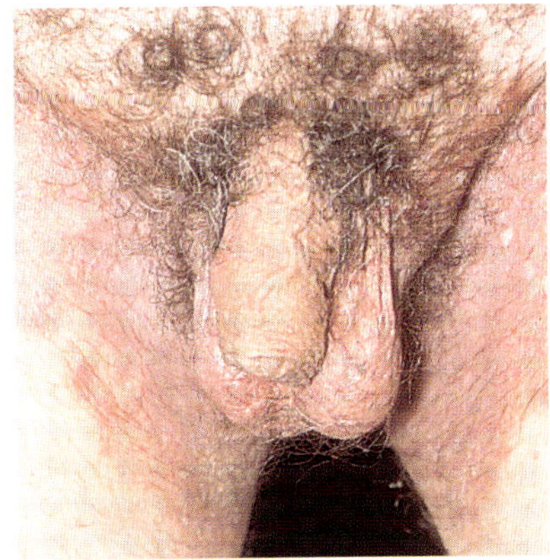

FIG. 37-6 *Clusters of vesicles and pustules, crusts, erosions, milia, and patches of hyperpigmentation.*

COURSE The disease itself is persistent and individual lesions of it are intractable, blisters resolving with erosions that heal slowly. Once a person develops Hailey-Hailey disease it is likely that lesions of it will come and go for a lifetime. Development of lesions cannot be prevented. Once they appear, they tend to persist for many weeks and months, new blisters appearing at the periphery of the centrifugally advancing process that leaves in its wake erosions, crusts, and, eventually, pigmentary changes. Maceration, an inevitable consequence of the disease having a decided predilection for intertriginous regions, complicates the picture further.

INTEGRATION: UNIFYING CONCEPT Hailey-Hailey disease is fundamentally an intraepidermal blistering disease characterized by the presence within the blister of acantholytic dyskeratotic cells. The histopathologic findings differ from those of pemphigus vulgaris because in Hailey-Hailey disease the epidermis is thicker, usually covered by scale-crusts, associated with acantholytic cells throughout at least half the thickness of it, and typified by acantholytic cells that also are dyskeratotic and often polygonal.

Moreover, in contrast to the situation in pemphigus vulgaris, the acantholytic cells are approximated closely to one another, a consequence of junctions between them being maintained even after desmosomal attachments have been lost. Vesicles and bullae of Hailey-Hailey disease tend to be flaccid. The constellation of histopathologic findings in Hailey-Hailey disease is specific for it, distinguishing it from all other intraepidermal blistering diseases that come into being by virtue of acantholysis.

THERAPY Topical or systemic antibiotics that eliminate secondary infection sometimes are palliative. Laser (pulsed CO_2) surgery and dermabrasion have been beneficial in some patients. Surgical excision of axillary and inguinal skin is said to be helpful in preventing development of new lesions.

DEFINITION An hemangioma is a benign neoplasm of blood vessels, a vascular malformation is an aberration in development of one or more major vascular structures, and an ectasia is a dilation of a preexisting end vessel.

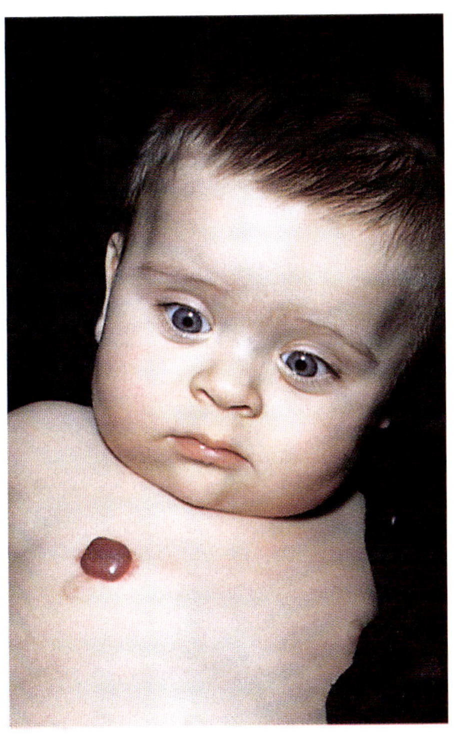

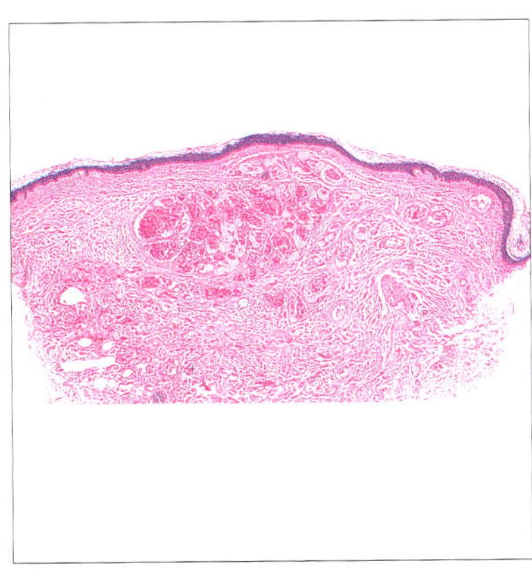

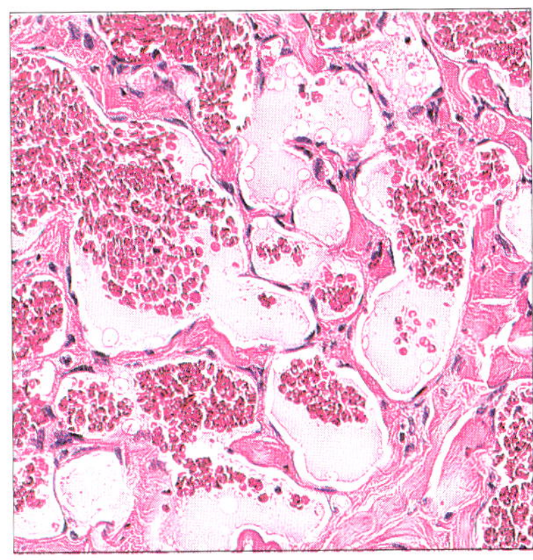

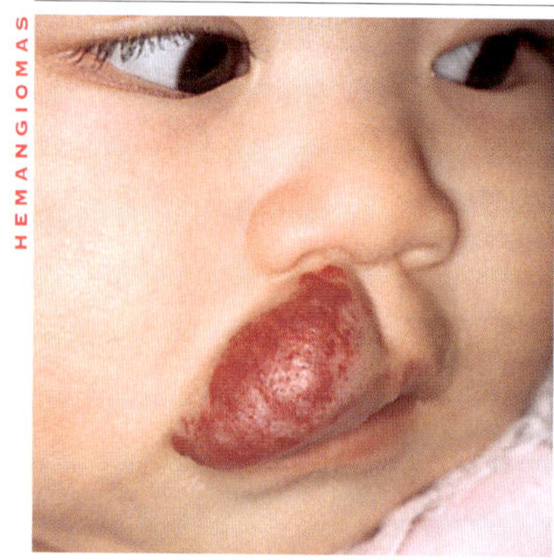

FIG. 38-1 *Strawberry hemangioma, involuting at one margin of the tumor in the form of a gray zone representing fibrosis.*

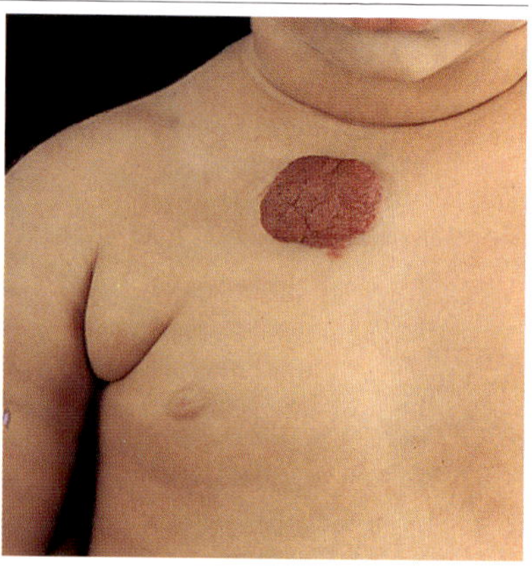

FIG. 38-2 *Strawberry hemangioma, tumor.*

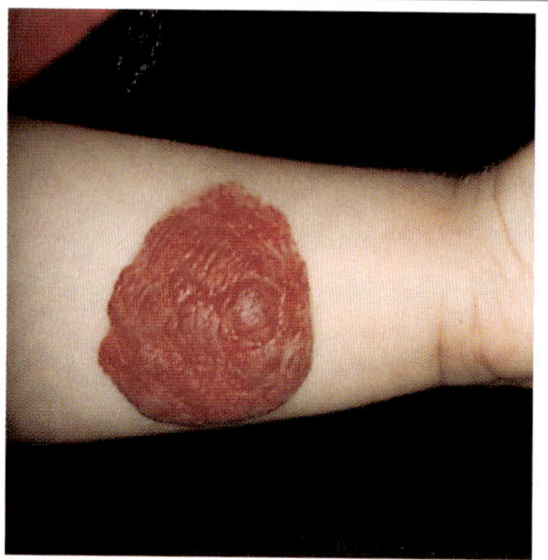

FIG. 38-3 *Strawberry hemangioma, tumorous plaque.*

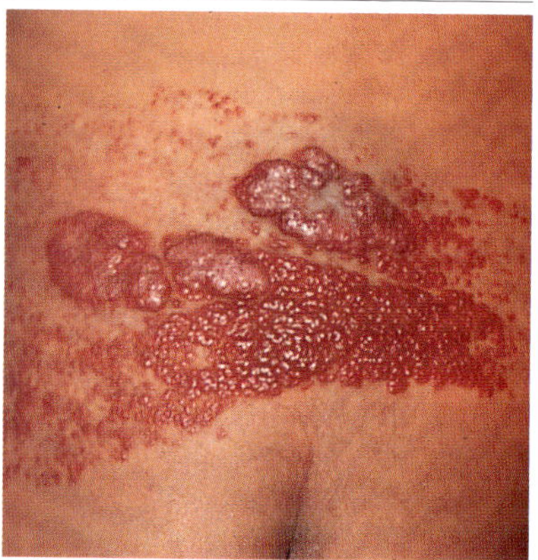

FIG. 38-4 *Strawberry hemangioma, papules, plaques, nodules, and zones of regression.*

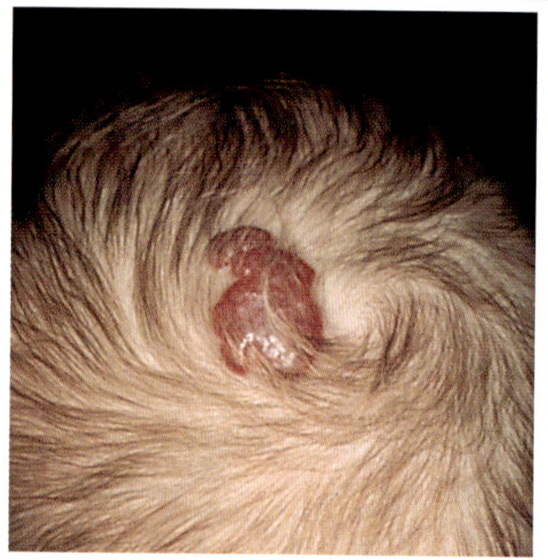

FIG. 38-5 *Strawberry hemangioma, tumor with foci of regression.*

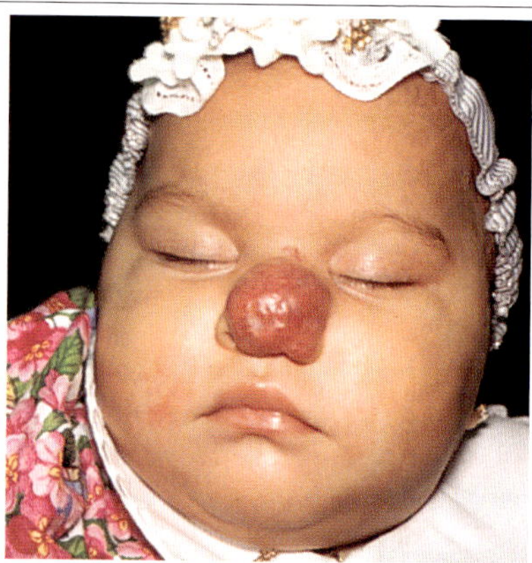

FIG. 38-6 *Strawberry hemangioma, tumor with zones of regression.*

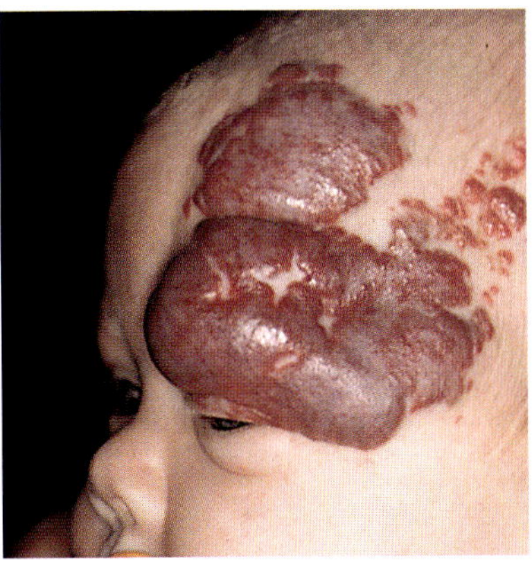

FIG. 38-7 *Strawberry hemangioma, papules and tumors within which are foci of regression.*

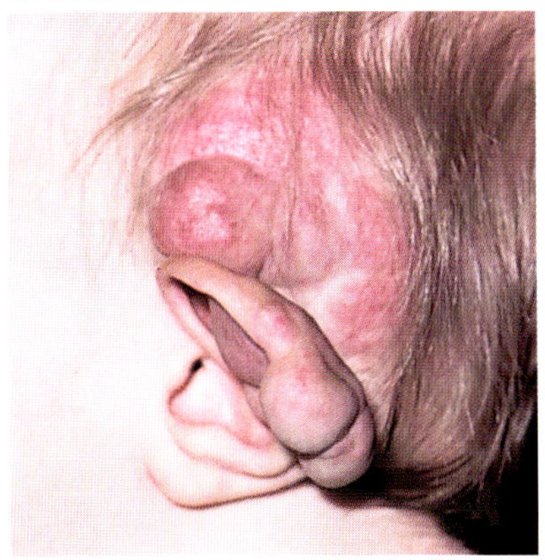

FIG. 38-8 *Strawberry hemangioma, nodules causing distortion of an ear.*

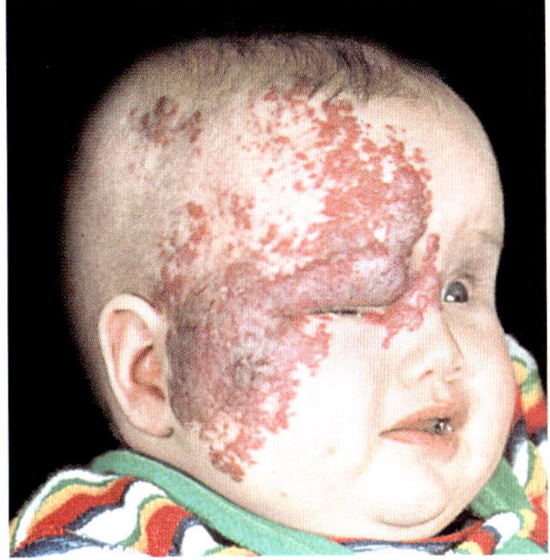

FIG. 38-9 *Strawberry hemangioma, papules, plaques, and tumors accompanied by many foci of regression.*

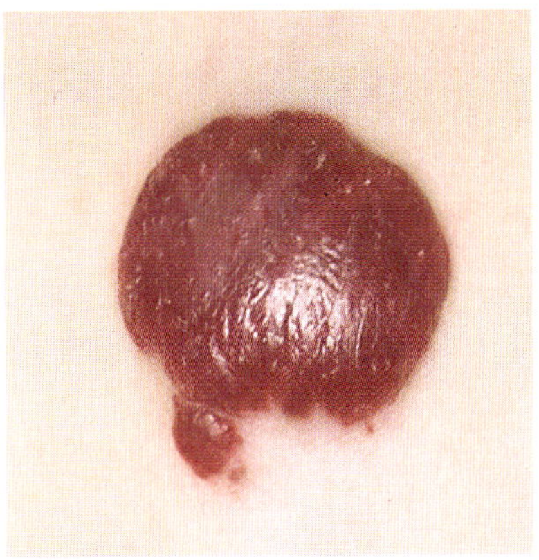

FIG. 38-10 *Strawberry hemangioma, tumor.*

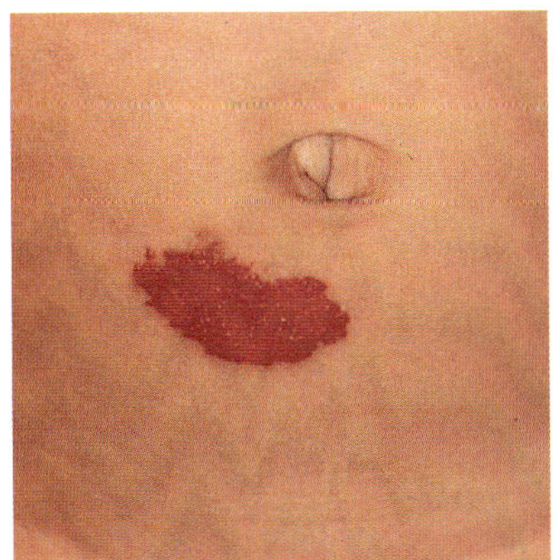

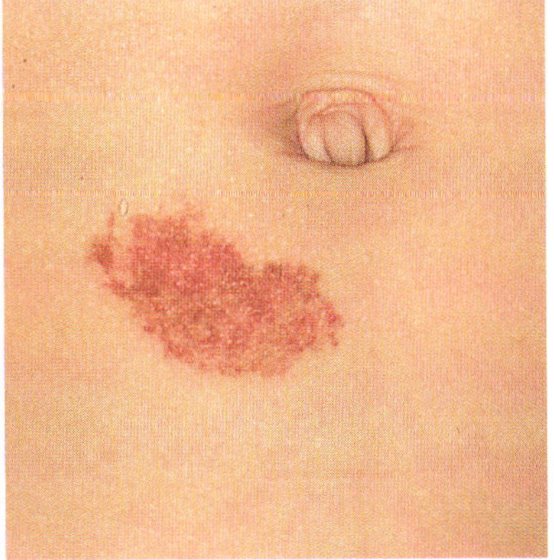

FIG. 38-11 (A, B) *Strawberry hemangioma; plaque at an early and later stage.*

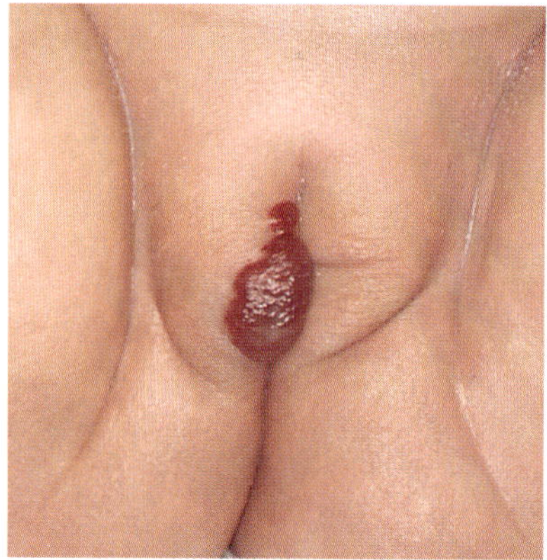

FIG. 38-12 *Strawberry hemangioma.*

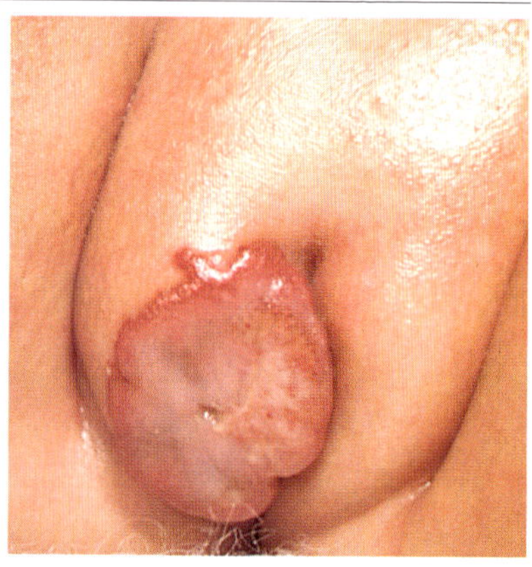

FIG. 38-13 *Strawberry hemangioma, tumor with ulceration and foci of regression.*

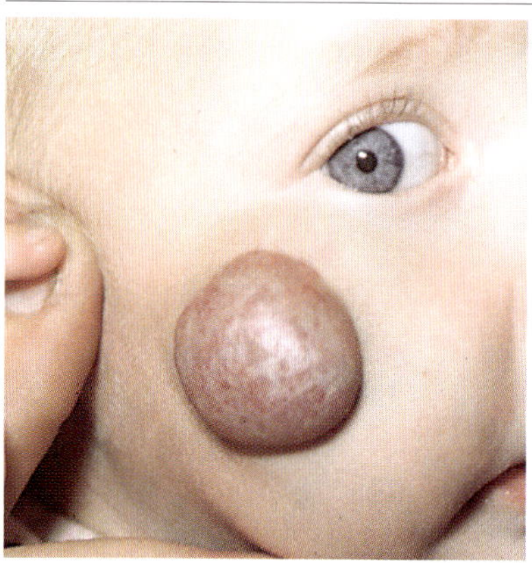

FIG. 38-14 *Strawberry hemangioma, tumor with zones of regression.*

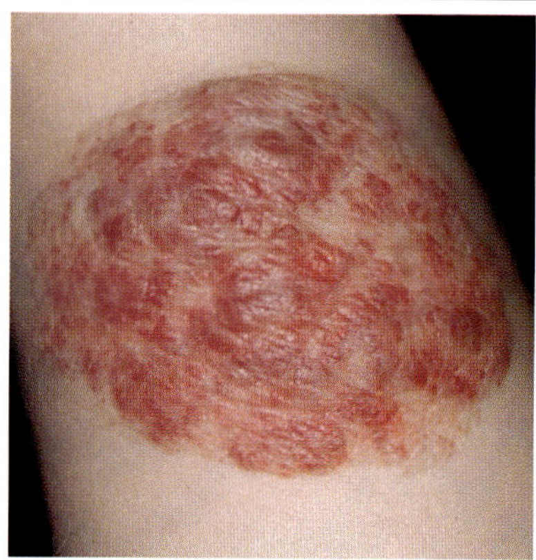

FIG. 38-15 *Strawberry hemangioma, plaque with zones of regression.*

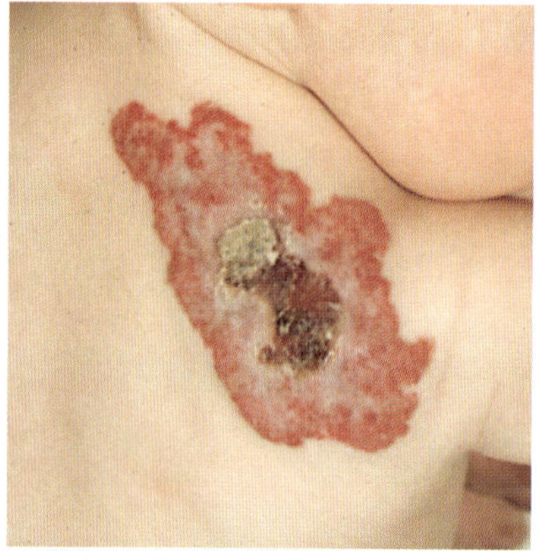

FIG. 38-16 *Strawberry hemangioma, plaque with crust and large zones of regression.*

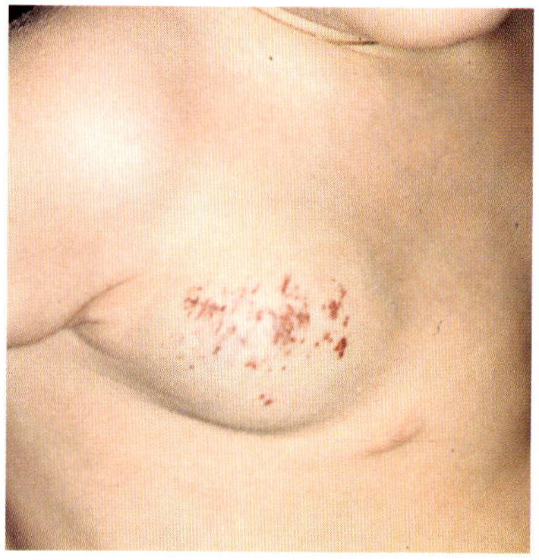

FIG. 38-17 *Cavernous hemangioma, tumor, as well as numerous papules, on the surface of a lesion that is resolving.*

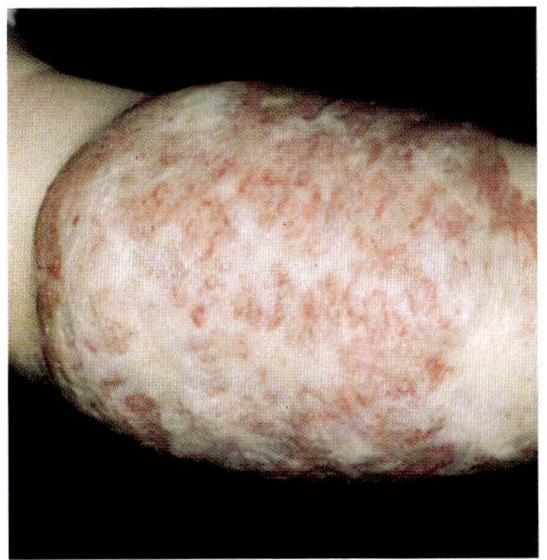

FIG. 38-18 *Cavernous hemangioma, tumor with large zones of regression.*

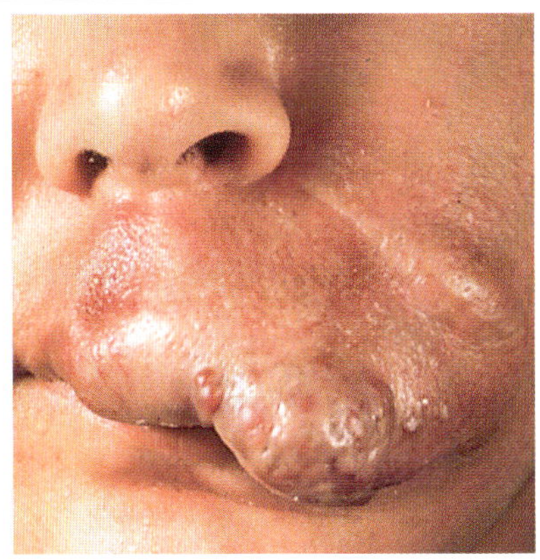

FIG. 38-19 *Cavernous hemangioma, tumor with partial regression and a permanently distorted lip.*

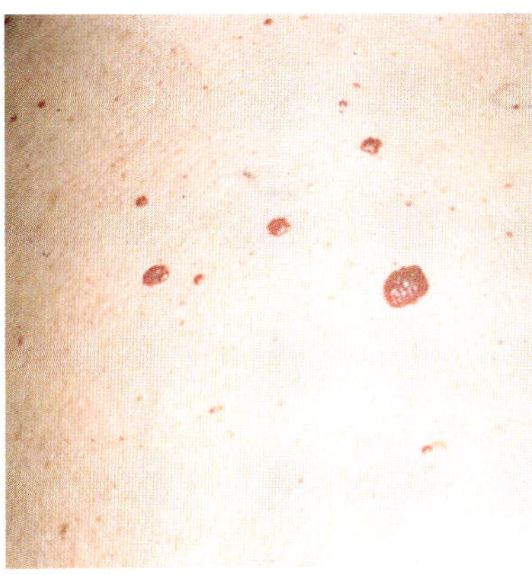

FIG. 38-20 *Cherry hemangiomas, papules.*

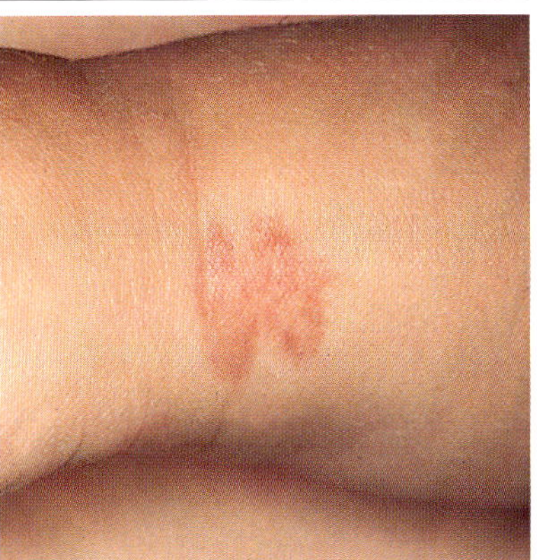

FIG. 38-21 *Tufted hemangioma, plaque.*

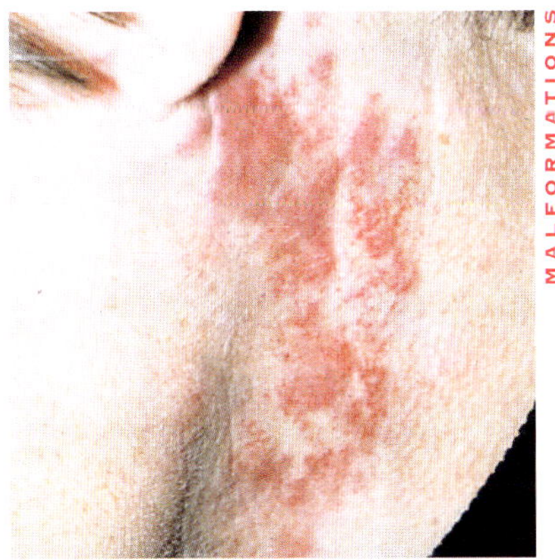

FIG. 38-22 *Tufted hemangioma, papules and plaques arranged in a reticulated pattern.*

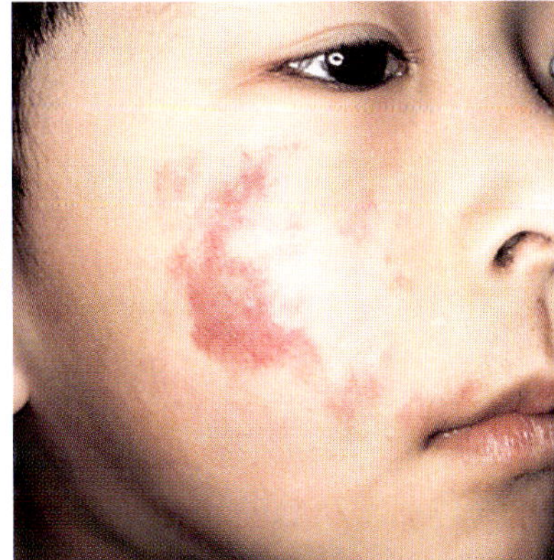

FIG. 38-23 *Nevus flammeus, macules and patches.*

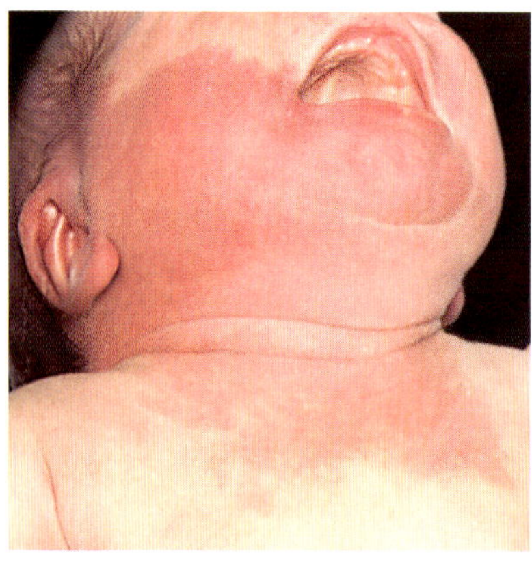

FIG. 38-24 *Nevus flammeus, macules and patches.*

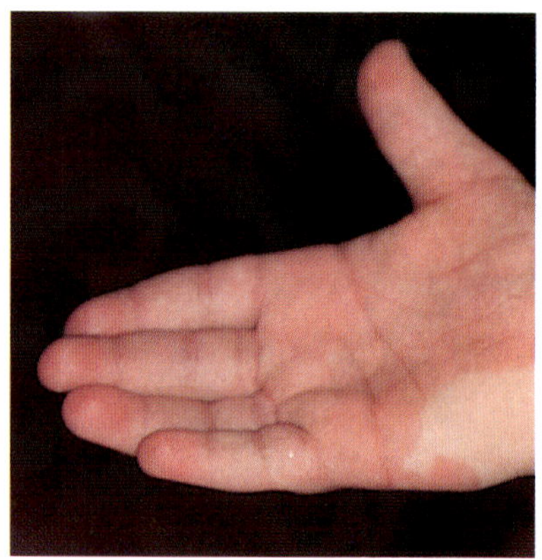

FIG. 38-25 *Nevus flammeus, patch.*

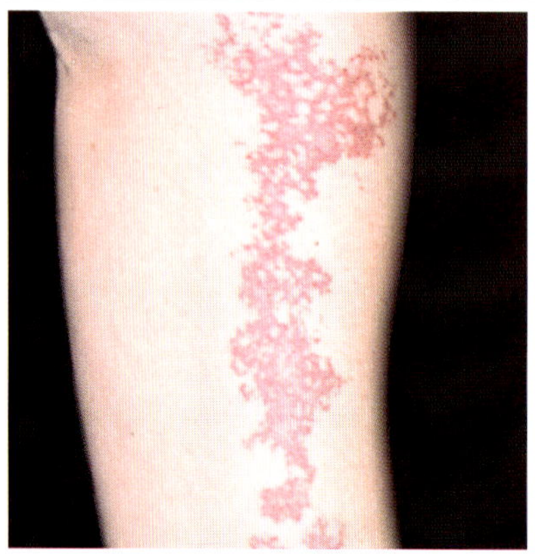

FIG. 38-26 *Nevus flammeus, reticulated in linear array.*

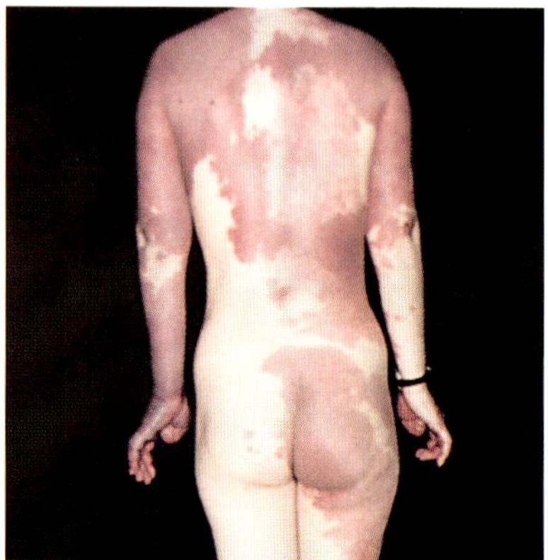

FIG. 38-27 *Nevus flammeus, macules and patches, systematized.*

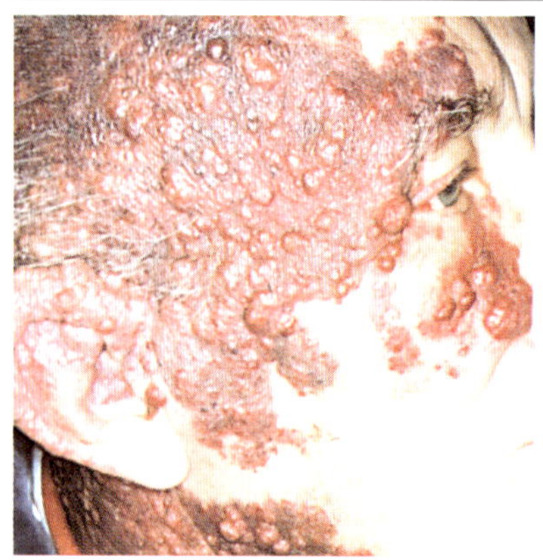

FIG. 38-28 *Nevus flammeus with papules and nodules atop it.*

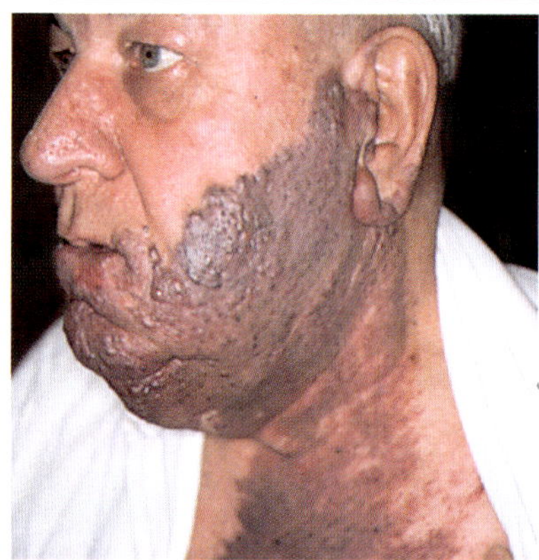

FIG. 38-29 *Nevus flammeus, joined by papules and nodules.*

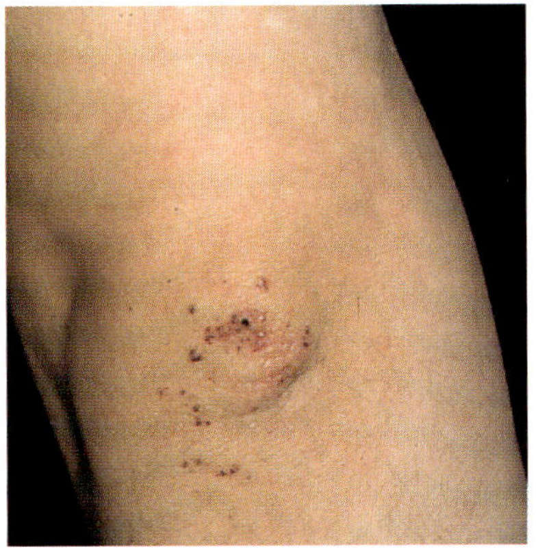

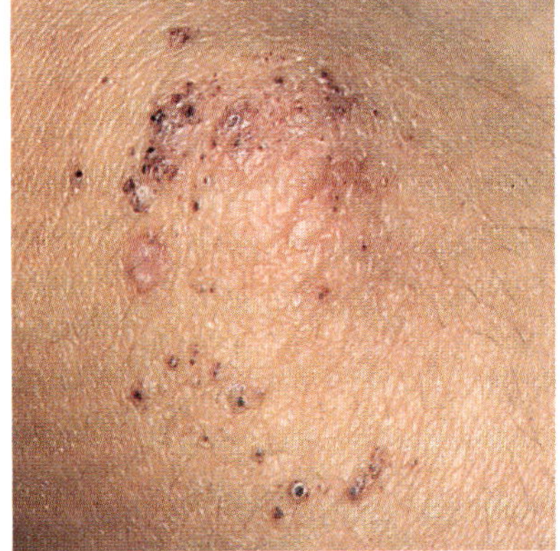

FIG. 38-30 (A, B) *Angioma serpiginosum.*

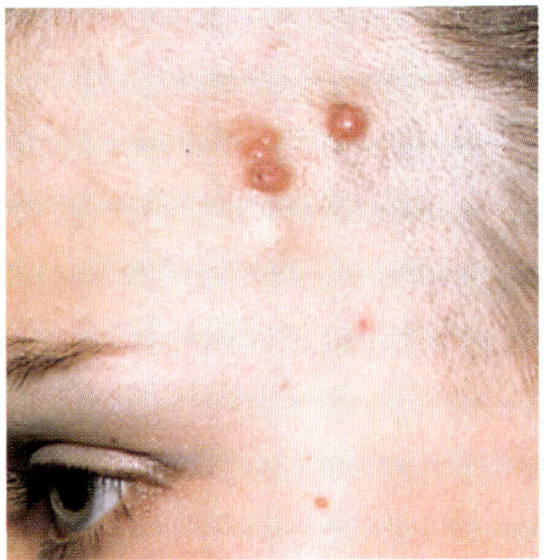

FIG. 38-31 *Angiolymphoid hyperplasia, papules.*

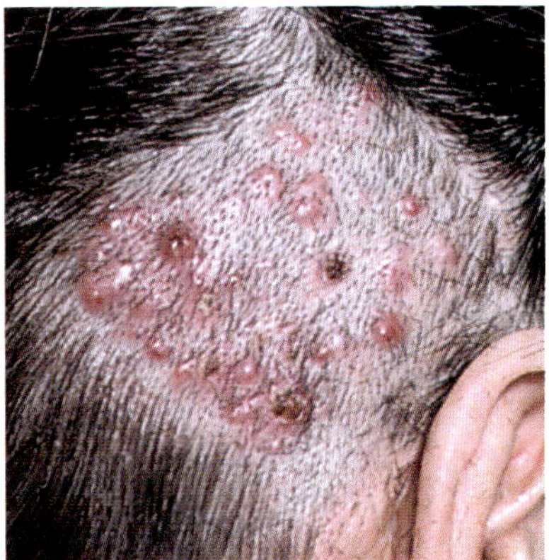

FIG. 38-32 *Angiolymphoid hyperplasia, papules, some of which are crusted.*

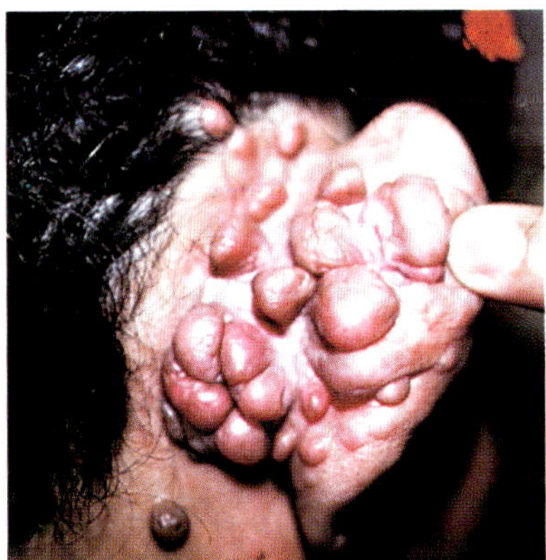

FIG. 38-33 *Angiolymphoid hyperplasia, papules and nodules.*

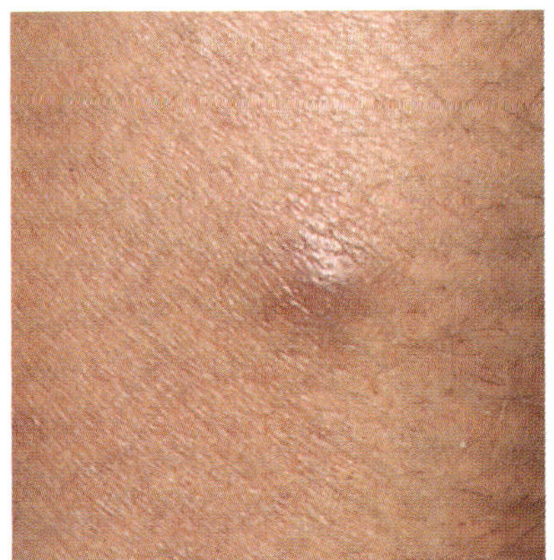

FIG. 38-34 *Arteriovenous shunt, papule.*

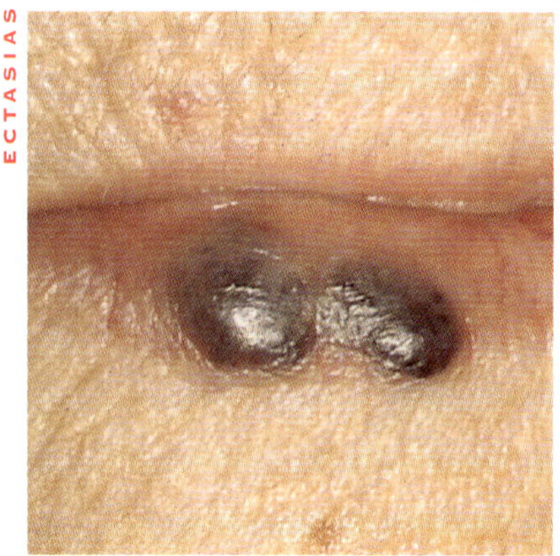

FIG. 38-35 *Venous lakes.*

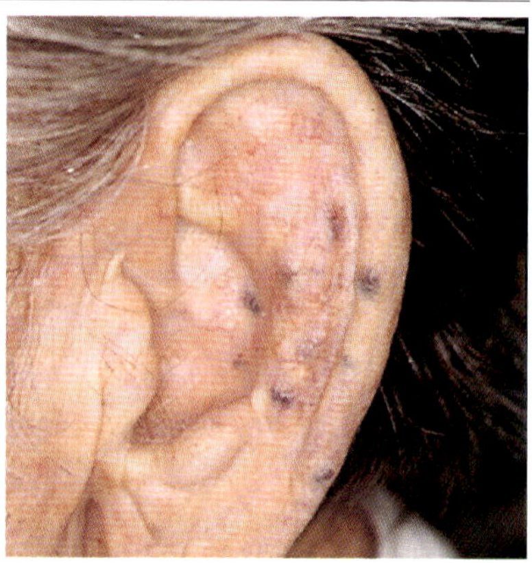

FIG. 38-36 *Venous lakes.*

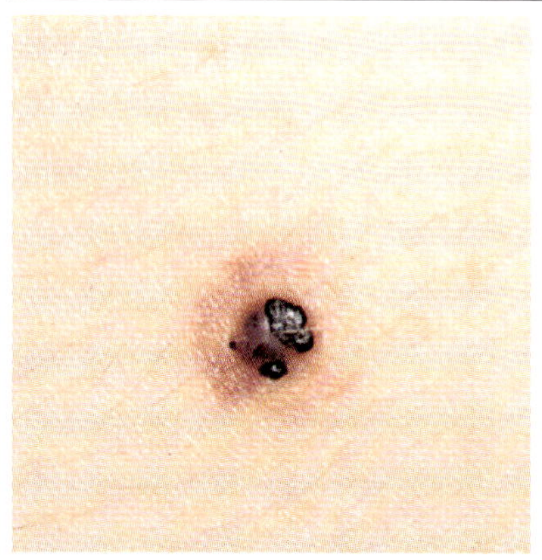

FIG. 38-37 *Thrombosed capillary aneurysm.*

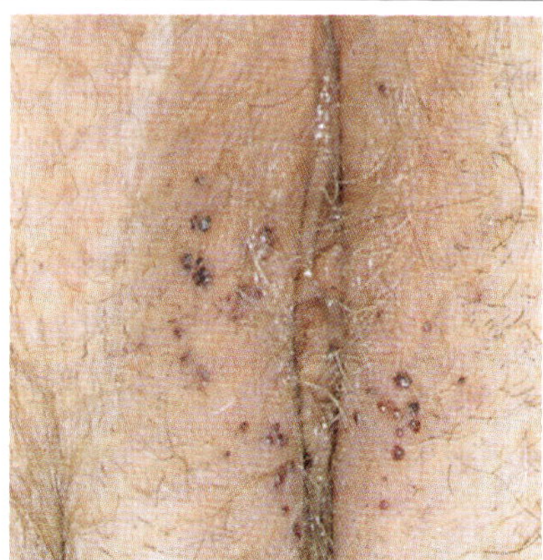

FIG. 38-38 *Angiokeratoma of Fordyce, papules.*

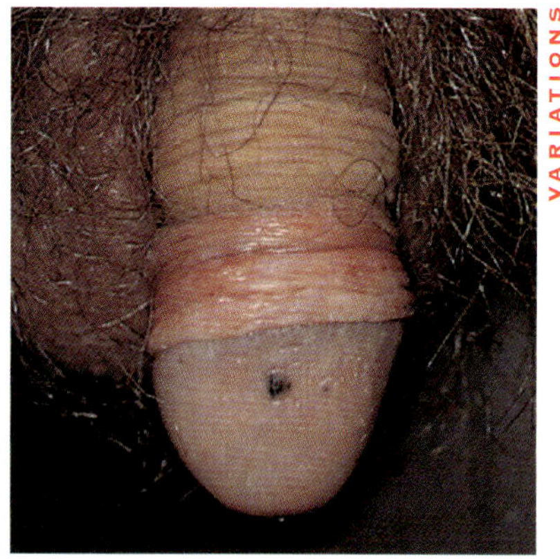

FIG. 38-39 *Angiokeratoma, solitary papule*

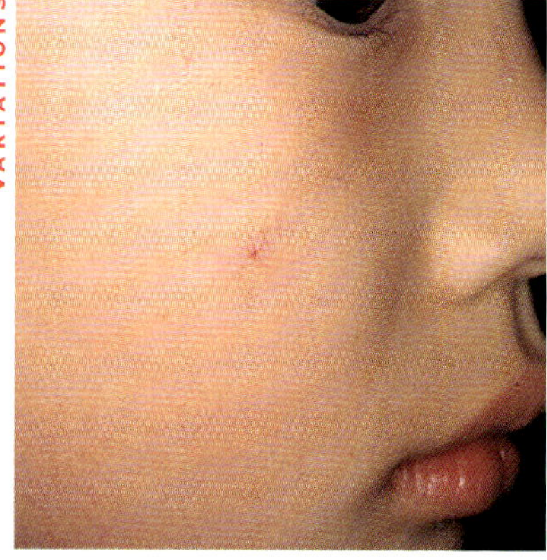

FIG. 38-40 *Spider angioma (nevus araneus).*

FIG. 38-41 *Glomangioma, papules.*

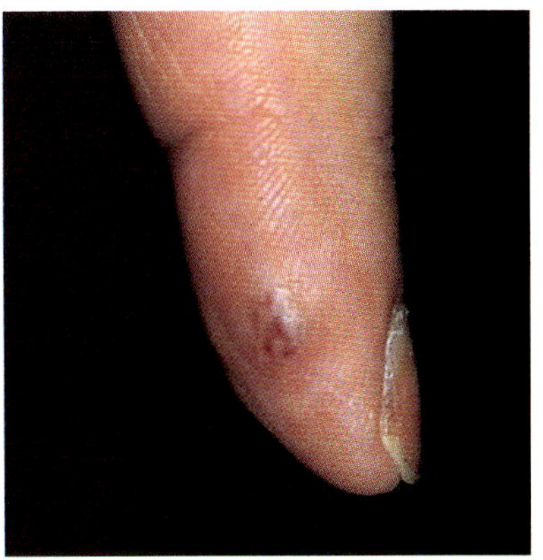

FIG. 38-42 *Glomus tumor, papule.*

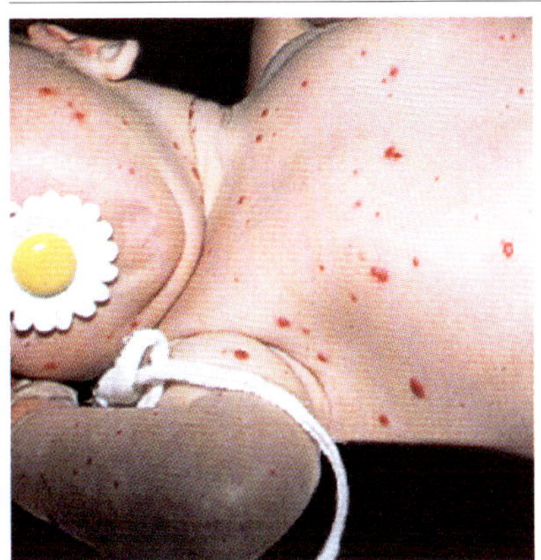

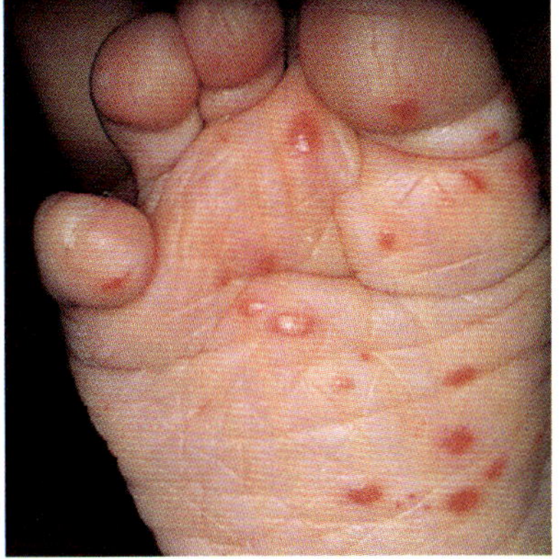

FIG. 38-43 (A, B) *Diffuse neonatal hemangiomatosis.*

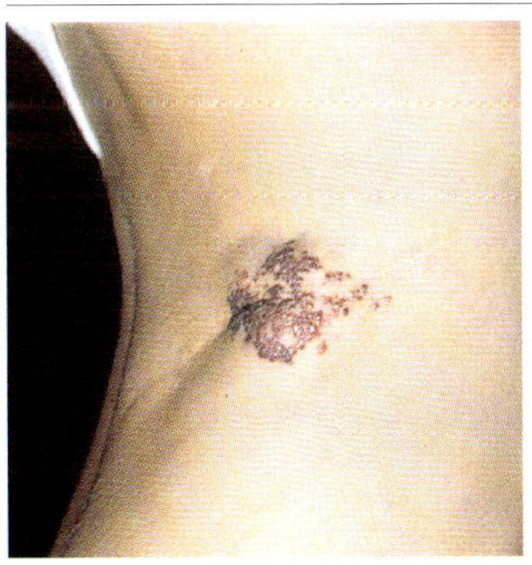

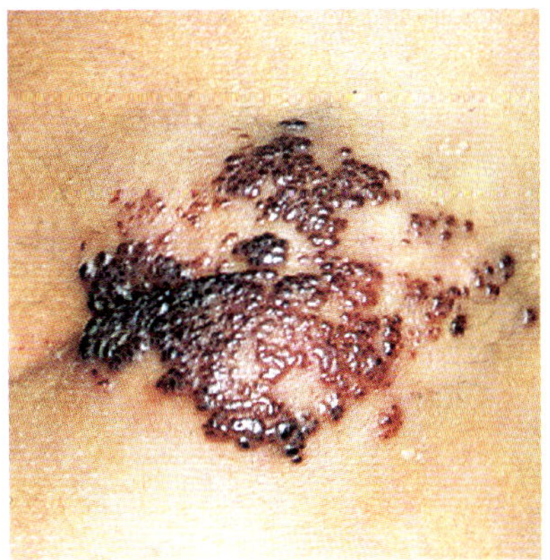

FIG. 38-44 (A, B) *Lymph-hemangioma circumscriptum, persistent after surgery.*

COURSE Except for strawberry hemangiomas in children that involute to become atrophic scars, hemangiomas in general tend to persist for a lifetime. Cherry hemangiomas, for example, develop in adulthood, and more and more of them appear with time. Although the color of a patch of nevus flammeus may lighten in time, the size of it remains about the same proportionate to the size of the person who bears it, and, furthermore, papules and sometimes nodules may develop upon it. Other vascular malformations and ectasias change little in the course of time.

INTEGRATION: UNIFYING CONCEPT For many reasons, it is extraordinarily difficult to present an integrated concept of vascular proliferations of the skin. Among them are lack of agreement about such basic issues as whether hemangiomas are hamartomas or benign neoplasms, and whether nevus flammeus consists of ectasias or qualifies as an hemangioma, or is ectasias in which hemangiomas develop. No comprehensive and comprehensible classification of hemangiomas has ever been set forth. To complicate matters further, the nature of a vascular malformation, such as angiolymphoid hyperplasia with eosinophilia, is poorly understood. It is known to be secondary to an arteriovenous shunt, but the reason for the presence within it of lymphoid follicles and numerous eosinophils is obscure. Furthermore, those infiltrates of inflammatory cells, although present often, are not found invariably in angiolymphoid hyperplasia. Last, the "angiokeratomas" of Fordyce, Mibelli, and Fabry are wholly different from one another, representing as they do different processes. In sum, at the moment, it is best to identify particular hemangiomas, vascular malformations, and ectasias with specificity on the basis of morphologic findings and to attempt to understand them as well as possible, but at the same time to adjust to the reality that until now no compelling unifying concept has been proposed for vascular proliferations and other vascular abnormalities in skin. We, too, are unable to do that.

THERAPY Hemangiomas that are present at birth tend to involute in months in the absence of therapy. Many modalities, however, are available for treatment of cutaneous vascular abnormalities, among them, surgery (resection, grafts, embolization, ligation of vessels), x-rays, cryosurgery, sclerosing agents, and camouflage by cosmetics. Recent advances in the technology of lasers have enhanced management of these lesions. For one example, the flashlamp-pumped pulsed-dye laser is effective in removing signs of nevus flammeus. Systemic corticosteroids and interferon can be employed successfully in the treatment of giant hemangioma.

HERPES SIMPLEX, ZOSTER, AND VARICELLA

DEFINITION Conditions caused by infection with different strains of herpesvirus and typified when fully developed by tense vesicles, herpes simplex consisting of grouped vesicles on an erythematous base, zoster being made up of vesicles, sometimes hemorrhagic ones, that course along a dermatome of an adult usually, and varicella being characterized by widespread discrete vesicles in children as a rule.

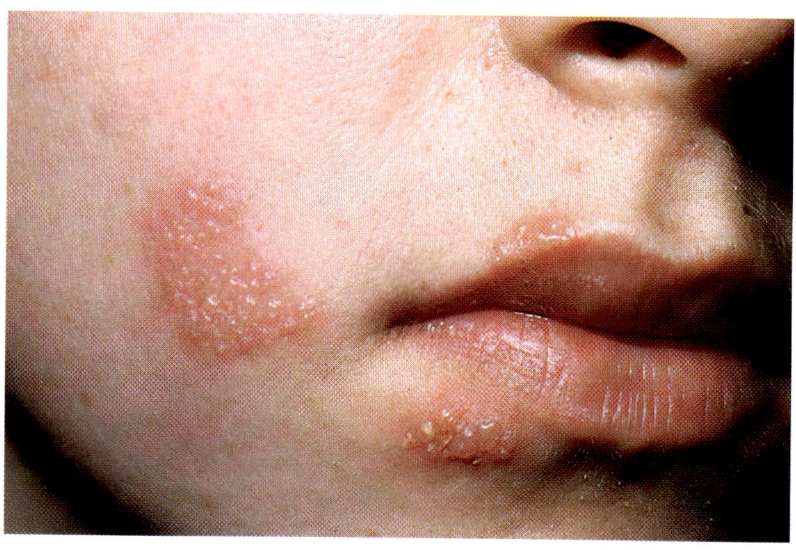

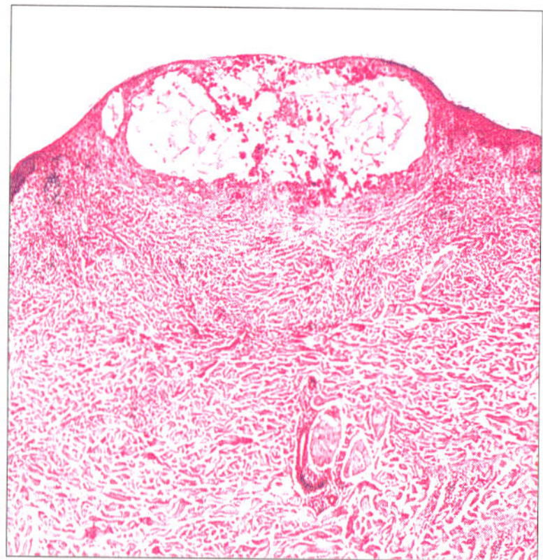

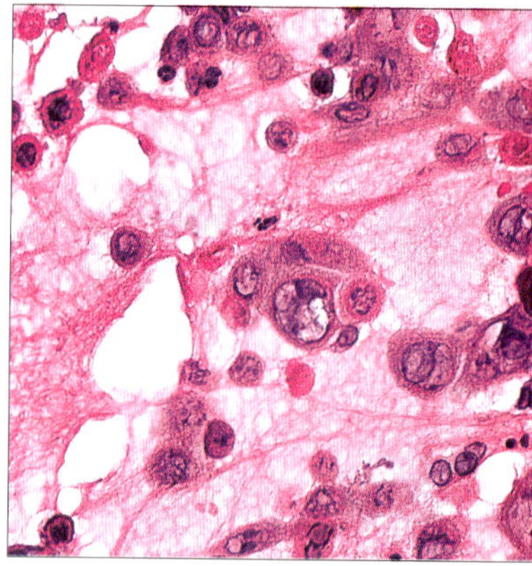

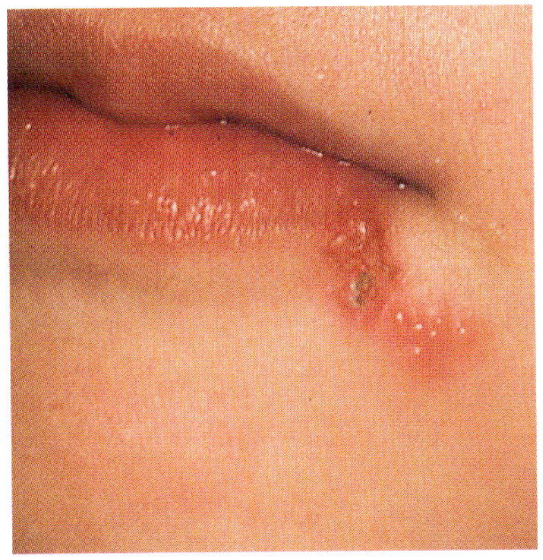

FIG. 39-1 *Vesicles on the lower lip, and grouped vesicles and crusts nearby.*

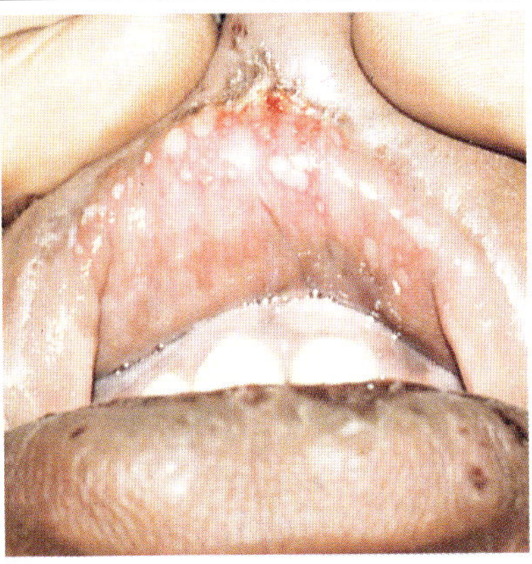

FIG. 39-2 *Pustules on the mucous membrane of the lips.*

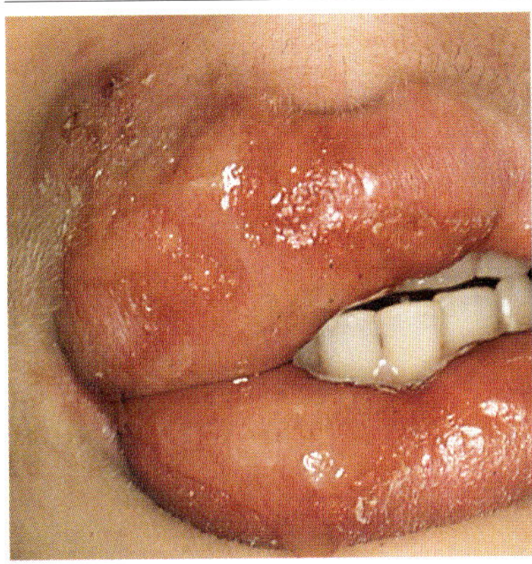

FIG. 39-3 *Vesicles and crusts in clusters on a markedly swollen lip.*

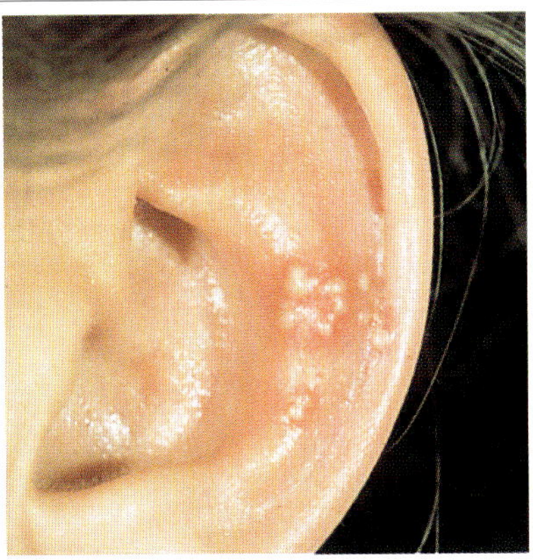

FIG. 39-4 *Grouped pustules on an ear.*

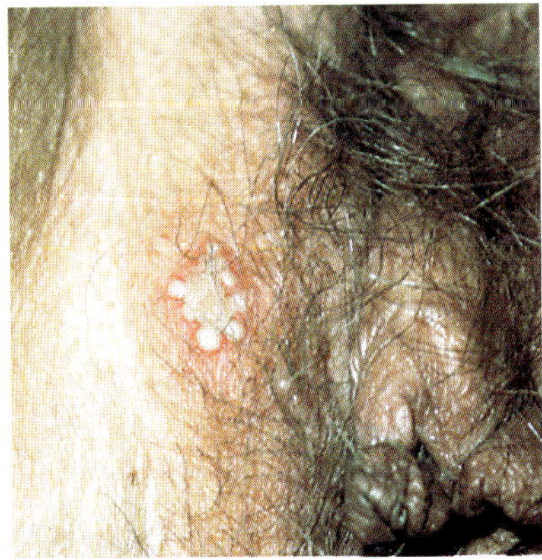

FIG. 39-5 *Grouped pustules have become confluent on a labium majus.*

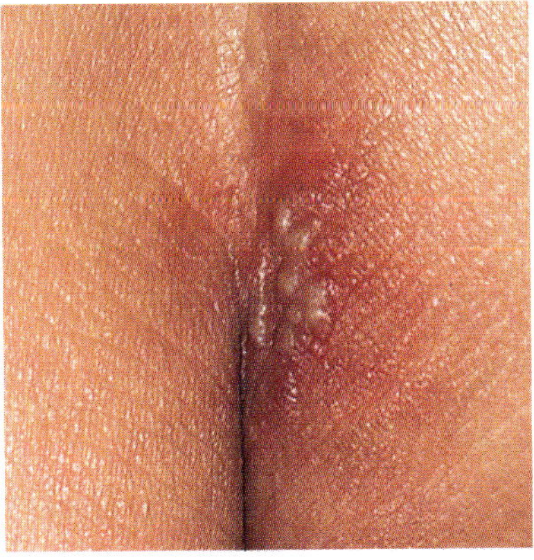

FIG. 39-6 *Grouped pustules on an erythematous base near an intergluteal fold.*

ARRANGEMENT

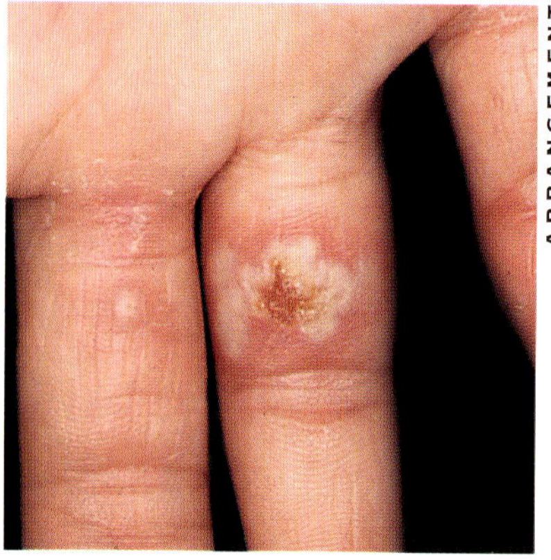

FIG. 39-7 *Pustules, an ulcer, and a crust.*

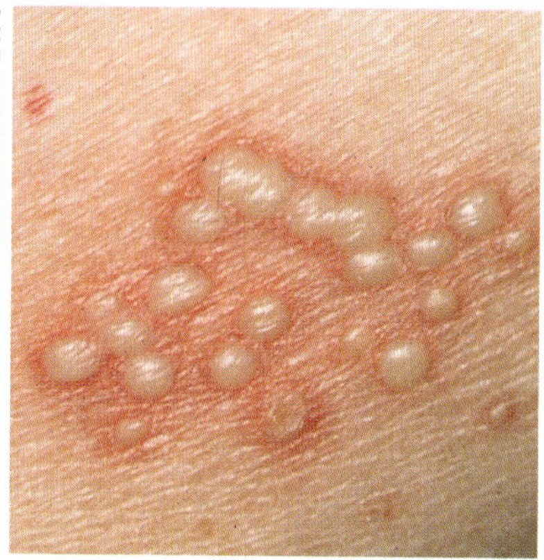

FIG. 39-8 *Grouped pustules on an erythematous base, a pattern referred to as "herpetiform."*

INDIVIDUAL LESIONS

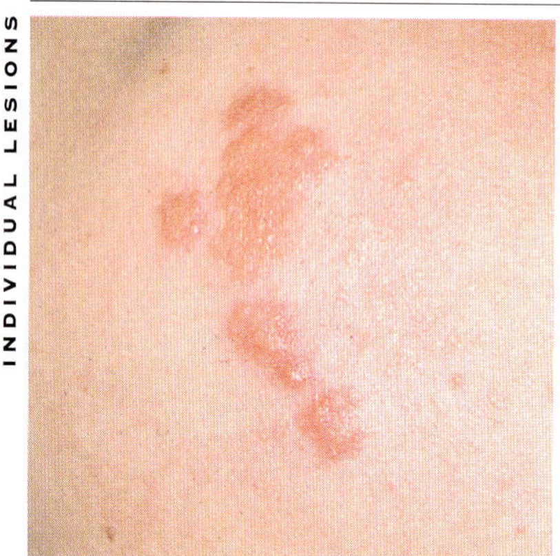

FIG. 39-9 *Papules and papulovesicles in herpetiform arrangement.*

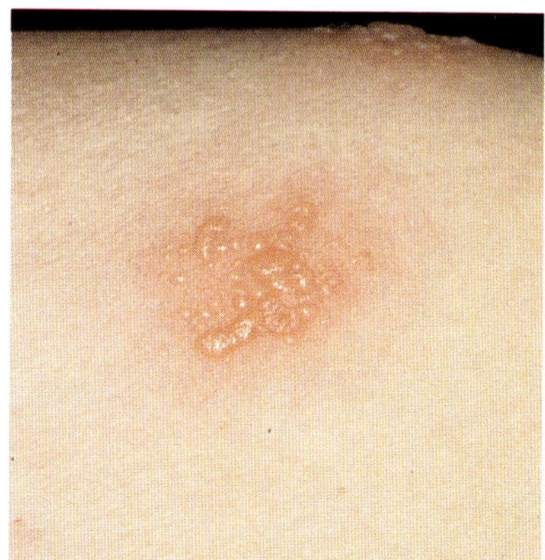

FIG. 39-10 *Tense vesicles grouped on an erythematous base.*

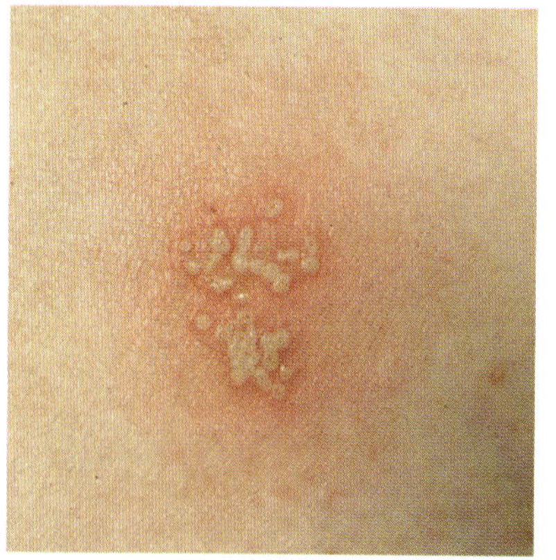

FIG. 39-11 *Grouped pustules on an erythematous base.*

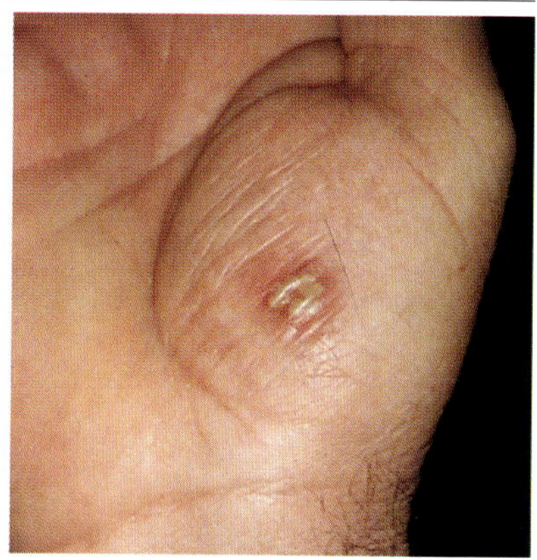

FIG. 39-12 *Grouped pustules in confluence on an erythematous base.*

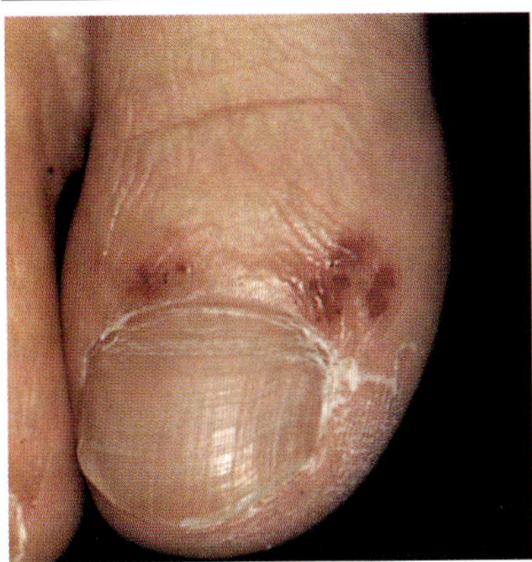

FIG. 39-13 *Hemorrhagic vesicles and crusts in herpetiform arrangement.*

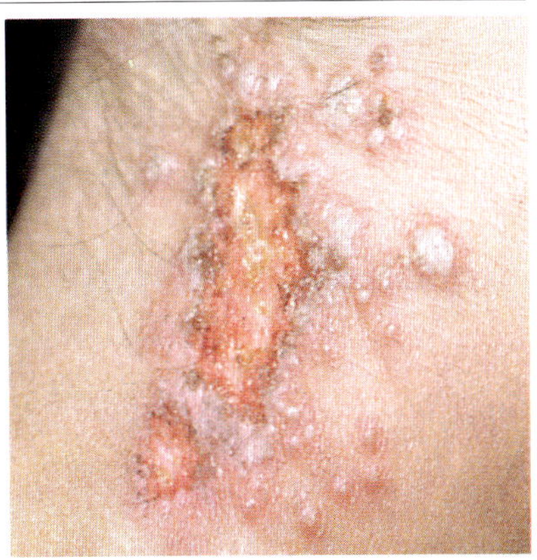

FIG. 39-14 *Papules, papulovesicles, pustules, erosions, and ulcers.*

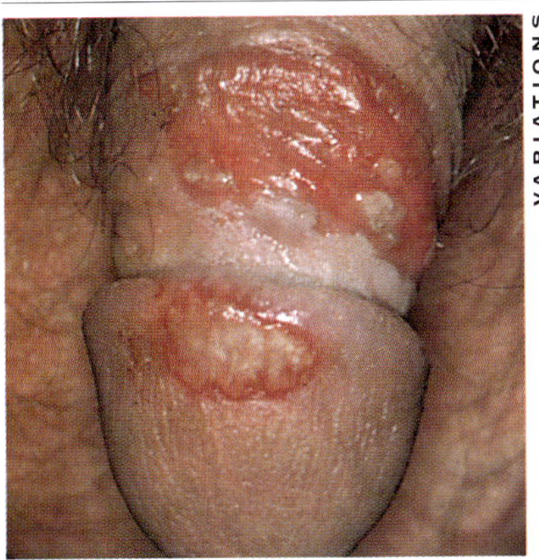

FIG. 39-15 *Ulcers with ragged margins.*

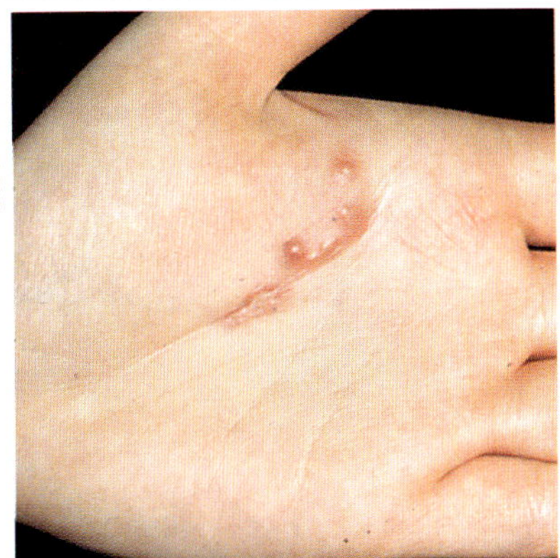

FIG. 39-16 *Papulovesicles in linear array.*

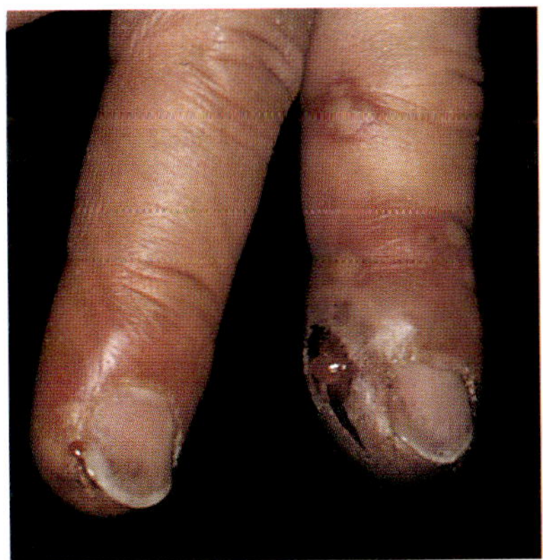

FIG. 39-17 *Herpetic whitlow (herpes simplex near the tip of a digit).*

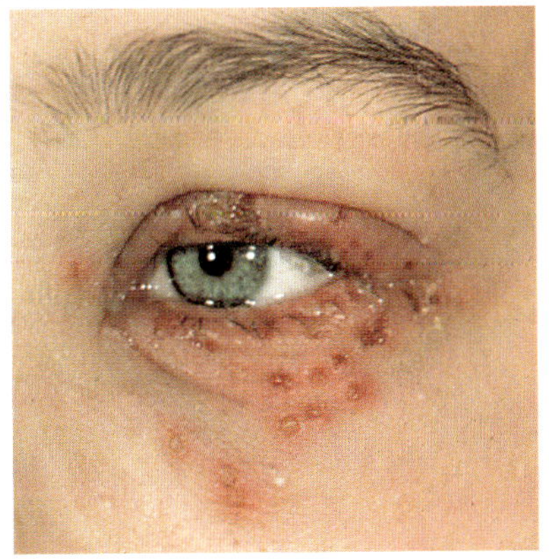

FIG. 39-18 *Eczema herpeticum (herpes simplex imposed on atopic dermatitis, i.e., skin that has been rubbed and scratched).*

VARIATIONS

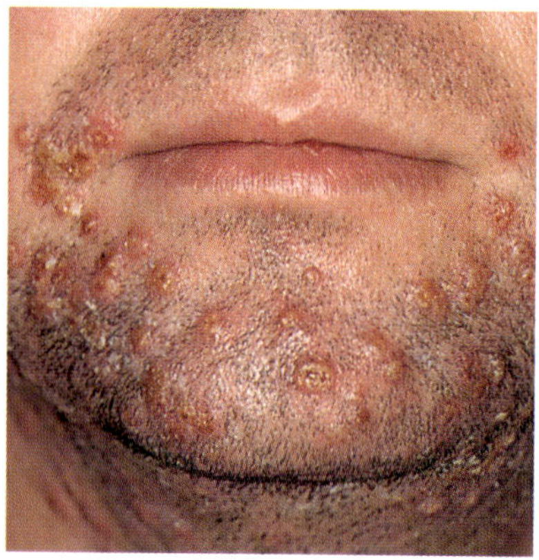

FIG. 39-19 *Eczema herpeticum (umbilicated vesicles and vesiculopustules of herpesvirus in a zone of atopic dermatitis).*

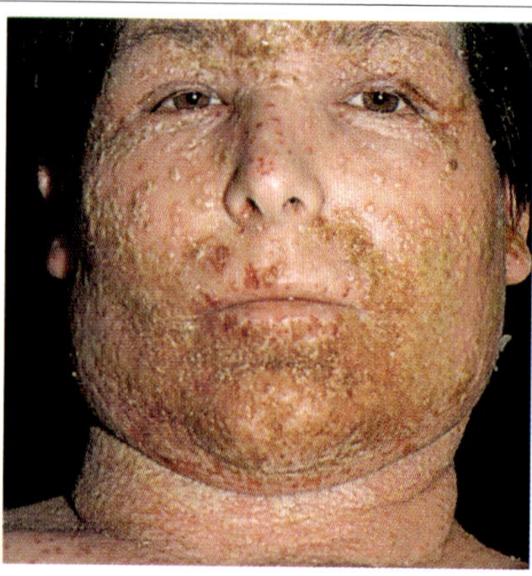

FIG. 39-20 *Eczema herpeticum (innumerable pustules of herpesvirus in skin that has become impetiginized).*

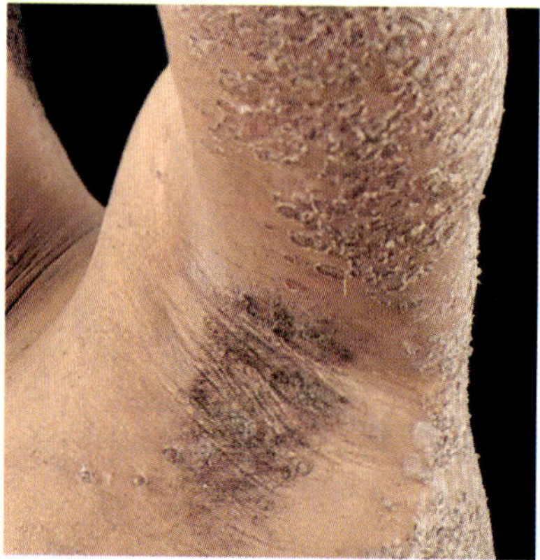

FIG. 39-21 *Eczema herpeticum (Kaposi's varicelliform eruption).*

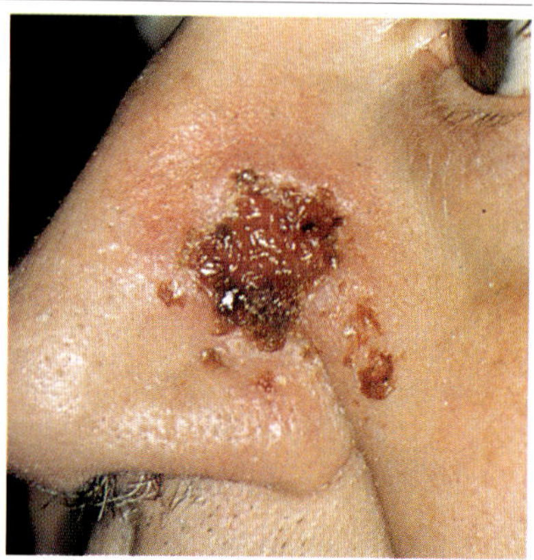

FIG. 39-22 *Ulcer covered by crust in a patient with chronic lymphocytic leukemia.*

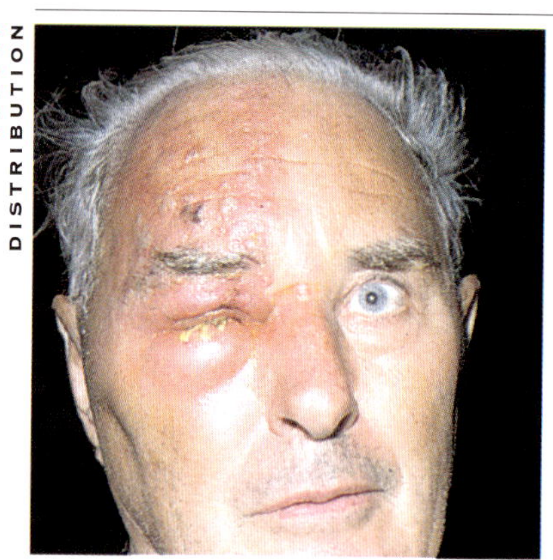

FIG. 39-23 *Vesicles and erosions on one side of the face.*

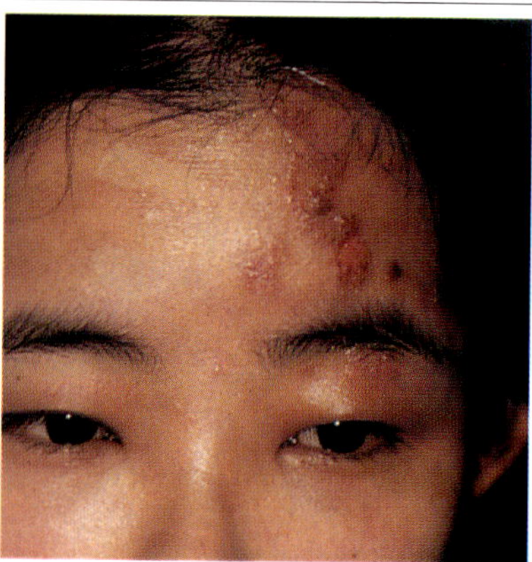

FIG. 39-24 *Vesicles, crusts, and periorbital edema on one side of the face.*

ZOSTER DISTRIBUTION

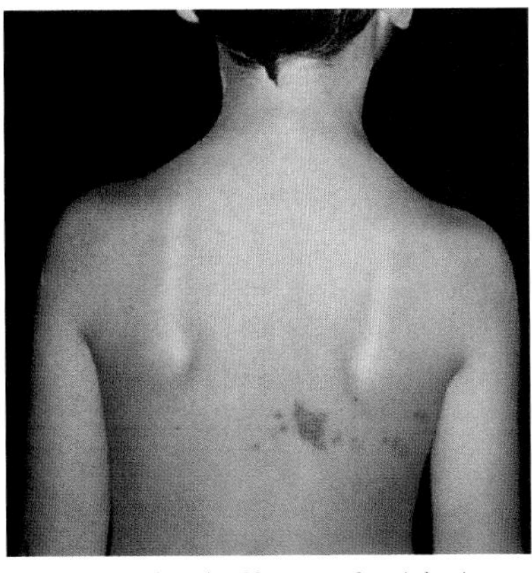 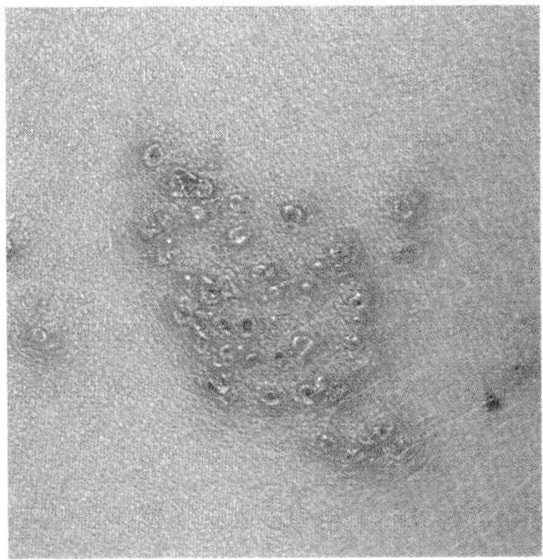

FIG. 39-25 (A, B) *Clusters of vesicles in zosteriform array.*

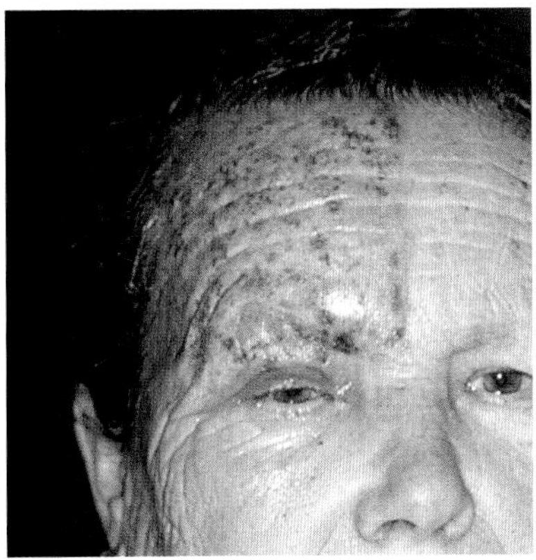 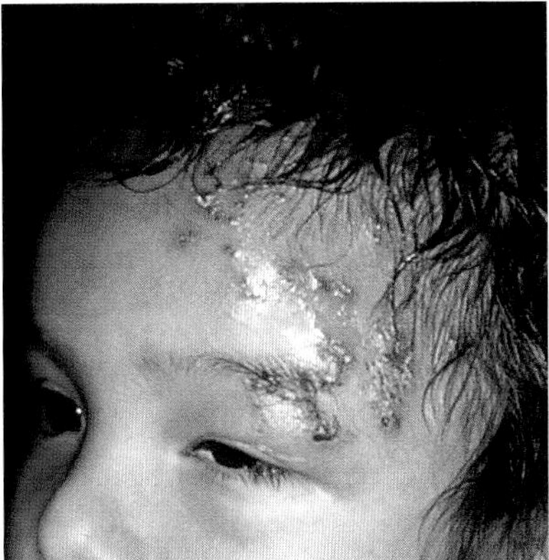

FIG. 39-26 *Crusts unilaterally.*

FIG. 39-27 *Papules and papulovesicles on one side of a face with marked periorbital edema.*

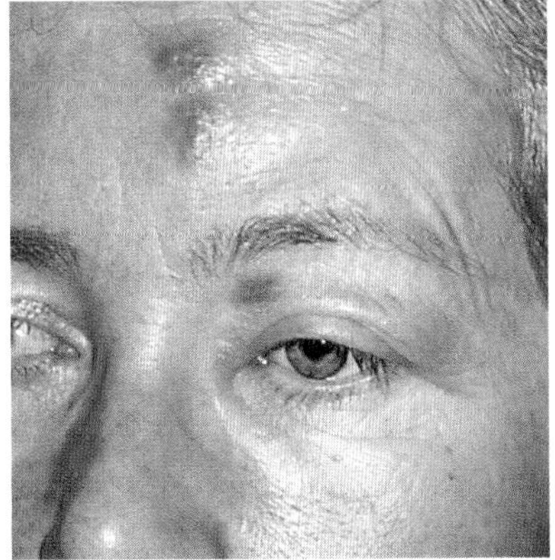 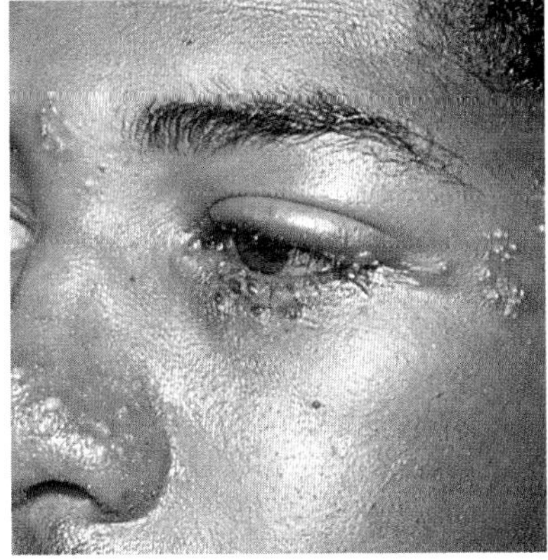

FIG. 39-28 *Vesicles, vesiculopustules, and crusts in unilateral distribution.*

FIG. 39-29 *Vesiculopustules in zosteriform arrangement along the trigeminal nerve. Nose involvement implies eye involvement, too.*

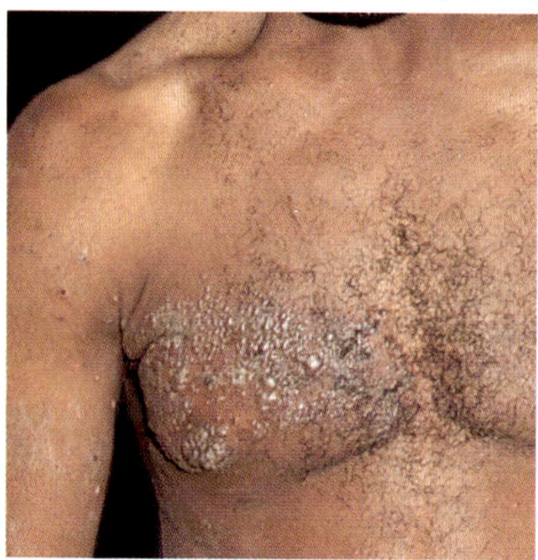

FIG. 39-30 *Vesicles and bullae on one side of the chest.*

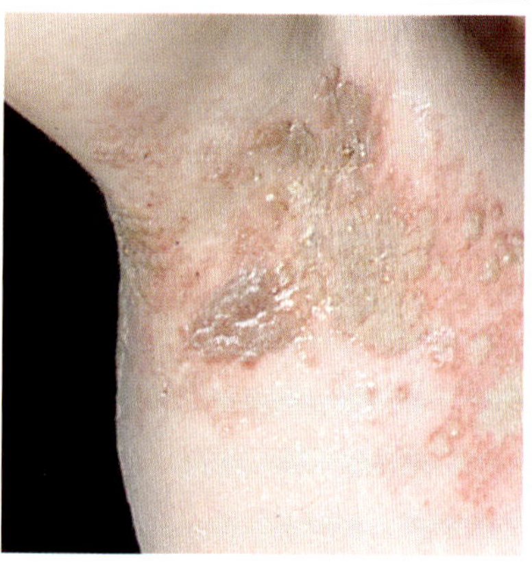

FIG. 39-31 *Vesicles and pustules unilaterally.*

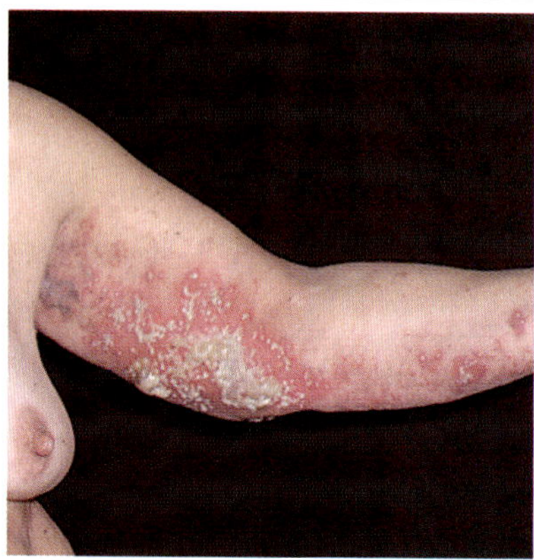

FIG. 39-32 *Vesicles and pustules on an erythematous base.*

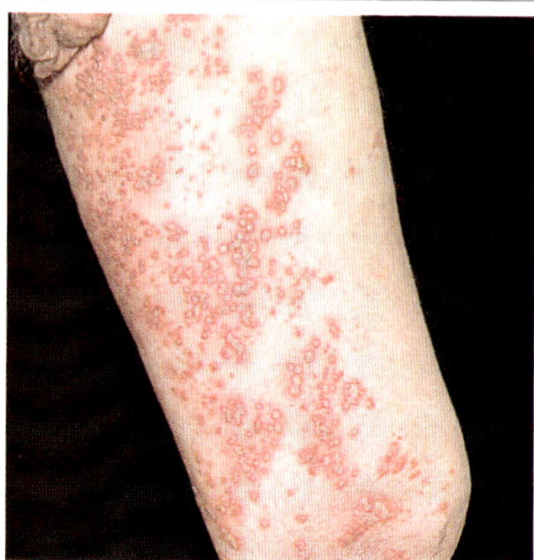

FIG. 39-33 *Vesiculopustules on a purpuric base.*

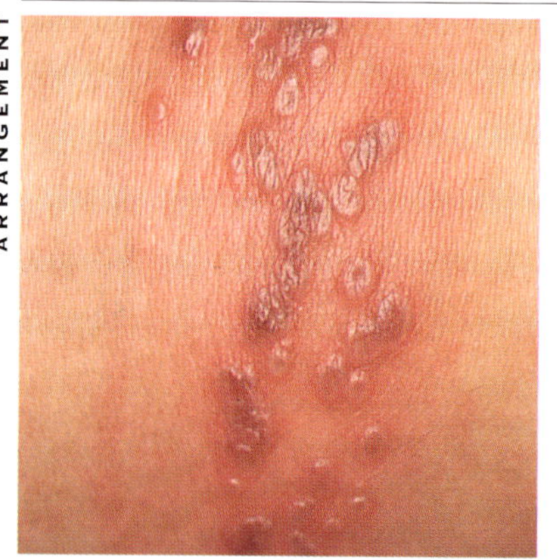

FIG. 39-34 *Clusters of umbilicated vesicles (herpetiform arrangement) on a hemorrhagic base.*

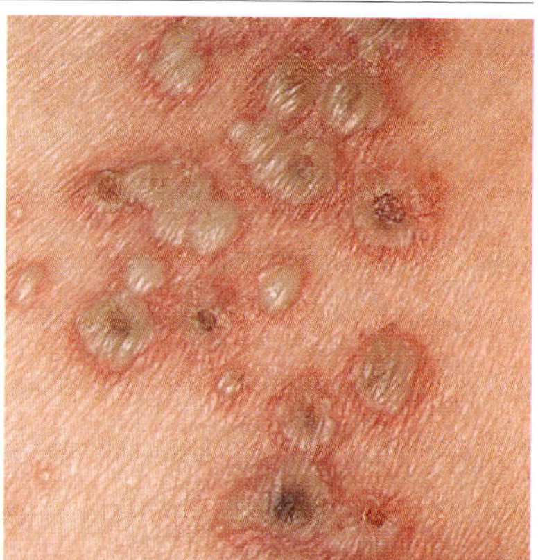

FIG. 39-35 *Clusters of pustules (herpetiform arrangement), some of them umbilicated and crusted on a red base.*

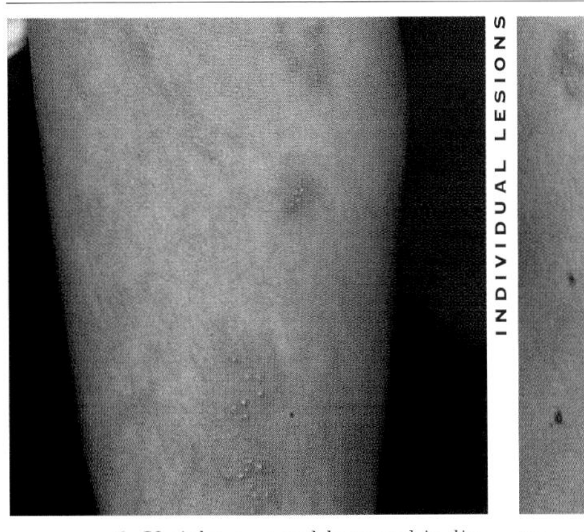

FIG. 39-36 *Vesicles on a red base and in linear array.*

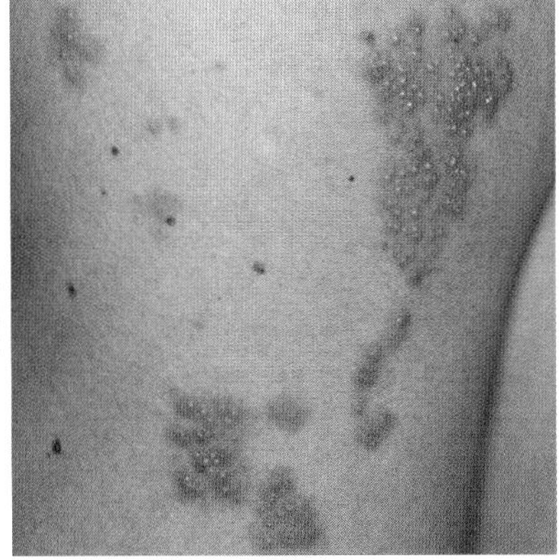

FIG. 39-37 *Papules and papulovesicles.*

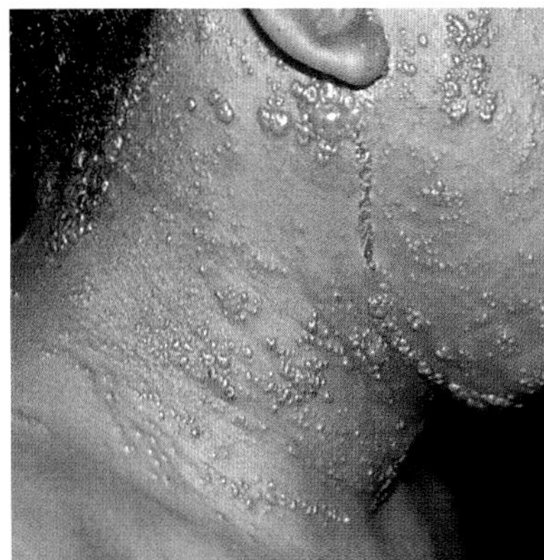

FIG. 39-38 *Papules and numerous tense vesicles.*

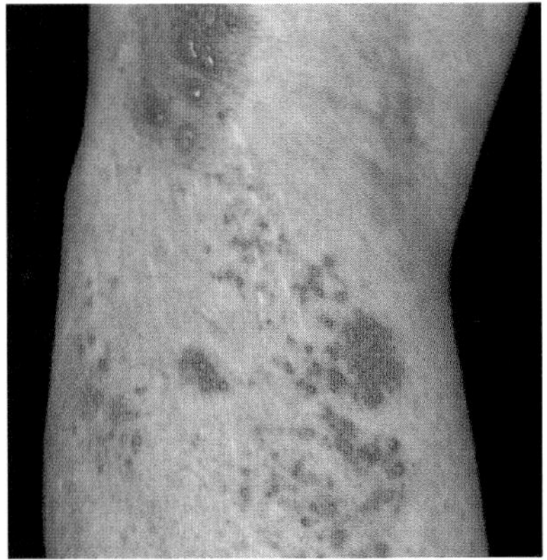

FIG. 39-39 *Papules and vesicles on a red base.*

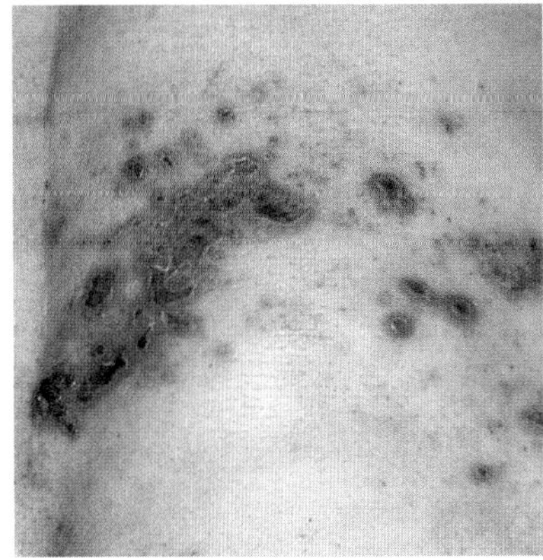

FIG. 39-40 *Ulcers covered by hemorrhagic crusts.*

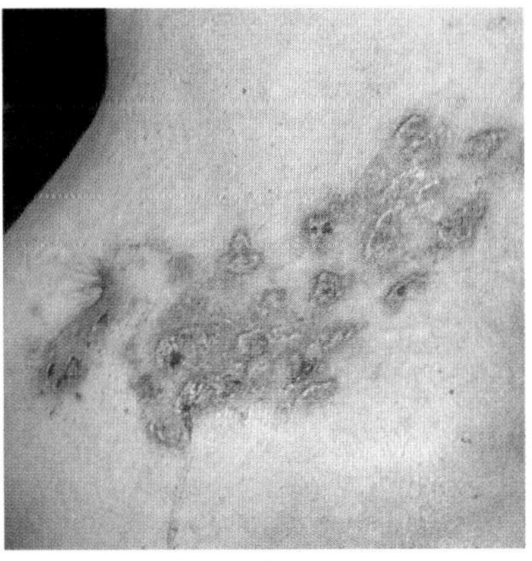

FIG. 39-41 *Ulcers and scars.*

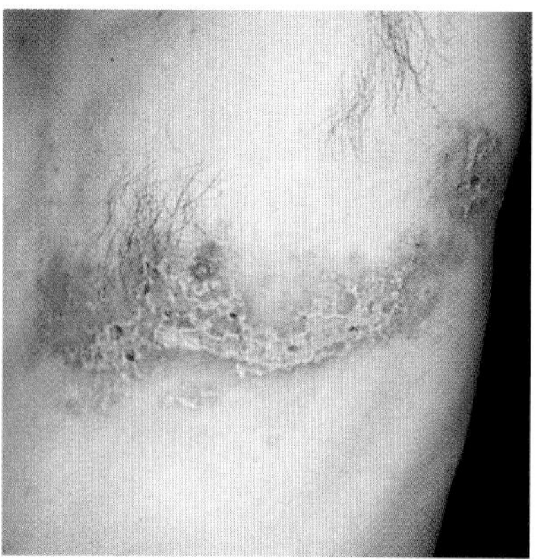

FIG. 39-42 *Scars and crusts.*

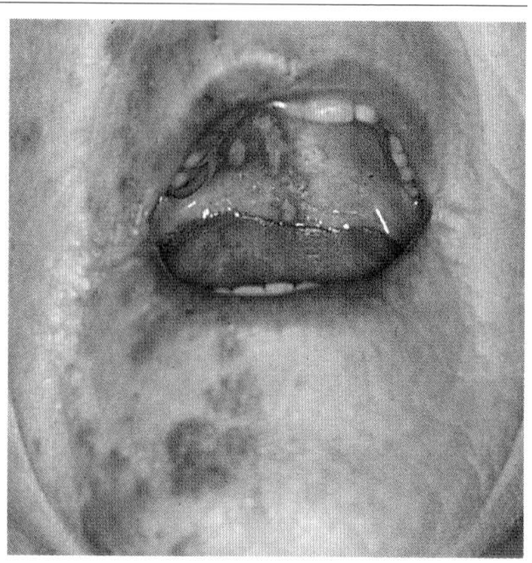

FIG. 39-43 *Papules on the face and ulcers on one half of the palate.*

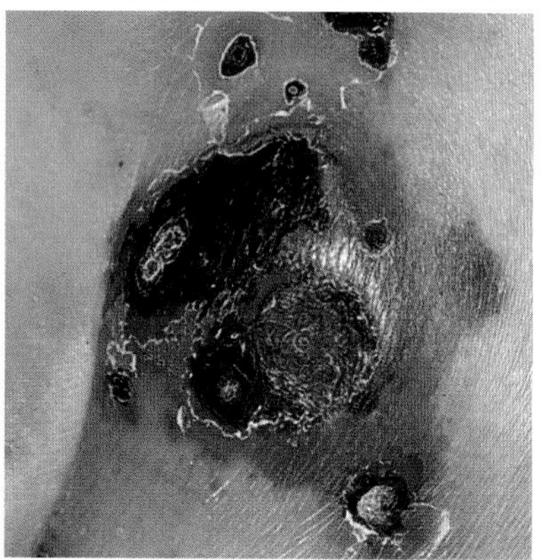

FIG. 39-44 *Eschars and purpura in an immunosuppressed patient.*

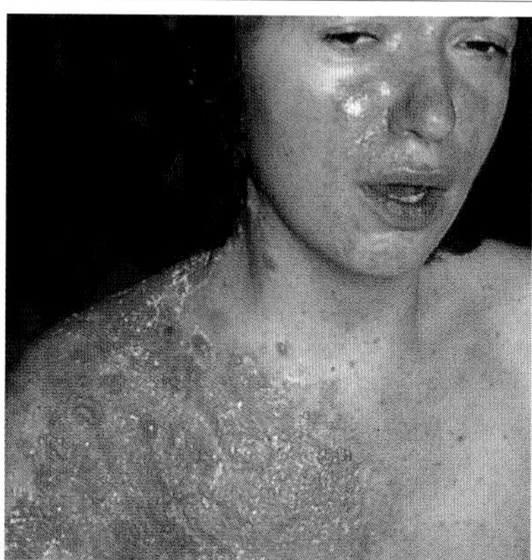

FIG. 39-45 *Widespread disseminated zoster.*

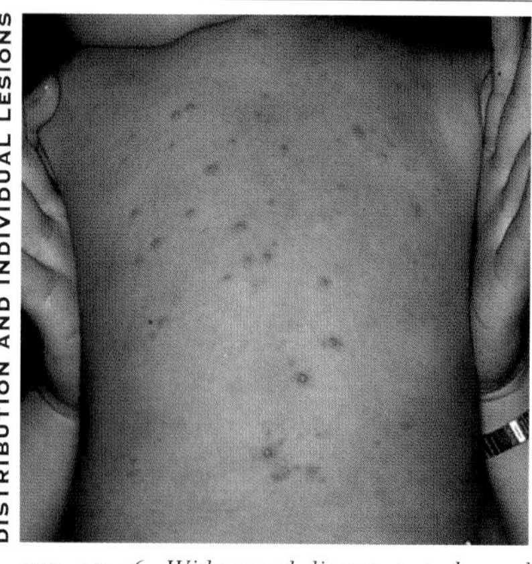

FIG. 39-46 *Widespread discrete papules and vesicles of varicella.*

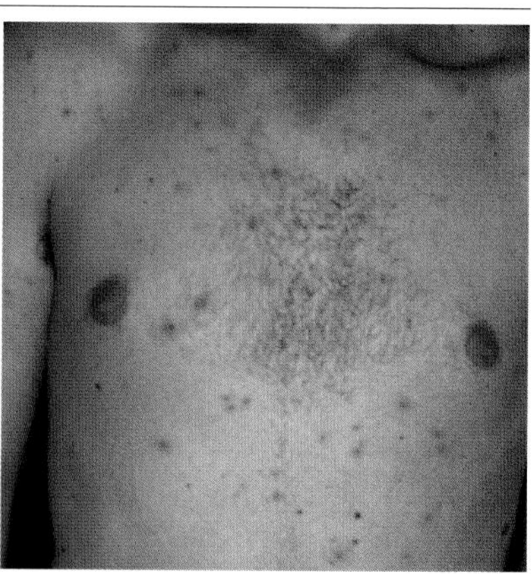

FIG. 39-47 *Widespread discrete papules and vesicles of varicella.*

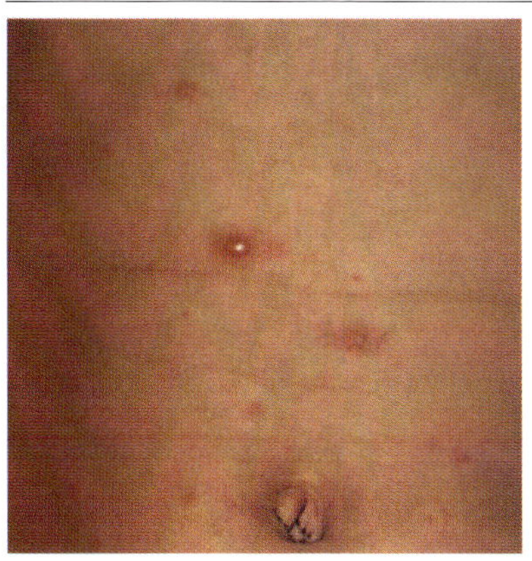

FIG. 39-48 *Papules and vesicles on a red base.*

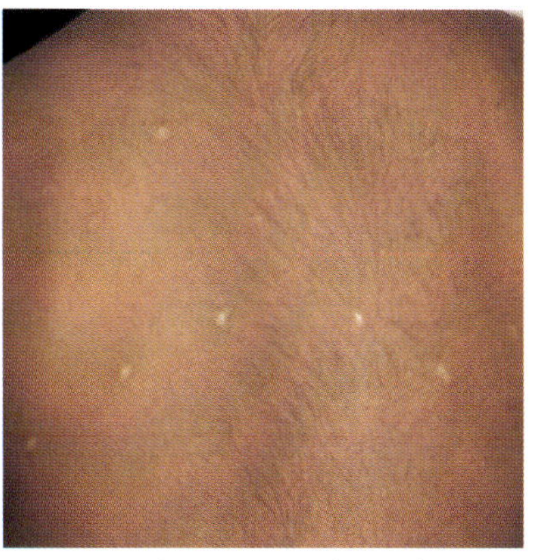

FIG. 39-49 *Hypopigmented macules represent residua of vesicles and crusts.*

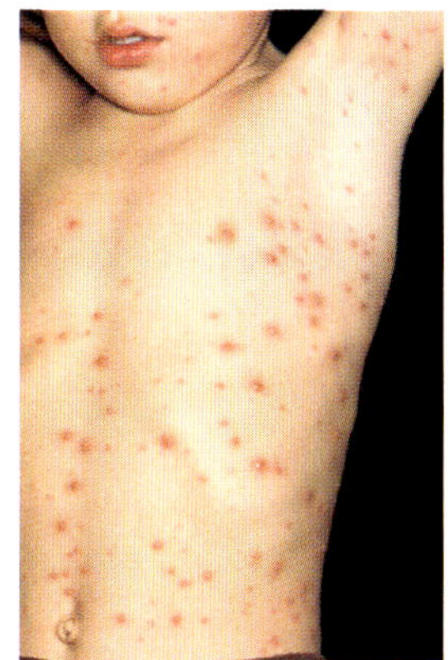

FIG. 39-50 *Papules and vesicles.*

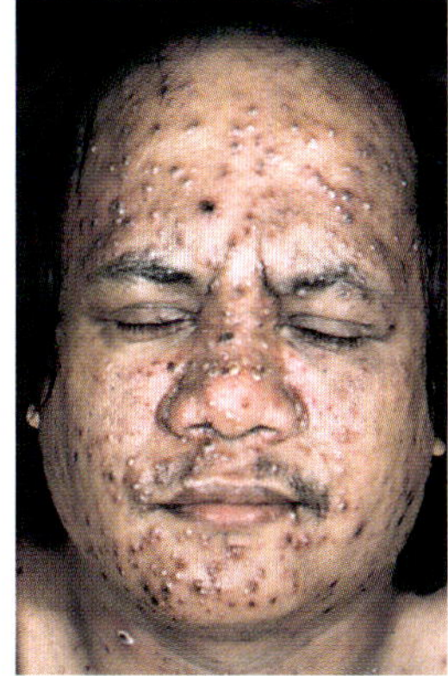

FIG. 39-51 *Papules, pustules with signs of necrosis, and crusts.*

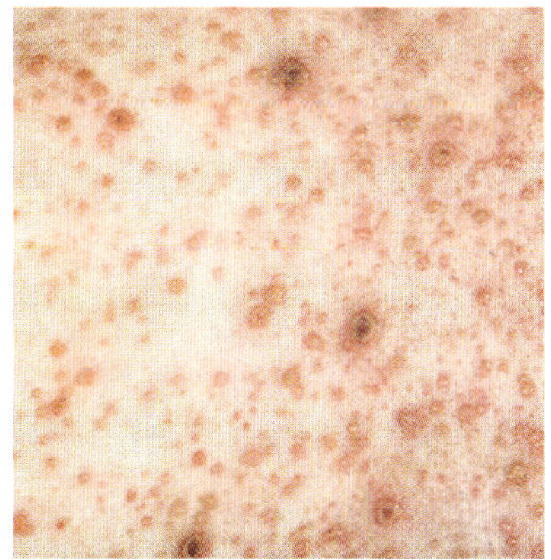

FIG. 39-52 *Papules, vesicles, and pustules, some with a necrotic center.*

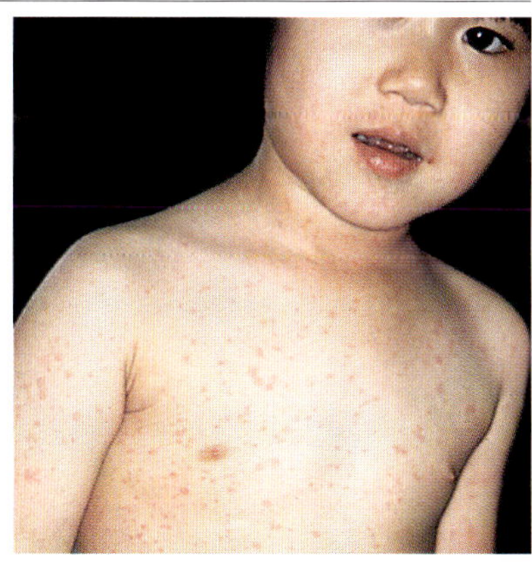

FIG. 39-53 (A) *Widespread papules and vesicles.*

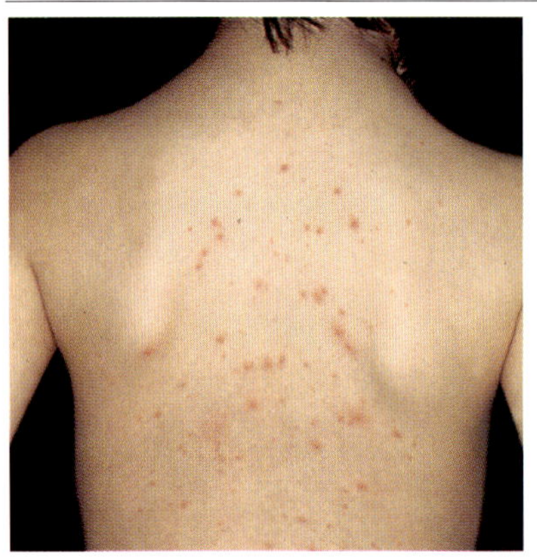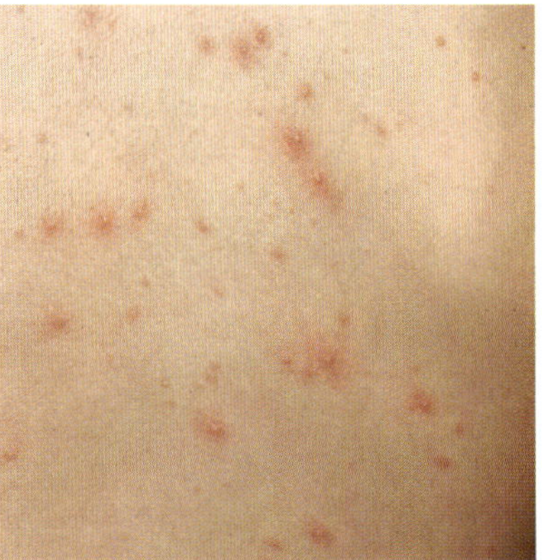

FIG. 39-53 (B, C) *Widespread papules and vesicles.*

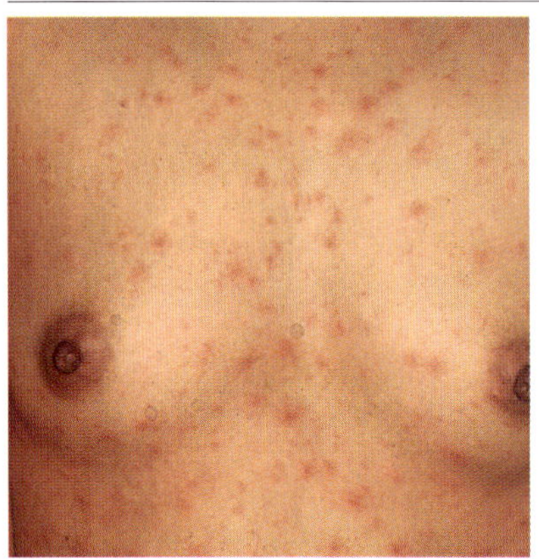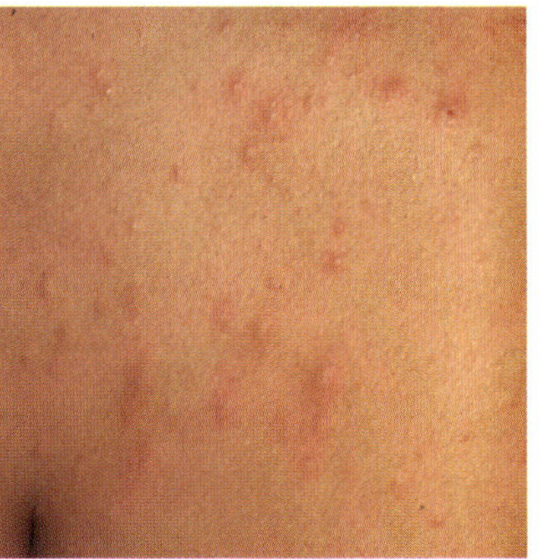

FIG. 39-54 (A, B) *Papules and papulovesicles.*

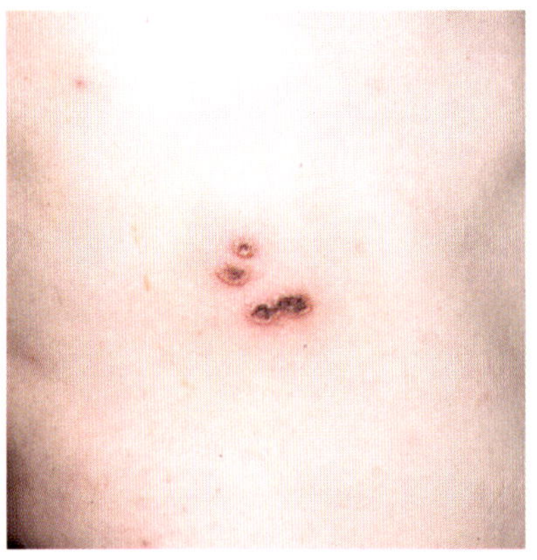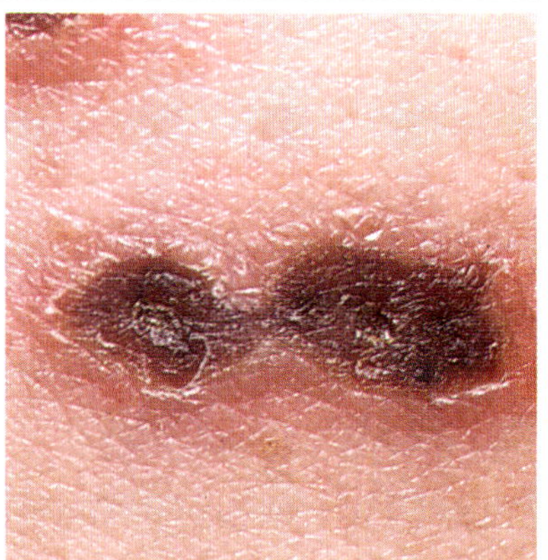

FIG. 39-55 (A, B) *Ulcerated, crusted papules of lesions that will resolve as scars.*

ADJUNCTIVE DIAGNOSTIC TESTS Tzanck preparation, that is, a search by conventional microscopy of scrapings from the undersurface of a roof of a vesicle, is undertaken for the presence of multinucleate keratinocytes that often are acantholytic, definitive signs of infection by herpesvirus. For rapid diagnosis of HSV1 and HSV2, monoclonal antibodies and immunofluorescence may be employed. Polymerase chain reaction is valuable for demonstration of DNA of herpesvirus.

COURSE As a rule, the course of varicella (chicken pox) is short, vesicles erupting and disappearing in about a week. Usually there are no residua, but some lesions may heal with permanent hypopigmentation and others with atrophic scars, reputedly as a consequence of scratching vesicles sufficiently intensely to produce ulcers. Vesicles of herpes simplex, especially those on a lip ("cold sores") or on genitalia, tend to last a bit longer than those of varicella, disappearing in most instances in less than two weeks. Vesicles of zoster, possibly because of their propensity to develop in patients who are immunosuppressed, often ulcerate and it may be many weeks, or even months, before those lesions heal with scars and altered pigmentation.

The neuralgia that oft-times accompanies zoster may parallel the course of the skin disease, or it may persist for years after the skin lesions have healed completely.

INTEGRATION: UNIFYING CONCEPT Morphologically, a vesicle of herpes simplex, zoster, and varicella cannot be distinguished from one another. Clinically, each begins tense and then becomes umbilicated. Histopathologically, each is characterized by intraepidermal vesiculation that results from ballooning and acantholysis.

In each of the three conditions under discussion here, there are characteristic nuclear changes specific for infection by herpesvirus, namely, steel-gray nuclei at the margin of which nucleoplasm is accentuated. Multinucleation is common. Cytoplasm is ballooned, and that phenomenon is followed inevitably by reticular alteration, which is succeeded invariably by necrosis of keratinocytes. Acantholytic cells appear concurrent with ballooning. The cytologic changes just described affect not only the epidermis, but structures of epithelial adnexa, in particular, folliculosebaceous units and eccrine ducts.

In short, although the herpesvirus responsible for herpes simplex (herpes simplex type 1 and herpes simplex type 2) is different from the one responsible for varicella-zoster (varicella-zoster virus), and the distribution of lesions in all three herpetic conditions is very different, the individual lesions of each of them are indistinguishable from one another morphologically, i.e., clinically and histopathologically. Although a clinician, at a glance, can identify herpes simplex, zoster, and varicella on the basis of distribution and arrangement of lesions, a histopathologist cannot.

THERAPY

Herpes simplex: Acyclovir-Zovirax and Valacyclovir-Valtrex are most effective when therapy is initiated early in the course of the infectious process.

Zoster: Systemic antiviral therapy (acyclovir) is indicated, particularly when an affected person is over 50 years of age. Soothing dressings are adjunctive.

Varicella: Antiviral therapy is appropriate in selected patients. Topical antipruritic agents may bring relief. A vaccine is available for prevention.

DEFINITION A proliferation of abnormal Langerhans' cells that may affect internal organs, e.g., the spleen, liver, and bone, sometimes with fatal outcome, as well as the skin, where lesions usually manifest themselves as purpuric papules or ulcers that may be localized (to the vulva, for example) or widespread.

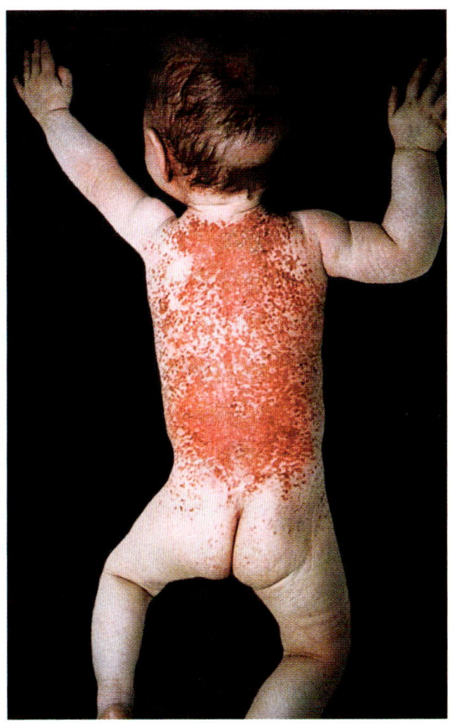

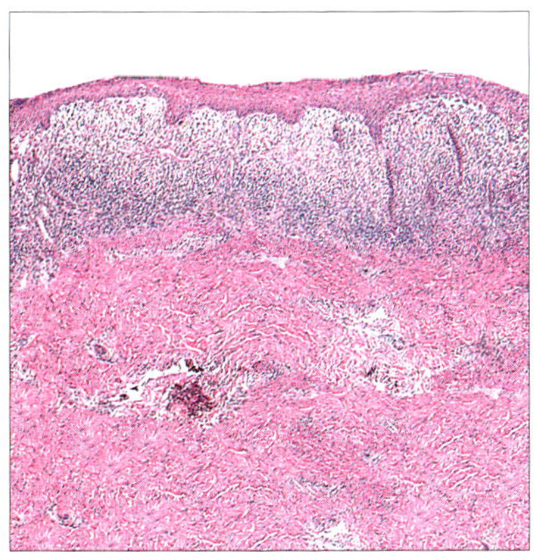

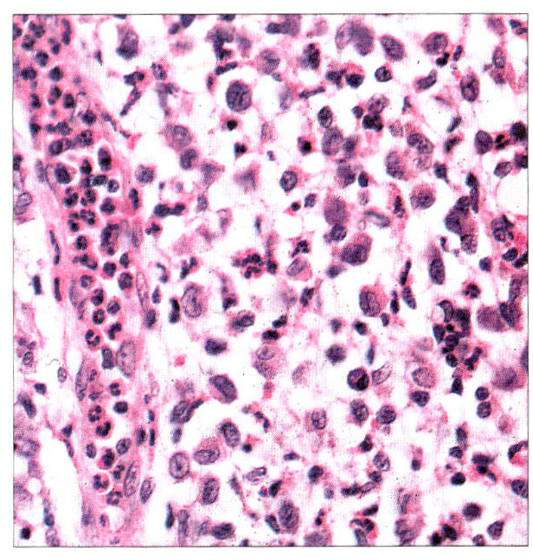

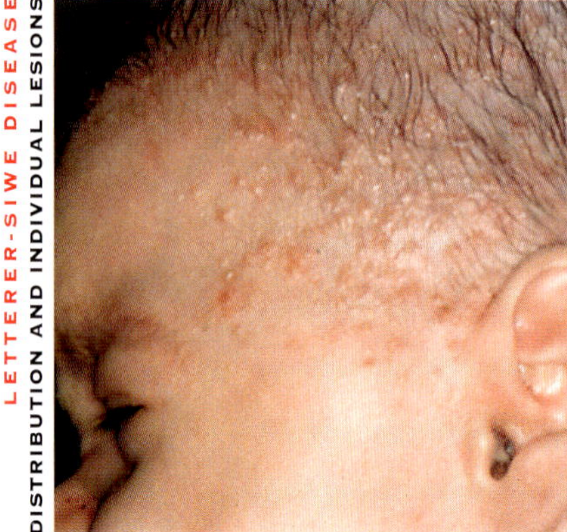

FIG. 40-1 *Papules on the scalp.*

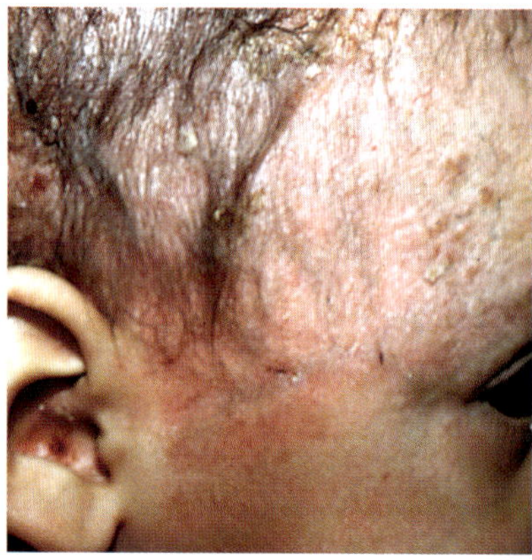

FIG. 40-2 *Scaly and crusted papules, some of them purpuric, on the face, including an ear, and the scalp.*

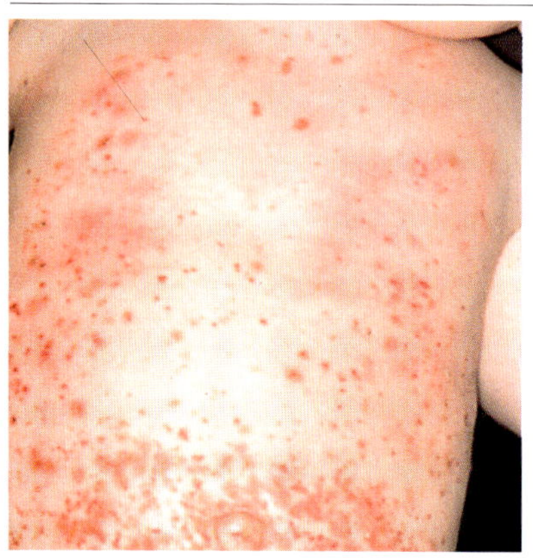

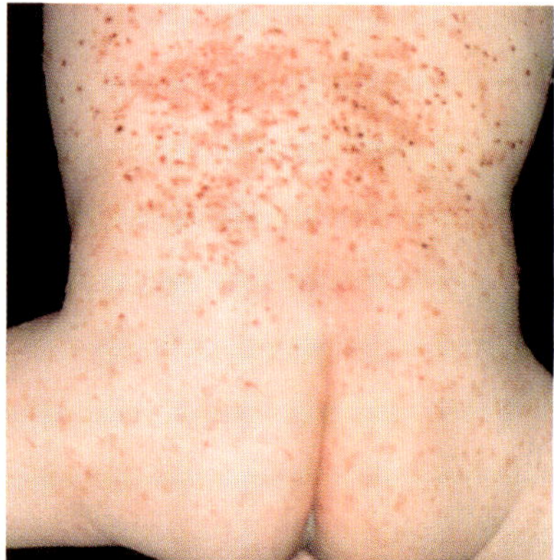

FIG. 40-3 (A, B) *Papules on the trunk and buttocks.*

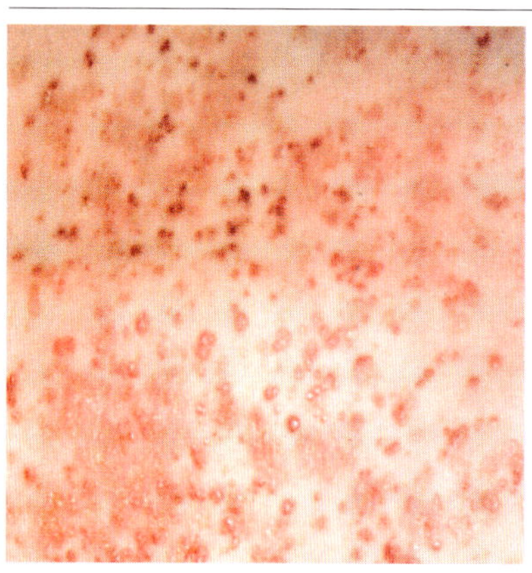

FIG. 40-3 (C) *Papules on the trunk.*

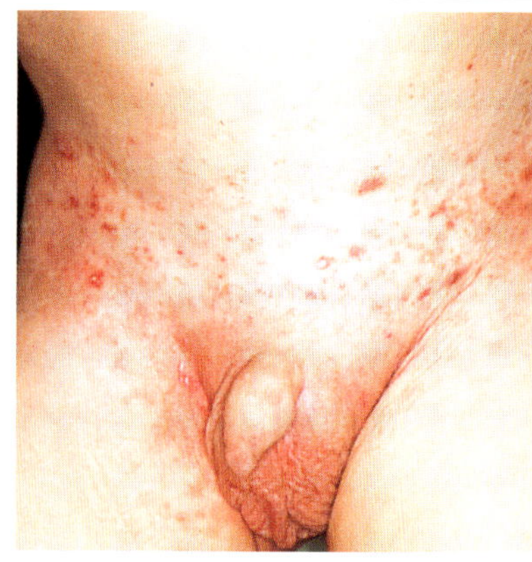

FIG. 40-4 *Papules on the abdomen and in the genital region.*

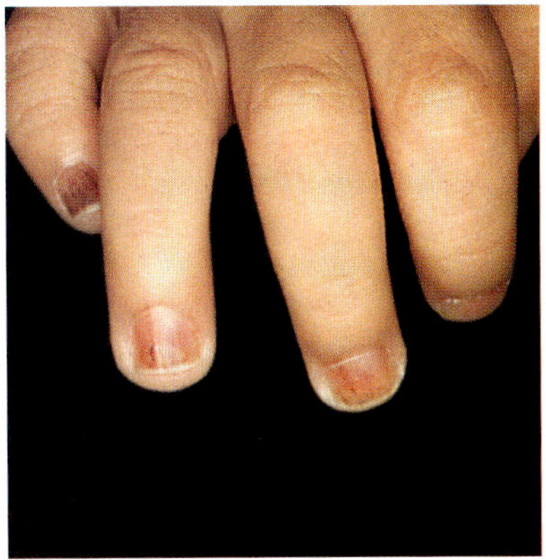

FIG. 40-5 *Purpuric vesicles and papules on the palm, a sign of poor prognosis in Letterer-Siwe disease.*

FIG. 40-6 *Hemorrhage in linear array in the nail unit.*

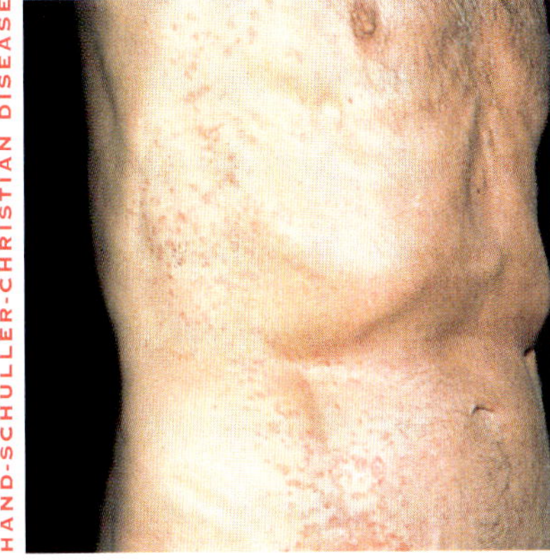
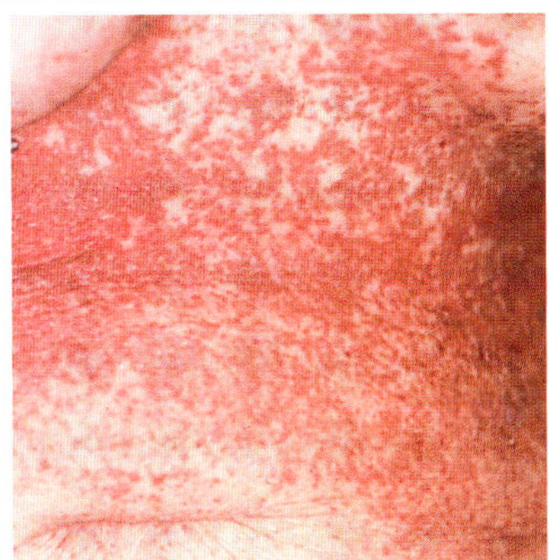

FIG. 40-7 *Widespread purpuric papules in an adult.*

FIG. 40-8 *Purpuric papules, some of which have become confluent to form plaques, on the trunk and breasts.*

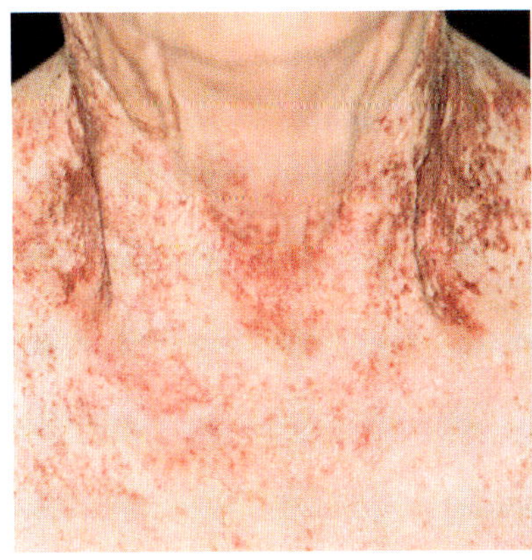
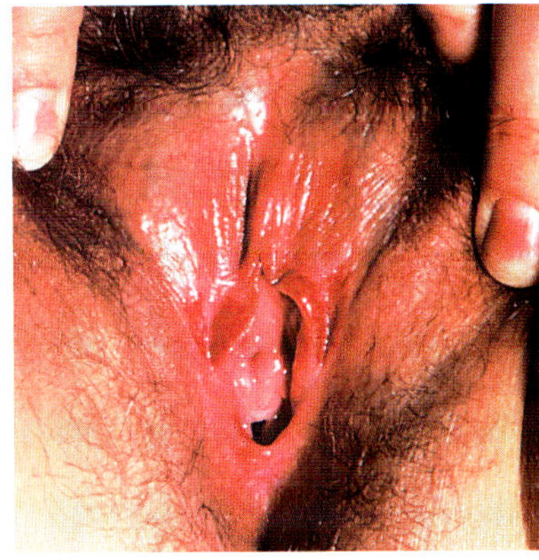

FIG. 40-9 *Purpuric papules, some of which are confluent.*

FIG. 40-10 *Deep ulcer with surrounding erythema on a labium majus.*

HAND-SCHÜLLER-CHRISTIAN DISEASE

ADJUNCTIVE DIAGNOSTIC TESTS Electron microscopy may be used to identify Langerhans' granules in cells of histiocytosis X, and positivity of those cells for CD1a antigen or S-100 protein is virtually confirmatory of the diagnosis.

COURSE Individual scaly or crusted papules of histiocytosis X usually last for months and even years. The disease itself persists for years and, in some patients, ends fatally. That dire ending is a consequence not of involvement of the skin, but of internal organs, such as the liver and the brain.

INTEGRATION: UNIFYING CONCEPT The common denominator of histiocytosis X is abnormal Langerhans' cells in the skin and internal organs, for example, the liver and spleen for the expression of the disease named eponymically for Letterer and Siwe, the pituitary gland for the manifestation of the disease named for Hand, Schüller, and Christian, and the bones for that presentation of the disease known as eosinophilic granuloma. Papules produced by proliferation of abnormal Langerhans' cells occur in the skin of neonates and children with Letterer-Siwe disease, and in adults with Hand-Schüller-Christian disease. Eosinophilic granuloma does not affect the skin.

Morphologically, the scaly or crusted papules of histiocytosis X are the same, irrespective of whether the disease involves very young persons (Letterer-Siwe) or older ones (Hand-Schüller-Christian). Furthermore, the abnormal Langerhans' cells present in the skin and in internal organs of all expressions of histiocytosis X have the same appearance. In sections stained by hematoxylin and eosin, those cells are typified by a large, lightly basophilic nucleus that often has a reniform or convoluted outline and by cytoplasm that is abundant and amphophilic.

Diagnosis of histiocytosis X by conventional microscopy is made by identification of the distinctive abnormal Langerhans' cells. In Letterer-Siwe disease, those cells tend to be arranged in band-like fashion in the upper part of the dermis and to be scattered as solitary units and in small collections within an epidermis that is covered by scale-crusts. A mixed infiltrate of lymphocytes, neutrophils, and eosinophils often accompanies the aberrant Langerhans' cells. In Hand-Schüller-Christian disease, by contrast, the abnormal Langerhans' cells tend to be distributed in nodular and diffuse arrangement throughout the dermis and sometimes in the upper part of the subcutaneous fat. Those cells, too, are often joined by lymphocytes, neutrophils, and eosinophils.

In sum, histiocytosis X is fundamentally a single pathologic process in which the prime abnormality is proliferation of abnormal Langerhans' cells. Although the clinical expressions of the process vary and are named according to those variations, to wit, Letterer-Siwe disease, Hand-Schüller-Christian disease, and eosinophilic granuloma, the cytologic appearance of the abnormal Langerhans' cells is the same in each of the clinical manifestations. The designation histiocytosis X is wrong because the cells that make up the process are not histiocytes (whose main function is phagocytosis); they are abnormal Langerhans' cells (whose main function is presentation of antigen to lymphocytes). So, too, is the appellation "Langerhans' cell granulomatosis" incorrect because the process seems to be neoplastic, not granulomatous, i.e., an inflammatory condition in which histiocytes, usually epithelioid ones, predominate at least in a focus.

THERAPY If localized, or even widespread, skin lesions may be treated with topical application of corticosteroids or with PUVA. Extracutaneous disease requires systemic chemotherapy, such as a vinblastine or methotrexate. Interferon-alpha is also efficacious.

DEFINITION Noninflammatory scaly disorders in which polygonal gray or brown scales tend to be elevated at their periphery, causing them to appear to be separated from contiguous scales, findings that are seen in three conditions, namely, ichthyosis vulgaris (and its look-alike, acquired ichthyosis), X-linked ichthyosis, and lamellar ichthyosis. Other conditions purported to be ichthyosis, among them nonbullous congenital ichthyosiform erythroderma, ichthyosis hystrix, and ichthyosis linearis circumflexa, do not fulfill the criteria just set forth.

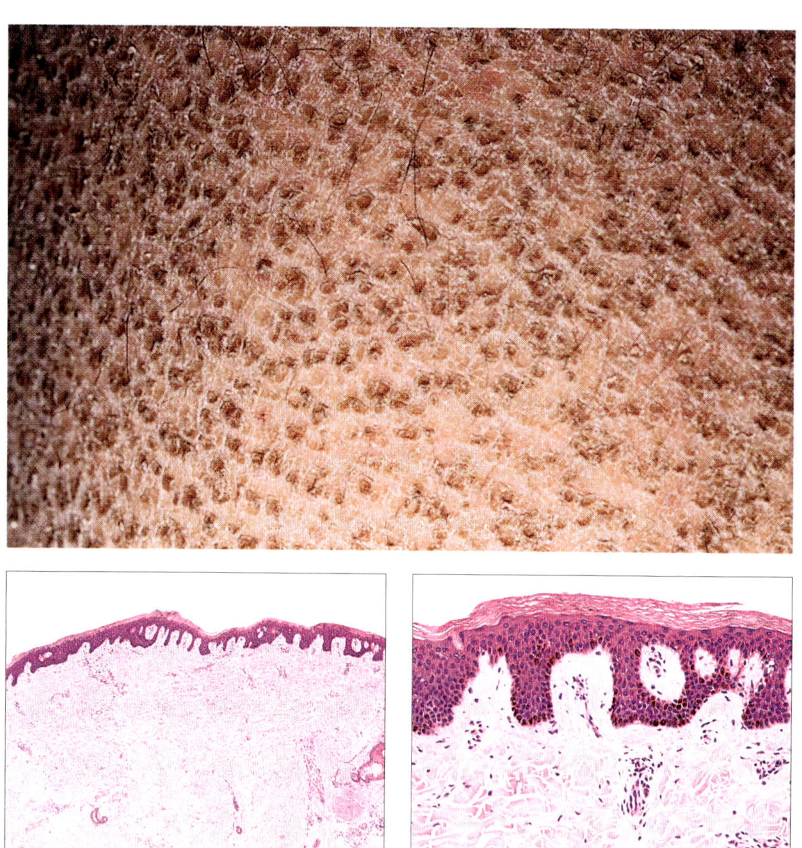

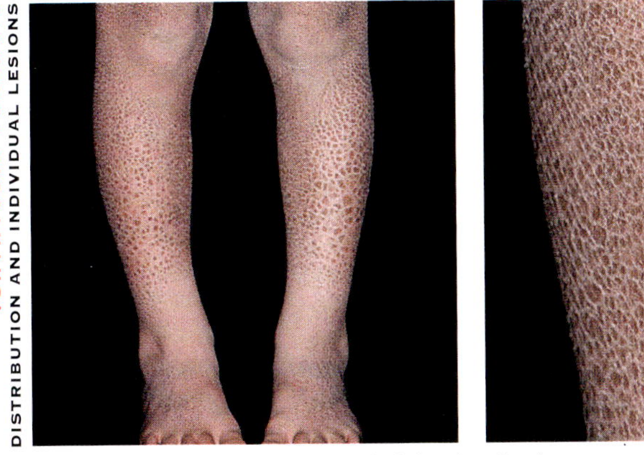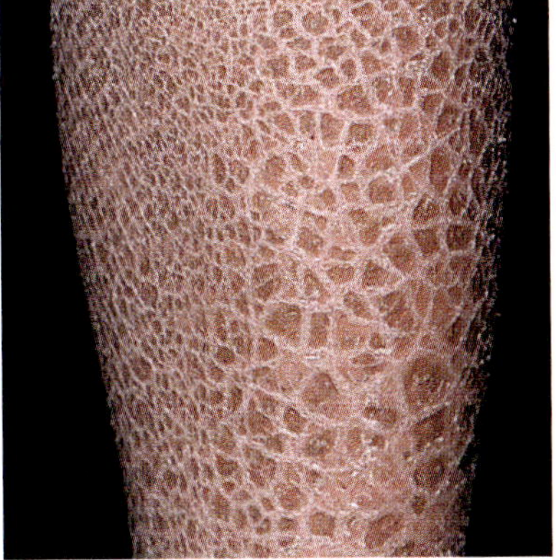

FIG. 41-1 (A, B) *Polygonal scales of ichthyosis vulgaris.*

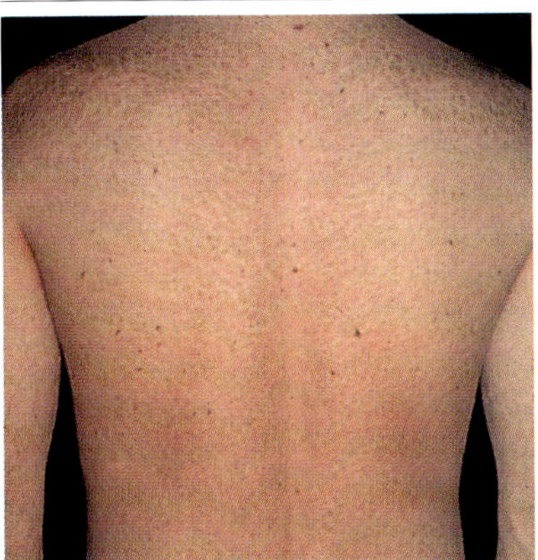

FIG. 41-2 (A, B) *Subtle scales of ichthyosis vulgaris.*

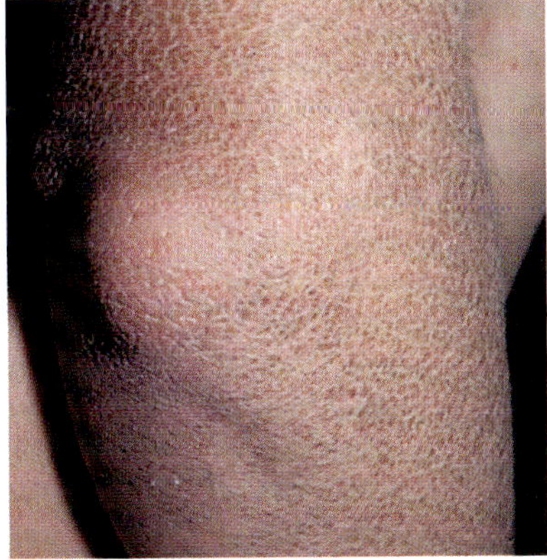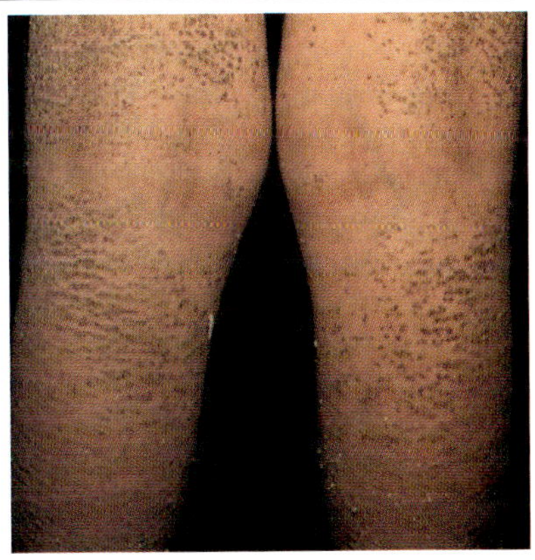

FIG. 41-3 *Typical scales of ichthyosis vulgaris.*

FIG. 41-4 *Sparing of popliteal fossae in ichthyosis vulgaris.*

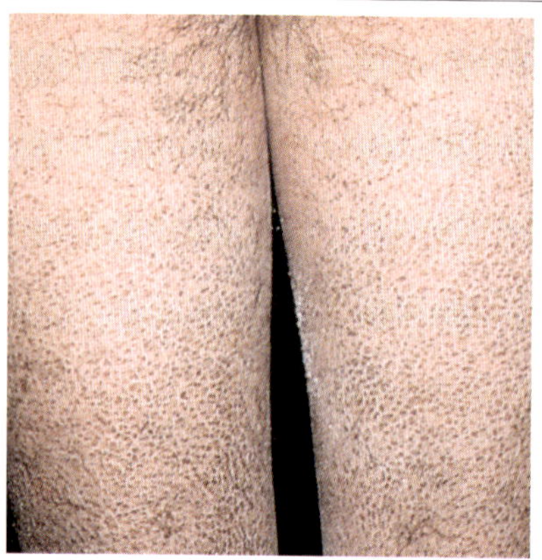

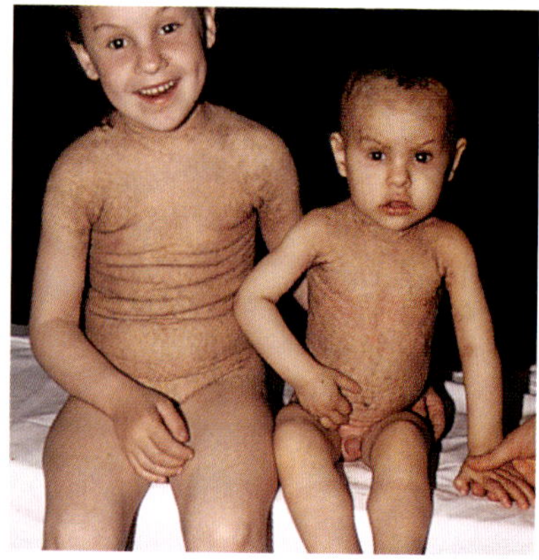

FIG. 41-5 *Moderately severe scales of ichthyosis vulgaris.*

FIG. 41-6 *Siblings with widespread ichthyosis vulgaris.*

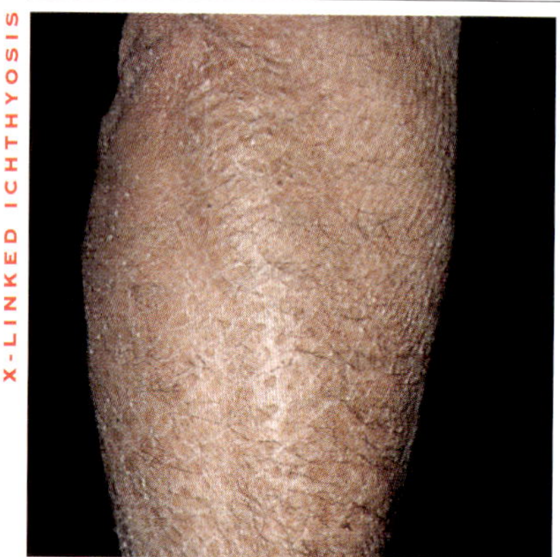

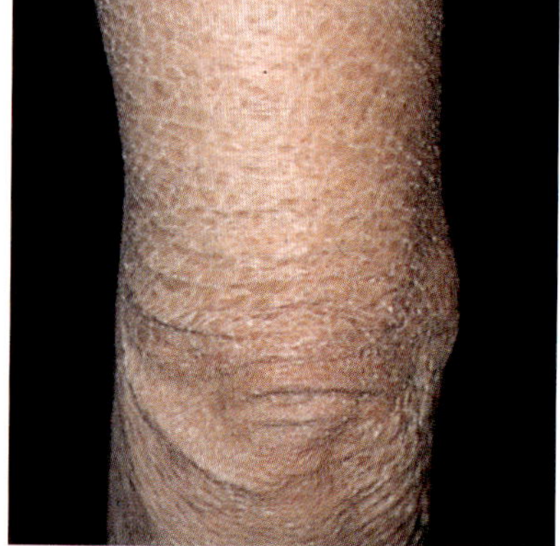

FIG. 41-7 (A, B) *Pigmented polygonal scales of X-linked ichthyosis.*

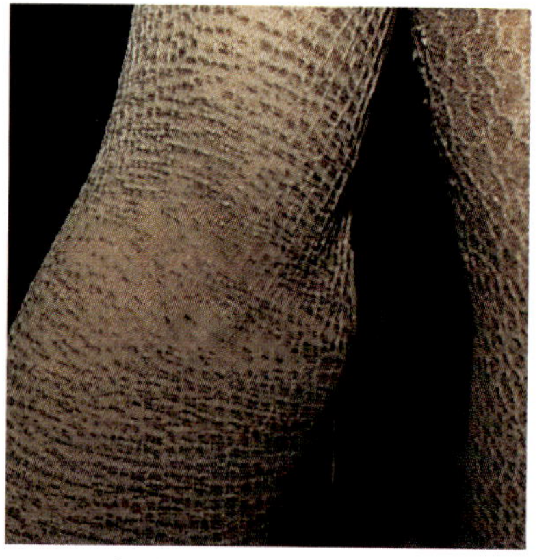

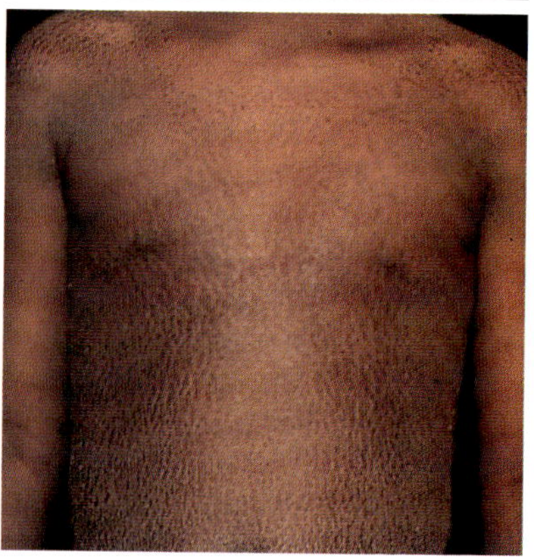

FIG. 41-8 *Involvement of an antecubital fossa in X-linked ichthyosis. Scales are more prominent than in ichthyosis vulgaris.*

FIG. 41-9 *Widespread involvement by X-linked ichthyosis.*

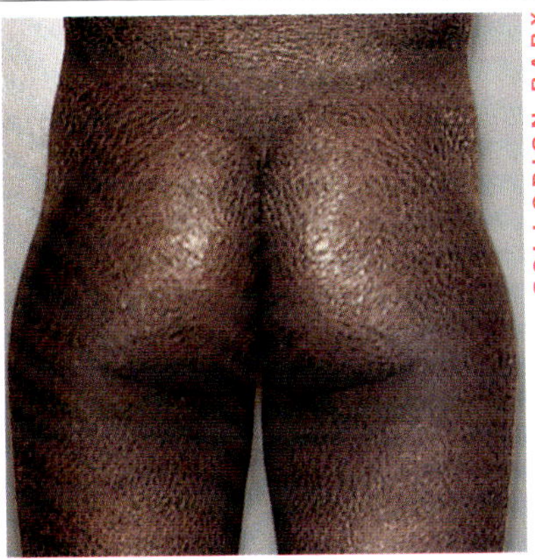

FIG. 41-10 *Widespread X-linked ichthyosis.*

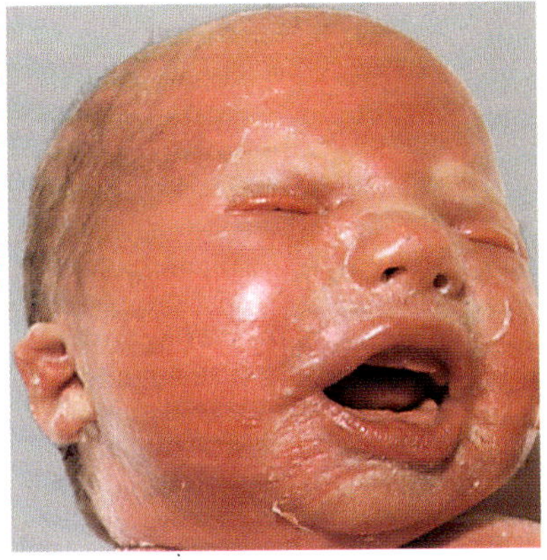

FIG. 41-11 *Collodion baby with incipient lamellar ichthyosis.*

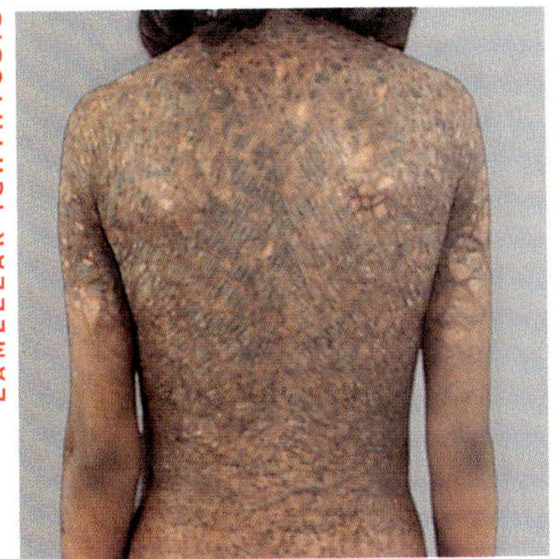

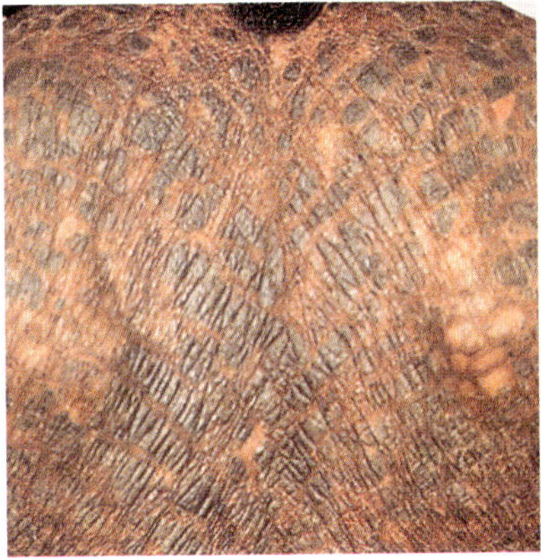

FIG. 41-12 (A, B) *Large, thick scales on the trunk and upper extremities of lamellar ichthyosis.*

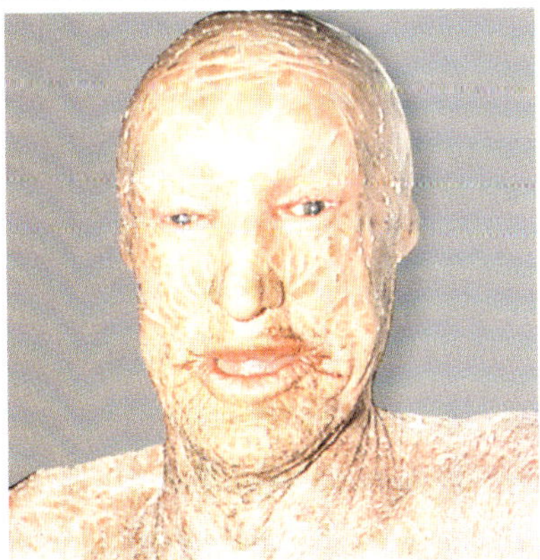

FIG. 41-13 *Ectropion and fissures associated with widespread, thick, polygonal scales of lamellar ichthyosis.*

COURSE The ichthyoses are either present at birth or appear shortly thereafter, and once present they persist for a lifetime. As a rule, the severity of ichthyosis lessens over the course of many decades, the scales becoming less pronounced. The true ichthyoses, however, never disappear completely.

INTEGRATION: UNIFYING CONCEPT The true ichthyoses, namely, ichthyosis vulgaris, X-linked ichthyosis, and lamellar ichthyosis are characterized by plate-like scales that tend to be adherent to the viable epidermis, desquamating only episodically. The clinical appearance of the scales, which bear only a vague resemblance to the scales of some fish (whence the name ichthyosis), is the feature that unites the "true" ichthyoses. Other unifying features are histopathologic findings, namely, laminated orthokeratosis and absence of infiltrates of inflammatory cells.

In short, each of the true ichthyoses is typified by orthokeratosis in which corneocytes are arranged mostly in laminated fashion. In general, the cornified layer of lamellar ichthyosis is thicker than that of X-linked ichthyosis which is thicker than that of ichthyosis vulgaris. Acquired ichthyosis is indistinguishable morphologically, i.e., clinically and histopathologically, from ichthyosis vulgaris. Certain other histopathologic differences enable the authentic ichthyoses to be distinguished from one another, for example, in ichthyosis vulgaris the granular zone is very thin, in X-linked ichthyosis the granular zone is prominent, and in lamellar ichthyosis the granular zone, like the cornified layer, is thickened markedly. A deficiency of the enzyme, sulphatase phosphate, is responsible for X-linked ichthyosis.

Many of the conditions conventionally termed "ichthyosis" are dramatically different from what we refer to as the "true" ichthyoses. For example, bullous congenital ichthyosiform erythroderma, known synonymously but inaccurately as epidermolytic hyperkeratosis, is a widespread epidermal nevus characterized by strikingly keratotic digitations.

Harlequin fetus is a severe aberration in cornification that differs from "true" ichthyosis by having armadillo-like horny plates separated from one another by fissures, rather than by having plate-like polygonal scales. Nonbullous congenital ichthyosiform erythroderma, which is wholly unrelated to bullous congenital ichthyosiform erythroderma and lamellar ichthyosis, is an inflammatory process in which mounds of parakeratosis are present in conjunction with slight spongiosis and psoriasiform hyperplasia.

In short, the true ichthyoses are noninflammatory processes typified by broad plate-like scales that consist of orthokeratotic corneocytes arranged in lamellar fashion. Despite the limitations of the term ichthyosis (the scales do not look exactly like those of many kinds of fishes), it is more precise than the synonym proposed for it, "disorders of cornification"; the latter designation is imprecise, including as it does such disparate conditions as psoriasis, pityriasis rubra pilaris, and Darier's disease, among many others such as the authentic ichthyoses.

THERAPY Ichthyosis vulgaris is best treated with emollients, alpha-hydroxy acids, or propylene glycol. Patients with severe ichthyosis deserve treatment with oral retinoids.

DEFINITION An infectious inflammatory process that consists of pustules that resolve with crusts in at least one locus and often several loci, usually on a face, and caused by streptococci or staphylococci.

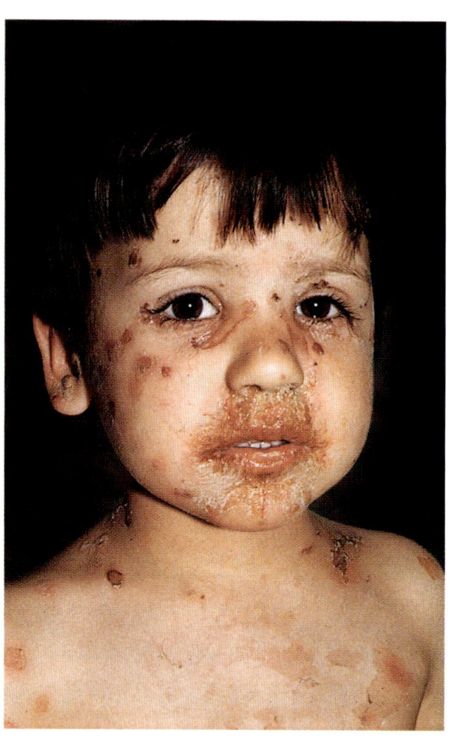

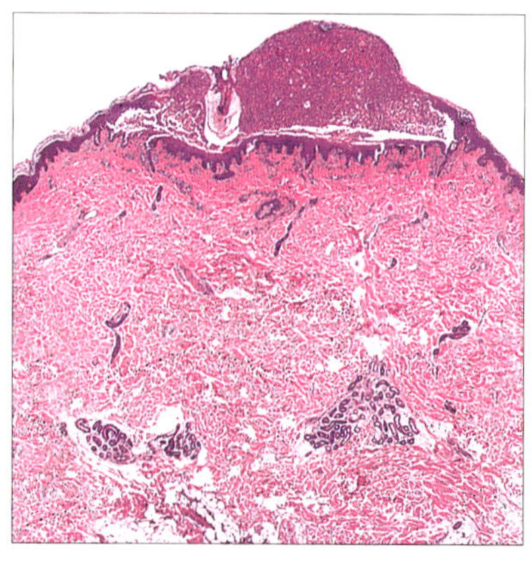

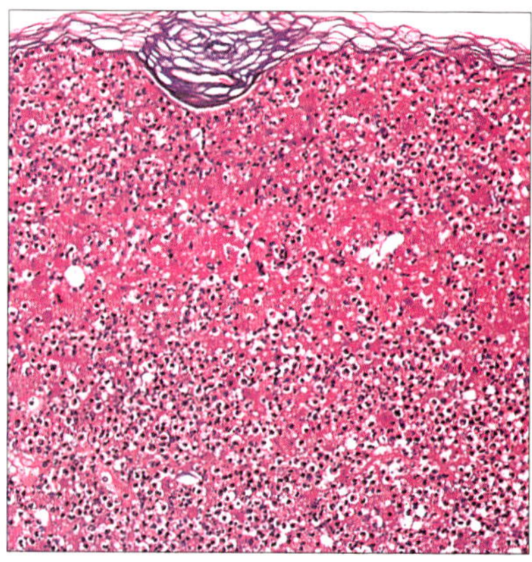

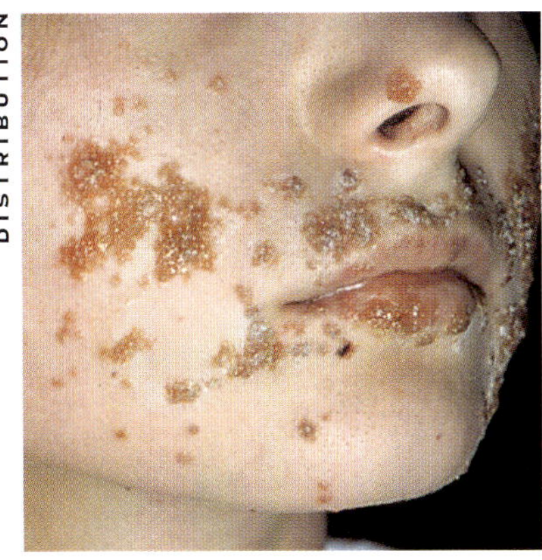

FIG. 42-1 *Erosions and crusts.*

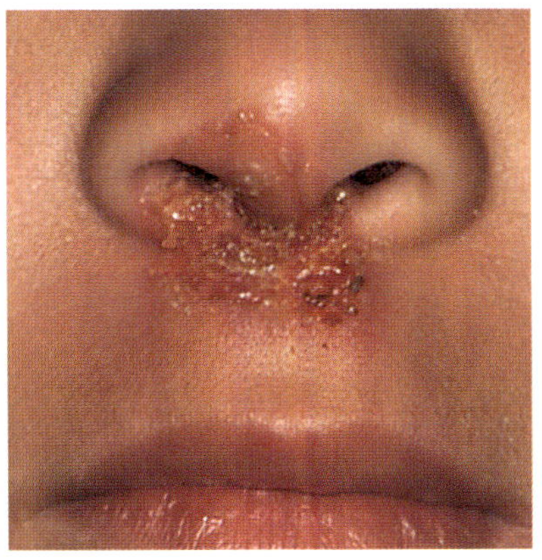

FIG. 42-2 *Crusts on the nose, nostrils, and upper lip.*

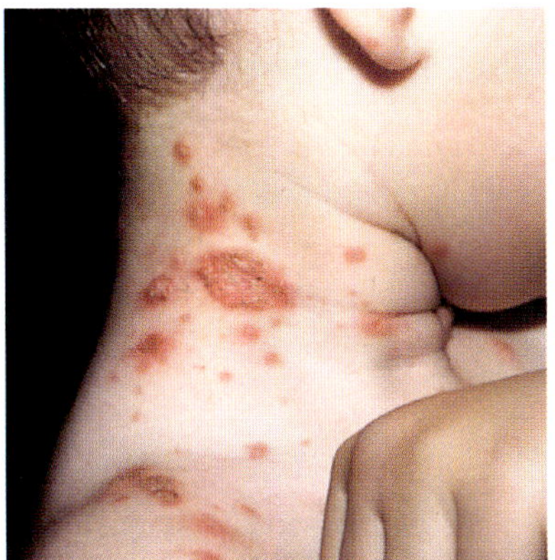

FIG. 42-3 *Erosions and crusts.*

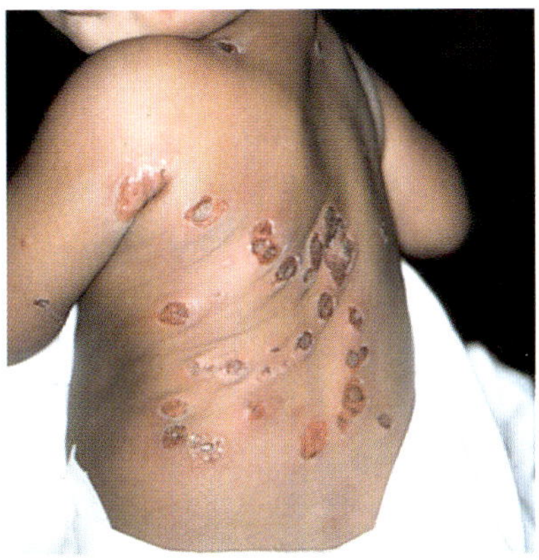

FIG. 42-4 *Papules and plaques covered by crusts on the chin, neck, and trunk.*

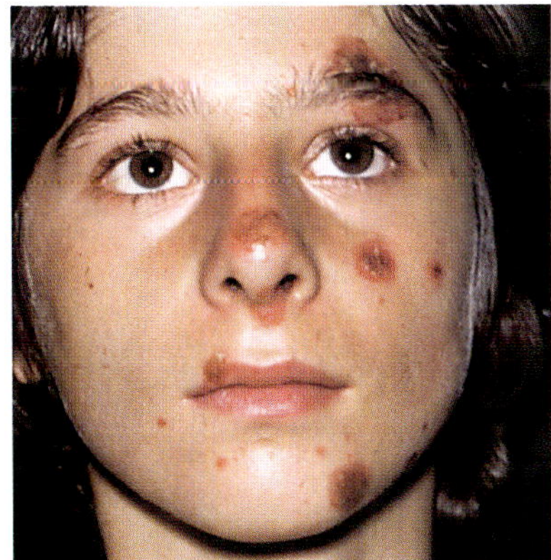

FIG. 42-5 *Papules and nummular plaques covered by crusts.*

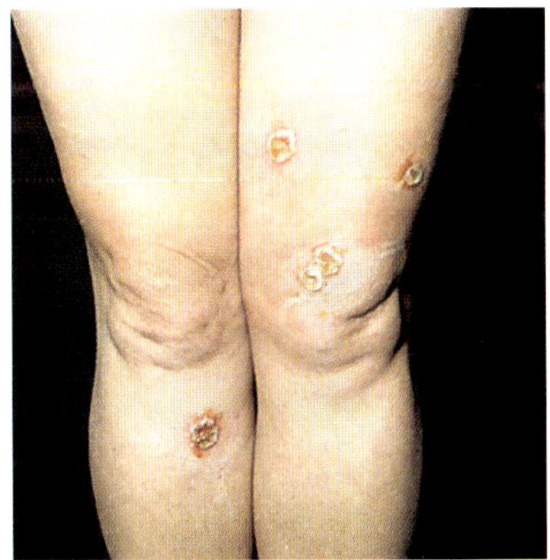

FIG. 42-6 *Pustules in annular configuration and crusts.*

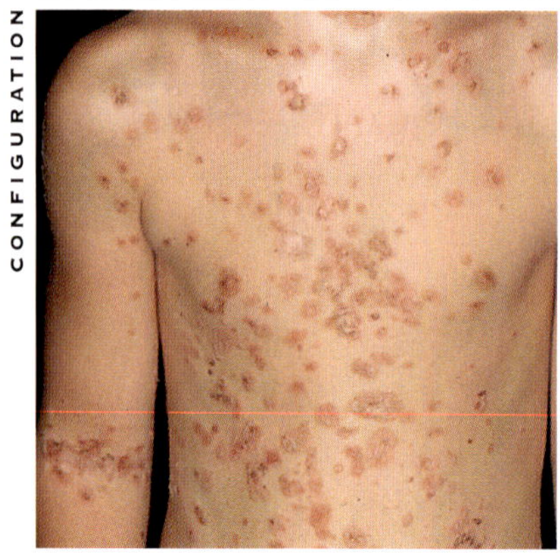

FIG. 42-7 *Crusts, some in annular configuration.*

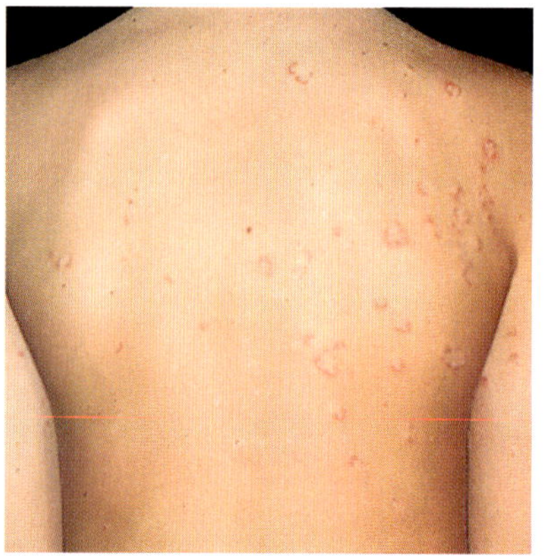

FIG. 42-8 *Crusts in arcuate and annular configuration.*

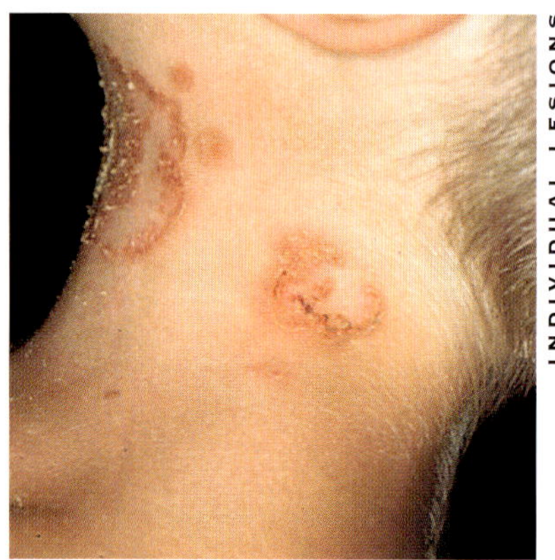

FIG. 42-9 *Crusts and scales with arcuate outlines.*

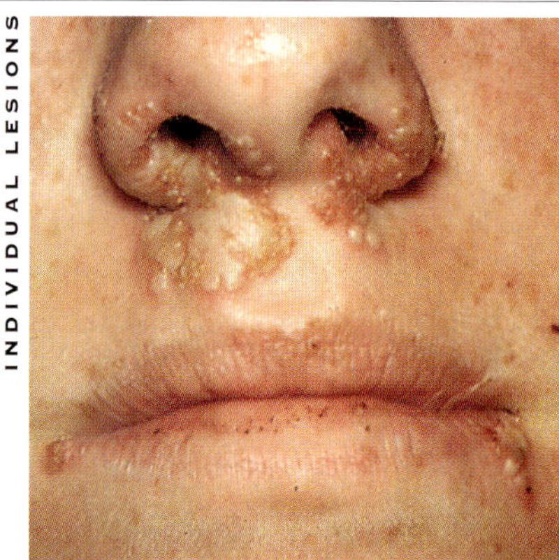

FIG. 42-10 *Grouped pustules and crusts.*

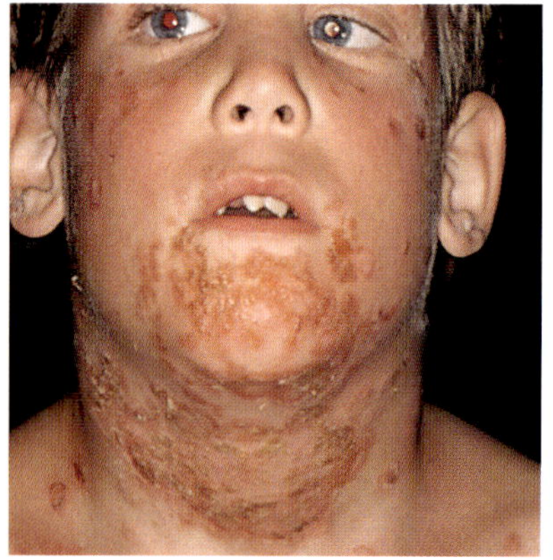

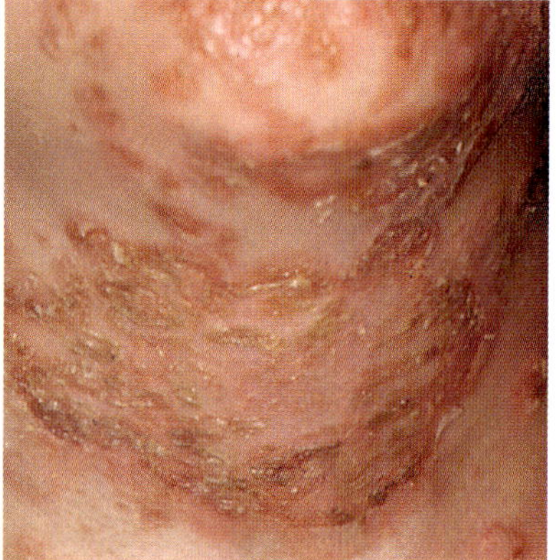

FIG. 42-11 (A, B) *Grouped crusts.*

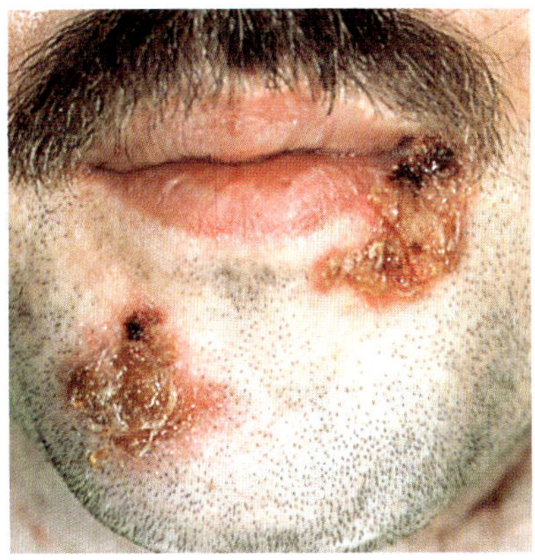

FIG. 42-12 *Nummular lesions of crusts atop erosions.*

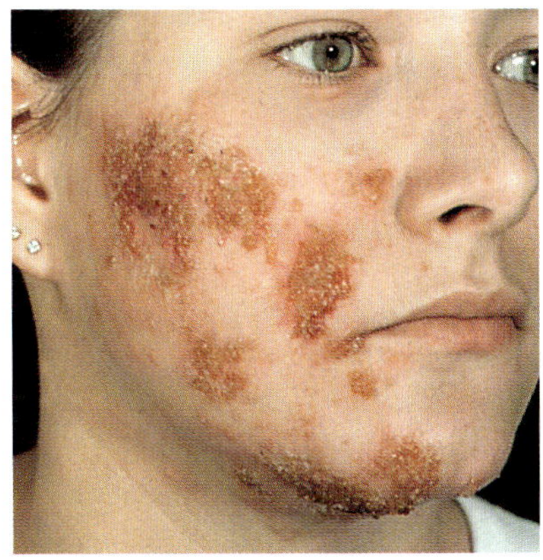

FIG. 42-13 *Many poorly circumscribed nummular plaques consisting of erosions covered by crusts.*

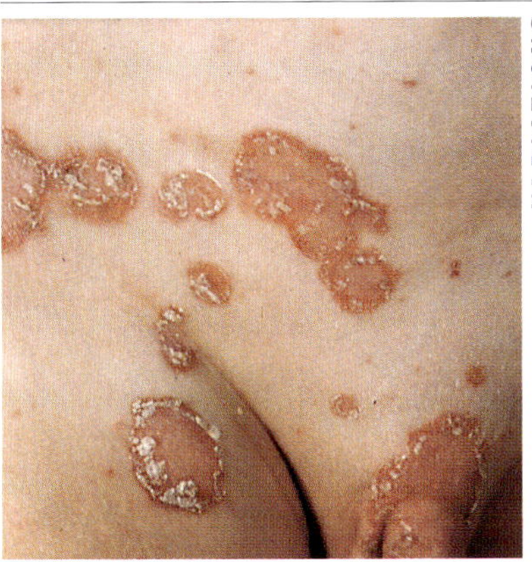

FIG. 42-14 *Crusts and scales at the periphery of papules and nummular patches and plaques.*

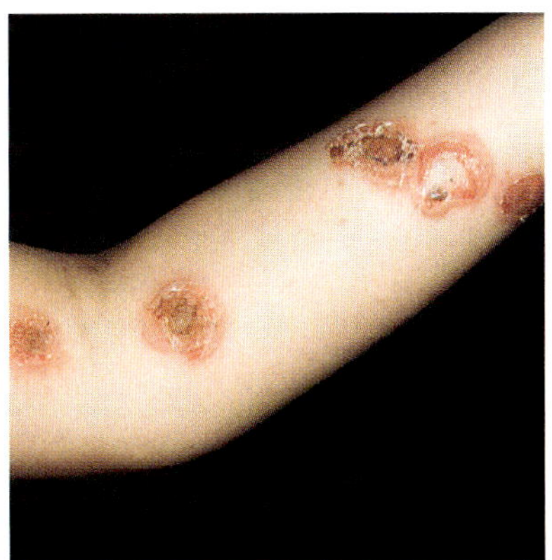

FIG. 42-15 *Bullous impetigo, streptococcal, resolving, with annular and nummular lesions consisting of erosions, crusts, and scales.*

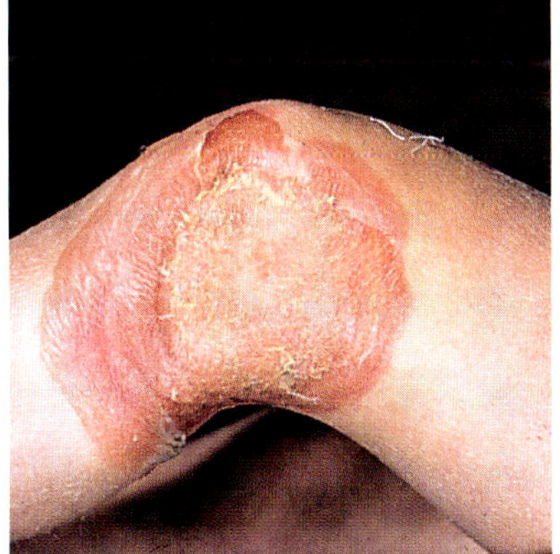

FIG. 42-16 *Blister of bullous impetigo, staphylococcal, at the periphery of a lesion whose center has resolved with crusts.*

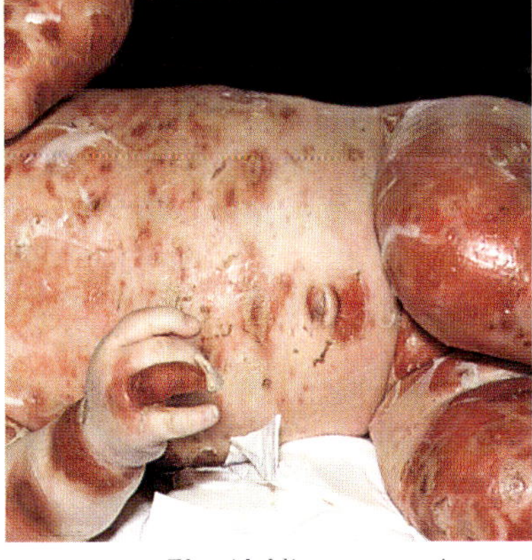

FIG. 42-17 *Flaccid blisters, extensive erosions, and scales of staphylococcal scalded-skin syndrome.*

COURSE Impetigo, whether pustular or bullous, is a self-limited infectious process. Pustules resolve as honey-colored crusts that fall off and leave behind macules of slightly altered pigmentation, the entire process usually lasting less than two weeks. Bullae may resolve more quickly, the blistering process ending in a week or so.

INTEGRATION: UNIFYING CONCEPT Both impetigo contagiosa and bullous impetigo are caused by gram-positive cocci, most often those of Staphylococcus aureus. In the case of impetigo contagiosa, bacteria within the epidermis induce neutrophils to be attracted chemotactically from capillaries in the papillary dermis to that surface epithelium, the result being a pustule clinically. In the case of bullous impetigo, staphylococci in the epidermis release an exotoxin, namely exfoliatin, which causes acantholysis and formation consequently of a blister in the upper part of the viable epidermis. In short, although both impetigo contagiosa and bullous impetigo are infectious processes caused by staphylococci, the mechanism of pustule and blister formation, respectively, are different.

Parenthetically, staphylococcal scalded-skin syndrome, caused by specific phage types of Staphylococcus aureus, differs clinically from both impetigo contagiosa and bullous impetigo. It occurs nearly exclusively in infants and consists of widespread flaccid blisters that soon become unroofed to reveal large zones of denudation. The histopathologic findings in staphylococcal scalded skin syndrome are indistinguishable from those in bullous impetigo (and pemphigus foliaceus), but the mechanism of blister formation is different; bacteria are not present within blisters, but at a distant site, and blisters result from the effects of an endotoxin manufactured by staphylococci and delivered through the bloodstream to every part of the skin.

THERAPY Topical antibiotics, such as mupirocin cream, are effective. For widespread lesions, antibiotics administered systemically are indicated.

DEFINITION A systemic disease, which manifests itself in the skin first as violaceous macules and patches that tend to progress to papules and plaques, and sometimes to nodules and tumors, all of which represent hyperplasia of endothelial cells.

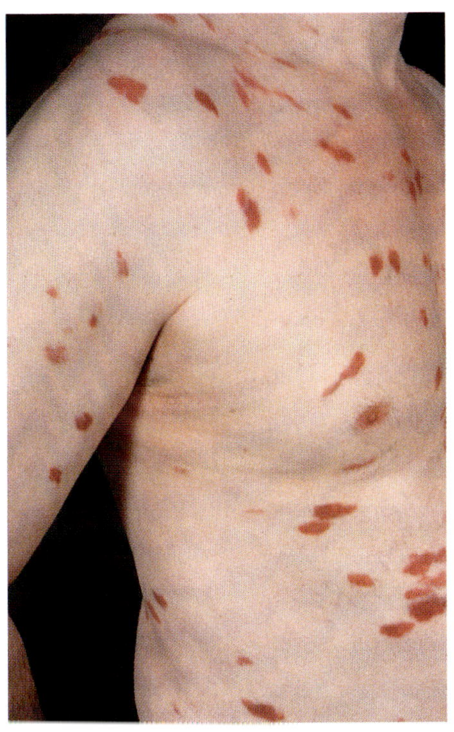

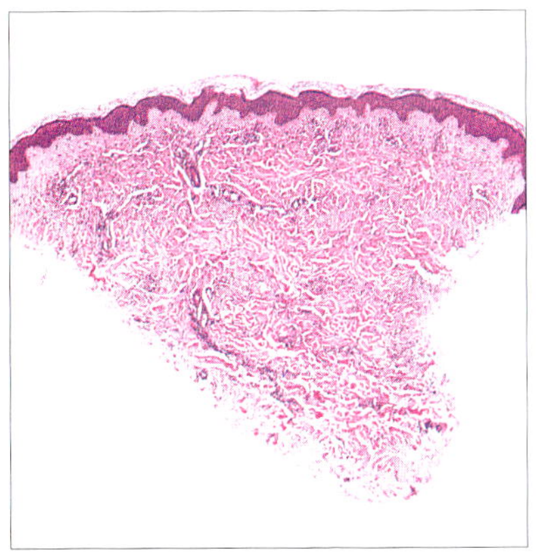

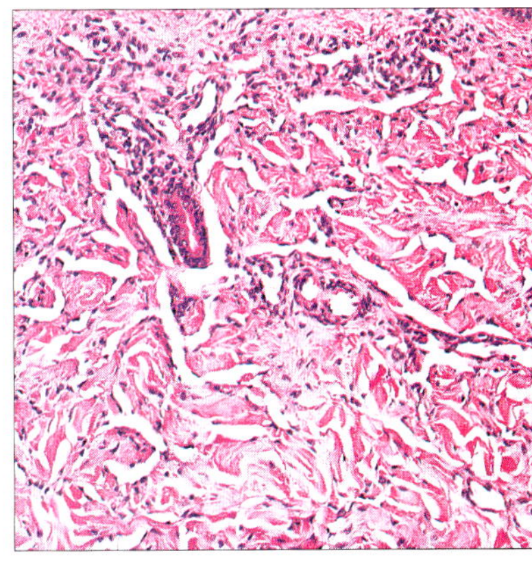

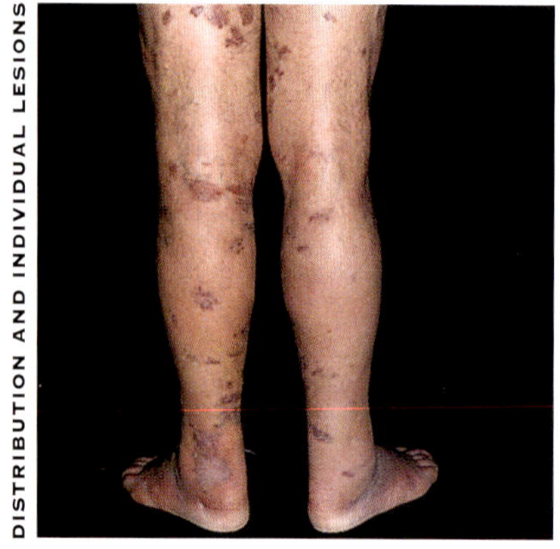

FIG. 43-1 *Papules and plaques on legs and feet.*

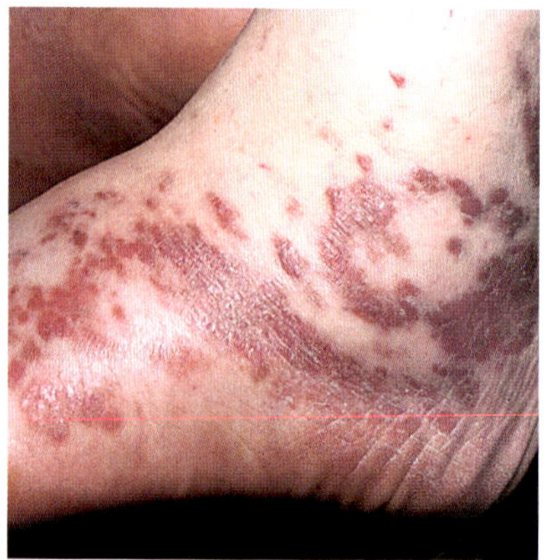

FIG. 43-2 *Macules, patches, papules, and plaques.*

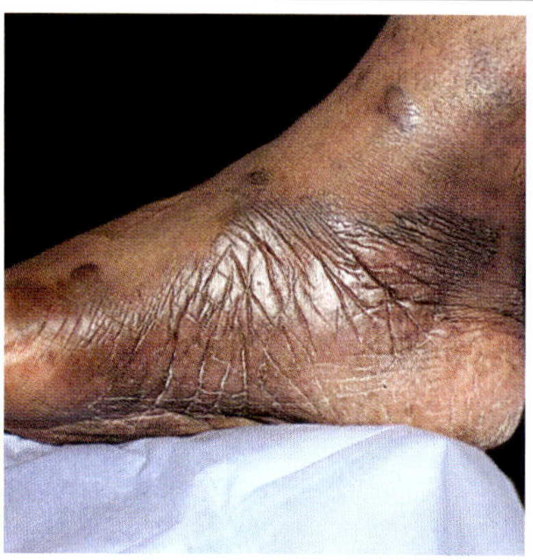

FIG. 43-3 *Macules, patches, papules, and plaques.*

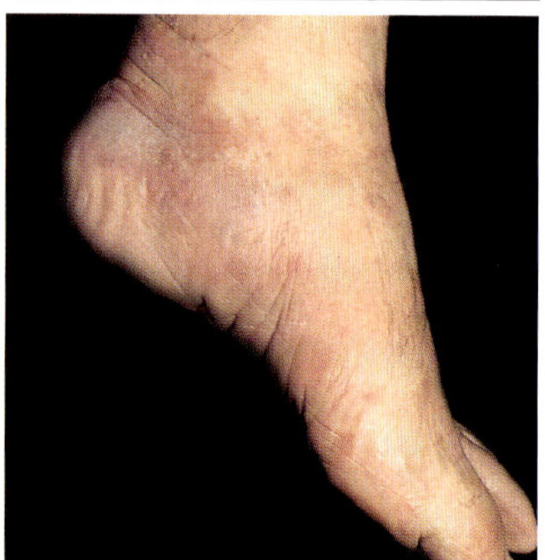

FIG. 43-4 *Subtle papules and plaques.*

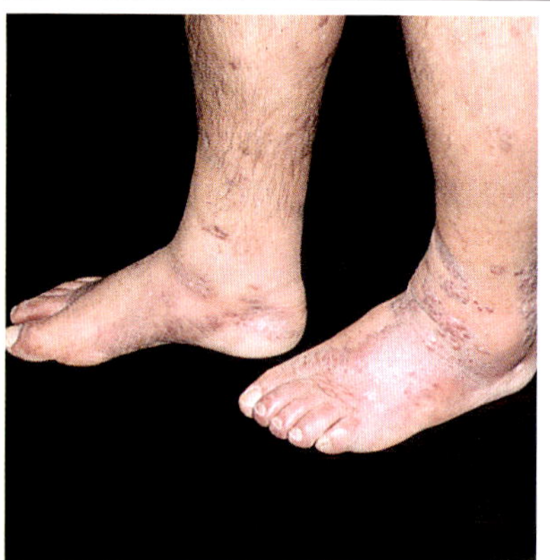

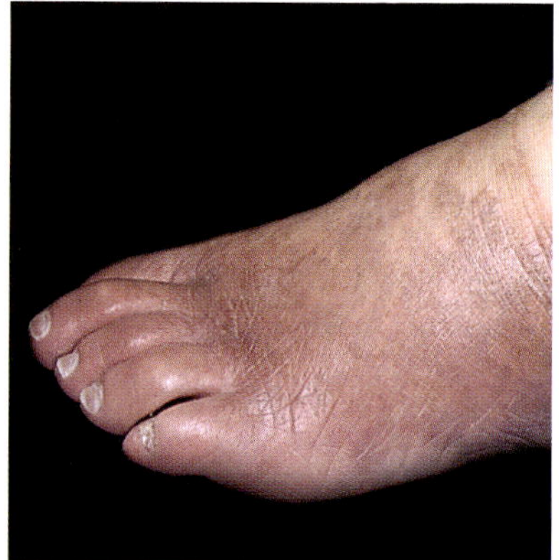

FIG. 43-5 (A, B) *Patches, papules, and plaques.*

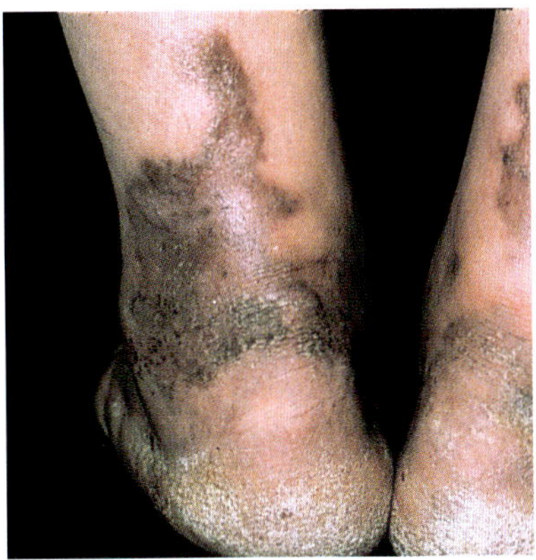

FIG. 43-6 *Plaques.*

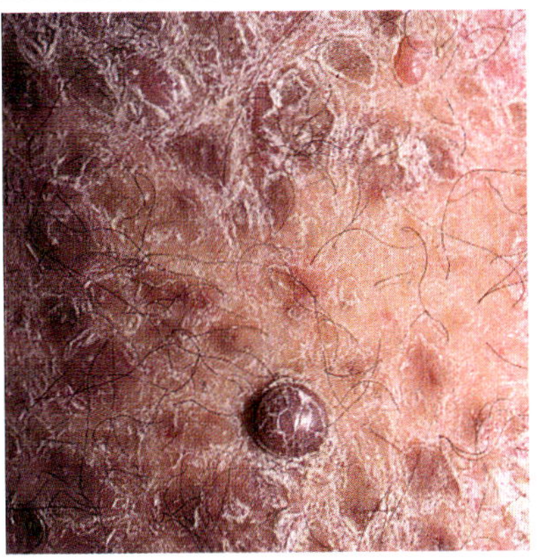

FIG. 43-7 *Papules, nodules, and plaques, many of them covered by scales.*

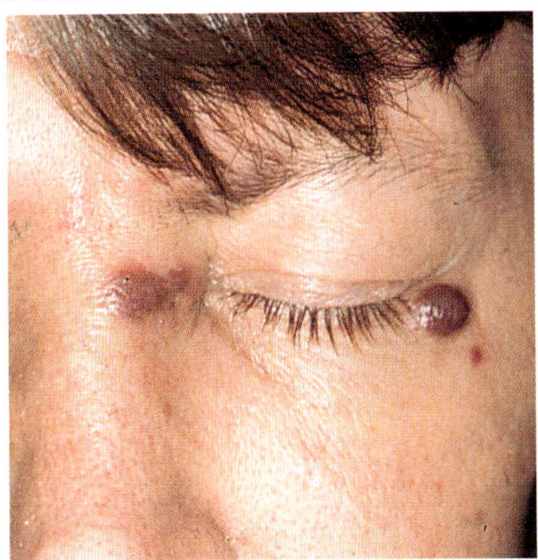
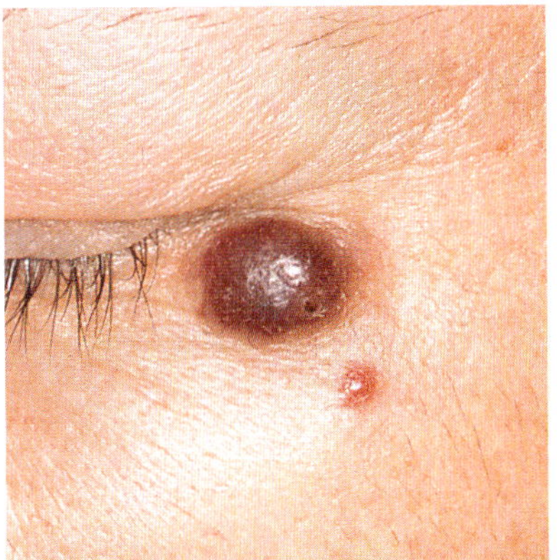

FIG. 43-8 (A, B) *Papules of different sizes and shapes.*

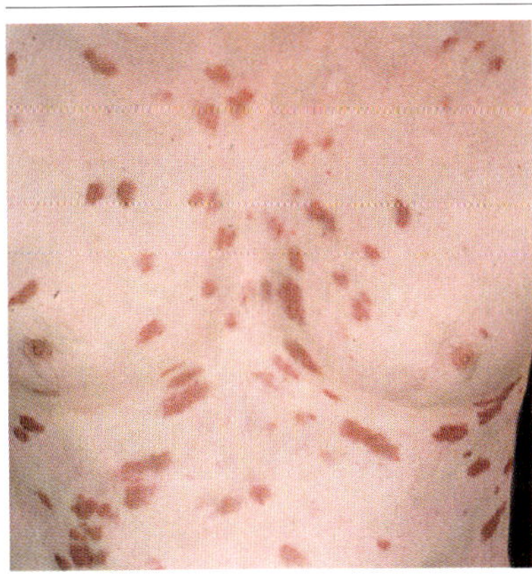

FIG. 43-9 *Papules and plaques, some of them elongated, distributed widely.*

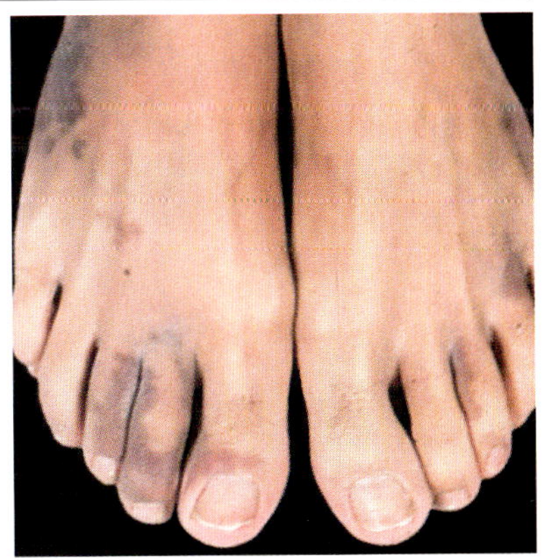

FIG. 43-10 *Patches, papules, and plaques.*

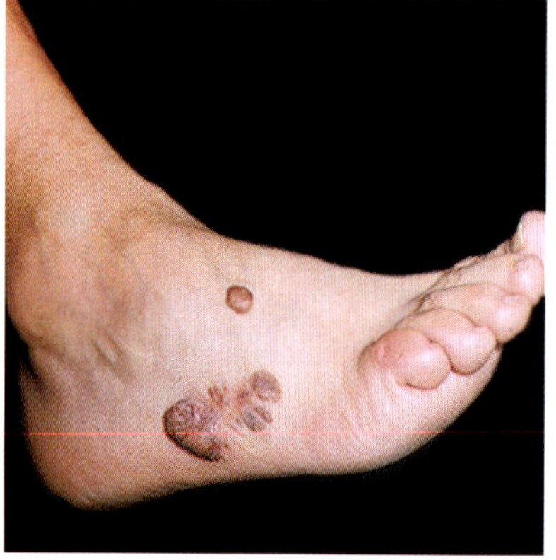

FIG. 43-11 *Papules, plaques, and nodules.*

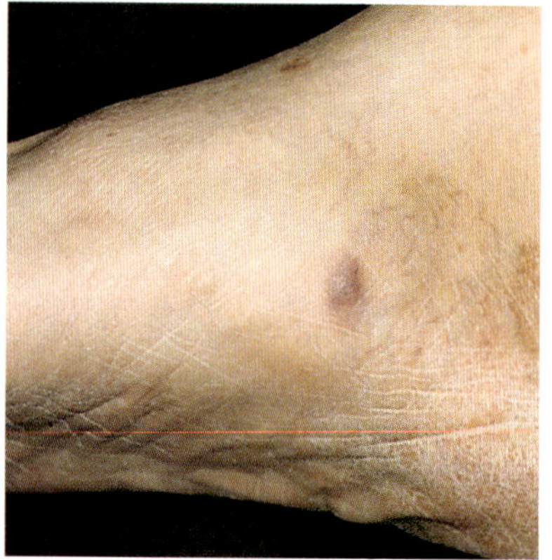

FIG. 43-12 *Papule.*

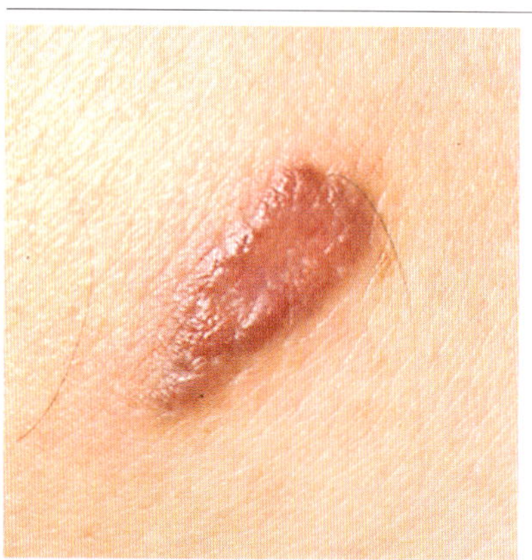

FIG. 43-13 *Plaque.*

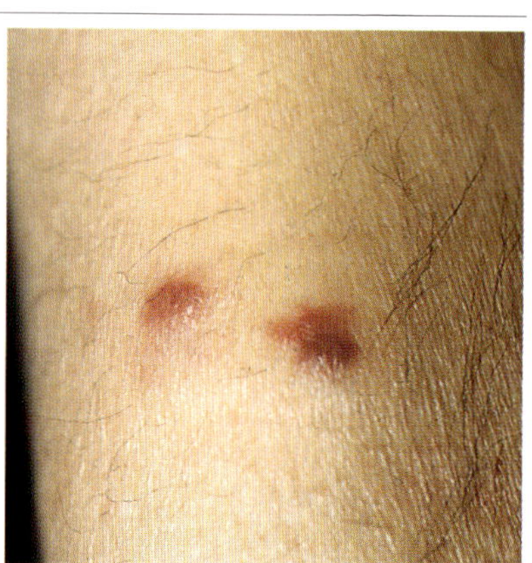

FIG. 43-14 *Two papules.*

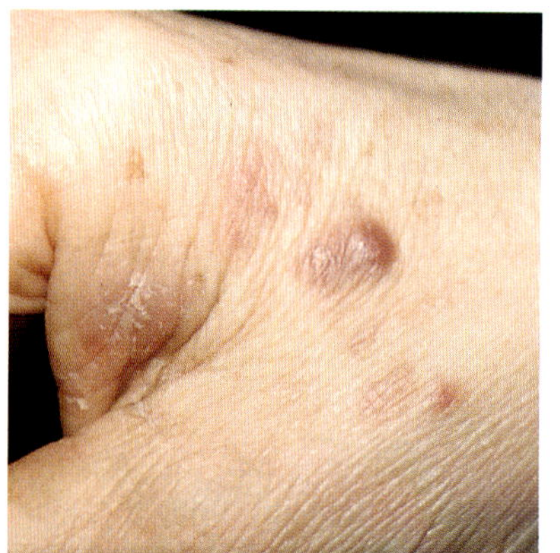

FIG. 43-15 *Macules and papules.*

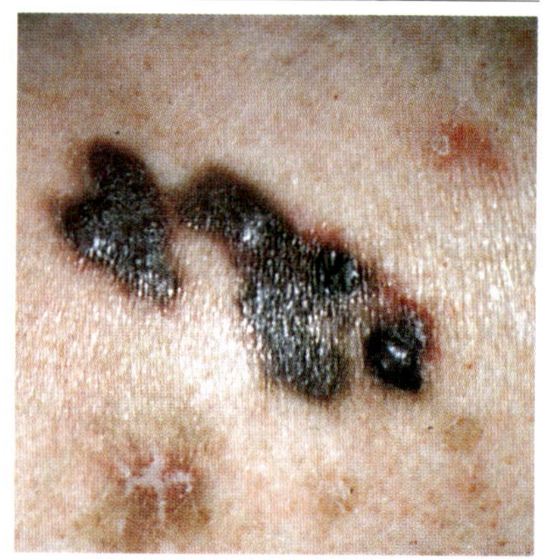

FIG. 43-16 *Plaque with peculiar geometric shape.*

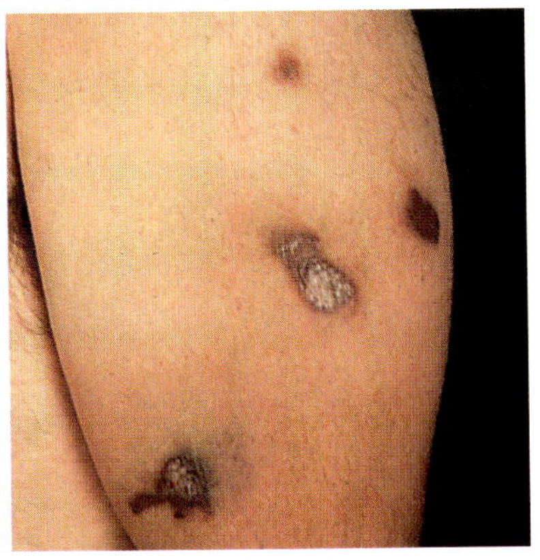

FIG. 43-17 *Papules and plaques, some keratotic.*

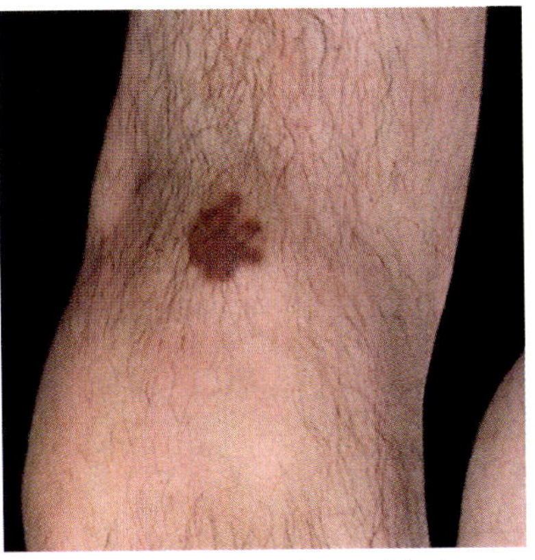

FIG. 43-18 *Plaque with a strikingly scalloped border.*

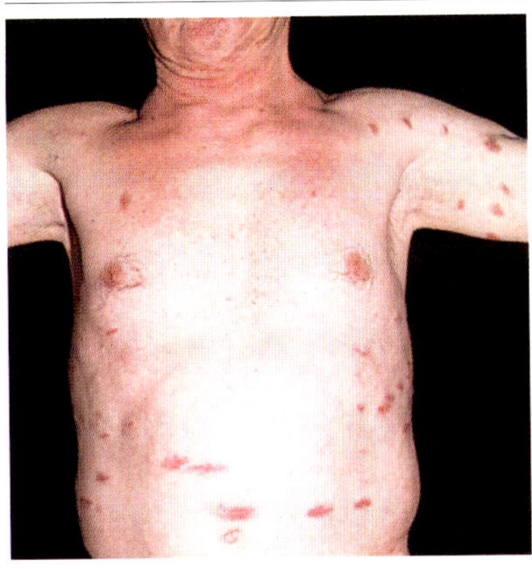
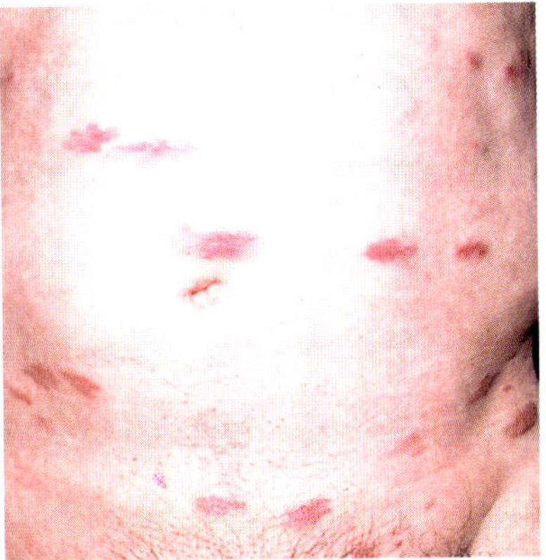

FIG. 43-19 (A, B) *Papules and plaques.*

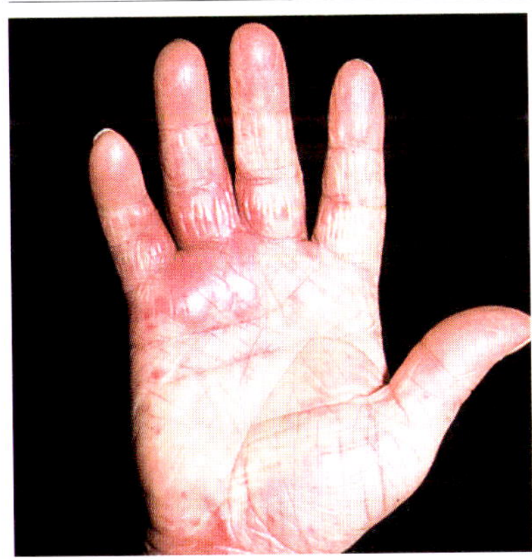

FIG. 43-20 *Papules and plaques.*

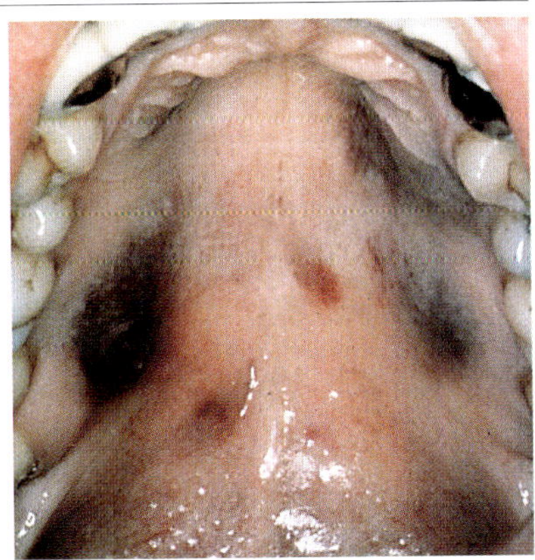

FIG. 43-21 *Macules and patches on the palate.*

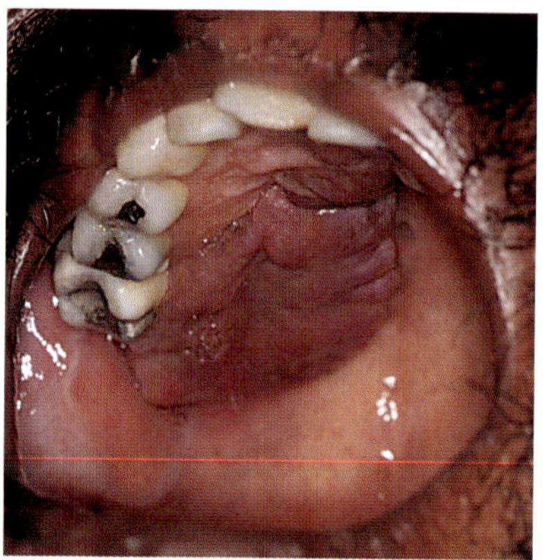

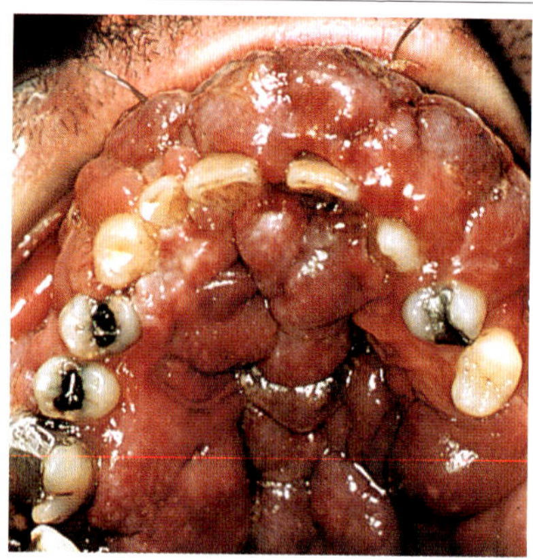

FIG. 43-22 *Tumor on the palate.*

FIG. 43-23 *A mass of nodules on the gingiva and the palate.*

COURSE In its stereotypical presentation, Kaposi's sarcoma, whether in southern Europeans or Ashkenazy Jews, in Africans, or in persons infected by HIV, progresses through stages. Lesions present themselves clinically in sequence, to wit, as macules and patches, papules and plaques, and nodules and tumors. Nodules and tumors of Kaposi's sarcoma may ulcerate. Some patients, however, have only macules and patches for many years; in others, lesions do not progress beyond the stage of papules and plaques. As a rule, the lesions of Kaposi's sarcoma persist and enlarge, at a pace that cannot be predicted. Furthermore, new lesions tend to appear. When, as sometimes happens, the immunologic status of a patient improves or a patient has been treated successfully with an anti-herpesvirus agent administered systemically, lesions of Kaposi's sarcoma may regress and even disappear.

INTEGRATION: UNIFYING CONCEPT The clinical and histopathologic findings of individual lesions of Kaposi's sarcoma are repeatable. Macules and patches consist of widely dilated, thin-walled blood vessels with jagged outlines that are situated around pre-existing venules of the superficial plexus, as well as of endothelial cells scattered as solitary units in the interstitium of the upper part of the reticular dermis. Patches and plaques of Kaposi's sarcoma are made up of a markedly increased number of thin-walled vessels like those present in macules and patches, but the newly-formed vessels are then present not only around venules of both the superficial and deep plexuses, but throughout the interstitium. Some endothelial cells are organized into incipient fascicles, and in some lesions those nascent fascicles may even be predominant. Erythrocytes are present in interstices between endothelial cells that make up fascicles. Nodules and tumors consist entirely of well-defined fascicles of spindle-shaped endothelial cells, the fascicles being arranged in a storiform pattern.

In short, Kaposi's sarcoma is the same morphologically in all populations affected by it, irrespective of cause. Human herpes simplex virus-8 has been identified in endothelial cells of Kaposi's sarcoma of all kinds, especially those with infection by HIV. All patients who develop Kaposi's sarcoma seem to be immunosuppressed and at increased risk for development of other proliferative processes, such as lymphomas.

Kaposi's sarcoma is not truly a sarcoma because it is not a malignant neoplasm, i.e., one that has the capability to kill by local destruction or by metastasis. Kaposi's sarcoma does neither. The lesions of Kaposi's sarcoma spring up, de novo, in many organs, where the changes progress in the same fashion as they do in macules and patches, papules and plaques, and nodules and tumors in the skin. Because the proliferation of endothelial cells in Kaposi's sarcoma may involute when the immunologic status of a patient improves, it is reasonable to classify Kaposi's sarcoma as a hyperplasia rather than as either a benign or malignant neoplastic process.

THERAPY A solitary lesion may be treated by excision, laser surgery, cryotherapy, or radiation therapy. Disease of internal organs is treated systemically with interferon alpha, antiretroviral drugs, or chemotherapy, for example, combinations of vinca alkaloids or combination chemotherapy.

DEFINITION Keratotic spikes that emerge from dilated ostia of follicles and are equidistant from one another. The term keratosis pilaris refers to the phenomenon when it presents itself without any distinct arrangement of individual lesions, whereas the designation lichen spinulosus is applied to the same lesions when they are arranged in a circle.

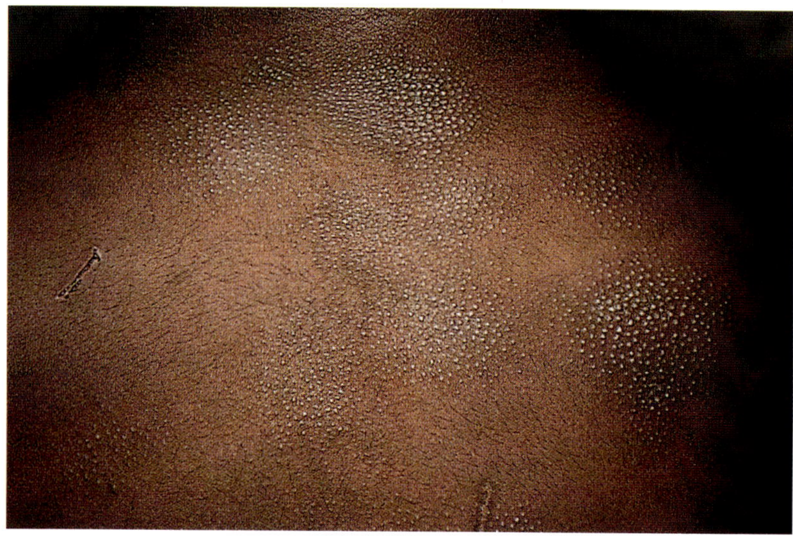

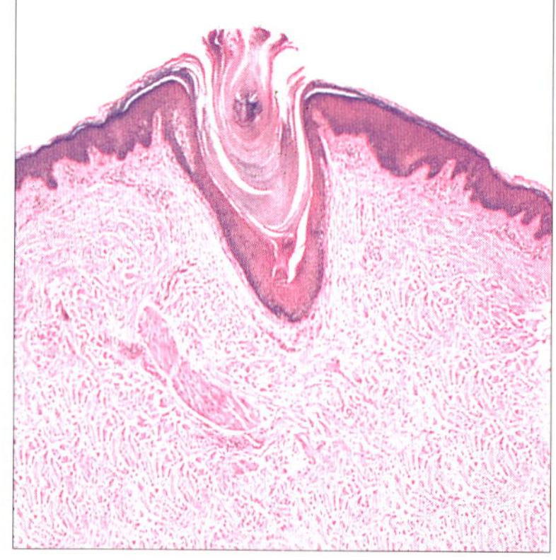

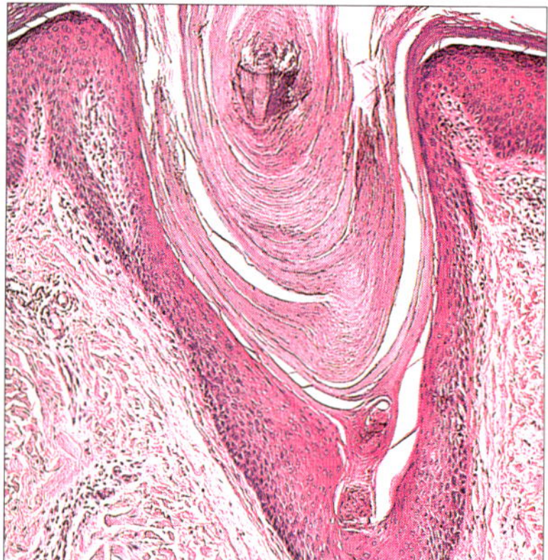

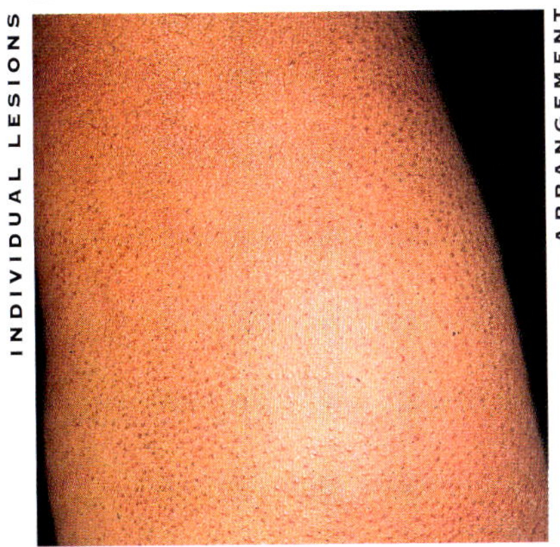

FIG. 44-1 *Closely-set tiny keratotic papules.*

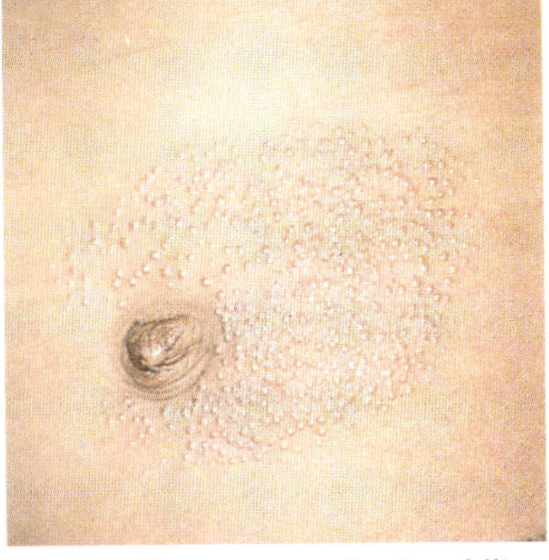

FIG. 44-2 *Keratoses emanating from follicular ostia and arranged in a nummular pattern on a pigmented base (lichen spinulosus).*

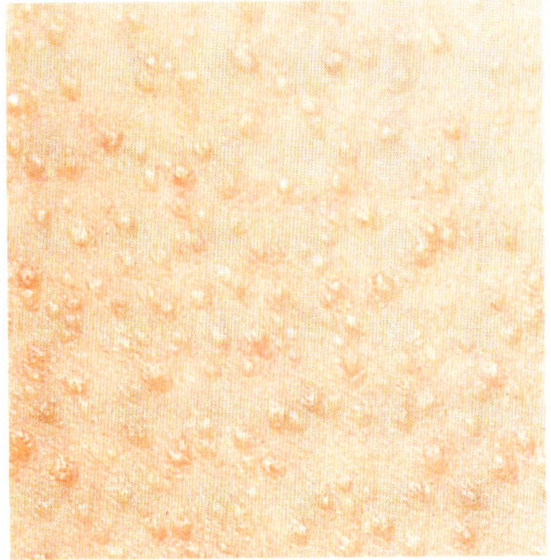

FIG. 44-3 *Widespread discrete papules (keratosis pilaris) more or less equidistant from one another.*

COURSE The keratotic spikes that project from infundibula slightly above the skin surface in keratosis pilaris/lichen spinulosus tend to persist for long periods of time, often years and sometimes for the lifetime of the person who bears them. New follicular keratoses may join those already extant.

INTEGRATION: UNIFYING CONCEPT Keratosis pilaris and lichen spinulosus are different names for the same pathologic process, the difference between them being only the manner in which lesions are arranged. In keratosis pilaris, the follicular keratoses tend to be present across a swath of skin, for example, the extensor surface of an arm or an entire trunk. In contrast, identical follicular keratoses of lichen spinulosus are arranged in a discrete circle. Each of the keratotic lesions of both conditions is characterized histopathologically by a plug of orthokeratotic corneocytes that fills and dilates an infundibulum. The apex of the plug of corneocytes protrudes just above the skin surface. When the plug causes a breach in the wall of an infundibulum, as happens episodically, an inflammatory process is set in motion, the result sometimes being parakeratotic cells within the infundibulum, and granulomas and even fibrosis around it.

A lesion of keratosis pilaris/lichen spinulosus differs from a comedo not only because the plug of corneocytes protrudes above the skin surface, but also because it is not accompanied by abundant sebaceous secretion and by numerous bacteria, yeasts, or mites.

Keratosis pilaris may appear in persons who have no other apparent abnormality, but it is common in persons who are atopic and in those with ichthyosis vulgaris.

THERAPY Lactic acid lotion or topical retinoids are beneficial.

DEFINITION An inflammatory disease caused by a trypanosome and that may involve skin and mucous membranes, as well as internal organs.

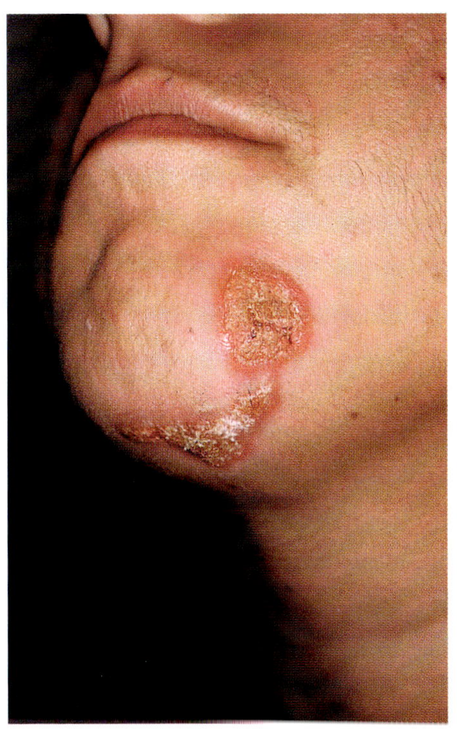

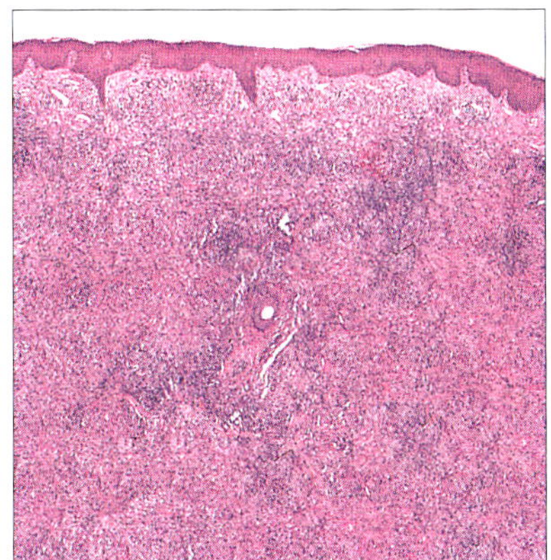

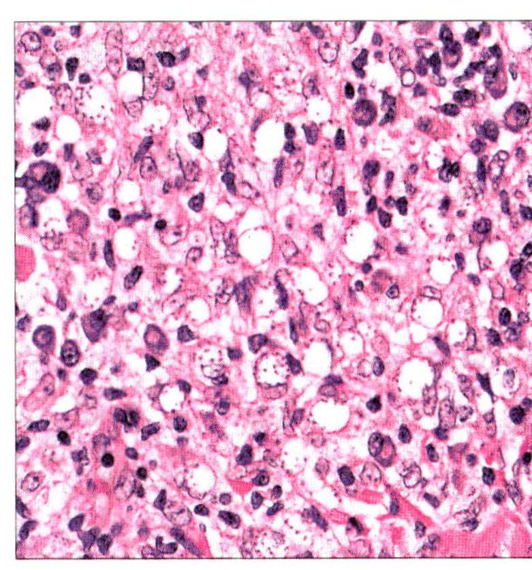

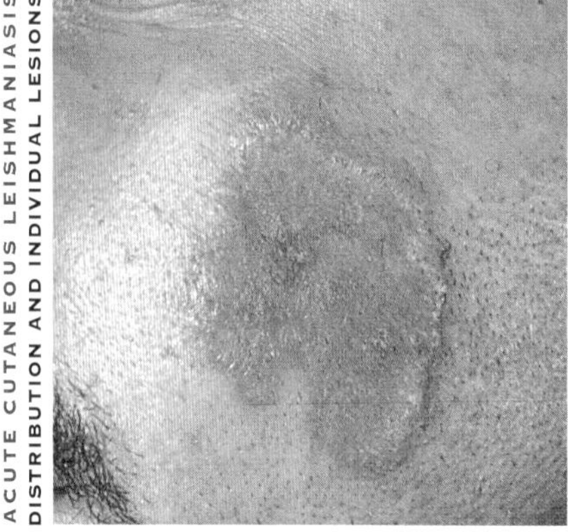

FIG. 45-1 *Plaque with distinctly elevated border on one side and no border on the other as a consequence of healing.*

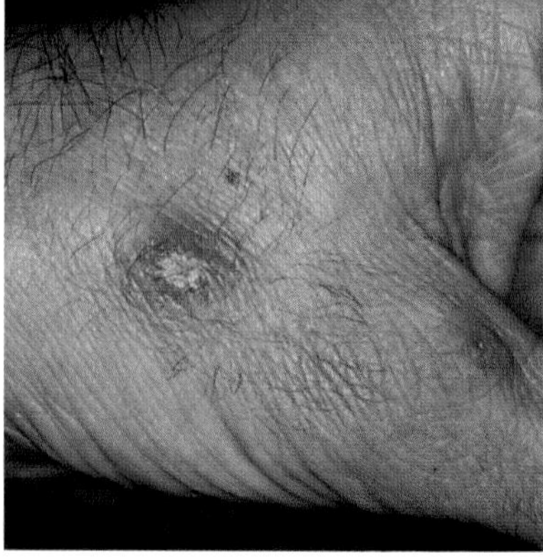

FIG. 45-2 *Crusted papule of acute cutaneous leishmaniasis.*

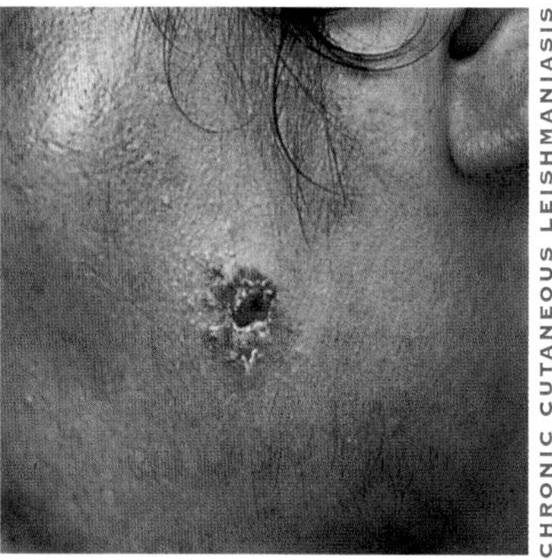

FIG. 45-3 *Papules around a crusted ulcer of acute cutaneous leishmaniasis.*

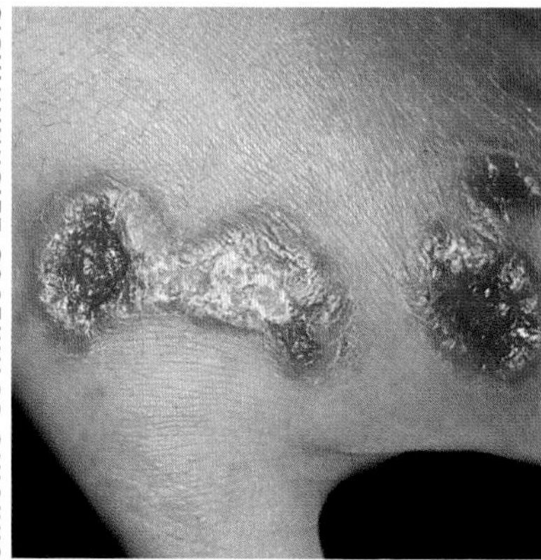

FIG. 45-4 *Scaly and ulcerated plaques of chronic cutaneous leishmaniasis.*

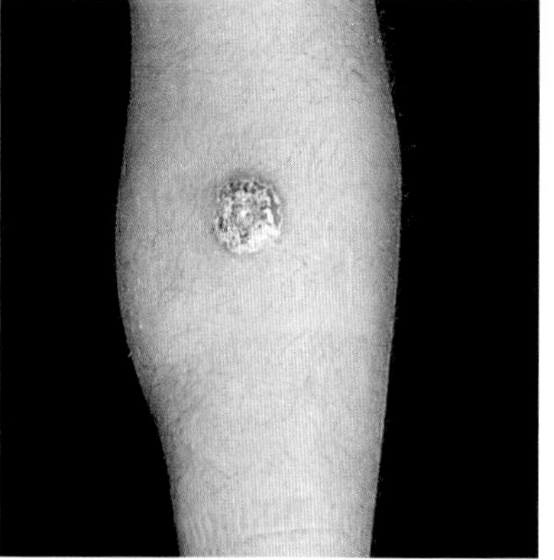

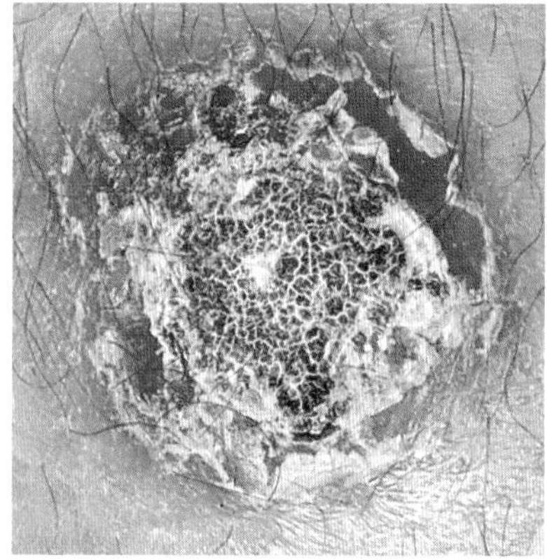

FIG. 45-5 (A, B) *A scaly plaque of chronic cutaneous leishmaniasis.*

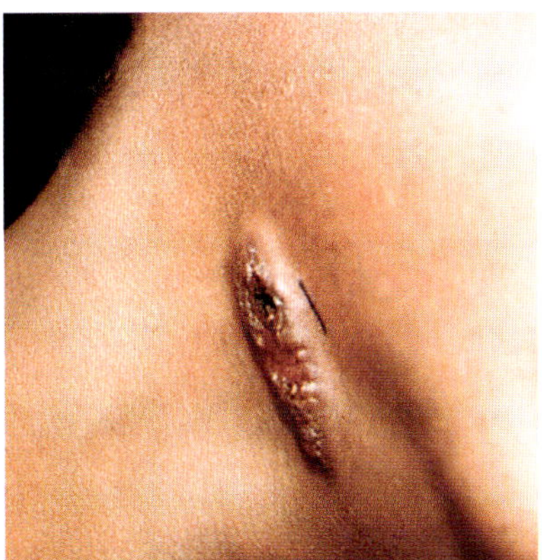

FIG. 45-6 *Linear ulcerated plaque covered by scales of chronic cutaneous leishmaniasis.*

ADJUNCTIVE DIAGNOSTIC TESTS Smears of tissue from lesions may be scoured by conventional microscopy in order to detect parasites. Those organisms also can be cultured. For specific identification of various species of leishmania, polymerase chain reaction may be useful.

COURSE The duration of a lesion of leishmaniasis varies according to the manifestation of the disease. For example, the ulcerated papule or nodule of Oriental sore usually heals in months with a scar, whereas that of the mucocutaneous type involutes more slowly, resolution being over years and also with scar. When a lesion of acute cutaneous leishmaniasis persists, it involutes in the center as an atrophic scar as new papules appear at the periphery of the scar. The process persists in that same fashion for decades.

INTEGRATION: UNIFYING CONCEPT There are four basic types of leishmaniasis, but only three are associated with skin lesions, namely, cutaneous leishmaniasis (acute and chronic), mucocutaneous leishmaniasis, and disseminated anergic cutaneous leishmaniasis. Visceral leishmaniasis, known also as kala-azar, is not associated with disease of the skin. The papules and nodules of acute cutaneous leishmaniasis, mucocutaneous leishmaniasis, and disseminated anergic cutaneous leishmaniasis are made up of dense, diffuse, dermal infiltrates of macrophages that, in sections stained by hematoxylin and eosin, are seen to contain innumerable gray-blue dots—the trypanosomes—within their cytoplasm. After many years, lesions of cutaneous leishmaniasis, considered at that stage to be chronic, come to resemble lupus vulgaris, clinically and histopathologically. Atrophic scars are surrounded by papules composed of collections of epithelioid histiocytes that are surrounded by numerous lymphocytes (tuberculoid granulomas).

The morphologic expression of leishmaniasis depends on a combination of the particular trypanosome responsible for the lesion and on the immunologic status of the host. The situation is analogous to that of leprosy. Acute cutaneous leishmaniasis is equivalent to lepromatous leprosy, disseminated anergic cutaneous leishmaniasis to diffuse lepromatous leprosy, and chronic cutaneous leishmaniasis to tuberculoid leprosy.

THERAPY Small lesions may be excised, subjected to cryotherapy, or injected with antimonials (Pentostam). They also may be treated systemically with ketoconazole or dapsone taken orally.

Widespread or systemic disease must be managed with Pentostam or amphotericin-B encapsulated in liposomes.

DEFINITION An inflammatory disease caused by Mycobacterium leprae. It can involve internal organs or be localized to the skin, where its clinical presentation is dependent on the immunologic status of the host. Persons who are competent immunologically have patches or plaques of tuberculoid leprosy, whereas those who are immunologically incompetent have nodules and tumors of lepromatous leprosy. When features of both tuberculoid and lepromatous leprosy are present together in one person, the disease is designated "borderline" or "dimorphous" leprosy. Early in the course, i.e., before it is yet apparent whether the disease will be tuberculoid or lepromatous, lesions present themselves as hypopigmented patches known properly as those of "indeterminate" leprosy.

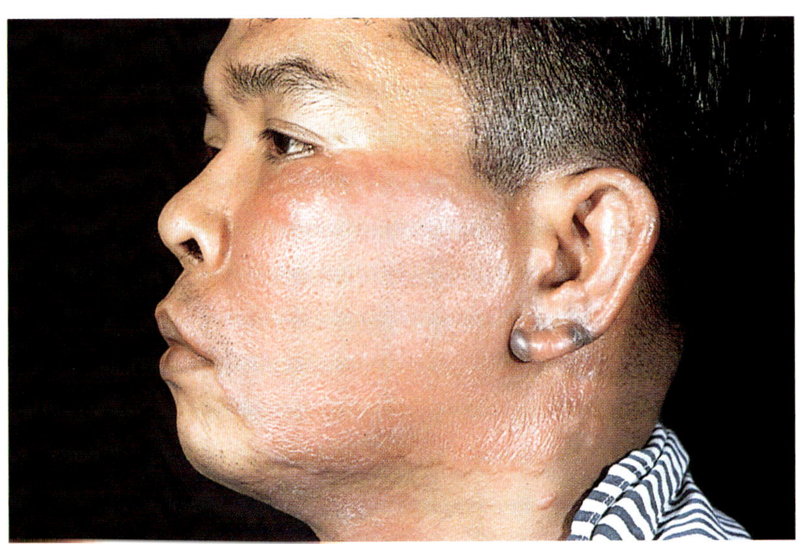

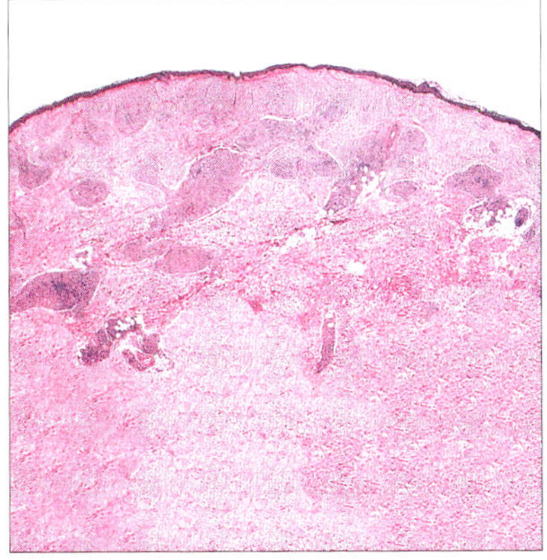

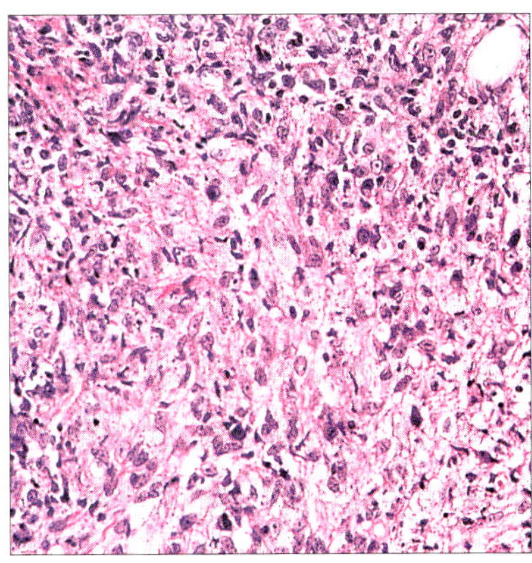

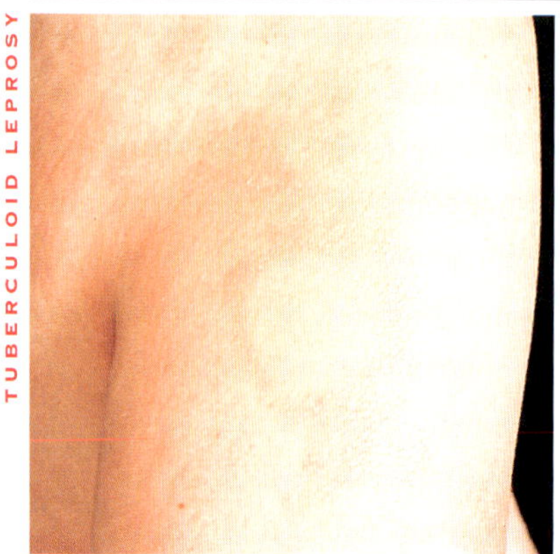

FIG. 46-1 *Slightly elevated plaques of tuberculoid leprosy, one of which is annular.*

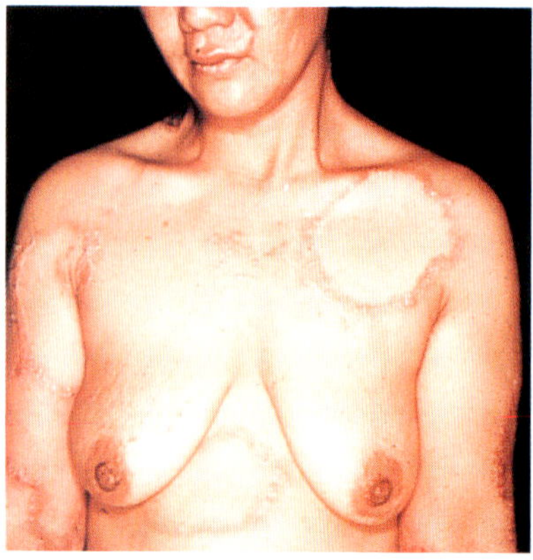

FIG. 46-2 *Annular plaques of tuberculoid leprosy with a hypopigmented center and hyperpigmented border.*

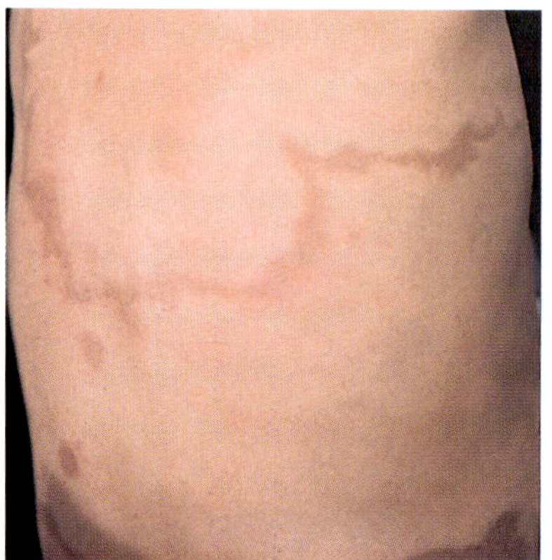

FIG. 46-3 *Plaques with serpentine outlines of borderline tuberculoid leprosy.*

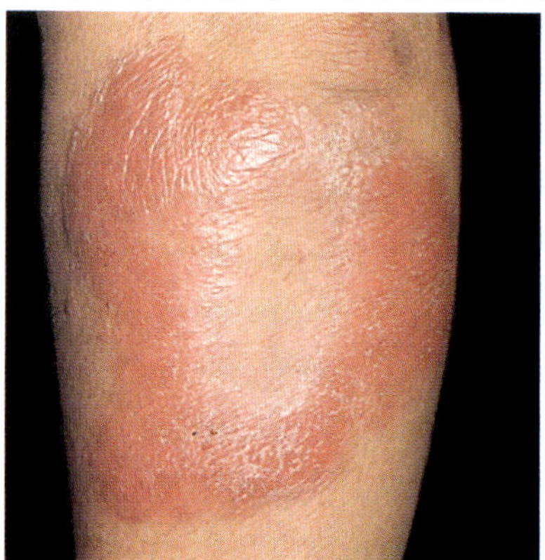

FIG. 46-4 *Smooth-surfaced plaque of tuberculoid leprosy.*

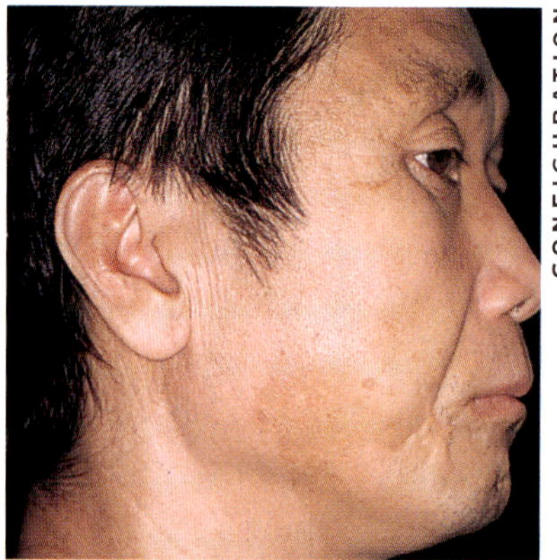

FIG. 46-5 *Hypopigmented macules in confluence (patches) of tuberculoid leprosy.*

CONFIGURATION

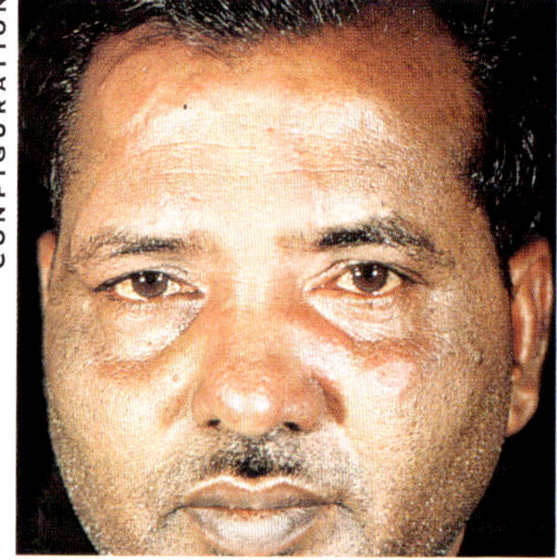

FIG. 46-6 *Annular plaques of tuberculoid leprosy.*

LEPROMATOUS LEPROSY

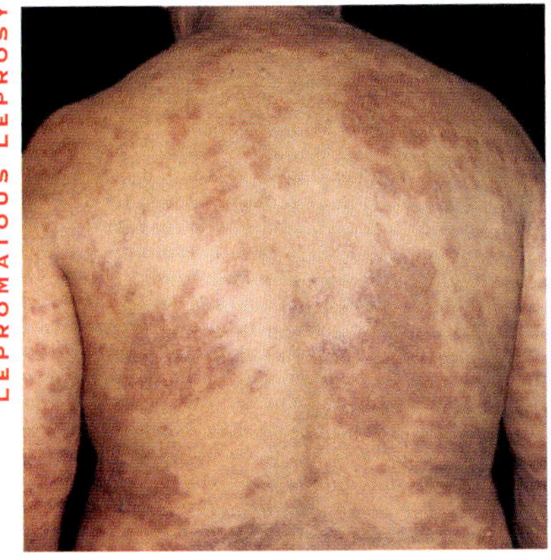

FIG. 46-7 *Papules and plaques of borderline lepromatous leprosy.*

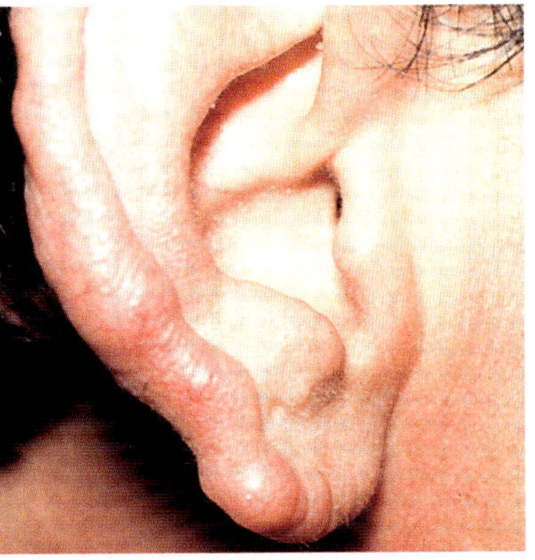

FIG. 46-8 *Papules of lepromatous leprosy.*

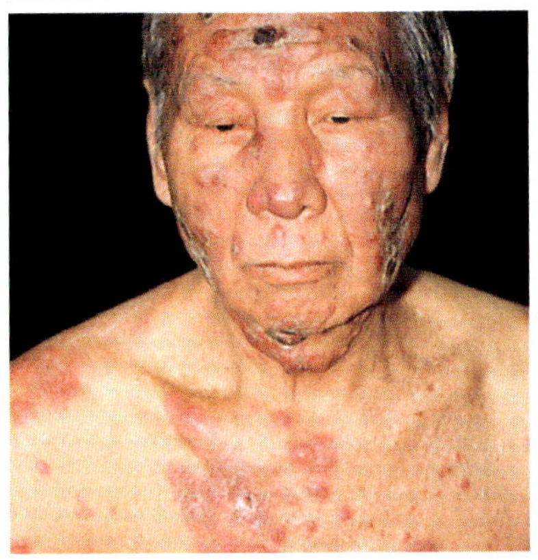

FIG. 46-9 *Crusted papules and plaques of lepromatous leprosy.*

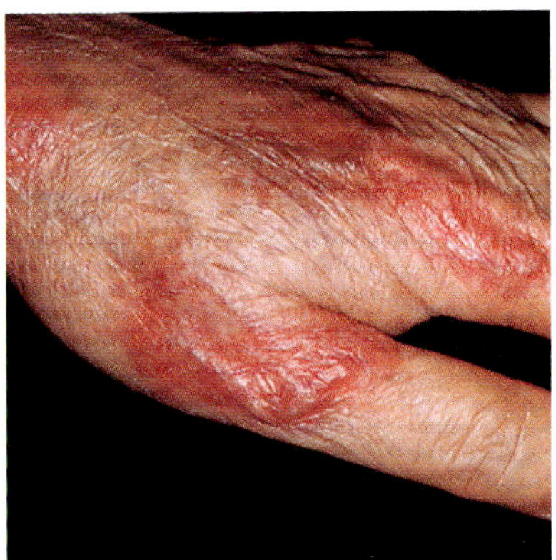

FIG. 46-10 *Plaques of lepromatous leprosy.*

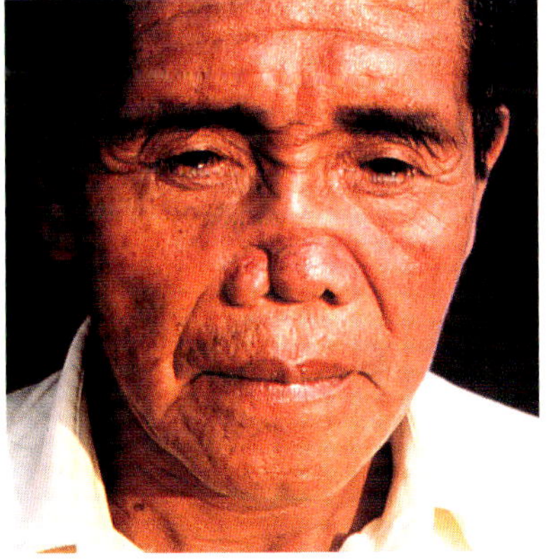

FIG. 46-11 *Destruction of nasal cartilage ("saddle nose") with hints of "leonine facies" of diffuse lepromatous leprosy.*

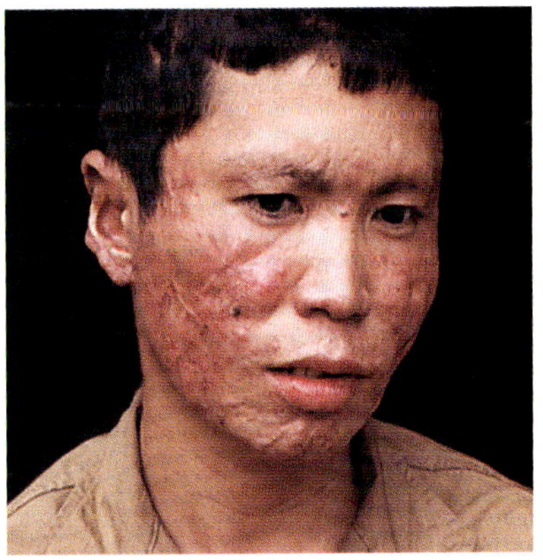

FIG. 46-12 *Nodules and plaques of lepromatous leprosy.*

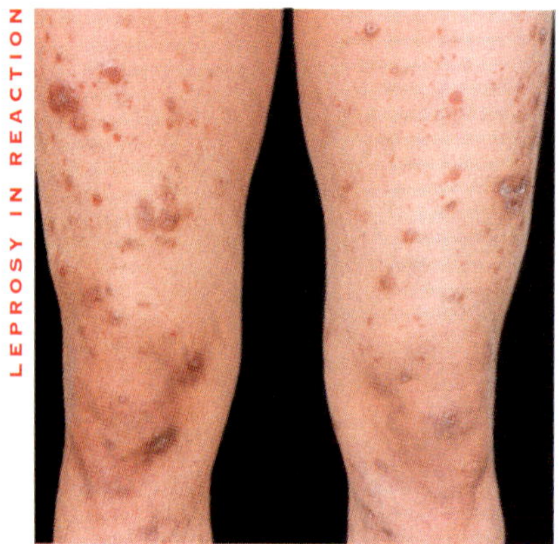

FIG. 46-13 *Papules, nodules, and plaques of lepromatous leprosy are red when leprosy is in reaction.*

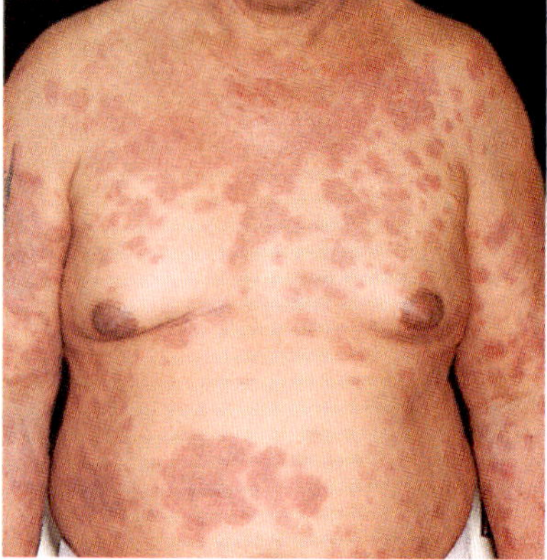

FIG. 46-14 *Confluent red patches and plaques of lepromatous leprosy in reaction.*

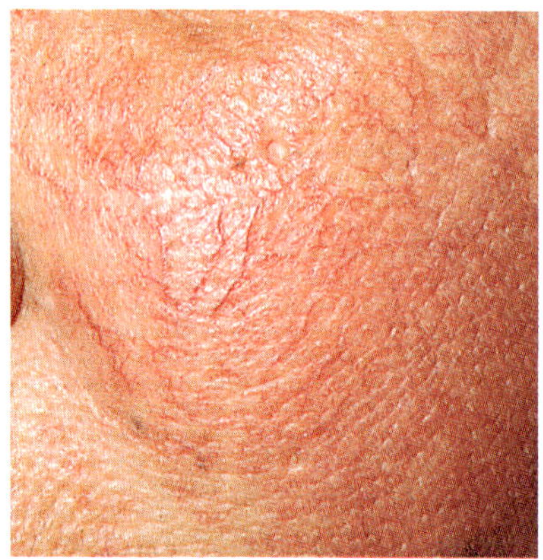

FIG. 46-15 *Plaque with erythema in leprosy in reaction.*

ADJUNCTIVE DIAGNOSTIC TESTS "Slit skin smears" and either Ziehl-Neelson or Fite-Farraco stains of tissue sections enable organisms, when they are present, to be detected by conventional microscopy.

COURSE Lesions of leprosy of all types tend to persist for many years. Macules tend to enlarge to become patches and plaques, and papules are given to eventuate in nodules and tumors. The usual course of leprosy of both lepromatous and tuberculoid types is sometimes interrupted by volcanic exacerbations known as "leprosy in reaction." In that circumstance, lesions already present become red and swollen.

INTEGRATION: UNIFYING CONCEPT Lesions of leprosy of all types represent infection by Mycobacterium leprae. How the disease expresses itself morphologically depends on the immunologic status of the individual infected. Patients with lepromatous leprosy are wholly unable to mount an immune response to the bacilli, thereby permitting them to proliferate wildly, whereas those with tuberculoid leprosy can mobilize an effective cell-mediated immune response to the organisms, which results in the eventual killing of them.

In general, papules, nodules, and tumors of lepromatous leprosy consist of nodular and diffuse infiltrates of foamy histiocytes within the dermis. Those foam cells, known historically as Virchow cells, come into being as a consequence of the ingestion by macrophages of myriad acid-fast leprae bacilli whose cell membrane is replete with lipid, thereby giving the cytoplasm a foamy appearance that in sections stained by hematoxylin and eosin exhibits a gray-blue cast. Unfortunately, for the most part, the macrophages are incapable of killing the organisms.

Specialized stains for acid-fast organisms, such as that devised by Fite, reveal innumerable bacilli in the cytoplasm of foamy macrophages. By contrast, plaques of tuberculoid leprosy are made up of clusters of epithelioid histiocytes (granulomas) surrounded by large numbers of lymphocytes (tuberculoid granulomas). Patients with dimorphous leprosy, as the name implies, have lesions that exhibit histopathologic findings of both lepromatous and tuberculoid leprosy. Macules and patches of indeterminate leprosy consist only of sparse superficial and deep perivascular and periadnexal infiltrates of lymphocytes and some histiocytes. A clue to diagnosis by conventional microscopy of indeterminate leprosy is the presence of mononuclear cells within cutaneous nerves, a finding shared by other types of leprosy and one responsible for neurologic defects associated with the disease.

Both diffuse lepromatous leprosy and tuberculoid leprosy may be associated with an explosive inflammatory response, leprosy in reaction, that imposes itself on the basic granulomatous process. Leprosy in reaction represents a tilt in immunologic balance in favor of the bacilli, rather than of the host. The major expressions of leprosy in reaction occur in persons with diffuse lepromatous leprosy and are termed "erythema nodosum leprosum" and "Lucio's phenomenon." Those reactions occur within lesions of diffuse lepromatous leprosy as a consequence of vasculitis affecting venules. If the vasculitis is sufficiently fulminant, as usually is the case in Lucio's phenomenon, ulceration is inevitable and the ulcers often are deep. Lesions of tuberculoid leprosy also may exacerbate floridly as a consequence of a patient being "in reaction."

THERAPY

Paucibacillary: Dapsone plus rifampin for one year.

Multibacillary: Dapsone plus rifampin plus clofazimine.

DEFINITION A granulomatous inflammatory process characterized clinically by closely-set, tiny, hypopigmented papules that have a predilection for
the trunk, dorsa of the hands and sides of the finger, and the penis of children
and young adults especially.

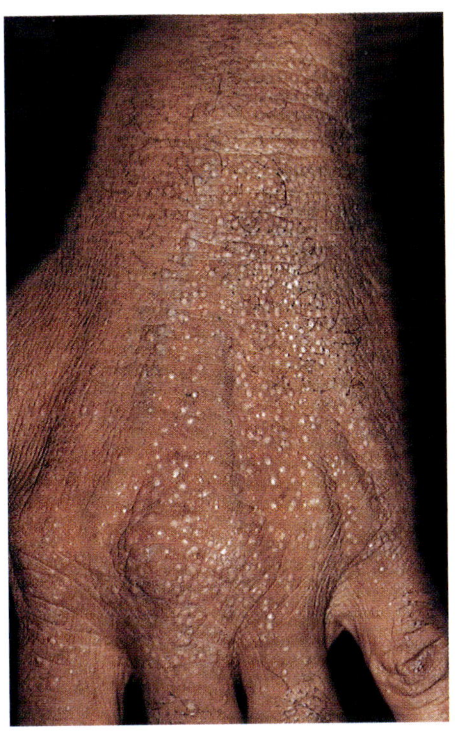

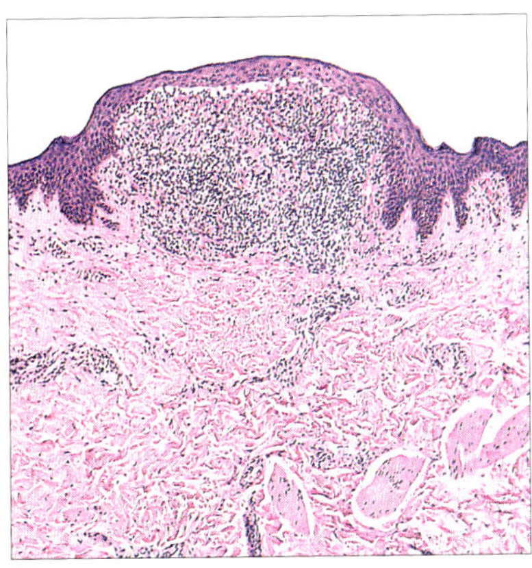

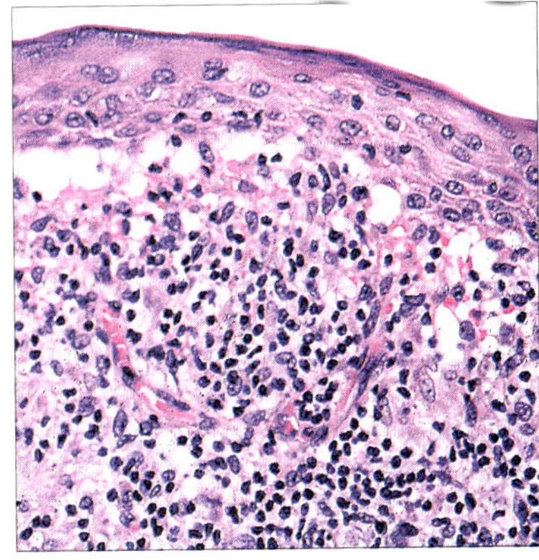

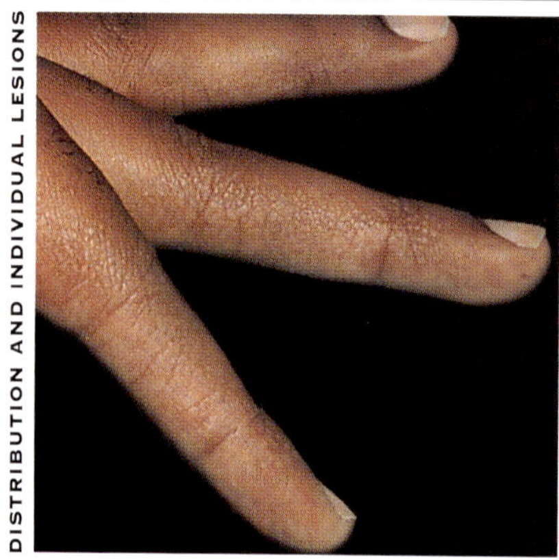

FIG. 47-1 *Closely-set tiny papules.*

FIG. 47-2 *Closely-set, smooth-surfaced, tiny papules nearly equidistant from one another in a line (Kobener phenomenon).*

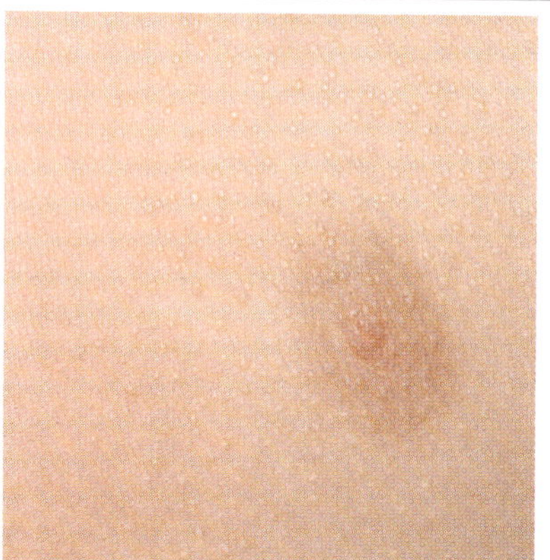

FIG. 47-3 *Discrete monomorphous papules.*

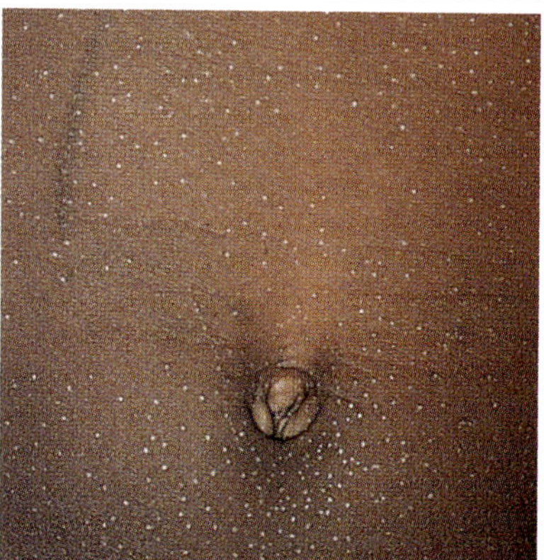

FIG. 47-4 *Tiny papules of relatively uniform size and shape.*

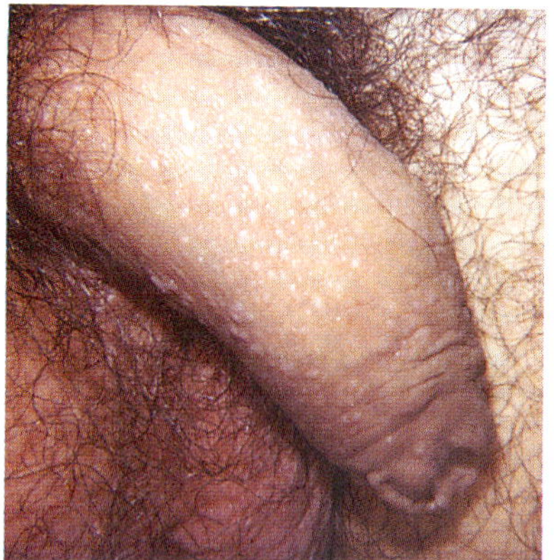

FIG. 47-5 *Tiny uniform papules.*

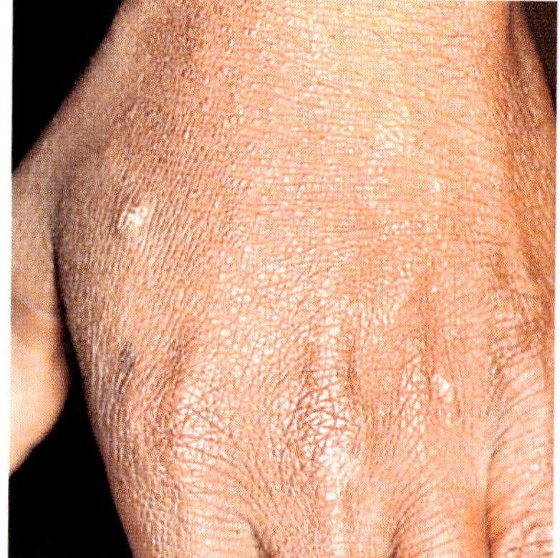

FIG. 47-6 *Tiny monomorphous papules set close to one another in groups.*

COURSE Papules of lichen nitidus erupt together at more or less the same time, last for many months or even a very few years, and gradually disappear. The course of the disease parallels that of the lesions themselves.

INTEGRATION: UNIFYING CONCEPT Lichen nitidus is a distinctive process that, contrary to old notions, is completely unrelated to lichen planus. Papules of lichen nitidus consist first of minute lichenoid infiltrates of lymphocytes confined to a single dermal papilla or to several contiguous papillae. In the course of weeks, the lymphocytes are joined by epithelioid histiocytes, and, in the ensuing weeks, those histiocytes, some of them multinucleate, come to predominate overwhelmingly. In short, lichen nitidus, unlike lichen planus, is a distinctive granulomatous dermatitis. When the surface of a papule of lichen nitidus is smooth, it is because corneocytes in the stratum corneum are orthokeratotic and arranged in basket-woven or laminated fashion. When the surface is covered by slight scale, it is because the corneocytes are parakeratotic.

The cause of lichen nitidus is not known.

THERAPY No treatment is necessary, but if a patient or the parents of a patient desire something be done, topical corticosteroids may be applied with slight benefit.

DEFINITION An inflammatory process consisting usually of violaceous papules that have a polygonal outline and flat top, and that tends to favor flexural surfaces of skin and the buccal mucosa of the oral cavity. It sometimes affects follicles and nail units as well.

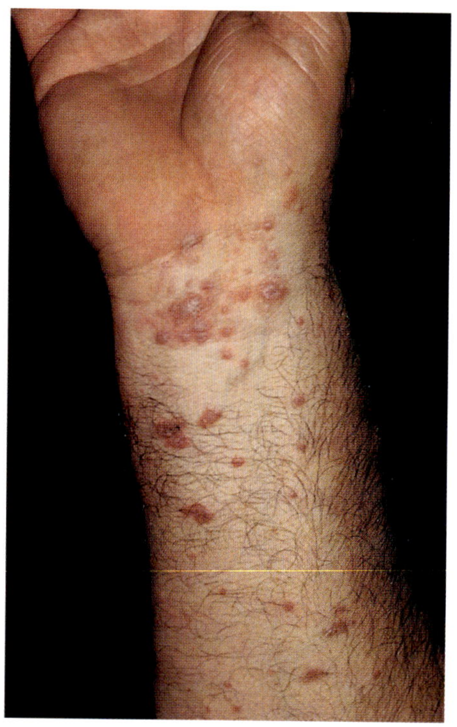

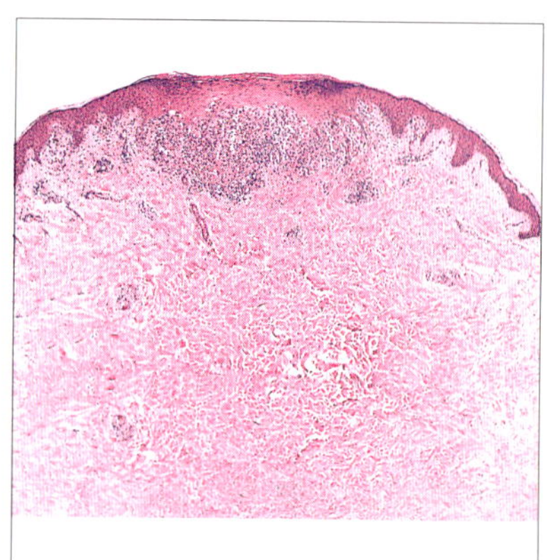

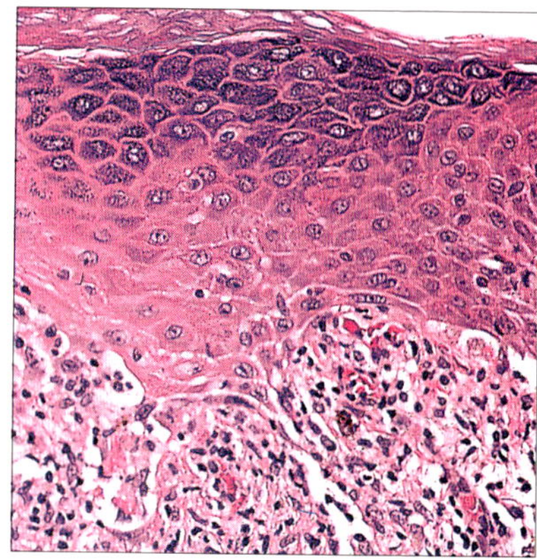

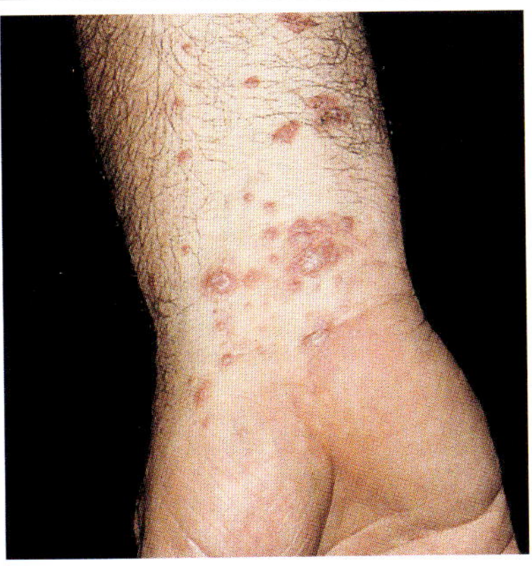

FIG. 48-1 *Keratotic papules, some of which have become confluent.*

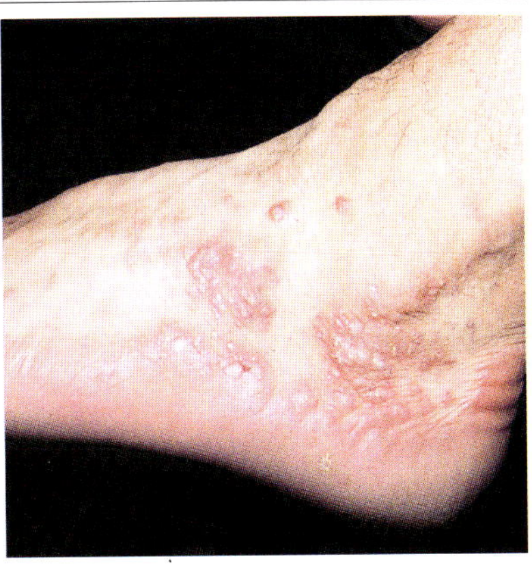

FIG. 48-2 *Keratotic papules and plaques.*

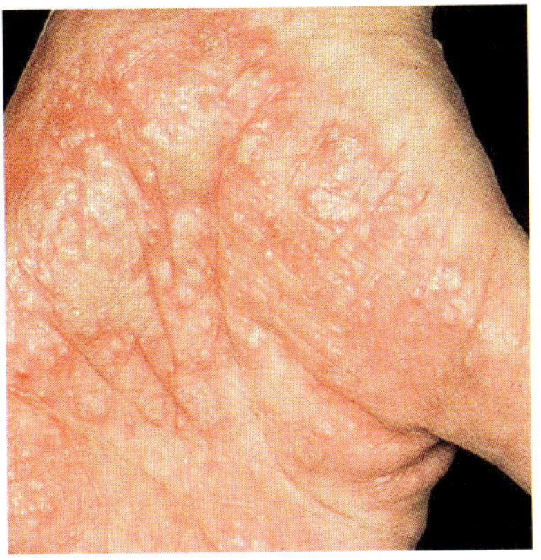

FIG. 48-3 *Papules and plaques.*

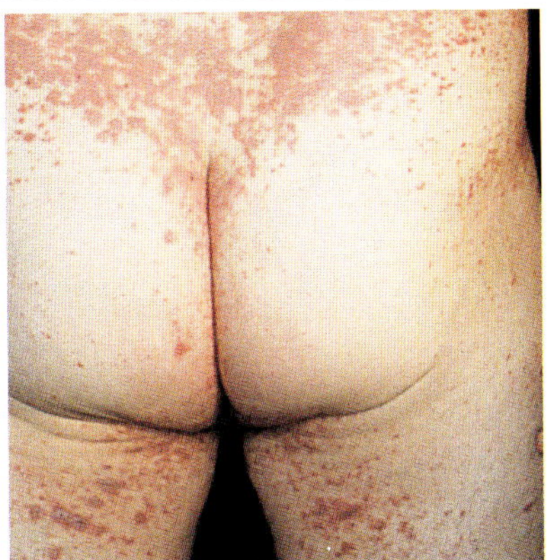

FIG. 48-4 *Discrete papules and plaques that have become confluent.*

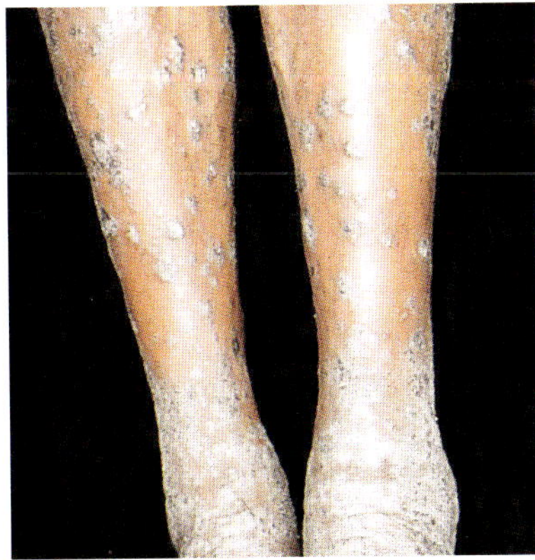

FIG. 48-5 *Papules and numerous plaques, some of which have become confluent.*

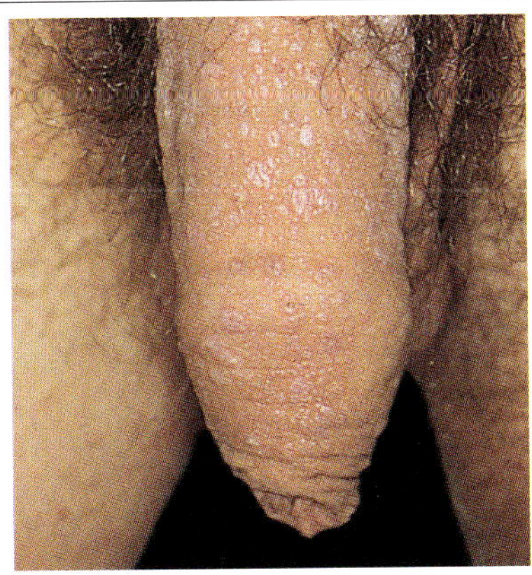

FIG. 48-6 *Papules, some of them annular.*

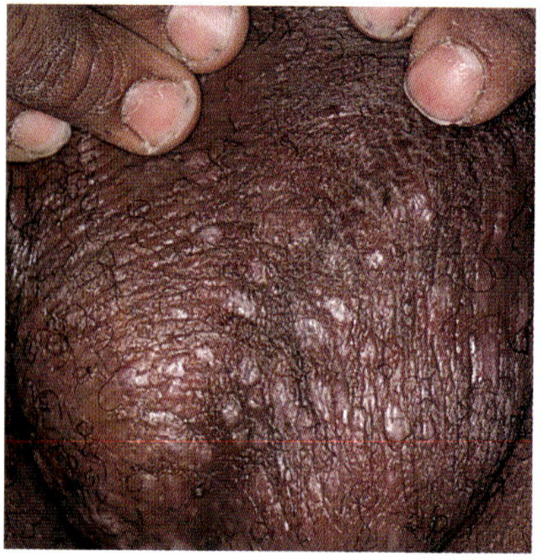

FIG. 48-7 *Lichenoid papules.*

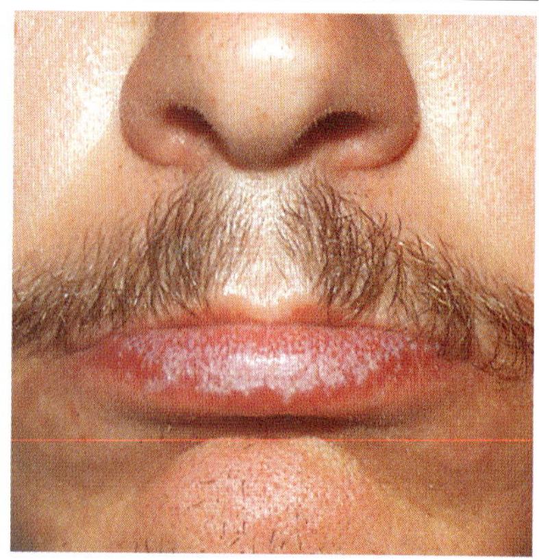

FIG. 48-8 *Papules on the lower lip, many of them having become confluent.*

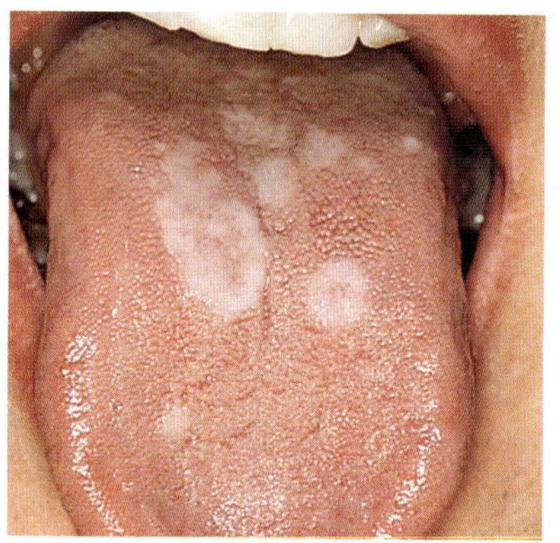

FIG. 48-9 *Papules and a plaque on the tongue.*

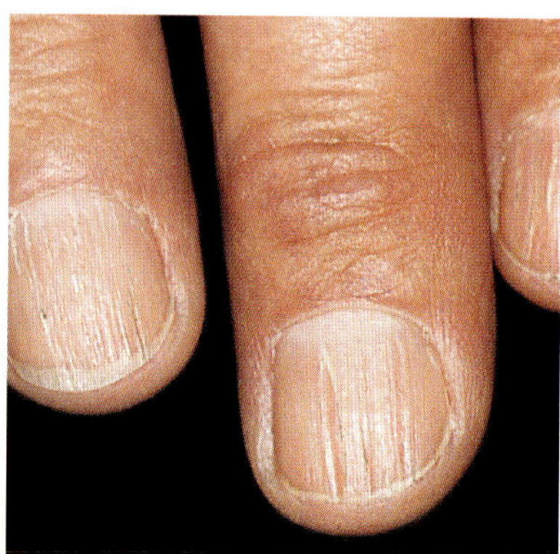

FIG. 48-10 *Longitudinal ridges of the nails.*

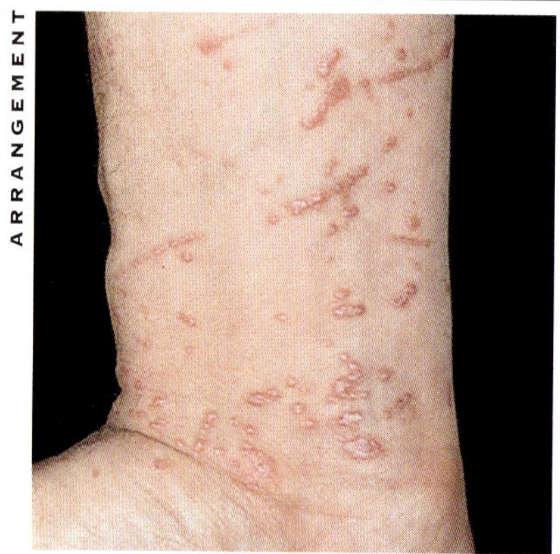

FIG. 48-11 *Papules, many of them in linear array, secondary to trauma (Koebner phenomenon).*

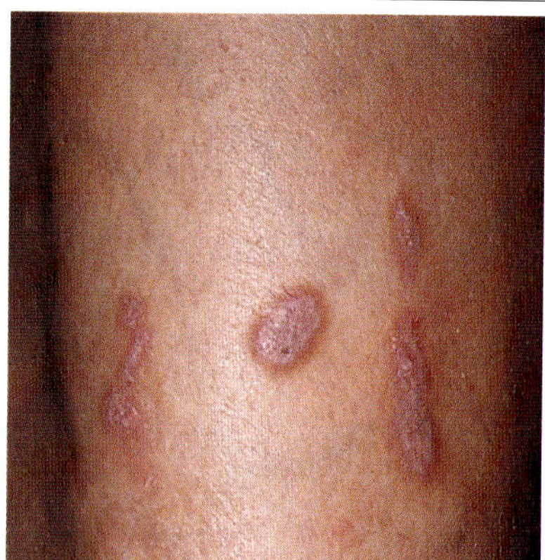

FIG. 48-12 *Papules, some of them arranged in a line.*

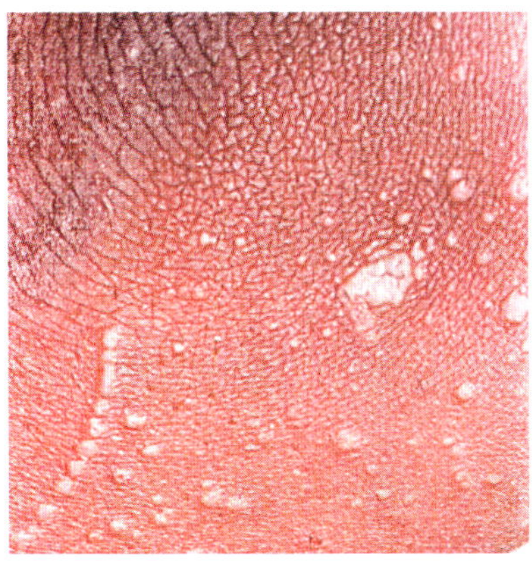

FIG. 48-13 *Papules arranged in a line (Koebner phenomenon).*

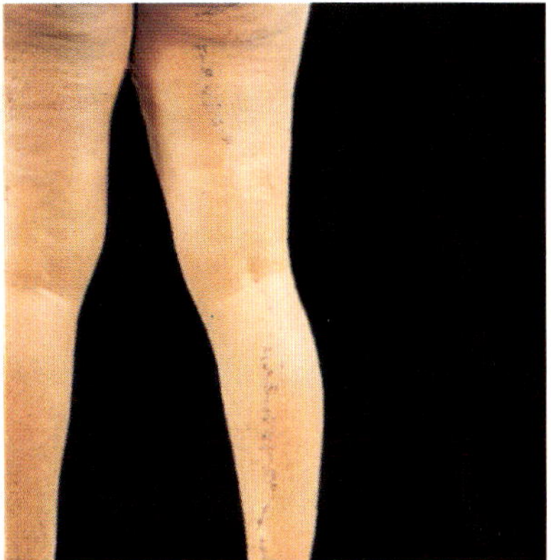

FIG. 48-14 *Flat-surfaced violaceous papules in linear arrangement (linear lichen planus).*

CONFIGURATION

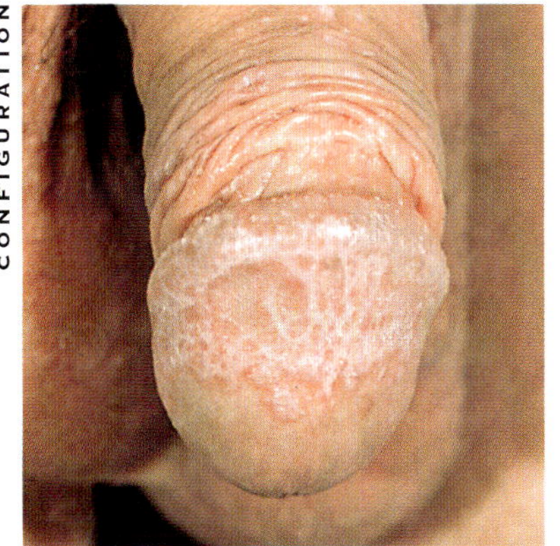

FIG. 48-15 *Reticulated pattern.*

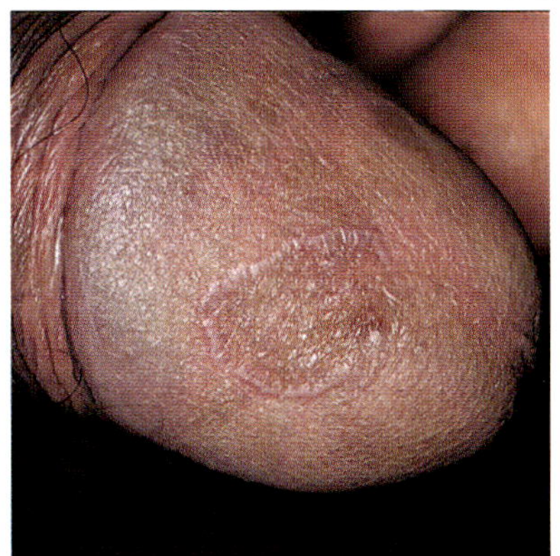

FIG. 48-16 *An annulus with a raised rim and a hyperpigmented center.*

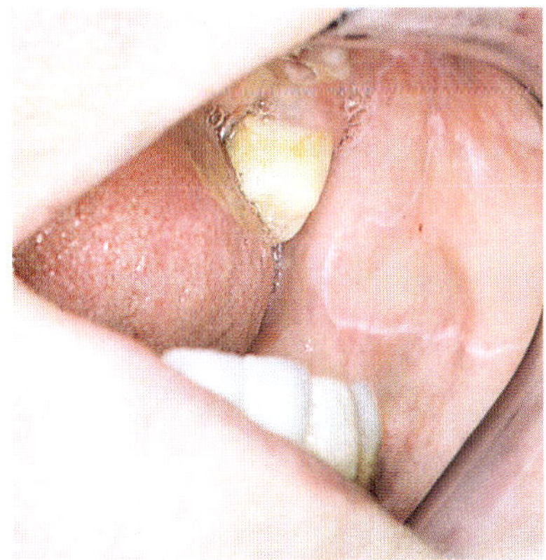

FIG. 48-17 *Annular lesion on the buccal mucosa.*

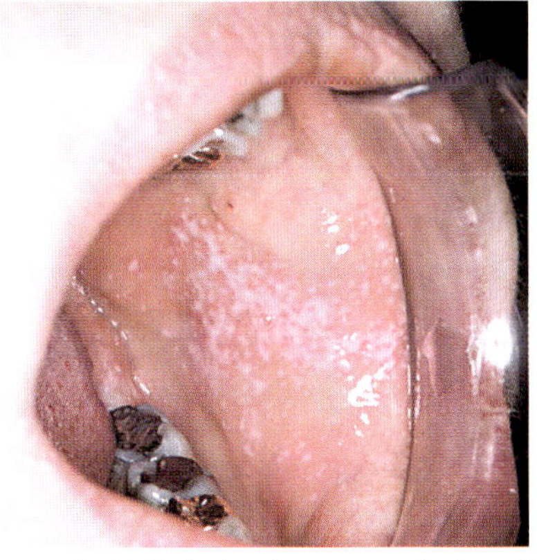

FIG. 48-18 *Reticulated pattern on the buccal mucosa.*

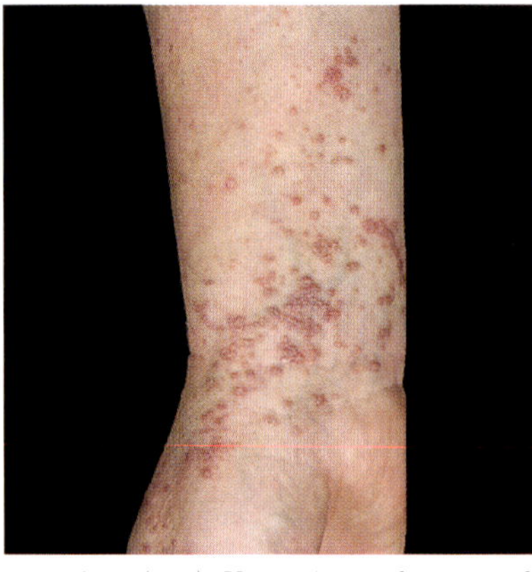 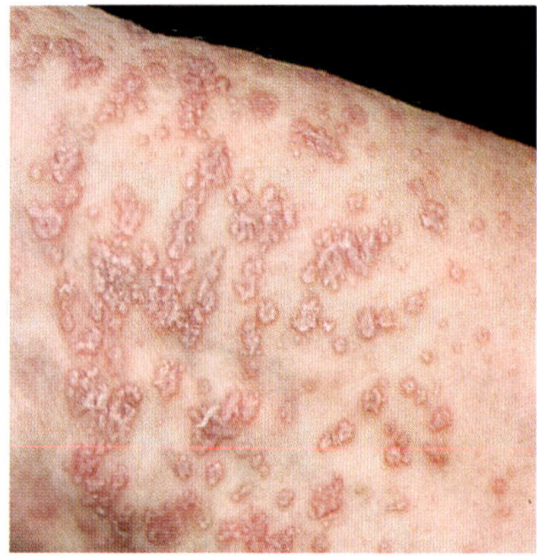

FIG. 48-19 (A, B) *Keratotic papules, some of which have become confluent to form vague outlines of rings and lines.*

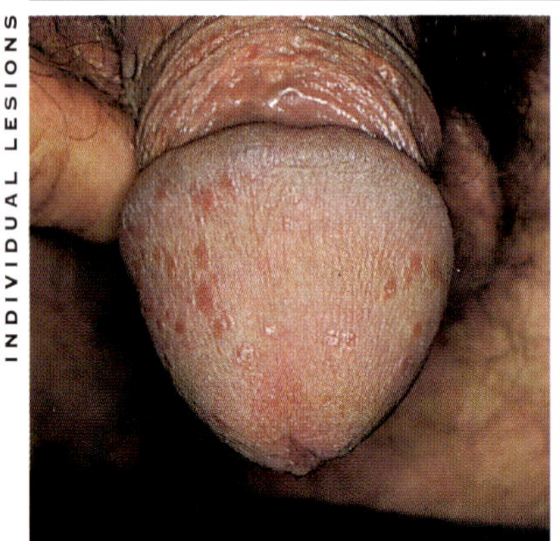 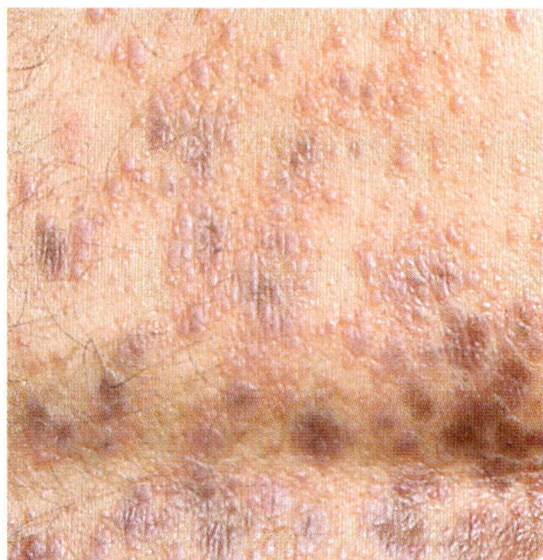

FIG. 48-20 *Subtle papules, some of them shiny.*

FIG. 48-21 *Nonkeratotic papules, some of which are darkly pigmented.*

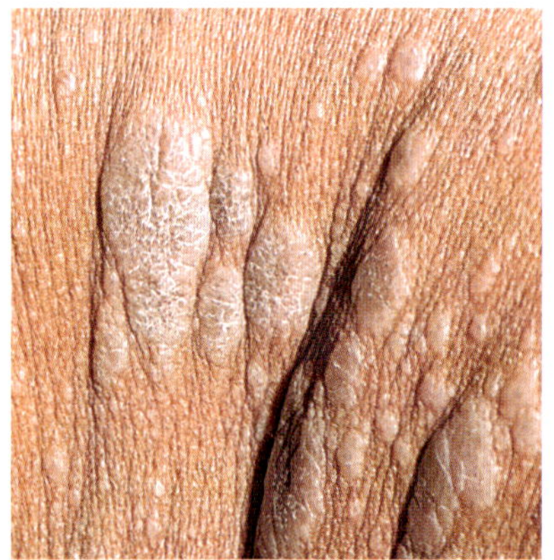 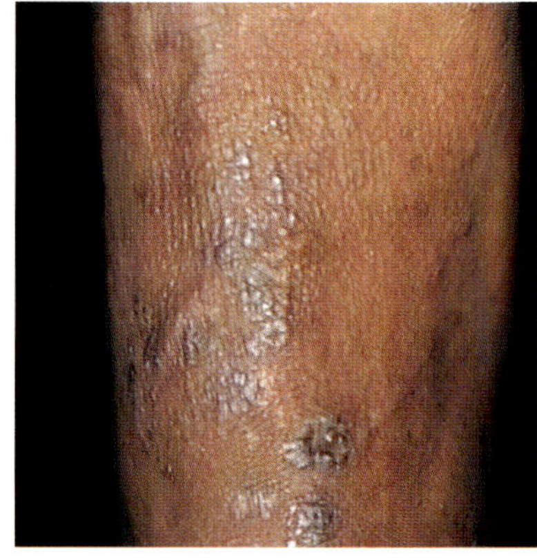

FIG. 48-22 *Discrete papules and plaques are variably keratotic.*

FIG. 48-23 *Lichenoid papules, some of them annular.*

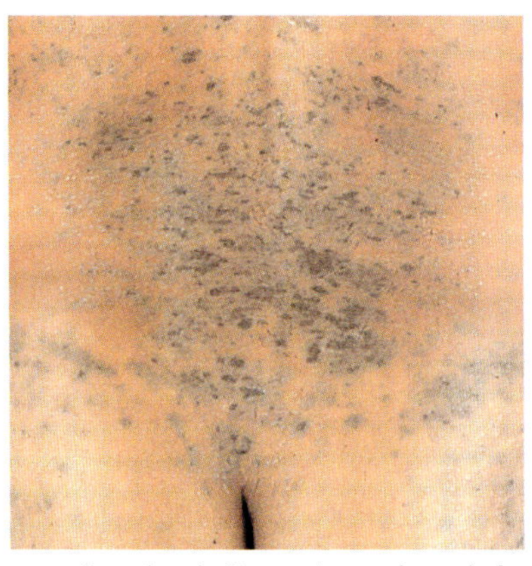
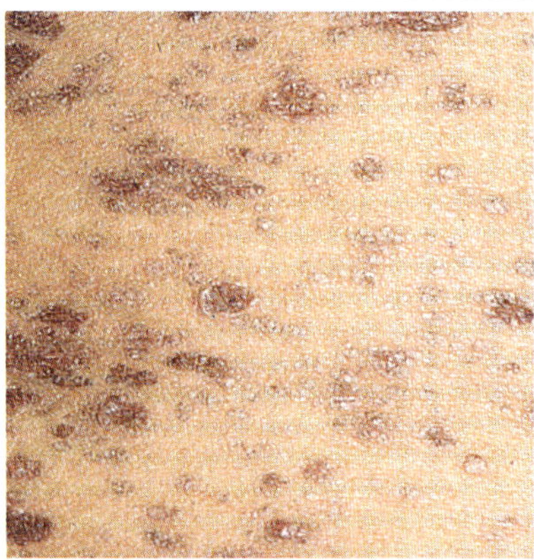

FIG. 48-24 (A, B) *Keratotic papules and plaques.*

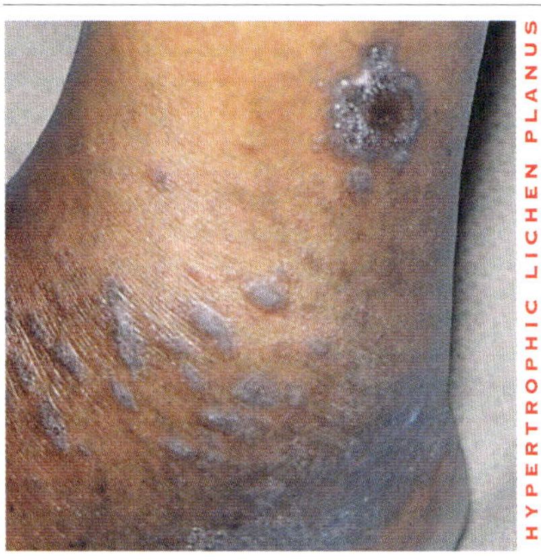
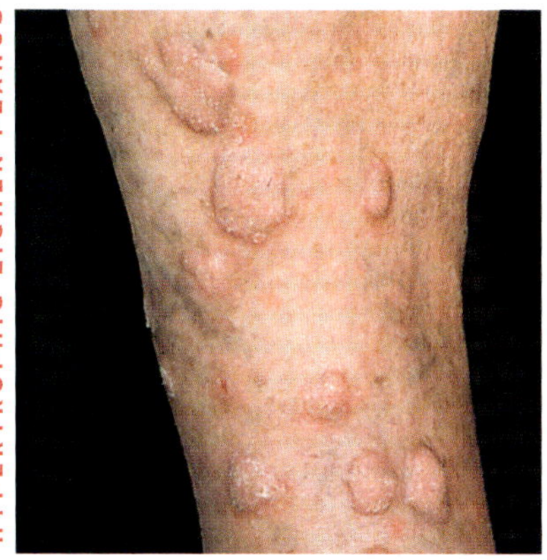

FIG. 48-25 *Pigmented, slightly keratotic papules and plaques.*

FIG. 48-26 *Markedly thickened keratotic plaques following prolonged rubbing.*

HYPERTROPHIC LICHEN PLANUS

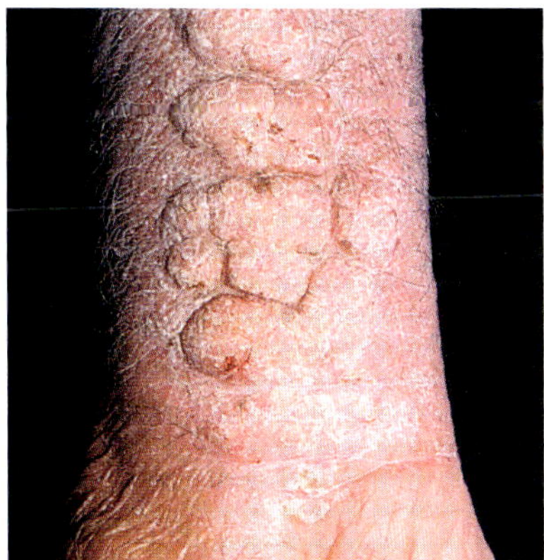
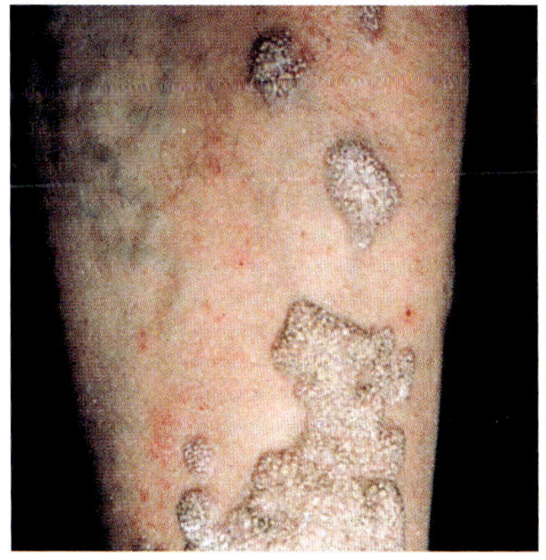

FIG. 48-27 *Markedly thickened keratotic plaques on a forearm rubbed for years.*

FIG. 48-28 *Markedly thickened, keratotic, pigmented papules and plaques.*

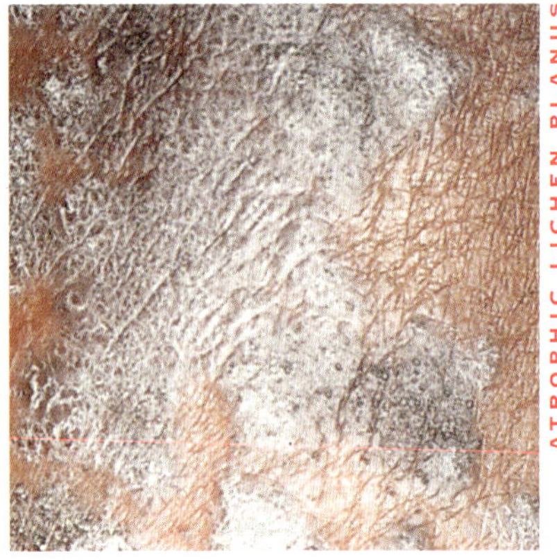

FIG. 48-29 *Keratotic pigmented papules and plaques.*

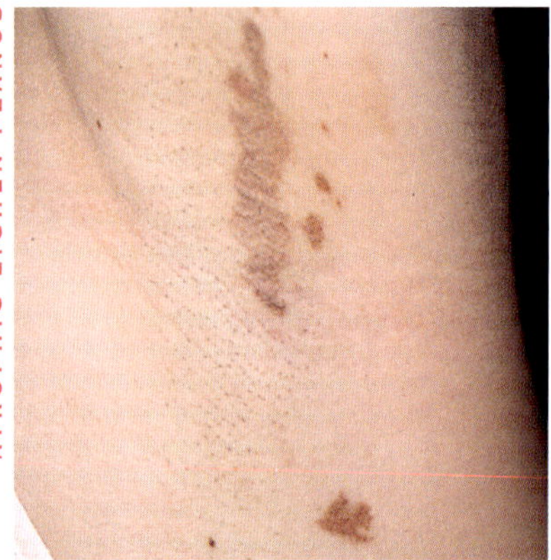

FIG. 48-30 *Hyperpigmented atrophic patch in linear configuration and similar satellite lesions, indicative of involution.*

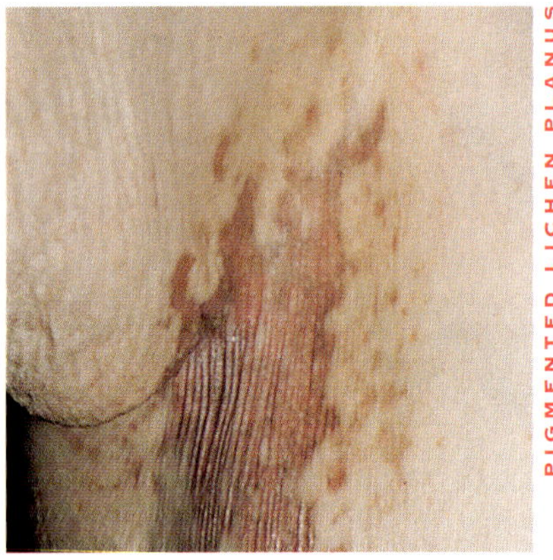

FIG. 48-31 *Atrophic pigmented macules and wrinkled pigmented patches of lesions that have largely resolved.*

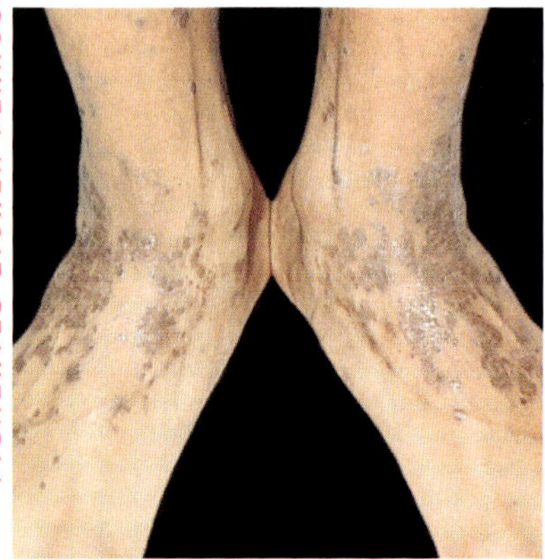

FIG. 48-32 *Papules, plaques, and flat pigmented lesions that have resolved.*

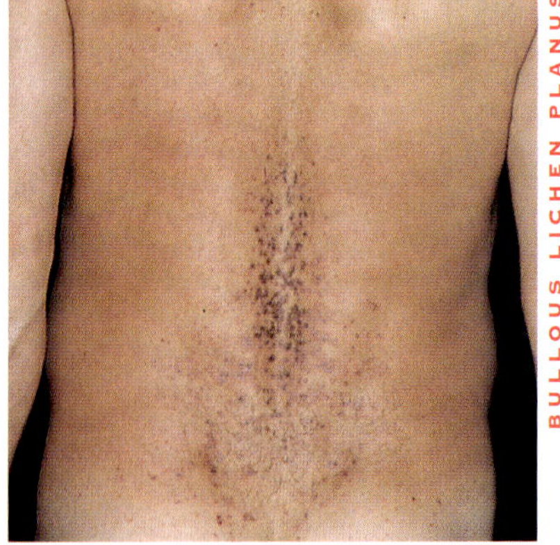

FIG. 48-33 *Pigmented macules and papules in the midline.*

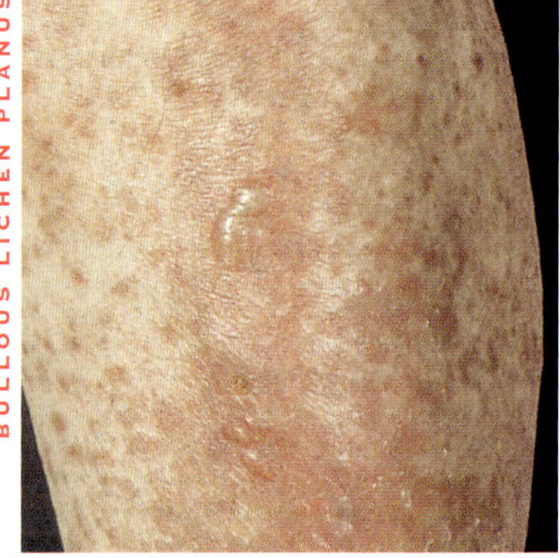

FIG. 48-34 *Vesicles atop some papules ("bullous" lichen planus).*

LICHEN PLANOPILARIS

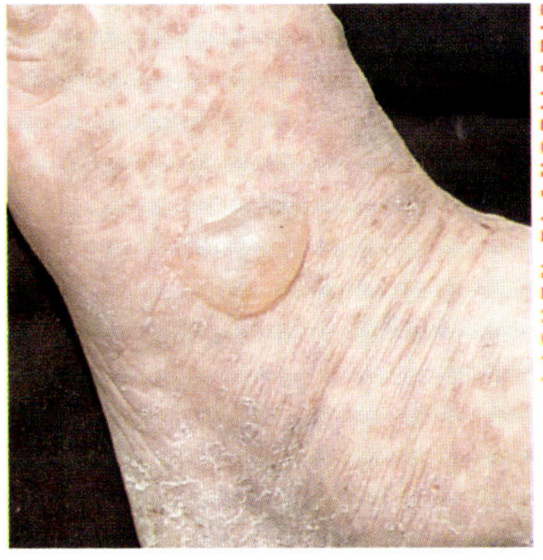

FIG. 48-35 *Bulla atop papules.*

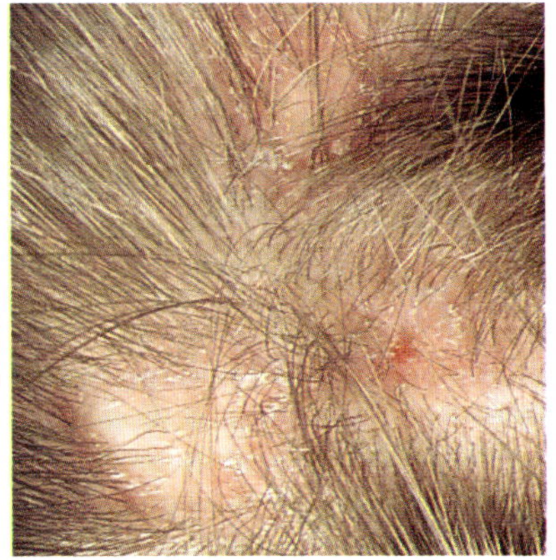

FIG. 48-36 *Reddish scaly patches of alopecia that represent still active lesions.*

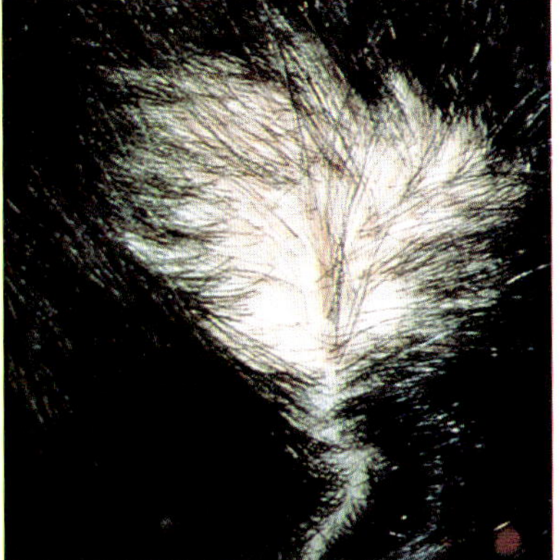

FIG. 48-37 *Patch of permanent alopecia.*

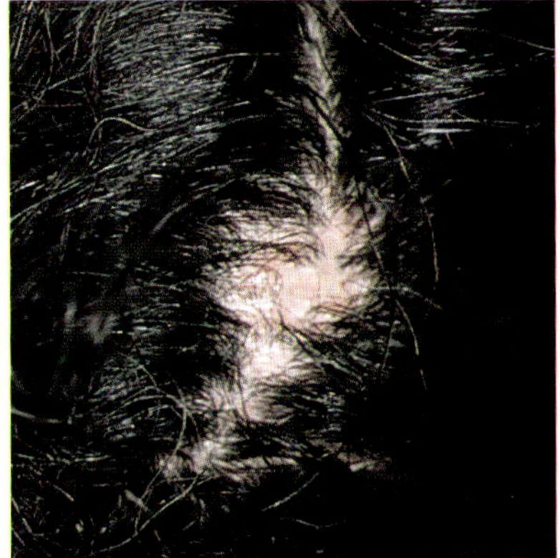

FIG. 48-38 *Patch of permanent alopecia associated with scales.*

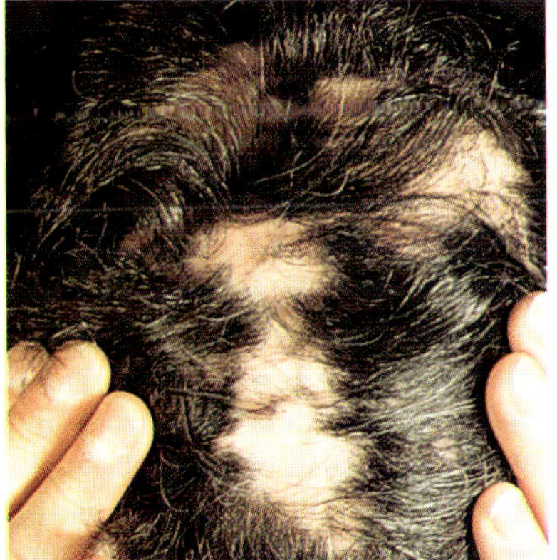

FIG. 48-39 *Noninflammatory zones of permanent alopecia.*

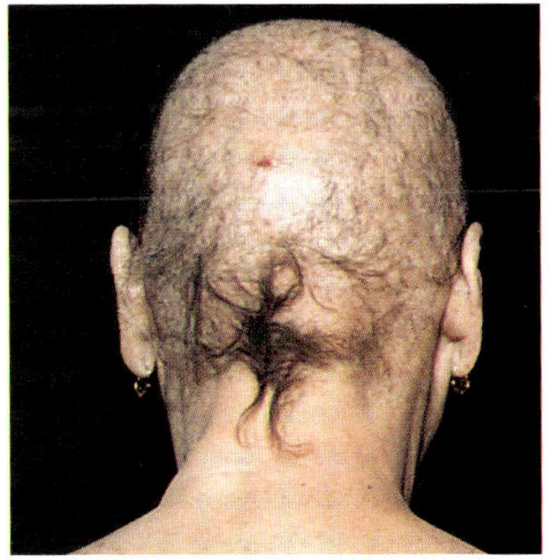

FIG. 48-40 *Diffuse permanent alopecia.*

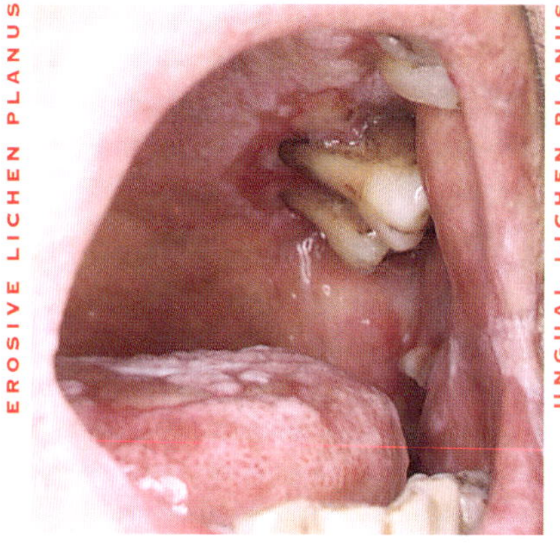

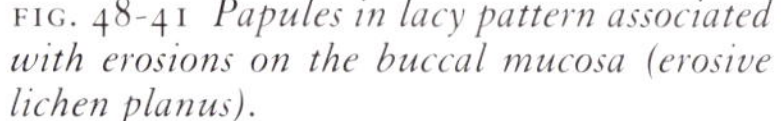

FIG. 48-41 *Papules in lacy pattern associated with erosions on the buccal mucosa (erosive lichen planus).*

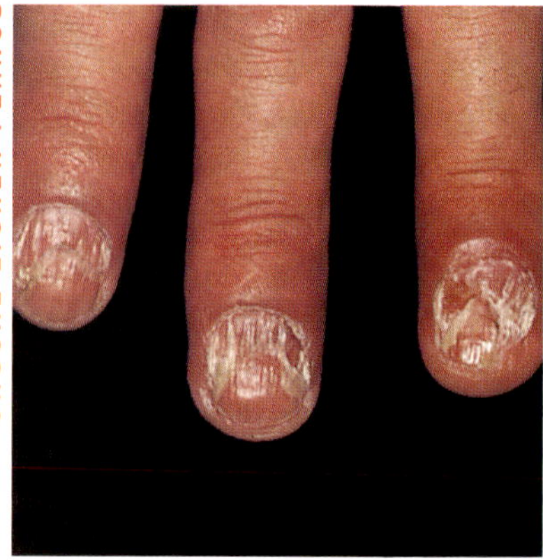

FIG. 48-42 *Onychodystrophy (pterygia of ungual lichen planus).*

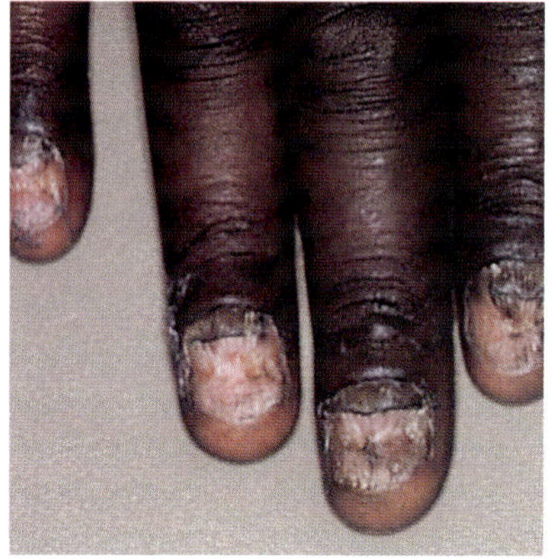

FIG. 48-43 *Onychodystrophy and partial loss of nails (ungual lichen planus).*

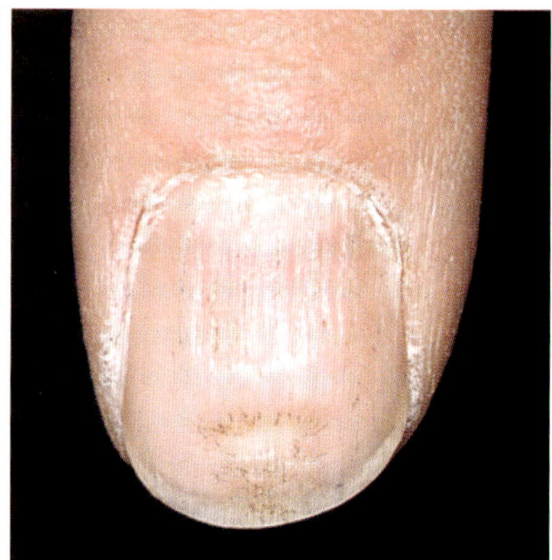

FIG. 48-44 *Longitudinally oriented ridges (ungual lichen planus).*

COURSE Just as is the case for all inflammatory diseases of the skin, lesions of lichen planus begin flat as pink or darker red macules and, very quickly, become violaceous papules. The papules sometimes become confluent to form plaques. In general, lesions of lichen planus tend to persist for months and usually begin to wane within a year. If lesions are rubbed persistently, as is the situation for what is called hypertrophic lichen planus, the condition may last for years. Vesicles of lichen planus come into being rapidly and also disappear rather quickly.

When lichen planus involves follicles, especially on the scalp, the effects of products of lymphocytes on that specialized epithelium can, in the course of years, destroy it, the result being permanent alopecia. When lichen planus involves the nail unit, the result may be the same; if the process destroys the nail matrix, the result, in a matter of years, is anonychia because there no longer is any possibility for development of nail plate. Short of complete loss of the nail plate by lichen planus there may be various distortions of it, a pterygium, for example.

INTEGRATION: UNIFYING CONCEPT Lichen planus is a single pathologic process that expresses itself differently as a consequence of either the particular epithelial component of the skin that is affected preferentially, i.e., epidermis, hair follicle, or nail unit (or any combination or constellation of them) or the dynamics of the process itself. When the process of lichen planus develops slowly in its stereotypical way, papules are expected. If, however, the process is accelerated dramatically, vesicles (so-called bullous lichen planus) come into being, and when that process is extensive and ulcerative on palms and soles or mucous membranes it is designated "erosive lichen planus." When conventional papules of lichen planus, especially those on the legs, are rubbed vigorously and persistently for months or years, lichen simplex chronicus is imposed on lichen planus (hypertrophic lichen planus). When the effects of lymphocytes over many months are severely destructive to the papillary dermis and epidermis, atrophy is inevitable (atrophic lichen planus). When severe destruction occurs secondary to longstanding effects of lymphocytes on follicles on a scalp, the outcome is permanent alopecia of lichen planopilaris, known also as pseudopelade of Brocq. When destruction of the nail matrix by the same mechanism is complete, the effect is anonychia.

When lesions are arranged in an annulus (annular lichen planus) or in a line (linear lichen planus), the basic process is still lichen planus. That is equally true when lesions occur on a mucous membrane; they are those of lichen planus. In short, there are many morphologic manifestations of the process of lichen planus.

THERAPY Topical corticosteroids, intralesional injections of corticosteroids, and even a short course of oral corticosteroids for acute widespread lesions may be appropriate. Other modes of treatment for widespread lesions are phototherapy (PUVA, UV-B) and retinoids. Painful oral lesions may be assuaged by topical corticosteroids in a coated base, a mouthwash that contains cyclosporin, or topical application of tacrolimus (FK506).

DEFINITION An inflammatory process that expresses itself as a cluster of closely-set smooth or scaly papules in linear array along the lines of Blaschko, and that usually resolves in months.

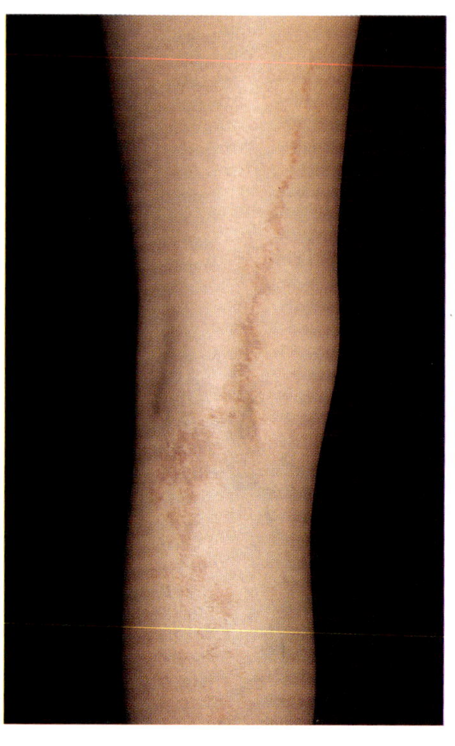

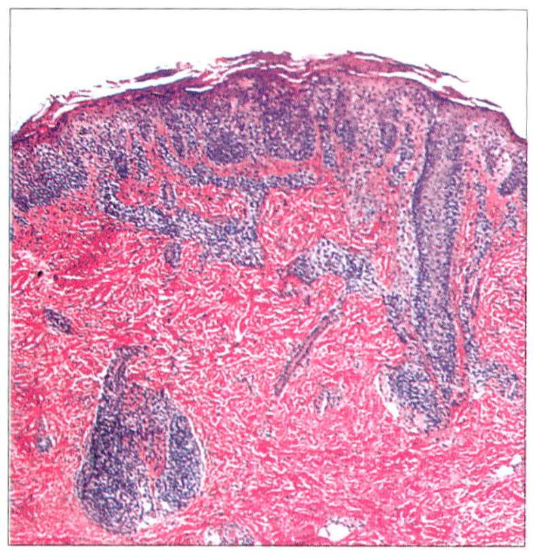

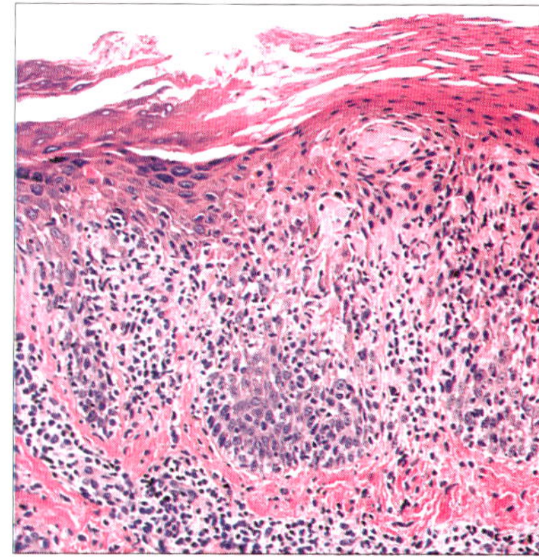

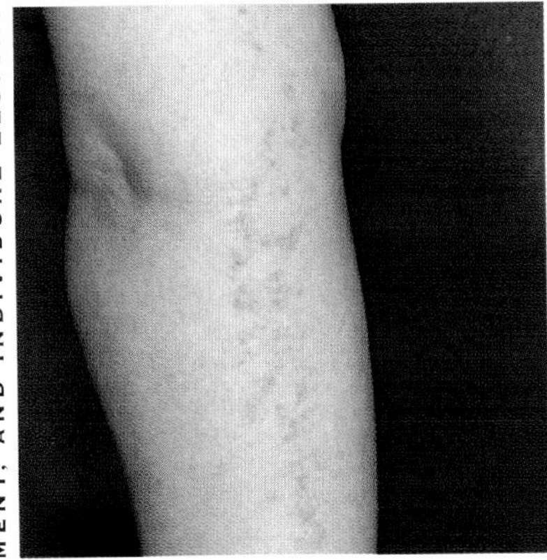

FIG. 49-1 *Papules in linear arrangement.*

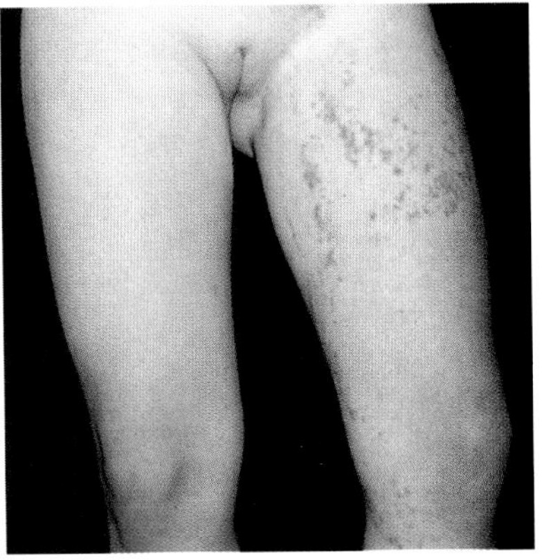

FIG. 49-2 *Closely-set papules that vaguely form lines.*

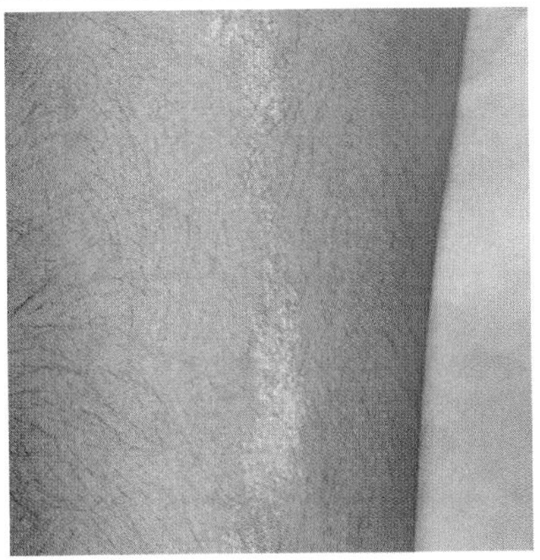

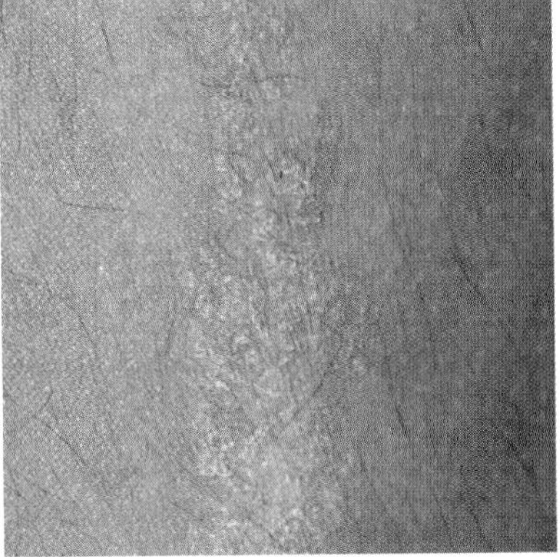

FIG. 49-3 (A, B) *Linear arrangement of papules.*

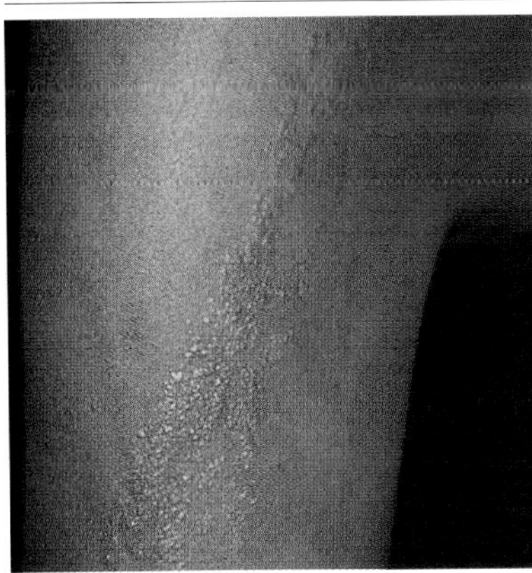

FIG. 49-4 *Closely-set scaly papules arranged in a line.*

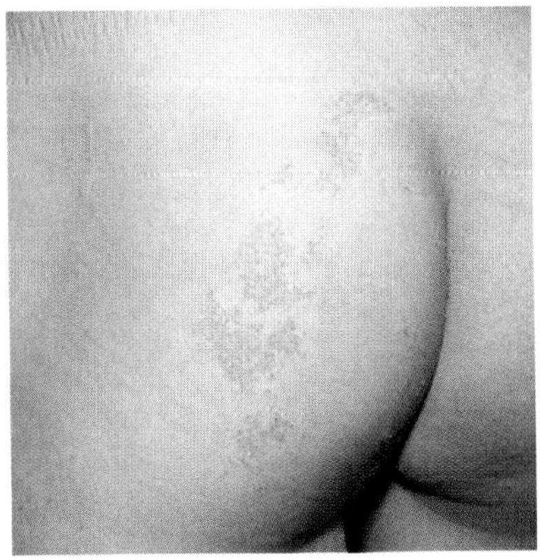

FIG. 49-5 *Tiny papules in groups and in linear array.*

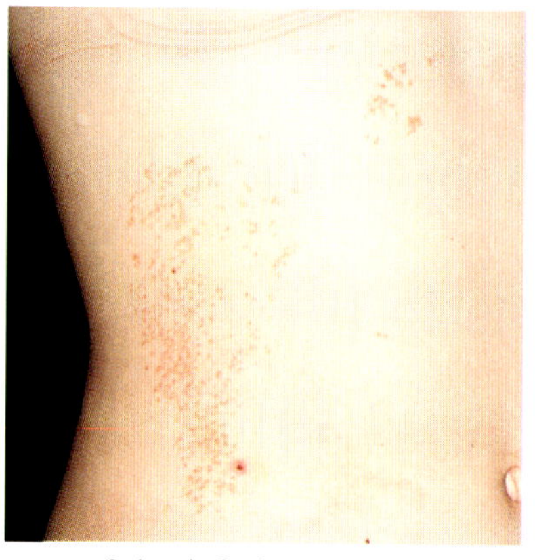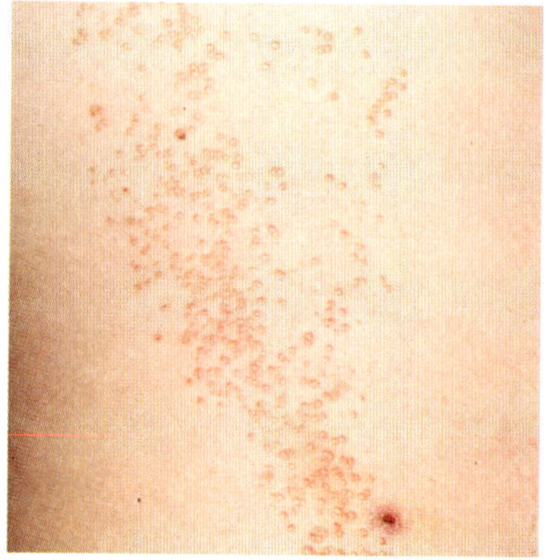

FIG. 49-6 (A, B) *Scaly papules in linear arrangement.*

COURSE The duration of individual papules of lichen striatus depends on the character of the histopathologic findings within it. For example, a lesion characterized by spongiosis and slight parakeratosis may disappear in weeks, whereas one typified by psoriasiform hyperplasia and lichenoid infiltrates of lymphocytes may persist for months. When granulomatous inflammation supervenes, a lesion may last for more than a year. As a rule, however, the entire course of lichen striatus is played out over a span of months.

INTEGRATION: UNIFYING CONCEPT Lichen striatus is an inflammatory process made up of many scaly papules that follow Blaschko's lines, especially on an extremity or the trunk. Because the pathologic process evolves and devolves over the course of months, a lesion that begins as a spongiotic dermatitis may progress to spongiotic psoriasiform dermatitis and, in time, to a spongiotic psoriasiform lichenoid dermatitis. Numerous individual necrotic keratinocytes, some of them in small clusters, are observed commonly in the epidermis.

When a particular papule of lichen striatus has been present for many months, it may exhibit in the upper part of the dermis, in addition to changes within the epidermis, foci of granulomatous inflammation in conjunction with predominant lymphocytes. Infiltrates of lymphocytes within the reticular dermis tend to be present around venules of both the superficial and deep plexuses, and to be aligned along epithelial and non-epithelial structures of adnexa. All of these findings, combined, contribute to the fact that lichen striatus presents itself histopathologically in protean but repeatable and recognizable ways.

The cause of lichen striatus is not known.

THERAPY Except for reassurance, no therapy is necessary. If treatment is advisable for other reasons, hydrocortisone cream may be applied.

DEFINITION A benign neoplasm of adipocytes that forms in the subcutaneous fat (as well as in other organs sometimes) and manifests itself clinically as either an elevated tumor or a tumor that cannot be visualized clinically, but that can be palpated, the skin overlying it in both circumstances being normal.

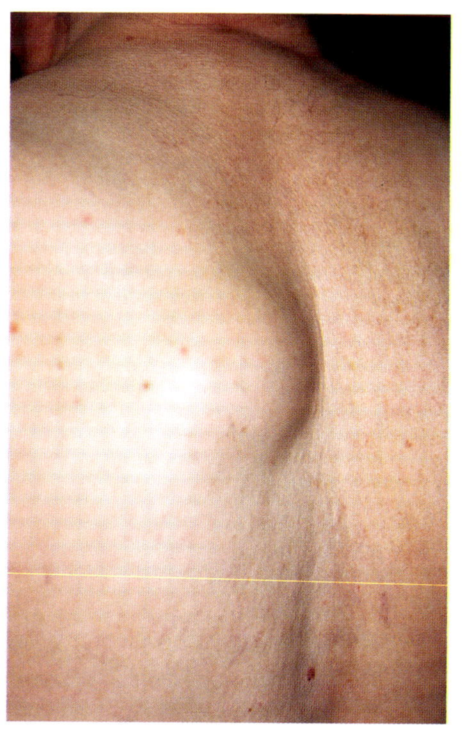

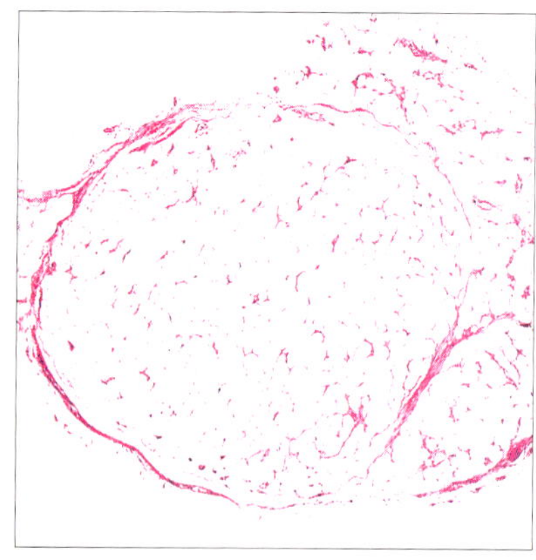

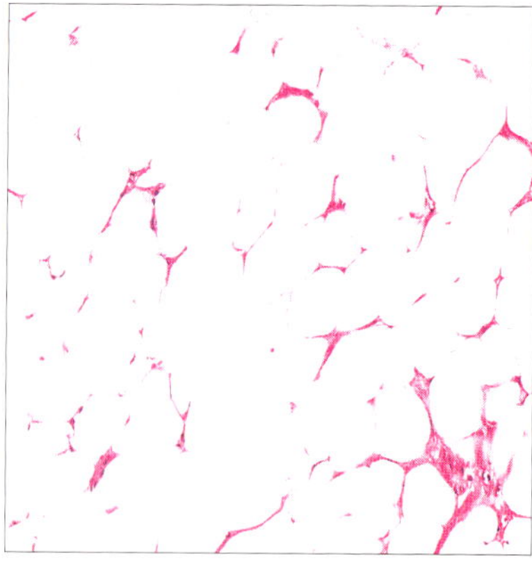

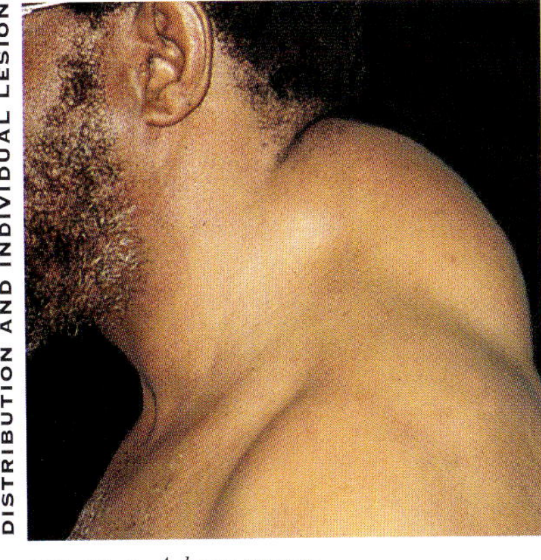

FIG. 50-1 *A huge tumor.*

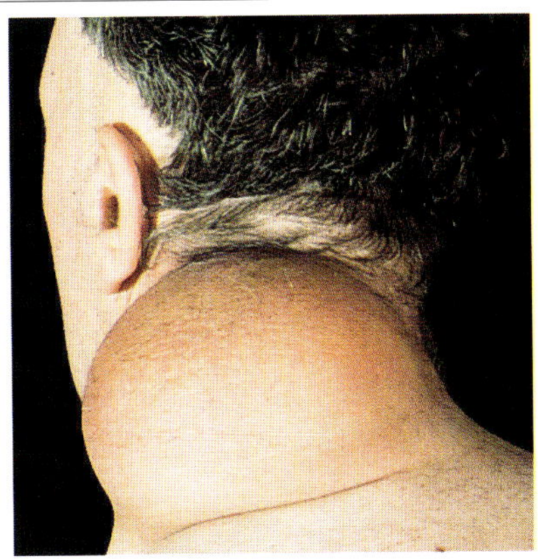

FIG. 50-2 *A mammoth tumor.*

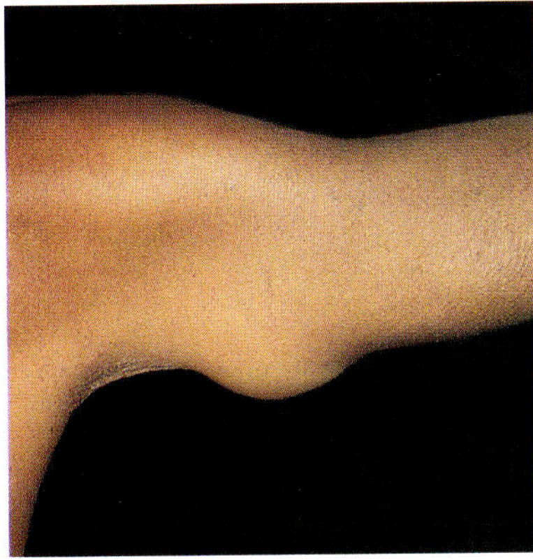

FIG. 50-3 *A large tumor.*

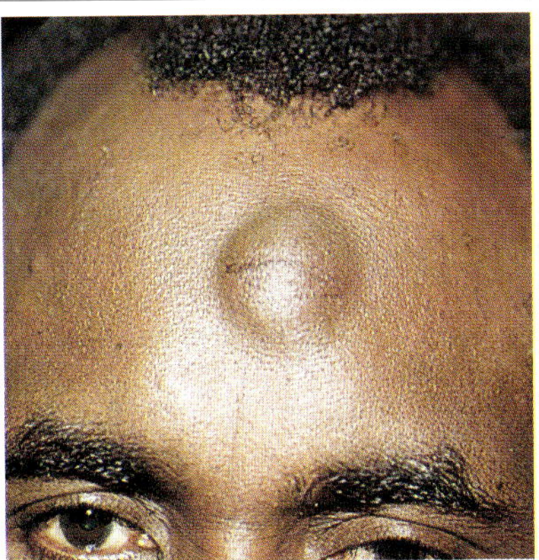

FIG. 50-4 *A tumor that could be misconstrued clinically as a cyst.*

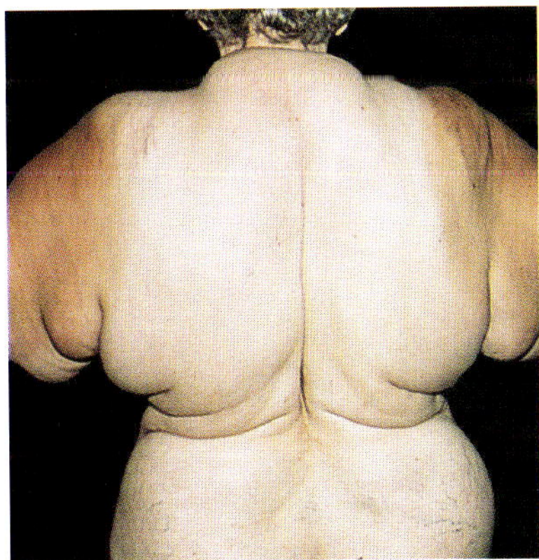

FIG. 50-5 *Benign symmetrical lipomatosis consists of massive lipomas.*

COURSE A lipoma, once it presents itself, remains there for the lifetime of a person who carries it. It may stay small or become larger, sometimes assuming gigantic dimensions.

INTEGRATION: UNIFYING CONCEPT Like all neoplasms in the skin and other organs, and like all pathologic processes in general, a lipoma, which is a distinctive benign neoplasm made up of adipocytes, may present itself in various guises. In addition to the predominant adipocytes in a lipoma, there may be numerous foci in which fascicles of oval-shaped adipocytes are present, a condition known as spindle-cell lipoma; there may be innumerable small blood vessels, some of them crowded, a phenomenon referred to as angiolipoma; there may be scatter of many multinucleate adipocytes, known picturesquely as "floret cells" because of their vague resemblance to a flower, a circumstance that is given the name "pleomorphic lipoma." A lipoma of any kind may be replete with mucin. Practically never does a lipoma eventuate in liposarcoma.

THERAPY Surgical excision is curative if a patient wants surgery for a not-too-large tumor. For those lipomas that are too large to be excised, liposuction may be employed.

LIVEDO VASCULITIS

DEFINITION A type of small-vessel vasculitis (venulitis) of the skin, occurring especially in the vicinity of the ankle, characterized at first by purpuric macules and patches that, in time, may become hemorrhagic blisters that ulcerate and heal with white, stellate scars (atrophie blanche).

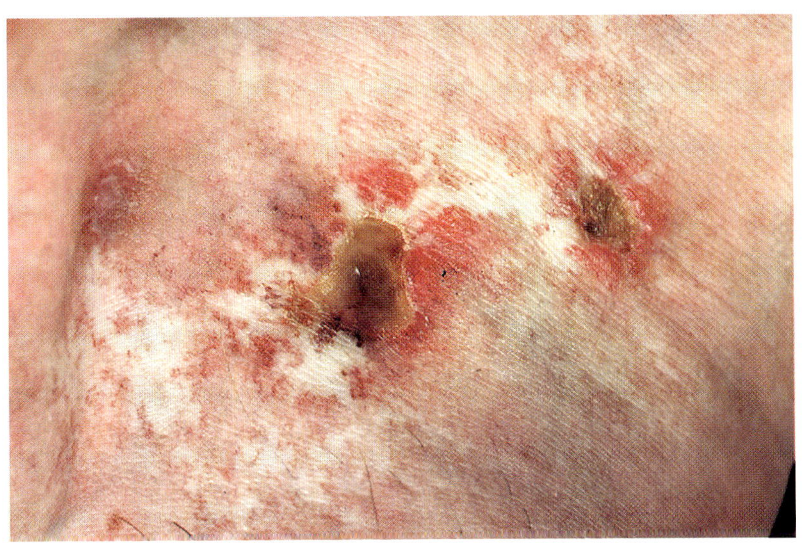

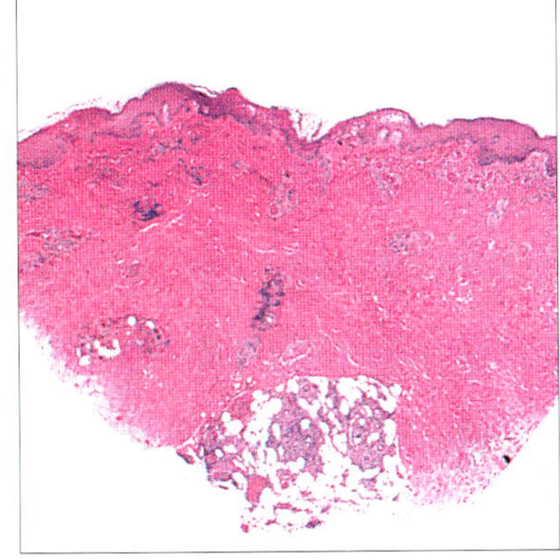

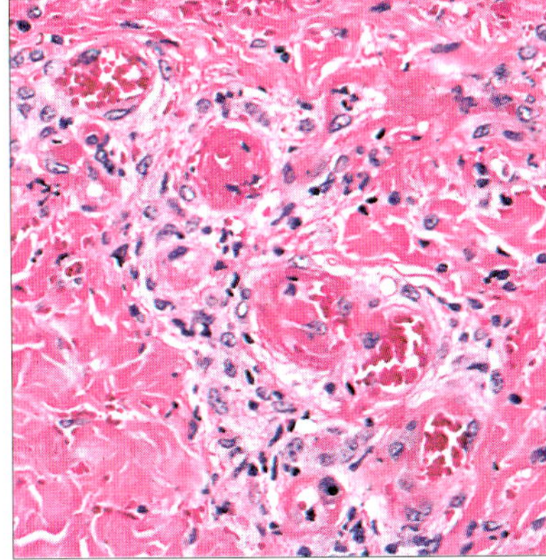

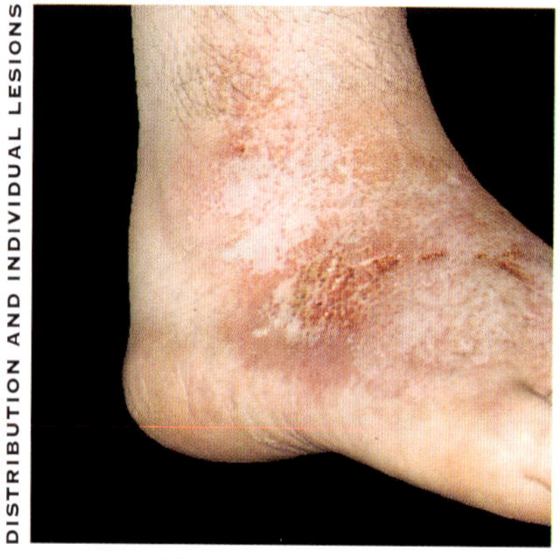

FIG. 51-1 *Purpuric and pigmented macules, patches, and white scars of livedo vasculitis.*

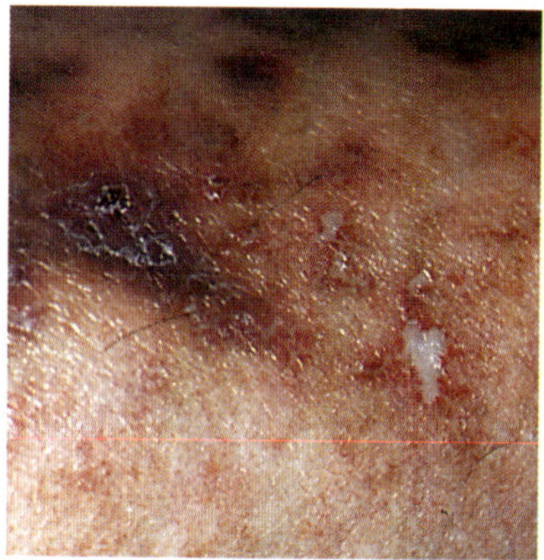

FIG. 51-2 *Reticulate hyperpigmentation and white atrophic scars of atrophie blanche, the end-stage of livedo vasculitis.*

ADJUNCTIVE DIAGNOSTIC TEST Search may be undertaken for antiphospholipid antibodies.

COURSE Livedo vasculitis progresses from reddish blue macules to papules to ulcerations that have jagged outlines, and, eventually, to white atrophic scars. Sometimes hemorrhagic blisters rather than purpuric papules occur in the sequence between macules and ulcers. Whatever the steps in chronologic course, however, the progression from dusky macules to white scars takes many months and usually years. Once the process begins, typically in young adult women, it may resolve completely in a few years, or worsen and then remit episodically for a lifetime.

INTEGRATION: UNIFYING CONCEPT Livedo vasculitis, as the name denotes, is a distinctive type of cutaneous vasculitis, in particular, the type characterized histopathologically by the presence in the reticular dermis of fibrin in the wall of venules and a thrombus within the lumen of them. Also present is a mixed infiltrate of inflammatory cells, neutrophils predominating early and lymphocytes later. As the process evolves, vesiculation may become manifest consequent usually to a combination of ballooning and spongiosis within the epidermis.

In time there is ulceration and, over a period of many months, sclerosis forms in the upper part of the dermis. That latter change, in combination with a thinned epidermis devoid of both discrete rete ridges and of melanin, presents itself clinically as white atrophic scars, whence the imprecise synonym for livedo vasculitis, atrophie blanche. In actuality, atrophie blanche is merely the end stage of the vasculitic process, devoid of infiltrates of inflammatory cells.

It is claimed that some lesions of livedo vasculitis are not truly vasculitic because they develop as a consequence of alterations in the coagulation cascade and are associated only with thrombi and not with notable infiltrates of inflammatory cells. Without the presence of inflammatory cells, an aberration consisting of fibrin within the wall or thrombi within the lumen of blood vessels (or both) does not qualify as vasculitis.

Of the three major types of small-vessel vasculitis in skin—allergic (leukocytoclastic) vasculitis, septic vasculitis, and livedo vasculitis, the latter is the least common and the most enigmatic because neither cause nor pathogenesis of it is known for sure.

There is no relationship between livedo vasculitis and livedo reticularis. The latter is not a vasculitis, but a kind of ectasia that does not change perceptibly in terms of its basic morphologic structure over time. The word "livedo" shared by both conditions means a bruise-like discoloration of the skin.

THERAPY Because a defect in fibrinolysis or abnormalities of adhesiveness of platelets may be responsible for livedo vasculitis in some patients, antiplatelet agents and fibrinolytic agents, such as salicylates and heparin in low dose, are recommended treatments.

LIVEDO RETICULARIS

DEFINITION Bluish red net-like pattern of macules and patches, a consequence of dilated small end vessels of the superficial plexus. When widespread, the condition may be a reflection of a variety of systemic abnormalities such as Sneddon's disease (livedo reticularis in conjunction with cerebral vascular thrombotic disease), periarteritis nodosa, and cryoglobulinemia.

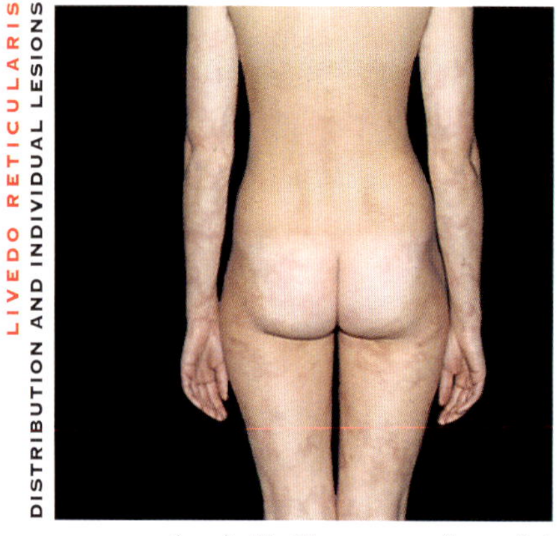
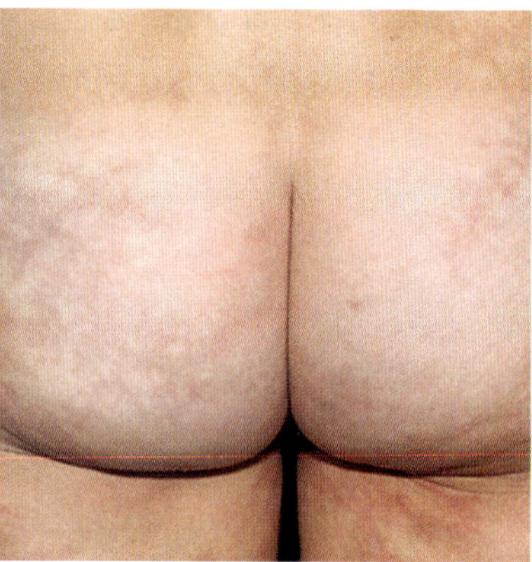

FIG. 51-3 (A, B) *Netlike pattern of superficial blood vessels in livedo reticularis.*

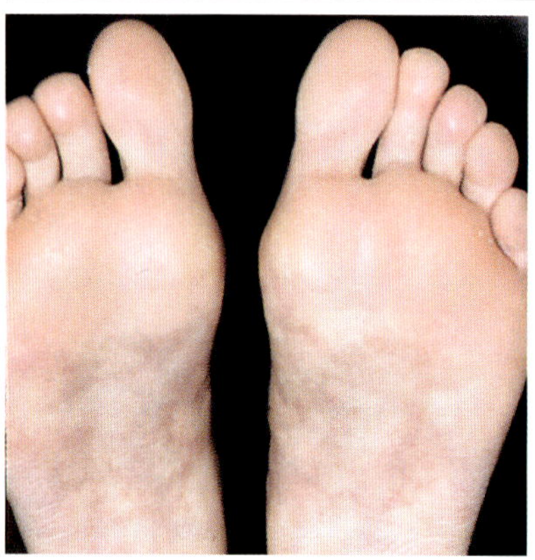

FIG. 51-3 (C) *Netlike pattern of superficial blood vessels in livedo reticularis on soles.*

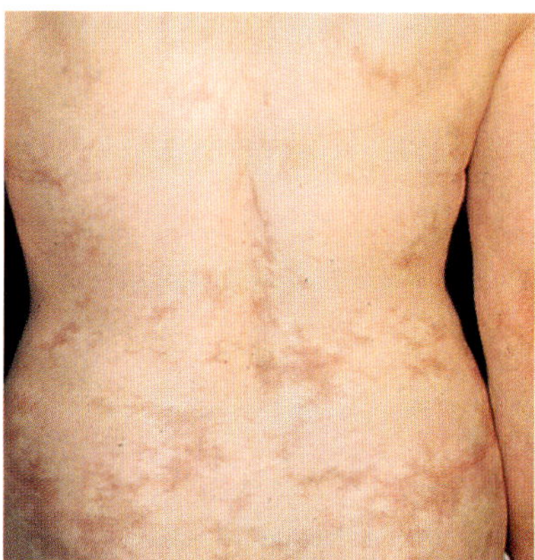

FIG. 51-4 *Widespread dusky erythematous patches with jagged outlines.*

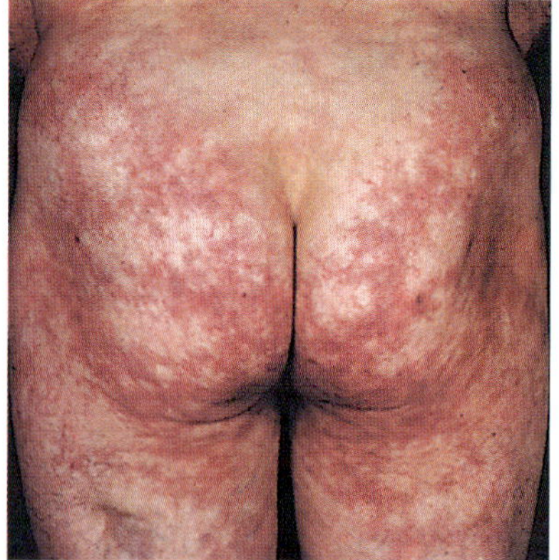

FIG. 51-5 *Dusky red patches with jagged outlines involving the trunk, buttocks, and legs extensively.*

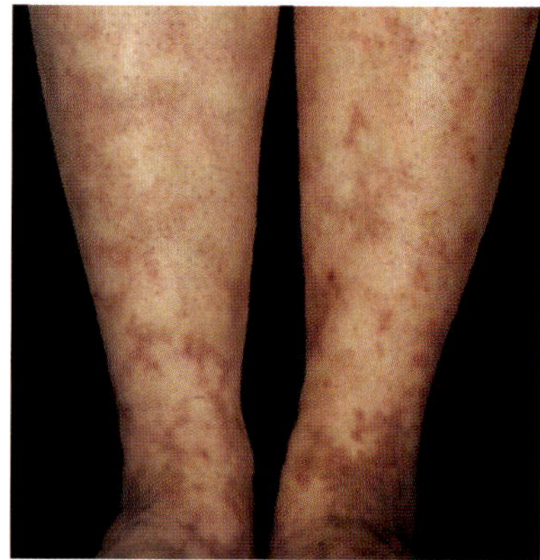

FIG. 51-6 *Reticulated pattern of dusky erythema in livedo reticularis.*

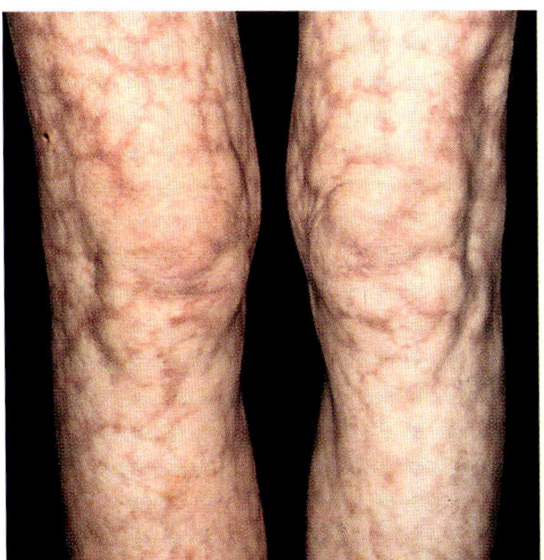

FIG. 51-7   *Distinctive netlike pattern of superficial vessels in livedo reticularis.*

COURSE   The netlike pattern formed by reddish blue lines of livedo reticularis on the legs corresponds to the course of the cutaneous vascular plexuses. The ectasias signify permanent dilation of venules, and they persist for a lifetime.

INTEGRATION: UNIFYING CONCEPT   The terminology of the condition under discussion here is not agreed on. In Europe, livedo reticularis refers to a distinctive cutaneous pattern in which a vascular network is associated with circular elements that are "closed" at the periphery. It is believed to be a physiological phenomenon and is synonymous with cutis marmorata. Livedo racemosa, by contrast, refers to a network with circular elements that are "open" at the periphery. By definition, that condition is associated with periarteritis nodosa, lupus erythematosus, Sneddon syndrome, or livedo vasculitis. The reason for the permanent ectasia in livedo reticularis and livedo racemosa is not known, but genetic factors are thought to be operative.

THERAPY   Livedo reticularis, occurring alone, does not require treatment, but if the condition is secondary to a systemic disease, that pathologic process should be identified and managed.

DEFINITION An inflammatory process that expresses itself in the skin in protean ways that are variations on a basic pathologic theme, and includes evanescent patches on the face ("butterfly blush"), scaly papules and plaques that resolve with atrophy and hyperpigmentation (classic discoid lupus erythematosus), arcuate, annular, and serpiginous lesions (subacute cutaneous lupus erythematosus), nonscaling plaques (tumid lupus erythematosus), subcutaneous nodules (lupus profundus), and blisters (bullous lupus erythematosus).

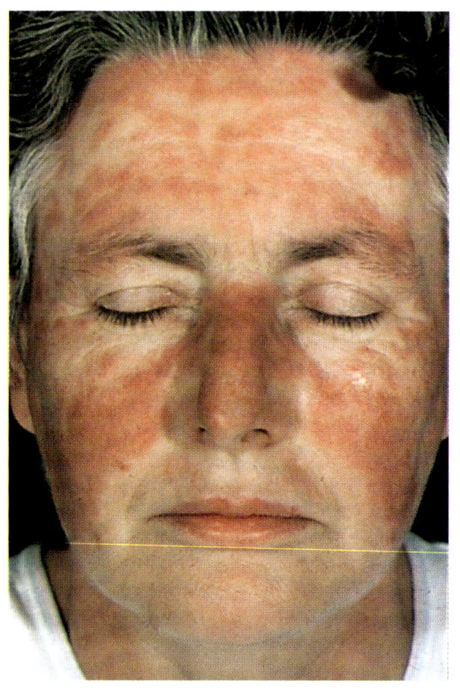

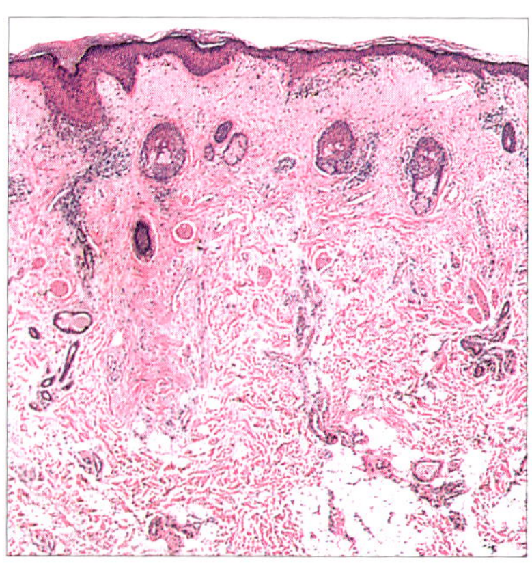

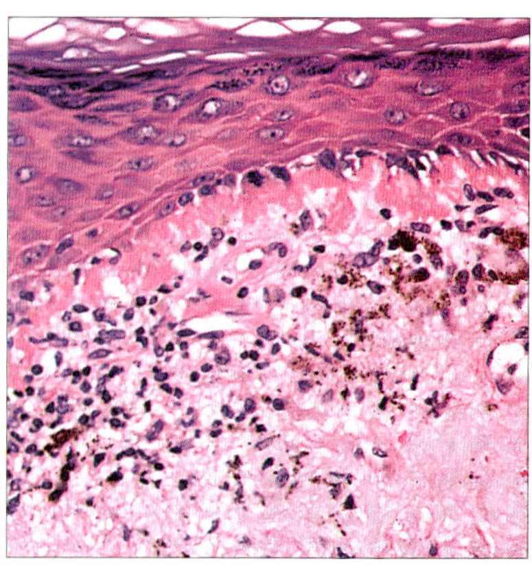

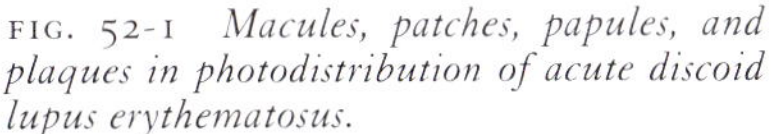

FIG. 52-1 *Macules, patches, papules, and plaques in photodistribution of acute discoid lupus erythematosus.*

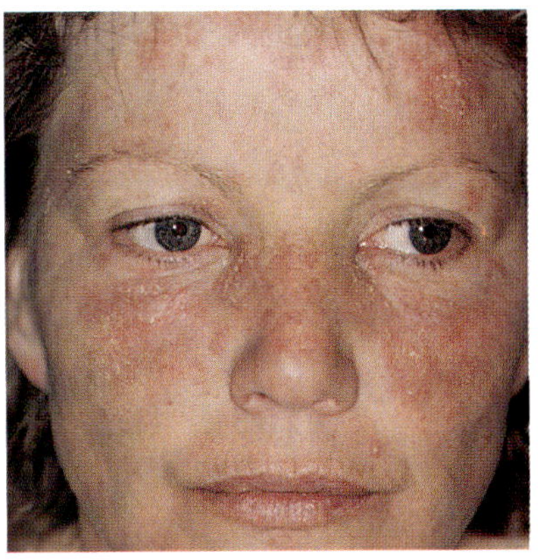

FIG. 52-2 *Plaques in photodistribution of acute discoid lupus erythematosus.*

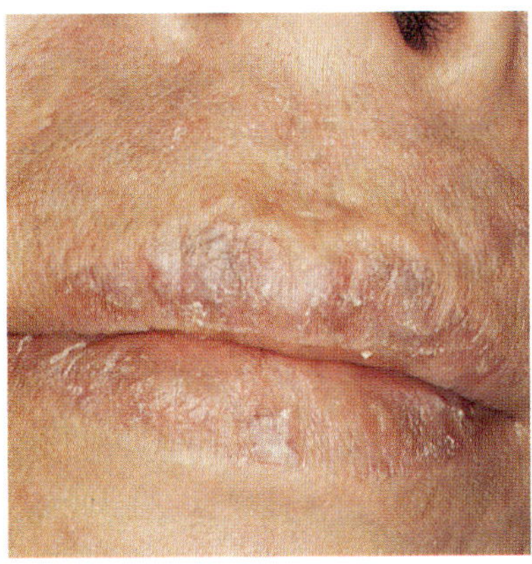

FIG. 52-3 *Atrophic scaly macules and papules of chronic discoid lupus erythematosus.*

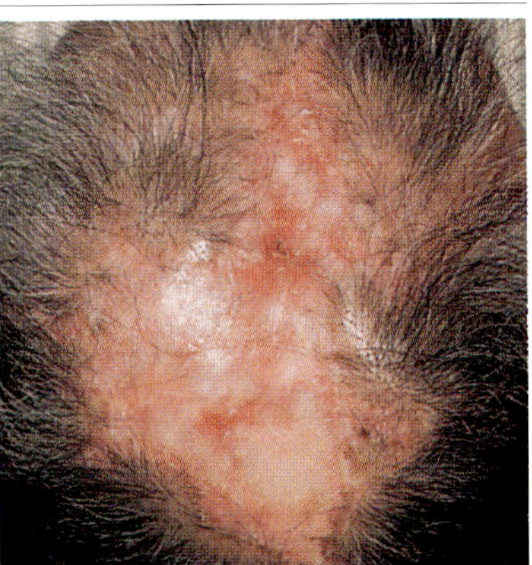

FIG. 52-4 *Atrophic hypopigmented patches of chronic discoid lupus erythematosus. The red lesions are active ones.*

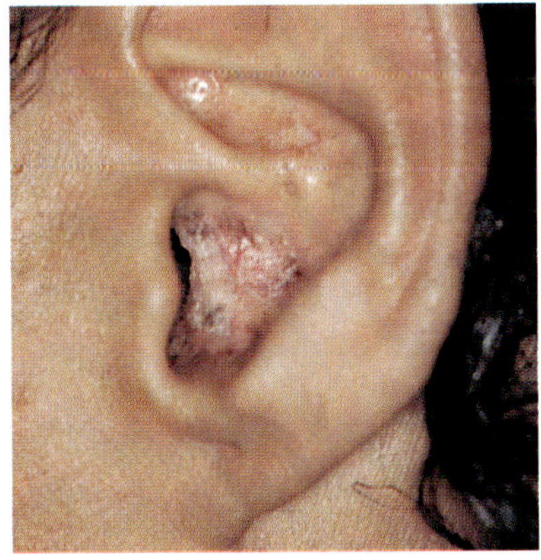

FIG. 52-5 *Atrophic, hyperpigmented and hypopigmented, keratotic lesions on a concha of chronic discoid lupus erythematosus.*

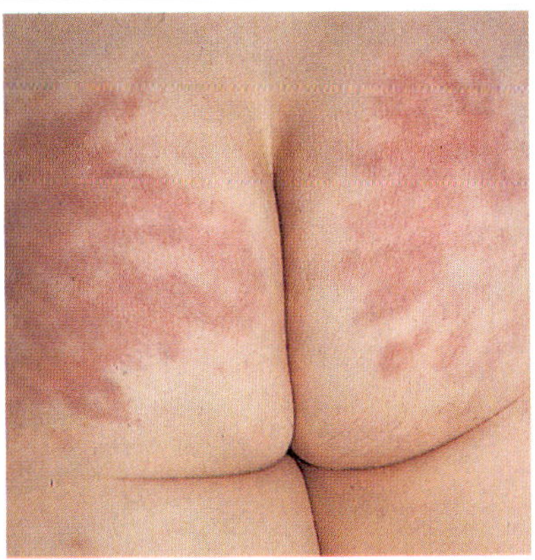

FIG. 52-6 *Patches and subtle plaques, some in striate, annular, and arcuate configuration, of acute discoid lupus erythematosus.*

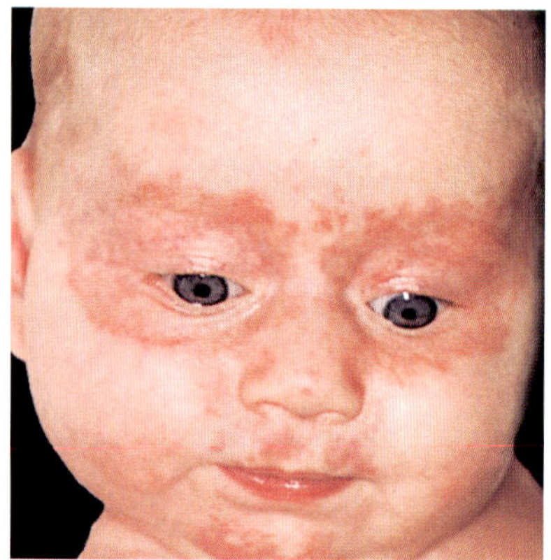

FIG. 52-7 *Macules, patches, and subtle papules and plaques of acute discoid lupus erythematosus in a neonate (neonatal L.E.).*

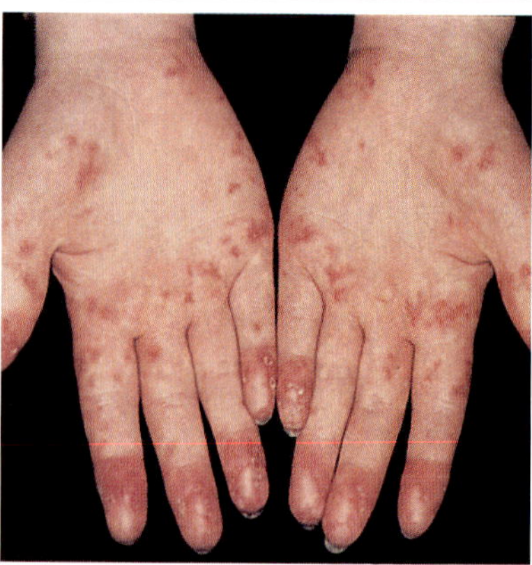

FIG. 52-8 *Erythematous scaly papules of sub-acute discoid lupus erythematosus on volar skin.*

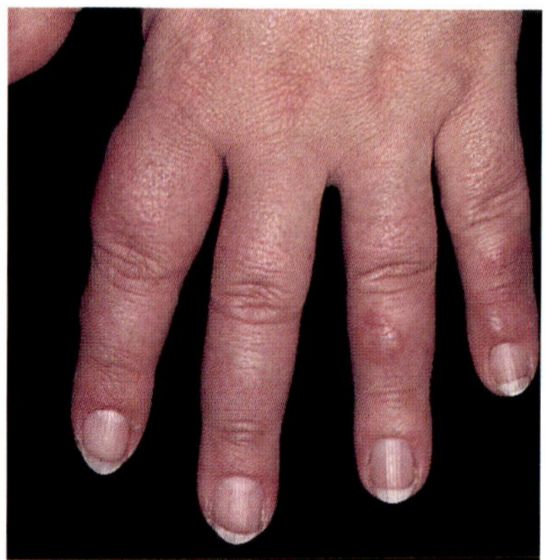

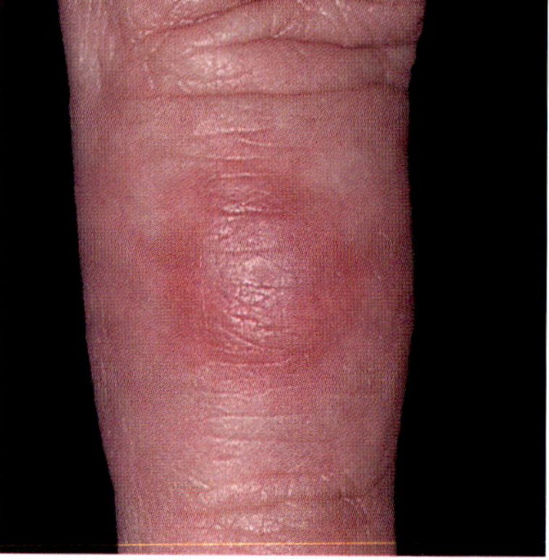

FIG. 52-9 (A, B) *Scaly macules, papules, and plaques of subacute discoid lupus erythematosus on the fingers.*

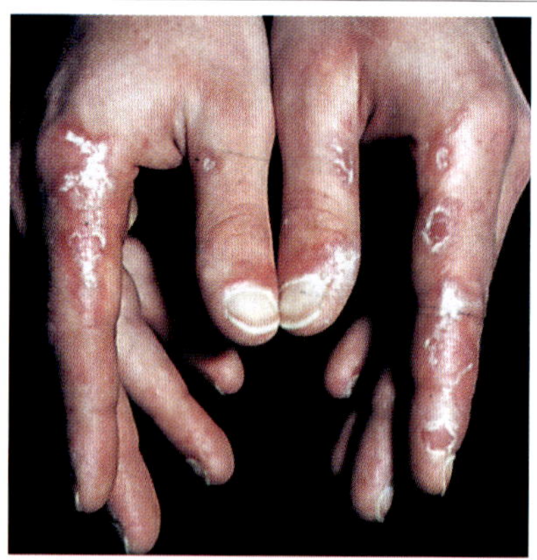

FIG. 52-10 *Keratotic papules and plaques of chronic discoid lupus erythematosus (hypertrophic lupus erythematosus).*

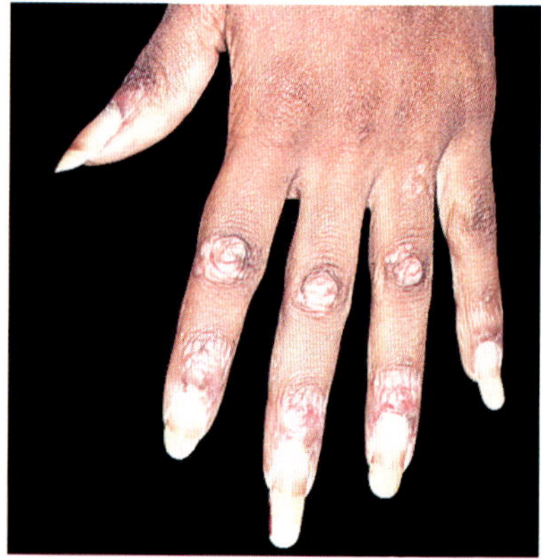

FIG. 52-11 *Keratotic papules of chronic discoid lupus erythematosus (hypertrophic lupus erythematosus).*

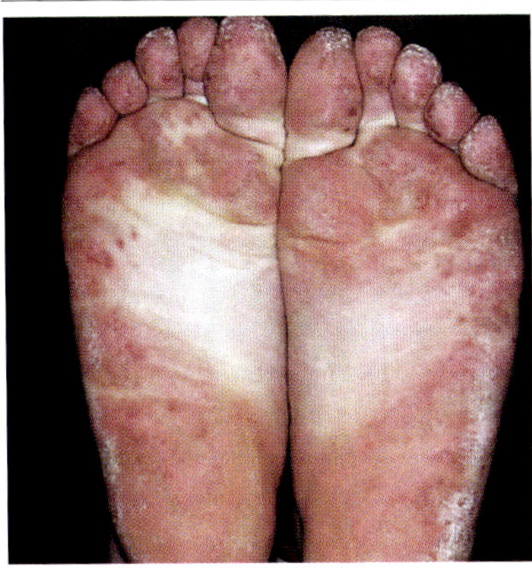

FIG. 52-12 *Scaly macules, patches, and subtle papules and plaques of subacute discoid lupus erythematosus.*

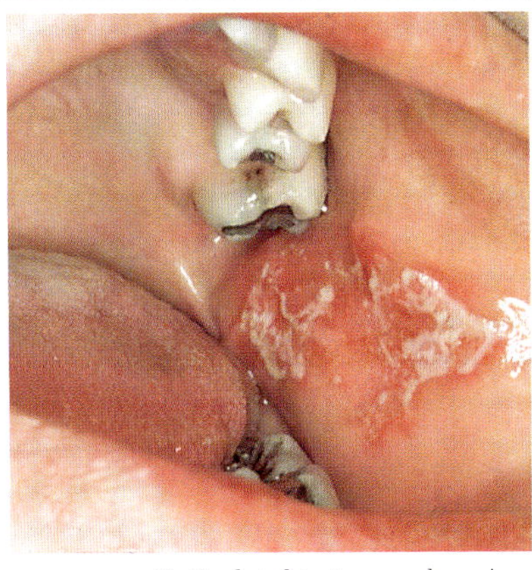

FIG. 52-13 *Reticulated pattern and erosions of acute discoid lupus erythematosus on the buccal mucosa.*

CONFIGURATION

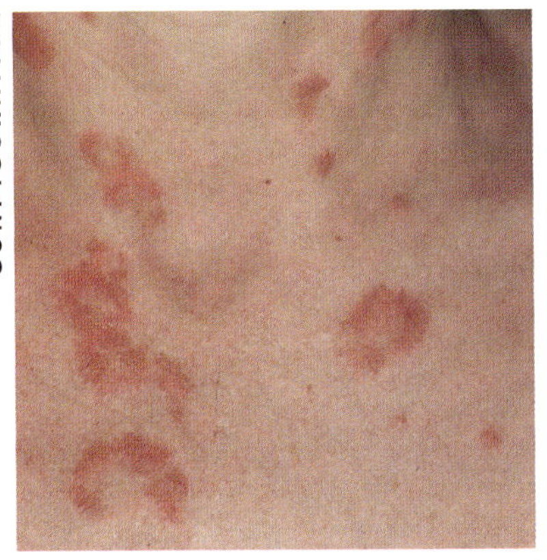

FIG. 52-14 *Arcuate and annular lesions of subacute cutaneous lupus erythematosus.*

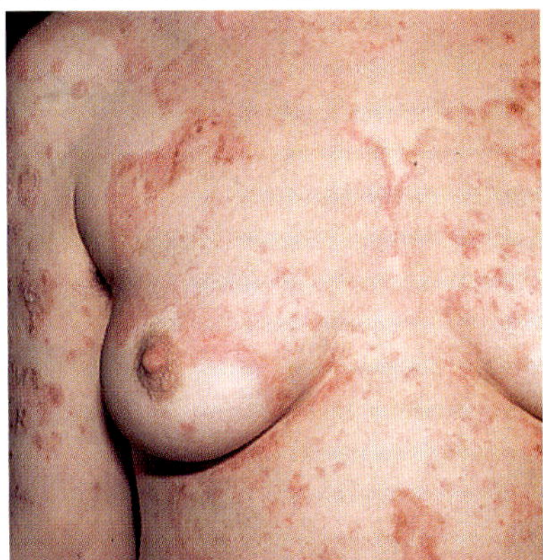

FIG. 52-15 *Arcuate, annular, and serpiginous plaques of subacute cutaneous lupus erythematosus.*

INDIVIDUAL LESIONS

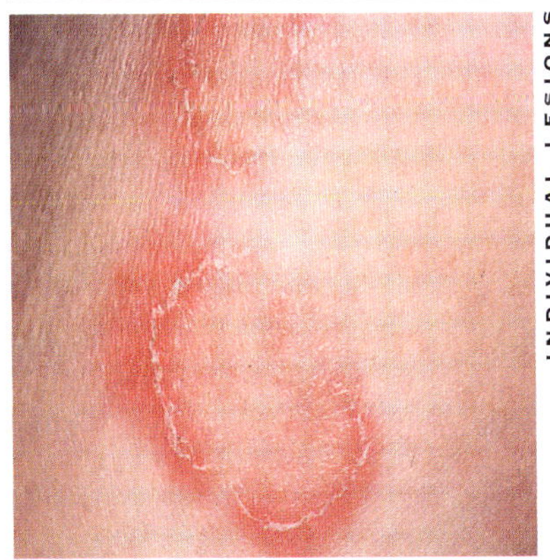

FIG. 52-16 *Arcuate plaques of subacute cutaneous lupus erythematosus.*

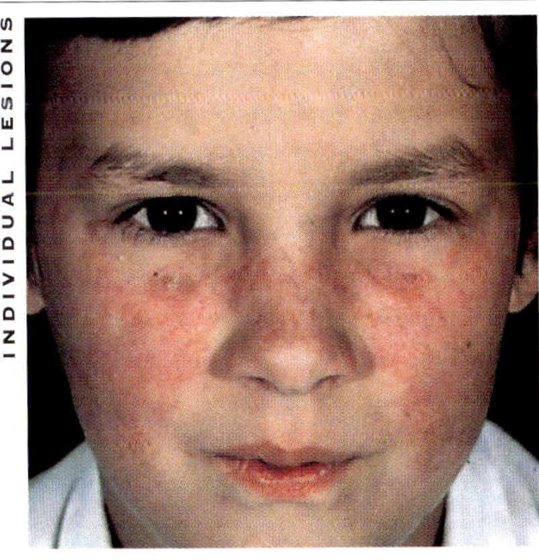

FIG. 52-17 *Patches and subtle plaques (acute discoid lupus erythematosus).*

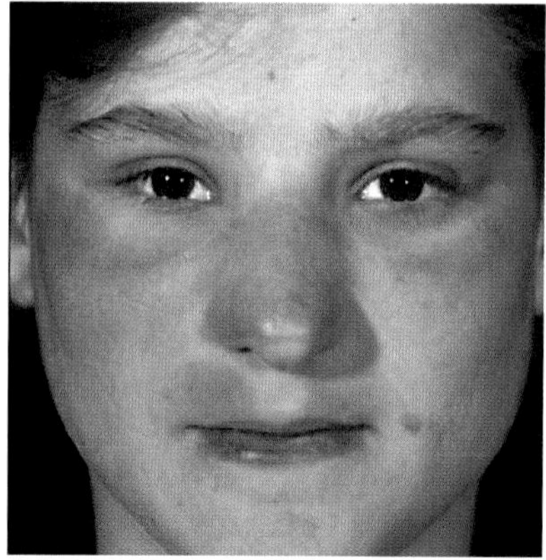

FIG. 52-18 *Patches and subtle plaques (acute discoid lupus erythematosus).*

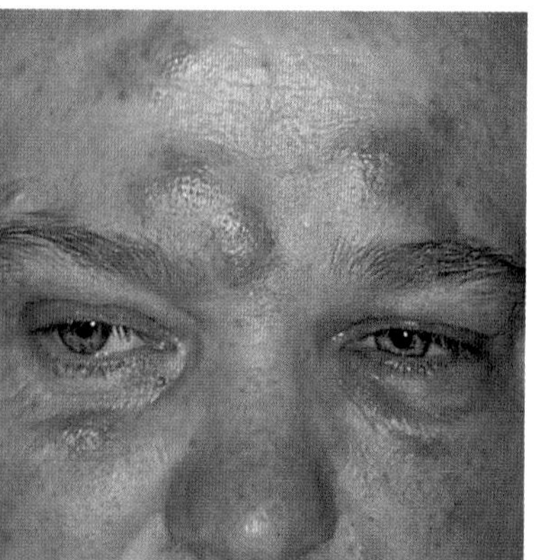

FIG. 52-19 *Plaques (tumid lupus erythematosus).*

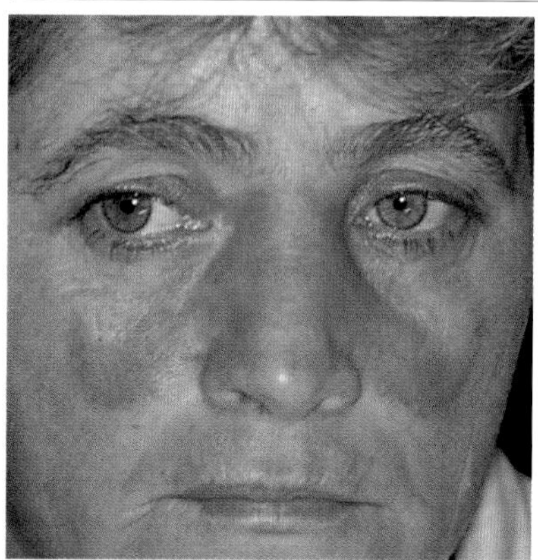

FIG. 52-20 *Plaques (subacute discoid lupus erythematosus).*

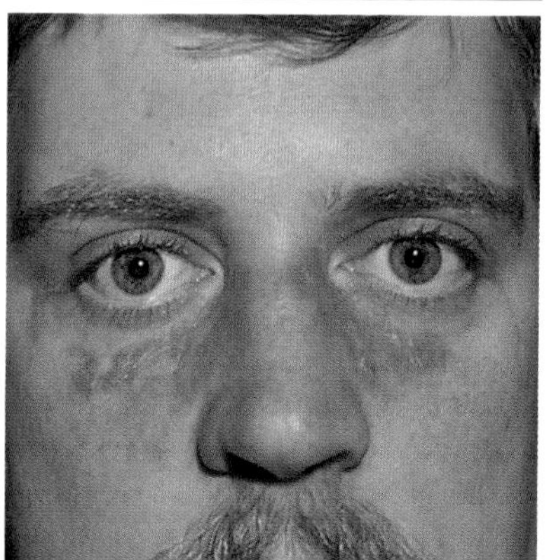

FIG. 52-21 *Slightly scaly papules and plaques (subacute discoid lupus erythematosus).*

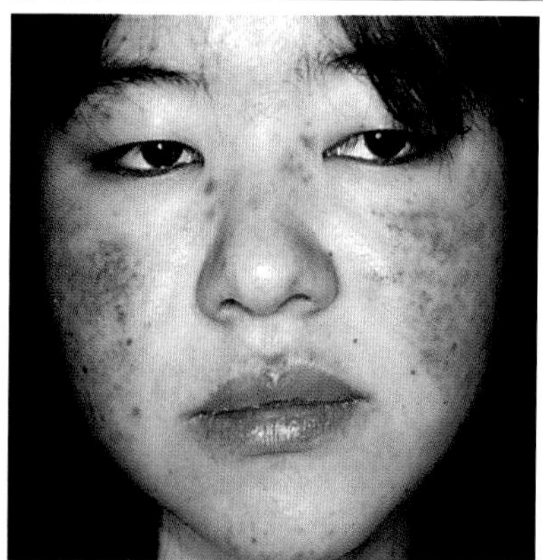

FIG. 52-22 *Hyper- and hypopigmentation, telangiectasia, and subtle atrophy (chronic discoid lupus erythematosus).*

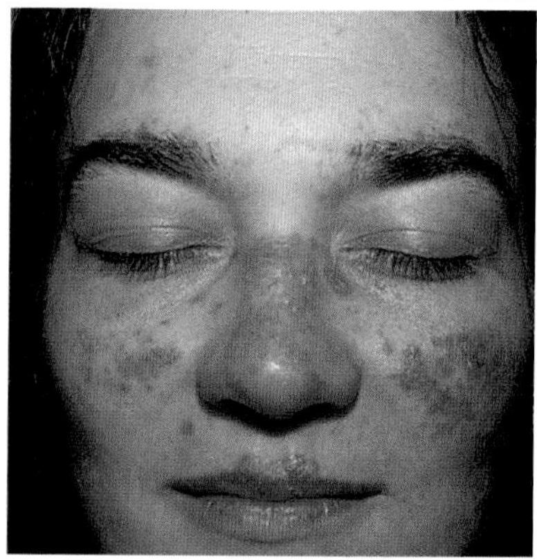

FIG. 52-23 *Keratotic papules and plaques (subacute discoid lupus erythematosus).*

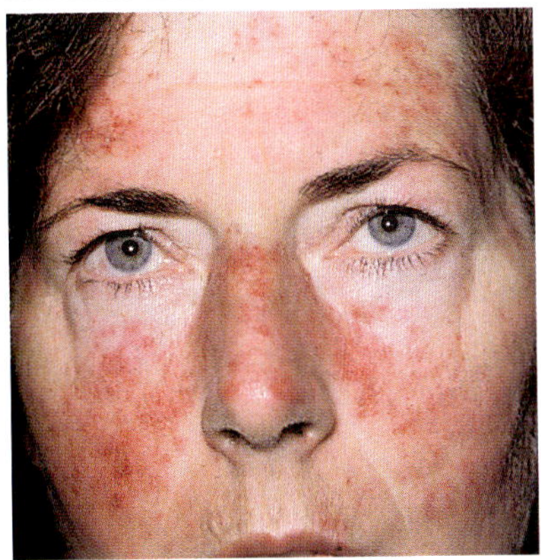

FIG. 52-24 *Macules, papules, and subtle plaques punctuated by telangiectases (subacute discoid lupus erythematosus).*

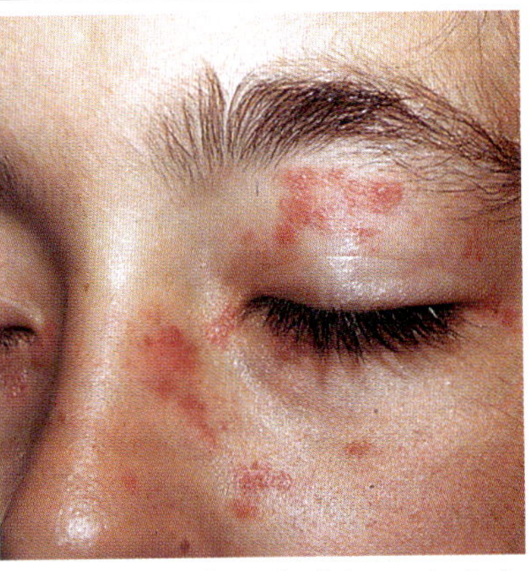

FIG. 52-25 *Macules and subtle papules (subacute discoid lupus erythematosus).*

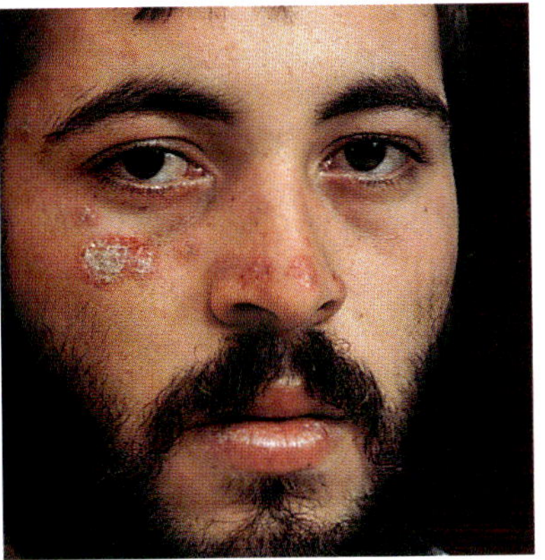

FIG. 52-26 *Scaly papules and plaques (subacute discoid lupus erythematosus).*

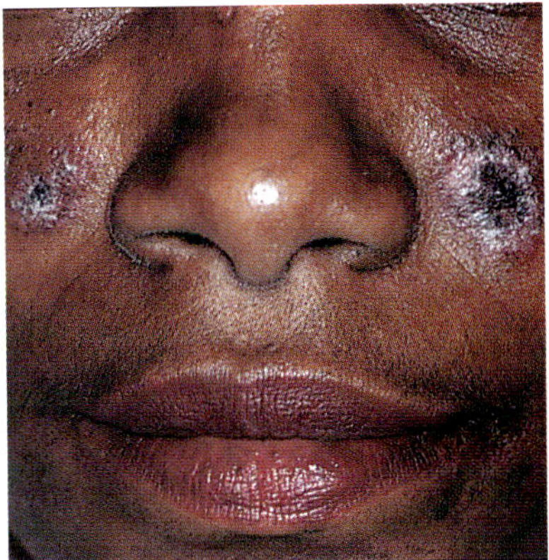

FIG. 52-27 *Scaly plaques with hyperpigmentation (subacute discoid lupus erythematosus).*

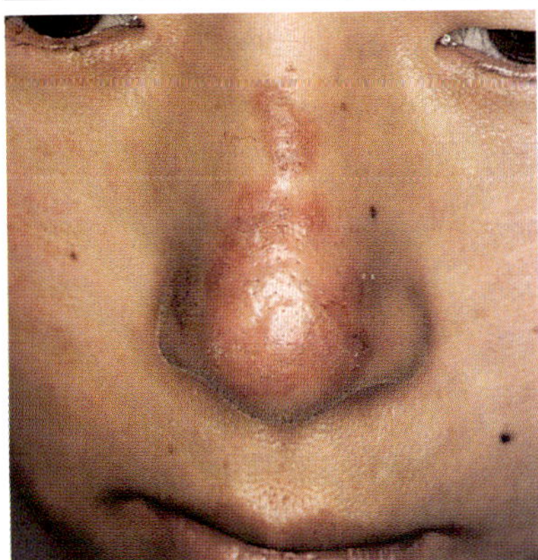

FIG. 52-28 *Papules and a plaque with patulous ostia of follicles (subacute discoid L.E.) and several Miescher's nevi.*

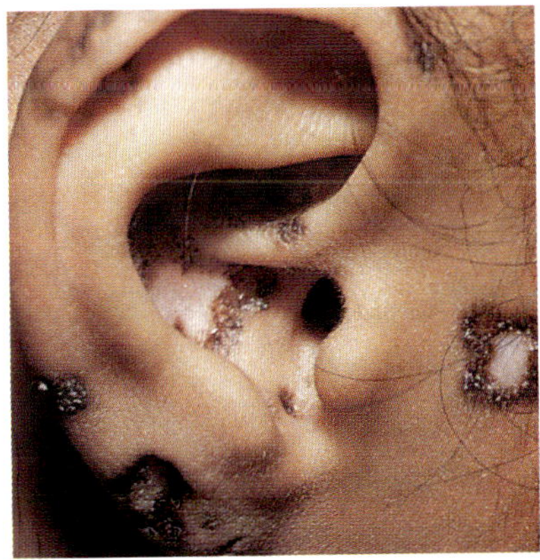

FIG. 52-29 *Papules with an atrophic hypopigmented center and hyperpigmented border (chronic discoid L.E.).*

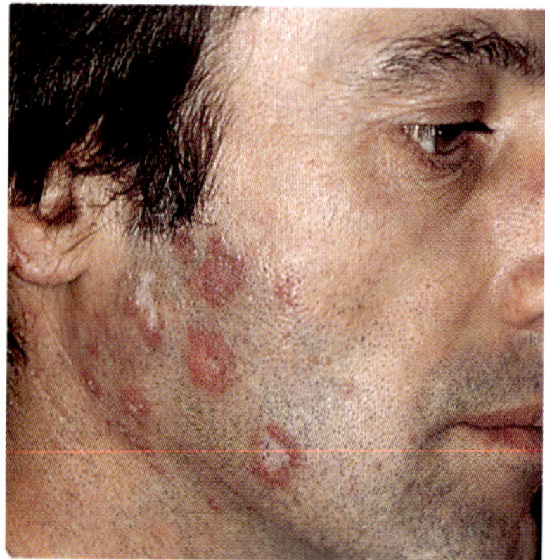

FIG. 52-30 *Arciform and annular plaques with an atrophic hypopigmented center (chronic discoid lupus erythematosus).*

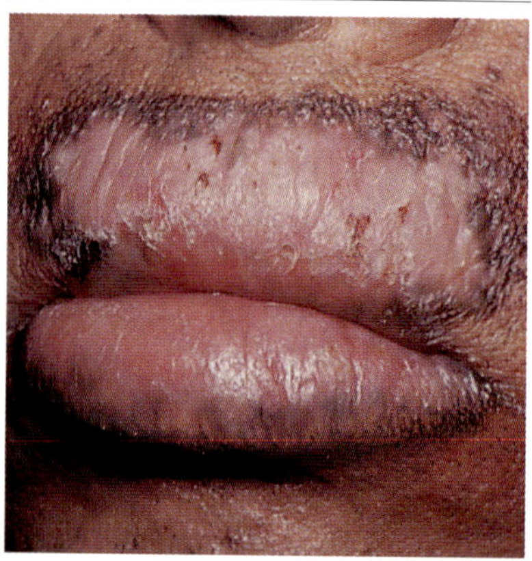

FIG. 52-31 *Scaly hypopigmented plaques with an erythematous border (chronic discoid lupus erythematosus).*

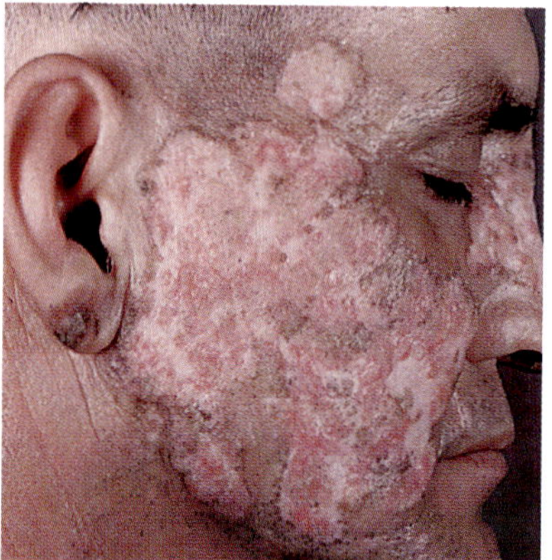

FIG. 52-32 *Plaques with hypopigmented center and hyperpigmented periphery (chronic discoid lupus erythematosus).*

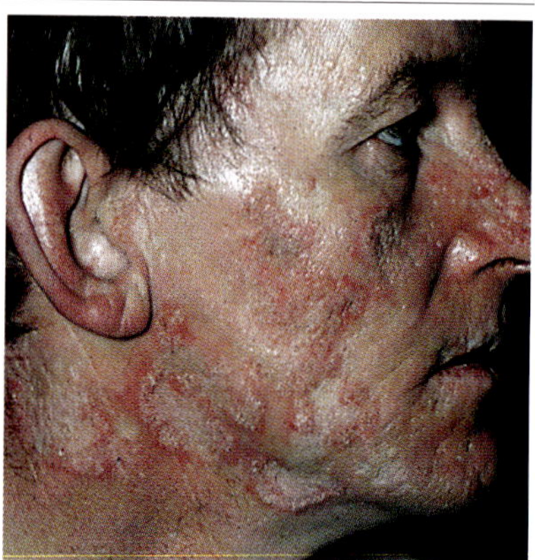

FIG. 52-33 *Hypopigmented patches with scalloped red, scaly, papular border (chronic discoid lupus erythematosus).*

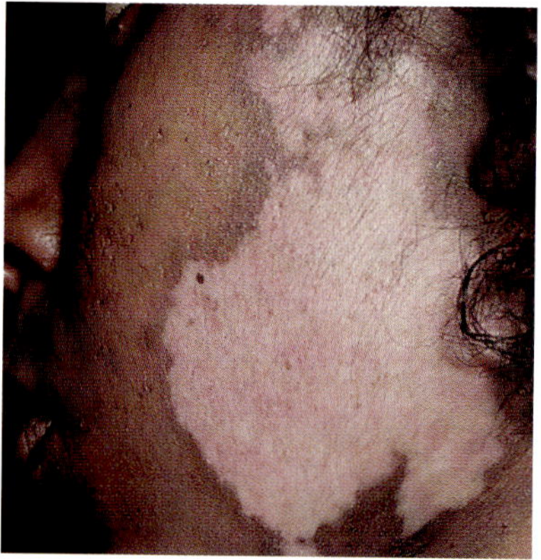

FIG. 52-34 *Atrophic hypopigmented patches with peripheral hyperpigmentation (chronic discoid lupus erythematosus).*

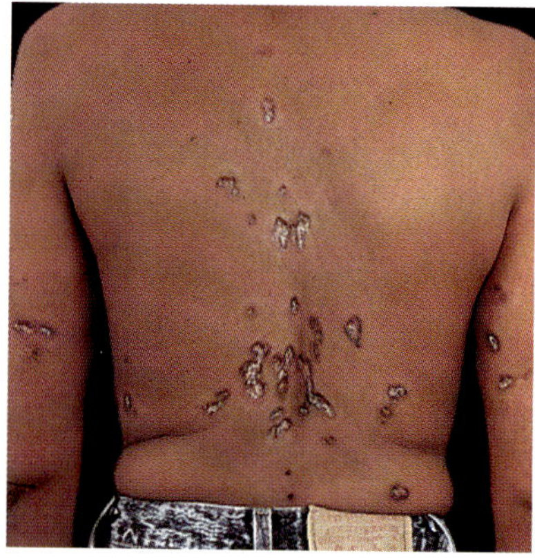

FIG. 52-35 *Hypopigmented scaly atrophic patches (chronic discoid lupus erythematosus).*

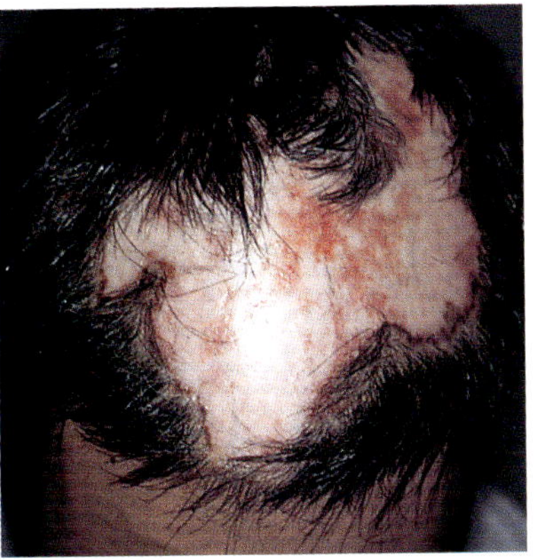

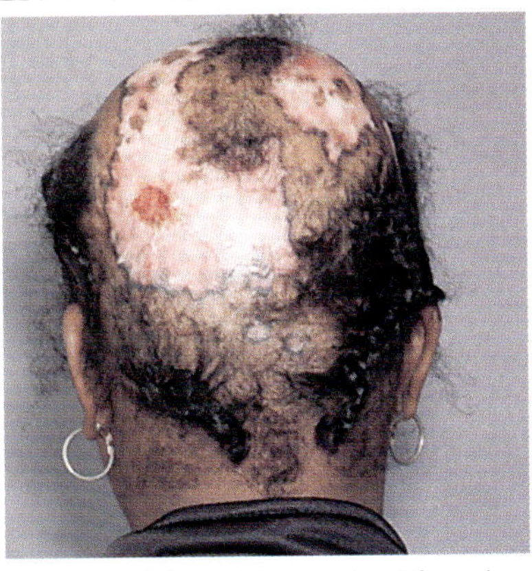

FIG. 52-36 *Permanent alopecia with scalloped border and scarring (chronic discoid lupus erythematosus).*

FIG. 52-37 *Cicatricial alopecia with erosions (chronic discoid lupus erythematosus).*

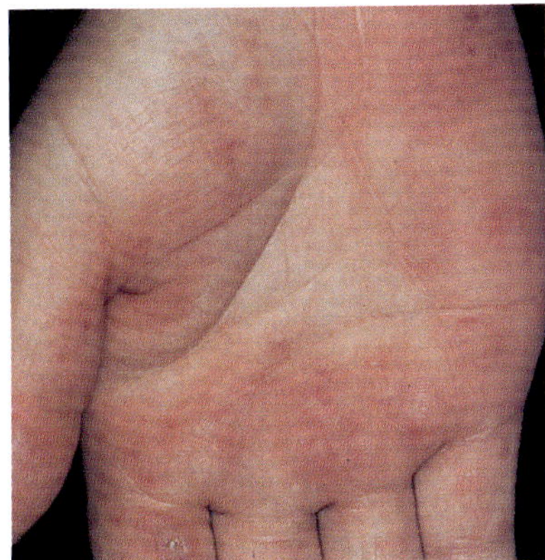

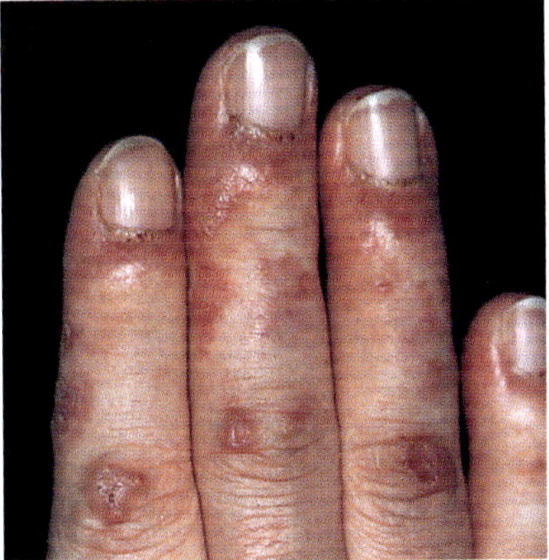

FIG. 52-38 (A, B) *Red papules, some of them scaly, on a palm, over joints, and along proximal nail folds (subacute discoid lupus erythematosus).*

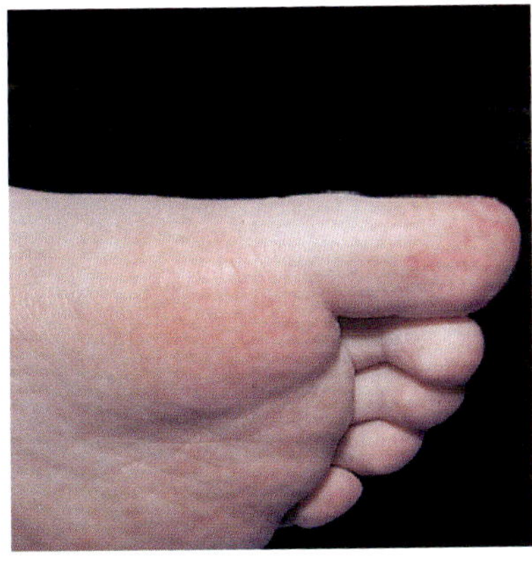

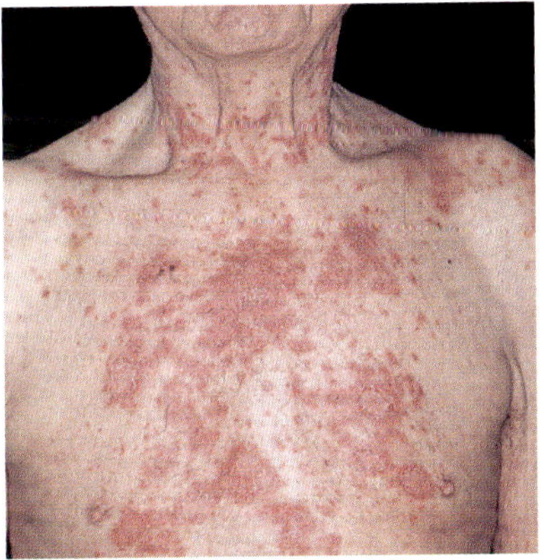

FIG. 52-39 *Erythematous slightly scaly papules, some with an atrophic center (chronic discoid lupus erythematosus).*

FIG. 52-40 *Erythematous slightly scaly papules and plaques with figurate outlines (subacute cutaneous L.E.).*

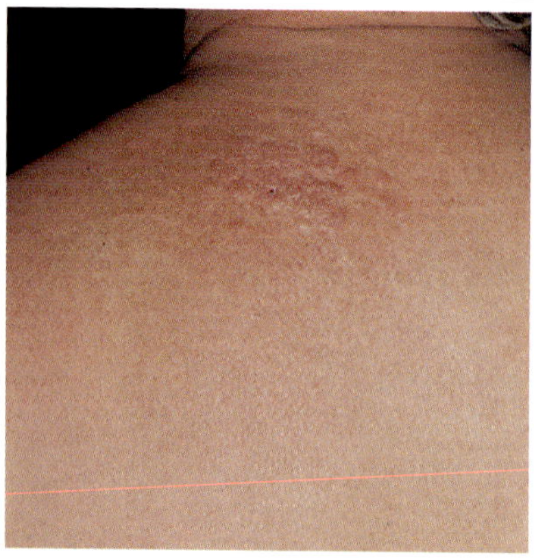 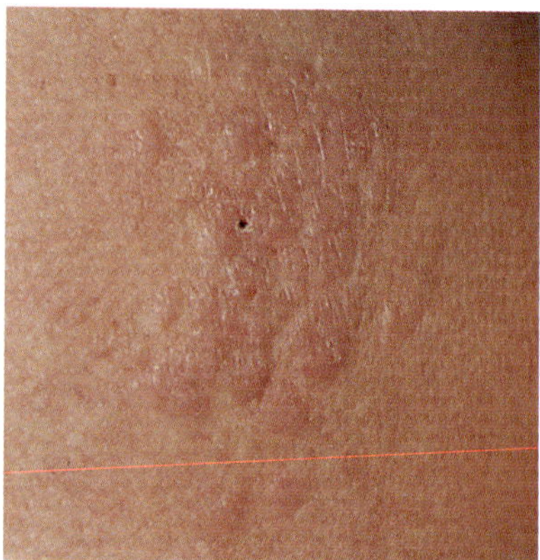

FIG. 52-41 (A, B) *Slightly erythematous nonscaly papules in a cluster (lupus erythematosus with mucinosis, a caricature of lupus tumidus).*

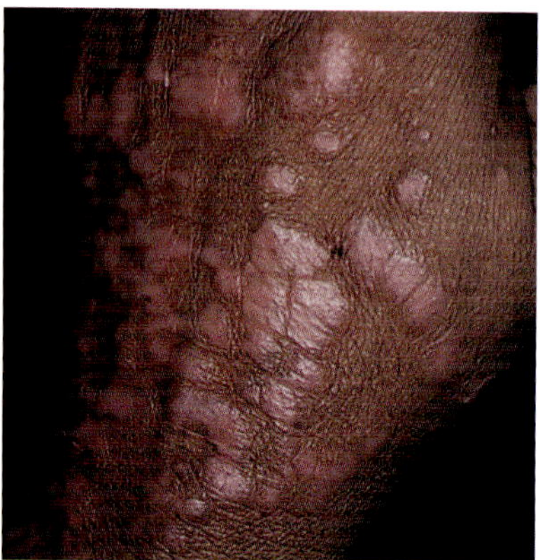

FIG. 52-42 *Hypopigmented papules and plaques (hypertrophic lupus erythematosus).*

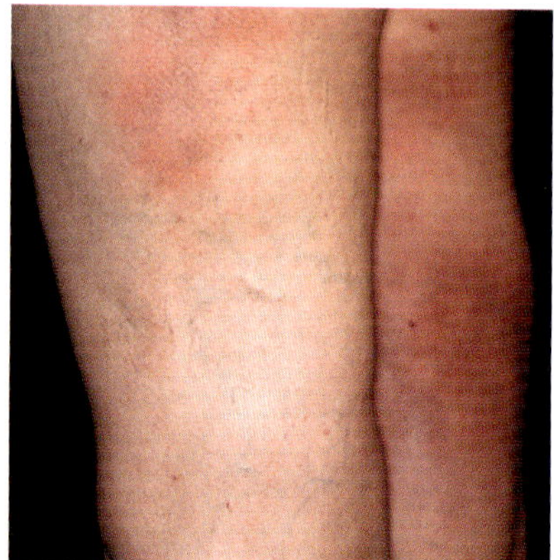

FIG. 52-43 *Indurated plaques with violaceous erythema (lupus profundus).*

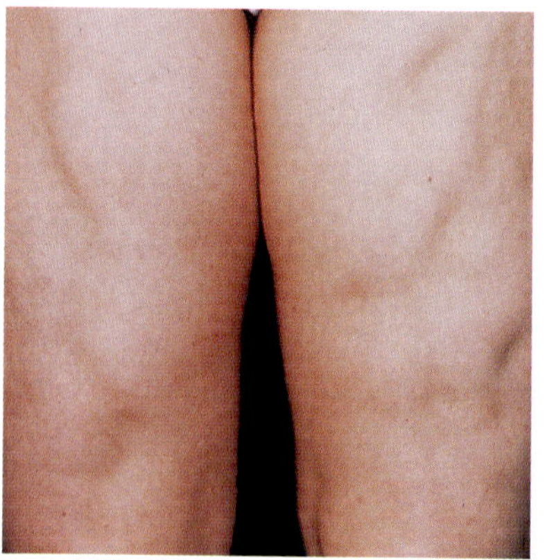

FIG. 52-44 *Deep gullies (lupus profundus).*

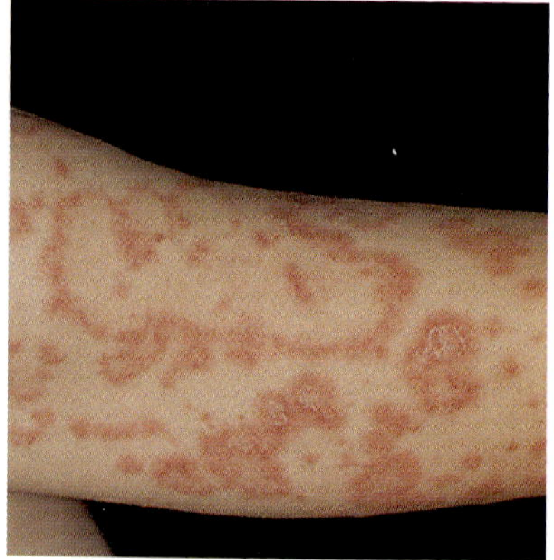

FIG. 52-45 *Scaly papules and plaques with arciform, annular, and serpiginous outlines (subacute cutaneous lupus erythematosus).*

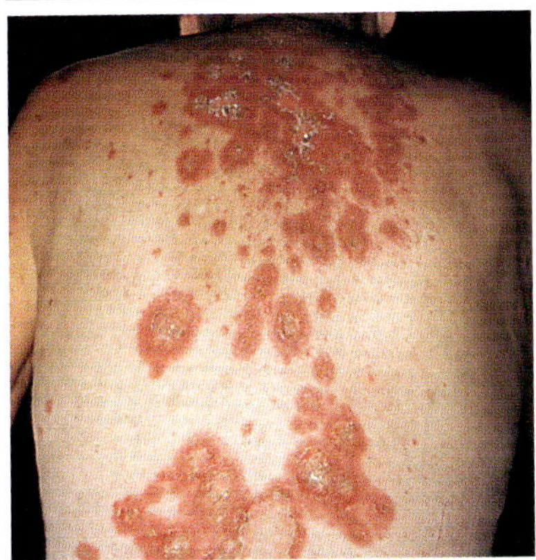

FIG. 52-46 *Scaly papules and plaques, some with annular configuration (subacute cutaneous lupus erythematosus).*

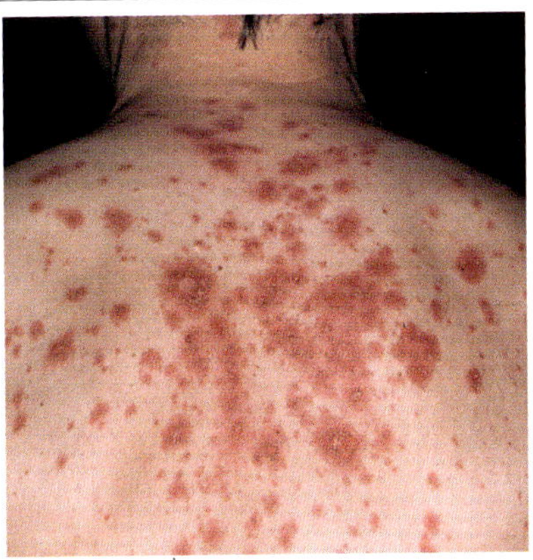

FIG. 52-47 *Macules, papules and plaques, some of the latter with a scalloped border (subacute cutaneous lupus erythematosus).*

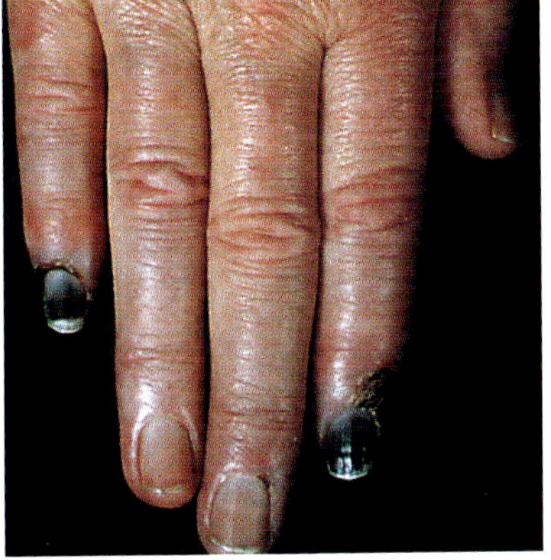

FIG. 52-48 *Hemorrhagic plaques of severe systemic lupus erythematosus consequent to infarction at fingertips (infarctive L.E.).*

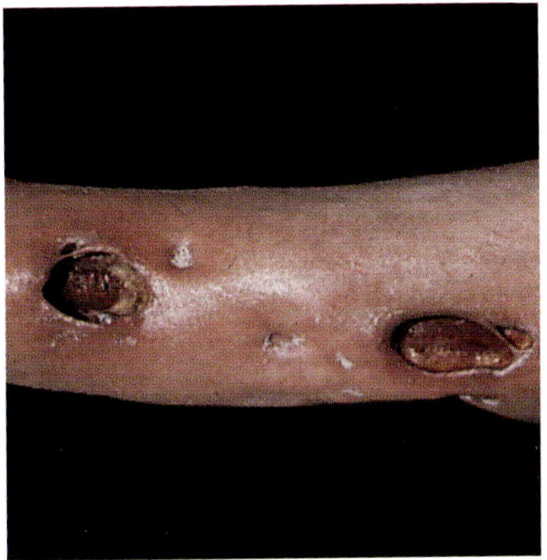

FIG. 52-49 *Sharply circumscribed deep ulcers secondary to large-vessel vasculitis of severe systemic lupus erythematosus.*

Lupus dermatitis and lupus panniculitis may be considered to be analogues of lupus nephritis, lupus arthritis, lupus carditis, lupus serositis, and lupus encephalitis, all of which are manifestations of a systemic disease that can occur at any age, even in newborns (neonatal lupus erythematosus).

ADJUNCTIVE DIAGNOSTIC TESTS Examination of sections of tissue from biopsy specimens of lesional and nonlesional skin (direct immunofluorescence) reveals immunoglobulins (IgG) and components of complement in a granular or continuous linear arrangement at the dermoepidermal junction (lupus band test).

Antinuclear antibodies can be demonstrated with immunoserological methods. The markers for lupus erythematosus are antibodies to double-stranded DNA, anti-SM, anti-Ro/SSA, and anti-La/SSB.

COURSE The chronologic sequence of lesions of lupus dermatitis varies dramatically depending on the specific type of lesion, e.g., a "butterfly blush" of acute discoid lupus erythematosus that often wanes within days or alopecia of chronic discoid lupus erythematosus that is permanent. From what has just been written, it is apparent that not every patch of discoid lupus erythematosus becomes a plaque that eventuates in a scar; lesions such as the "butterfly blush" may disappear without residua and others may resolve with only postinflammatory pigmentary changes. Blisters of bullous lupus erythematosus involute quickly as crusts and heal with pigmentary alterations, but usually without scars.

INTEGRATION: UNIFYING CONCEPT Perhaps no subject in dermatology, with the possible exception of mycosis fungoides, is as confusing to students as that of lupus erythematosus. The names given to lesions in the skin are dizzying, among them, acute, subacute, and chronic discoid lupus erythematosus, subacute cutaneous lupus erythematosus, neonatal lupus erythematosus, bullous lupus erythematosus, lupus profundus, lupus tumidus, localized discoid lupus erythematosus, cutaneous lupus erythematosus, systemic lupus erythematosus, and so on.

One way to think about cutaneous/subcutaneous lesions of lupus erythematosus is as a single pathologic process, to wit, lupus dermatitis/panniculitis. When reddish patches of acute discoid lupus erythematosus appear on malar eminences ("butterfly blush"), they are characterized histopathologically by a sprinkling of neutrophils in the upper part of the dermis, immediately beneath the epidermis. When that process is accelerated exponentially, a lesion of bullous lupus erythematosus comes into being characterized by a subepidermal blister that houses countless neutrophils and nuclear "dust" of them. Bullous lupus erythematosus is simply a caricature of acute discoid lupus erythematosus.

If the erythematous patches of acute discoid lupus erythematosus do not wane within days or weeks but persist and advance to become subtle plaques, the stage of subacute discoid lupus erythematosus has been reached. It is typified by a superficial perivascular infiltrate of lymphocytes, as well as by lymphocytes scattered along the dermoepidermal junction in conjunction with vacuolar alteration, and a thinned, slightly hyperkeratotic epidermis. An increase in the amount of mucin in the reticular dermis is an expected finding in discoid lupus erythematosus at nearly all stages of it.

If the plaques persist and become broader and thicker, a fully-developed lesion of subacute discoid lupus erythematosus is the result. It consists of a superficial and deep perivascular infiltrate of lymphocytes, lymphocytes along the dermoepidermal junction in concert with vacuolar alteration there, a thickened basement membrane beneath a thinned hyperkeratotic epidermis, and, often, plugs of corneocytes in widened infundibula.

When, after years, a lesion of subacute discoid lupus erythematosus involutes with hyperpigmentation and hypopigmentation, atrophy, and telangiectases (poikiloderma), all that is seen is sclerosis in the upper part of the dermis, the virtual absence of adnexal structures, a markedly thickened epidermal basement membrane, and a thinned, slightly hyperkeratotic epidermis, a state known as "chronic discoid lupus erythematosus." When the infiltrates of lymphocytes of discoid lupus erythematosus affect lobules in the subcutaneous fat, as well as the dermis, the condition is called lupus profundus. When the infiltrate of lymphocytes affects the dermis, but not the dermoepidermal junction and the epidermis, in association with copious quantities of mucin, the lesions are known as those of lupus tumidus (sometimes referred to confusingly histopathologically as "lymphocytic infiltration of Jessner and Kanof," and bewilderingly clinically, in the company of a netlike pattern, as "reticular erythematosus mucinosis"). When mucin in the reticular dermis is so abundant that it causes prominent papules and plaques to form, the condition is known as mucinous lupus erythematosus. When lesions, especially on the trunk, have arcuate, annular, and serpiginous outlines, but show the characteristic histopathologic features of discoid lupus erythematosus, they are designated "subacute cutaneous lupus erythematosus." Neonatal lupus erythematosus is simply lupus dermatitis in a neonate, early lesions being like those of acute discoid lupus erythematosus and late lesions like those of chronic discoid lupus erythematosus.

Rather than dicing the cutaneous and subcutaneous expressions of lupus erythematosus into artificial compartments, it is preferable to conceive of those manifestations as part of a single pathologic process, to wit, lupus dermatitis/panniculitis. The process is analogous to lupus arthritis, lupus encephalitis, lupus serositis, lupus carditis, and lupus nephritis, all of which represent manifestations of a systemic disease, systemic lupus erythematosus.

Whereas lupus nephritis may prove to be fatal, lupus dermatitis does not. A single lesion of discoid lupus erythematosus on an ear or of several lesions of tumid lupus erythematosus may be of little more than cosmetic concern, but, it is, nonetheless, an expression of a systemic disease. When, however, lesions of discoid lupus erythematosus are widespread, as occurs, for example, after a severe sunburn in a person clad in a bikini, or if lesions are bullous (referred to conventionally as bullous systemic lupus erythematosus), the implication of those changes is that vital organs are affected concurrently and severely by the same systemic disease, and that the prognosis is grave.

THERAPY For lupus dermatitis, protection against the rays of the sun is paramount. Topical corticosteroids, intralesional injections of corticosteroids, and cryotherapy are helpful for lesions that are not widespread, and antimalarials (hydroxychloroquine and chloroquine), systemic corticosteroids, thalidomide, retinoids, and dapsone are beneficial for widespread lesions.

For systemic lupus erythematosus in which there are signs or symptoms of disease of internal organs, systemic corticosteroids and nonsteroidal anti-inflammatory agents are recommended. In patients who are seriously ill, azathioprine and cyclophosphamide may be added to the regimen, all of which should be supervised by a team of specialists in diagnosis and management of lupus erythematosus.

LYMPHOMAS (OTHER THAN MYCOSIS FUNGOIDES AND LYMPHOMATOID PAPULOSIS)

DEFINITION Malignant neoplasms of B-lymphocytes especially that present themselves usually as papules, nodules, and tumors, sometimes solitary but at other times numerous, and often in clusters on any anatomic site. When "primary," B-cell lymphomas of the skin seem to be wholly cutaneous with no evidence of extracutaneous manifestations after complete staging has been performed. The major categories of primary cutaneous B-cell lymphomas are follicle center-cell lymphoma with preferential location on the head and back, immunocytoma (and marginal-zone lymphoma) situated on the trunk, buttocks, and extremities, and large B-cell lymphoma with predilection for the legs of older patients.

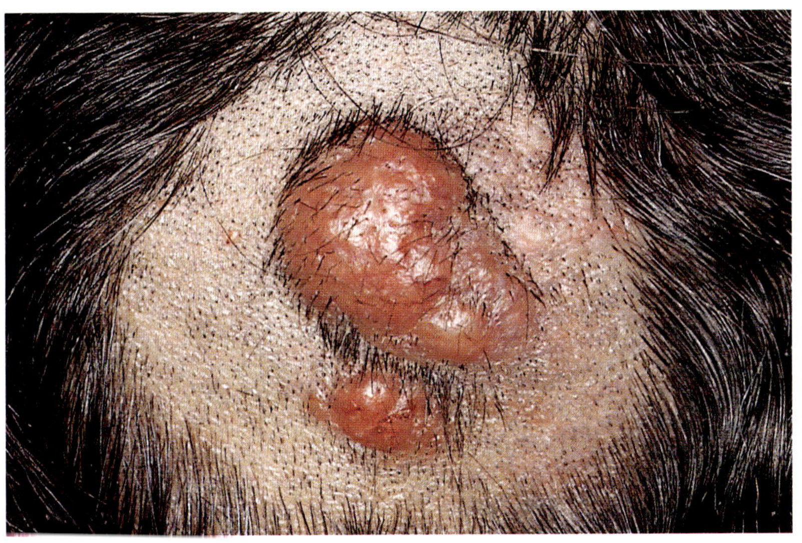

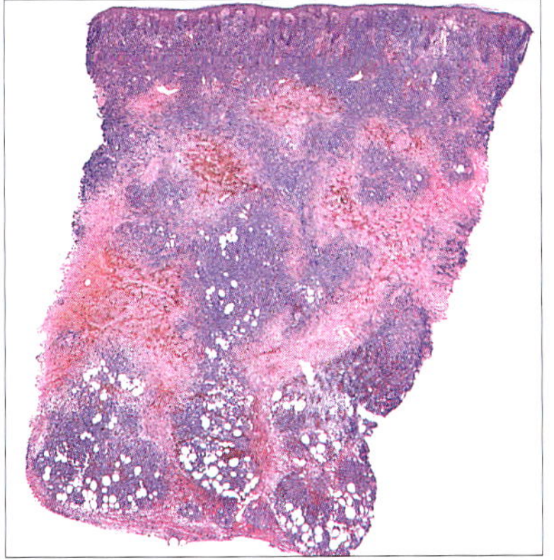

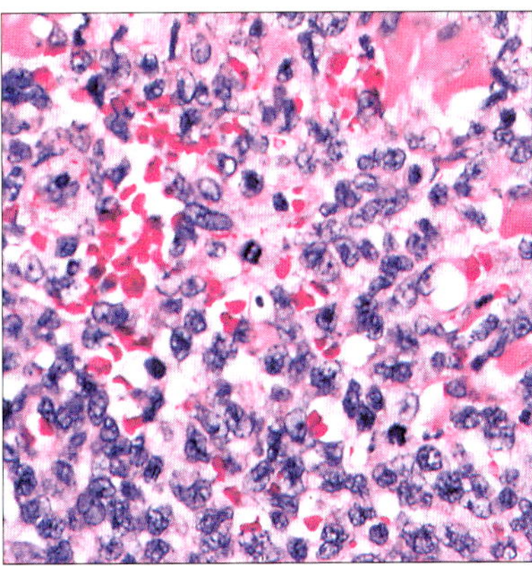

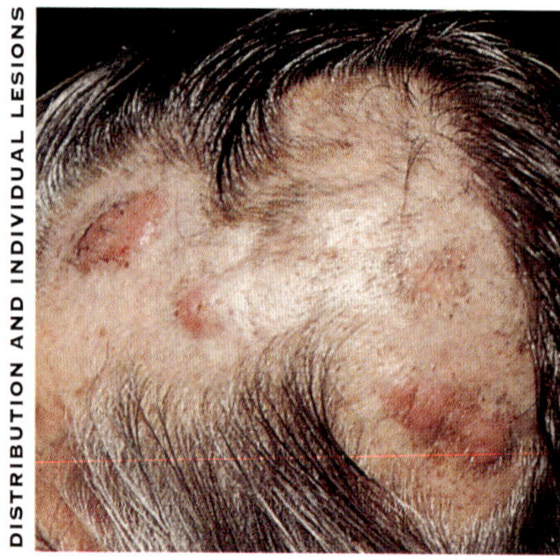

FIG. 53-1 *Papules and nodules (follicle center-cell lymphoma).*

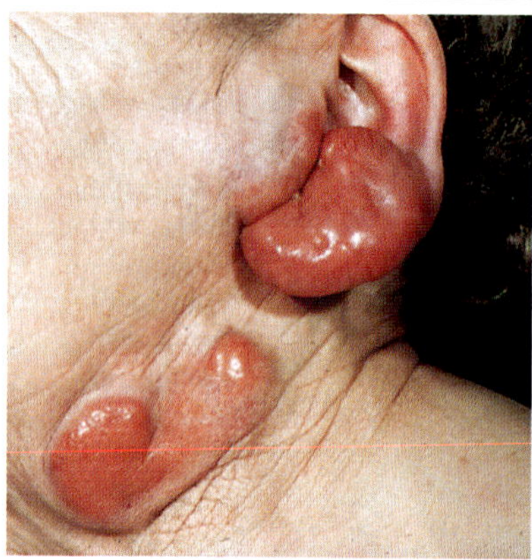

FIG. 53-2 *Tumors (follicle center-cell lymphoma).*

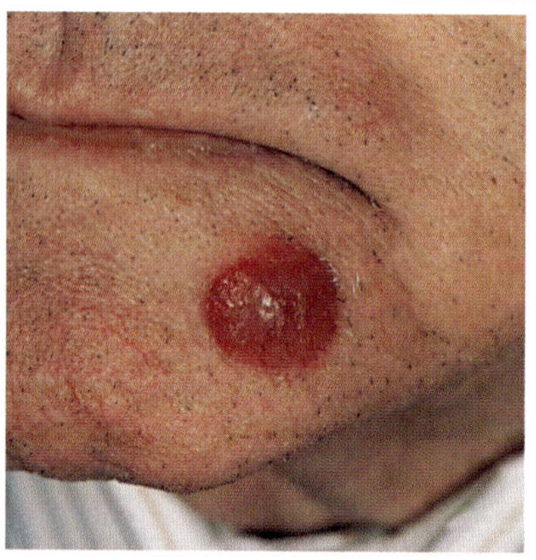

FIG. 53-3 *Tumor (follicle center-cell lymphoma).*

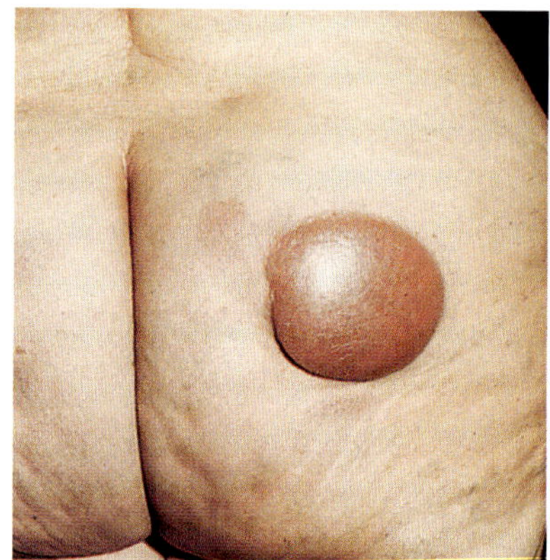

FIG. 53-4 *A huge tumor in conjunction with patches and plaques (immunocytoma).*

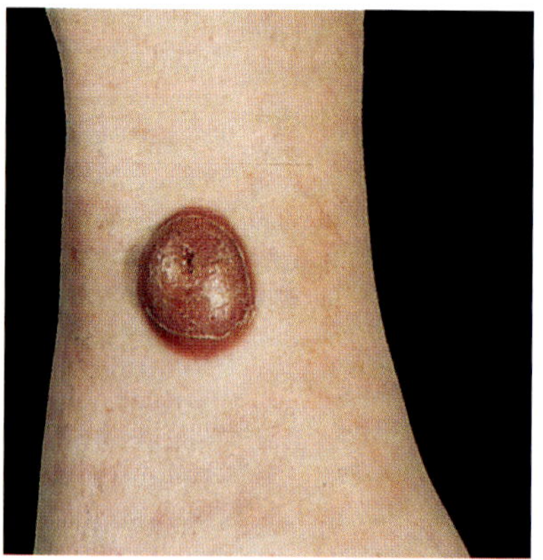

FIG. 53-5 *Tumor (large-cell lymphoma).*

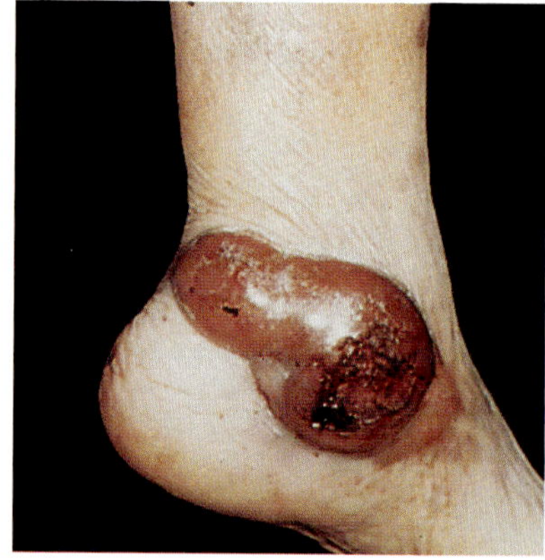

FIG. 53-6 *Papules and a gigantic ulcerated tumor (large-cell lymphoma).*

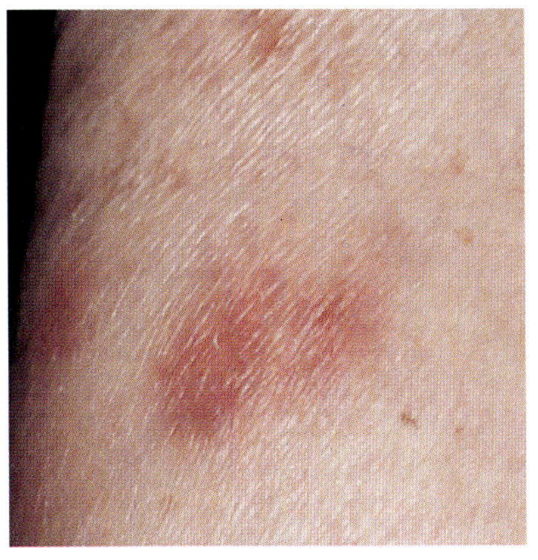

FIG. 53-7 *Papules and a plaque on the leg (early stage of large-cell lymphoma).*

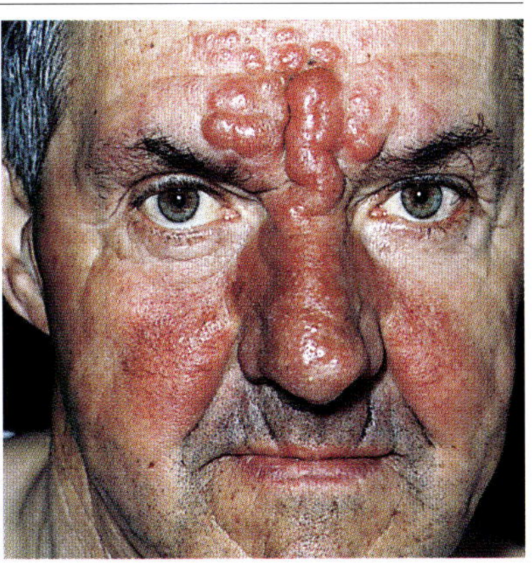

FIG. 53-8 *Papules and nodules (chronic lymphocytic leukemia, B-cell type).*

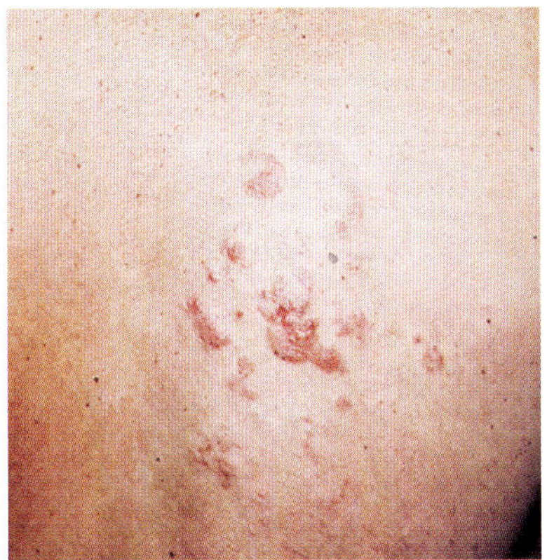

FIG. 53-9 *Smooth-surfaced papules and nodules in a cluster (marginal zone lymphoma).*

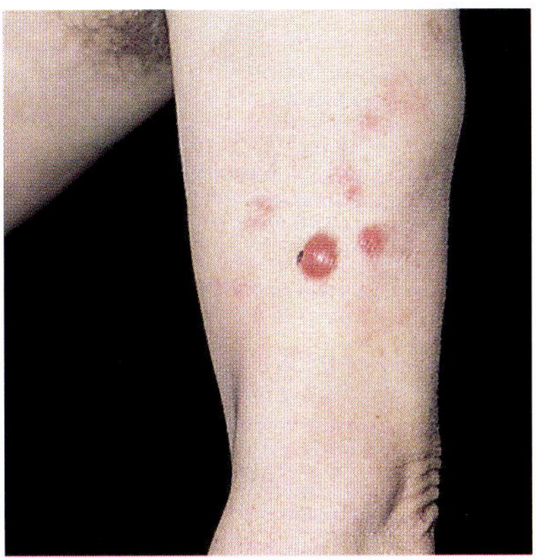

FIG. 53-10 *Macules, papules, and a nodule (marginal-zone lymphoma).*

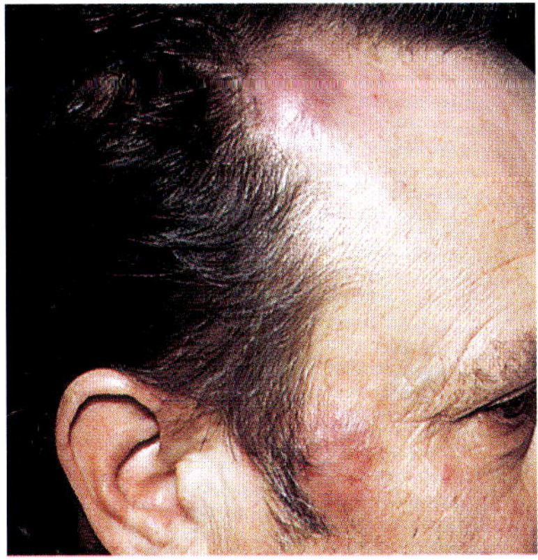

FIG. 53-11 *Smooth-surfaced plaque and nodule (follicle center-cell lymphoma).*

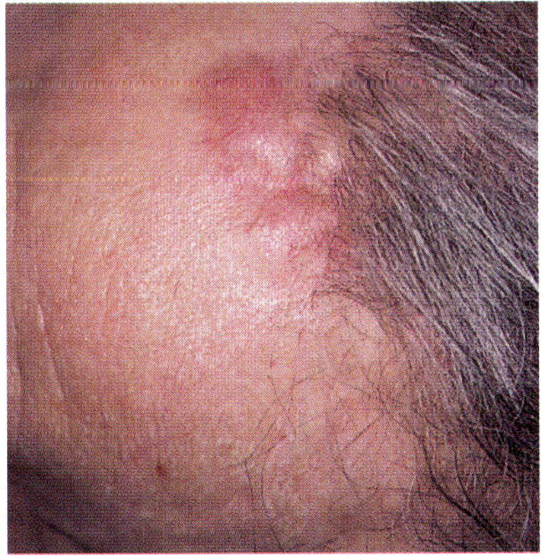

FIG. 53-12 *Smooth-surfaced nodules (follicle center-cell lymphoma).*

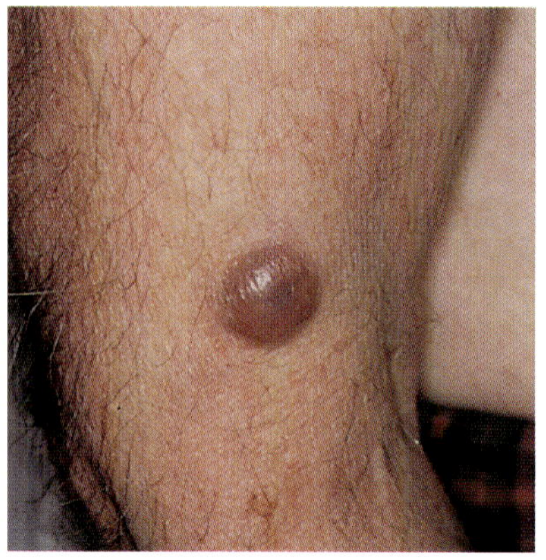

FIG. 53-13 *Smooth-surfaced nodule (large-cell lymphoma of an extremity).*

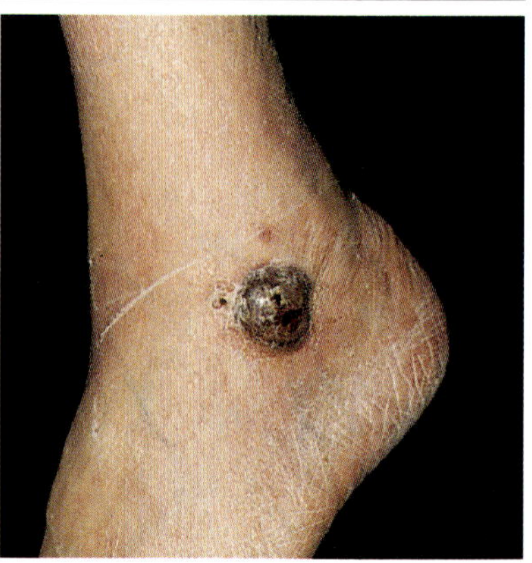

FIG. 53-14 *Tumor (large-cell lymphoma of an extremity).*

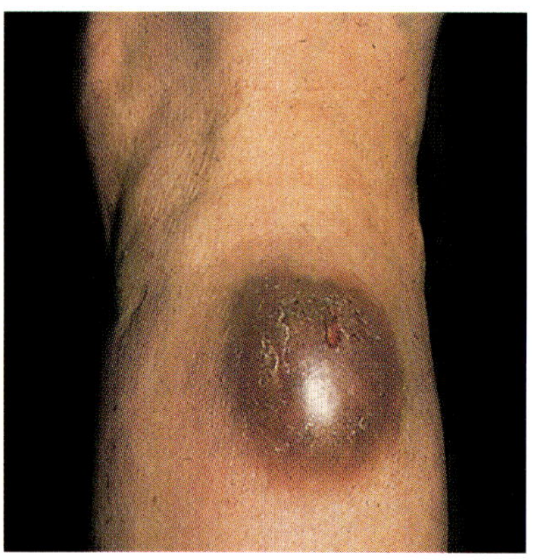

FIG. 53-15 *Isolated tumor (large-cell lymphoma of an extremity).*

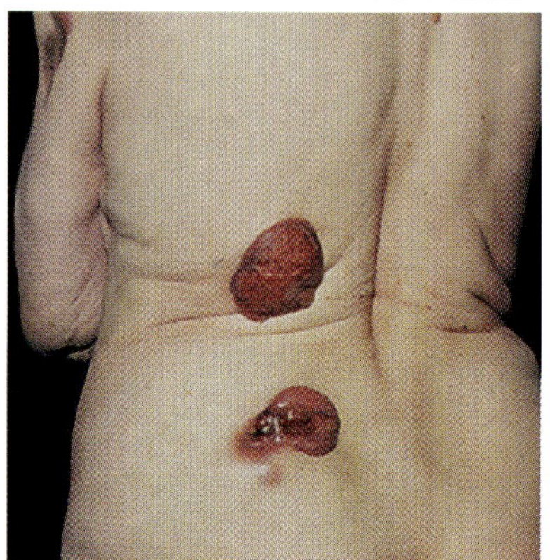

FIG. 53-16 *Ulcerated nodules and tumors (involvement of the skin by a nodal B-cell lymphoma).*

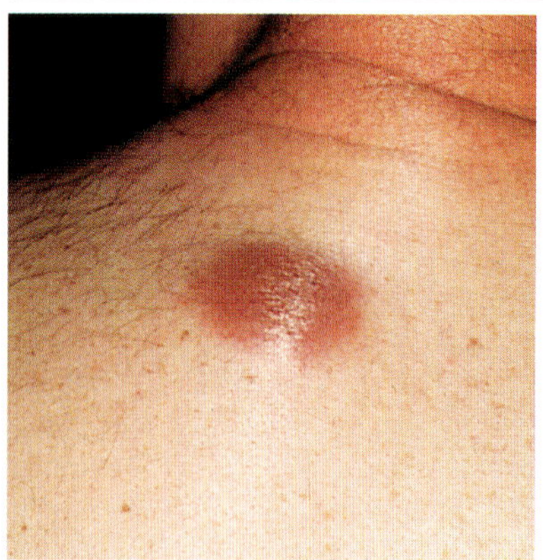

FIG. 53-17 *Low-domed, rust-colored tumor (marginal zone lymphoma).*

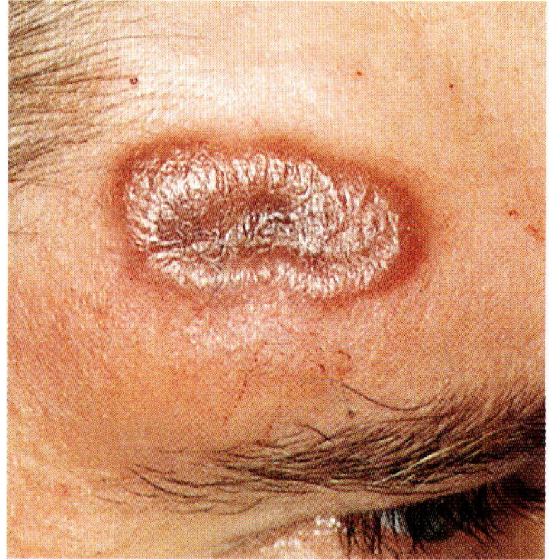

FIG. 53-18 *Markedly indented tumorous plaque (large-cell anaplastic lymphoma, CD30 positive).*

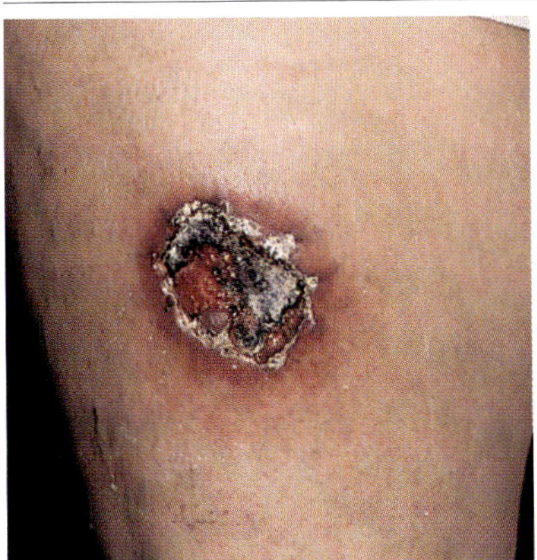

FIG. 53-19   *Ulcerated nodule with ragged margins (pleomorphic T-cell lymphoma).*

Cutaneous T-cell lymphomas other than mycosis fungoides present themselves as macules and patches, papules and plaques, and nodules and tumors that may appear on any anatomic site. Included among them are anaplastic large-cell lymphoma and panniculitis-like T-cell lymphoma. Anaplastic large-cell lymphoma of T-cell type usually occurs as a solitary, rapidly growing tumor. Most of the neoplastic lymphocytes express the CD30 antigen. Panniculitis-like T-cell lymphoma is a distinct type derived from activated cytotoxic T-cells and characterized by plaques and subcutaneous tumors on the extremities and the trunk.

ADJUNCTIVE DIAGNOSTIC TESTS   Assessment of immunophenotypic and molecular genetic attributes is necessary in order to establish a specific diagnosis. Staging procedures are requisite to determine whether there is overt evidence of systemic disease.

COURSE   Large-cell anaplastic lymphoma (CD30 positive) usually has a good prognosis and may even undergo complete regression in the absence of treatment. Panniculitis-like T-cell lymphoma may be indolent or end quickly with death after a fulminant course.

The prognosis of primary cutaneous B-cell lymphoma usually is excellent, in contrast to that for nodal lymphomas. Only large-cell lymphomas of B-cell type have a less favorable prognosis.

INTEGRATION: UNIFYING CONCEPT Attempts to classify cutaneous lymphomas other than mycosis fungoides have been numerous and uniformly unsuccessful. Those classifications initially were known by the names of persons responsible for them, such as Rappaport, and Lukes and Collins. Next they were named according to a city, to wit, Kiel, where Lennert and his students conducted extensive studies of the subject. More recently, they have been designated for societies in which coworkers come from a particular continent, such as EORTC (European Organization for Research and Treatment of Cancer), or from different continents, e.g., REAL (Revised European American Lymphoma).

In brief, however, it can be said that all of the classifications have failed because they have focused mostly on cytologic features of lymphoma, rather than on an effort to truly integrate the clinical, histopathologic, and biologic attributes. Unlike the situation with mycosis fungoides, where the clinical, histopathologic, and biologic aspects have been integrated neatly, in regard to other lymphomas even nomenclature still is in dispute. Nonetheless, the B-cell lymphomas, for instance, still can be recognized for what they are by their distinctive characteristics and predilections, such as the type that favors the head and back (follicle center-cell lymphoma), the extremities, trunk, and buttocks (immunocytoma, marginal zone lymphoma), and the leg (large B-cell lymphoma).

Even though a particular type of lymphoma cannot always be identified clinically on the basis of findings in a particular papule, nodule, or tumor (those solid lesions in different lymphomas often look alike clinically), it surely can be categorized precisely when all morphologic attributes—clinical, histopathologic, and cytopathologic—are wedded to biologic behavior. In this respect, the lymphomas under consideration here are different from those of mycosis fungoides because by inspection grossly of only a single lesion they cannot be diagnosed with confidence. By contrast, a patch of parapsoriasis en plaques can be diagnosed with surety, as can a plaque of pagetoid reticulosis or a pendulous tumor of granulomatous slack skin, thereby permitting a diagnosis of mycosis fungoides.

In sum, each of the cutaneous lymphomas discussed in this chapter has the same individuality as do mycosis fungoides and lymphomatoid papulosis, and a student of this atlas and of the subject of lymphomas in general should make an effort to become cognizant of those specificities and, in the process, become able to diagnose them with exactness.

THERAPY Many patients with what are thought to be "primary" cutaneous B-cell lymphomas have an excellent prognosis. Discrete lesions, if few, can be excised surgically or exposed to radiotherapy. Widespread lesions may be managed systemically with interferon or chemotherapy.

In large-cell anaplastic lymphoma, local treatment is by excision or irradiation. Panniculitis-like T-cell lymphoma requires chemotherapy according to standard regimens.

DEFINITION A distinctive type of lymphoma characterized by the presence mostly of papules, some of them purpuric, that may ulcerate and heal with a scar, and by lesions that tend to come and go for years, eventually disappearing entirely or, on occasion, becoming nodular and even tumorous, which is an indication of likelihood of detectable lymphomatous involvement of some organs besides the skin.

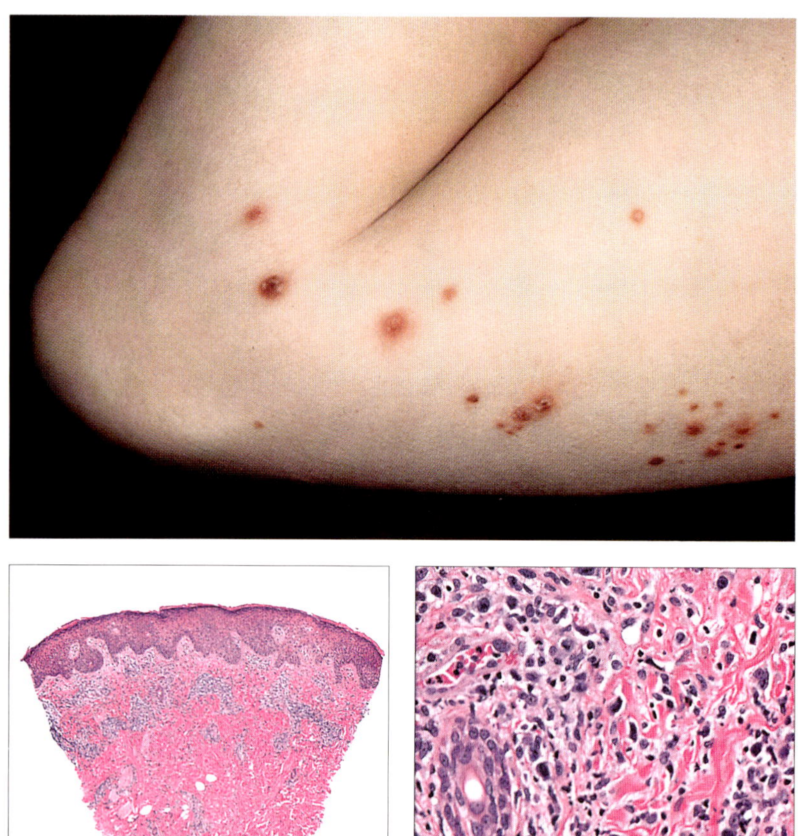

DISTRIBUTION

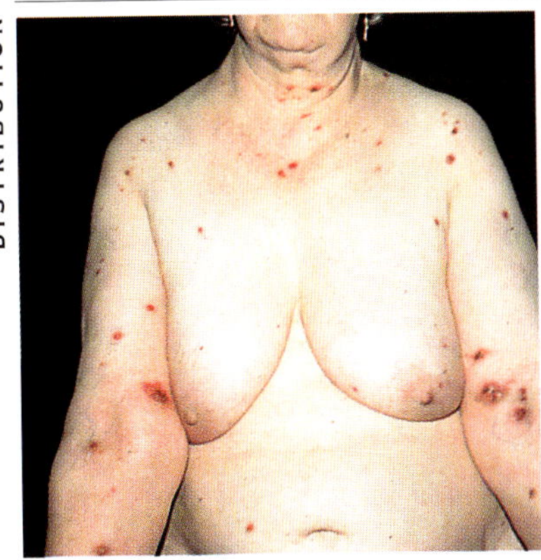

FIG. 54-1 *Widespread papules.*

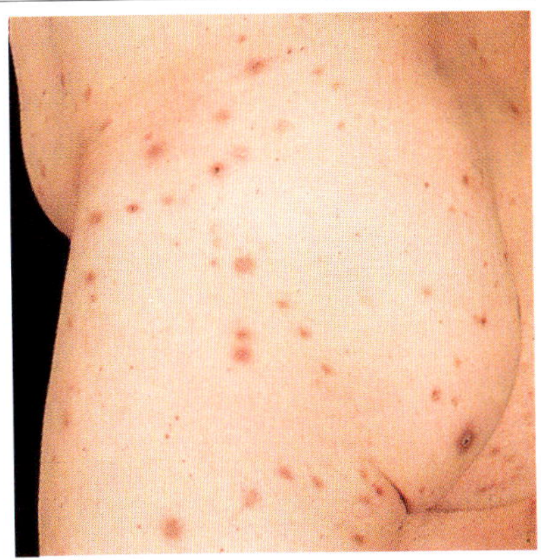

FIG. 54-2 *Papules.*

ARRANGEMENT

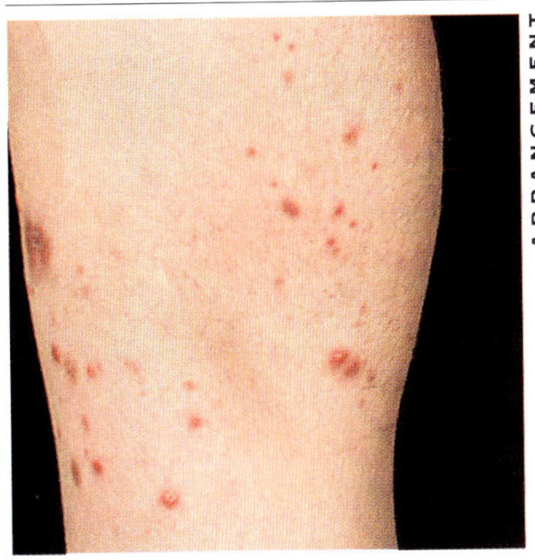

FIG. 54-3 *Papules and subtle papulovesicles.*

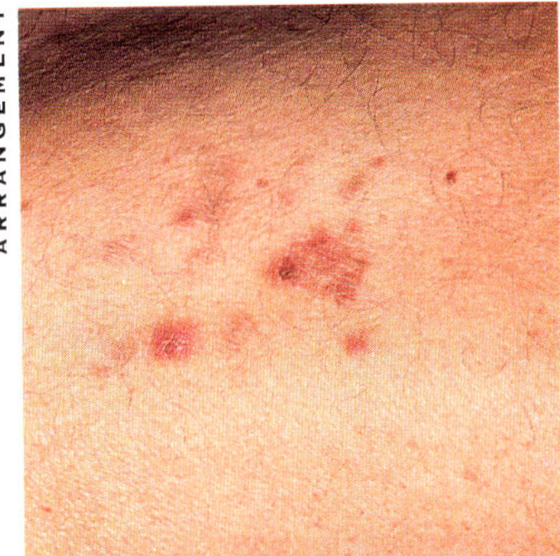

FIG. 54-4 *Papules, in a cluster, at different stages of evolution and devolution.*

INDIVIDUAL LESIONS

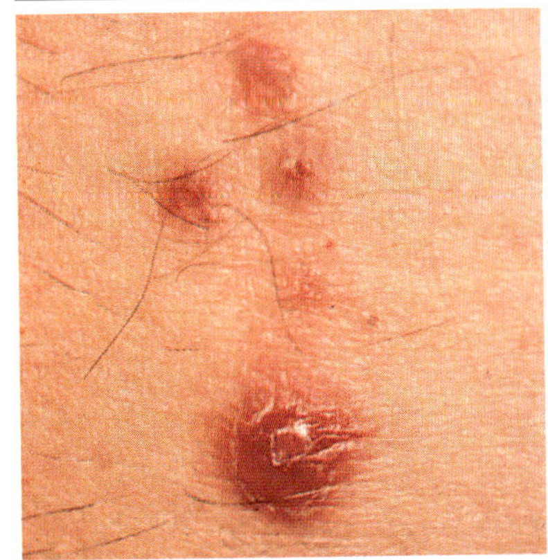

FIG. 54-5 *Cluster of papules, the largest scaly one being the oldest.*

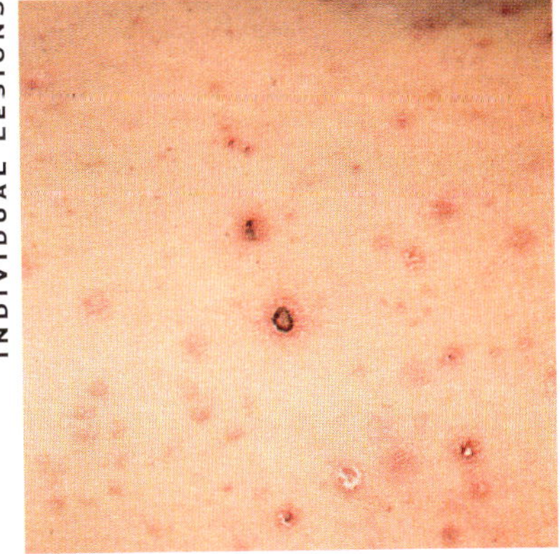

FIG. 54-6 *Papules in different stages, e.g., smooth, scaly, or ulcerated with a hemorrhagic crust.*

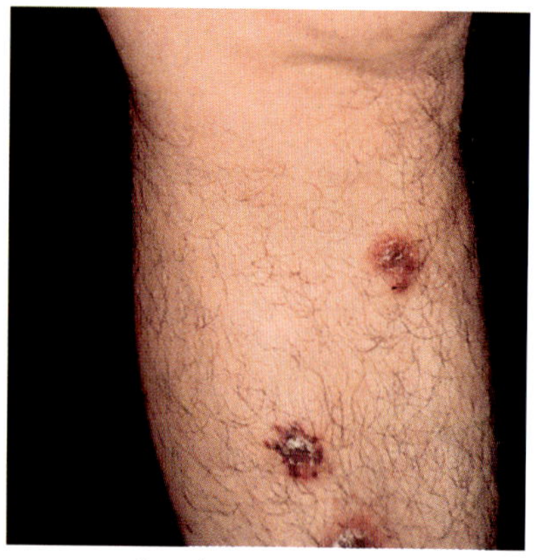

FIG. 54-7 *Papules with hemorrhagic crusts.*

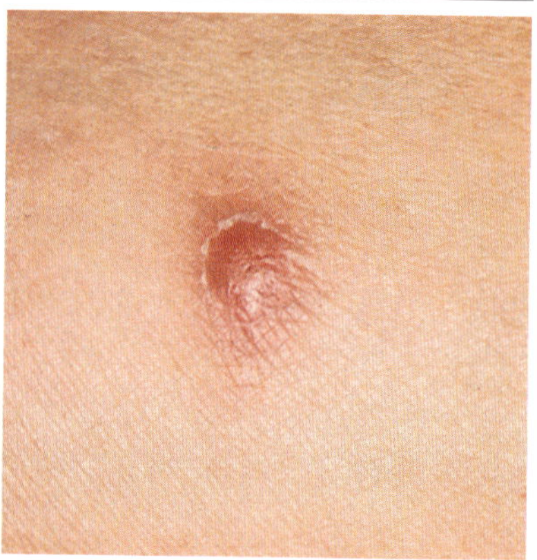

FIG. 54-8 *Smooth-surfaced papule with peripheral scale.*

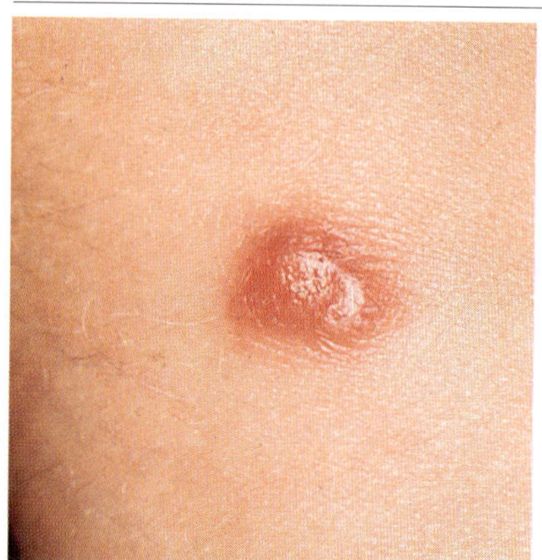

FIG. 54-9 *Scaly papule.*

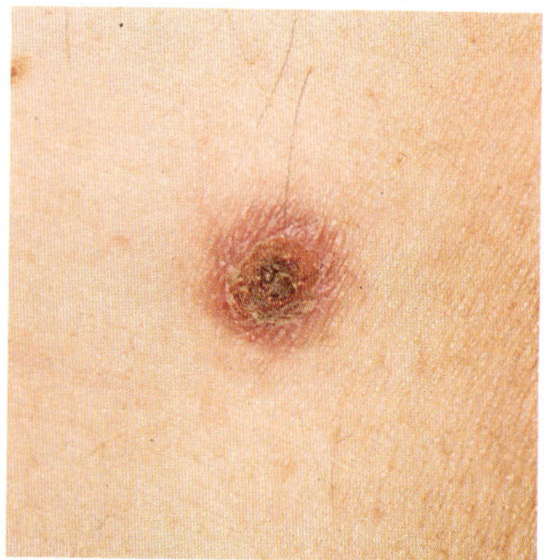

FIG. 54-10 *Scaly, crusted papule.*

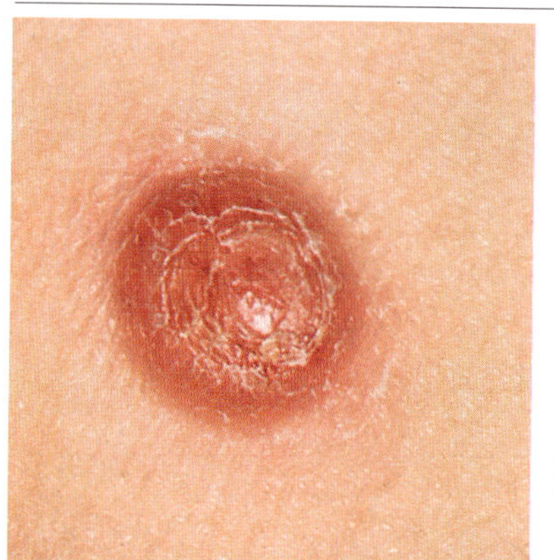

FIG. 54-11 *Papule with scale.*

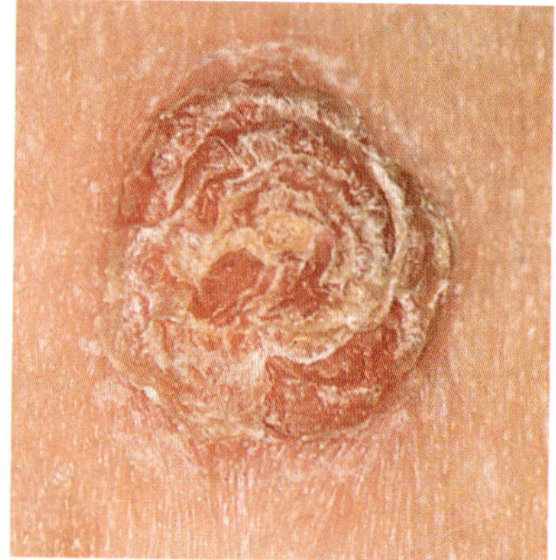

FIG. 54-12 *Papule with prominent scale-crust.*

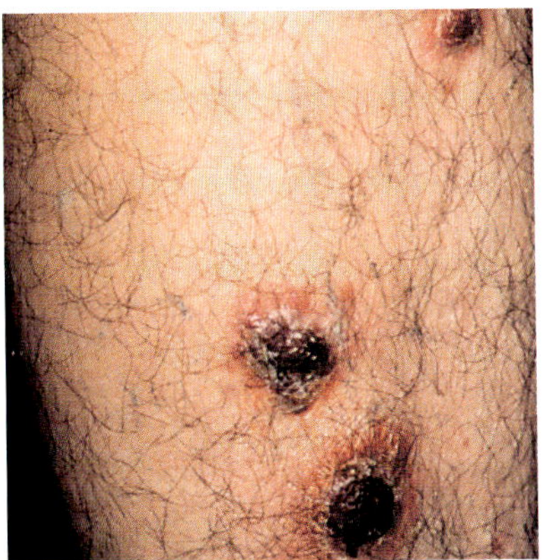

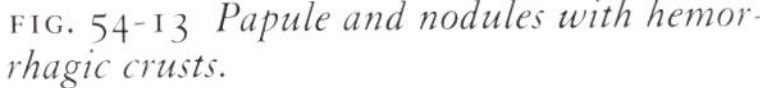

FIG. 54-13 *Papule and nodules with hemor-rhagic crusts.*

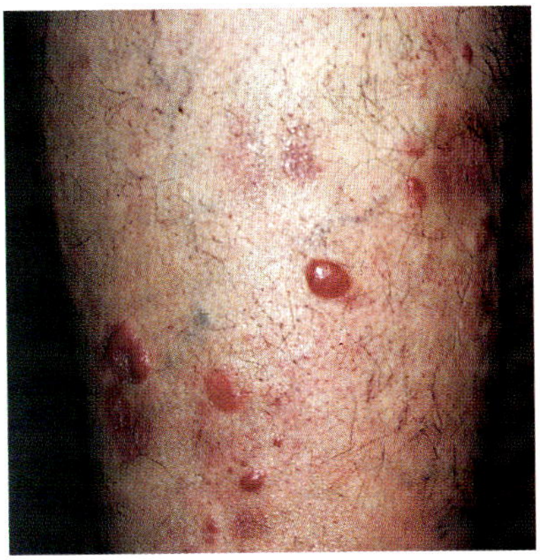

FIG. 54-14 *Smooth-surfaced papules and pigmented macules, the latter representing lesions that have involuted.*

ADJUNCTIVE DIAGNOSTIC TEST Immunohistopathologic staining of sections of tissue achieves the purpose of demonstrating CD30 positive large T-lymphocytes.

COURSE Papules of lymphomatoid papulosis may last for weeks and involute without noticeable residua. If, however, papules ulcerate, the lesions last for months and heal with scars. The disease may play itself out in months, but in some people it lasts for decades. As lesions resolve, new ones appear. A sign of worsening prognosis is enlargement of papules to nodules and even to tumors. That phenomenon implies that the lymphoma may then be detectable in internal organs as well as in the skin, but even then patients seem to live in harmony with the disease rather than die of it.

INTEGRATION: UNIFYING CONCEPT Lymphomatoid papulosis, like mycosis fungoides, is a systemic lymphoma, from the outset of which involvement of internal organs is sufficiently negligible that it goes unnoticed and undetected. Most people with the disease are ostensibly well for a lifetime and die of unrelated causes. In fact, papules of lymphomatoid papulosis, even those that come and go for years, usually heal with few residua—pigmentary alteration or, at most, a scar.

It was the appearance of well-being of patients with lymphomatoid papulosis after about a score of years that prompted MacCauley to consider it a pseudomalignancy. In his original publication about the subject in 1968, he asserted that the condition, despite the presence invariably of strikingly abnormal lymphocytes within papules, was akin in his estimation to keratoacanthoma. Since then, it has become clear that keratoacanthoma is really one type of squamous-cell carcinoma and that lymphomatoid papulosis is truly one expression of lymphoma.

Papules of lymphomatoid papulosis are formed of infiltrates that assume a wedge shape within the dermis and are composed, in part, of strikingly abnormal lymphocytes in both perivascular and interstitial arrangement. It is common for some abnormal lymphocytes to be in mitosis. The abnormal lymphocytes usually are joined by small lymphocytes, plasma cells, neutrophils, and eosinophils, but at times they monopolize the infiltrate. The papillary dermis may be edematous, and vesicles may form within and beneath the epidermis. When a lesion ulcerates, fibrosis in the upper part of the dermis ensues.

Lesions of lymphomatoid papulosis sometimes are present concurrently with lesions that show typical features of other lymphomas, such as mycosis fungoides and Hodgkin's disease. Not only is lymphomatoid papulosis different from those other lymphomas in terms of clinical and histopathologic findings, but the lymphocytes responsible for it express the CD30 antigen.

Despite differences among lymphomatoid papulosis, mycosis fungoides, and Hodgkin's disease, clinically, histopathologically, and immunocytochemically, the fact that they sometimes occur together in one patient, albeit uncommonly, indicates that they are related to one another. It seems that a single lymphomatous process may express itself differently, morphologically and immunocytochemically, and when that happens the manifestations of that process are given different names such as lymphomatoid papulosis, mycosis fungoides, and Hodgkin's disease. It is likely that various lymphomatous processes that now go by different names are related to one another.

Because the individual lesions of lymphomatoid papulosis bear some resemblance to those of Mucha-Habermann disease, it was thought by some authors that they were simply variations on a single theme. In actuality, Mucha-Habermann disease is an inflammatory process, in contrast to lymphomatoid papulosis, which is a lymphomatous one. The two diseases are wholly unrelated to one another.

THERAPY PUVA with maintenance treatment for as long as lesions continue to appear, oral methotrexate, and interferon are suitable ways of managing the disease.

DEFINITION Hamartomas ("congenital" melanocytic nevi) and benign neoplasms ("acquired" melanocytic nevi) of various specific types, all of which are composed of abnormal melanocytes and manifested clinically as lesions of different colors, shapes, and sizes, among them, macules and patches, papules and plaques, and nodules and tumors.

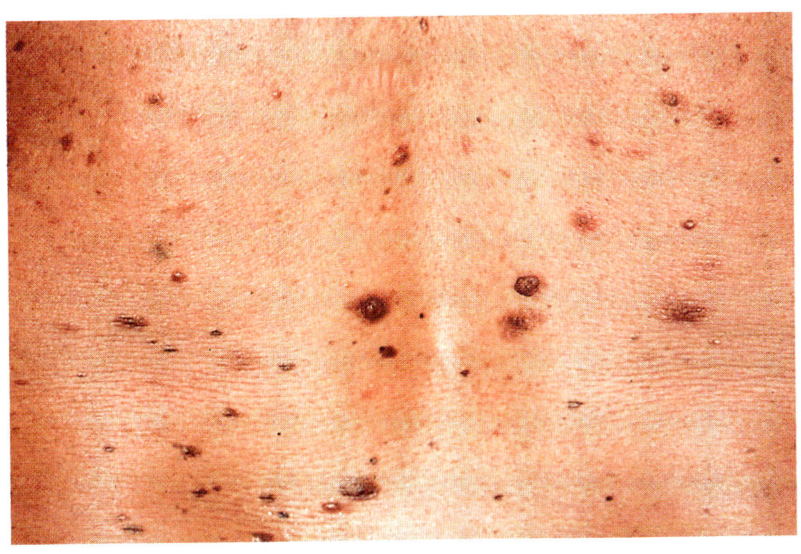

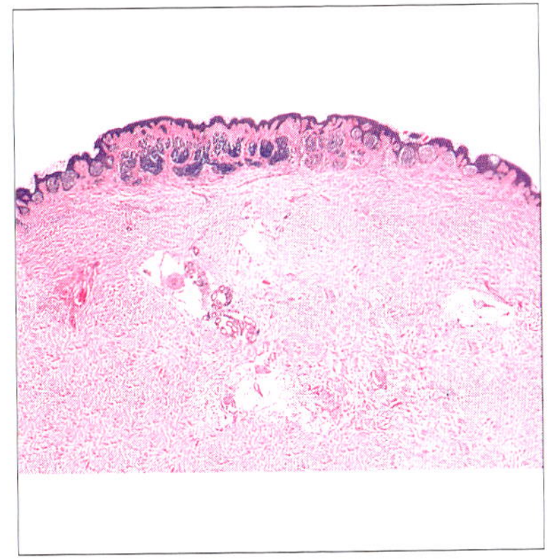

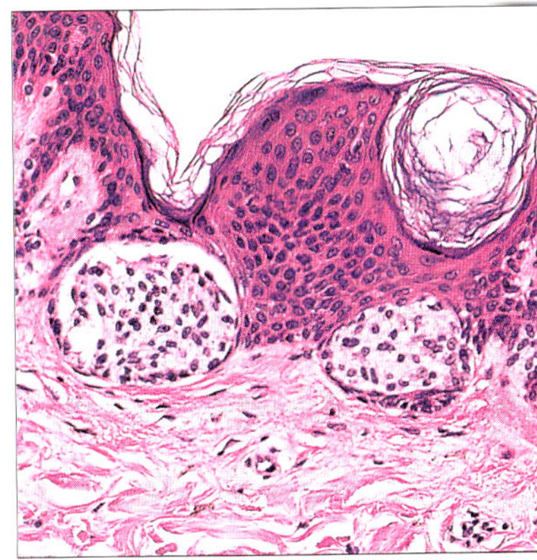

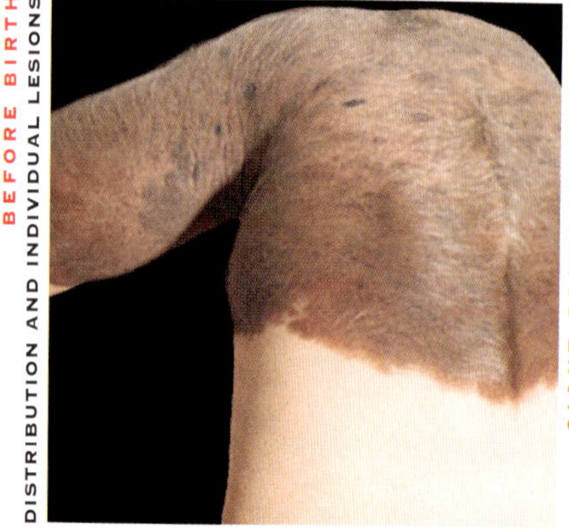

FIG. 55-1 *Giant congenital hairy nevus, garment type.*

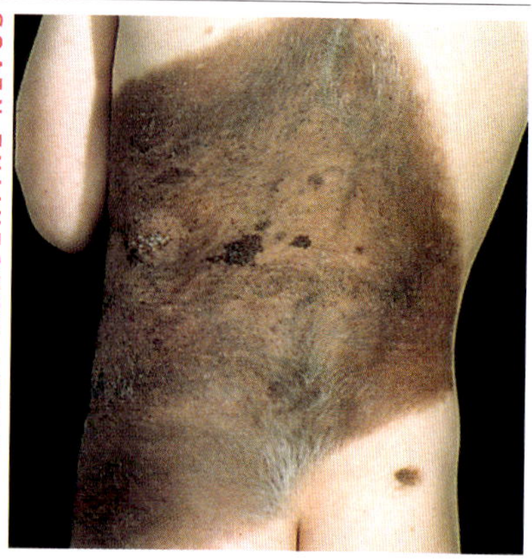

FIG. 55-2 *Giant congenital nevus.*

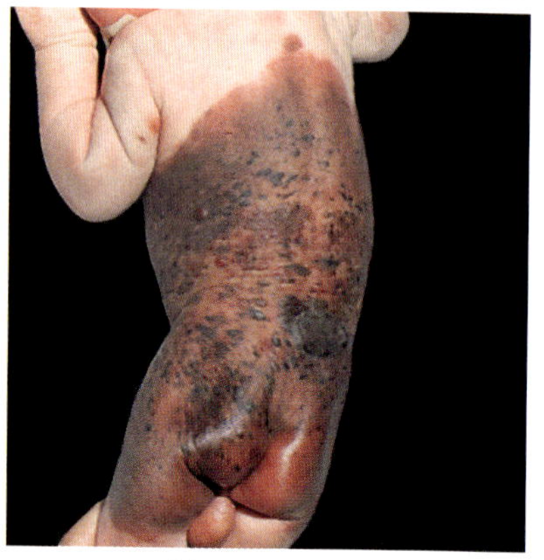

FIG. 55-3 *Giant congenital nevus with numerous nodules and tumors.*

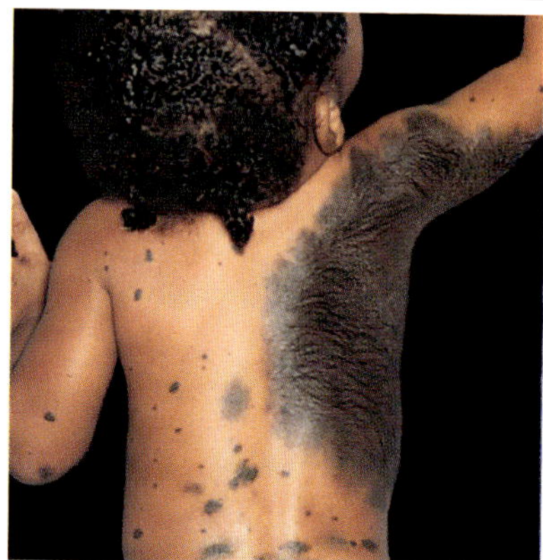

FIG. 55-4 *Giant hairy congenital nevus consisting of large and small lesions.*

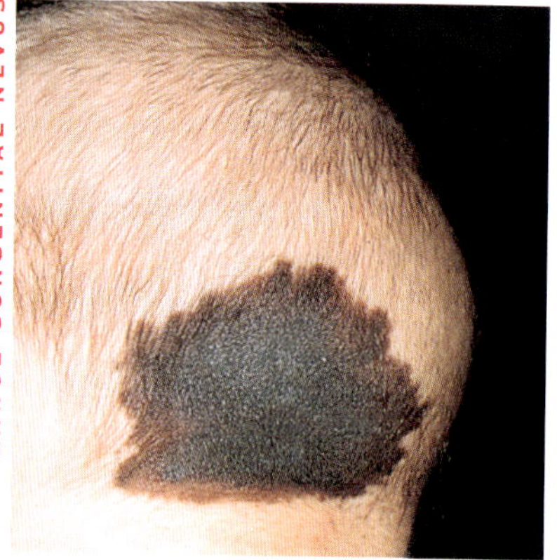

FIG. 55-5 *Large congenital nevus on the scalp.*

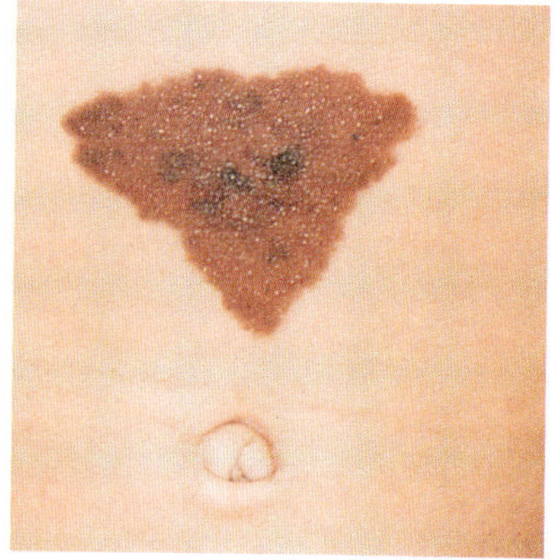

FIG. 55-6 *Large congenital nevus with pyramidal shape.*

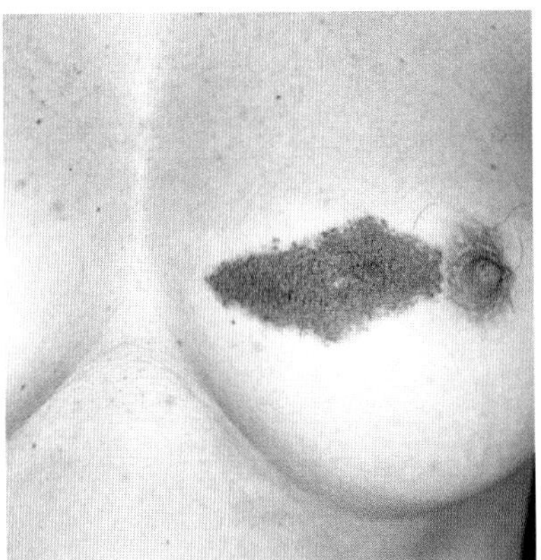

FIG. 55-7 *Large congenital nevus.*

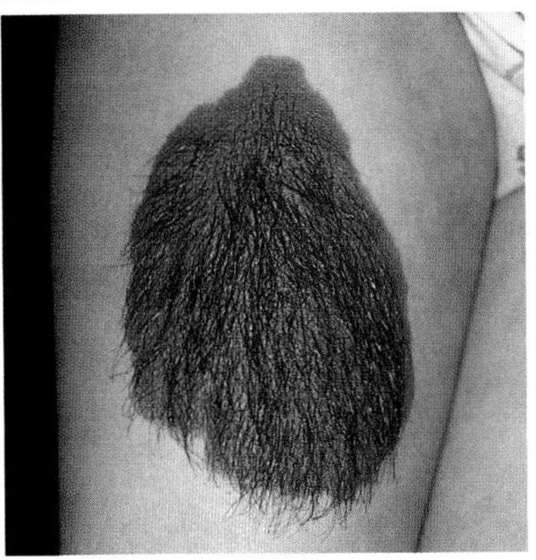

FIG. 55-8 *Large congenital hairy nevus.*

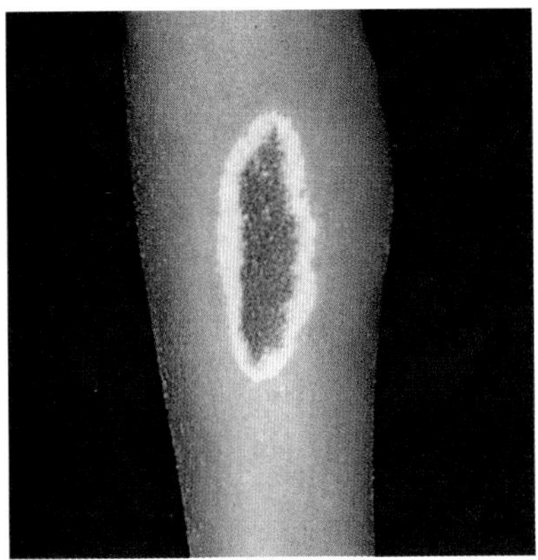

FIG. 55-9 *Large congenital nevus with halo.*

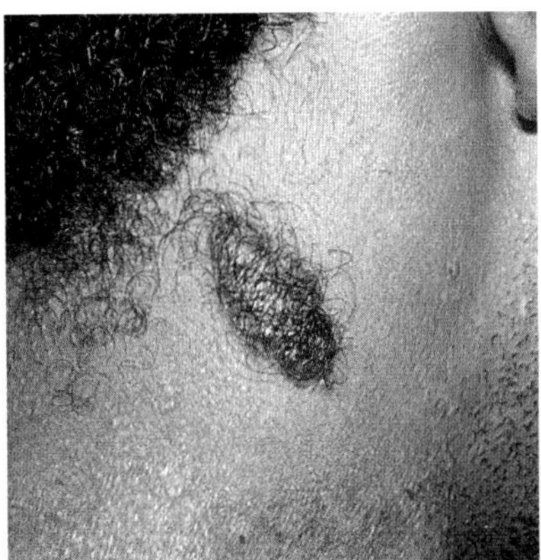

FIG. 55-10 *Large congenital nevus sporting many terminal hairs.*

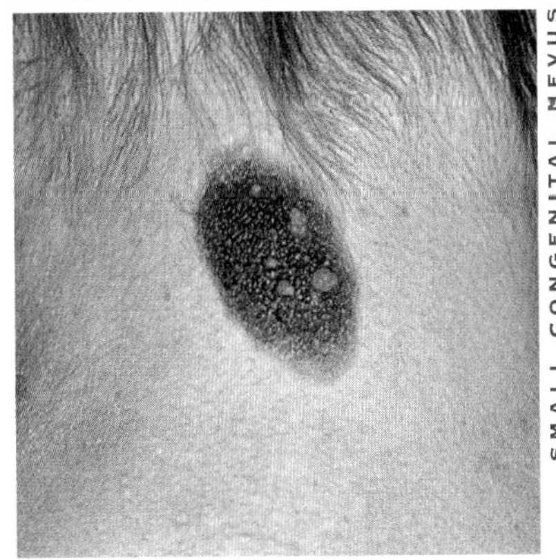

FIG. 55-11 *Large congenital nevus with prominent papillations.*

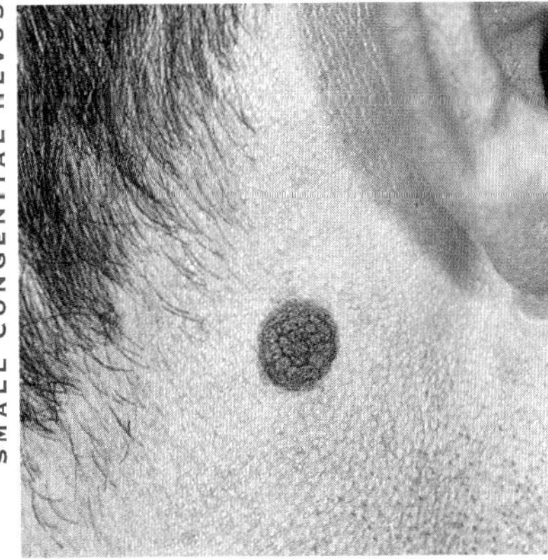

FIG. 55-12 *Small congenital nevus with a mammillated surface.*

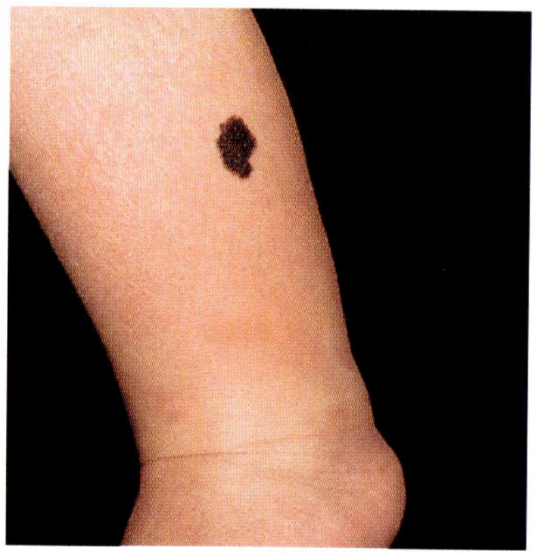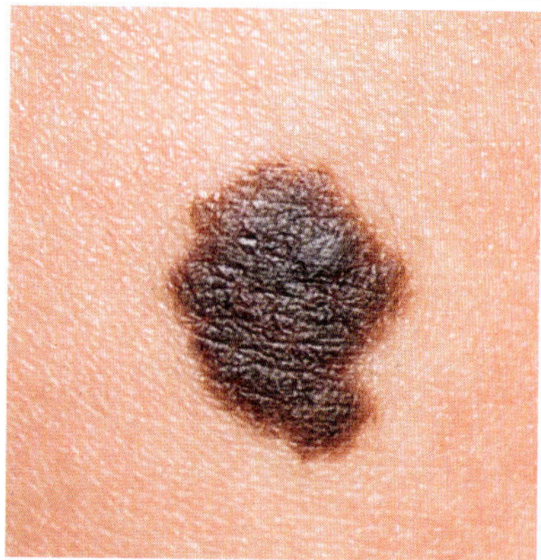

FIG. 55-13 (A, B) *Small congenital nevus with peculiar shape but uniform color.*

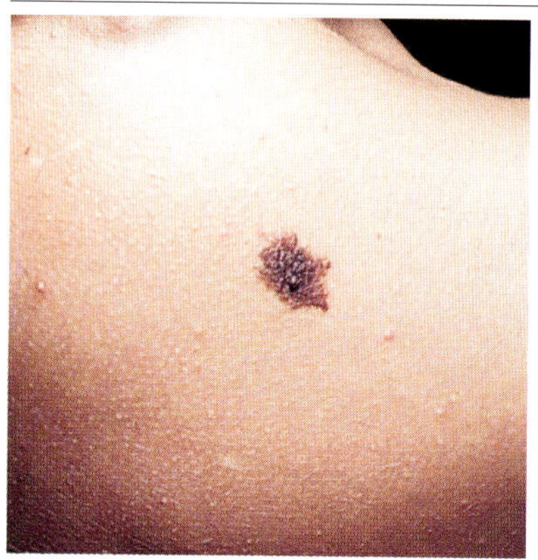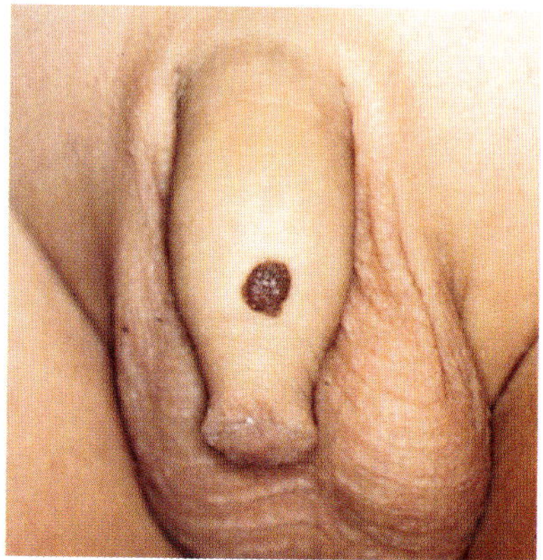

FIG. 55-14 *Small congenital nevus, asymmetrical with jagged outline.*

FIG. 55-15 *Small congenital nevus, sharply circumscribed and uniform in color.*

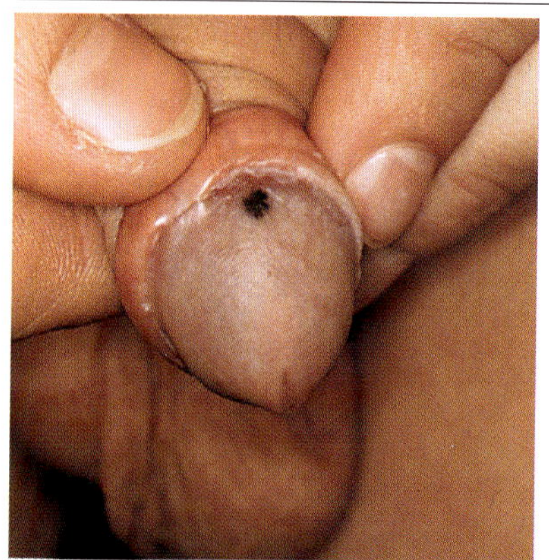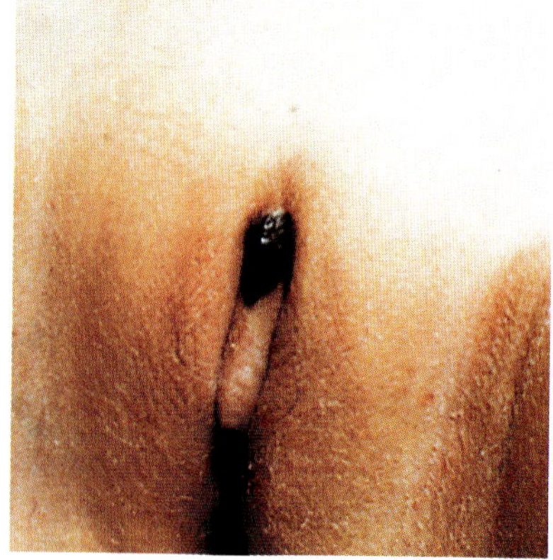

FIG. 55-16 *Small congenital nevus.*

FIG. 55-17 *Small congenital nevus.*

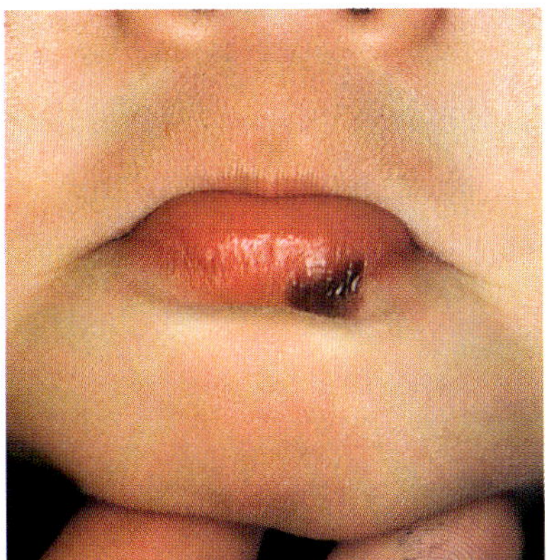

FIG. 55-18 *Small congenital nevus on both skin and a mucocutaneous surface.*

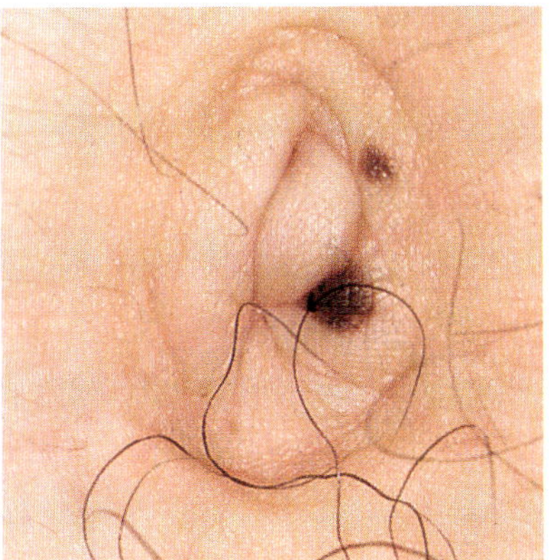

FIG. 55-19 *Two small congenital nevi on the umbilicus.*

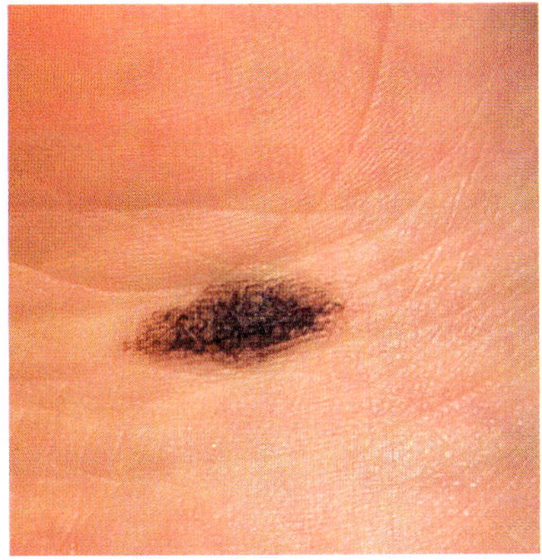

FIG. 55-20 *Small congenital nevus with delicate lines of pigment at its periphery on a palm.*

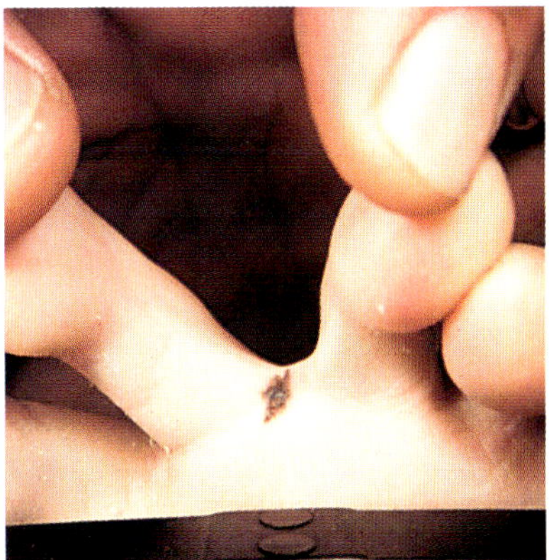

FIG. 55-21 *Small interdigital congenital nevus of fusiform shape.*

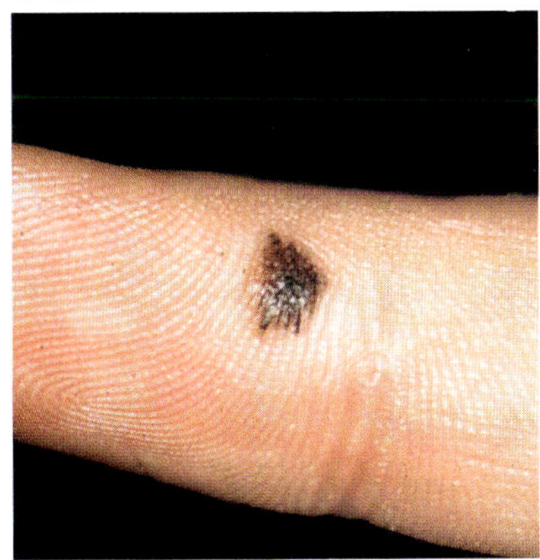

FIG. 55-22 *Small congenital nevus with strikingly notched outline on volar skin.*

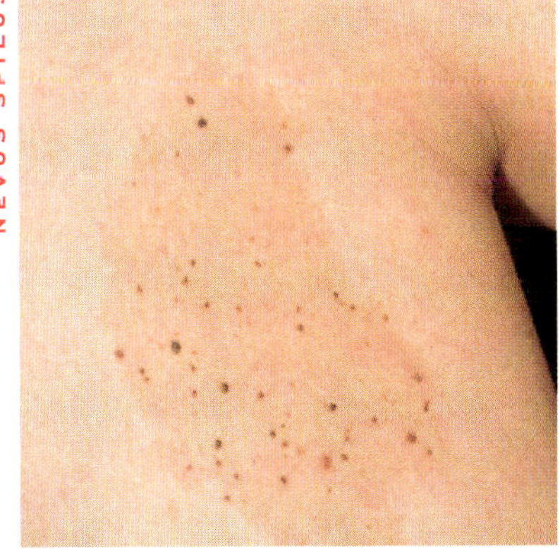

FIG. 55-23 *Congenital speckled lentiginous nevus (nevus spilus) characterized by brown papules on a fawn-colored patch.*

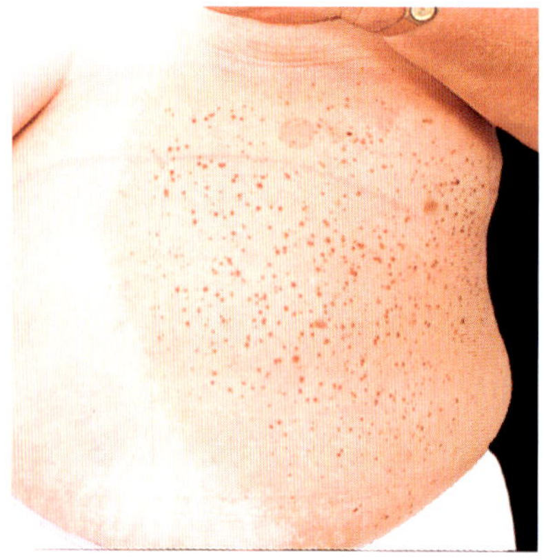

FIG. 55-24 *Congenital speckled lentiginous nevus (nevus spilus) of great breadth.*

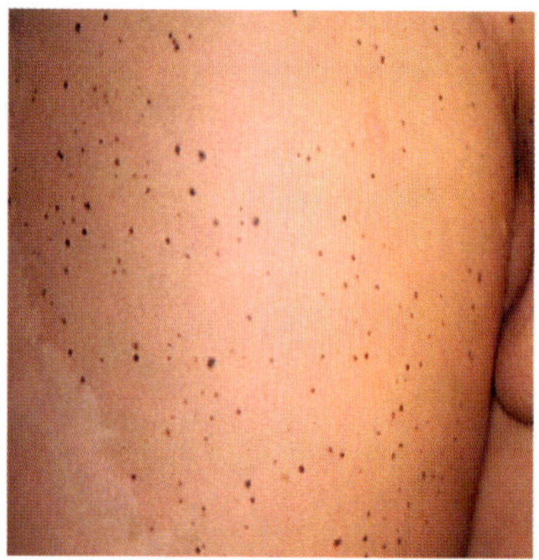

FIG. 55-25 *Congenital speckled lentiginous nevus.*

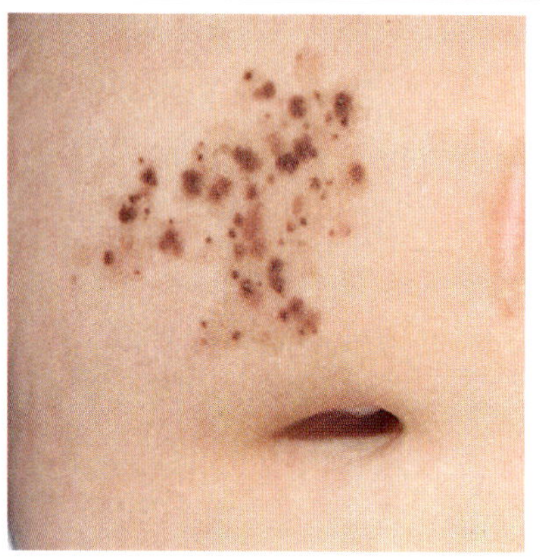

FIG. 55-26 *Congenital speckled lentiginous nevus with papules on a fawn-colored patch.*

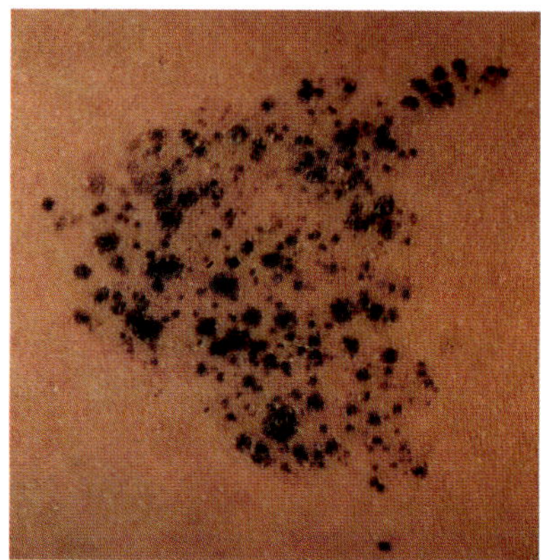

FIG. 55-27 *Congenital speckled lentiginous nevus.*

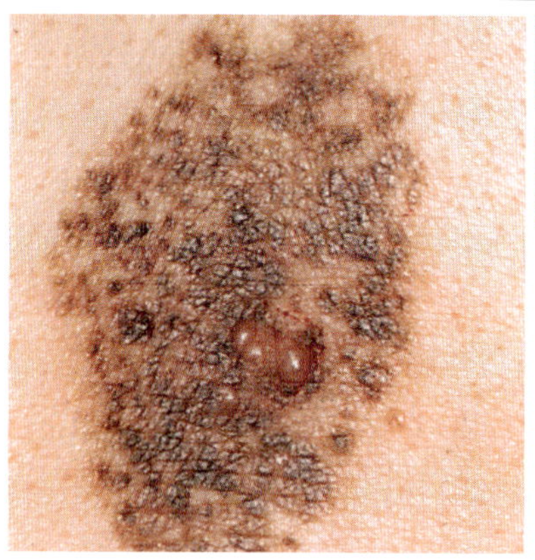

FIG. 55-28 *Congenital speckled lentiginous nevus with globoid papules of Spitz's nevus.*

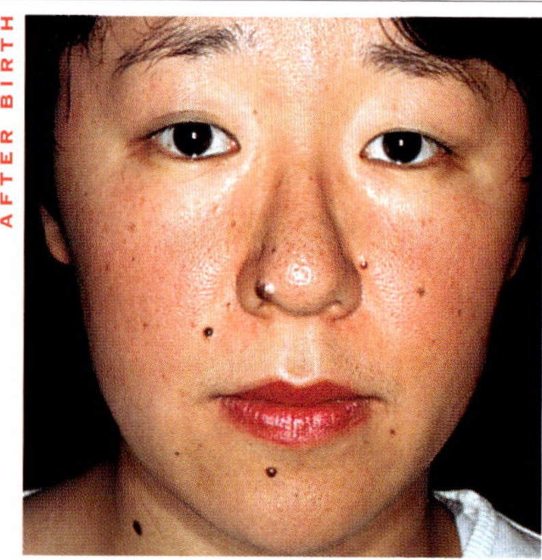

FIG. 55-29 *Miescher's nevi in the form of numerous papules on the face.*

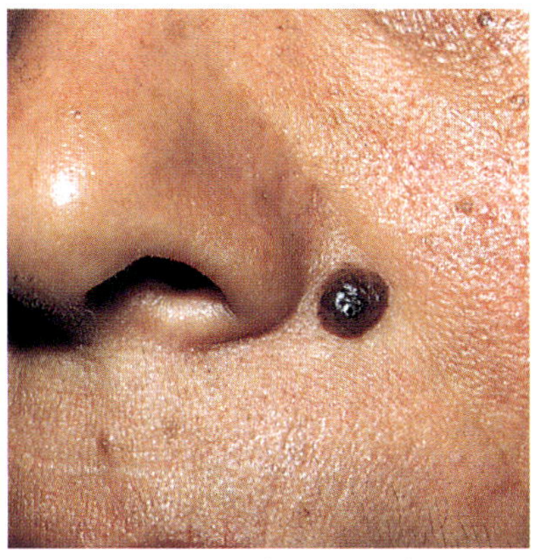

FIG. 55-30 *Miescher's nevi at an early stage on the upper lip and nose.*

FIG. 55-31 *Miescher's nevi on the face—a small one on the lip and a larger darker one near the paranasal fold.*

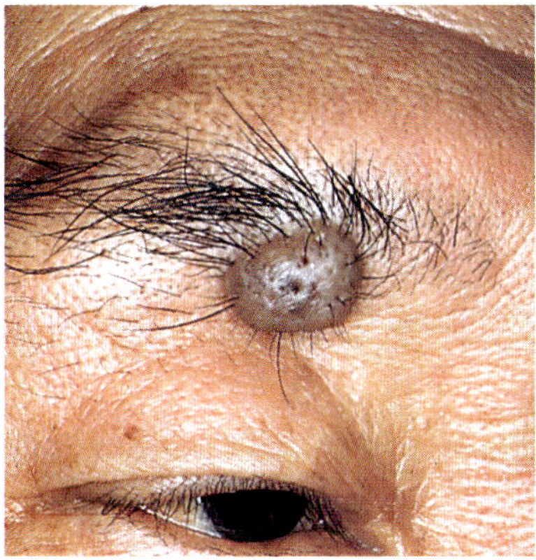

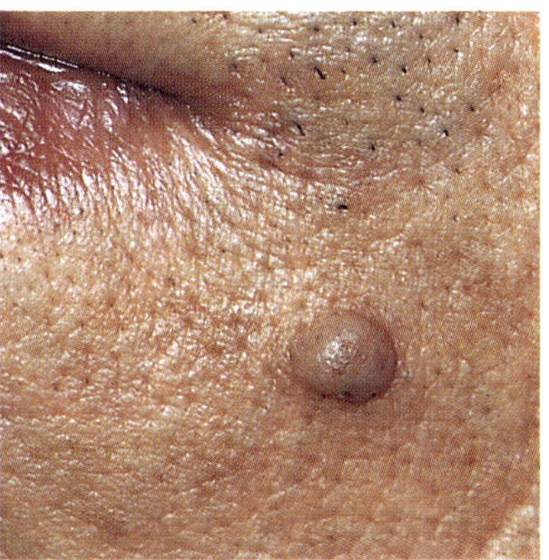

FIG. 55-32 *Miescher's nevus sporting terminal hairs on an eyebrow.*

FIG. 55-33 *Miescher's nevus on the chin; it is devoid of pigment, a consequence of its being long-standing.*

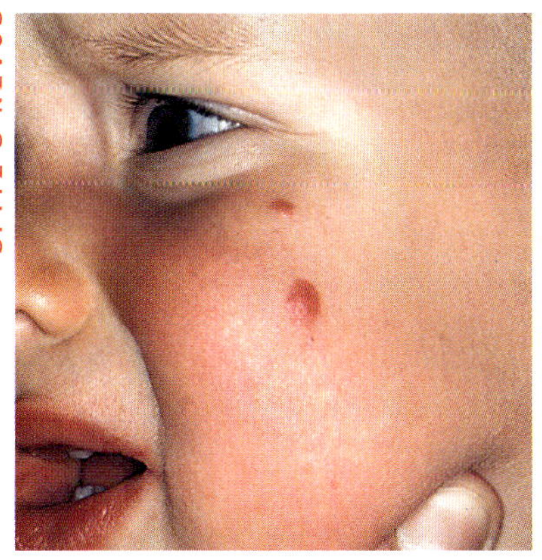

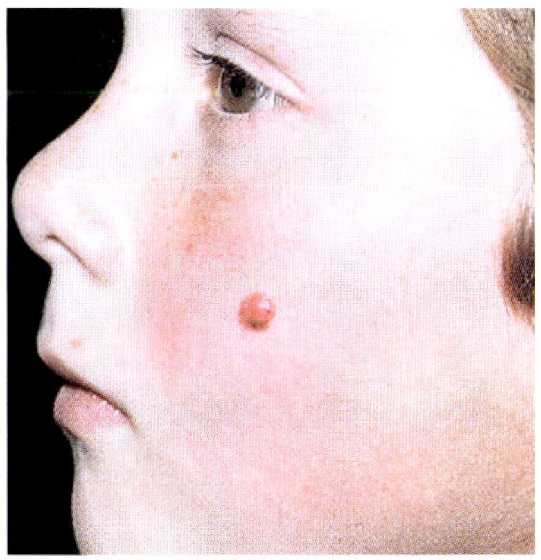

FIG. 55-34 *Two pink papules of Spitz's nevus on the cheek.*

FIG. 55-35 *Pink papule with a focally brown border of a Spitz's nevus on the cheek.*

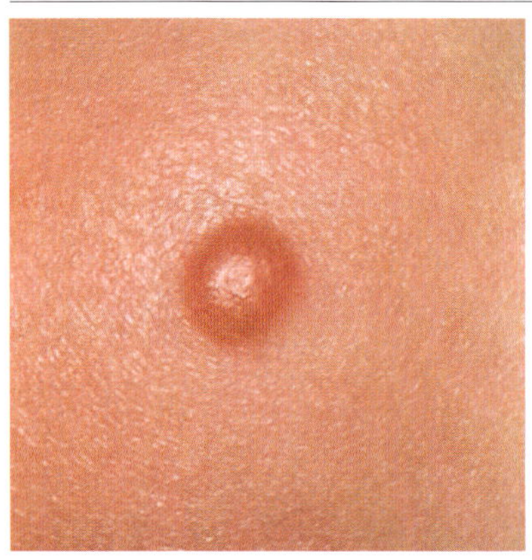

FIG. 55-36 *Pink papule of Spitz's nevus.*

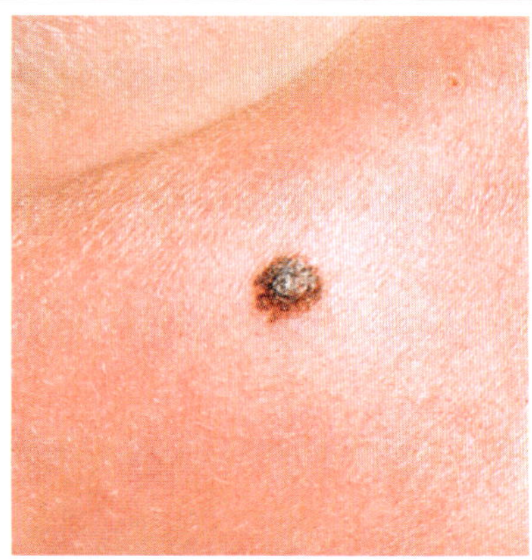

FIG. 55-37 *Brown papule with scalloped border of a Spitz's nevus on the cheek.*

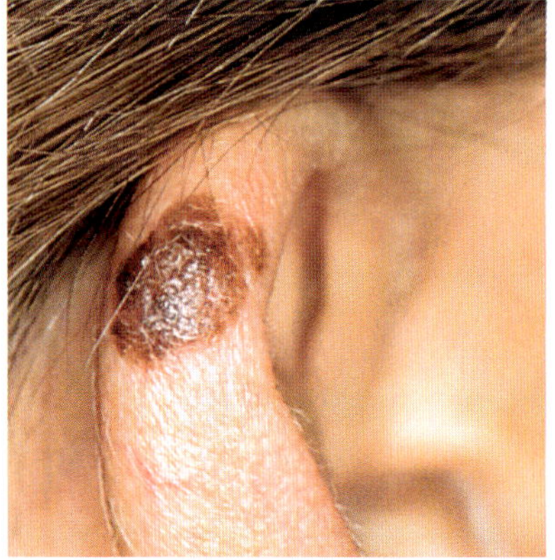

FIG. 55-38 *Papule of Spitz's nevus with various shades of brown.*

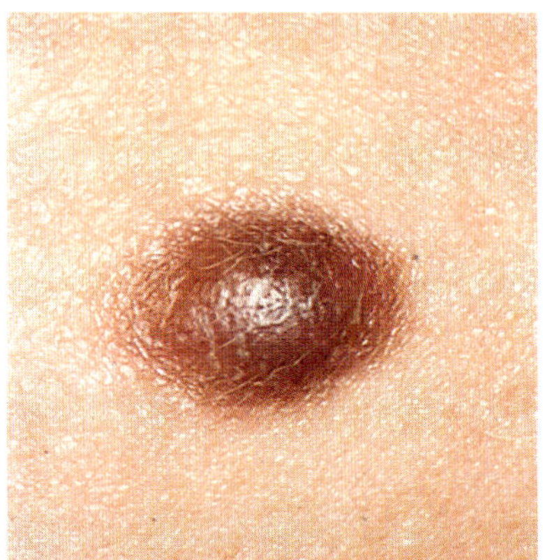

FIG. 55-39 *Brown nodule of Spitz's nevus.*

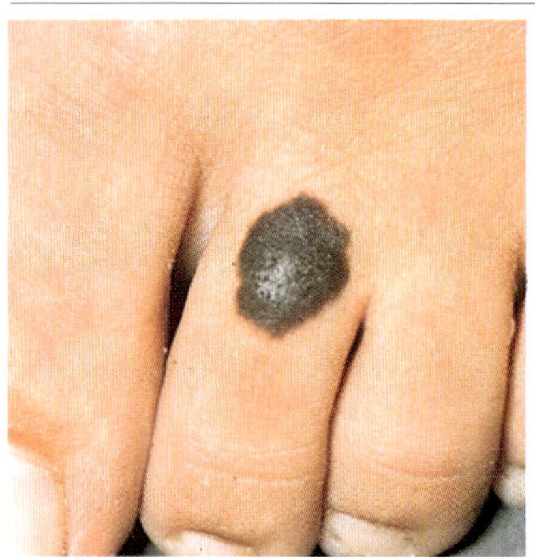

FIG. 55-40 *Blue-black plaque with scalloped border of Spitz's nevus.*

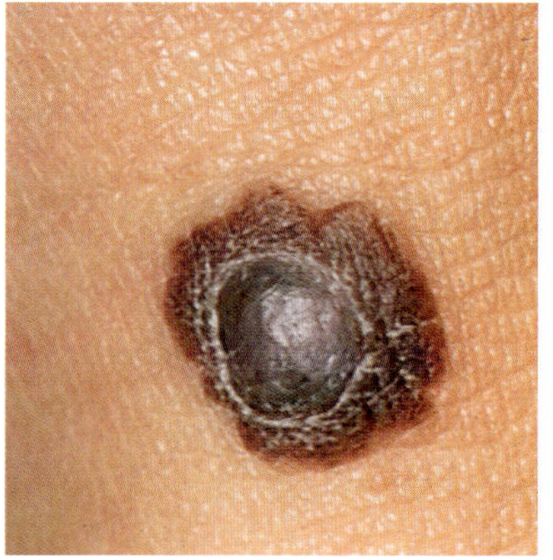

FIG. 55-41 *Combined nevus with a Spitz's component in the center and a conventional superficial congenital nevus at the periphery.*

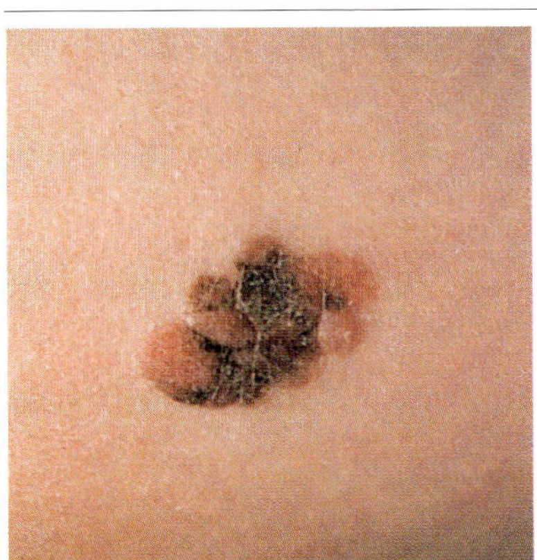

FIG. 55-42 *Spitz's nevus in the form of a multilobulated plaque of several colors and with a scalloped border.*

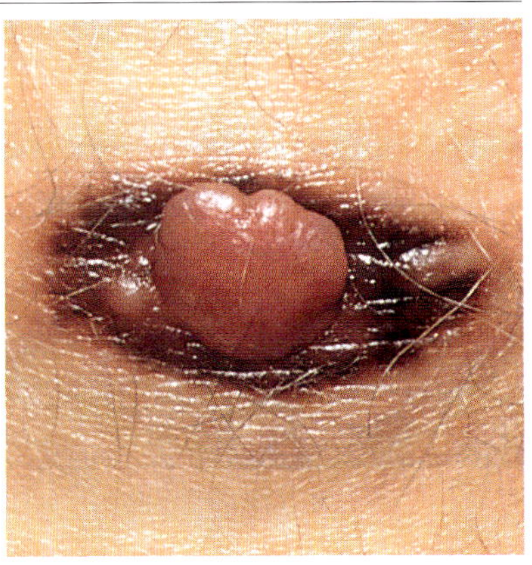

FIG. 55-43 *Combined nevus with a Spitz's component in the center mostly and a superficial type of congenital nevus at the periphery.*

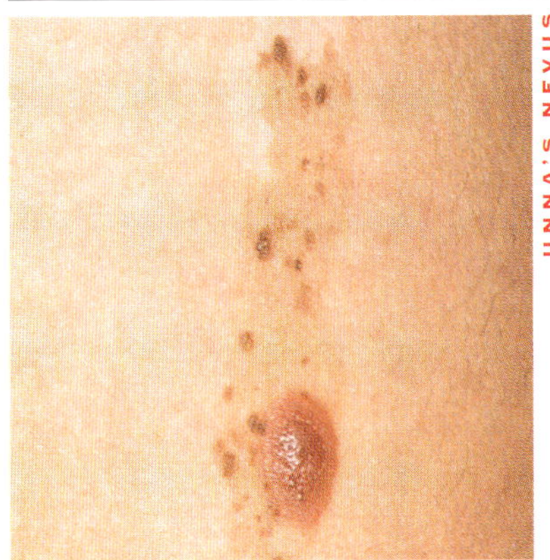

FIG. 55-44 *Nodule of Spitz's nevus within a congenital speckled lentiginous nevus (nevus spilus).*

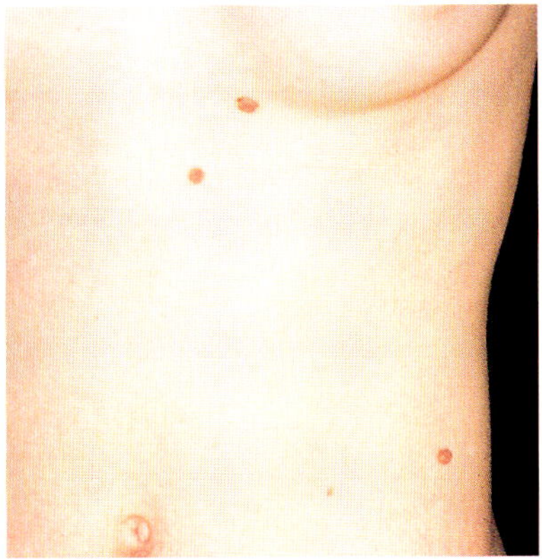

FIG. 55-45 *Tan papule of Unna's nevus near a hip and three Clark's nevi.*

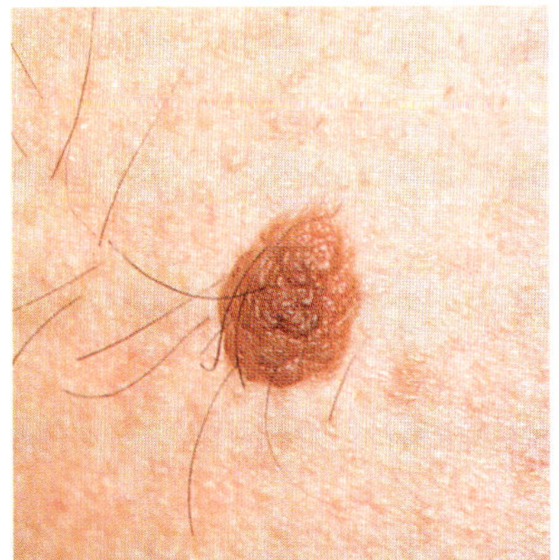

FIG. 55-46 *Brown papule with mammillated surface of Unna's nevus.*

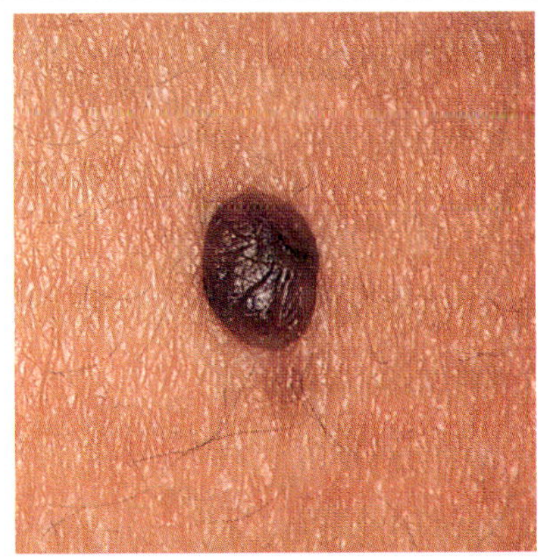

FIG. 55-47 *Dome-shaped lesion of Unna's nevus on the trunk.*

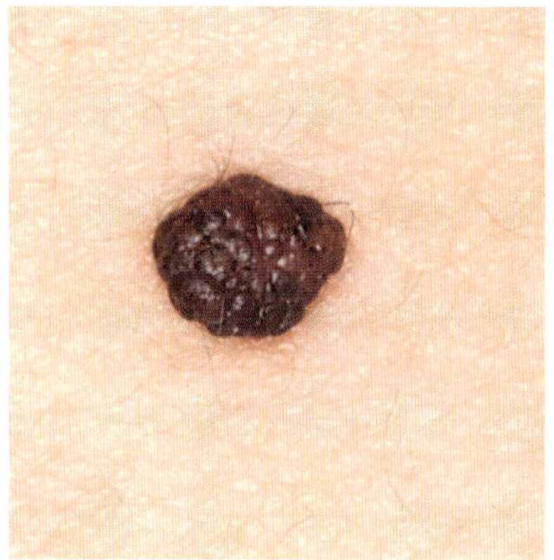

FIG. 55-48 *Frambesiform papule of Unna's nevus on the trunk.*

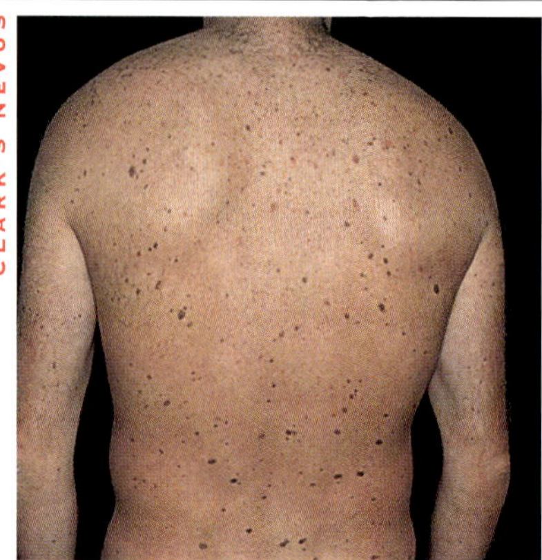

FIG. 55-49 *Macules and papules of Clark's nevus in a patient who already had four melanomas.*

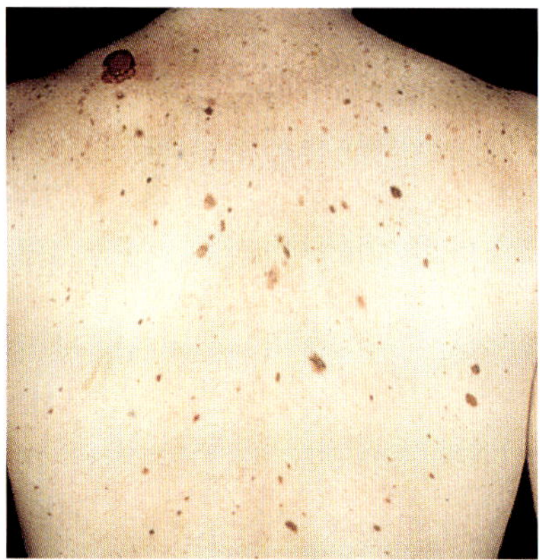

FIG. 55-50 *Many Clark's nevi and a sessile ulcerated melanoma near the neck.*

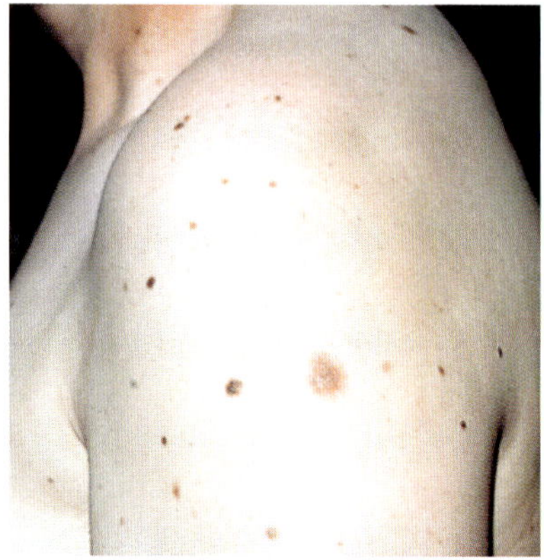

FIG. 55-51 *Clark's nevi, some of which are tiny macules and papules, and others larger papules and a plaque.*

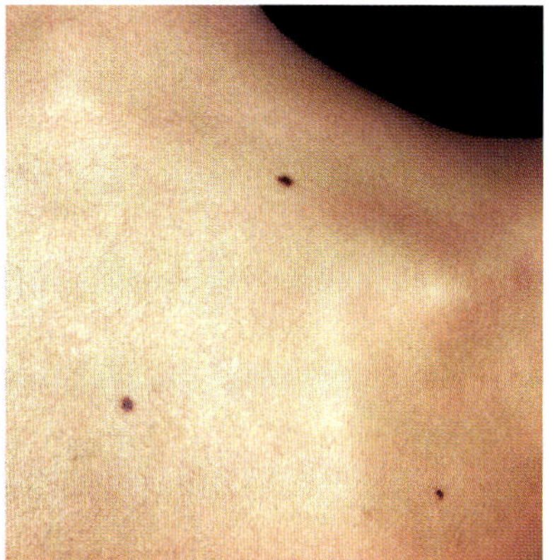

FIG. 55-52 *Three Clark's nevi on the back.*

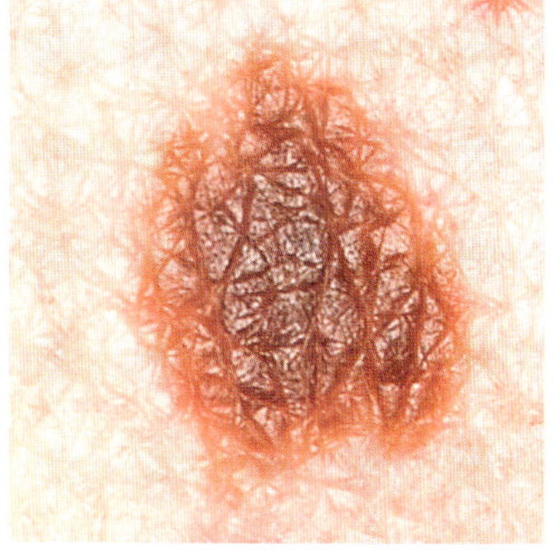

FIG. 55-53 *Clark's nevus with accentuation of skin markings.*

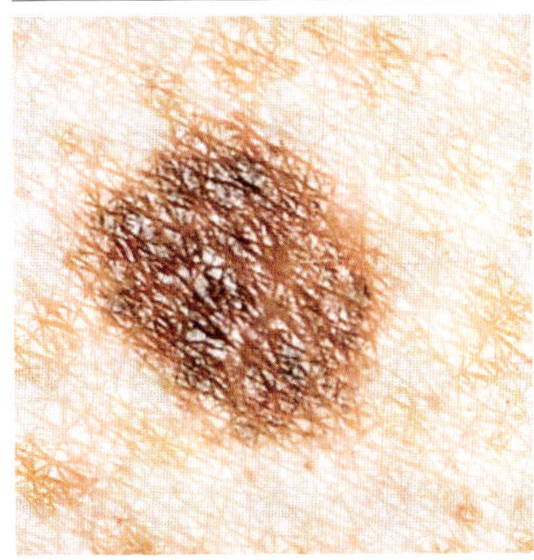

FIG. 55-54 *Clark's nevus as a macule with variegation in color.*

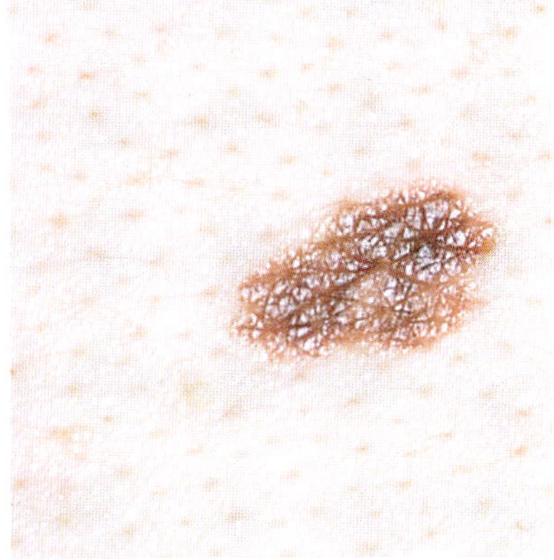

FIG. 55-55 *Clark's nevus with a subtly mammillated surface.*

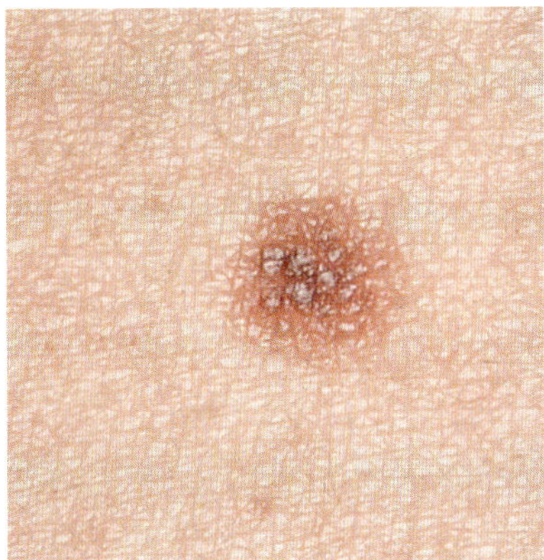

FIG. 55-56 *Clark's nevus with a mammillated surface.*

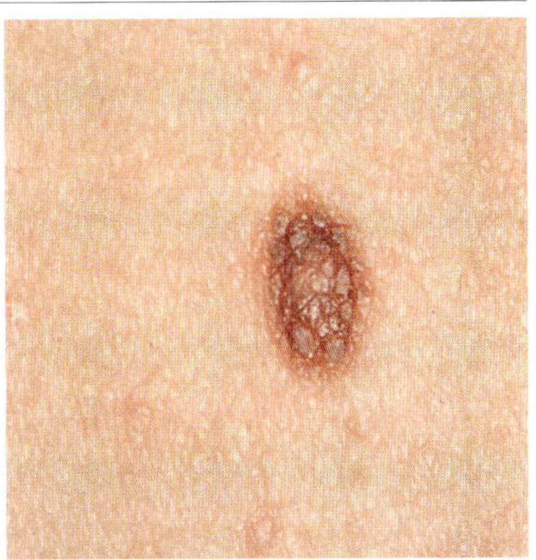

FIG. 55-57 *Clark's nevus characterized by relative symmetry, sharp circumscription, and mammillated surface.*

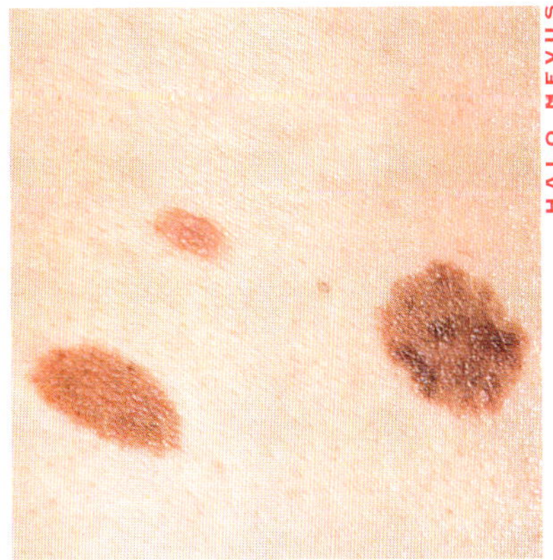

FIG. 55-58 *Clark's nevi at different stages of evolution.*

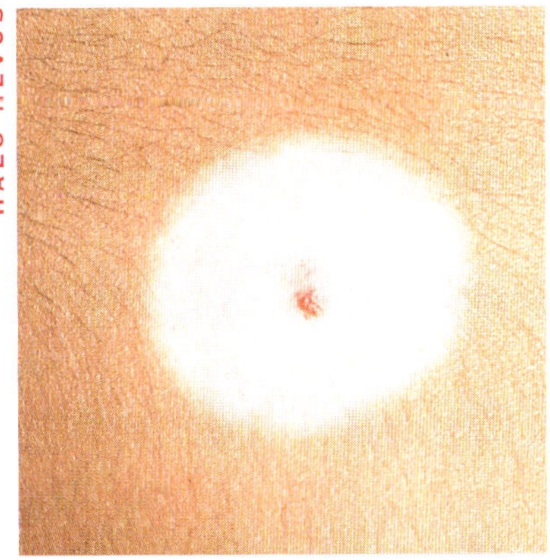

FIG. 55-59 *Halo nevus of Clark's type with a tiny papular center and a depigmented patch at the periphery.*

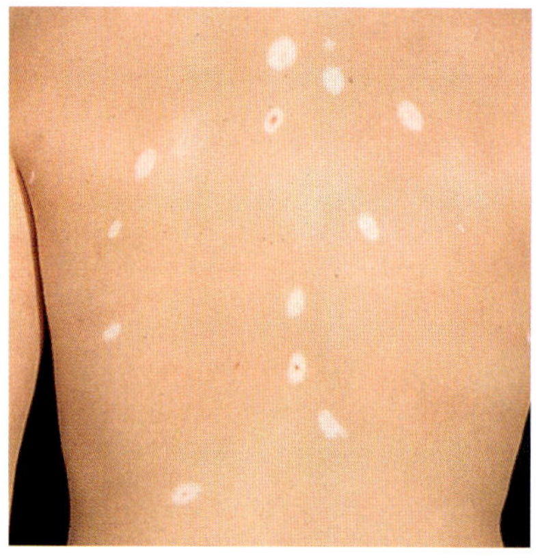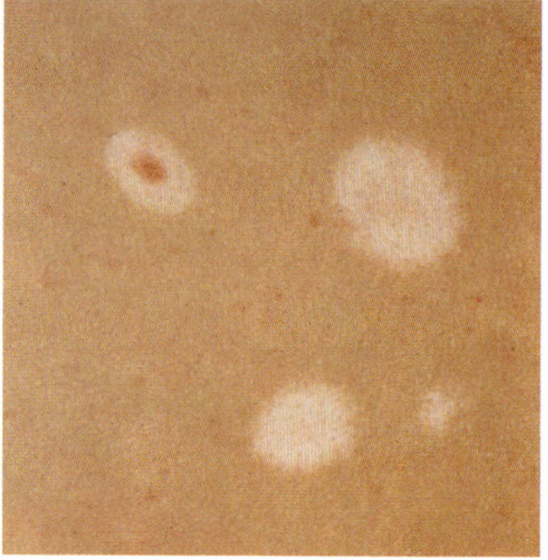

FIG. 55-60 (A, B) *Halo nevi of Clark's type in different stages of devolution, some of them regressed completely.*

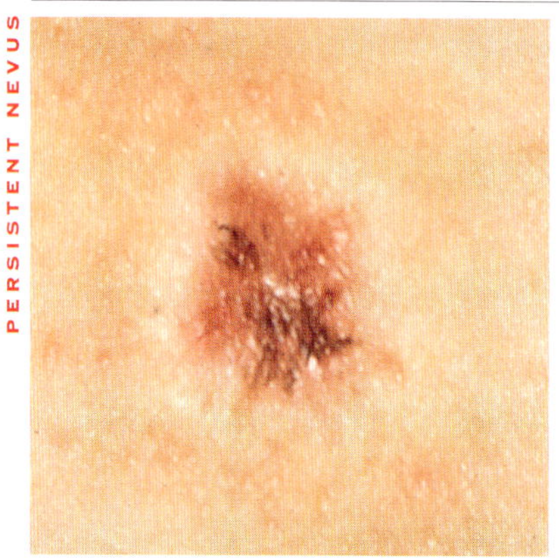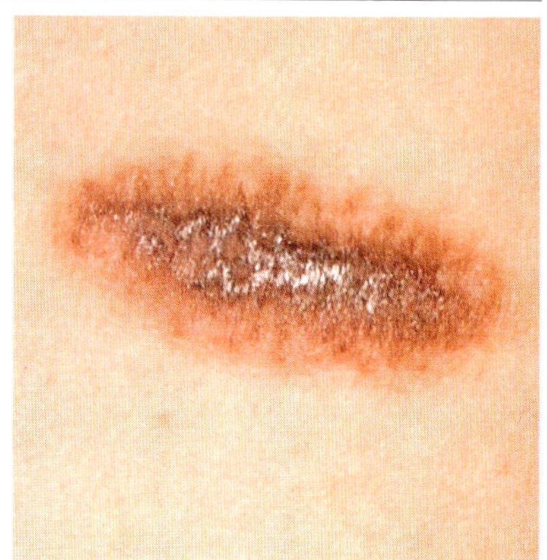

FIG. 55-61 *A recurrent (persistent) nevus in a scar may, as in this situation, simulate melanoma.*

FIG. 55-62 *Recurrent melanocytic nevus along a scar.*

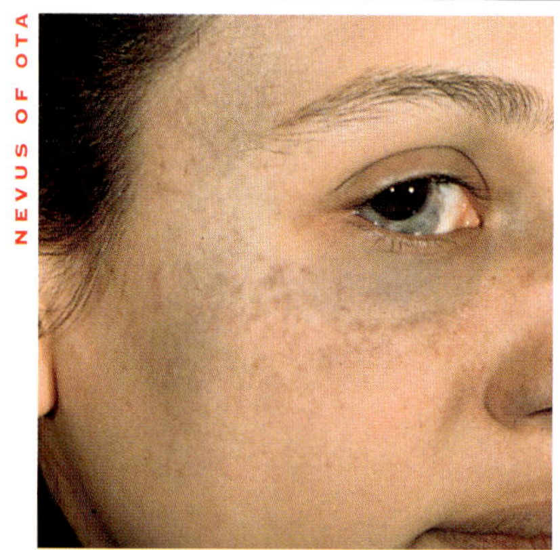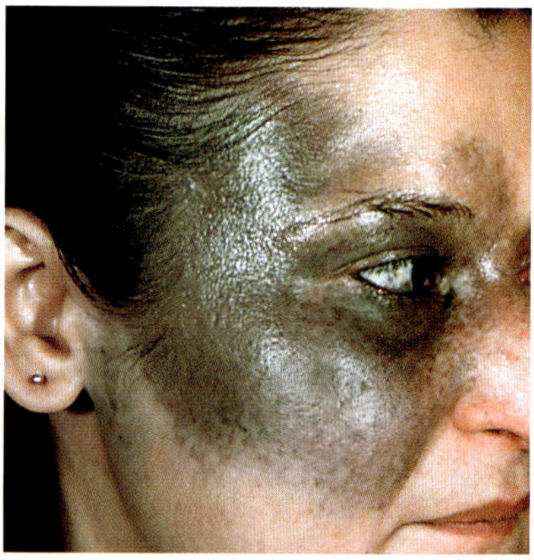

FIG. 55-63 *Nevus of Ota effecting skin and sclera.*

FIG. 55-64 *Nevus of Ota involving skin and sclera.*

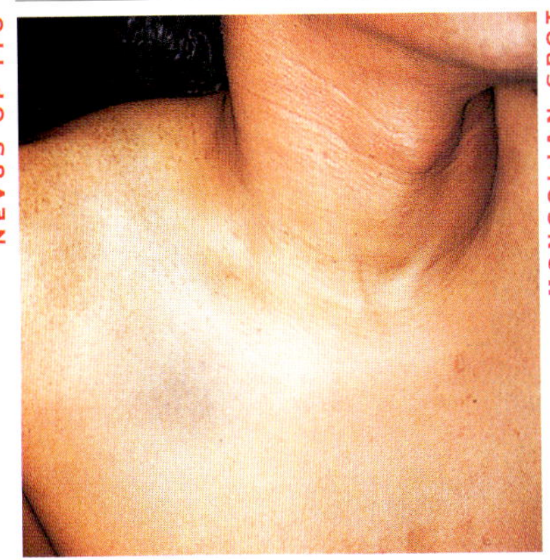

FIG. 55-65 *Nevus of Ito.*

FIG. 55-66 *Mongolian spot.*

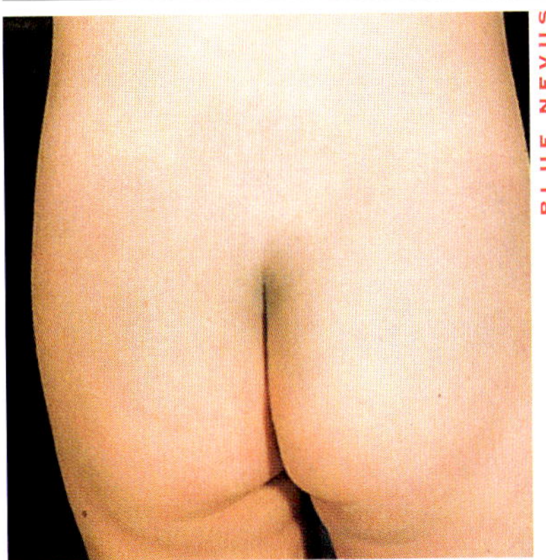

FIG. 55-67 *Mongolian spot.*

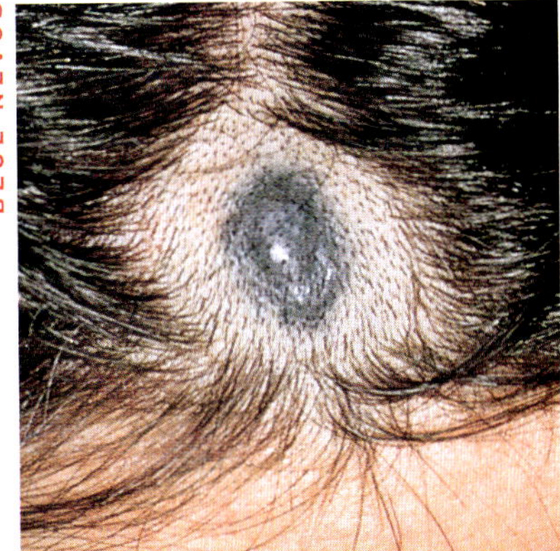

FIG. 55-68 *Blue nodule.*

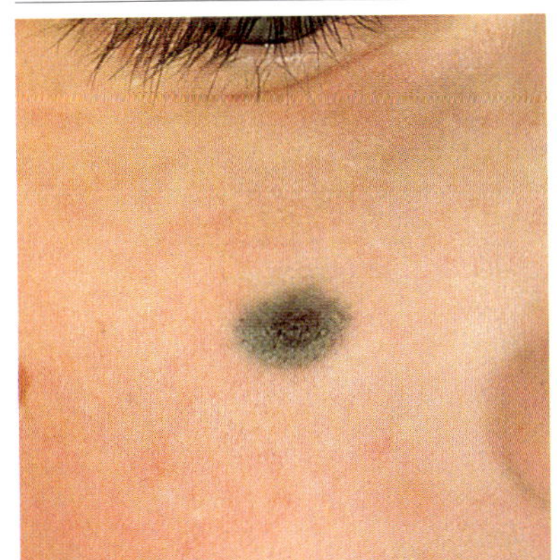

FIG. 55-69 *Blue papule.*

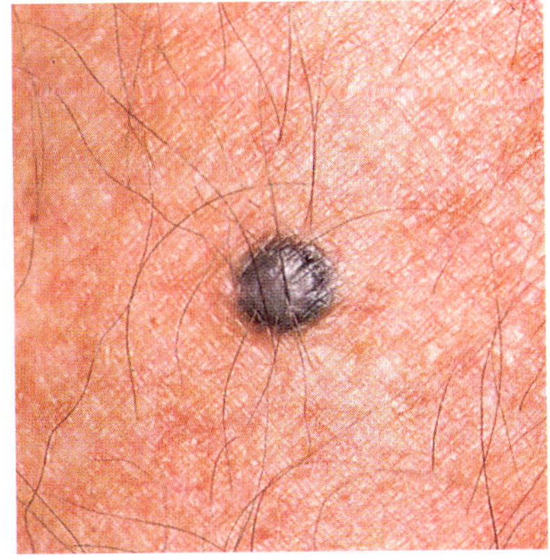

FIG. 55-70 *Blue-brown papule.*

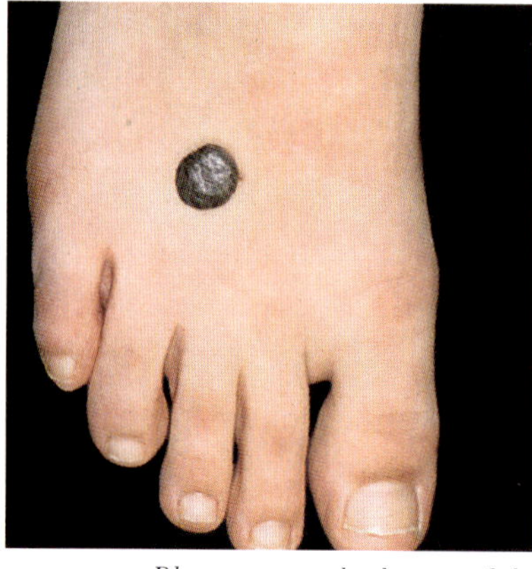

FIG. 55-71 *Blue nevus on the dorsum of the foot.*

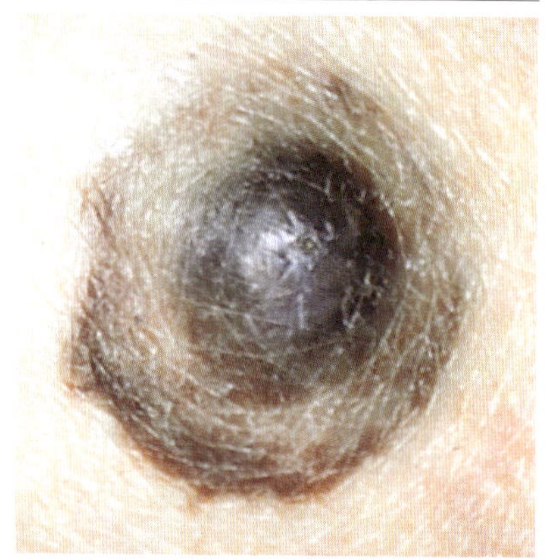

FIG. 55-72 *Blue nevus with target shape.*

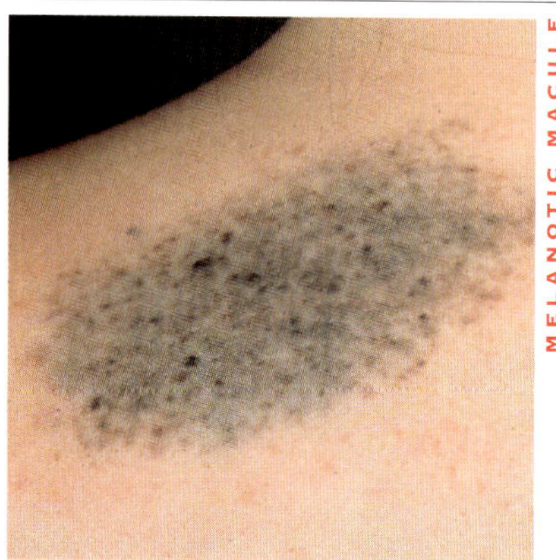

FIG. 55-73 *Blue nevus, agminated type, in which a plaque is composed of closely-set papules.*

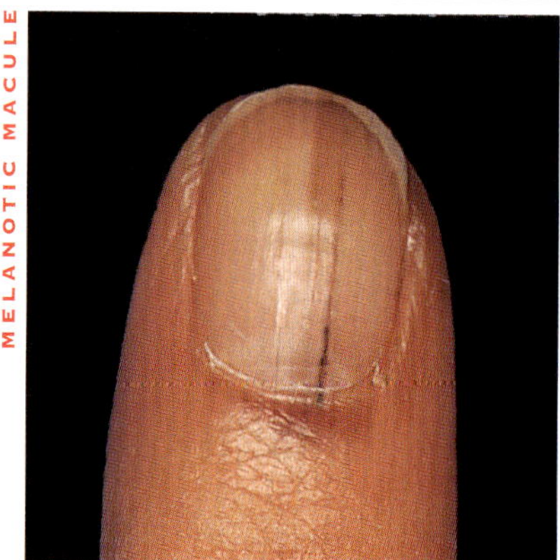

FIG. 55-74 *Melanotic macule in a streak, the commonest expression of melanonychia striata.*

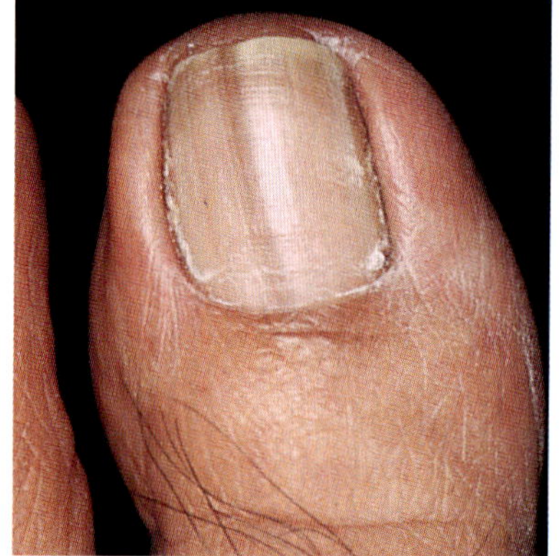

FIG. 55-75 *Melanotic macule in a streak (melanonychia striata).*

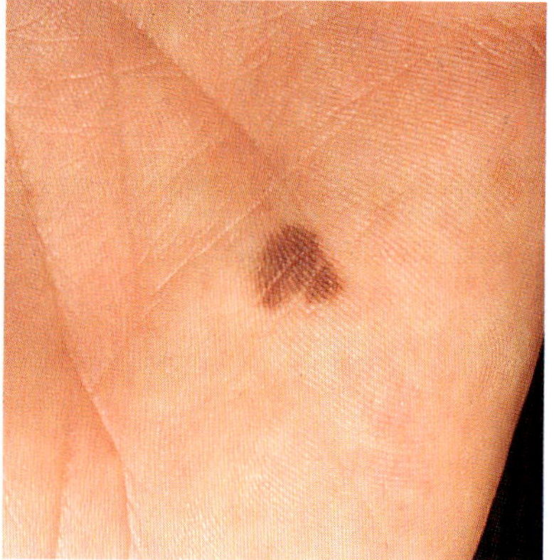

FIG. 55-76 *Melanotic macule (volar).*

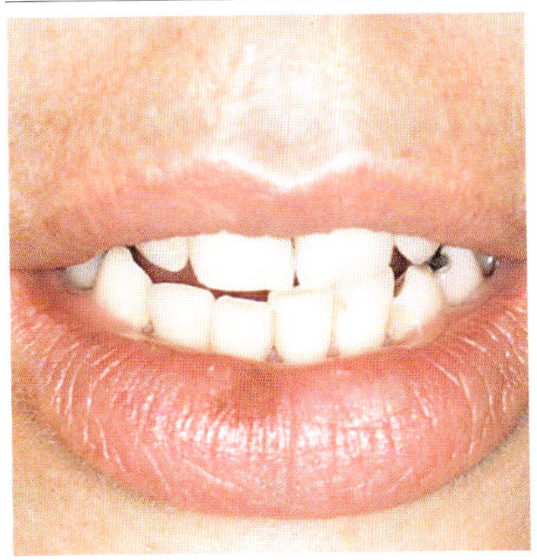

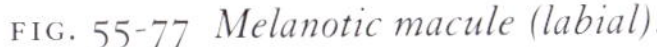

FIG. 55-77 *Melanotic macule (labial).*

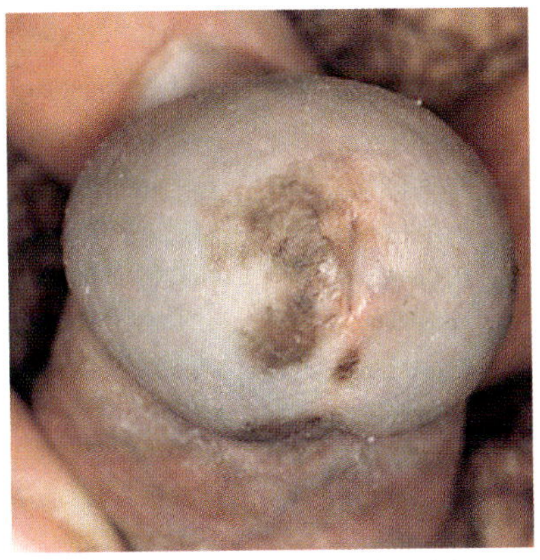

FIG. 55-78 *Melanotic macule (penile).*

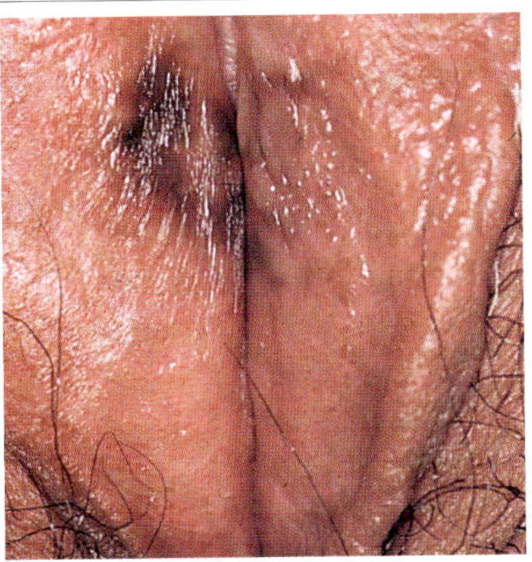

FIG. 55-79 *Melanotic macule (vulvar).*

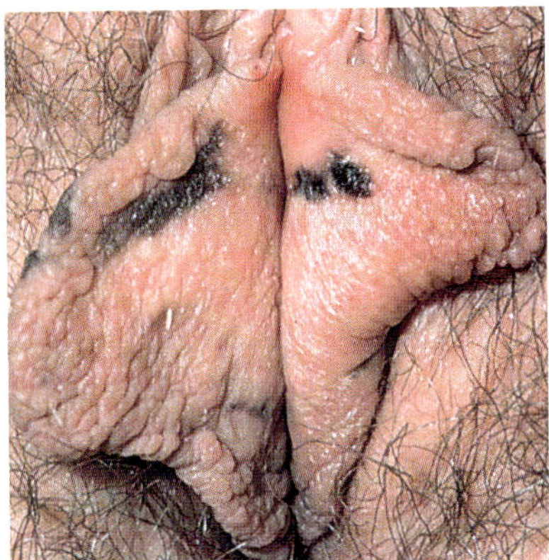

FIG. 55-80 *Melanotic macule (vulvar).*

ADJUNCTIVE DIAGNOSTIC TESTS Dermoscopy (dermatoscopy, epiluminescence microscopy) enhances capability for differentiating a nevus from a melanoma, as well as for distinguishing pigmented lesions made up of melanocytes from those composed of other kinds of cells, for example, pigmented keratinocytes and structures such as blood vessels.

COURSE All kinds of melanocytic nevi, whether they be hamartomas such as giant congenital hairy nevi, or benign neoplasms, such as acquired Spitz's nevi, behave in a biologically benign way—that is, they arise, grow to a certain size, and, for practical purposes, stop enlarging. Few other statements can be made as generalizations about melanocytic nevi because there are so many types of them and those types are so different from one another. A Clark's nevus, for example, is either flat or slightly elevated and usually is a shade of brown. In contrast, Spitz's nevus, when fully developed, may be a plaque, a papillated polyp, or a sessile papule. The colors of Spitz's nevi vary greatly, from black in the plaque of the "pigmented spindle-cell type" to orange or red in the papule that develops quickly in children. A papule of Miescher's nevus or Unna's nevus usually is uniform in color. In contrast, a patch punctuated by subtle papules of nevus spilus is multicolored in shades of brown. Many more examples of contrasts could be given.

Melanocytic nevi may develop at any time in the course of a life, even in elderly people in whom Clark's nevi may become manifest. Once a nevus appears, it tends to persist. The notion that nevi usually disappear completely in time is erroneous; melanocytic nevi, over time, become less pigmented and therefore become less noticeable. Apart from a halo nevus, in which lymphocytes destroy melanocytes of the nevus, nevi do not usually vanish.

INTEGRATION: UNIFYING CONCEPT The common denominator of all melanocytic nevi is the presence of abnormal melanocytes that may appear in the epidermis, the dermis, or the subcutaneous fat, or in any combination of those sites. In fully-formed lesions they are arranged in roundish groups called "nests" or in elongated aggregations designated "fascicles." By this definition, a so-called common blue nevus does not qualify as an authentic melanocytic nevus, because none of the markedly pigmented, bipolar dendritic melanocytes that compose it are arranged in either nests or fascicles; by contrast, in a so-called cellular blue nevus, the oval and spindle-shaped melanocytes that make it up are organized in fascicles. In most expressions of melanocytic nevi, the constituent melanocytes have small, monomorphous nuclei. In Spitz's nevus, however, nuclei of melanocytes may be large and pleomorphic.

Melanocytic nevi of every type may be identified for what they are, clinically and histopathologically, with specificity. Each has its own distinctive morphologic appearance. For example, a Miescher's nevus on a face is dome shaped and characterized histopathologically by a wedge-shaped infiltrate of melanocytes of the nevus that extends throughout much, if not all, of the dermis. By contrast, an Unna's nevus looks clinically like an acrochordon, and consists of nests of melanocytes like those of Miescher's nevus; nests of it are present throughout the extent of the entire exophytic portion of the lesion.

A small congenital nevus (superficial type) is characterized by angiocentricity and adnexocentricity of monomorphous melanocytes of the nevus, as well as by splaying of those melanocytes between collagen bundles in the upper part of the reticular dermis. By contrast, a large (including gigantic) congenital nevus (deep type) is typified by a dense, diffuse infiltrate of melanocytes of the nevus that sweeps through the reticular dermis, into septa of the subcutaneous fat, and sometimes into the wall of veins there. In short, each type of melanocytic nevus—deep penetrating nevus, Clark's nevus, Spitz's nevus, nevus spilus, giant hairy nevus, and so on—has its own distinctive morphologic features, and each behaves in a biologically benign way.

The classification of melanocytic nevi as "congenital" or "acquired" has serious limitations. Many types of melanocytic nevi that fulfill criteria, clinically and histopathologically, for a congenital nevus, such as congenital speckled lentiginous nevus (nevus spilus) are not present at birth; some of them even appear at puberty or later. Miescher's nevus and Unna's nevus, for example, fulfill certain histopathologic criteria for a congenital nevus. Both are associated with splaying of monomorphous melanocytes between collagen bundles in the reticular dermis, but neither type of nevus is present at birth.

Some dermatologists and dermatopathologists refer to what are thought to be congenital nevi and are presumed to be present at birth but that actually appear after birth as "congenital pattern-like nevi" or "tardive" congenital nevi; those terminological evasions are not illuminating. Some types of melanocytic nevi, like Spitz's nevi, may be present at birth (as solitary, agminated, or systematized lesions), but the overwhelming majority of Spitz's nevi make their appearance after birth.

A melanoma can develop in every type of melanocytic nevus. The phenomenon is uncommon, however, compared with melanomas that develop de novo—that is, not in association with a pre-existing nevus. Only about 20 percent of all melanomas in Caucasians begin in association with a preexisting melanocytic nevus, and hardly any melanomas in Asians and Africans arise in conjunction with a nevus. For that reason it may be inferred that about 95 percent of all melanomas in the world begin de novo and not in contiguity with a nevus. A Clark's so-called dysplastic nevus is the type with which melanoma is affiliated most commonly, but that phenomenon probably occurs in less than 0.01 percent of all Clark's nevi and may be due to the fact that Clark's nevus is more common by far than any other type of nevus. Rarely does a melanoma arise in association with an Unna's, Miescher's, or Spitz's nevus, but not uncommonly a melanoma is found in continuity with a superficial type of congenital nevus. Rare, too, is the phenomenon of melanoma beginning in a deep type of congenital nevus. A "malignant blue nevus" is really a melanoma that has begun in a pre-existing blue nevus, and a "malignant Spitz's nevus" is actually a melanoma that was misdiagnosed originally as a Spitz's nevus.

Melanotic macules are not related to melanocytic nevi; the melanocytes increased in number in the basal layer of a hyperpigmented epidermis are disposed as solitary units only, never in nests. Those melanocytes have small monomorphous nuclei and often prominent thin dendrites that are shown to better advantage with the Fontana-Masson silver stain. The melanocytes are equidistant from one another.

Melanotic macules represent a single pathologic process, irrespecitve of whether they appear on an oral lip ("labial lentigo"), on genital skin ("melanosis of the vulva or penis"), in the nail unit ("melanonychia striata," which is by far the leading reason for a pigmented streak in a nail), or elsewhere on the integument. A melanoma has never been reported to develop in continuity with a melanotic macule.

THERAPY Any pigmented lesion, including nevi of various kinds and melanotic macules, that is thought clinically to possibly be a melanoma should be biopsied, preferably by complete excision. Nevi and melanotic macules may be removed for cosmetic reasons and that procedure, too, should be complete excision with narrow margins.

DEFINITION A malignant neoplasm of melanocytes that, in the skin, begins as a macule and may become a patch or a papule. A flat lesion of melanoma tends to be asymmetrical, poorly circumscribed with a scalloped, jagged, or notched border, and variegate, mostly shades of brown. A patch may become a plaque or upon it may develop a papule, nodule, or tumor. A papule may develop into a nodule or tumor. The surface of an elevated lesion of melanoma tends to be uneven. When a melanoma is no longer flat, it has capability to metastasize and cause death.

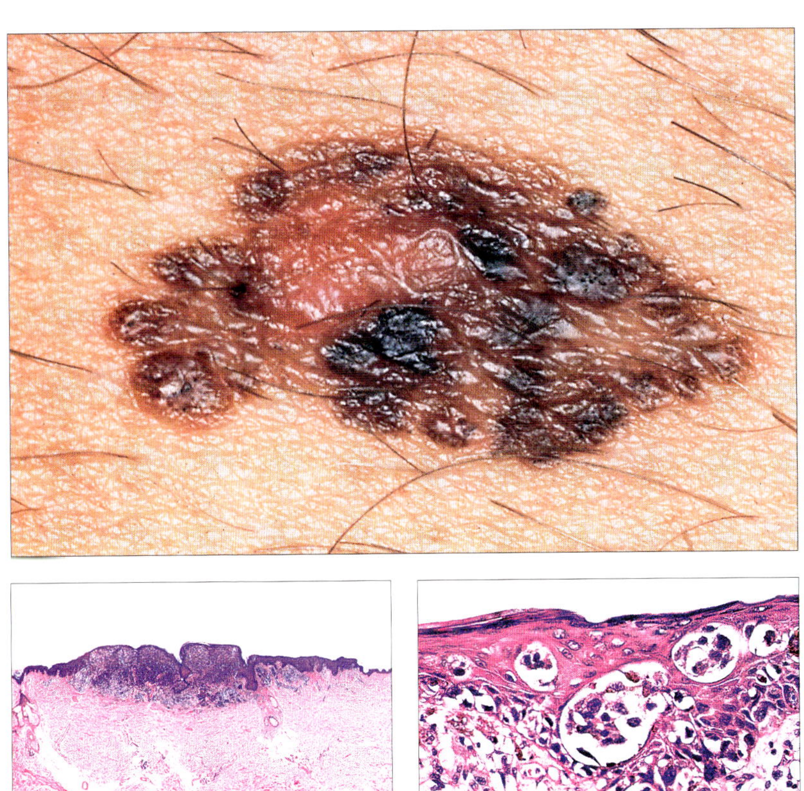

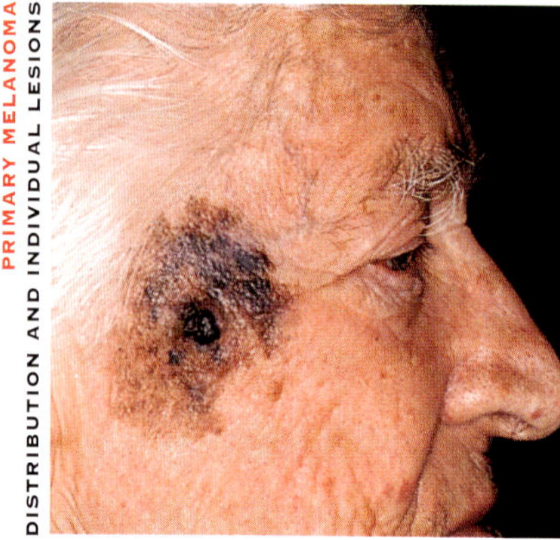
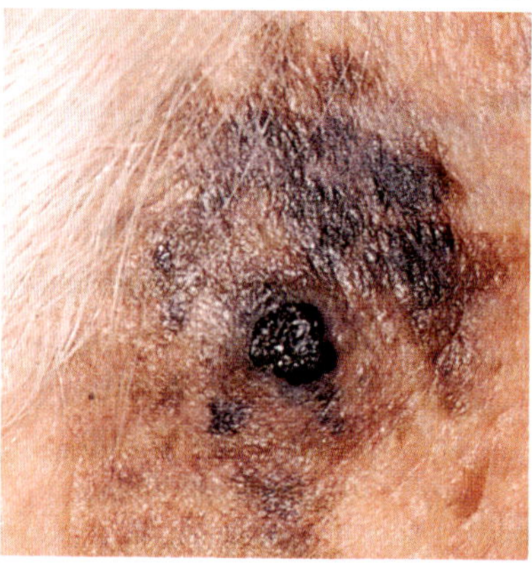

FIG. 56-1 (A, B) *Broad, asymmetrical, unevenly pigmented patch/plaque with a nodule and a notched border.*

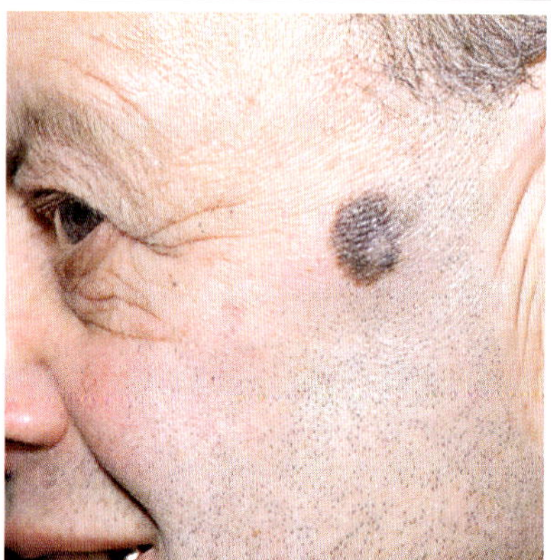
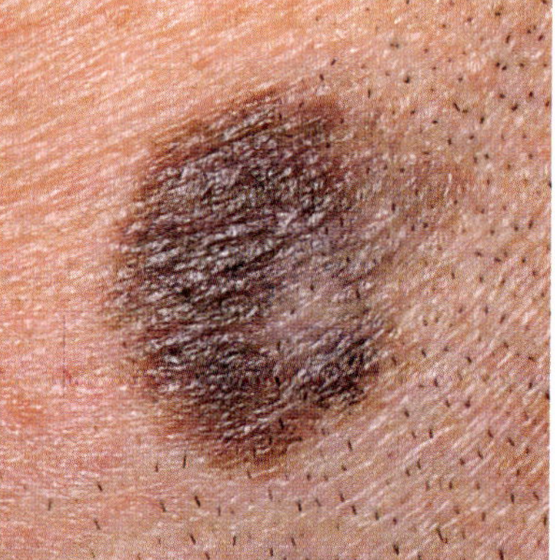

FIG. 56-2 (A, B) *Asymmetrical plaque of relatively uniform size, except for a hypopigmented focus of regression.*

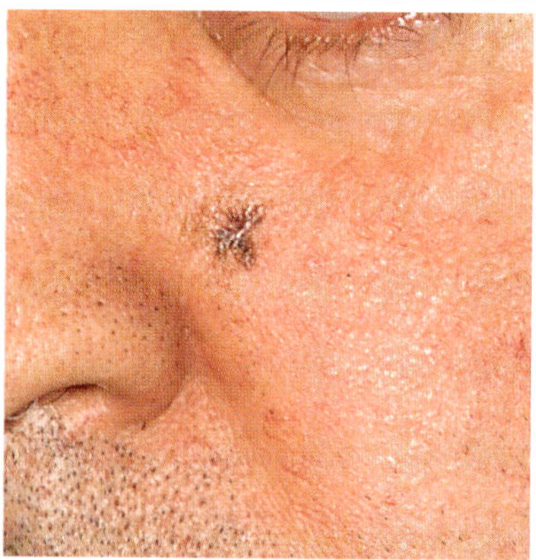
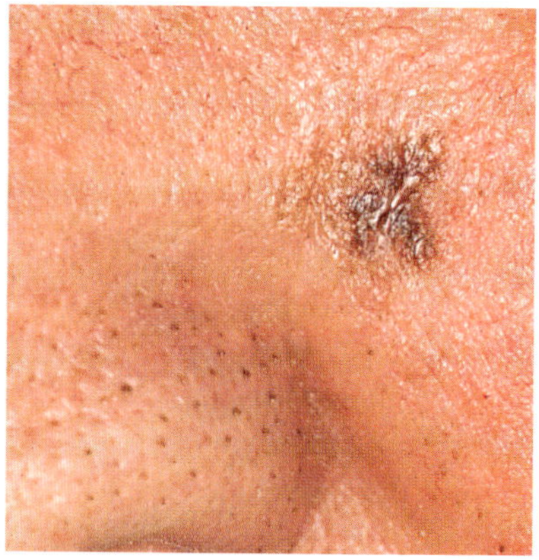

FIG. 56-3 (A, B) *Asymmetrical macule with strikingly scalloped border. The scale is due, in part, to associated seborrheic dermatitis.*

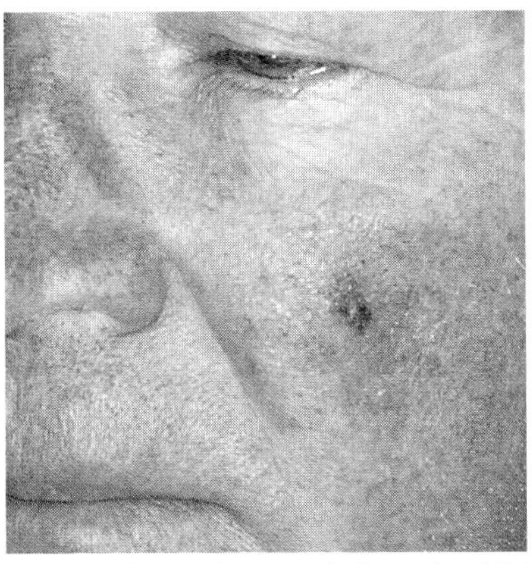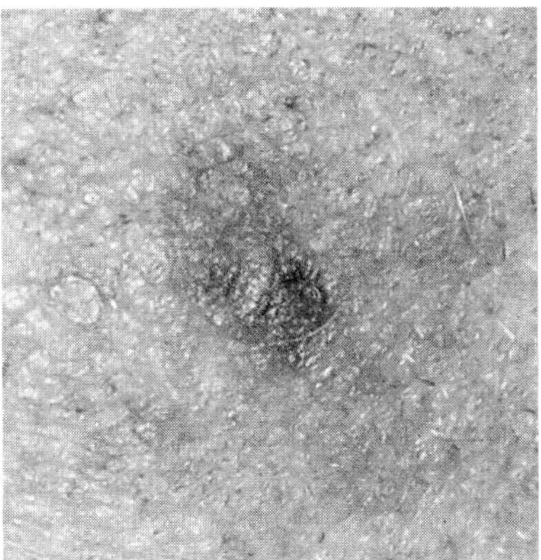

FIG. 56-4 (A, B) *Asymmetrical papule with jagged outline.*

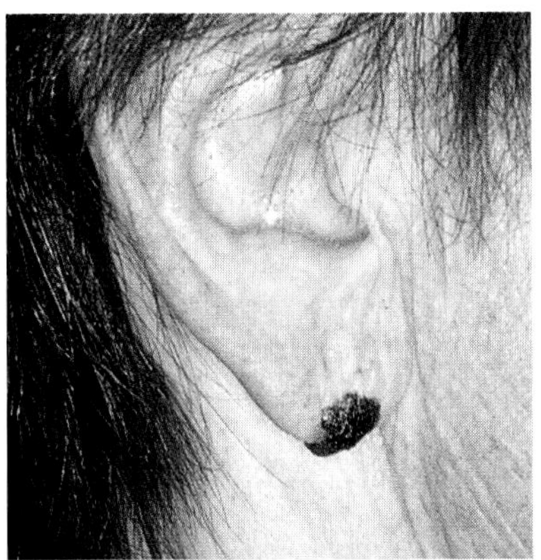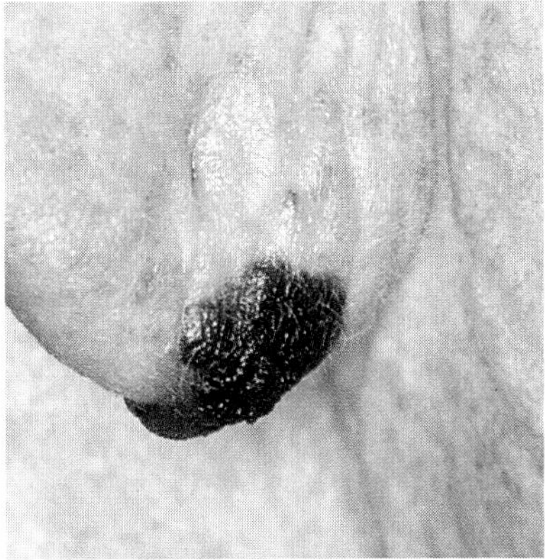

FIG. 56-5 (A, B) *Plaque whose border is crenulated and whose surface is uneven.*

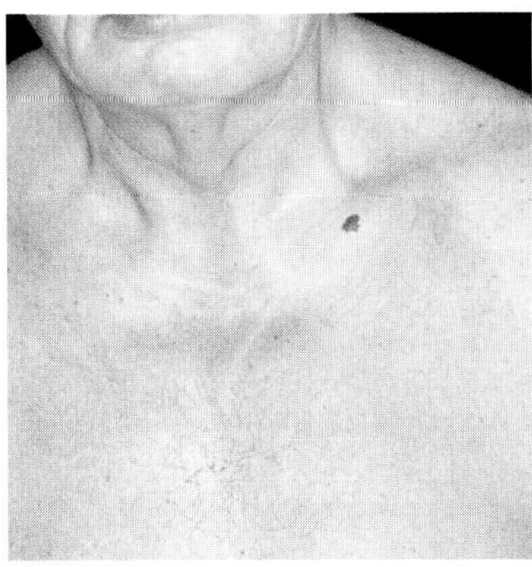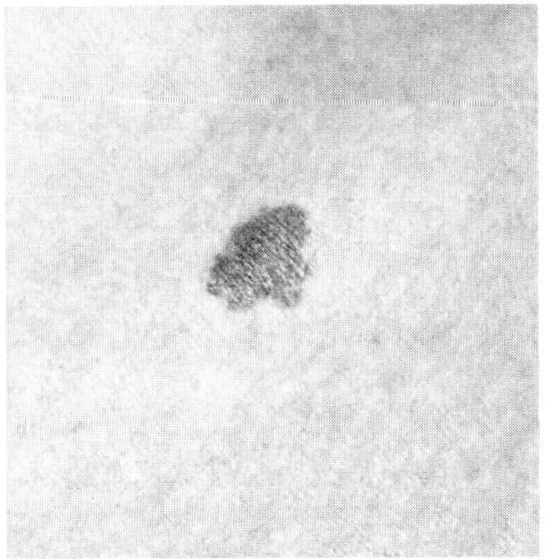

FIG. 56-6 (A, B) *Asymmetrical macule with scalloped border.*

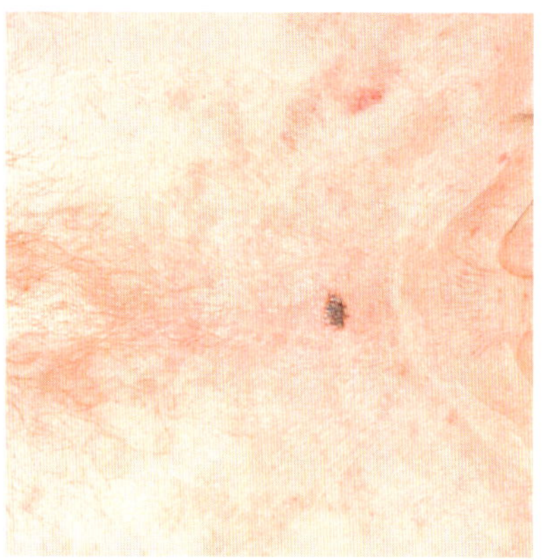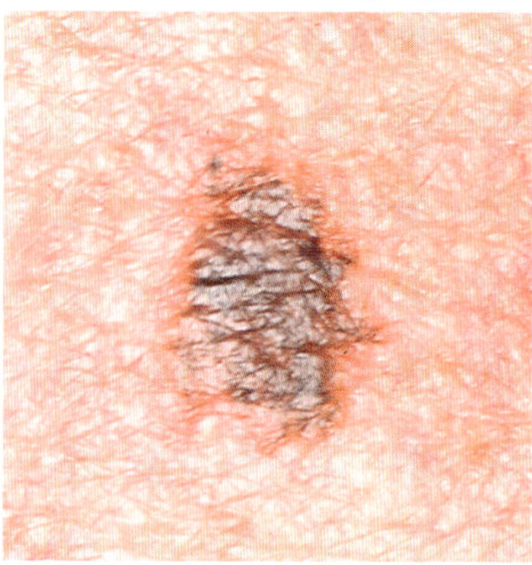

FIG. 56-7 (A, B) *Asymmetrical, poorly circumscribed macule on the chest.*

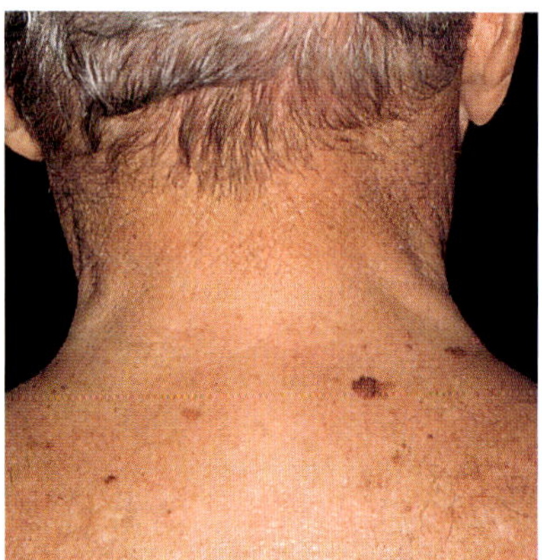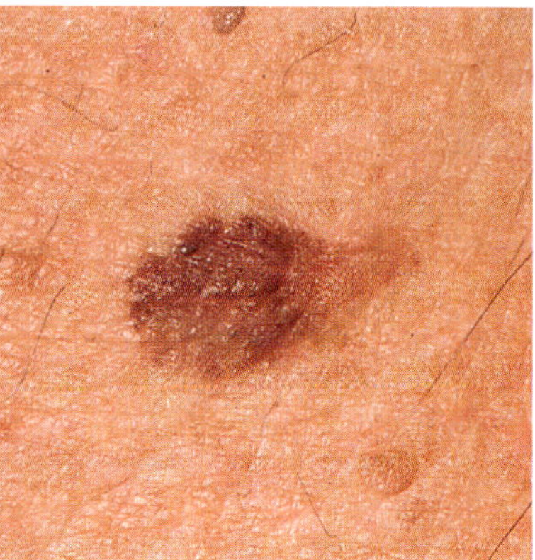

FIG. 56-8 (A, B) *Asymmetrical papule with scalloped border and uneven distribution of pigment.*

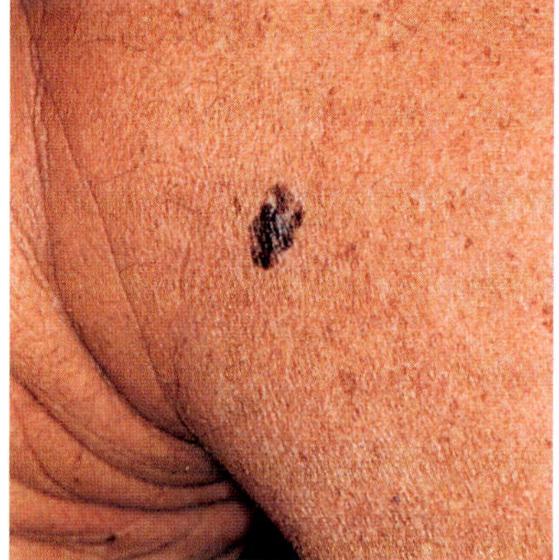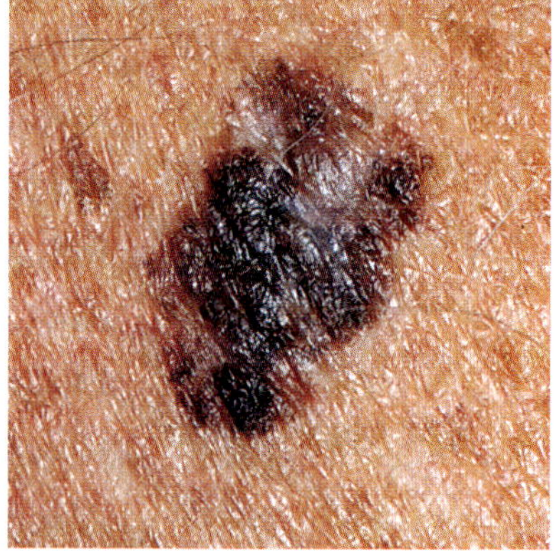

FIG. 56-9 (A, B) *Asymmetrical plaque with marked variegation in color, including white as a sign of regression focally.*

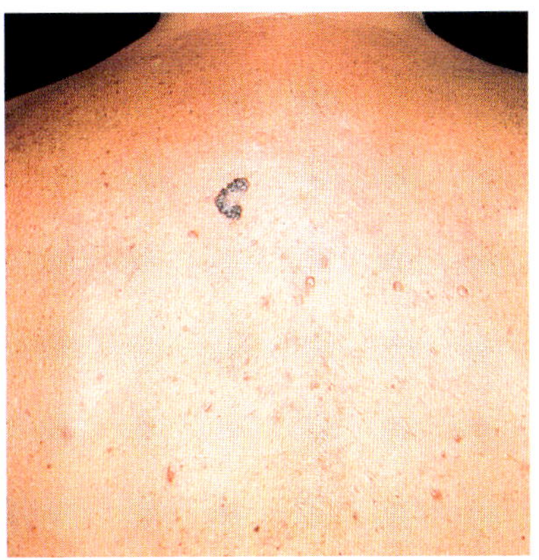 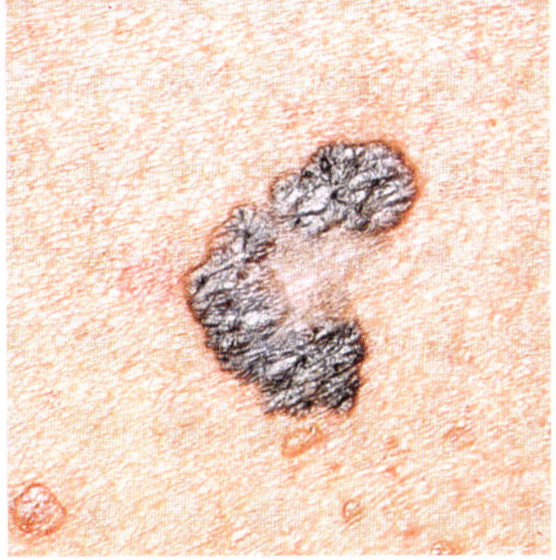

FIG. 56-10 (A, B) *Arciform plaque with scalloped border and a central zone of regression. The numerous papules beneath it are melanocytic nevi of Clark's type.*

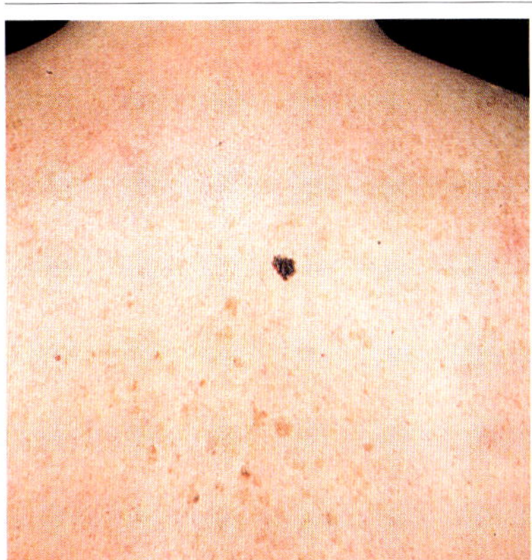 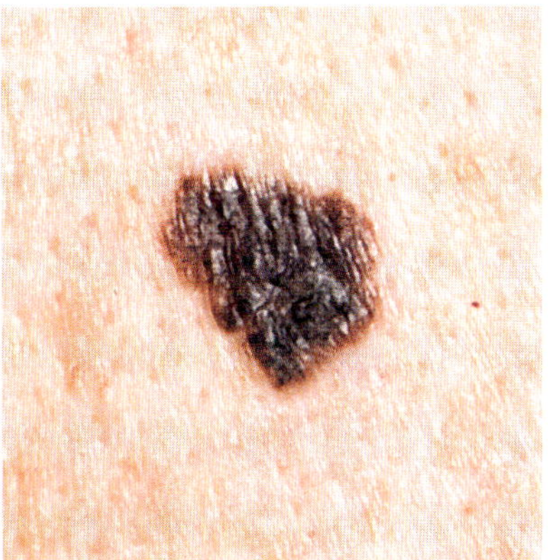

FIG. 56-11 (A, B) *Asymmetrical papule with scalloped border and uneven surface.*

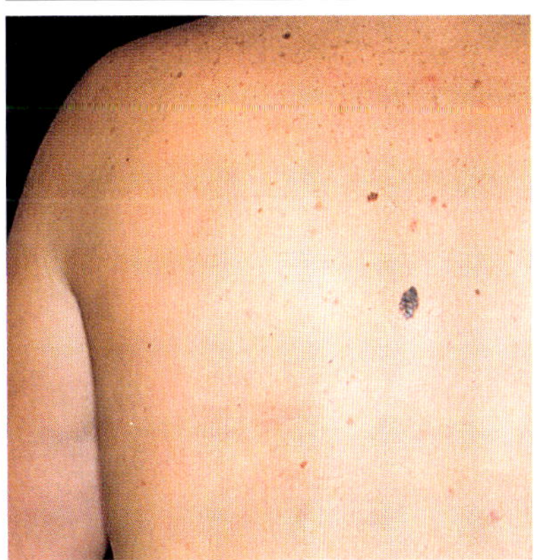 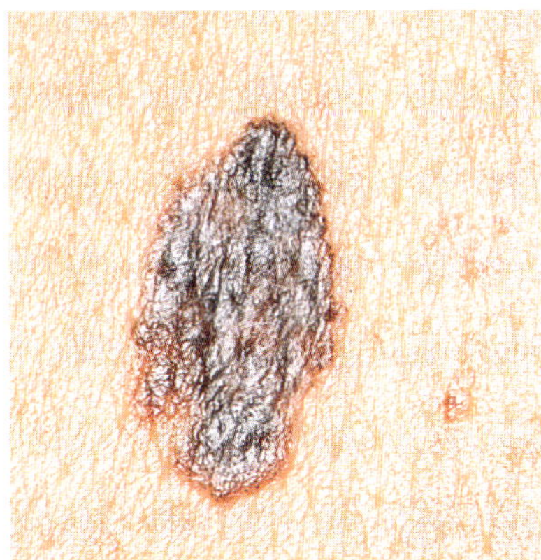

FIG. 56-12 (A, B) *Asymmetrical plaque with crenulated border and uneven surface. There also are many Clark's nevi.*

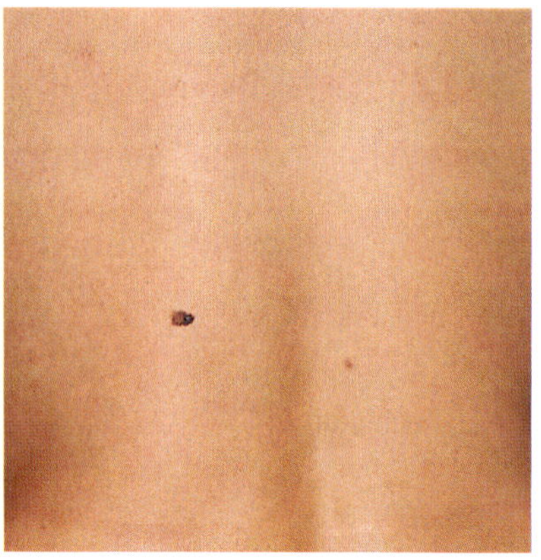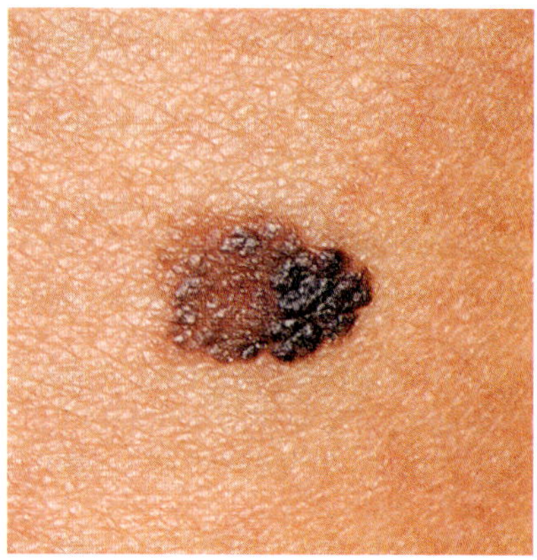

FIG. 56-13 (A, B) *Asymmetrical plaque with a markedly uneven surface. There is no sign of damage to skin by the effects of sunlight.*

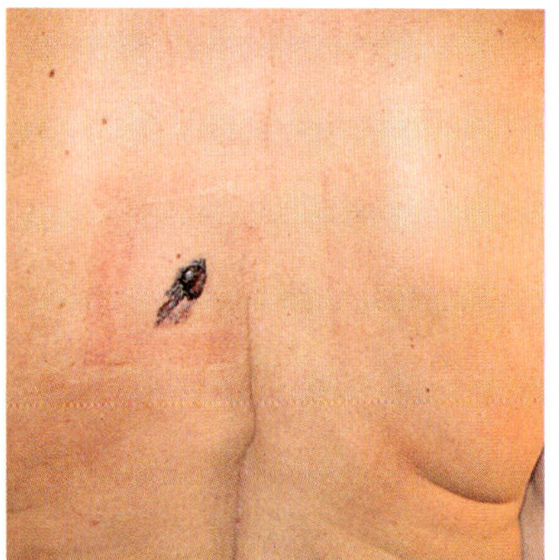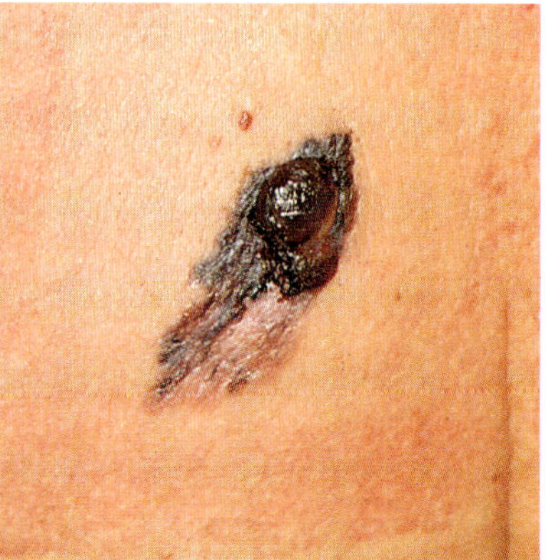

FIG. 56-14 (A, B) *Asymmetrical lesion in which a patch is associated with a plaque and an eroded nodule.*

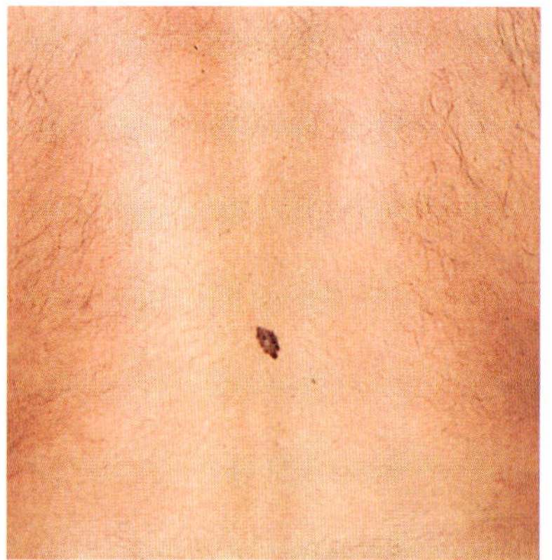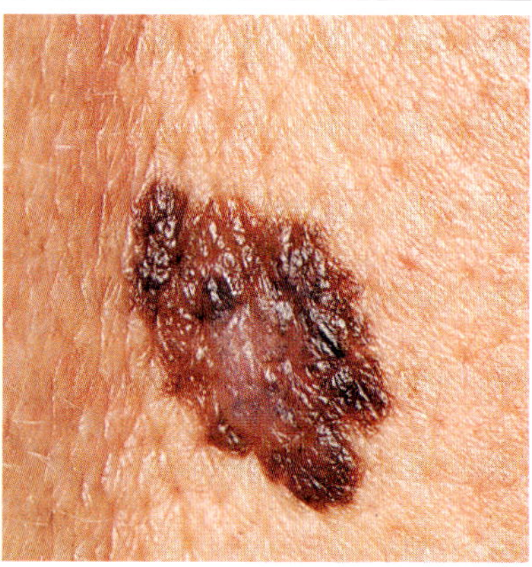

FIG. 56-15 (A, B) *Asymmetrical plaque with scalloped border, uneven surface, and a central zone of regression on a back. Note the absence of nevi.*

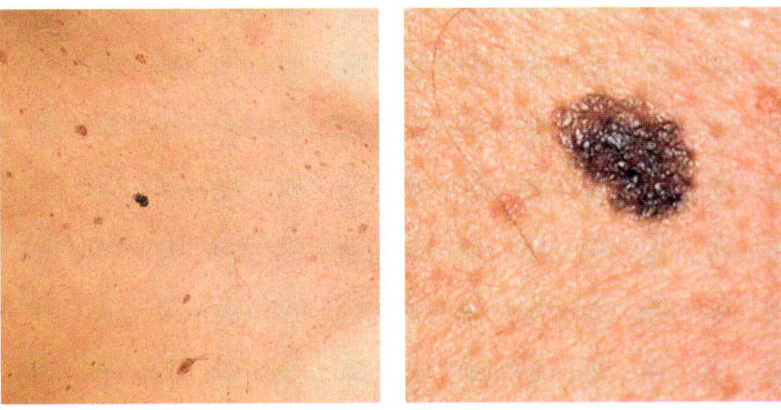

FIG. 56-16 (A, B) *Asymmetrical plaque whose border is crenulated and whose surface is uneven on the back. Numerous Clark's nevi also are present.*

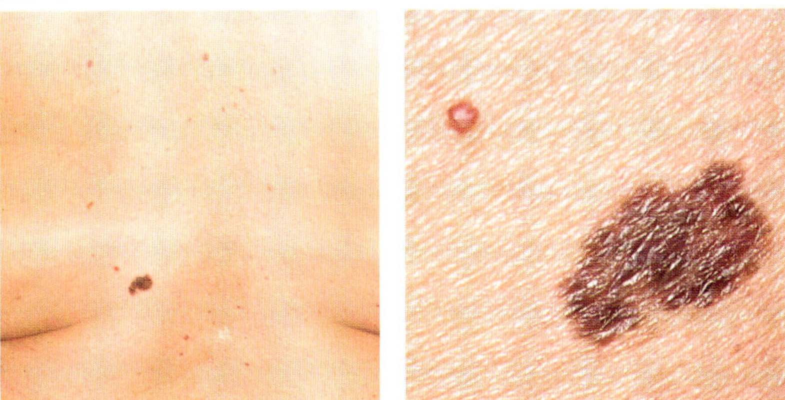

FIG. 56-17 (A, B) *Asymmetrical slightly elevated plaque. The pink lesion is a cherry hemangioma.*

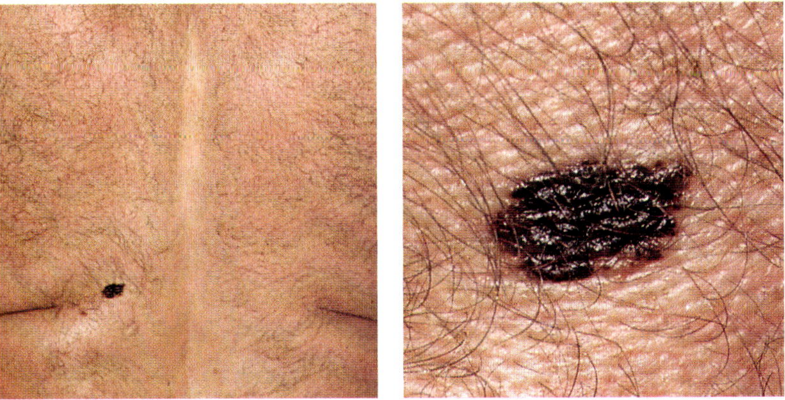

FIG. 56-18 (A, B) *Slightly raised plaque with scalloped border and preserved skin markings.*

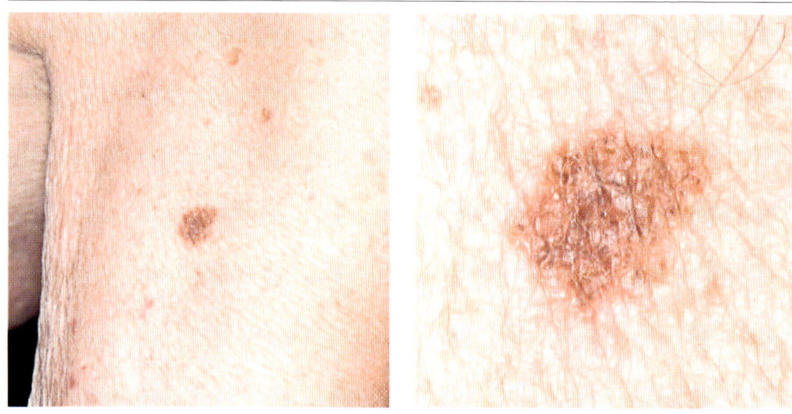

FIG. 56-19 (A, B) *Macule with ill-defined margin and an uneven surface.*

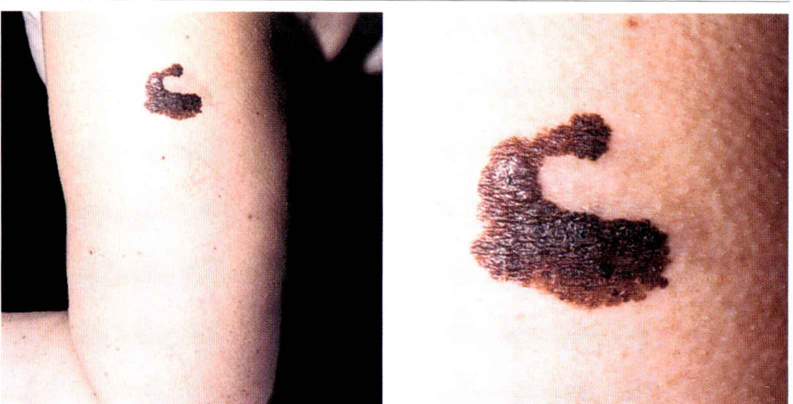

FIG. 56-20 (A, B) *Arciform plaque with markedly scalloped border and a central zone of regression.*

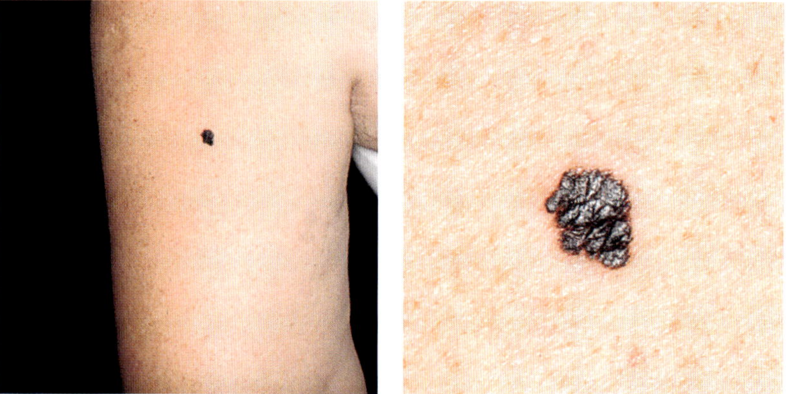

FIG. 56-21 (A, B) *Papule with markedly scalloped border.*

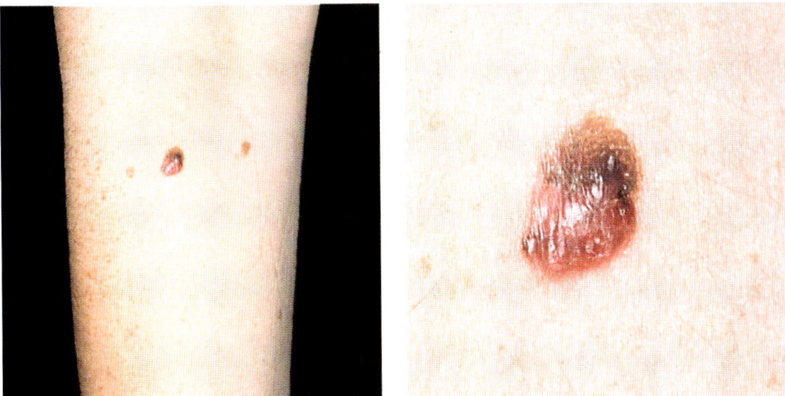

FIG. 56-22 (A, B) *Asymmetrical papule with uneven surface and variegate color. Clark's nevi also are present.*

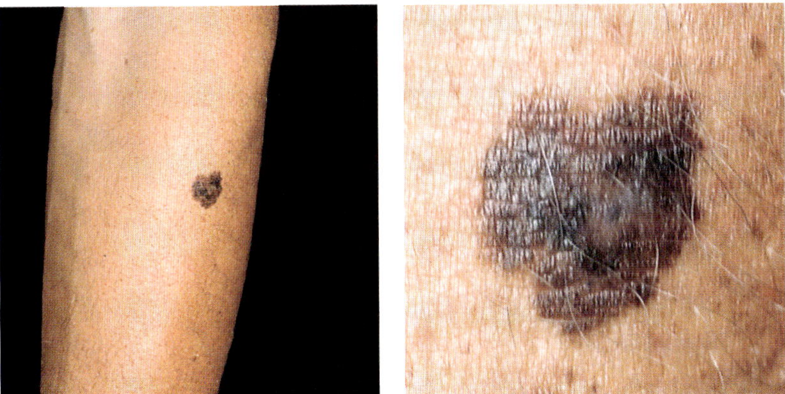

FIG. 56-23 (A, B) *Plaque with scalloped border and a central zone of partial regression.*

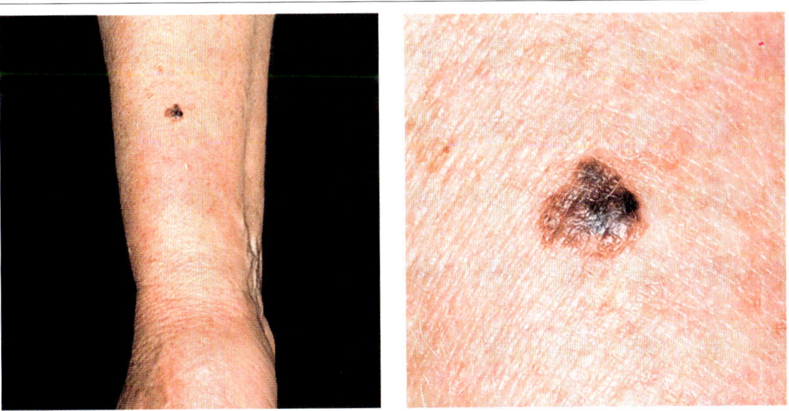

FIG. 56-24 (A, B) *Asymmetrical papule with an uneven surface.*

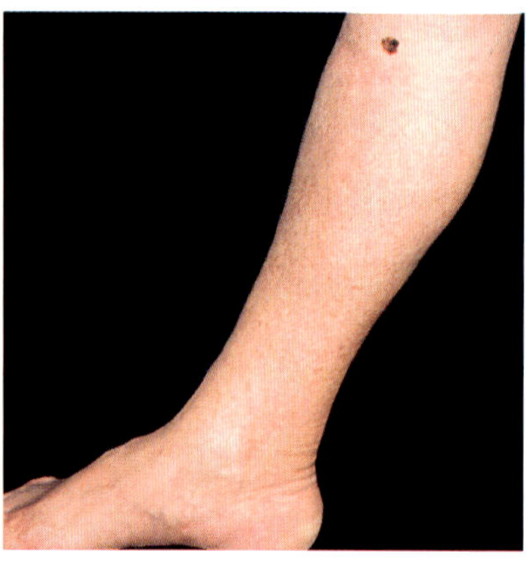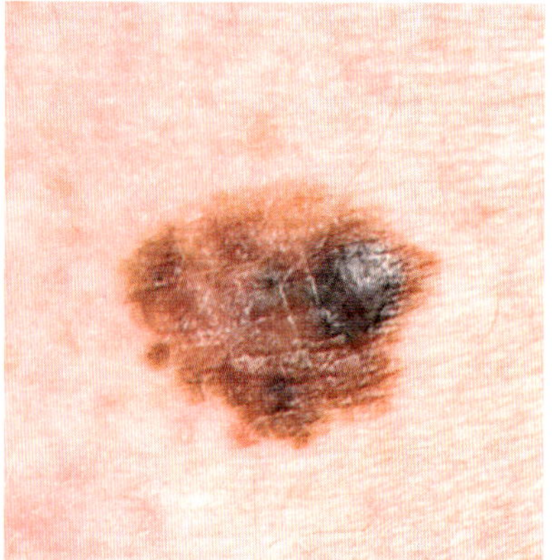

FIG. 56-25 (A, B) *Asymmetrical patch with a small papule upon it, notched borders, and an uneven surface.*

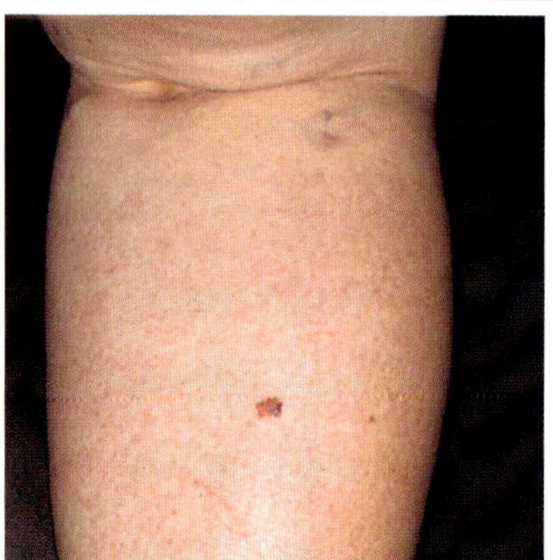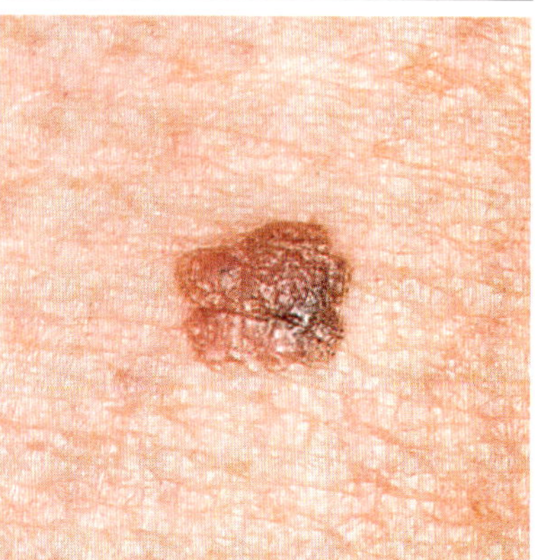

FIG. 56-26 (A, B) *Asymmetrical papule with notched border and uneven surface.*

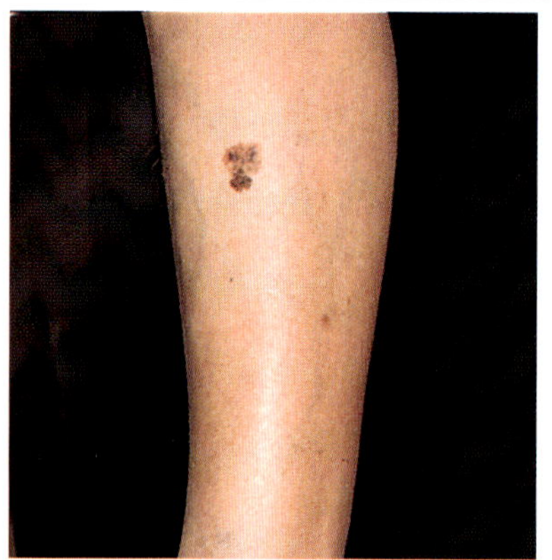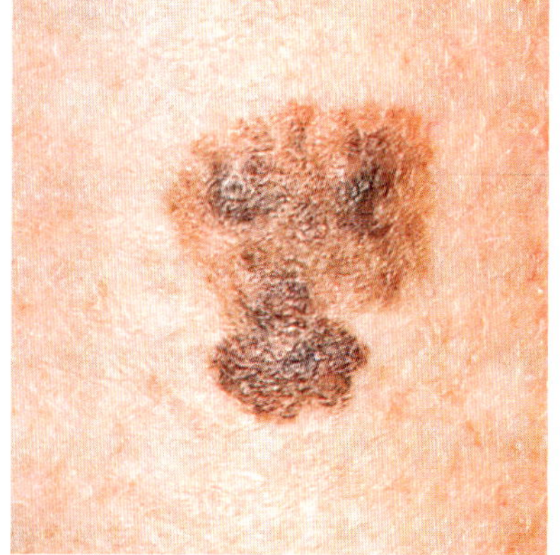

FIG. 56-27 (A, B) *Asymmetrical plaque with scalloped border and uneven surface.*

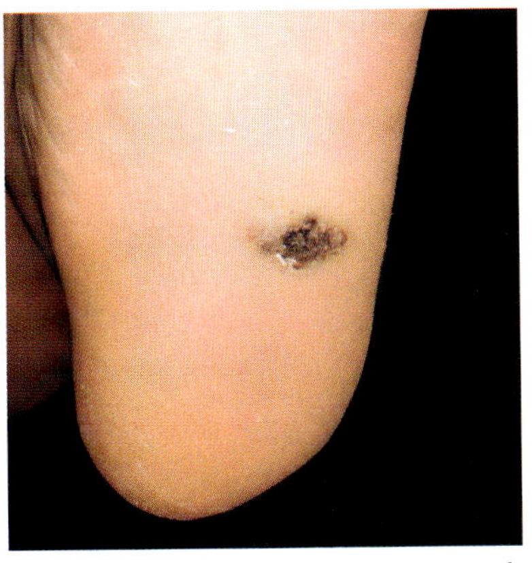 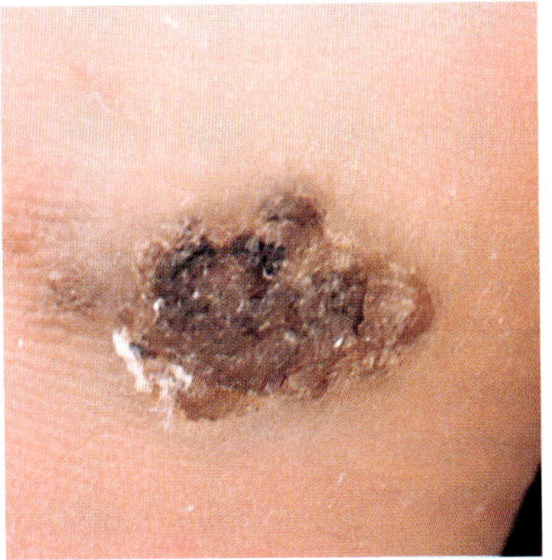

FIG. 56-28 (A, B) *Asymmetrical plaque with notched border and uneven surface.*

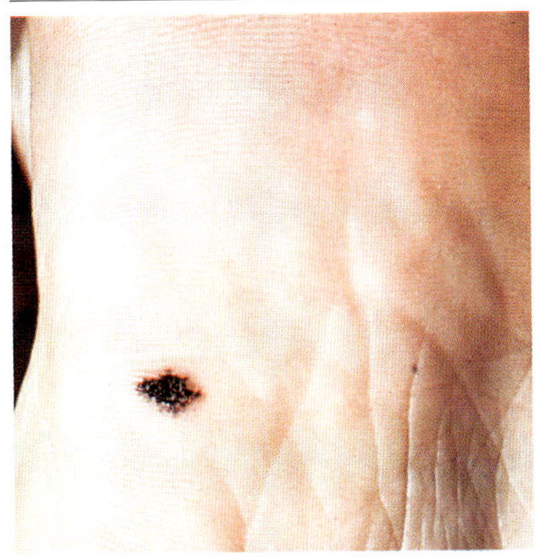 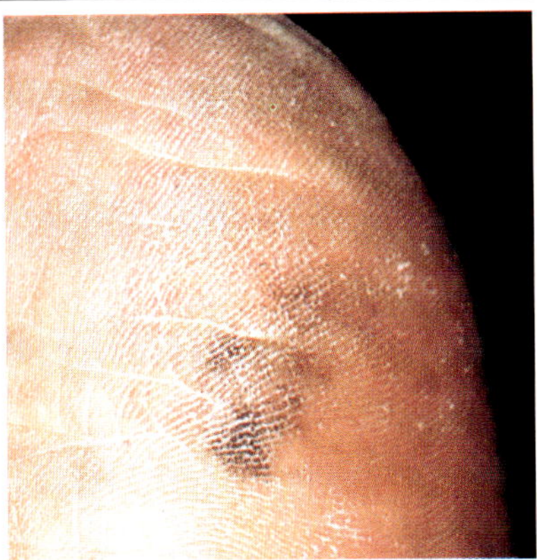

FIG. 56-29 *Asymmetrical fusiform black papule.*

FIG. 56-30 *Asymmetrical variegated patch.*

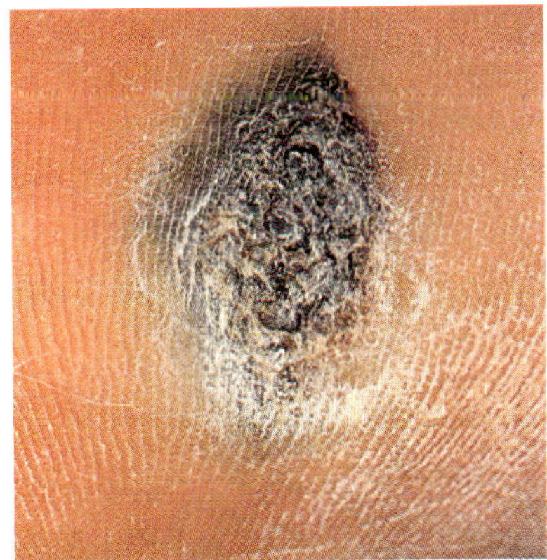 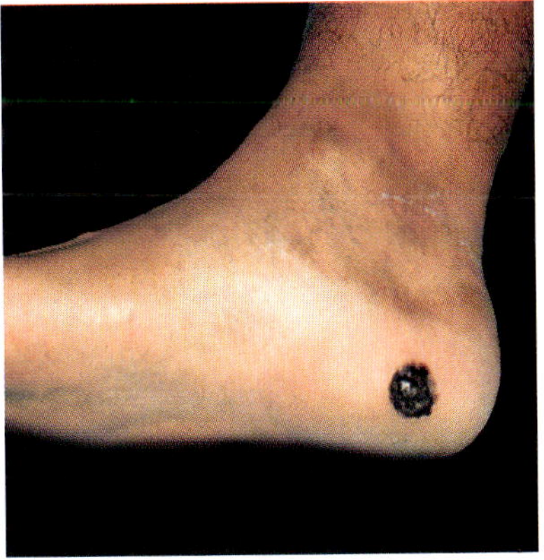

FIG. 56-31 *Asymmetrical blue-black plaque with an uneven surface.*

FIG. 56-32 *Tumor in an African-American.*

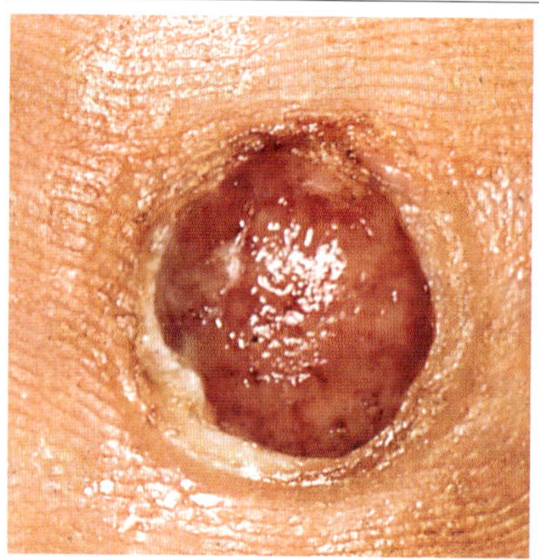

FIG. 56-33 *Sessile ulcerated nodule (amelanotic melanoma).*

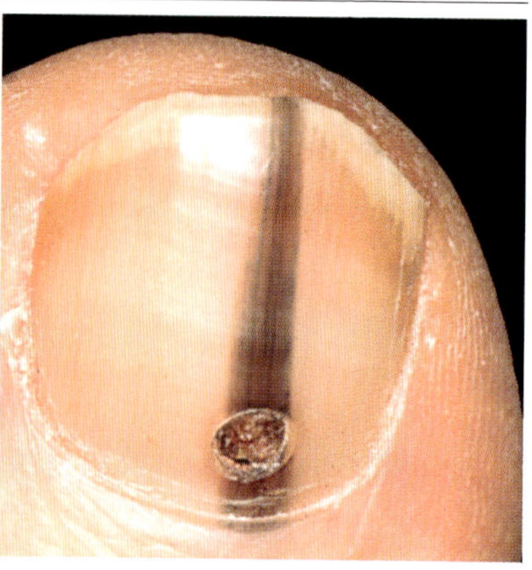

FIG. 56-34 *Pigmented streak (melanonychia striata) that is broader at its base and that displays streaks within it (melanoma in situ).*

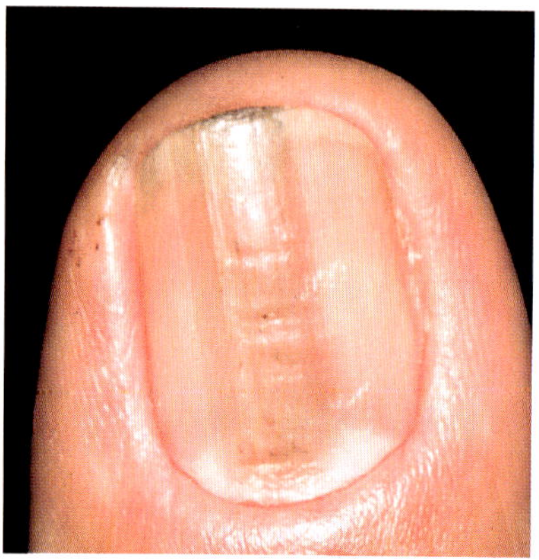

FIG. 56-35 *Pigmented band (melanoma in situ).*

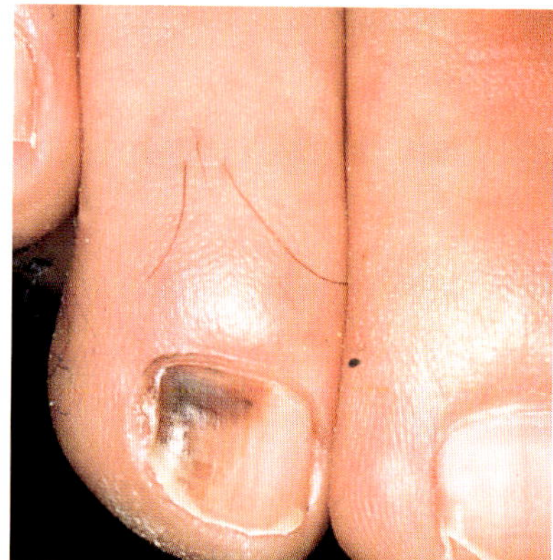

FIG. 56-36 *Pigmented macule and ill-defined streak (melanoma in situ).*

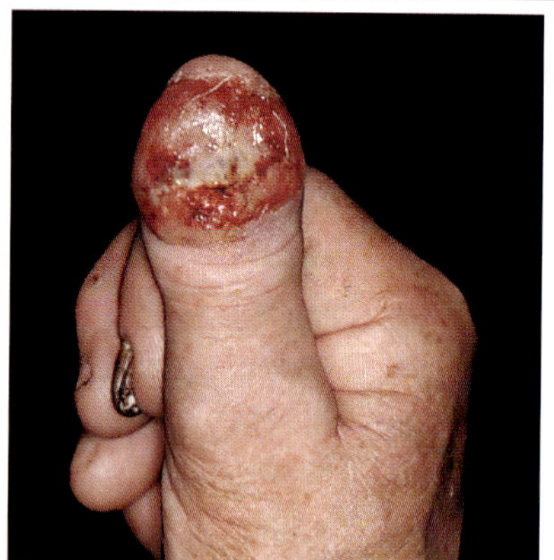

FIG. 56-37 *Ulcerated tumor that has destroyed the nail plate.*

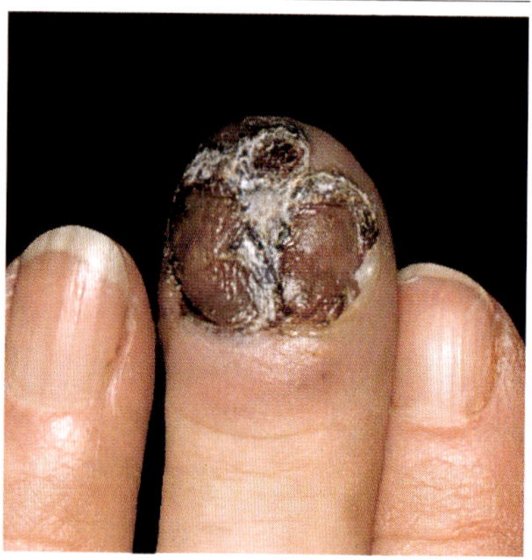

FIG. 56-38 *Ulcerated nodule with loss of the nail plate.*

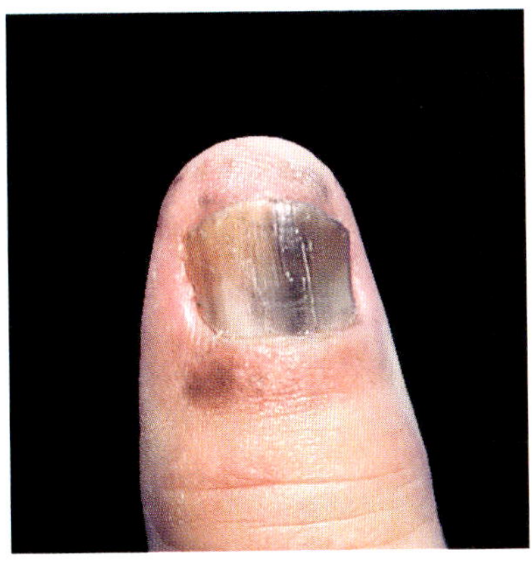

FIG. 56-39 *Asymmetrical uneven pigmentation subungually and in the posterior nail fold (Hutchinson's sign).*

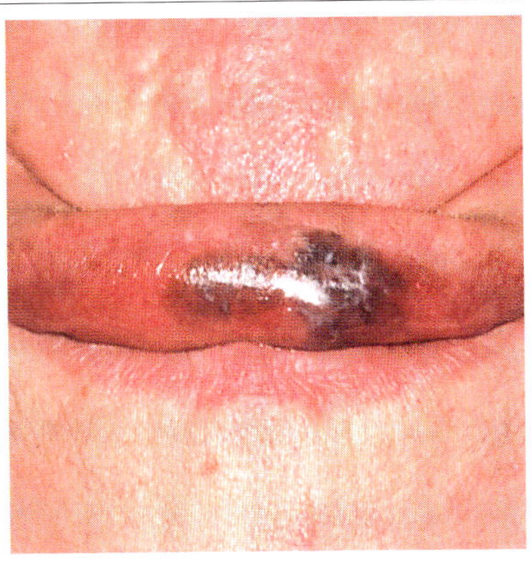

FIG. 56-40 *Asymmetrical pigmented patch with variation in color and a scalloped border.*

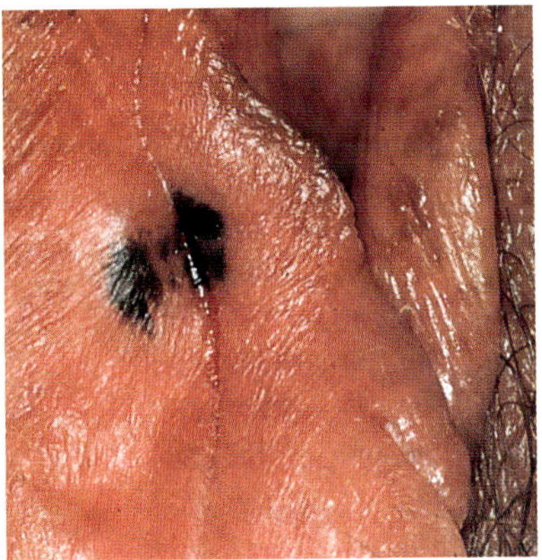

FIG. 56-41 *Asymmetrical black patch on the vulva.*

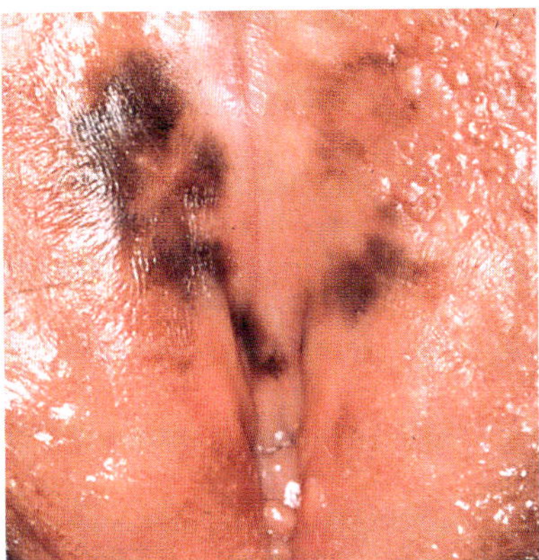

FIG. 56-42 *Asymmetrical pigmented patches with variegation in color and a hypopigmented zone of regression.*

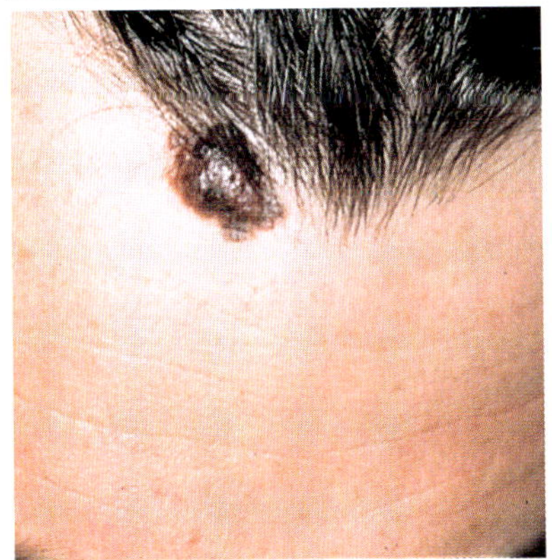

FIG. 56-43 *Nodule surrounded by macular pigmentation in scalloped outline.*

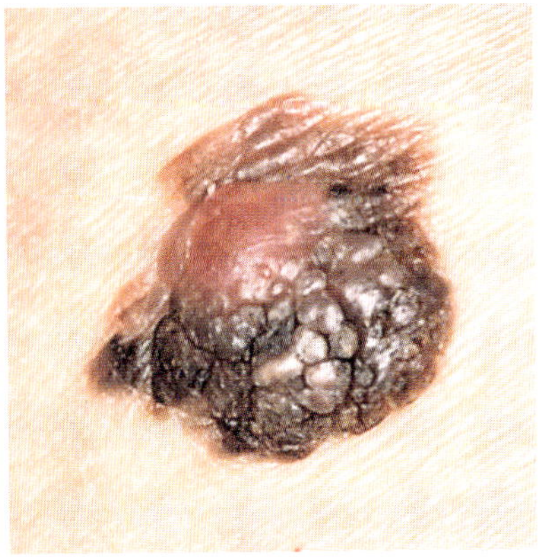

FIG. 56-44 *Asymmetrical plaque on which are red and brown papules.*

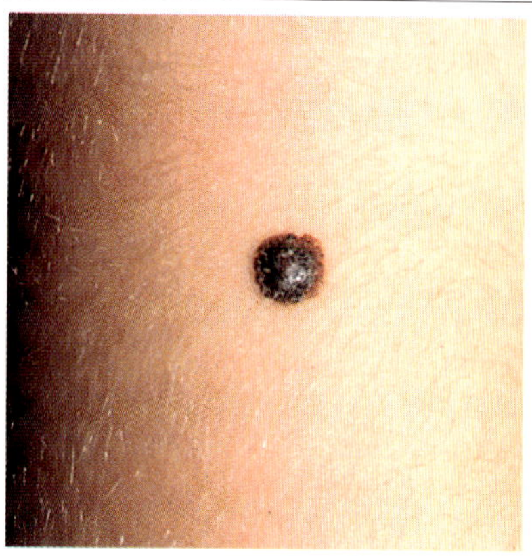

FIG. 56-45 *Papule with a subtle scalloped macular border at its upper margin.*

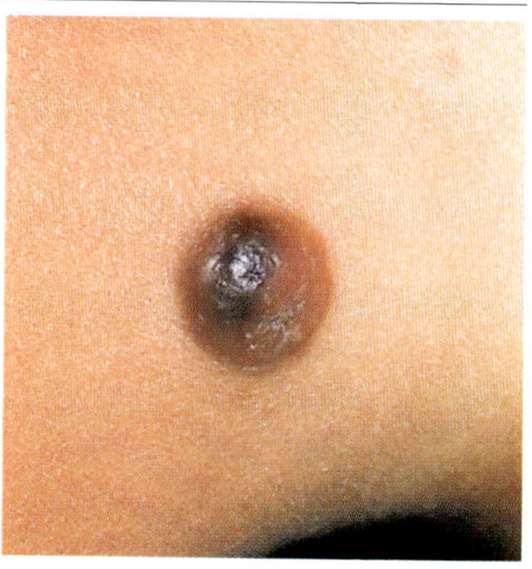

FIG. 56-46 *Nodule, variegate in shades of brown, in a 13-year-old girl dead two years later of metastatic melanoma.*

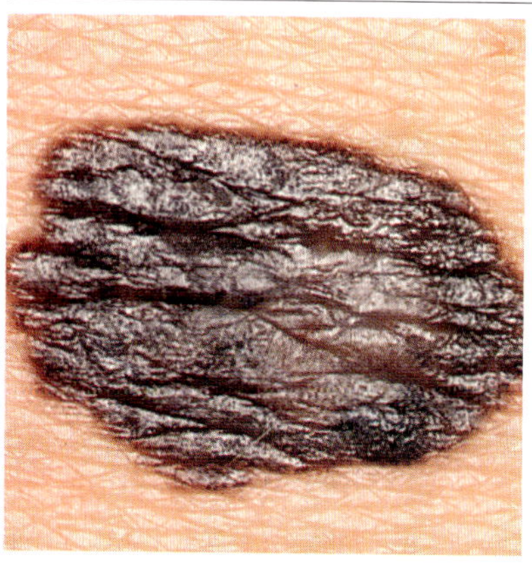

FIG. 56-47 *Plaque with scalloped margins, an uneven surface, and an eccentric zone of partial regression.*

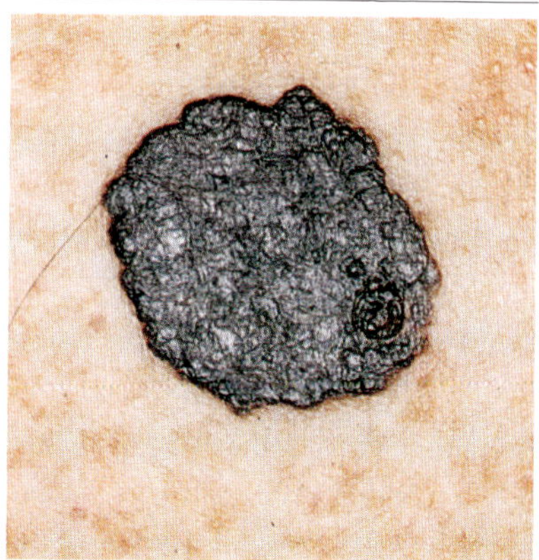

FIG. 56-48 *Plaque with scalloped margin and an uneven surface.*

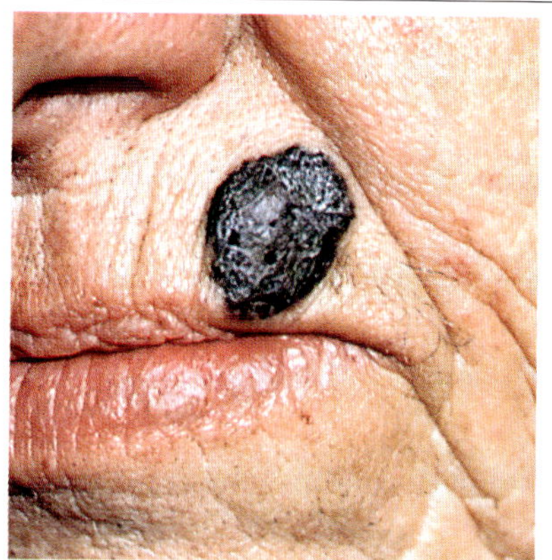

FIG. 56-49 *Black tumor.*

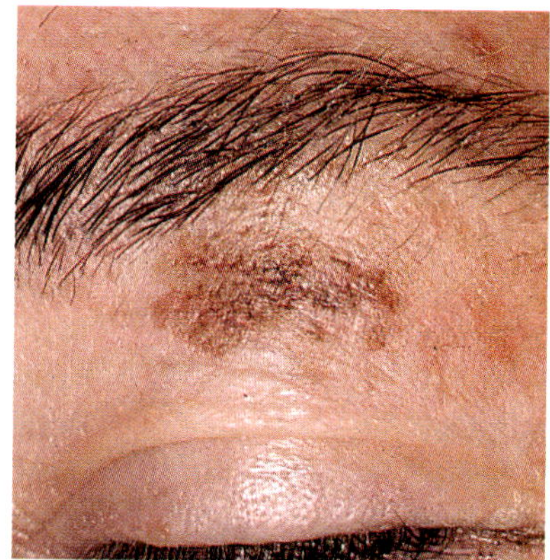

FIG. 56-50 *Asymmetrical, poorly circumscribed patch with shades of brown.*

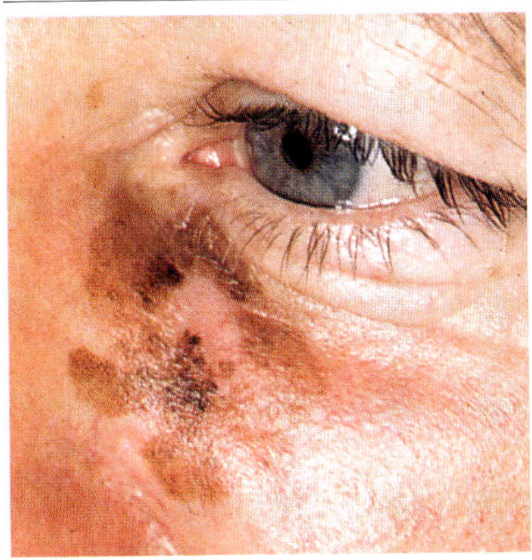

FIG. 56-51 *Asymmetrical patch with mottled pigmentation and signs of regression in the center.*

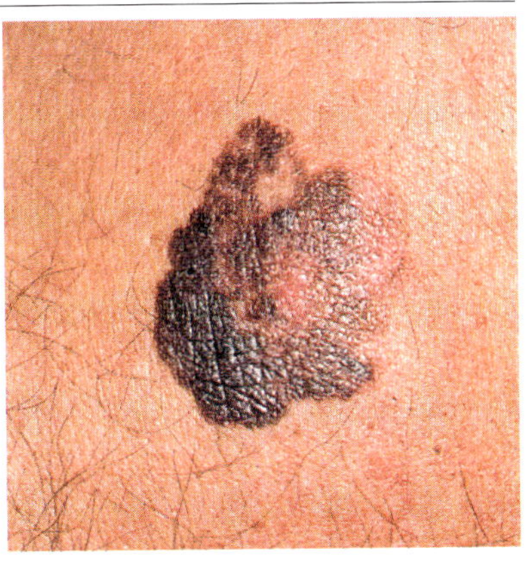

FIG. 56-52 *Asymmetrical patch/plaque and signs of regression on the trunk.*

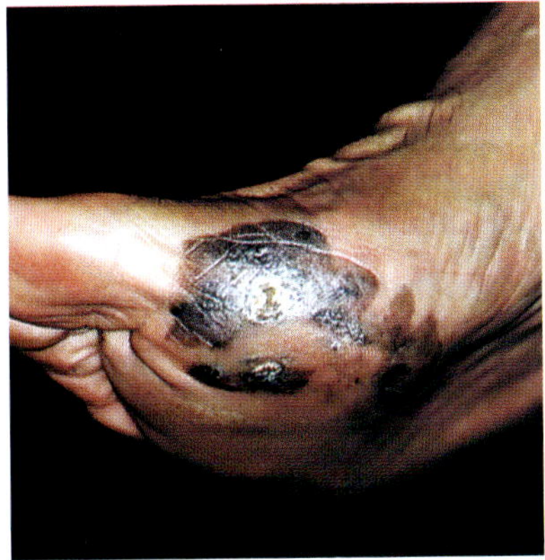

FIG. 56-53 *Asymmetrical patch/plaque and signs of regression on the foot.*

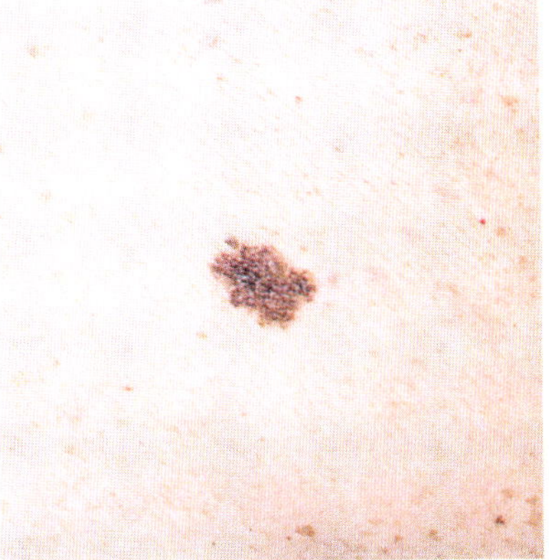

FIG. 56-54 *Asymmetrical brown patch with uneven pigmentation throughout it.*

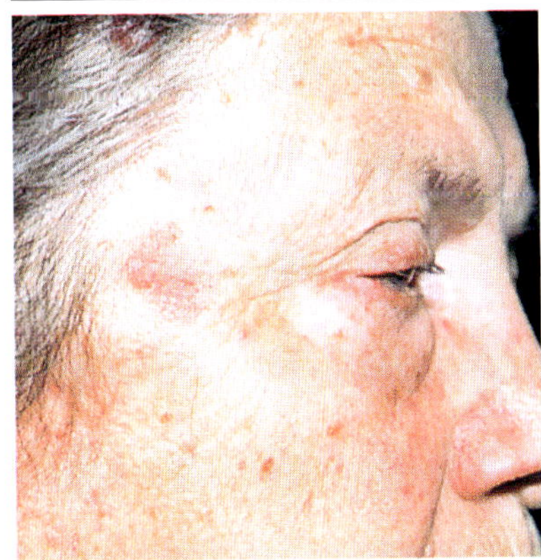

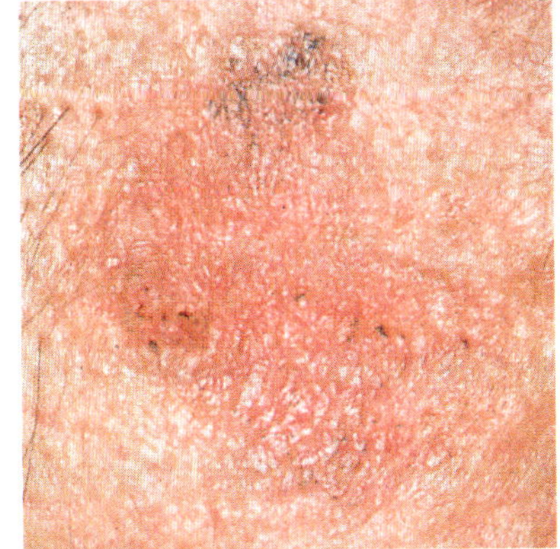

FIG. 56-55 (A, B) *Asymmetrical reddish patch with scalloped border and pigment at the superior pole.*

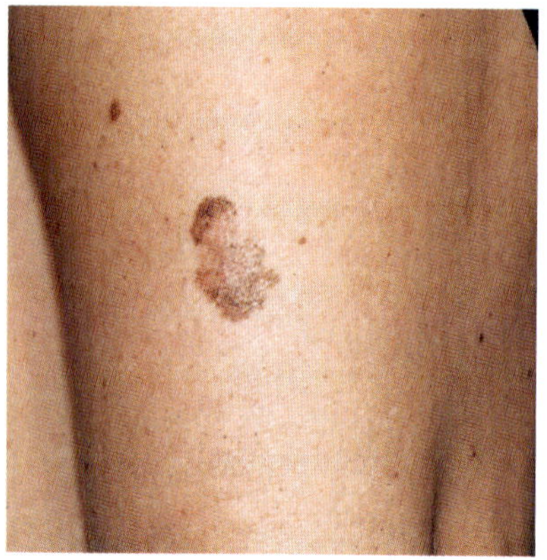

FIG. 56-56 *Asymmetrical patch with scalloped border and variegation of pigment. There are several Clark's nevi.*

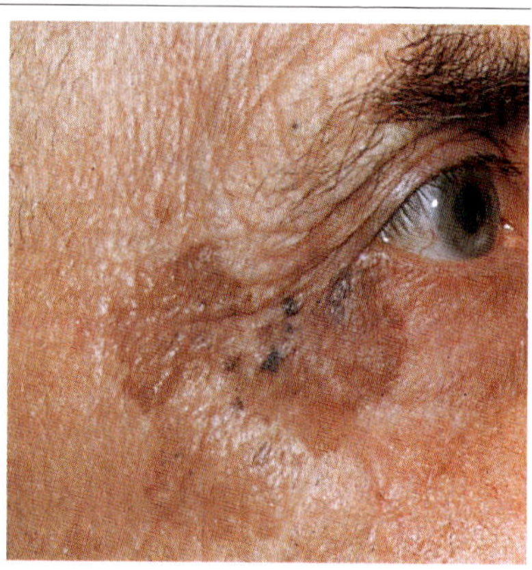

FIG. 56-57 *Asymmetrical patch with marked variation in shades of brown and foci of black.*

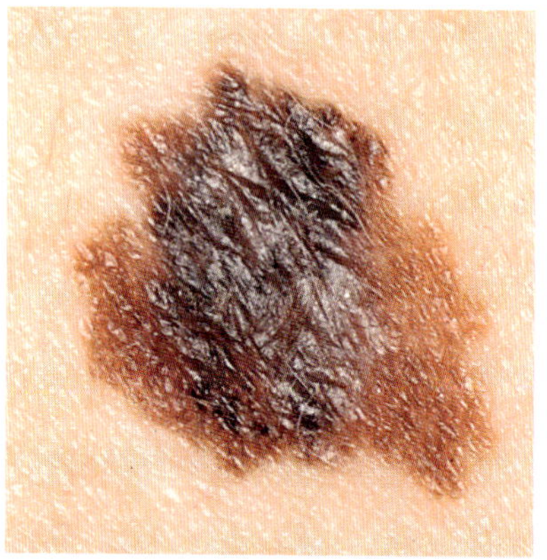

FIG. 56-58 *Asymmetrical plaque whose periphery is largely macular and scalloped, and whose surface is uneven.*

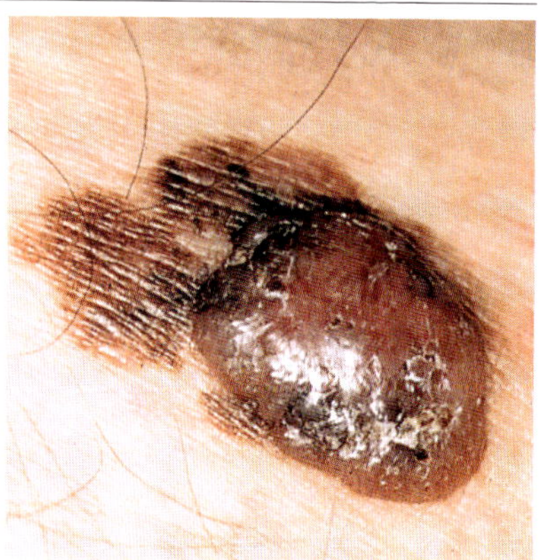

FIG. 56-59 *Tumor upon a patch/plaque that has notched borders and an uneven surface.*

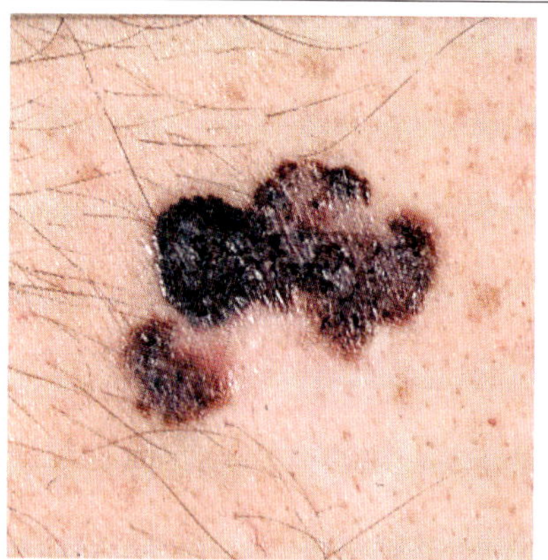

FIG. 56-60 *The white concave zone and the gray zones represent foci of regression of melanoma.*

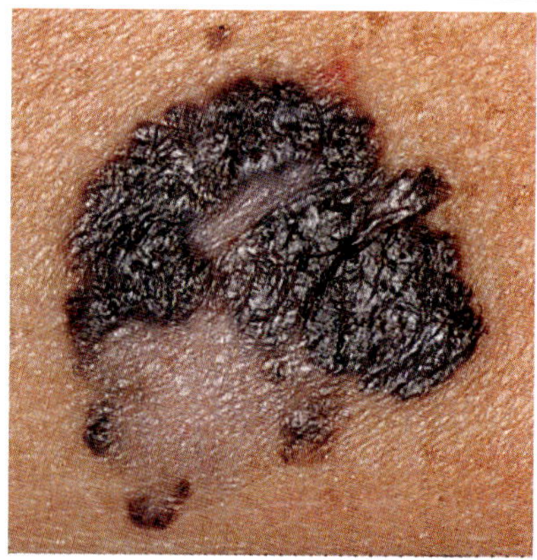

FIG. 56-61 *Zones of hypopigmentation within the asymmetrical plaque represent regression of melanoma.*

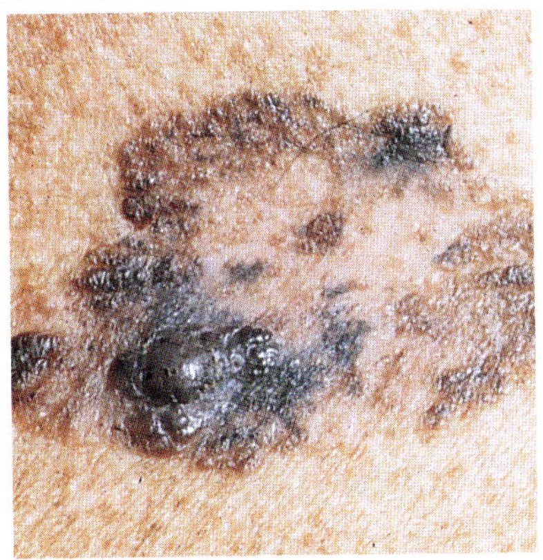

FIG. 56-62 *The flat, whitish zone represents focal regression of melanoma.*

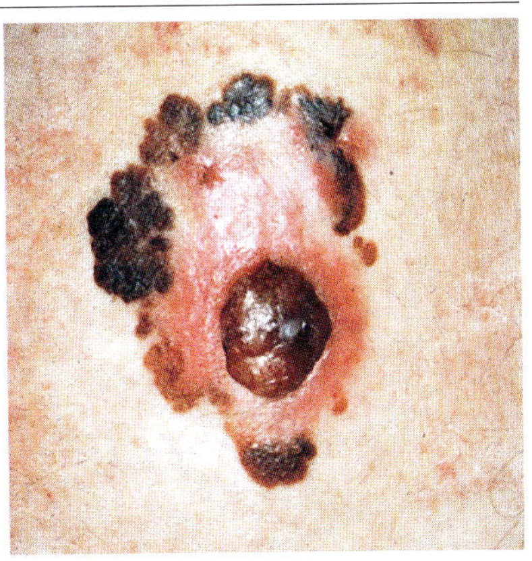

FIG. 56-63 *Extensive regression seen as a broad zone of red and white within a melanoma.*

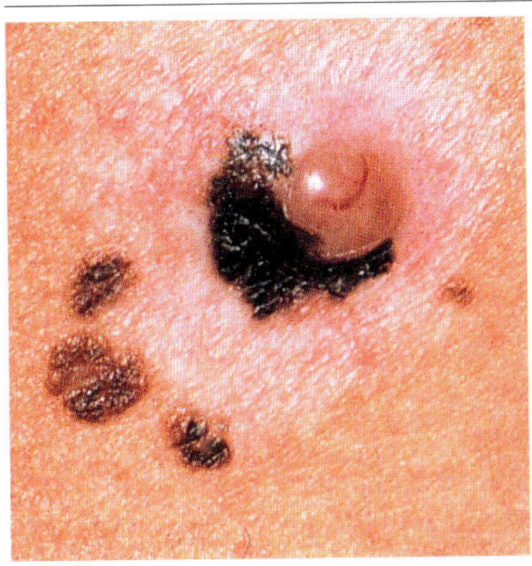

FIG. 56-64 *Zones of regression result in the appearance of islands of melanoma that seem now to be separate from one another.*

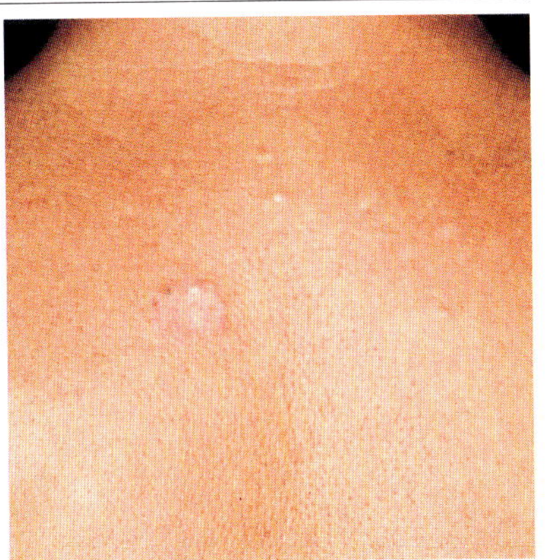

FIG. 56-65 *Nearly complete regression of melanoma in the form of a white plaque.*

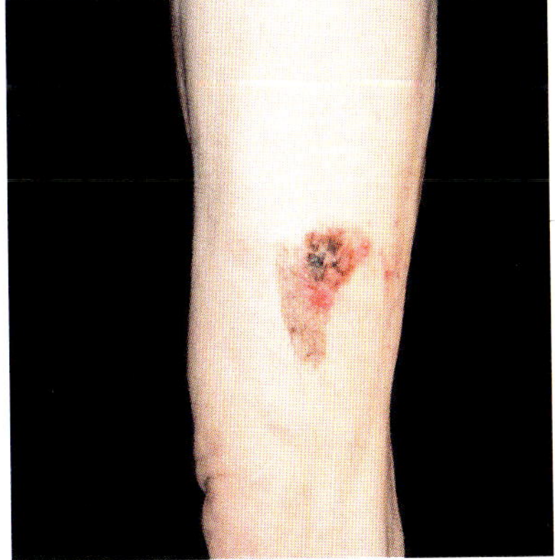

FIG. 56-66 *Asymmetrical pigmented patch/plaque with varied hues at the superior pole of a congenital melanocytic nevus.*

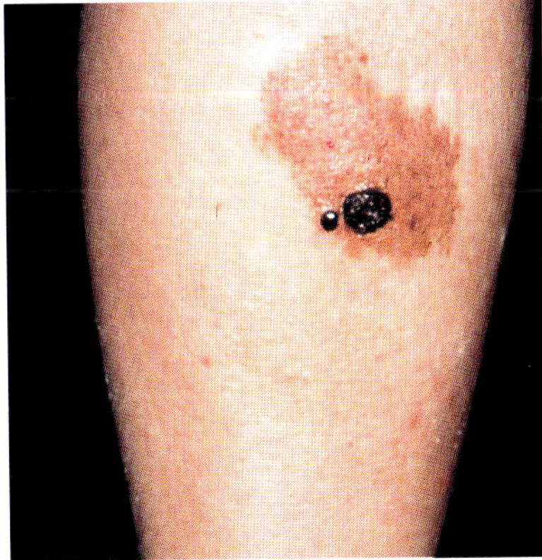

FIG. 56-67 *A black papule and nodule of melanoma at the periphery of a congenital melanocytic nevus.*

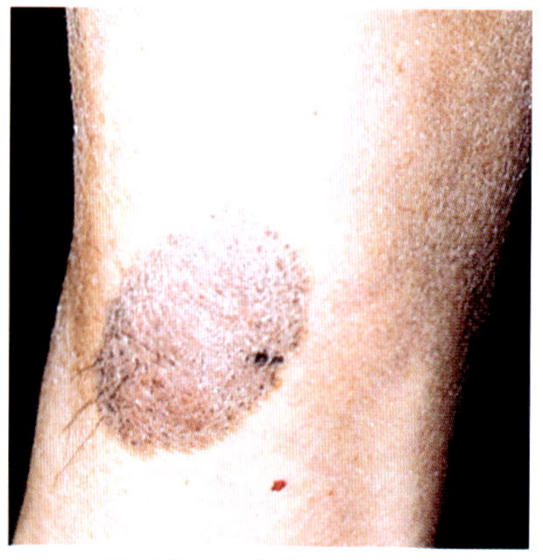

FIG. 56-68 *The small black area at 3 o'clock represents a tiny melanoma that began in association with a congenital nevus.*

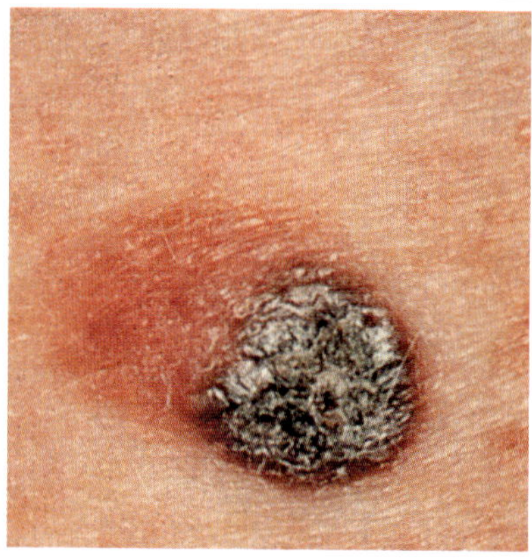

FIG. 56-69 *Melanoma on the right, Clark's nevus on the left.*

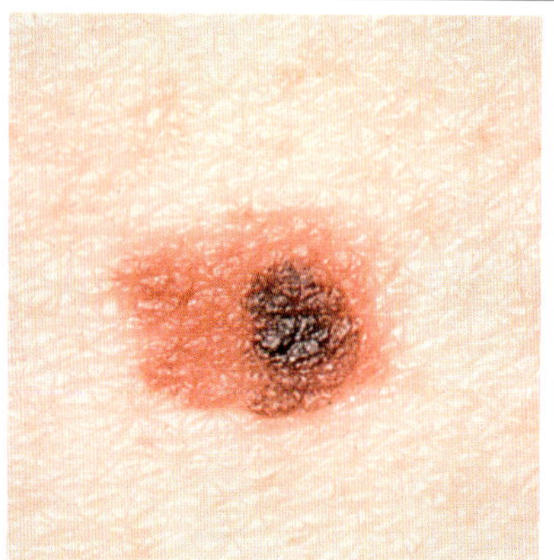

FIG. 56-70 *Melanoma mostly on the right, Clark's nevus on the left.*

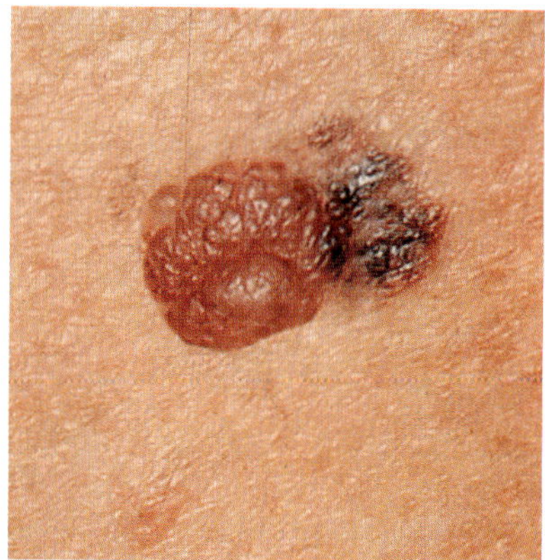

FIG. 56-71 *Melanoma on the right, Unna's nevus on the left, a combination encountered rarely.*

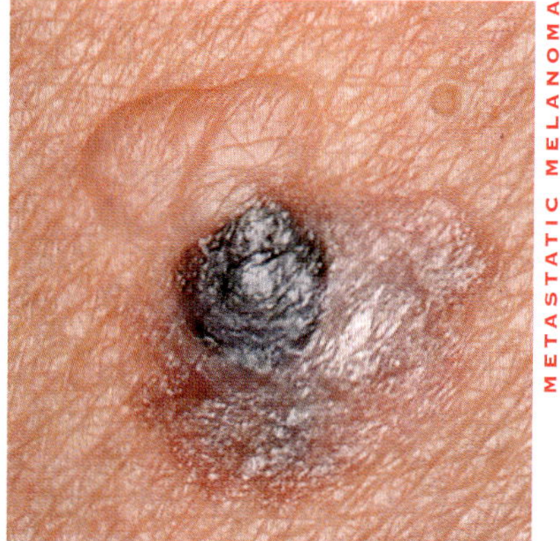

FIG. 56-72 *Melanoma in the center of a skin-colored, plaque-like nevus.*

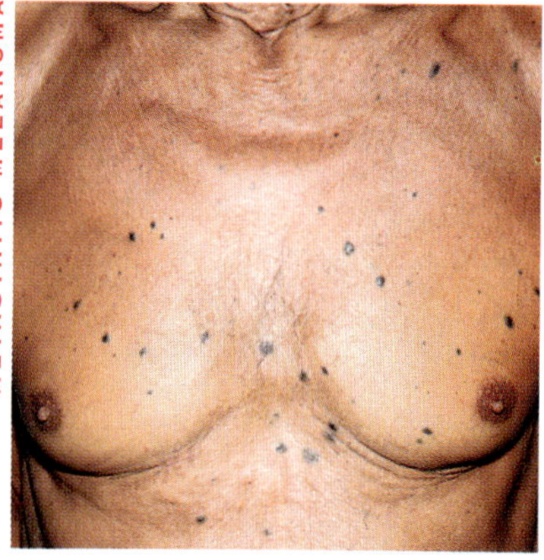

FIG. 56-73 *Dark-blue papules of metastatic melanoma.*

METASTATIC MELANOMA

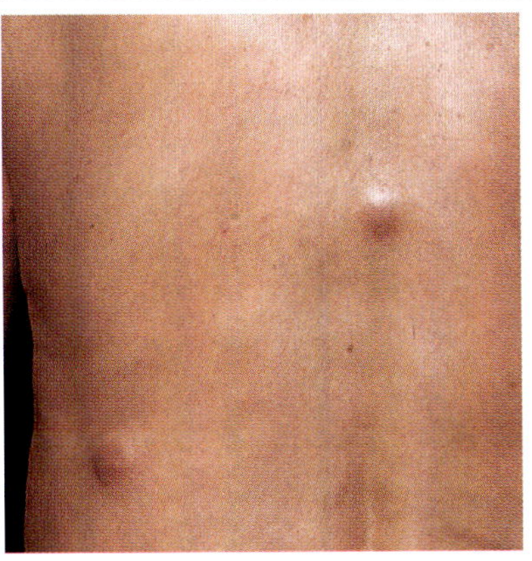

FIG. 56-74 *Skin-colored nodules of metastatic melanoma.*

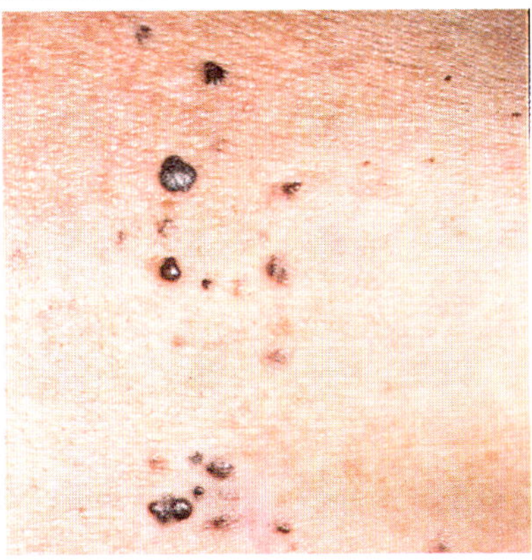

FIG. 56-75 *Pigmented papules of metastatic melanoma near a scar.*

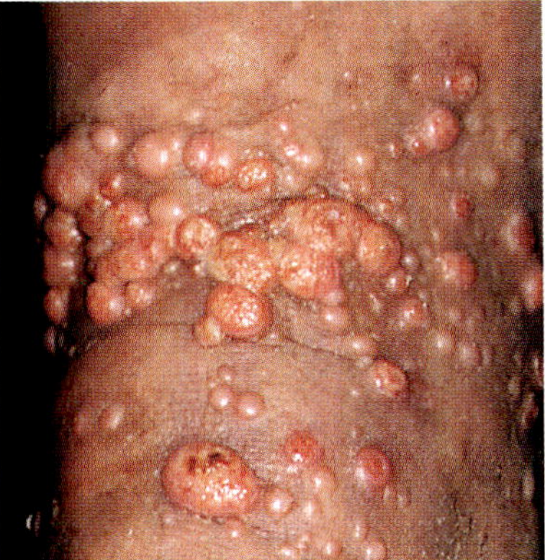

FIG. 56-76 *Smooth-surfaced and ulcerated papules and nodules of metastatic melanoma.*

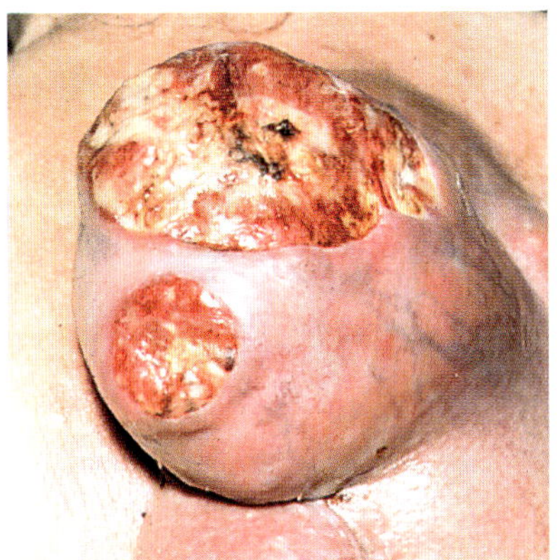

FIG. 56-77 *Huge ulcerated tumor of metastatic melanoma.*

ADJUNCTIVE DIAGNOSTIC TESTS Dermoscopy (dermatoscopy, epiluminescence microscopy) may enhance accuracy of diagnosis. The procedure is performed by covering the lesion with oil and a glass slide in order to render the stratum corneum translucent. Subsequently the lesion is illuminated by incident light and viewed through a hand lens or a digital epiluminescence microscope. The pattern formed by elements of the lesion enables specific diagnosis to be rendered in the vast majority of cases.

Sentinel-node biopsy is currently popular for gauging whether metastasis has occurred and determining how therapy should be carried out. Because the technique is predicated on the idea that melanoma metastasizes mostly by lymphatics, it is likely that the method will not stand the test of time; melanoma often metastasizes through blood vessels.

COURSE For practical purposes, all melanomas on all anatomic sites begin as macules that, at the outset, often are fawn colored or tan and in time become broader and darker. At a very early stage in its evolution, such as when a lesion is less than 3.0 mm in greatest diameter, a melanoma cannot be identified with surety clinically, i.e., by "naked eye" examination alone. As the macule becomes broader, more asymmetrical, more scalloped or notched at its periphery, and more variegate in shades of brown, it becomes recognizable clinically as melanoma. Because melanoma is a malignant neoplasm, it grows persistently and irrepressibly, even if imperceptibly. A macule of melanoma may become a patch and remain a patch for the lifetime of a patient. A macule of melanoma may become a papule, which, in turn, may become a nodule or a tumor. That sequence of papule to nodule to tumor may develop upon a patch of melanoma. A patch may become a plaque and upon a plaque may develop a nodule or a tumor.

Melanomas on all anatomic sites may undergo partial or complete regression. Partial regression manifests itself clinically as a zone of hypopigmentation within the melanoma, either at its center or its periphery. Complete regression of melanoma expresses itself as an off-white macule or patch, sometimes with a bluish cast. It is likely that total regression of primary cutaneous melanoma actually occurs after there has been metastasis of it to a regional lymph node. From there sensitized lymphocytes return to the skin and destroy the primary melanoma.

INTEGRATION: UNIFYING CONCEPT Morphologically, that is, clinically and histopathologically, melanomas are the same on all anatomic sites. The designations "lentigo maligna melanoma," "superficial spreading melanoma," and "acrolentiginous melanoma" are simply terms for melanomas on different anatomic sites, namely, sun-damaged skin of the face, especially for lentigo maligna melanoma, of the trunk and extremities above the acra for superficial spreading melanoma, and of the acra, including nail units, for acrolentiginous melanoma. In short, the so-called histogenetic classification of melanoma is really a classification predicated entirely on anatomic site and has nothing whatever to do with histogenesis.

The stereotypical expression clinically of melanoma on all anatomic sites is a lesion characterized by asymmetry, notched or scalloped borders, and variegation in shades of brown. The stereotypical expression histopathologically of melanoma on all anatomic sites is a neoplasm that is asymmetrical, poorly circumscribed, and characterized further by nests of melanocytes within the epidermis that are not equidistant from one another, vary in size and shape, and have become confluent in foci, the result of the confluence sometimes being formation of aggregations with peculiar geometric shapes. Melanocytes disposed as solitary units within the epidermis predominate over nests in some high-power fields. Some solitary melanocytes and nests of melanocytes are present well above the dermoepidermal junction, at times including the upper reaches of the epidermis, even the cornified layer. Findings like those in the epidermis are present far down epithelial structures of adnexa. Within the dermis, nests of melanocytes do not become smaller with progressive descent, and nuclei of melanocytes do not become smaller either. Nests of melanocytes within the dermis also vary in size and shape and have become confluent in foci, sometimes forming aggregations with bizarre geometric outlines and sheets of cells. The base of the neoplasm is uneven. Melanin is sometimes more plentiful at the base than at the surface of the neoplasm. Last, nuclei of melanocytes are atypical; some neoplastic melanocytes within the dermis are in mitosis, and some neoplastic melanocytes may be necrotic. These criteria, in constellation, serve to enable a morphologist to distinguish melanoma from nevi of all kinds. Moreover, the criteria for melanoma, clinically and histopathologically, are the same on all anatomic sites. Parenthetically, those criteria are the very opposite of those of melanocytic nevi.

Time was when proponents of the current "histogenetic classification" of melanoma contended that lentigo maligna melanoma had a better prognosis than other types of melanoma. The assertion has been withdrawn even by advocates of that classification. There are, however, some differences, in general, in behavior of melanoma according to anatomic site. For example, when thicknesses are matched, melanomas of the scalp and genitalia have a poorer prognosis than melanomas on a breast or an upper extremity. Nevertheless, the prognosis for primary cutaneous melanoma in a particular individual cannot be gauged with confidence on the basis of any single criterion, such as thickness, levels, anatomic site, sex, and age of patient, or on the basis of any combination of those criteria. Attemps to gauge prognosis of melanoma accurately are akin to divination.

It is not yet known what factors determine capability of a melanoma to metastasize. Some very thin melanomas—less than 0.4 mm in thickness, for example—are known to have metastasized, whereas some very thick melanomas—more than 4.0 mm in thickness, for example—seem not to have metastasized prior to complete excision. When, at last, it is learned what factors are responsible for metastasis of melanoma, among them the immunologic status of the person who bears the melanoma, the measuring sticks used currently, such as thickness, will seem woefully inadequate.

The vast majority of melanomas in the world, including those that begin in Africans and Asians, as well as in Caucasians, develop de novo. Virtually all of them in Asians and Africans arise de novo and tend to be situated on a palm or sole, an indication of the importance of genetic factors in the development of melanoma. Approximately 20 percent of melanomas in Caucasians develop in association with a preexisting nevus, but hardly ever in Asians and Africans.

The type of nevus with which melanoma is most closely associated is Clark's (dysplastic) nevus. In that circumstance, the melanoma almost always begins at the periphery of the nevus and evolves in the very same way as does a melanoma that arises de novo. A melanoma may develop rarely in conjunction with another type of melanocytic nevus, such as that of Unna or Miescher, or sometimes in congenital nevi of different sizes, and not necessarily at the periphery, but, as a rule, the melanocytes of the nevus do not "convert" or "transform" into those of melanoma. An exception is melanoma that originates in the substance of a very large congenital melanocytic nevus, such as the one designated pilar neurocristic hamartoma.

THERAPY Surgical excision with margins sufficient to remove the neoplasm completely is the treatment for primary cutaneous melanoma. Lymph node dissection is indicated when lymph nodes are suspected of harboring metastases of melanoma. Prophylactic lymph node dissection, although not yet abandoned completely, does not enhance survival. Chemotherapy, interferon, vaccination, and gene therapy are experimental methods for advanced metastatic disease, and benefit has yet to be demonstrated with consistency. The same can be stated for the technique of "sentinel-node biopsy." In short, there is no consistently effective treatment available for metastatic melanoma.

Wide and deep excision of primary melanoma is not indicated and never has been; the purpose of surgery is to extirpate the primary melanoma in its entirety.

The most important rule for management of primary melanoma is detection and identification of it at a stage when it is still curable with certainty by simple excision, that is, when it is flat clinically and in situ histopathologically.

DEFINITION Pigmented macules and patches mostly in the middle third of the face, vertically and horizontally, distributed symmetrically and occurring mainly in postpubescent women as a consequence of the combined effects of estrogen and ultraviolet light on melanocytes.

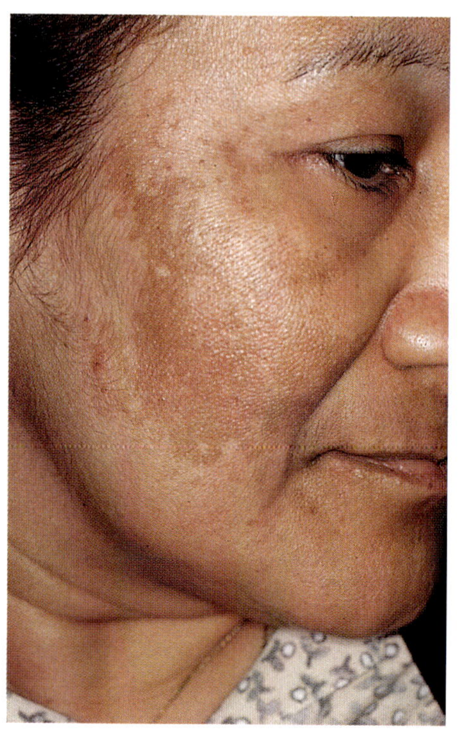

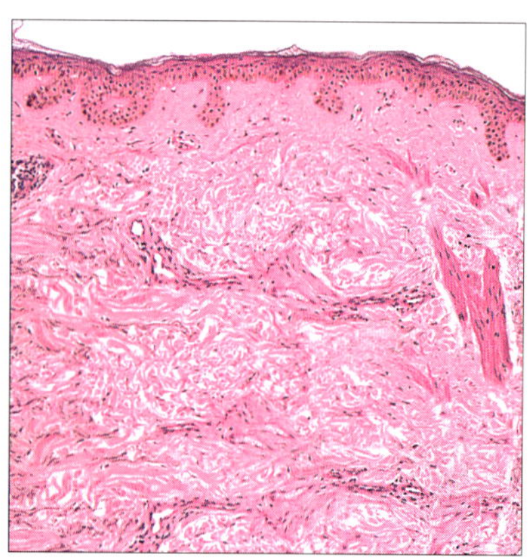

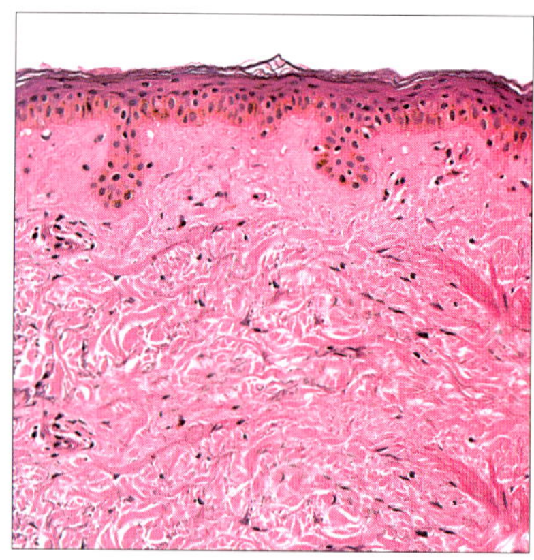

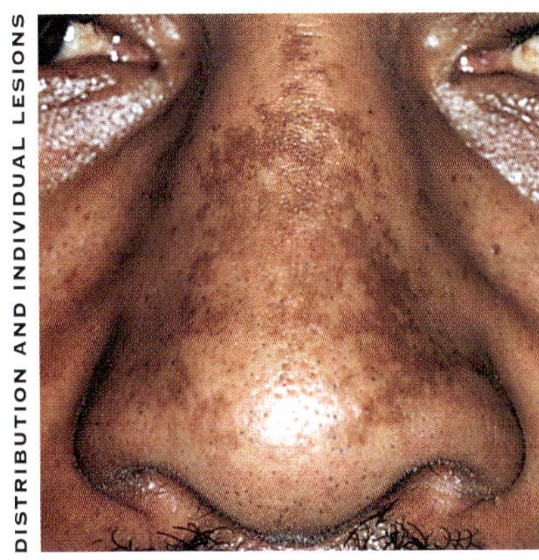

FIG. 57-1 *Mottled pigmentation.*

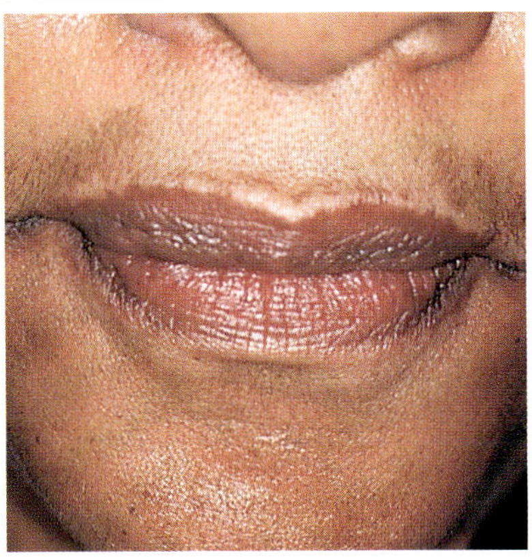

FIG. 57-2 *Pigmented patches in symmetrical distribution.*

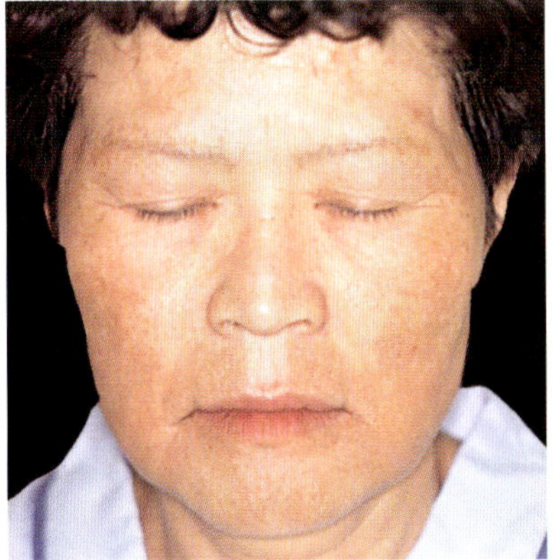

FIG. 57-3 *Pigmented patches.*

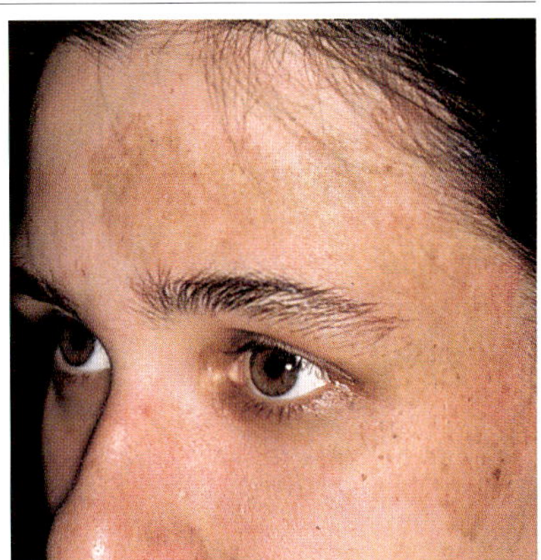

FIG. 57-4 *Pigmented patches.*

COURSE The pigmented macules and patches of melasma that appear during the first trimester of pregnancy disappear within a very short time after parturition. By contrast, the melasma that develops secondary to the effects of birth control pills does not leave soon after that hormone has been discontinued; it often persists for years. The melasma that makes itself known in middle-aged women also tends to last for the rest of a lifetime. During the course of pregnancy and while birth control pills are being taken, the lesions of melasma darken progressively.

INTEGRATION: UNIFYING CONCEPT Melasma results from the effects of estrogen coupled with ultraviolet light on melanocytes. Although there is no increased number of epidermal melanocytes in a lesion of melasma, the amount of melanin made by melanocytes—especially those melanocytes situated in the middle third of the face and forehead—increases markedly. The findings of melasma histopathologically are those of epidermal hyperpigmentation.

THERAPY Chemicals and medications that combine with ultraviolet light to induce the condition should not be used again. Broad-spectrum sun screens, topical hydroquinone preparations, retinoic acid, azelaic acid (which inhibits tyrosinase), chemical peels (trichloroacetic acid, alpha-hydroxy acids), and laser surgery are beneficial.

DEFINITION A hyperplasia of infundibular epithelium consequent to the effects of infection by a pox virus and manifesting itself clinically as one or more skin-colored, smooth-surfaced, dome-shaped papules, each with a central umbilication filled with horny material.

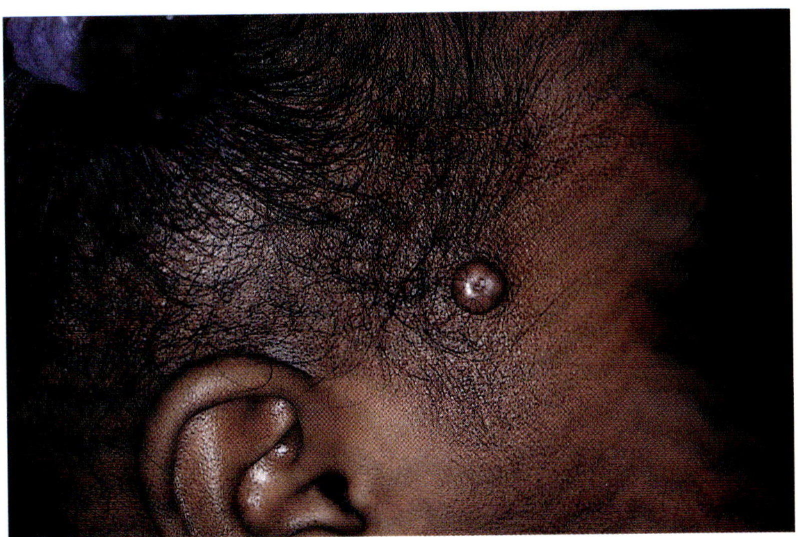

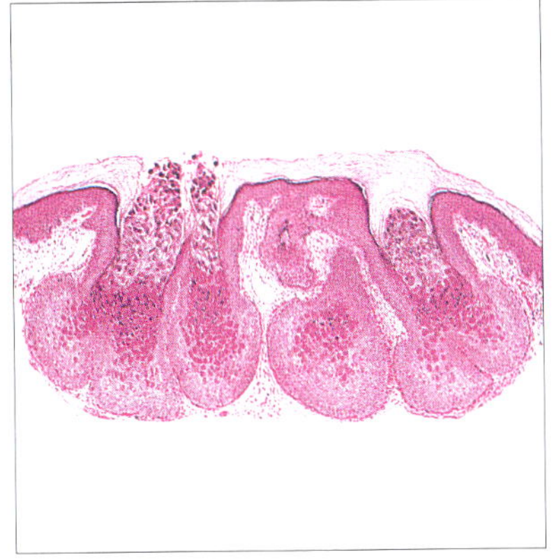

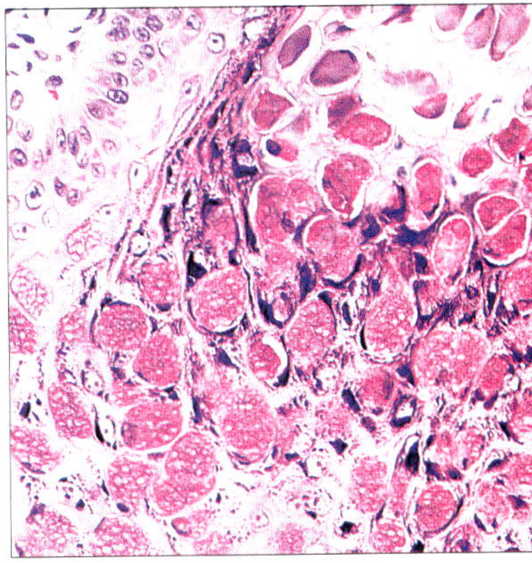

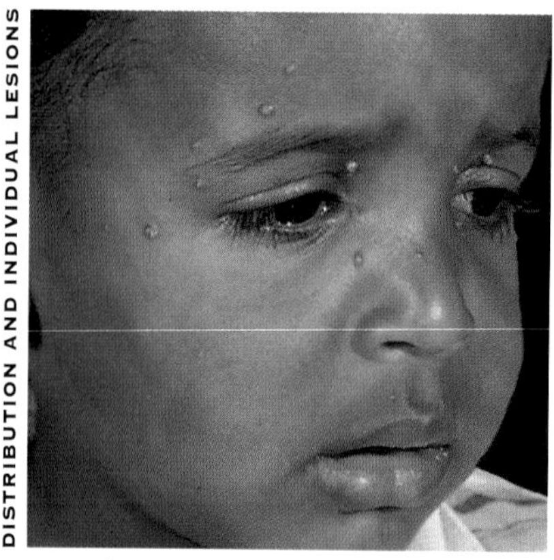

FIG. 58-1 *Umbilicated papules.*

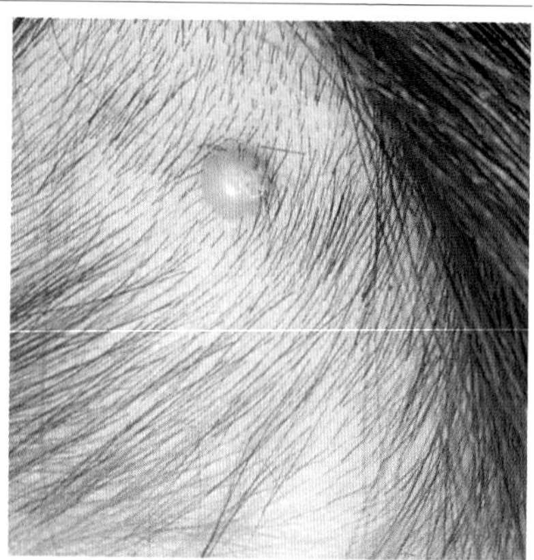

FIG. 58-2 *Papule with horny material in its center.*

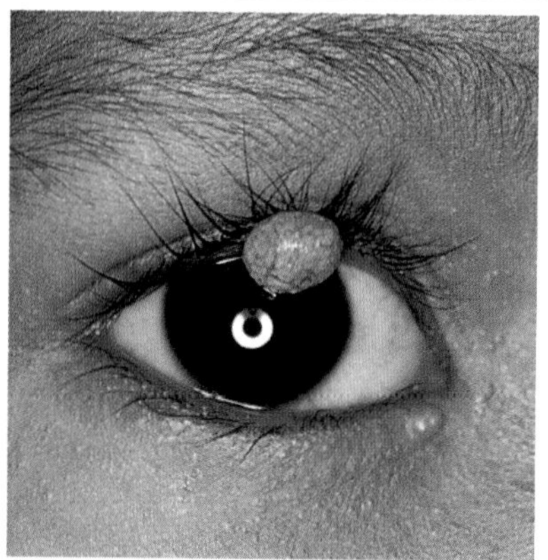

FIG. 58-3 *Papules of different sizes.*

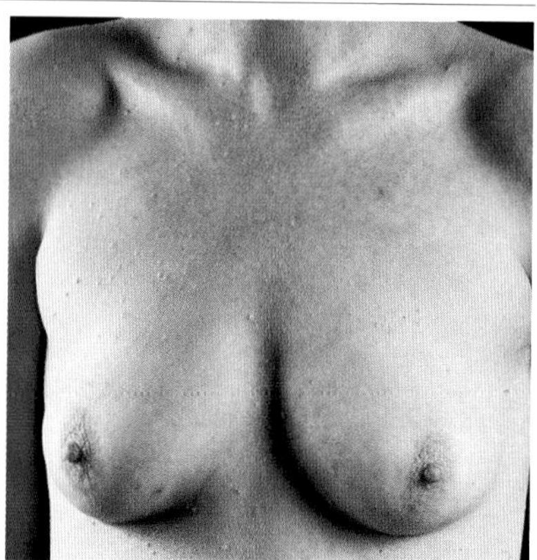

FIG. 58-4 *Widespread tiny papules.*

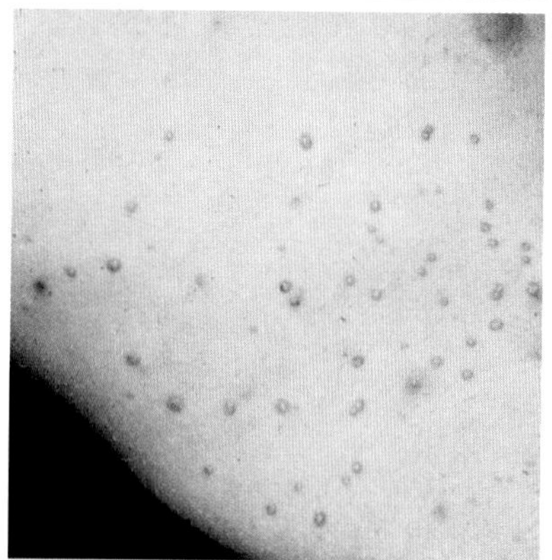

FIG. 58-5 *Widespread papules.*

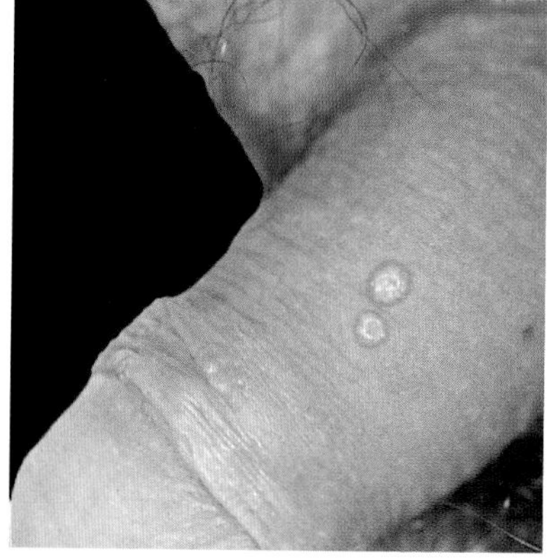

FIG. 58-6 *Umbilicated papules with horny material in their center.*

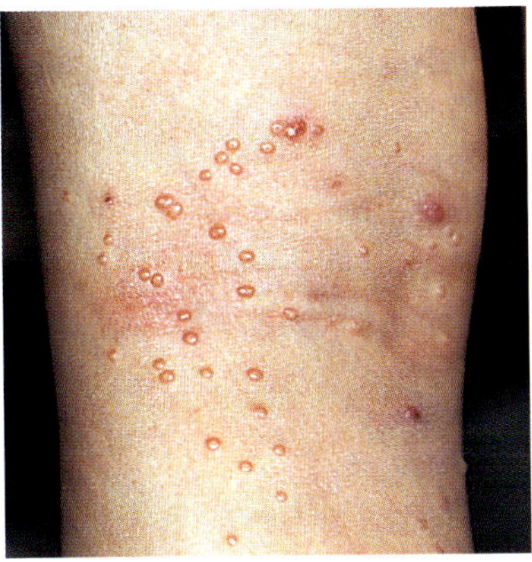

FIG. 58-7 *Numerous papules, some of them inflamed secondary to rupture of a crater, in a person with atopic dermatitis.*

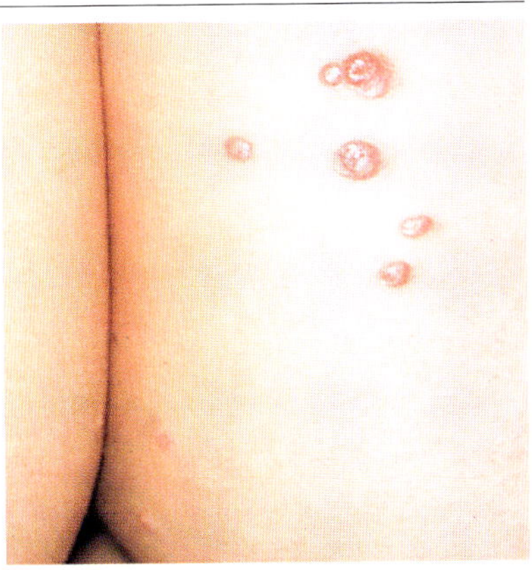

FIG. 58-8 *Smooth-surfaced, dome-shaped papules, some of them umbilicated.*

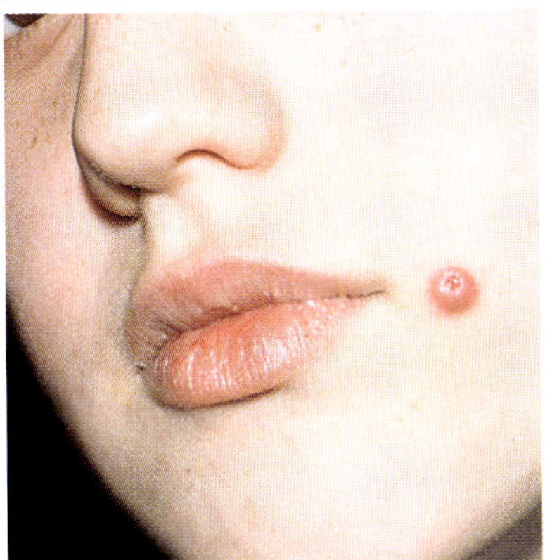

FIG. 58-9 *Umbilicated dome-shaped papule.*

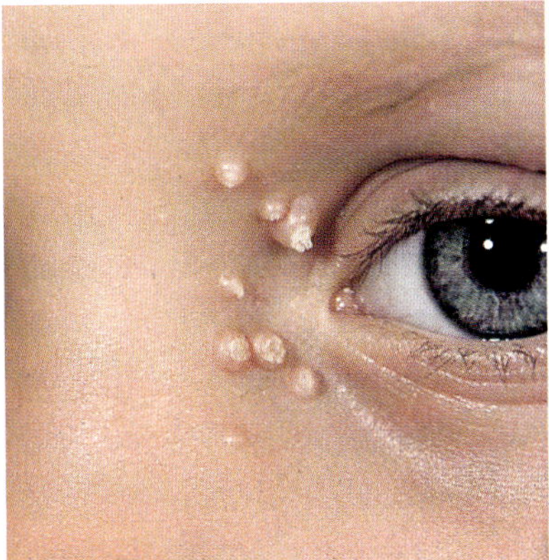

FIG. 58-10 *Warty papules, with a central keratotic plug, arranged in a cluster.*

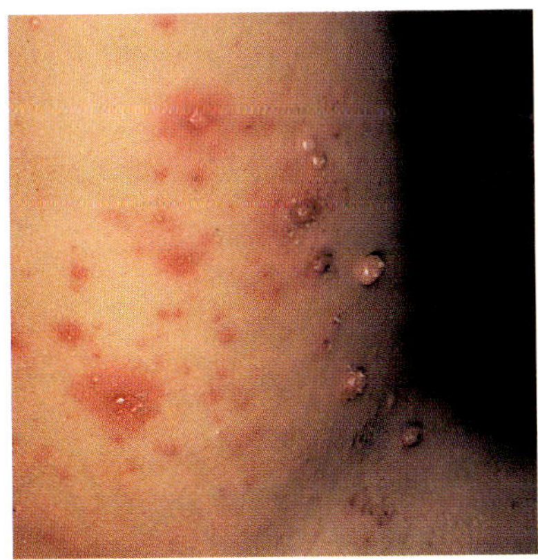

FIG. 58-11 *Erythematous zones around some papules, a sign that horny material from dilated infundibula has been extruded.*

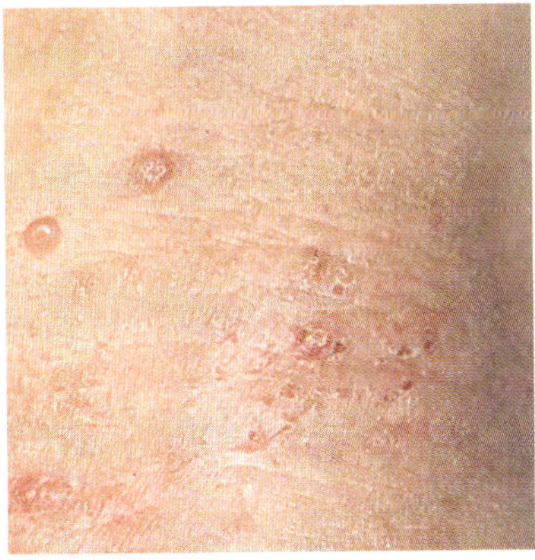

FIG. 58-12 *Umbilicated papules in a zone of lichen simplex chronicus in a patient who is atopic.*

COURSE Lesions of molluscum contagiosum tend to be umbilicated papules that, over the course of months, involute and disappear in much the same manner as verruca vulgaris, the latter being caused by a papillomavirus rather than a pox virus. The lesions of molluscum contagiosum may last for years if a person is immunosuppressed.

INTEGRATION: UNIFYING CONCEPT Molluscum contagiosum is caused by a pox virus that has a predilection for infundibular epithelium. For that reason the lesion is crateriform clinically, the crater being made up of contiguous widely-dilated infundibula that are chock-full of corneocytes. Nearly all of those epithelial cells, including corneocytes, contain within them large packets of virus called molluscum bodies. Those bodies are evidences histopathologically of millions of virions that have proliferated in the cytoplasm of affected epithelial cells, which, as a consequence of maturation, have become corneocytes. By microscopy it is apparent that only epithelium is infected by the virus of molluscum contagiosum and the upper part of follicular epithelium in particular, to wit, the infundibulum. It is rare for molluscum contagiosum to appear on non-hair-bearing skin, such as a palm or sole.

It is the clinical similarity of solitary keratoacanthoma, a type of squamous-cell carcinoma that is crateriform and emanates from infundibular keratinocytes, to molluscum contagiosum, a hyperplasia that is crateriform and consists of infundibular keratinocytes, that prompted the old designation "molluscum sebaceum" for keratoacanthoma.

THERAPY Removal of papules by curettage or cryotherapy.

DEFINITION An inflammatory process in which lesions may erupt (pityriasis lichenoides et varioliformis acuta) and evolve rapidly from erythematous macules and papules to become purpuric papules, papulovesicles that may be hemorrhagic, ulcers, eschars, and, eventually, scars. Alternatively, the macules may evolve more slowly (pityriasis lichenoides chronica) to become scaly papules. In some patients, rapidly developing and slowly evolving lesions may be present concurrently, e.g., purpuric papules and scaly papules may coexist.

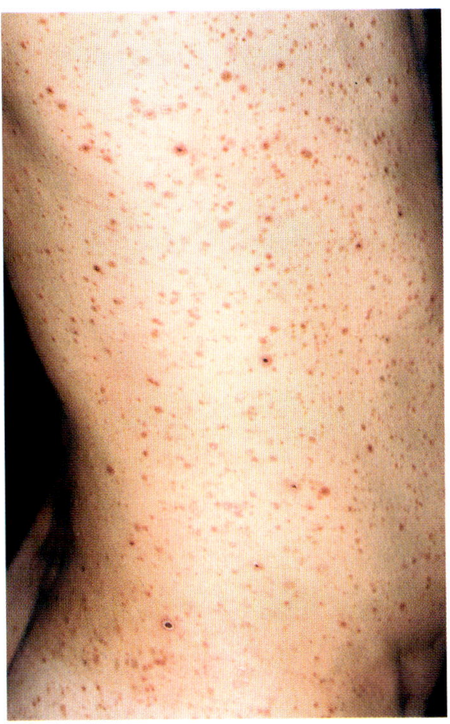

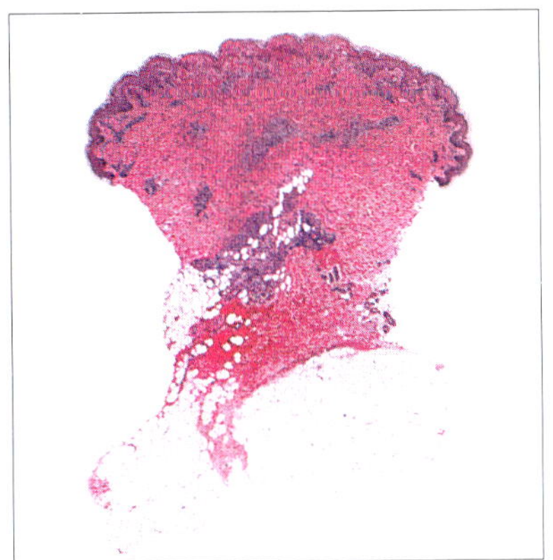

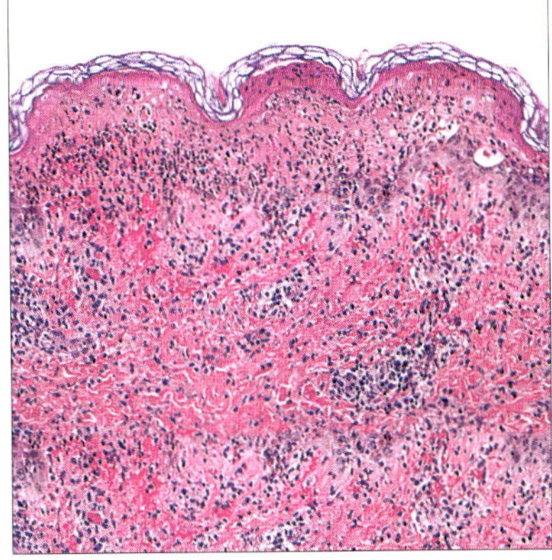

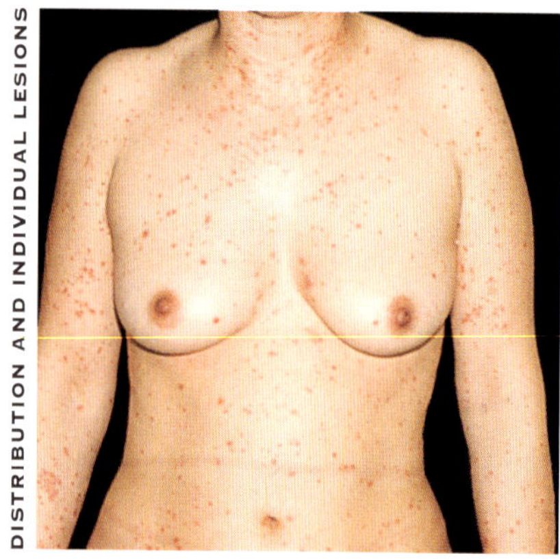

FIG. 59-1 *Widespread purpuric papules.*

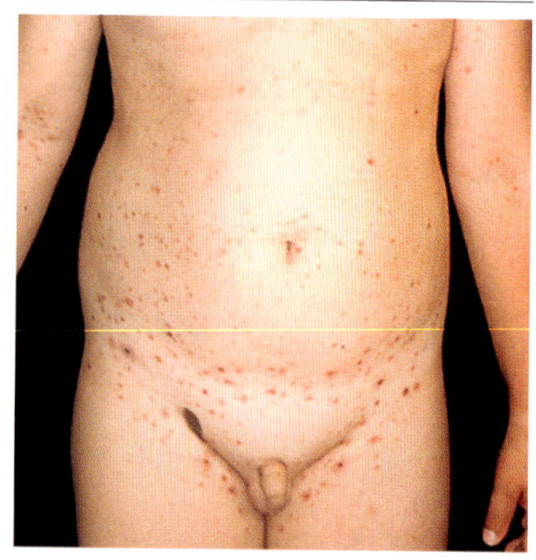

FIG. 59-2 *Widespread purpuric papules.*

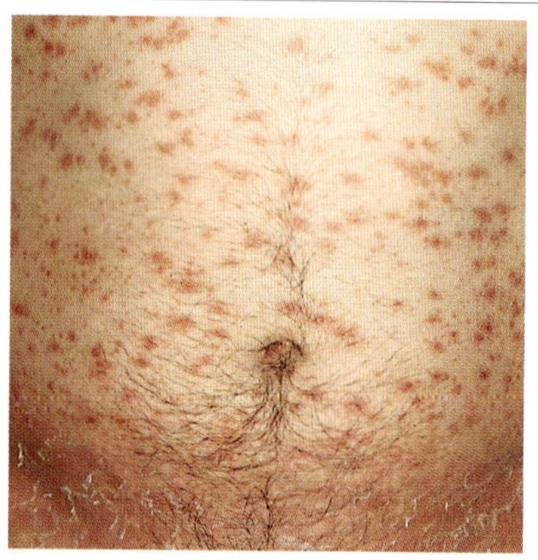

FIG. 59-3 *Purpuric papules, some covered by hemorrhagic crusts.*

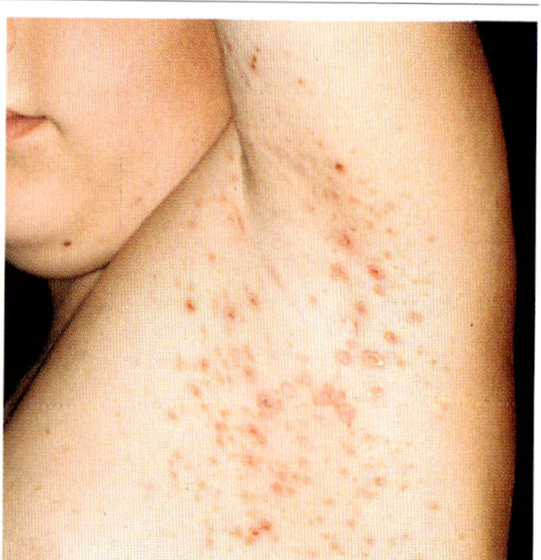

FIG. 59-4 *Discrete papules.*

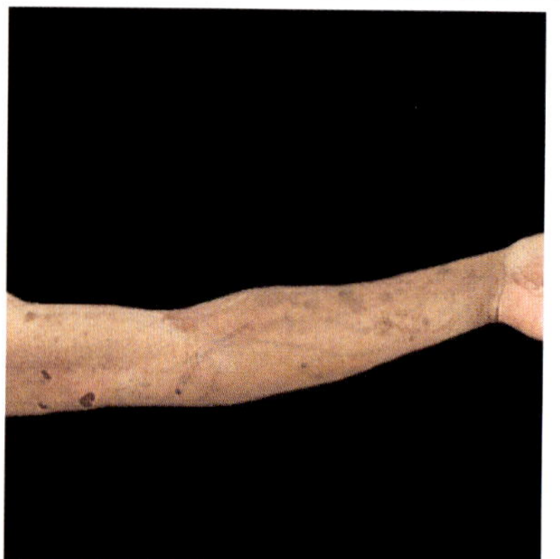

FIG. 59-5 *Discrete purpuric papules, one of them covered by a hemorrhagic crust.*

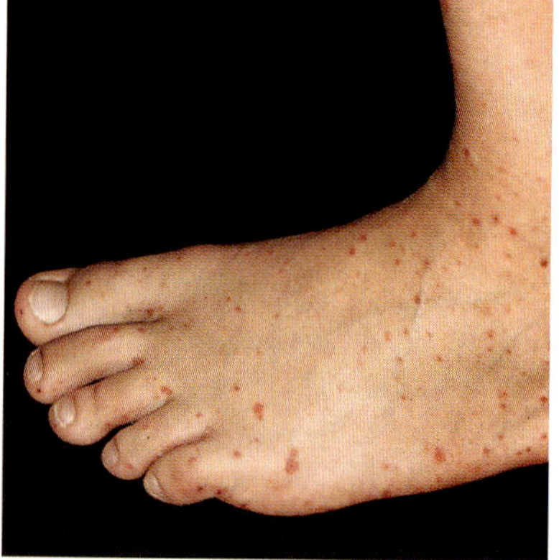

FIG. 59-6 *Purpuric papules.*

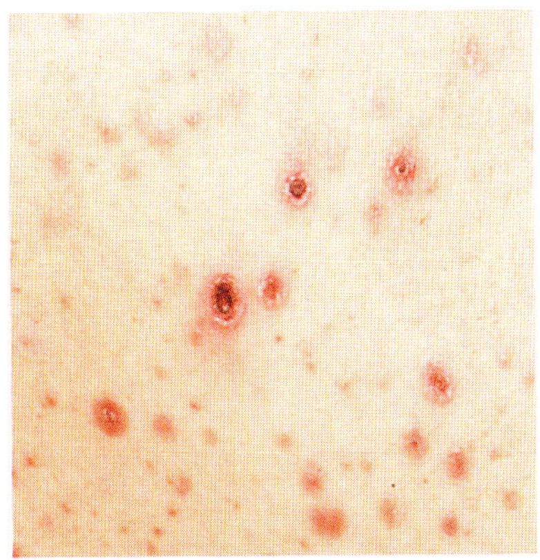

FIG. 59-7 *Smooth-surfaced erythematous papules, scaly papules, and hemorrhagic crusted papules.*

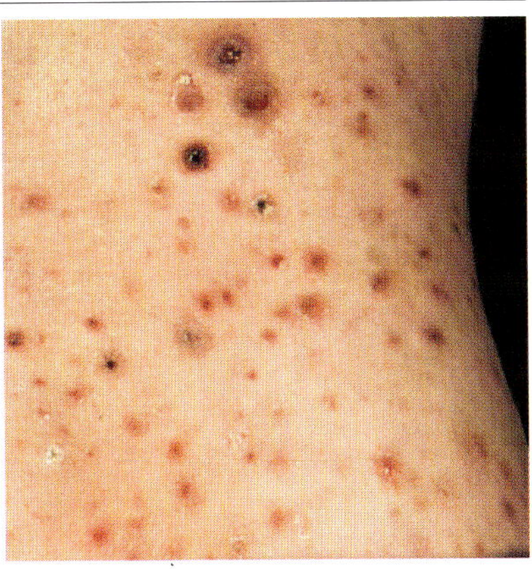

FIG. 59-8 *Erythematous papules, purpuric papules, scaly and crusted papules, and scale-crusts.*

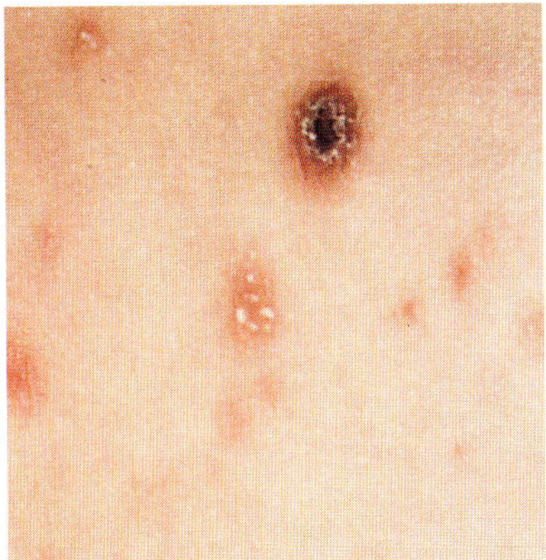

FIG. 59-9 *Smooth-surfaced, scaly, and crusted papules.*

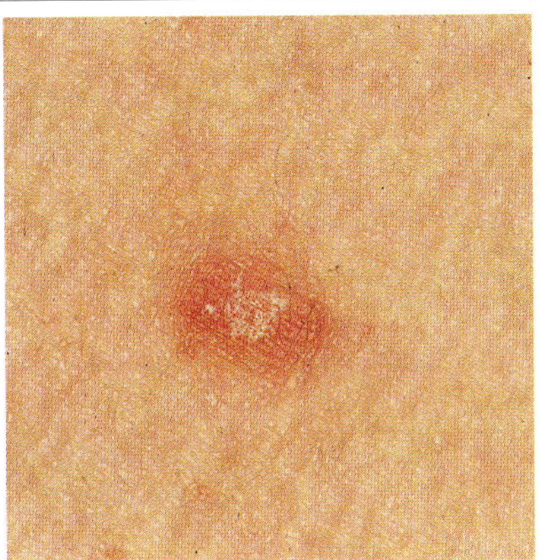

FIG. 59-10 *Scaly papule.*

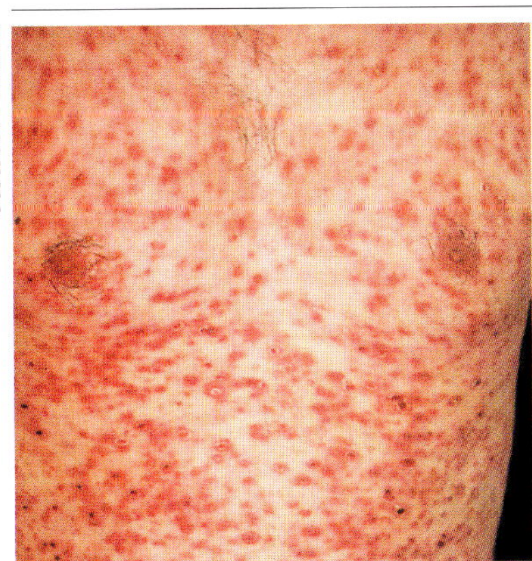

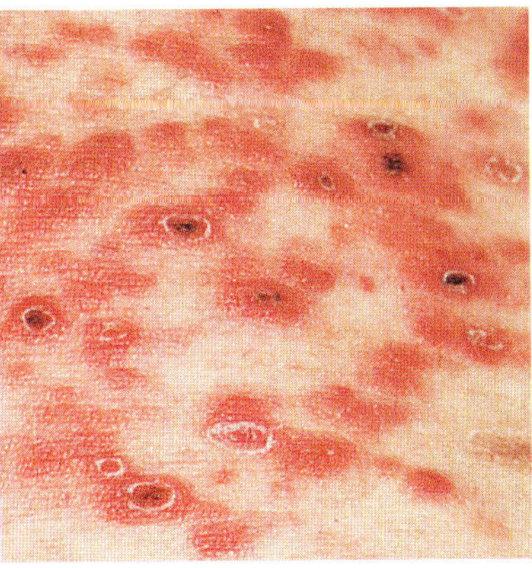

FIG. 59-11 (A, B) *Innumerable widespread purpuric papules, many ulcerated and covered by hemorrhagic crusts, of pityriasis lichenoides acuta.*

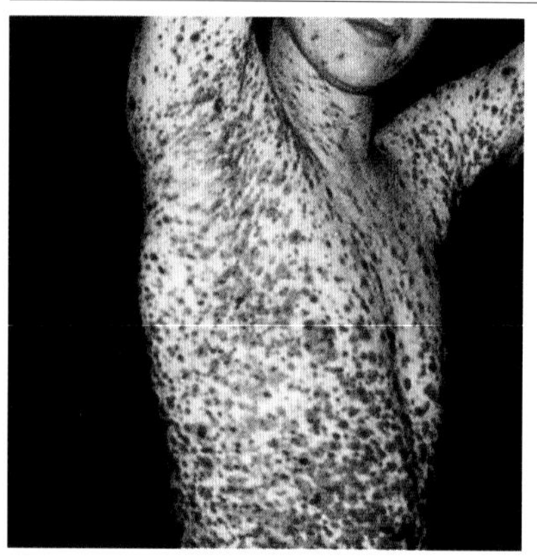

FIG. 59-12 *Hemorrhagic macules, patches, and papules, many ulcerated and covered by hemorrhagic crusts ("fulminant").*

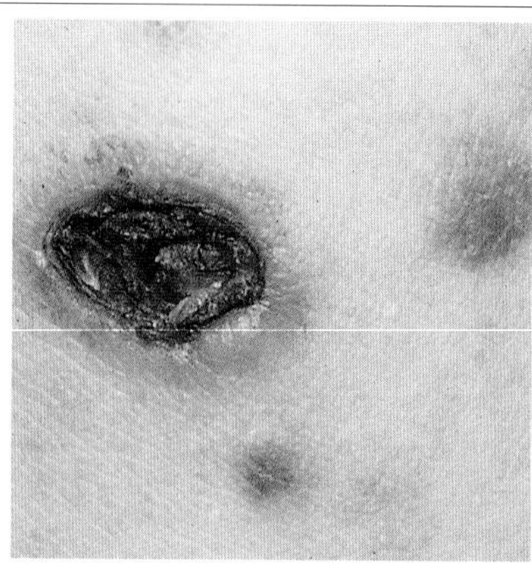

FIG. 59-13 *Smooth-surfaced papules and an ulcerated papule covered by an eschar of pityriasis lichenoides acuta.*

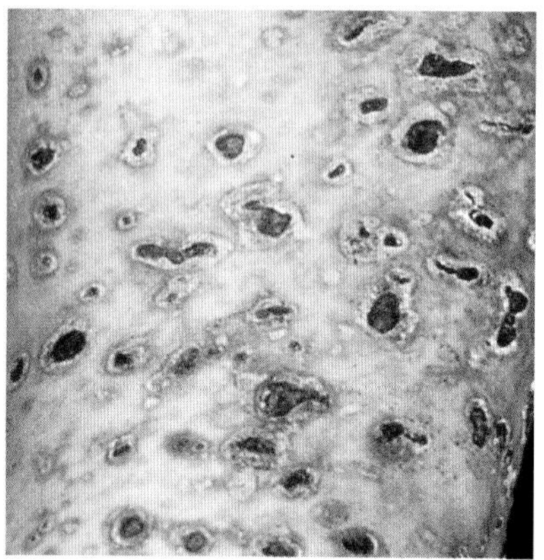

FIG. 59-14 *Ulcers, eschars, and scars of pityriasis lichenoides acuta.*

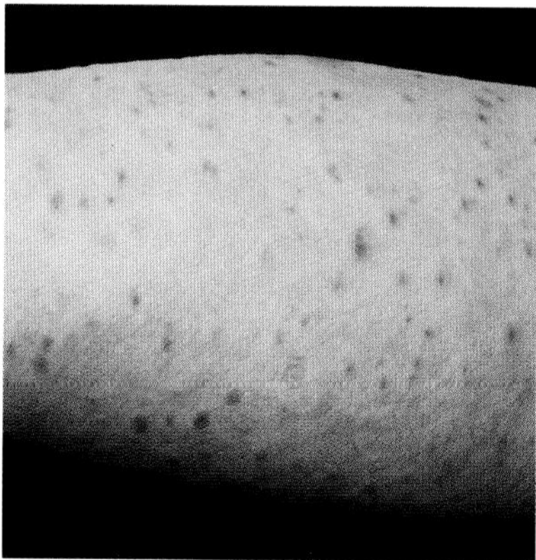

FIG. 59-15 *Discrete papules of pityriasis lichenoides chronica.*

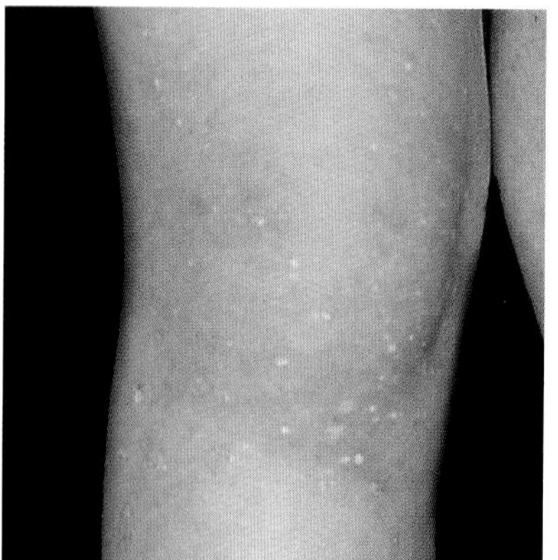

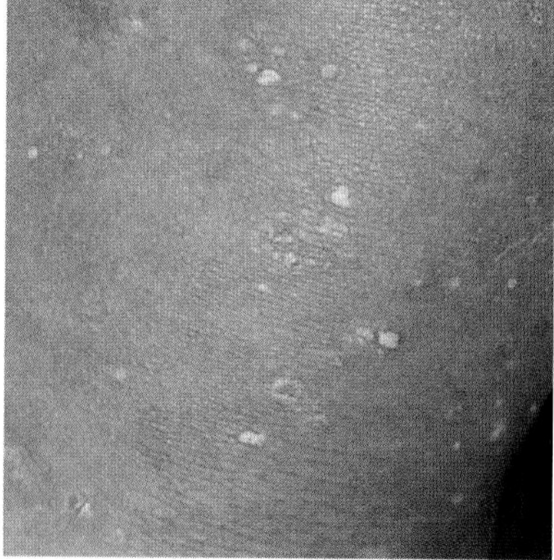

FIG. 59-16 (A, B) *Many papules covered by chalk-white scales of pityriasis lichenoides chronica.*

COURSE Lesions of Mucha-Habermann disease evolve in two very different ways, namely, as an efflorescence and at a petty pace. The former (acuta) begins as pink macules that quickly become reddish papules. They tend to transform rapidly into papulovesicles, which become necrotic and ulcerate to form eschars that heal with scars. Sometimes the process is so fulminant that hemorrhagic vesicles, and even hemorrhagic bullae, monopolize.

The expression of Mucha-Habermann disease characterized by rapid development of lesions that often culminate in vesicles is known formally as "pityriasis lichenoides et varioliformis acuta." An exaggeration of the process results in "fulminant" Mucha-Habermann disease with widespread hemorrhagic blisters that ulcerate deeply and become covered by an eschar. Patients with this severely necrotizing form of the disease may die of it.

In contrast, slowly evolving lesions of Mucha-Habermann disease (chronica) begin as pink macules that progress very slowly into redder papules that become scaly. In time they progress to scaly brown papules that, after many months, become hyperpigmented macules. The slowly evolving expression of Mucha-Habermann disease is known as "pityriasis lichenoides chronica."

In short, rapidly-evolving lesions of Mucha-Habermann disease can become vesicles within days, eschars within a few weeks, and scars thereafter. Slowly evolving lesions of Mucha-Habermann disease play out their lives as scaly papules over many months and sometimes years. The disease itself is unpredictable in terms of longevity; its acute expression is sometimes finished in weeks, whereas its chronic manifestation sometimes sputters for years.

INTEGRATION: UNIFYING CONCEPT Clinically and histopathologically, Mucha-Habermann disease is a single distinctive pathologic process. It is not unique in being associated with lesions that may be accelerated to become blisters or decelerated to remain scaly papules. The same is true of lichen planus, which may become vesicular (bullous lichen planus) or be scaly papules, of psoriasis, which may become pustular (pustular psoriasis) or be scaly papules or plaques, and of lupus erythematosus (lupus dermatitis), which may be bullous (bullous lupus erythematosus) or simply scaly papules and plaques.

Papules of pityriasis lichenoides acuta are characterized histopathologically by a wedge-shaped, superficial and deep, perivascular infiltrate of lymphocytes, and by lymphocytes scattered along the dermoepidermal junction in association with vacuolar alteration. Individual necrotic keratinocytes are present throughout an epidermis that displays ballooning and spongiosis. Parakeratosis that may house neutrophils is also present. If extravasated erythrocytes are numerous, the lesions will be purpuric. If ballooning and spongiosis eventuate in vesiculation, a papulovesicle is the result. When epidermal necrosis is extensive and ulceration supervenes, an eschar comes into being. If ulceration is deep enough, a scar results.

Pityriasis lichenoides chronica is typified histopathologically by a superficial perivascular infiltrate of lymphocytes, lymphocytes in association with vacuolar alteration along the dermoepidermal junction, only a few necrotic keratinocytes within the epidermis, just a hint, if that, of ballooning and spongiosis, and subtle mounds of parakeratosis. The lesions of this scaly clinical presentation never progress to vesiculation, ulceration, eschars, or scars.

Not surprisingly, some patients with pityriasis lichenoides show acute and chronic lesions concurrently. The fulminant expression of the process is simply a caricature of pityriasis lichenoides acuta.

Despite some similarities in the clinical appearance between Mucha-Habermann disease and lymphomatoid papulosis, the two are unrelated. Mucha-Habermann disease is an inflammatory process, whereas lymphomatoid papulosis is a lymphoma.

THERAPY Oral erythromycin or tetracyclines, as well as PUVA, are indicated for the acute form, and methotrexate for fulminant examples.

DEFINITION A systemic lymphoma of T-lymphocytes that manifests itself first in the skin as macules and then patches that often are scaly. Most people with the disease have only scaly macules and patches for a lifetime, but some patients may develop papules, plaques, nodules, tumors, and ulcerated tumors. As a rule, only those with extensive nodular and tumorous lesions die of the systemic effects of the disease.

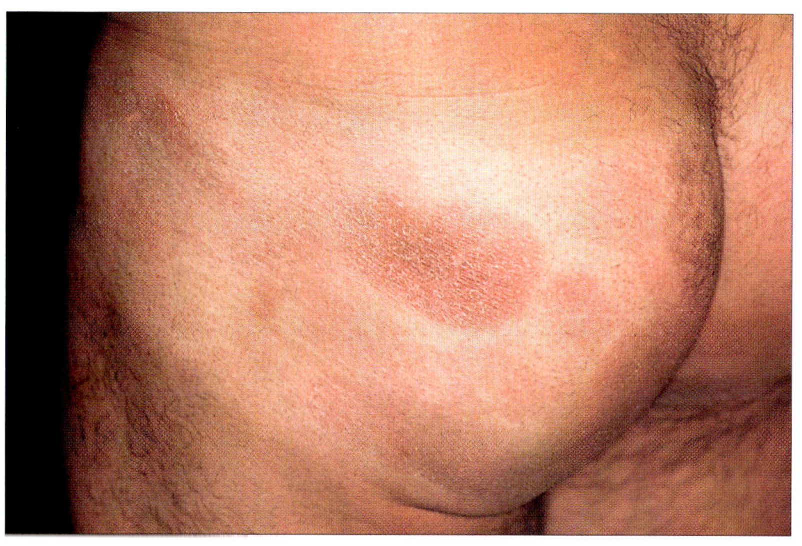

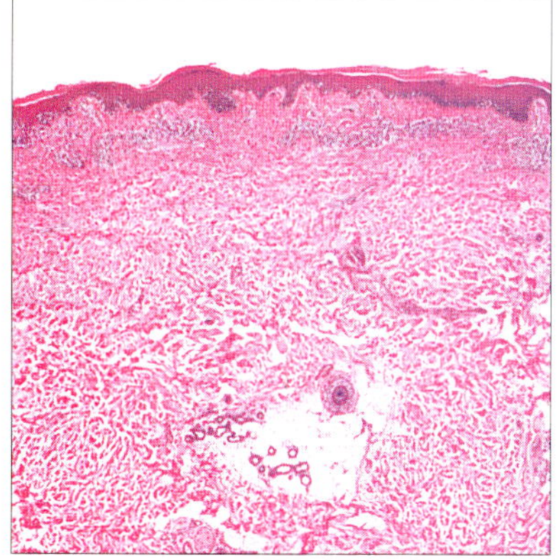

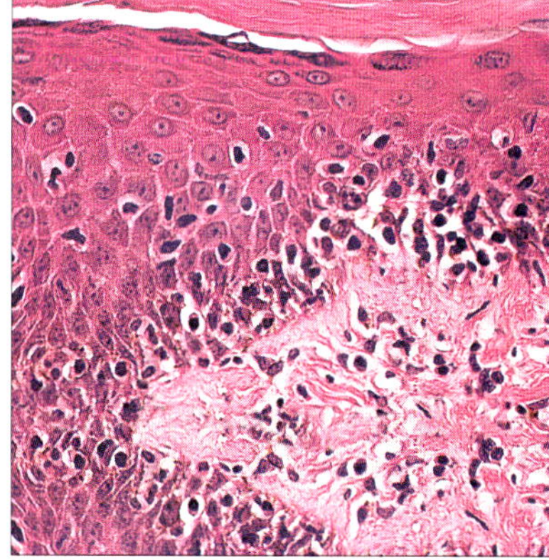

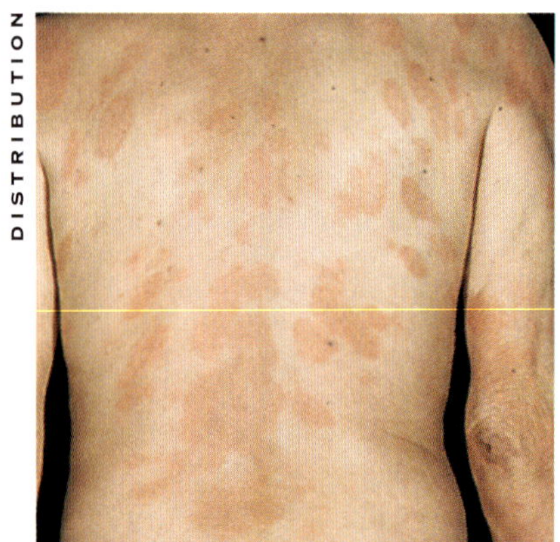

FIG. 60-1 *Widespread macules, patches, and subtle plaques.*

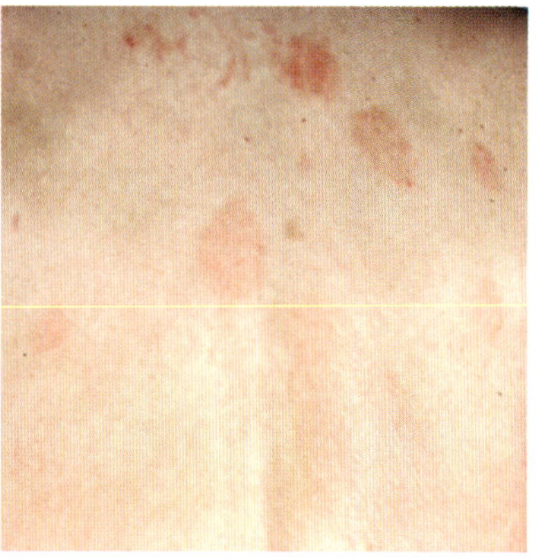

FIG. 60-2 *Patches and plaques.*

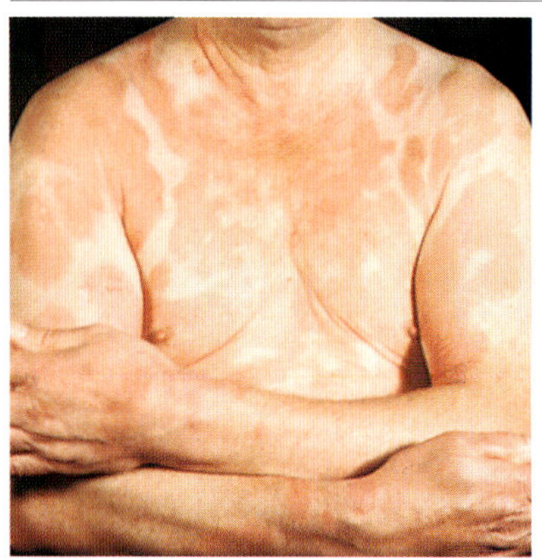

FIG. 60-3 *Patches and plaques.*

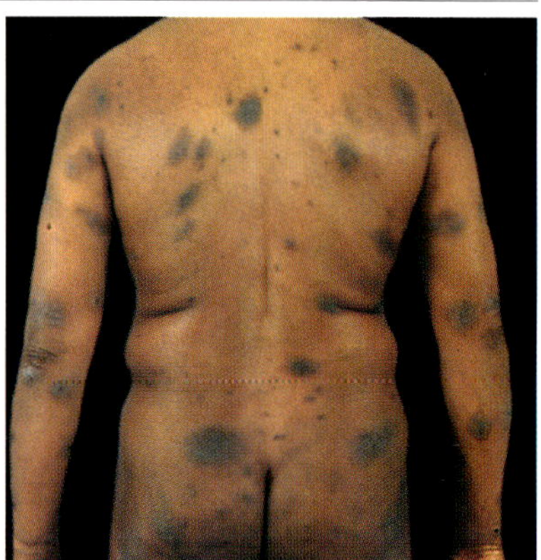

FIG. 60-4 *Hyperpigmented plaques.*

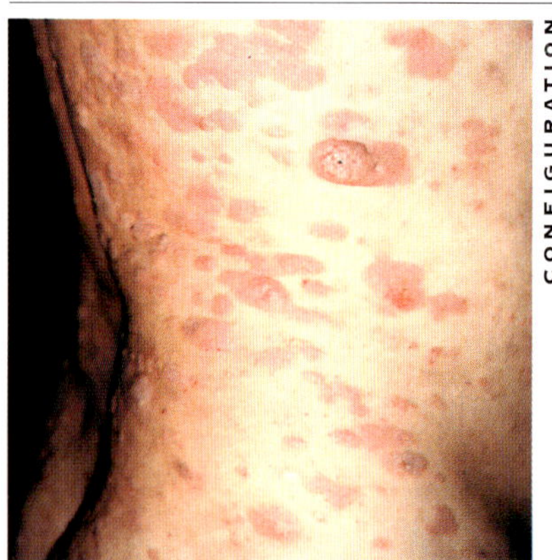

FIG. 60-5 *Widespread elongated plaques reminiscent of "digitate dermatosis," which is mostly patches; a single process.*

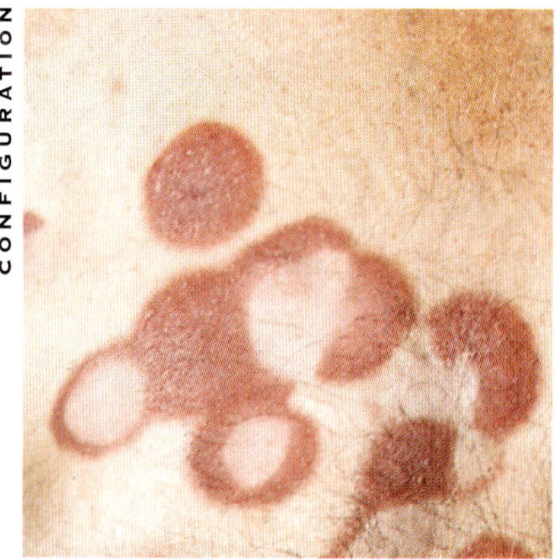

FIG. 60-6 *Bizarre geometric shapes of plaques—serpiginous, arcuate, and annular.*

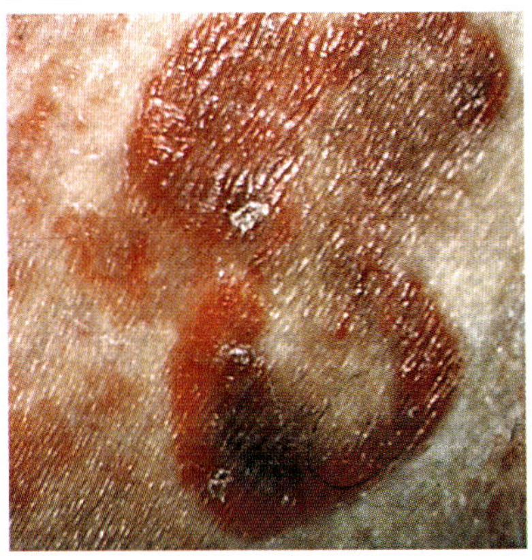

FIG. 60-7 *Peculiar geometric shapes of plaques.*

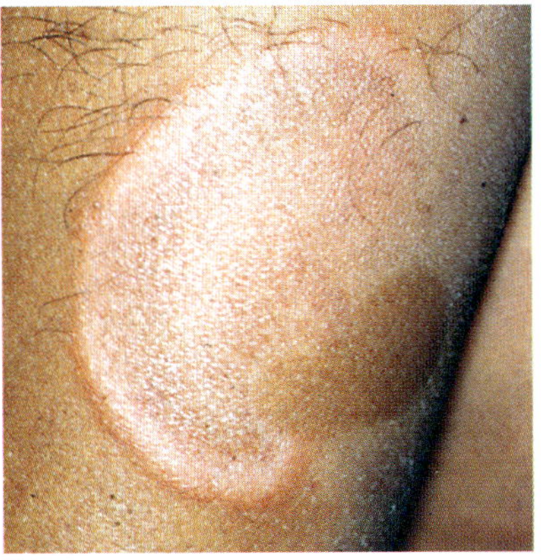

FIG. 60-8 *Arciform scaly plaque with hyperpigmented patch.*

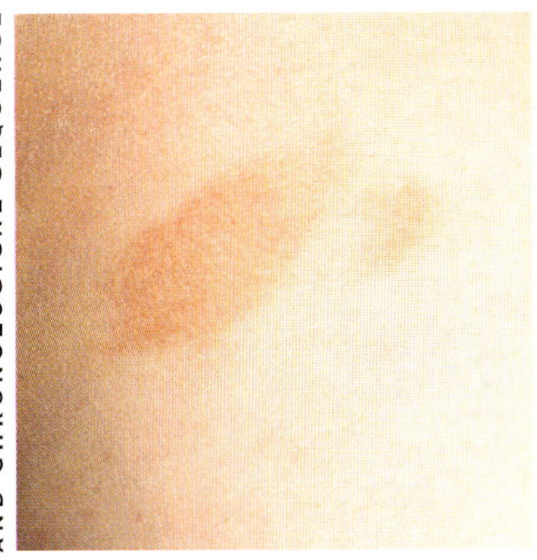

FIG. 60-9 *Slightly scaly patches.*

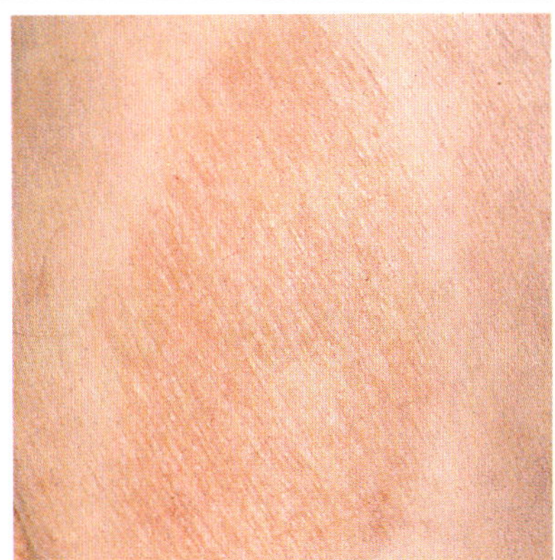

FIG. 60-10 *Slightly scaly patch.*

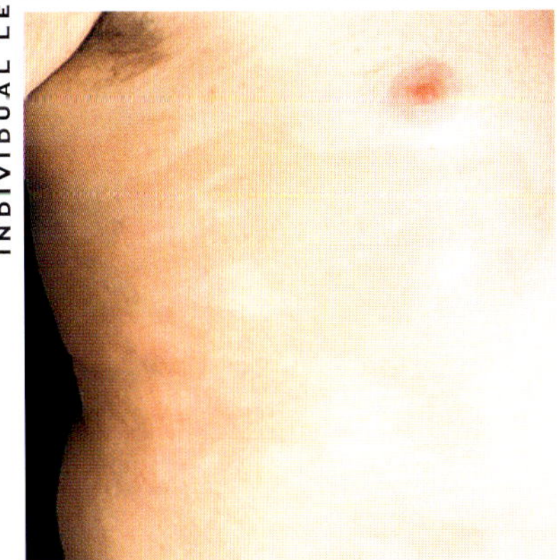

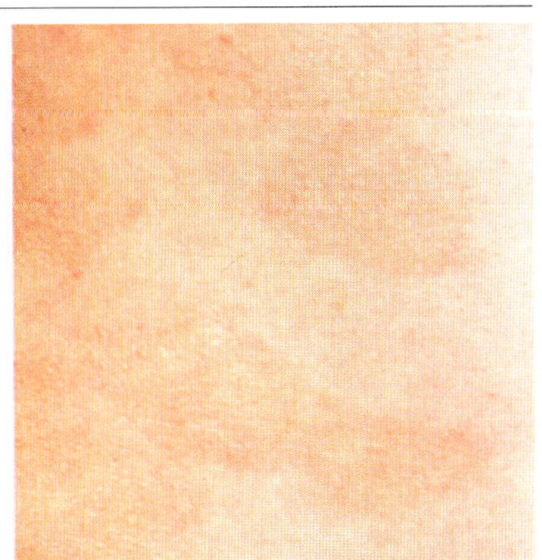

FIG. 60-11 (A, B) *Patches with delicate scale.*

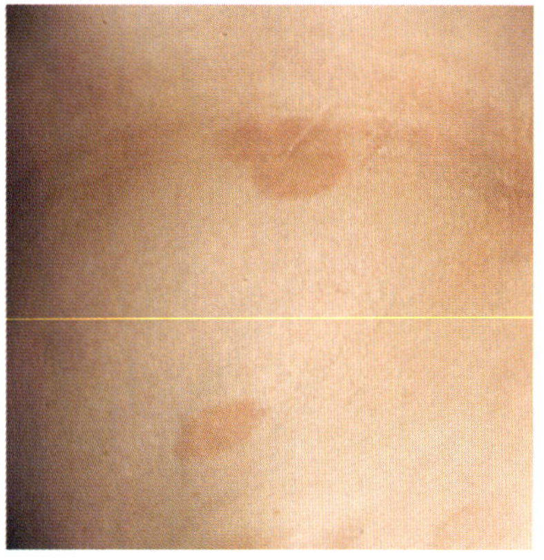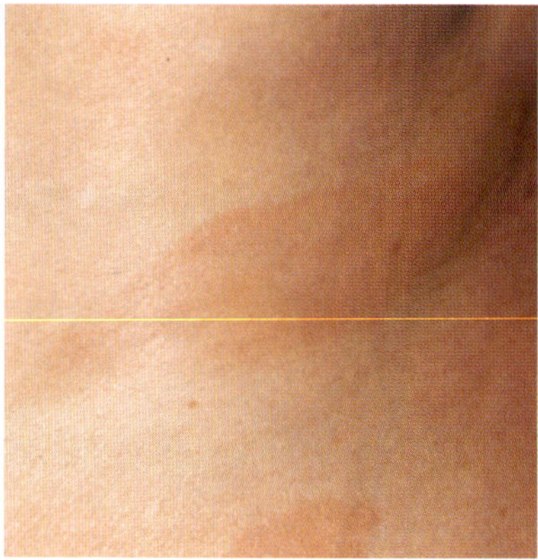

FIG. 60-12 (A, B) *Patches with delicate scale.*

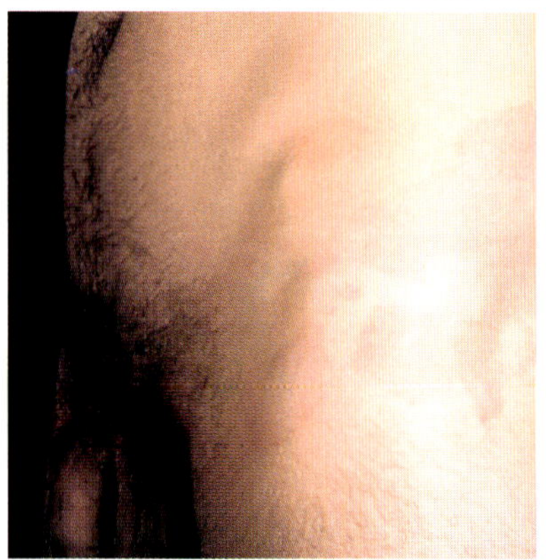

FIG. 60-13 *Patches and incipient plaques.*

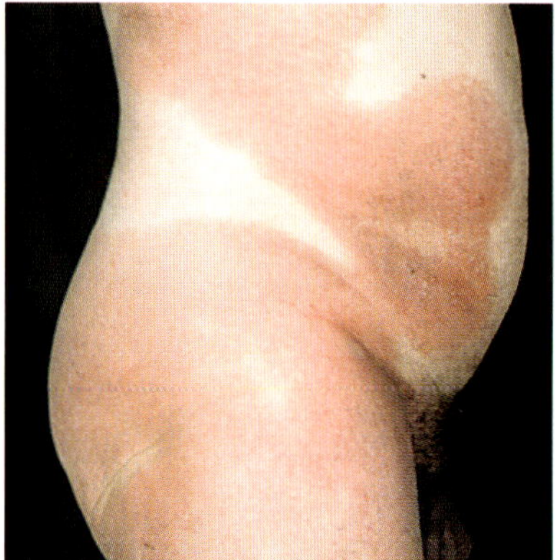

FIG. 60-14 *Patches and plaques.*

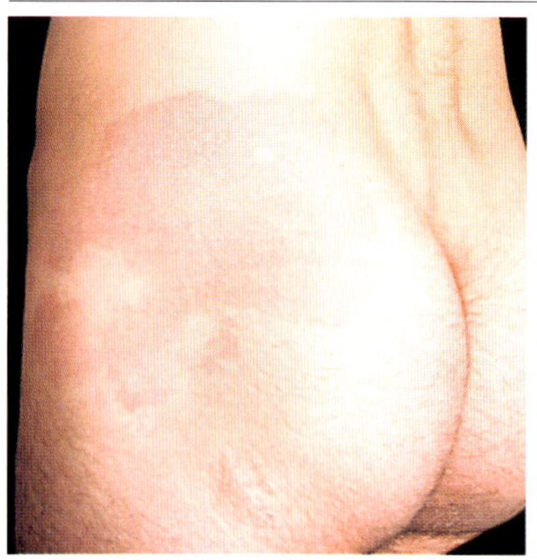

FIG. 60-15 *Plaques. The buttocks are a favorite site for patches and plaques of mycosis fungoides.*

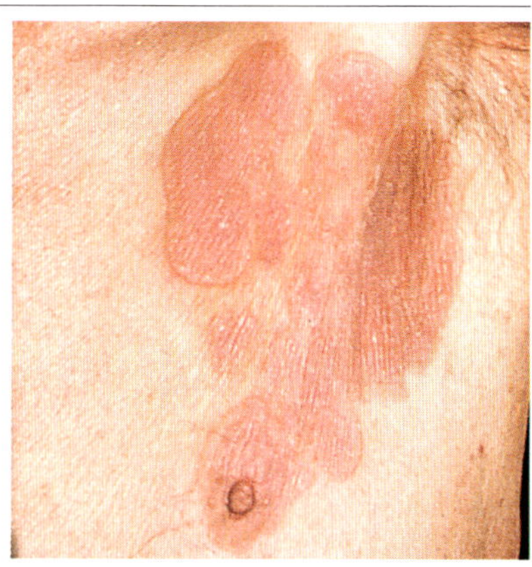

FIG. 60-16 *Plaques, one of which involves the areola.*

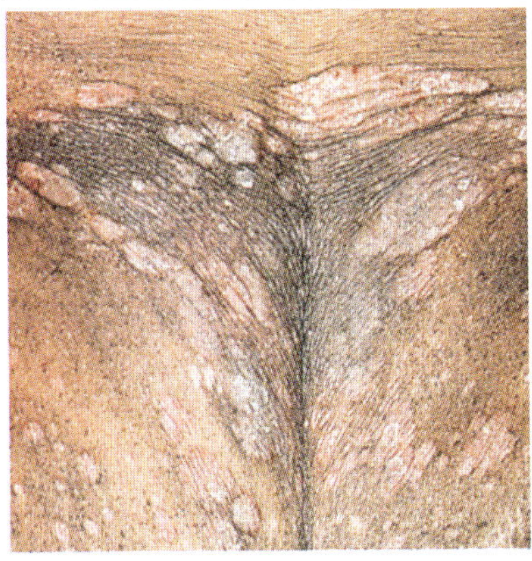

FIG. 60-17 *Papules and plaques that have become confluent to assume polycyclic outlines.*

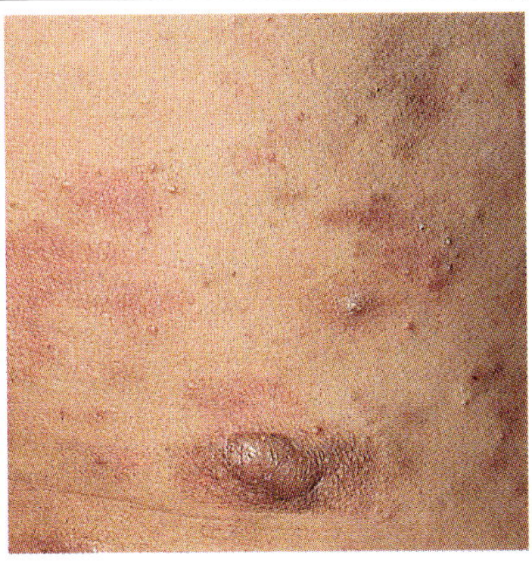

FIG. 60-18 *Papules, plaques, and a nodule.*

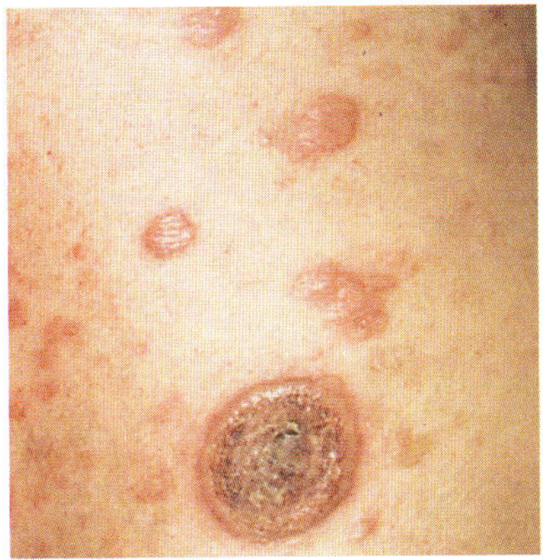

FIG. 60-19 *Papules, plaques, and a plaque-like tumor.*

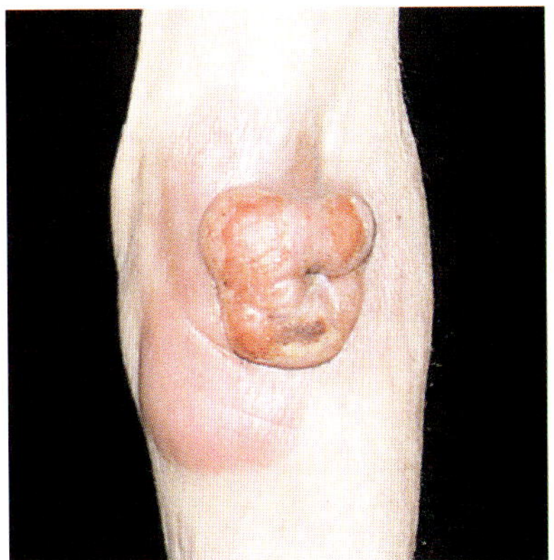

FIG. 60-20 *Plaques and a multilobate tumor.*

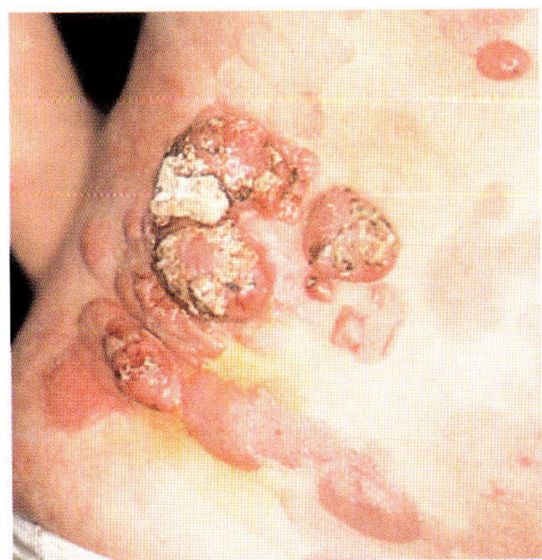

FIG. 60-21 *Patches, plaques, nodules, and tumors.*

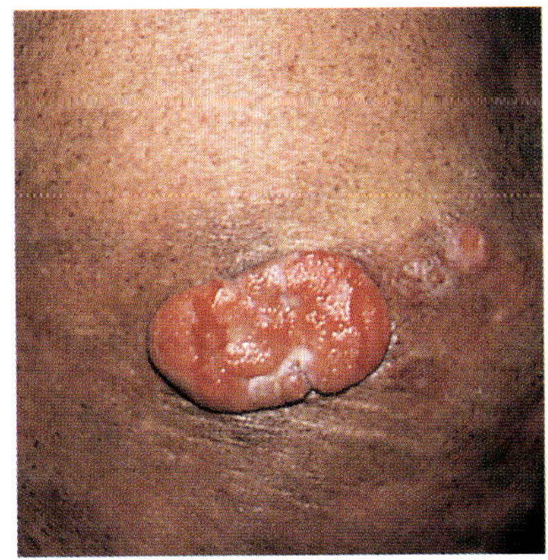

FIG. 60-22 *Ulcerated papules and a tumor.*

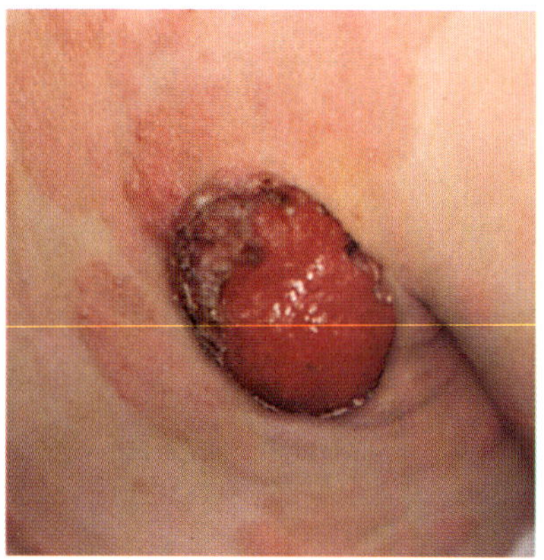
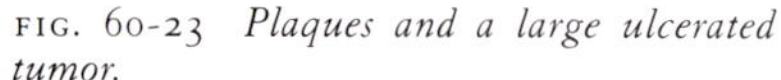

FIG. 60-23 *Plaques and a large ulcerated tumor.*

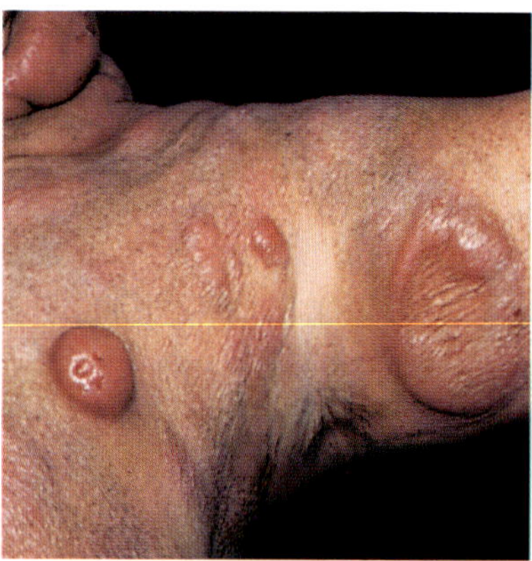

FIG. 60-24 *Plaques, nodules and tumors.*

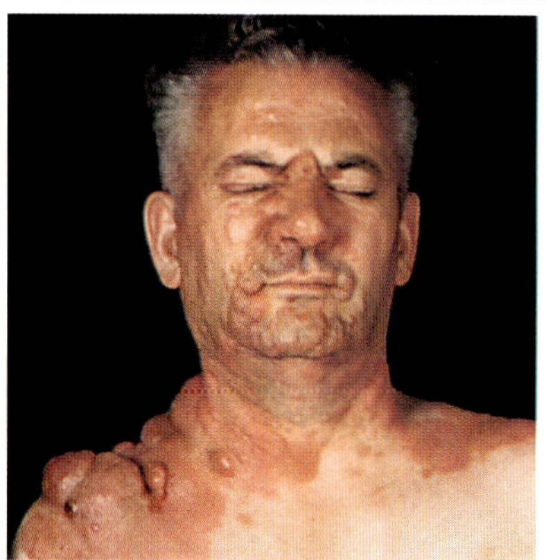

FIG. 60-25 *Plaques, nodules and tumors.*

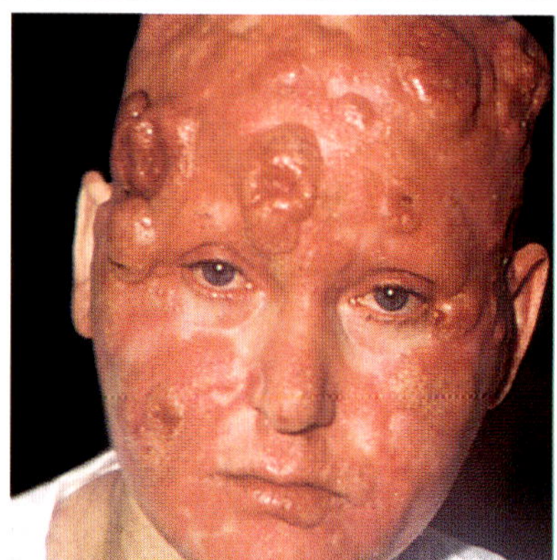

FIG. 60-26 *Papules, plaques, nodules, and tumors.*

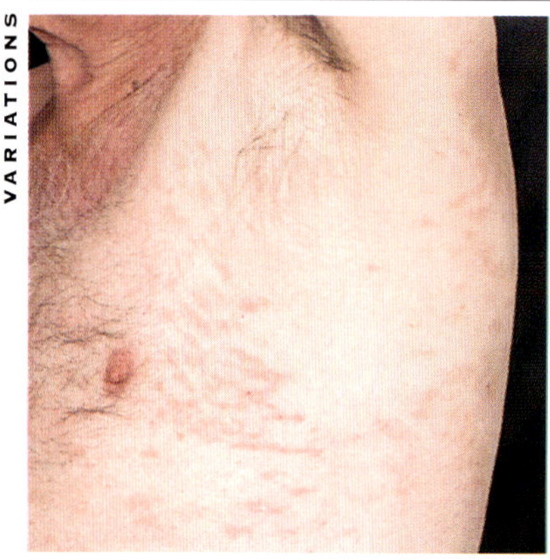

FIG. 60-27 *Slightly erythematous linear lesions distributed along lines of cleavage (digitate dermatosis).*

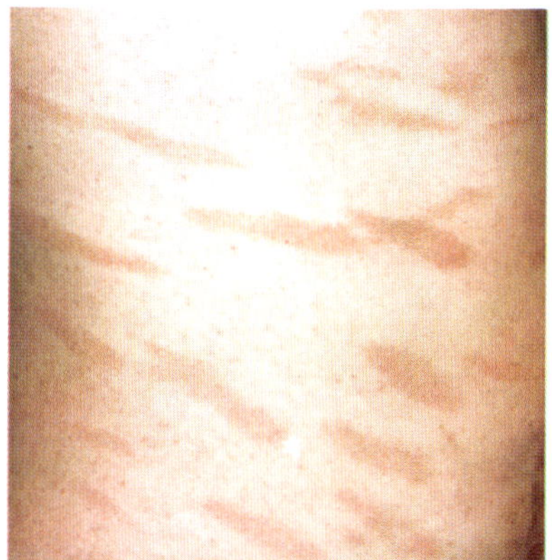

FIG. 60-28 *Ellipsoid patches and subtle plaques (digitate dermatosis).*

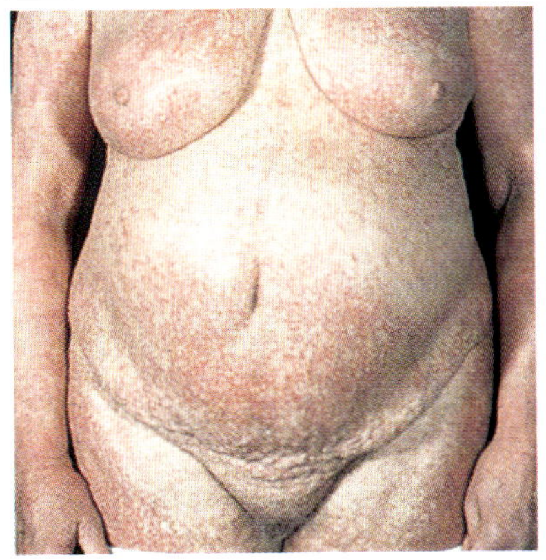
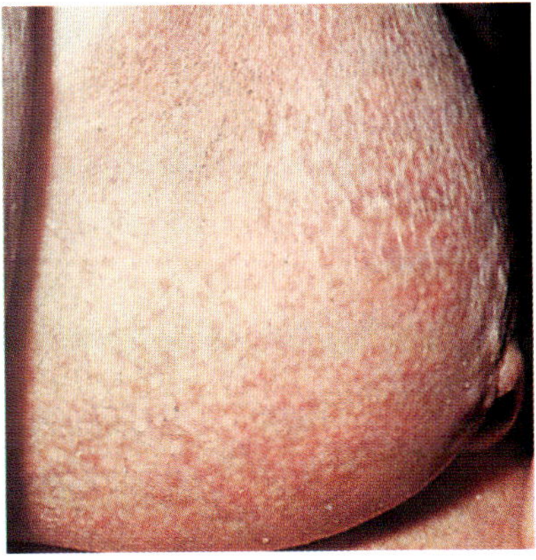

FIG. 60-29 (A, B) *Macules and patches in reticulated pattern (parakeratosis variegata).*

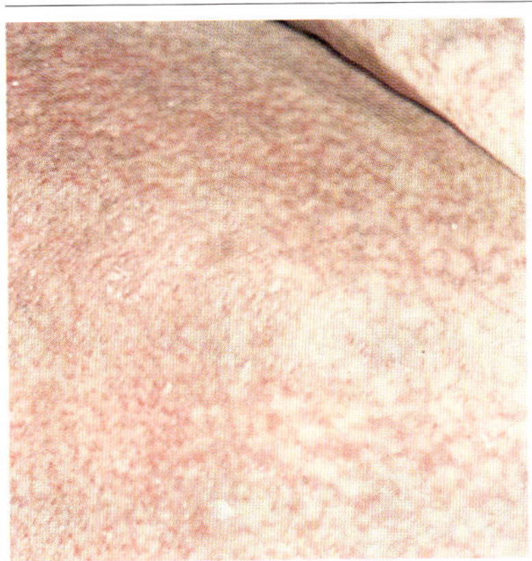

FIG. 60-29 (C) *Netlike pattern of parakeratosis variegata.*

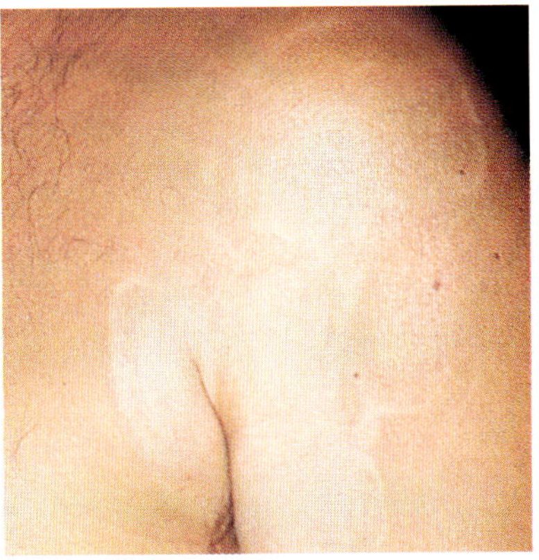

FIG. 60-30 *Hypopigmented patches surrounded by arciform plaques (hypopigmented mycosis fungoides).*

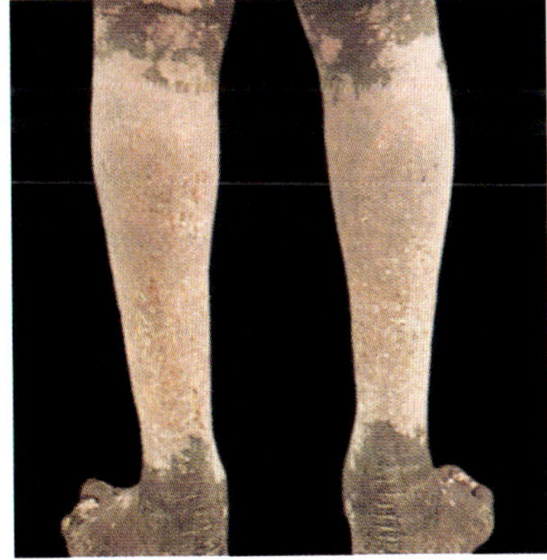

FIG. 60-31 *Hypopigmented scaly patches in a dark-skinned person (hypopigmented mycosis fungoides).*

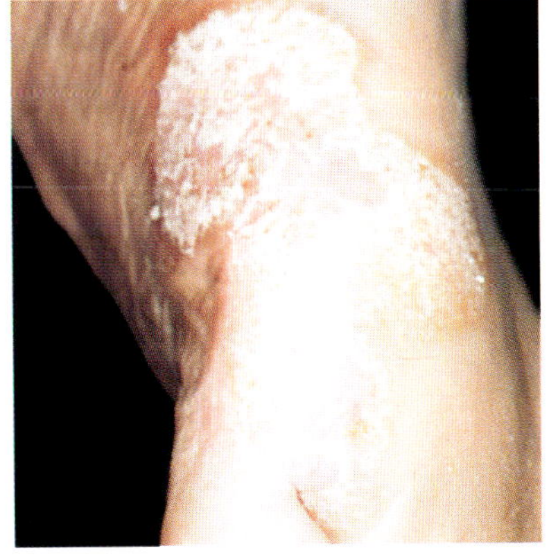

FIG. 60-32 *Keratotic plaque on the foot (pagetoid reticulosis, Woringer-Kolopp disease).*

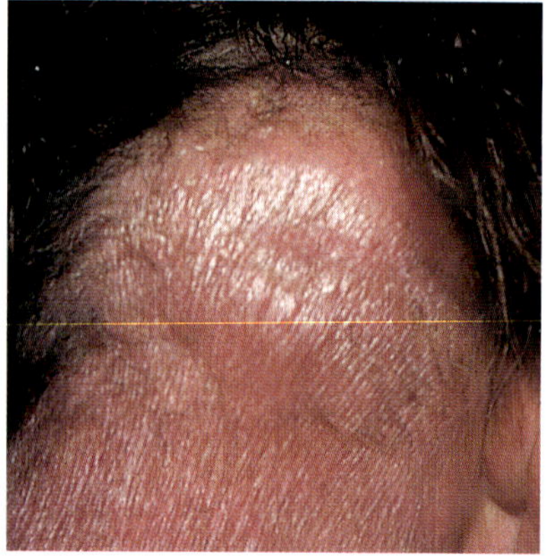

FIG. 60-33 *Large plaque accompanied by alopecia (mycosis fungoides with follicular mucinosis).*

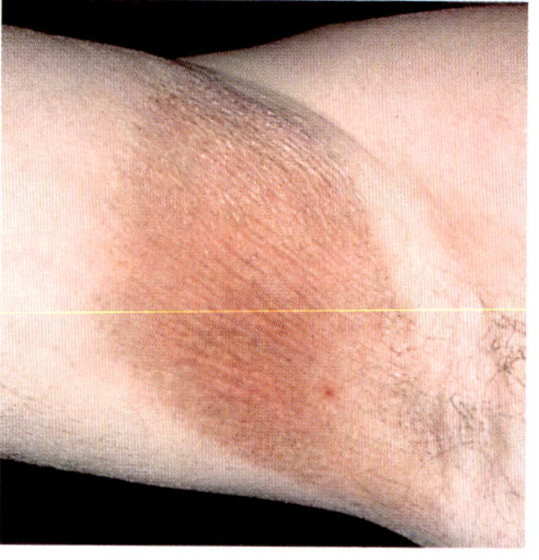

FIG. 60-34 *Rust-colored plaque, a stage in the evolution of granulomatous slack skin.*

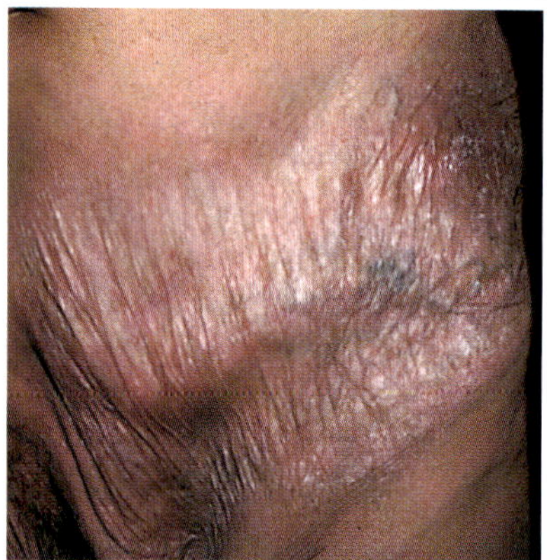

FIG. 60-35 *Huge, atrophic, somewhat pendulous lesion with atrophic surface (granulomatous slack skin).*

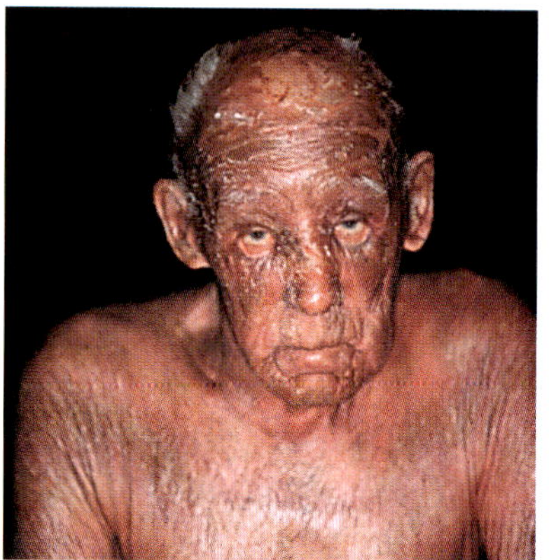

FIG. 60-36 *Exfoliative erythroderma (Sézary syndrome) with signs of the effects of persistent, vigorous rubbing.*

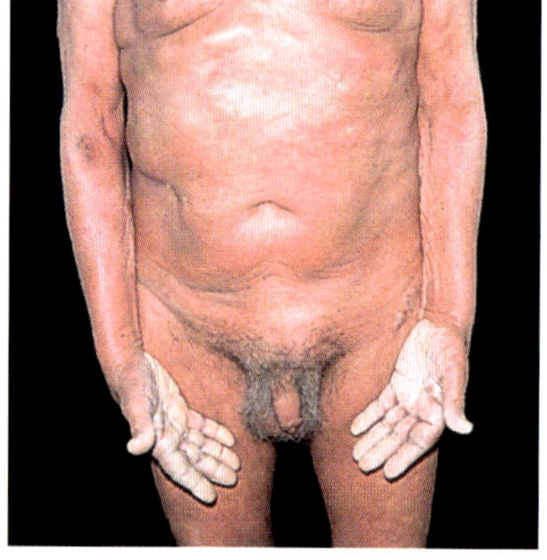

FIG. 60-37 *Exfoliative erythroderma with marked hyperkeratosis of palms (Sézary syndrome).*

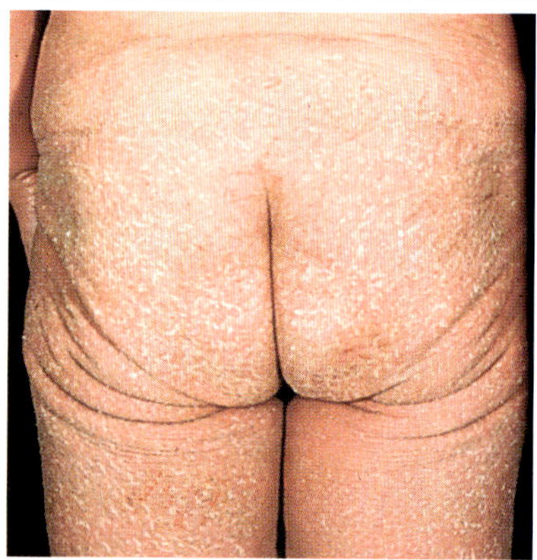

FIG. 60-38 *Exfoliative erythroderma (Sézary syndrome).*

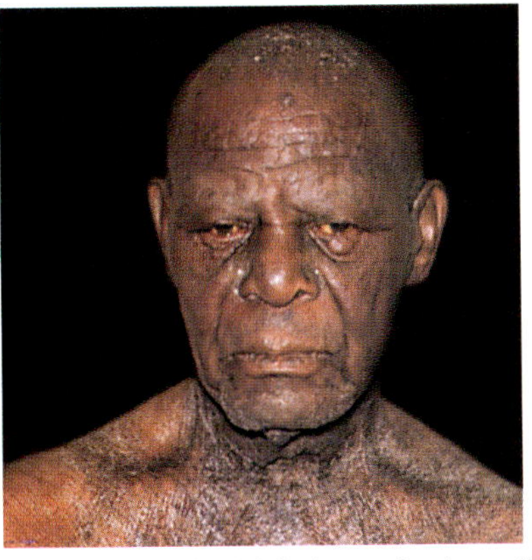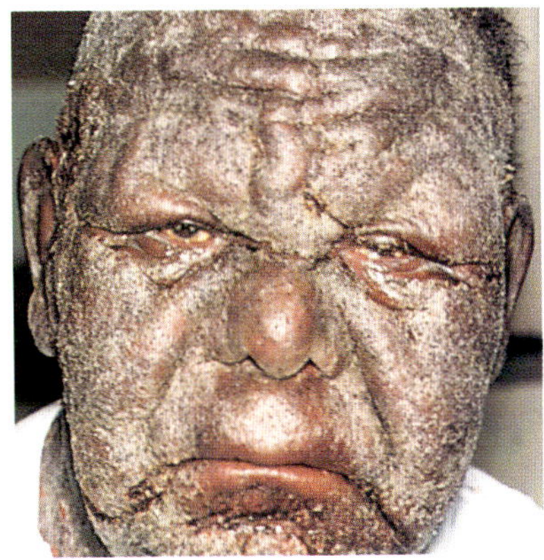

FIG. 60-39 (A, B) *Exfoliative erythroderma (Sézary syndrome); on the right, the same patient two years later with a leonine face.*

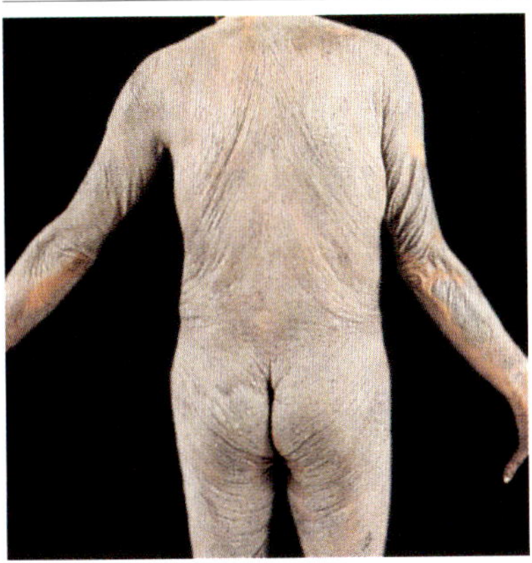

FIG. 60-40 *Exfoliative erythroderma in a patient with mycosis fungoides.*

ADJUNCTIVE DIAGNOSTIC TESTS Assessment of peripheral blood and examination for staging may be undertaken in order to determine the extent of systemic disease.

COURSE Most patients with mycosis fungoides have only patches of the disease for a lifetime. Some patients, however, have subtle plaques in addition to patches. Only uncommonly do nodules and tumors develop in patients with mycosis fungoides. Once a patch of mycosis fungoides develops, it tends to persist; rarely does a lesion of mycosis fungoides of any kind disappear in the absence of therapy. Patients who have nodules and tumors usually have patches and plaques as well. Once thick lesions of mycosis fungoides have come into being, whether they be thick plaques, nodules, or tumors, the prognosis changes from good or excellent to poor. Patients with mycosis fungoides who have very thick lesions usually die of systemic lymphoma.

INTEGRATION: UNIFYING CONCEPT Mycosis fungoides is a systemic lymphoma that usually manifests itself first in the skin as macules and then patches. The macules and ellipsoid patches take the form of what is known usually as "digitate dermatosis," and the larger patches of what is called "parapsoriasis en plaques." When patches have a yellowish hue, they are designated "xanthoerythroderma perstans," and when they have a reticulated pattern, they are referred to as "parakeratosis variegata." When, in time, patches become atrophic, they are termed "poikiloderma vasculare atrophicans." Digitate dermatosis also is referred to as "small-plaque parapsoriasis," and all the other expressions of mycosis fungoides just alluded to are known as "large-plaque parapsoriasis."

All of this terminology is confusing to students of the subject, because all of the lesions, clinically and histopathologically, are really those of mycosis fungoides and should be identified straightforwardly as mycosis fungoides. That diagnosis in itself does not denote a fatal end, any more than does a diagnosis of lupus erythematosus or melanoma. The fact is that the overwhelming majority of patients with mycosis fungoides (and with lupus erythematosus or melanoma) do not die of that malignant neoplastic process.

All of the lesions called small-plaque and large-plaque parapsoriasis have in common superficial perivascular infiltrates of lymphocytes and lymphocytes aligned as solitary units in the basal layer of the epidermis, in the spinous zone in conjunction with scant spongiosis, and sometimes in the upper reaches of the epidermis, such as the granular zone. That constellation of findings is diagnostic of mycosis fungoides. Sometimes lymphocytes within the epidermis are larger than those within the dermis. Wiry bundles of collagen in haphazard array are often present in the upper part of the dermis in association with patchy lichenoid infiltrates of lymphocytes. In short, there is no need to invoke terms like small- and large-plaque parapsoriasis, digitate dermatosis, parapsoriasis en plaques, xanthoerythroderma perstans, parakeratosis variegata, and poikiloderma vasculare atrophicans; the diagnosis is mycosis fungoides.

Other distinctive clinical expressions of mycosis fungoides include plaques of pagetoid reticulosis near an ankle, pendulous lesions of granulomatous slack skin near axillary and inguinal regions, and the erythroderma of Sézary syndrome. There is no need for any of those terms, except as descriptive modifiers of the diagnosis of mycosis fungoides, just as is the case for nodules and tumors of mycosis fungoides that are referred to universally as simply those of mycosis fungoides. In short, what has just been described represents the spectrum of morphologic findings of the systemic lymphoma called mycosis fungoides.

The original concept of mycosis fungoides, as it was set forth by Alibert in 1806 was limited and incorrect. Alibert conceived of mycosis fungoides as a disease that consisted of papules, nodules, and tumors, but not of macules, patches, and plaques, and as a condition that, in his view, led inevitably to death. For almost two centuries, Alibert's was the accepted concept of mycosis fungoides among dermatologists, general pathologists, and dermatopathologists. Furthermore, it was asserted repeatedly that mycosis fungoides could not be diagnosed, clinically or histopathologically, when lesions were flat. Small- and large-plaque expressions were said to be "pre-mycosis fungoides" that in a small percentage of patients "converted" or "transformed" into authentic mycosis fungoides. In actuality, mycosis fungoides is mycosis fungoides from the very outset. Not only can mycosis fungoides be diagnosed with specificity when lesions are flat, but most patients with mycosis fungoides have only flat lesions for a lifetime. Practically never do those patients die of mycosis fungoides.

In conclusion, mycosis fungoides should not be thought of as an invariably fatal disease, but as that kind of systemic lymphoma that manifests itself first in the skin as flat lesions which usually remain flat for a patient's lifetime.

THERAPY Topical nitrogen mustard, PUVA, or topical corticosteroids (alone or in combination) are beneficial for flat lesions. Chlorambucil combined with prednisone is recommended for treatment of Sézary syndrome. Radiotherapy, interferon (in combination with PUVA), photopheresis, or chemotherapy is advisable for plaques, nodules, tumors, and erythroderma.

DEFINITION A granulomatous inflammatory process characterized clinically by patches that become yellowish plaques and that in time resolve with atrophy and telangiectases. The condition usually occurs in persons with diabetes.

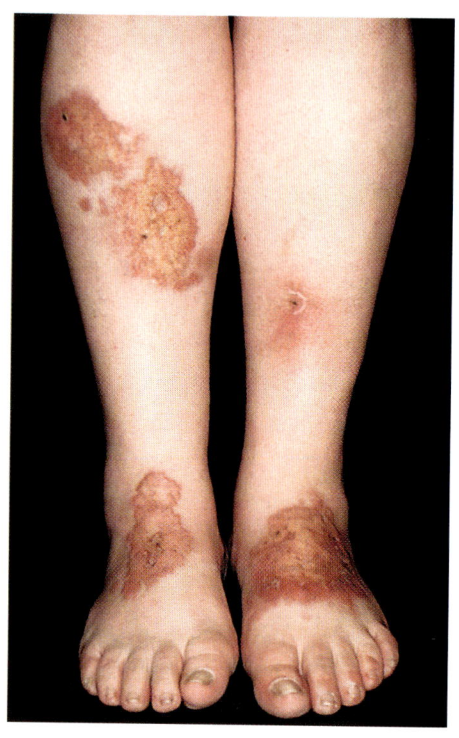

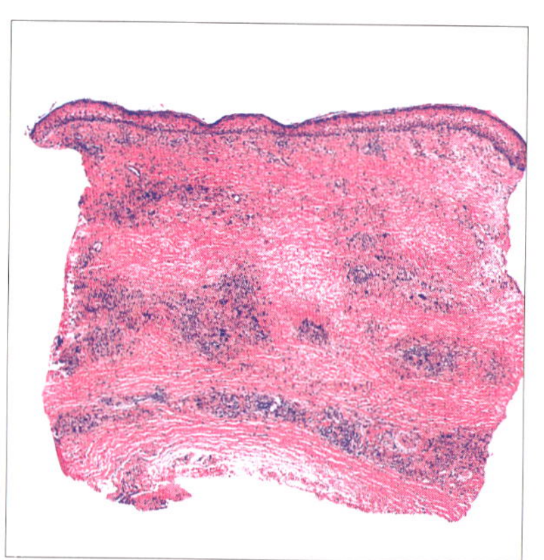

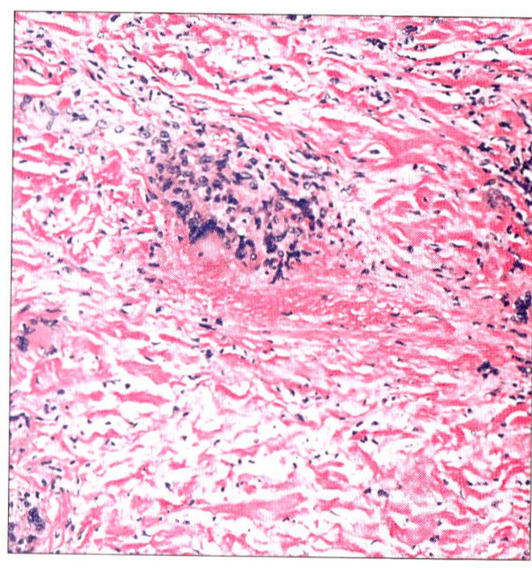

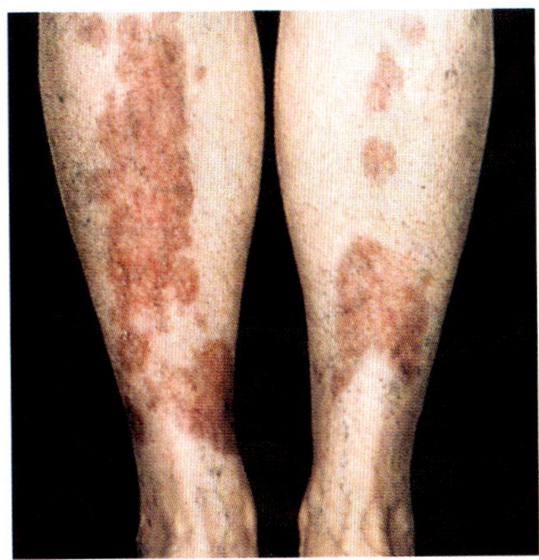

FIG. 61-1 *Atrophic hyperpigmented patches with a slightly yellow hue.*

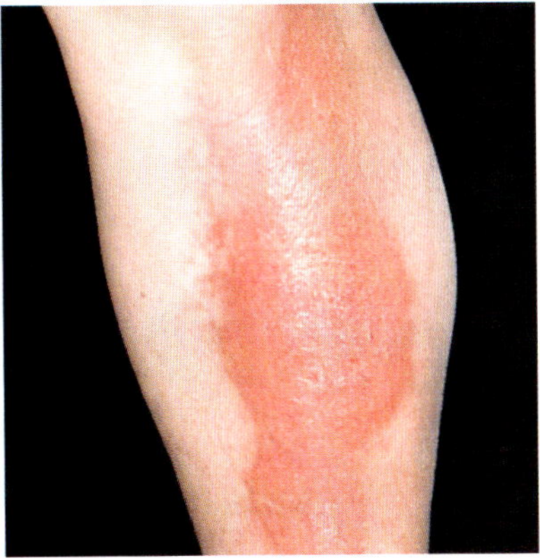

FIG. 61-2 *Typical location of an evolving, mostly smooth-surfaced, reddish yellow plaque.*

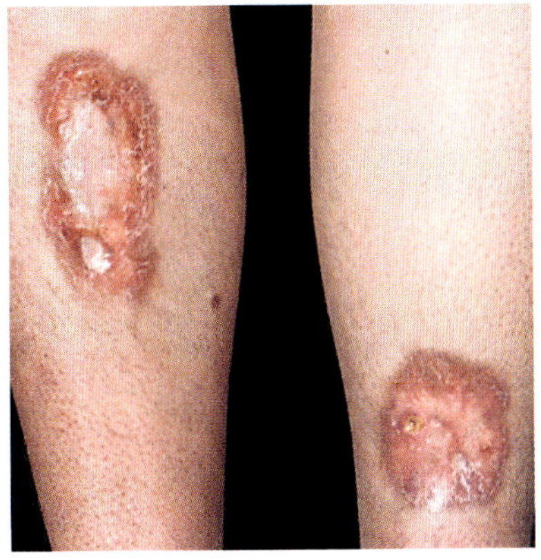

FIG. 61-3 *Late lesions marked by plaque-like hyperpigmented scaly borders, and an atrophic yellow center.*

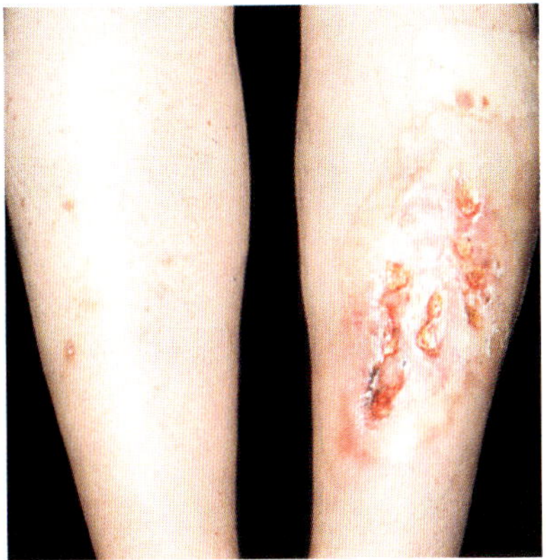

FIG. 61-4 *Very late yellowish atrophic plaque punctuated by large, deep ulcers.*

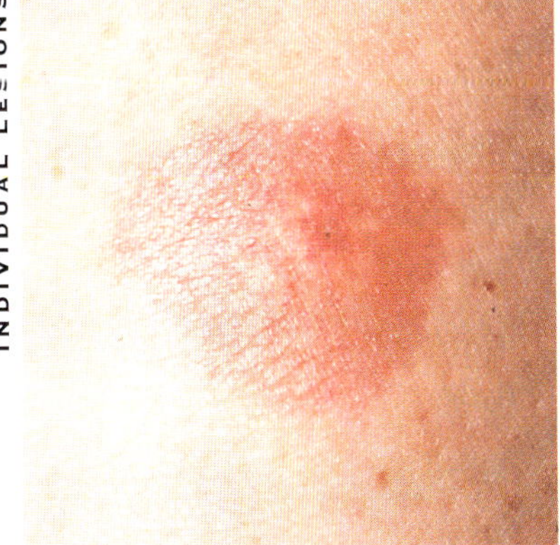

FIG. 61-5 *An early smooth-surfaced patch with a vaguely yellow cast.*

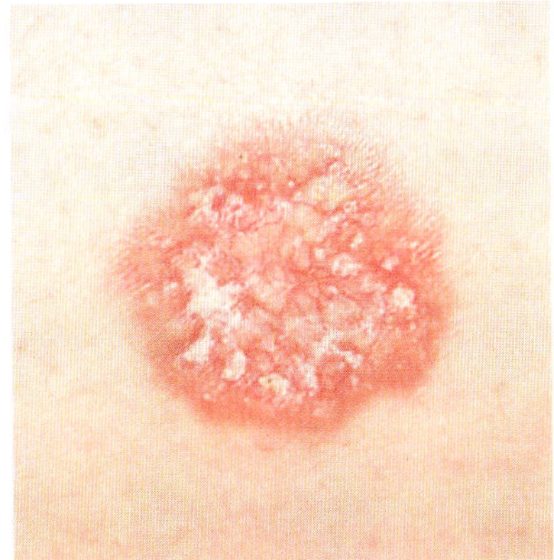

FIG. 61-6 *A plaque whose border is smooth and whose center is white and yellow, telangiectatic, scarred, and scaly.*

ADJUNCTIVE DIAGNOSTIC TESTS Examinations should be undertaken to detect diabetes mellitus.

COURSE Necrobiosis lipoidica begins, like virtually all inflammatory diseases, as a macule that becomes either a patch or a papule and eventually a plaque. For years the plaque expands slowly centrifugally and, in time, assumes a yellowish cast. Ulceration may supervene. After many years, the plaque involutes as an atrophic patch that maintains its yellowish cast and is joined by innumerable telangiectases.

INTEGRATION: UNIFYING CONCEPT An evolving reddish macule/patch of necrobiosis lipoidica is characterized by a small-vessel vasculitis mediated by neutrophils. A mixed-cell infiltrate of neutrophils, lymphocytes, and plasma cells is present around blood vessels of the superficial and deep plexuses, as well as within the interstitium of the reticular dermis. As the lesion becomes a plaque, vasculitic changes no longer are apparent. In addition to perivascular and interstitial infiltrates of lymphocytes and plasma cells, there are zones in the reticular dermis of degeneration of collagen, which are surrounded by epithelioid histiocytes aligned in a palisade. In time, as a plaque continues to evolve, the zones of degenerated collagen are replaced by thick bundles of collagen that continue to be encircled by epithelioid histiocytes. Later still, the granulomatous infiltrate wanes, and by the time the lesion has become an atrophic patch, all that remains are altered bundles of collagen in the reticular dermis, telangiectases in the upper part of the dermis, and deposits of lipid. The lipid deposits are not detectable in sections stained by hematoxylin and eosin, but only in fresh tissue stained by oil red O or Sudan black, where they can be observed just beneath the thinned epidermis.

Necrobiosis lipoidica is a distinctive pathologic process that often is a manifestation of the diabetic state. Many patients with necrobiosis lipoidica have overt diabetes, and many who do not have latent diabetes.

THERAPY Intralesional injection of corticosteroids is effective for active lesions, that is, those evidenced by redness and elevation. That treatment prevents progression of the process and hastens regression of it. Corticosteroids should not be applied to, or injected into, atrophic patches because they only worsen the atrophy.

DEFINITION A constellation of lesions that represent disorders of melanocytes (e.g., axillary "freckles" and café au lait "spots") and of proliferations of Schwann cells (e.g., papules, nodules, and tumors of neurofibroma). The cutaneous lesions may be accompanied by neoplasms with neural differentiation that are situated in nerves (e.g., acoustic neuroma) and in the brain (e.g., gliomas), as well as by manifestations of various kinds in the eyes (e.g., Lisch nodules) and bones (e.g., scoliosis).

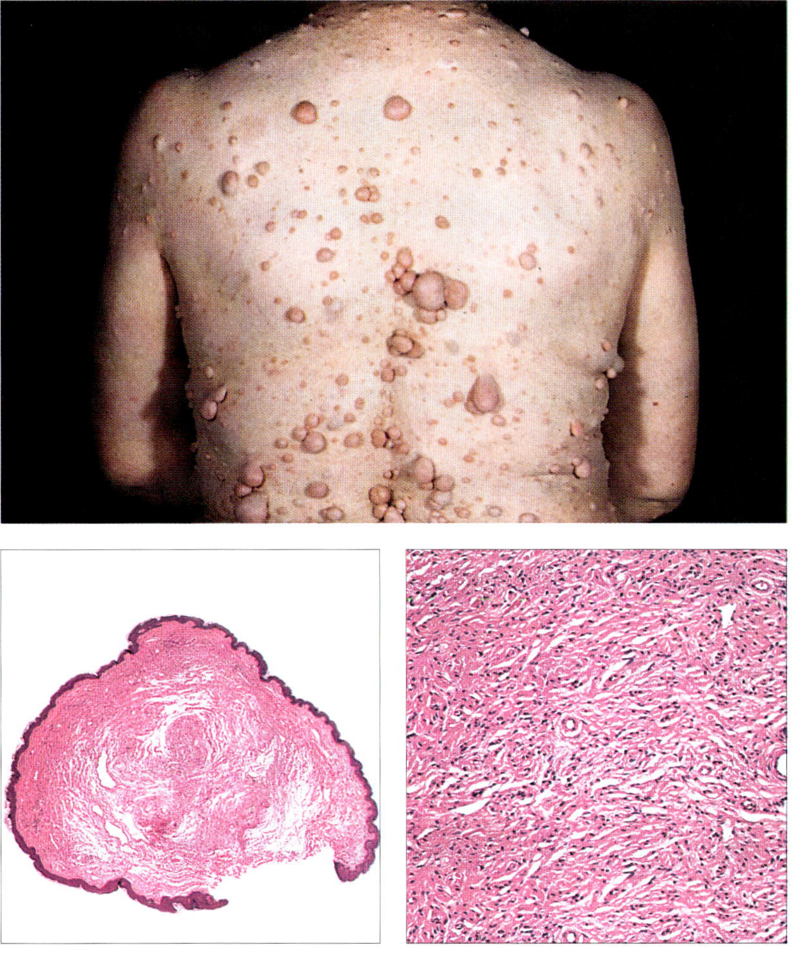

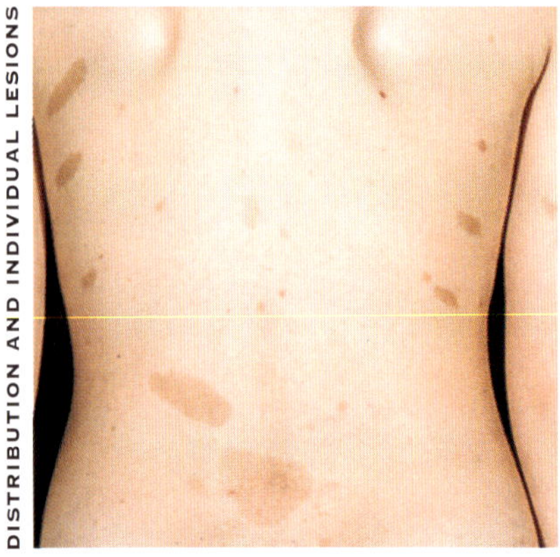

FIG. 62-1 *Café au lait spots. When patients have several such lesions, it is likely that they have neurofibromatosis.*

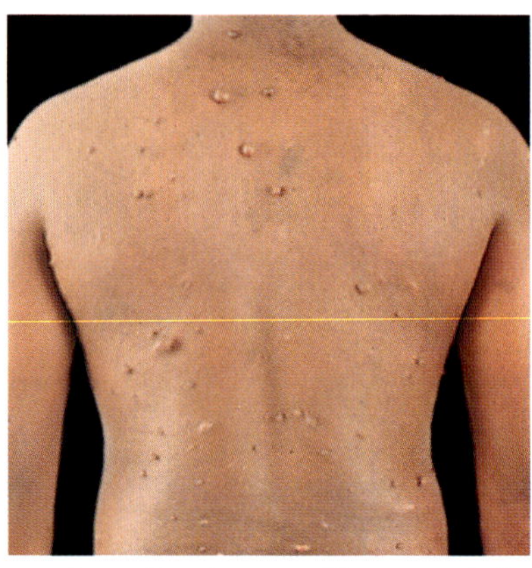

FIG. 62-2 *Papular neurofibromas and pigmented macules.*

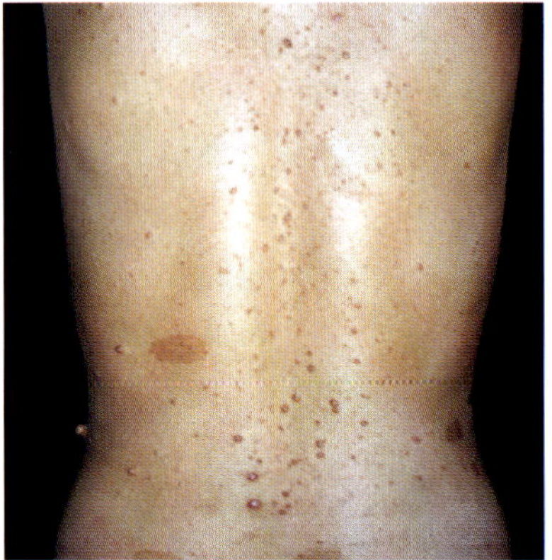

FIG. 62-3 *Café au lait spots and papular neurofibromas.*

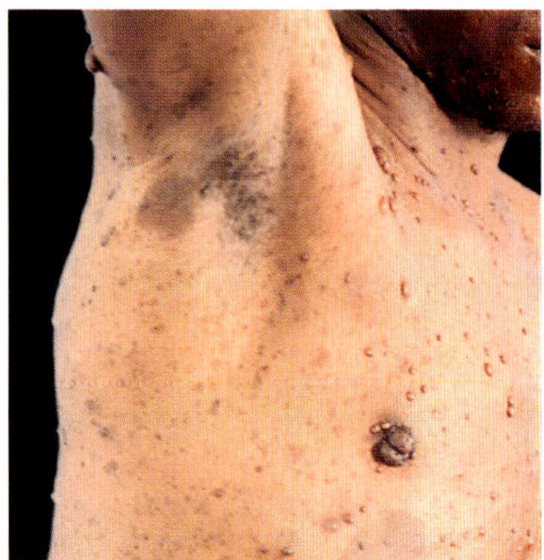

FIG. 62-4 *Café au lait spots and neurofibromas.*

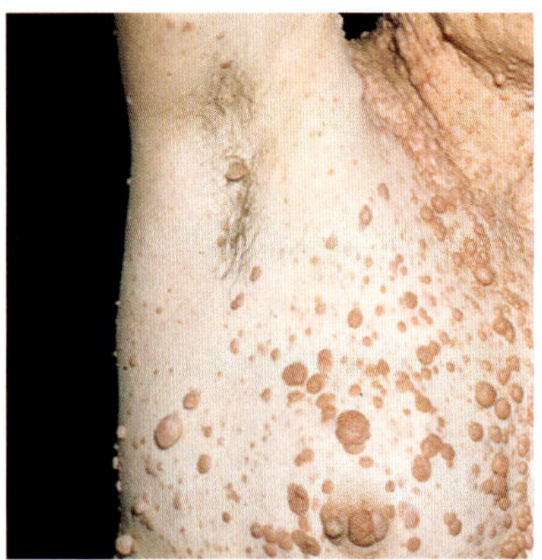

FIG. 62-5 *Papular, nodular, and tumorous lesions of neurofibroma.*

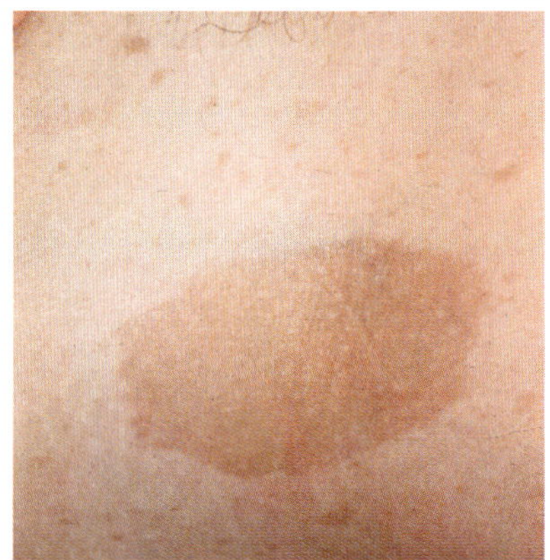

FIG. 62-6 *Pigmented patch (café au lait spot) surrounded by pigmented macules.*

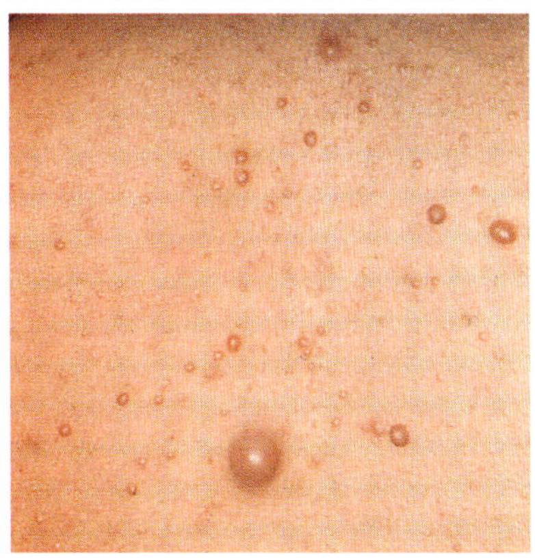

FIG. 62-7 *Papules and a nodule of neurofibroma.*

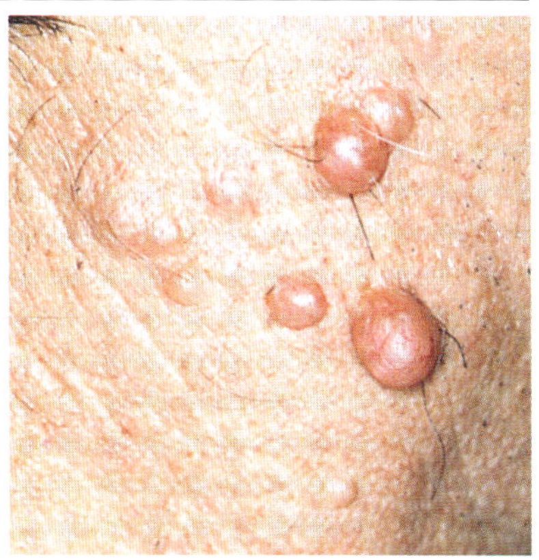

FIG. 62-8 *Papules, nodules, and tumors of neurofibroma.*

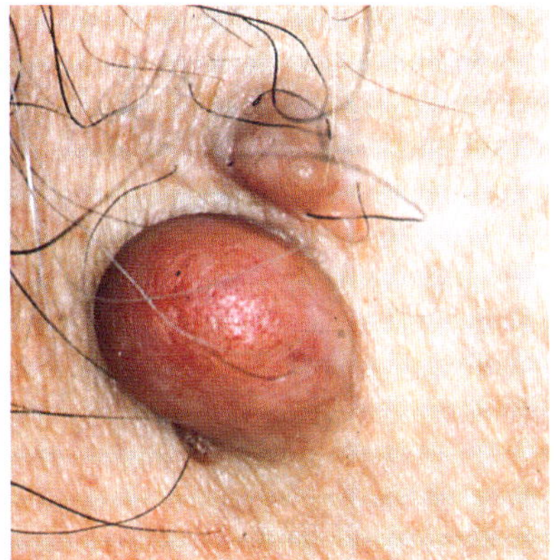

FIG. 62-9 *Nodule and tumor of neurofibroma.*

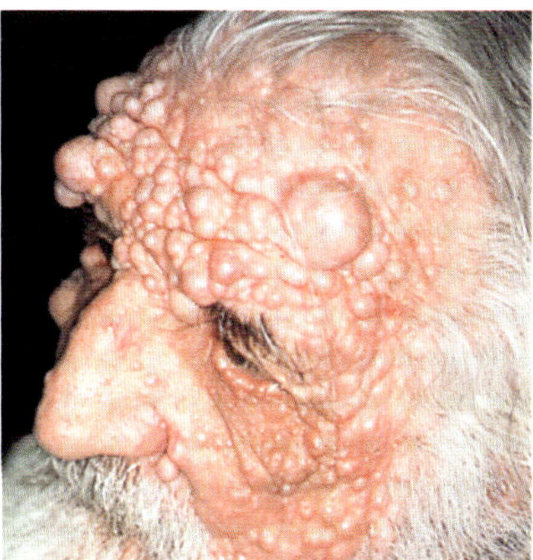

FIG. 62-10 *Closely-set, smooth-surfaced papules, nodules, and tumors of neurofibromatosis.*

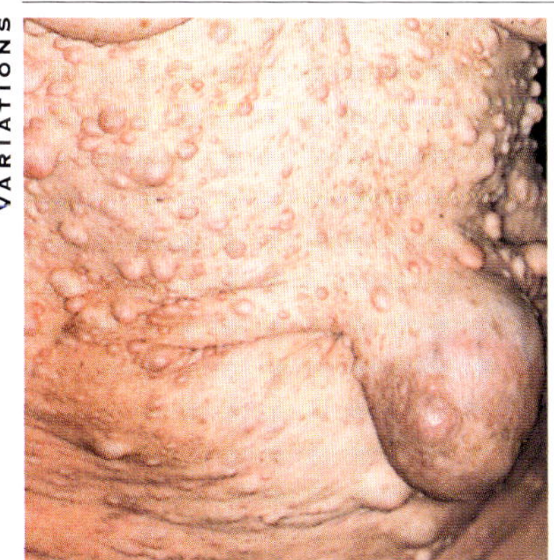

FIG. 62-11 *Papules, nodules, and tumors, one of them gigantic (plexiform), of neurofibroma.*

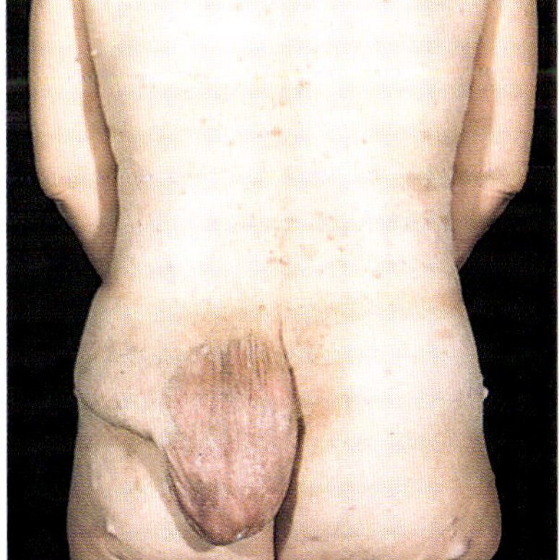

FIG. 62-12 *Gigantic plexiform neurofibroma in the setting of papular and nodular neurofibromas and café au lait spots.*

VARIATIONS

ADJUNCTIVE DIAGNOSTIC TESTS Investigations for staging have value in assessing systemic manifestations of neurofibromatosis.

COURSE Once a papule of neurofibromatosis appears, it is certain to be there for the lifetime of a person. The papule may remain a papule or, more likely, become a nodule and even a tumor. Some tumors may become pendulous. As a rule, patients with neurofibromatosis have countless neurofibromas of different sizes. What has just been stated in regard to the course of neurofibromas applies equally to that of café au lait spots and axillary "freckles," i.e., they persist.

INTEGRATION: UNIFYING CONCEPT Each soft papule, nodule, or tumor of neurofibromatosis consists of a neurofibroma, a benign neoplasm made up mostly of delicate fibrillary wavy bundles of collagen that are joined by countless Schwann cells, each of which possesses a thin wavy nucleus. In addition, there are many fibrocytes that have oval nuclei, and mast cells that have oblong nuclei when cut along the long axis and round nuclei when cut in cross section.

In addition to neurofibromas, patients with neurofibromatosis usually have pigmented macules and patches, the former referred to, imprecisely, as "axillary freckles," and the latter, picturesquely, as "café au lait spots." The histopathologic findings in both the macules and the patches are the same, namely, a slightly increased number of melanocytes that sometimes produce giant melanosomes, which they convey through dendrites, along with ordinary granules of melanin, to adjacent keratinocytes. The result is an epidermis that is slightly hyperpigmented.

Neurofibromatosis is a systemic disease in which neurofibromas may be present not only in the skin, but also in large nerves and in the brain. The process also involves other organs, such as the eyes and the bones. Neurofibromatosis is considered to be one of the phakomatoses. Several different types of neurofibromatosis have been identified, a situation analogous to that in Ehlers-Danlos syndrome.

The genetic defects that underlie neurofibromatosis have been cloned and characterized. At least two types can be recognized, both of them inherited in autosomal-dominant fashion. Neurofibromatosis type I is characterized by numerous neurofibromas, café au lait spots, axillary and inguinal "freckling," and pigmented hamartomas of the iris (Lisch nodules). Extracutaneous manifestations also are found in that type of neurofibromatosis.

The hallmark of neurofibromatosis type II is bilateral vestibular schwannomas. The manifestations in the skin are much less prominent than in neurofibromatosis type I.

Parenthetically, it should be mentioned that a single neurofibroma showing clinical features like those pictured in this chapter usually has no implication of neurofibromatosis.

THERAPY Simple excision of papules and nodules, and of those tumors that lend themselves to that procedure, is worthwhile if a patient so desires for cosmetic reasons. Genetic counseling is advisable for persons with neurofibromatosis. Routine follow-up is recommended for early detection of various complications.

DEFINITION A hamartoma of epidermis, epithelial structures of adnexa, and presumably dermal elements, typified, when fully formed, by a papillated or verrucous yellowish plaque situated usually on the scalp. The condition may present itself as a solitary lesion or as multiple lesions that follow Blaschko's lines and, when systematized, is almost always associated with other congenital abnormalities.

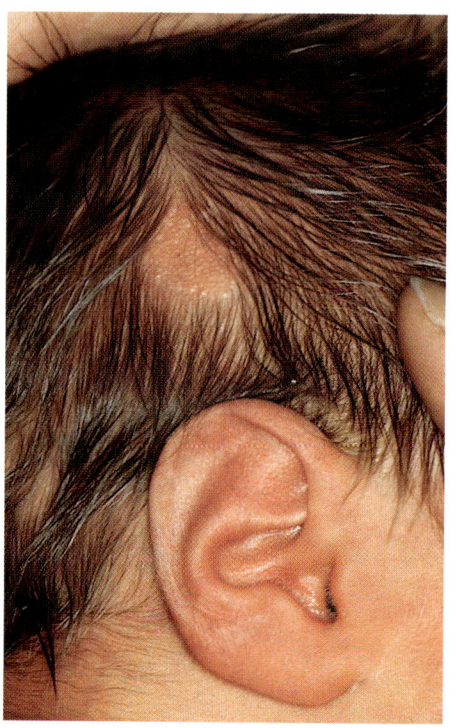

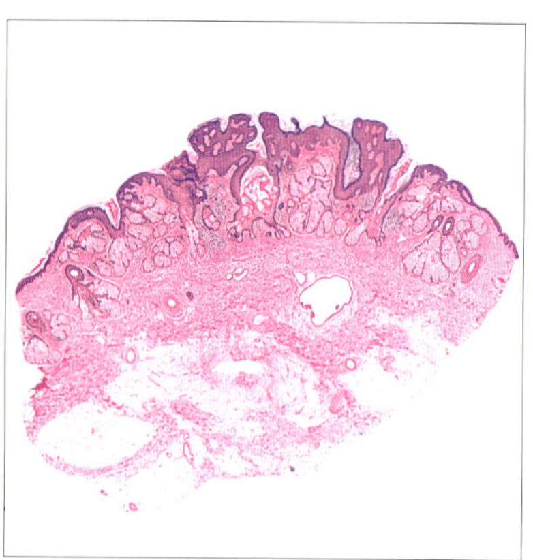

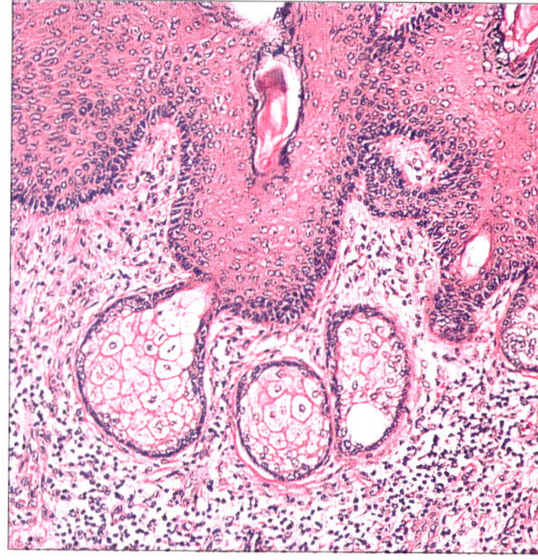

DISTRIBUTION

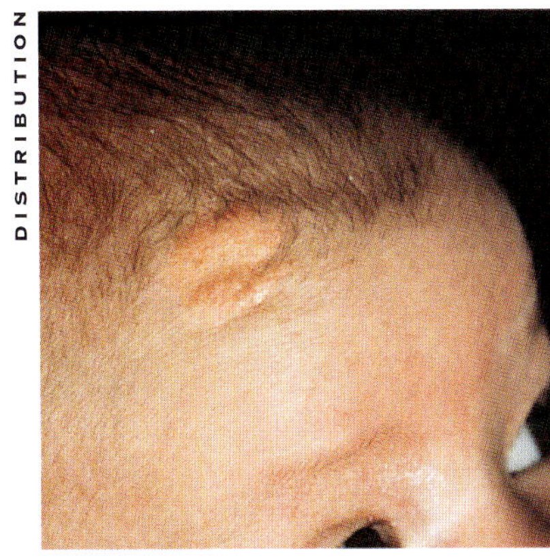

FIG. 63-1 *A yellowish plaque.*

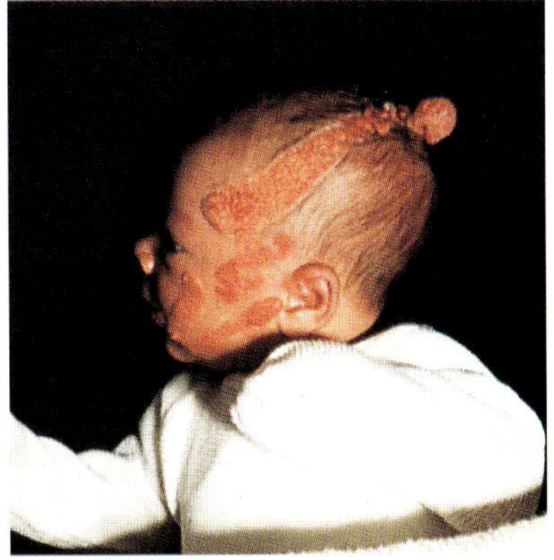

FIG. 63-2 *Numerous linear yellow lesions, some of them exuberantly exophytic.*

CONFIGURATION

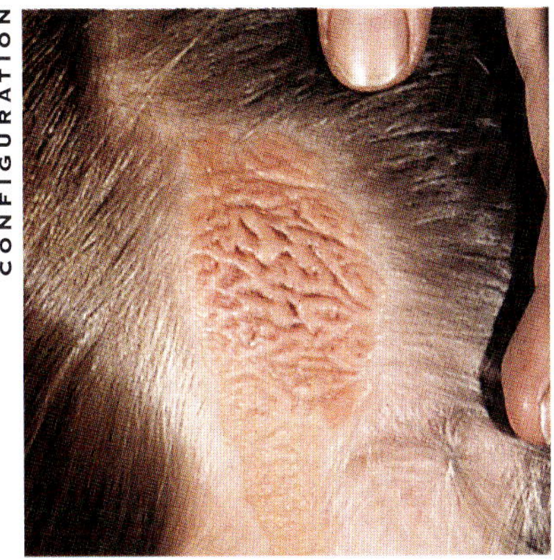

FIG. 63-3 *A linear plaque with a surface that is partially cerebriform and partially gently mammillated.*

ARRANGEMENT

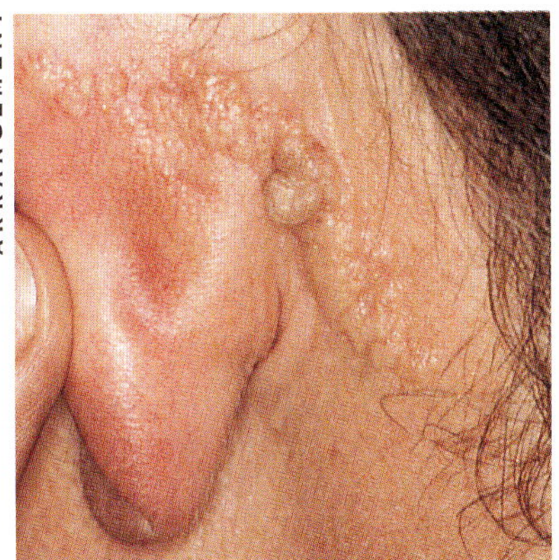

FIG. 63-4 *Papules in linear array.*

INDIVIDUAL LESIONS

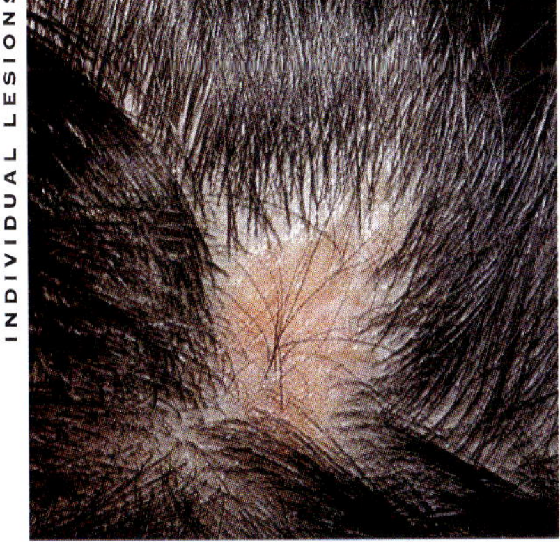

FIG. 63-5 *A slightly elevated, flat-surfaced, alopecic plaque.*

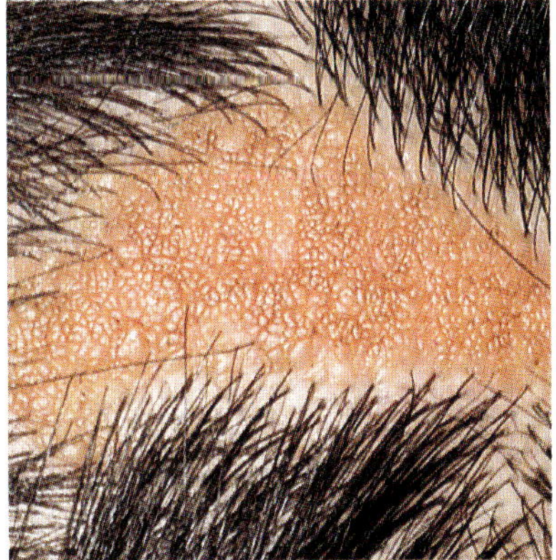

FIG. 63-6 *A gently mammillated alopecic plaque.*

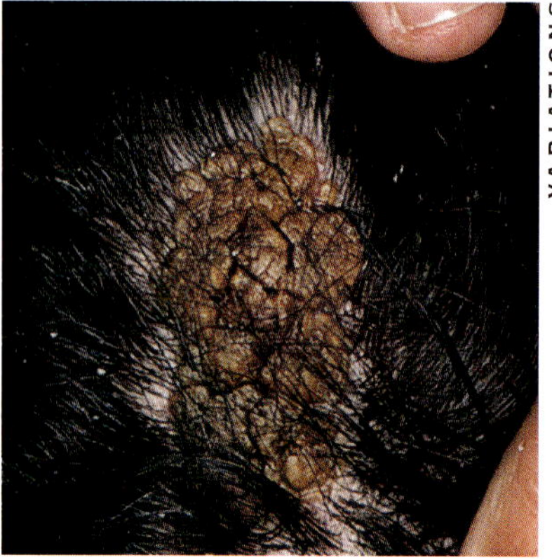

FIG. 63-7 *A verrucous alopecic plaque.*

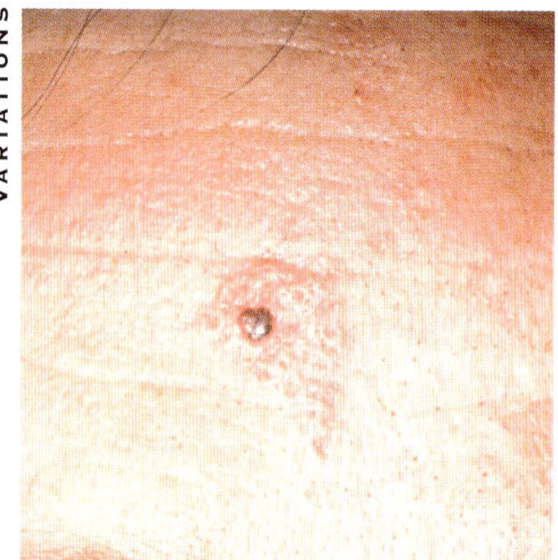

FIG. 63-8 *A pigmented papule of trichoblast-oma in a plaque of nevus sebaceus.*

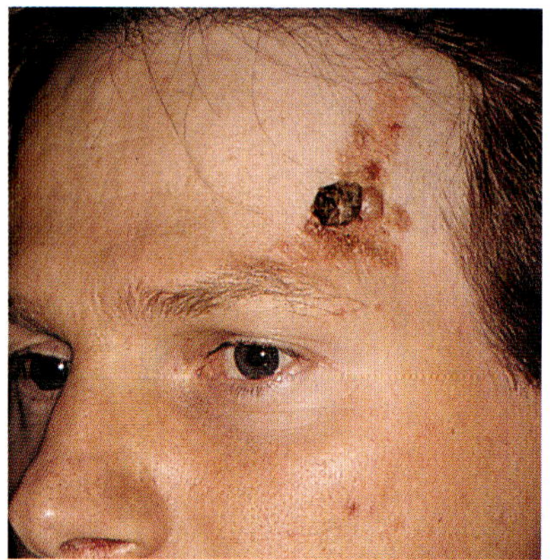

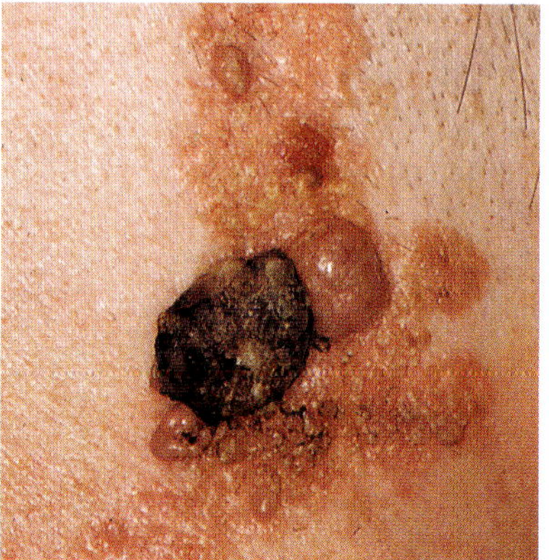

FIG. 63-9 (A, B) *A black nodule and a rust-colored nodule of trichoblastoma in a plaque of nevus sebaceus.*

COURSE A lesion of nevus sebaceus usually is present at birth and typically on the scalp, where it appears as an alopecic, slightly yellowish macule. For years it remains flattish and grows at the same pace as the growth of the child who bears it. At puberty, however, the lesion tends to become mammillated and more yellow. As time goes on, the surface may become increasingly papillated and may even become verrucous.

Benign neoplasms develop commonly in fully-formed lesions of nevus sebaceus, chief among them trichoblastomas that are often markedly pigmented hemispherical papules. Much less often a malignant neoplasm arises in a nevus sebaceus, usually a trichoblastic (basal-cell) carcinoma. Trichoblastomas are at least 10 times more common than basal-cell carcinomas in lesions of nevus sebaceus. Once a lesion of nevus sebaceus has come into being, it persists for a lifetime.

INTEGRATION: UNIFYING CONCEPT Nevus sebaceus is the quintessential example of an organoid nevus, i.e., a hamartoma that, in the skin, consists of various elements indigenous to the organ. The components of nevus sebaceus are epidermal in the form of gentle mammillation, prominent papillation, or even digitations. They are sebaceous in the form of clusters of pyriform lobules of sebocytes, and follicles as primitive germs and a papilla situated just beneath surface epithelium (and absence of terminal follicles within the substance of the hamartoma itself). The apocrine component takes the form of numerous tubular structures that reside within the dermis and sometimes the subcutaneous fat.

A variety of cysts, cystic hamartomas, and benign and malignant neoplasms may develop within a nevus sebaceus. Even in a newborn, it is not uncommon for a benign neoplasm of apocrine character, namely, syringocystadenoma papilliferum, to be present in association with nevus sebaceus. An apocrine cyst, called apocrine hidrocystoma, is often present in a nevus sebaceus, as are cystic hamartomas like steatocystoma. The commonest neoplasm that occurs in nevus sebaceus is not basal-cell carcinoma, as has been asserted for almost three-quarters of a century, but trichoblastoma, the benign analogue of basal-cell carcinoma. Among the malignant neoplasms that sometimes appear in nevus sebaceus, in addition to basal-cell carcinoma, are sebaceous carcinoma and apocrine carcinoma.

THERAPY Simple surgical excision is preferable if the decision is made to remove the lesion. It is not necessary, however, to extirpate every nevus sebaceus, as was advocated in times past when trichoblastomas that often develop in them were thought to be basal-cell carcinomas. In fact, however, a malignant neoplasm may arise in the course of a nevus sebaceus, just as a melanoma may originate in conjunction with a melanocytic nevus. Not all nevi need to be excised, and so it is, too, for nevus sebaceus.

DEFINITION An arteritis in the subcutaneous fat manifested clinically at first by one or more red nodules that, in time, become ulcerated and heal with scars, usually on the posterior aspect of the legs of short, thick-legged women. No cause is usually found, but when Mycobacterium tuberculosis is shown to be the agent responsible, the condition then is termed "erythema induratum."

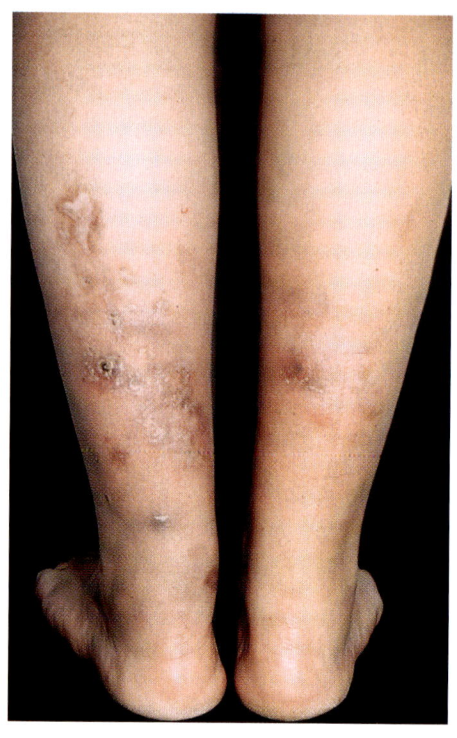

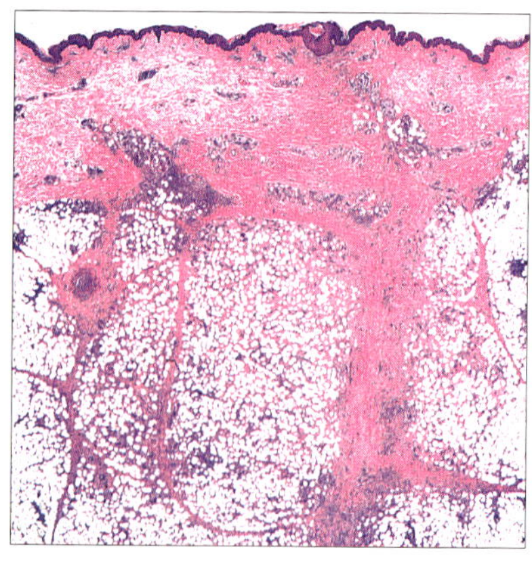

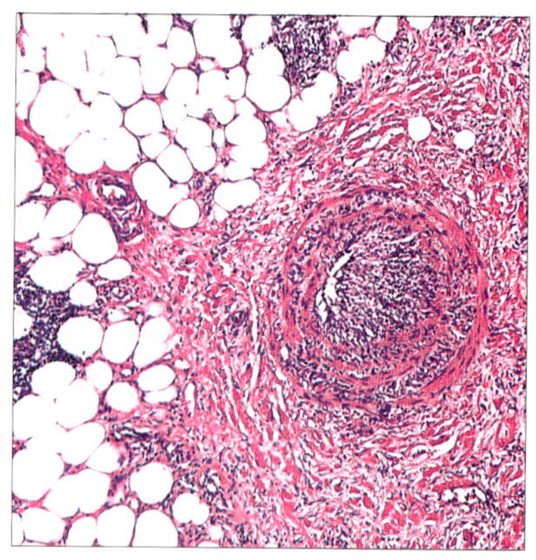

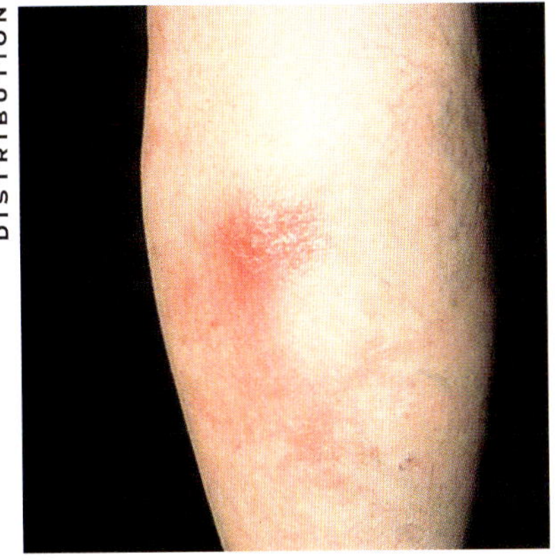

FIG. 64-1 *Poorly-circumscribed red plaque and nodule on the calf.*

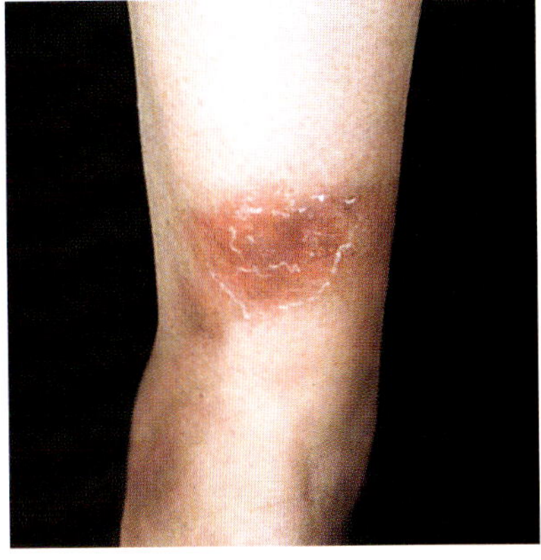

FIG. 64-2 *A plaque with a nodular component associated with collarettes of scale adjacent to a smooth-surfaced nodule.*

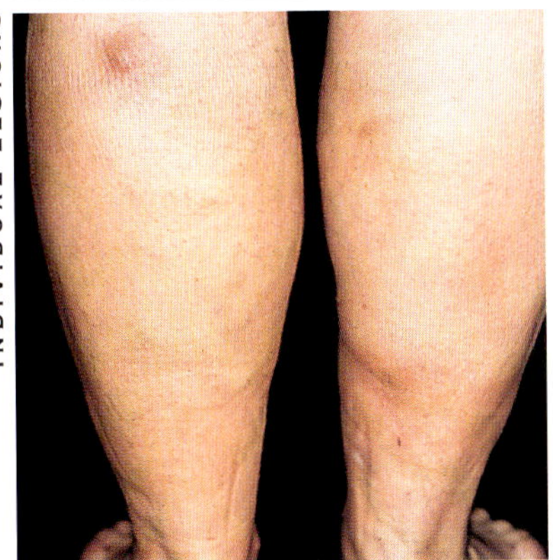

FIG. 64-3 *Nodule on the upper part of the calf and a plaque on the lower part of the other leg.*

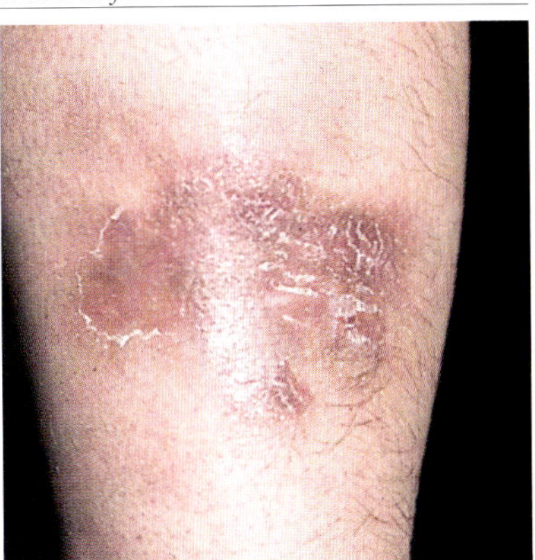

FIG. 64-4 *Red scaly plaques and nodules that have become confluent (evolving lesions).*

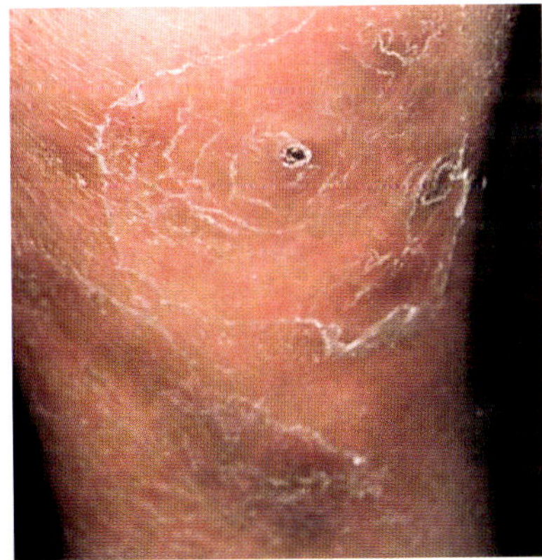

FIG. 64-5 *Nodules covered by scales and crusts.*

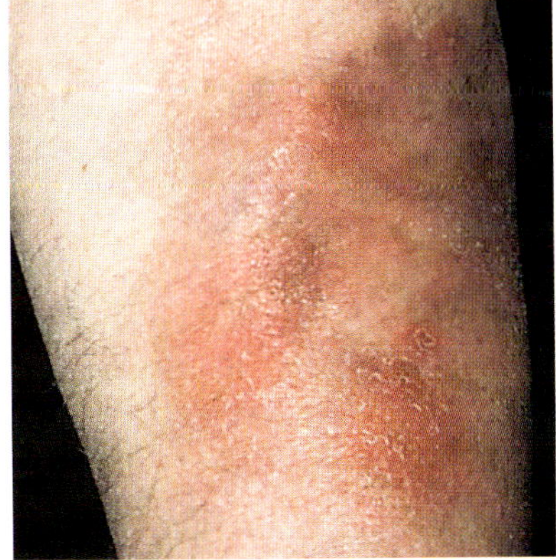

FIG. 64-6 *Pigmented scaly nodules that have become confluent (resolving lesions).*

ADJUNCTIVE DIAGNOSTIC TESTS Assessment should be undertaken for the presence of tuberculosis, namely, a Mantoux skin test and a chest x-ray. Demonstration of Mycobacterium tuberculosis DNA can be accomplished in sections of tissue of biopsy specimens by polymerase chain reaction.

COURSE The earliest lesion of nodular vasculitis is a reddish macule that soon becomes papular and nodular, and within weeks usually proceeds to ulceration. In the ensuing months, the lesion heals as a depressed scar accompanied by altered pigmentation.

INTEGRATION: UNIFYING CONCEPT Nodular vasculitis is fundamentally an arteritis. As a consequence of severe compromise of the function of a muscle-rich vessel situated in a septum in the subcutaneous fat, infarction occurs with resultant necrosis of large numbers of adipocytes in fat lobules. Other sequelae include suppuration as a consequence of the chemotactic effects of necrotic adipocytes on neutrophils, and, in time, foci of granulomatous inflammation, followed, still later, by fibrosis. Sometimes all of the stages are present concurrently in tissue sections of a single biopsy specimen. When infarction is extensive, the lesion ulcerates and necrotic fat pours to the surface of the skin. The ulcer heals with a scar within the dermis.

Nodular vasculitis almost always occurs on the calf or calves of short, thick-legged women. Tall, thin-legged women never develop the condition. The cause of nodular vasculitis usually cannot be determined, but if it is shown to be the tubercle bacillus, the condition is then designated erythema induratum. In short, erythema induratum is simply nodular vasculitis caused by Mycobacterium tuberculosis.

THERAPY If the underlying cause is tuberculosis (erythema induratum), treatment should be directed at elimination of the Mycobacteria by means of antituberculous agents.

For nontubercular lesions, treatment should include bed rest and the administration of anti-inflammatory drugs that are either corticosteroids or nonsteroidal ones. Other modalities that may be employed include potassium iodide and methotrexate.

DEFINITION An inflammatory process of unknown cause consisting of pruritic coin-shaped lesions of different sizes and made up of vesicles that soon are scratched away, leaving erosions, ulcerations, and crusts as residua.

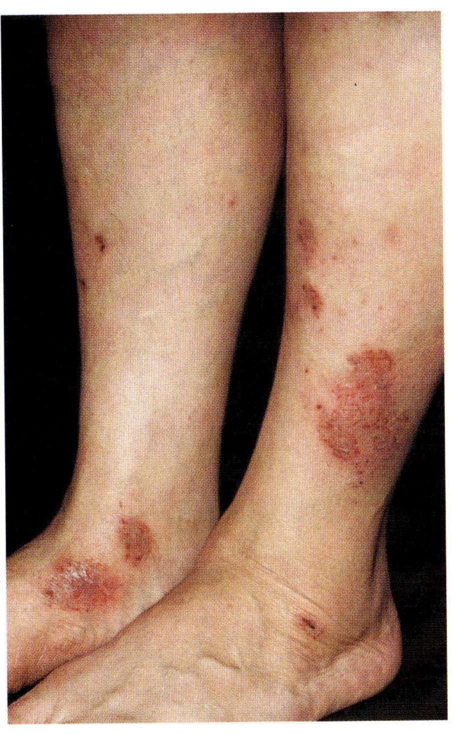

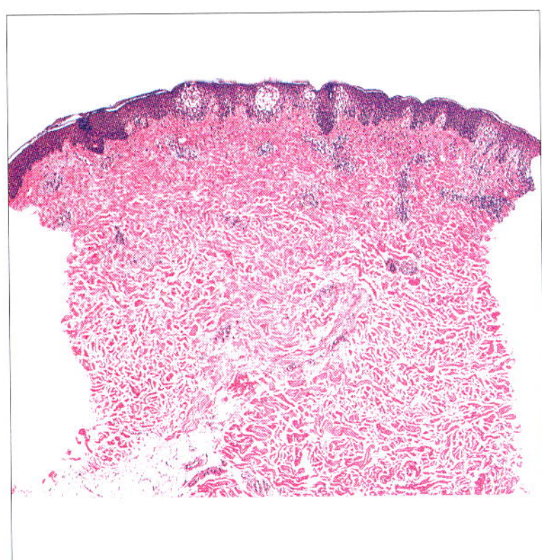

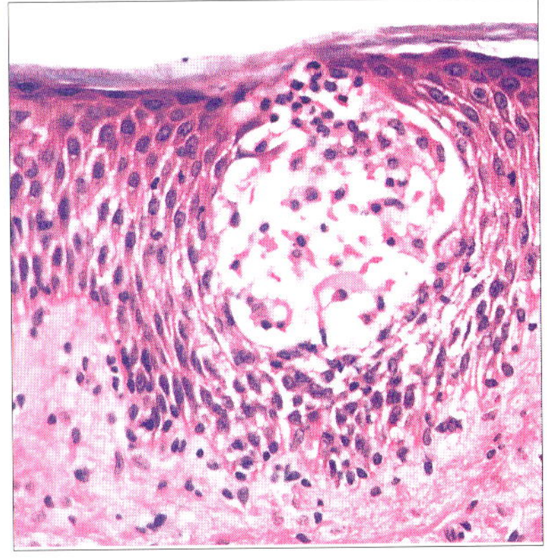

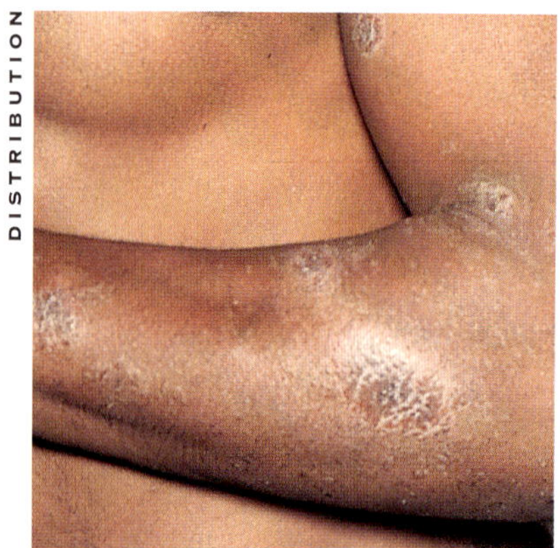

FIG. 65-1 *Nummular plaques covered by scale-crusts, as well as papules topped by scales.*

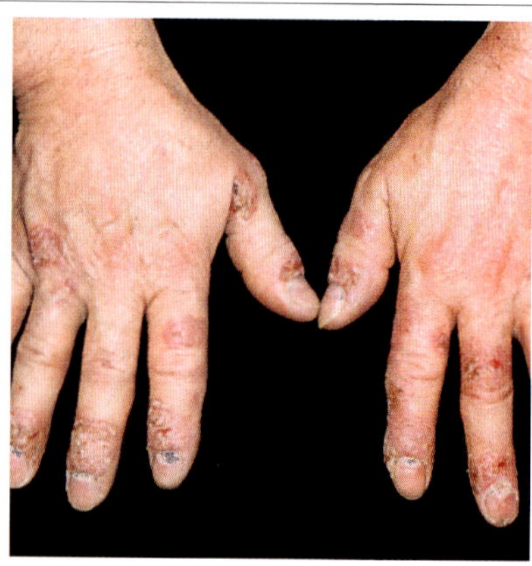

FIG. 65-2 *Eroded, crusted, nummular plaques.*

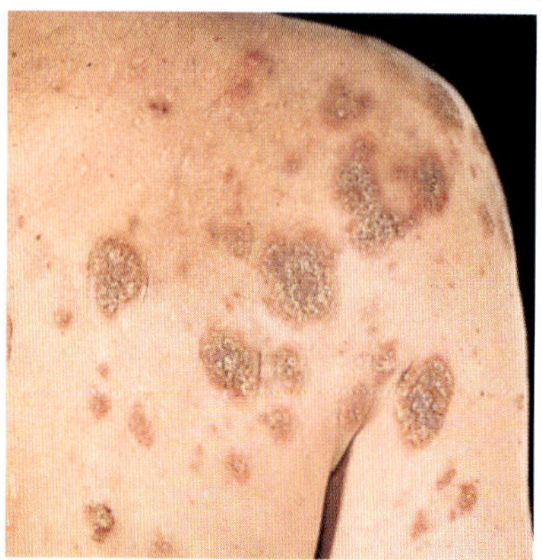

FIG. 65-3 *Crusted papules and nummular plaques.*

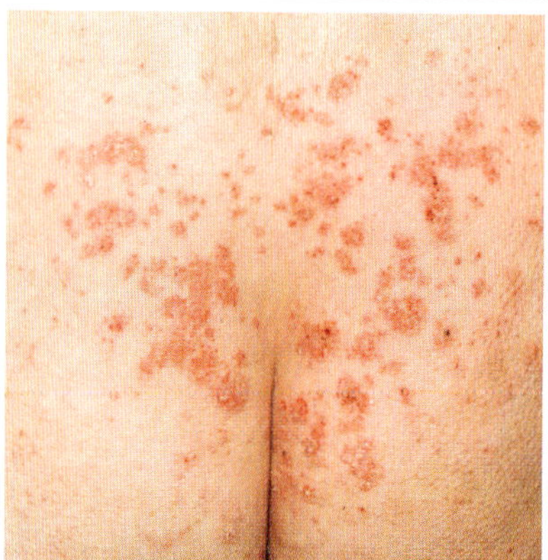

FIG. 65-4 *Scaly, crusted papules and nummular plaques.*

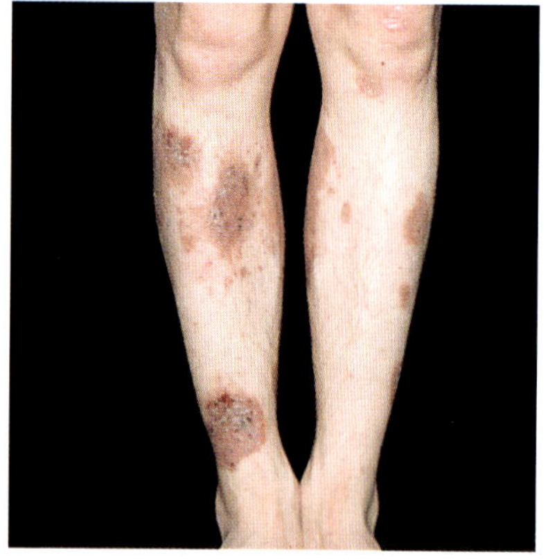

FIG. 65-5 *Small and large nummular plaques covered by hemorrhagic crusts. The erosions follow animated scratching.*

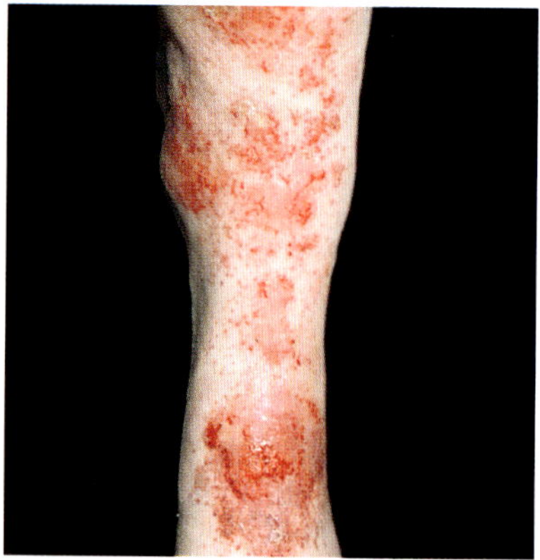

FIG. 65-6 *Nummular plaques punctuated by erosions produced by excoriation.*

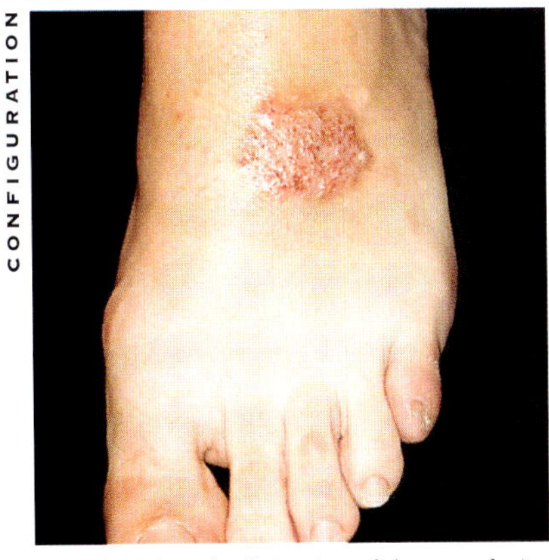 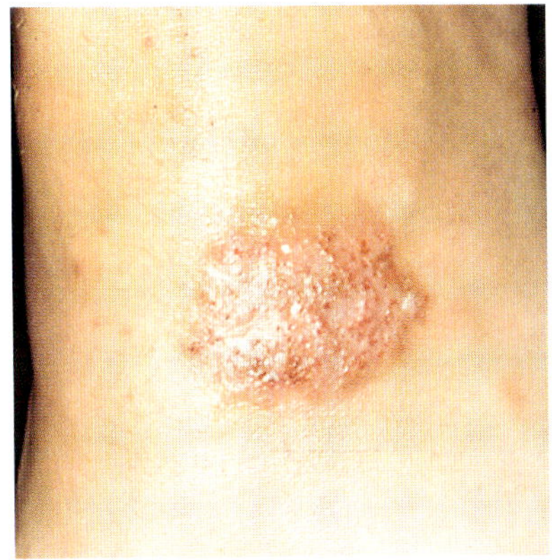

FIG. 65-7 (A, B) *Coin-shaped (nummular) plaque made up of tiny vesicles and crusts. There also are signs of excoriation.*

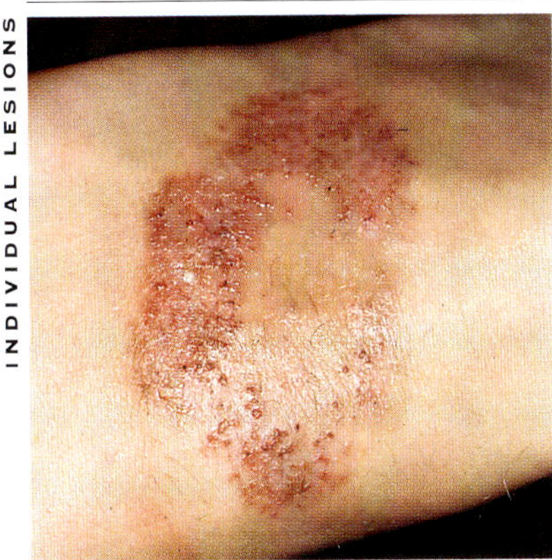 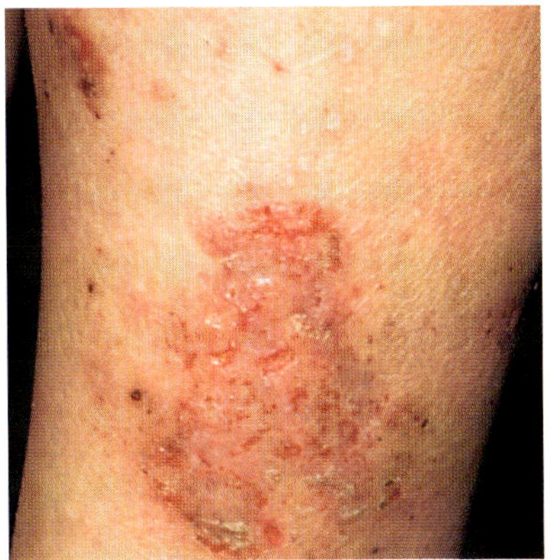

FIG. 65-8 *Vesicles eroded secondary to excoriation, with pustules consequent to impetiginization.*

FIG. 65-9 *Ill-defined nummular plaques whose surface is dotted by erosions and ulcerations secondary to furious scratching.*

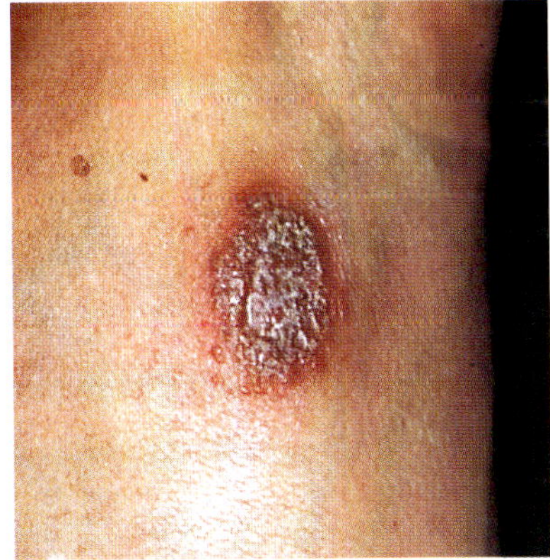 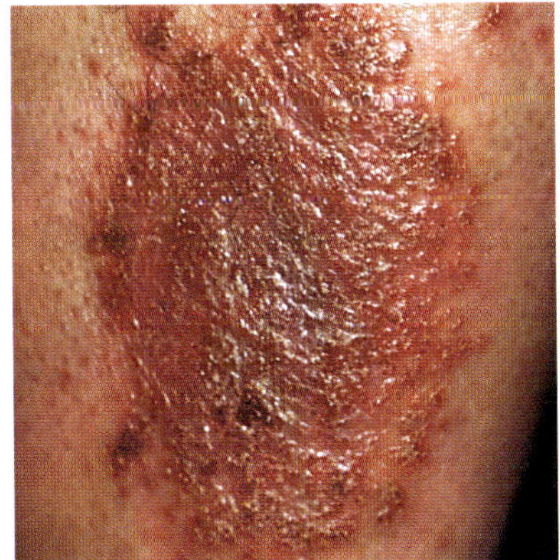

FIG. 65-10 *Coin-shaped plaque covered by scales and crusts.*

FIG. 65-11 *Poorly delimited nummular plaque composed of tiny papules and papulovesicles covered by scales and crusts.*

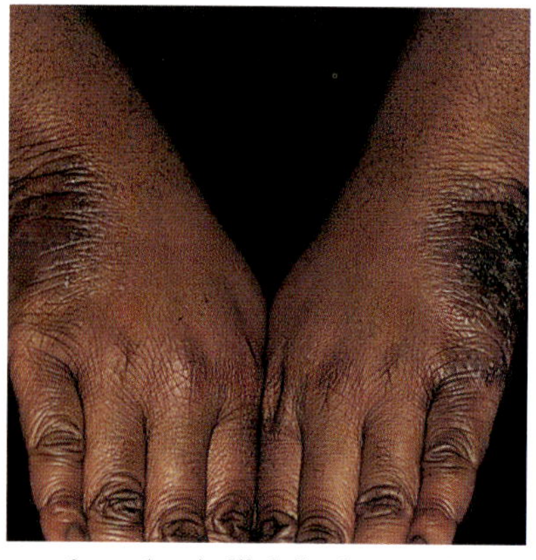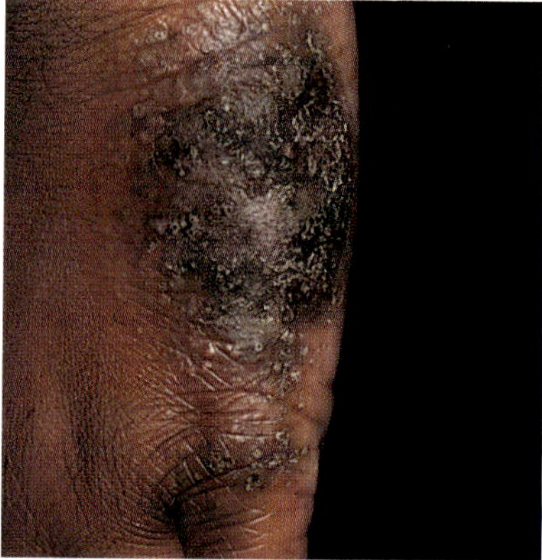

FIG. 65-12 (A, B) *Ill-defined nummular plaques covered by scales and crusts.*

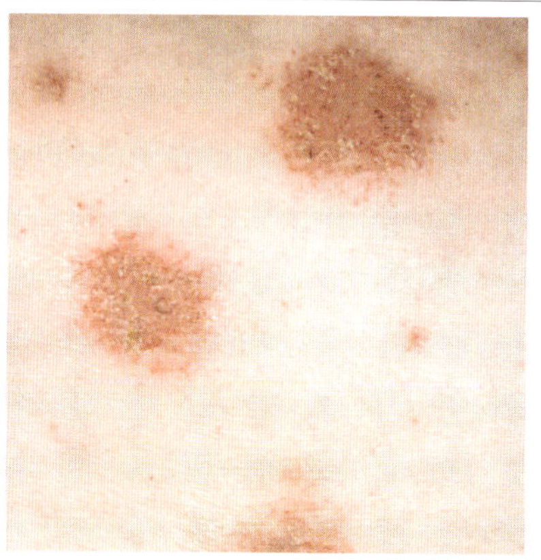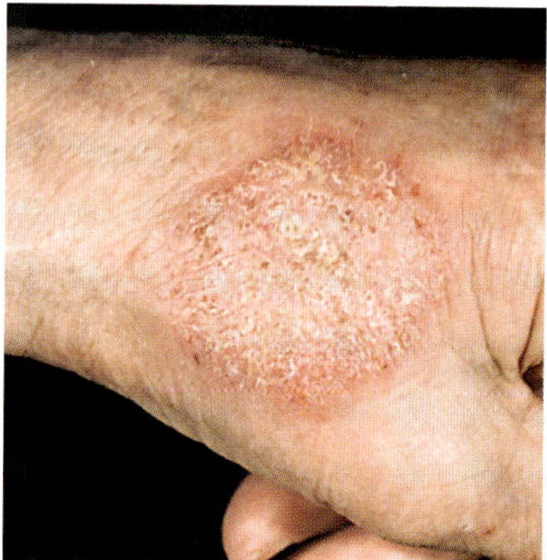

FIG. 65-13 *Longstanding lesions of nummular dermatitis with evidence of lichen simplex chronicus.*

FIG. 65-14 *Large nummular plaque surmounted by scales and scale-crusts.*

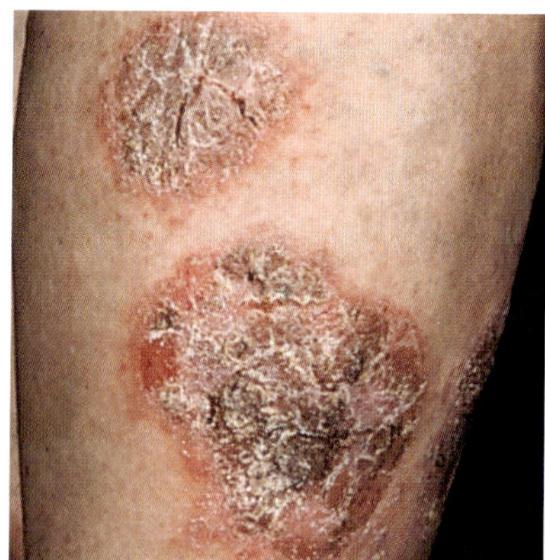

FIG. 65-15 *Nummular plaques covered by thick scale-crusts and associated with erosions and fissures.*

ADJUNCTIVE DIAGNOSTIC TEST Patch tests enable an allergic contactant to be identified when the cause is truly allergic. Usually no cause is proven.

COURSE Nummular dermatitis usually begins as a pink macule that rapidly becomes vesicular. A macule and then a patch of nummular dermatitis is studded with vesicles. Such pristine lesions are not often seen, because the condition is inordinately pruritic and animated excoriation by a person afflicted quickly destroys the vesicles. By the time patients with nummular dermatitis visit a physician, they usually sport impetiginized crusted plaques, and signs of persistent rubbing (lichen simplex chronicus) and of excoriations (erosions and ulcerations). Vesicular lesions of nummular dermatitis may resolve in weeks without much residuum. If, however, lesions are rubbed and scratched intensely, individual plaques may last for months. Sometimes macules of nummular dermatitis become papules prior to vesiculation.

The course of nummular dermatitis itself is unpredictable; sometimes lesions erupt and disappear in a short time. In other instances, lesions continue to appear and to resolve. The process, marked by exacerbations and remissions, tends to go on for years.

INTEGRATION: UNIFYING CONCEPT Nummular dermatitis is fundamentally a spongiotic vesicular dermatitis that is indistinguishable histopathologically from allergic contact dermatitis, dyshidrotic dermatitis, and an id reaction. It can be differentiated clinically from those conditions by virtue of the coin shape that clusters of papules and vesicles, initially, and scale-crusts, later, assume. Although the cause of nummular dermatitis is not known, the fact that it sometimes occurs together with signs of allergic contact dermatitis and, occasionally with an id reaction, prompts the inference that delayed hypersensitivity may play a part in its development.

Longstanding lesions of nummular dermatitis may not be identifiable for what they are, clinically or histopathologically, because the fundamental process has been obscured by findings of lichen simplex chronicus, sometimes accompanied by signs of excoriation. Only the coin shape of lesions can provide a hint of the original spongiotic nature. The "distinctive exudative discoid and lichenoid chronic dermatosis" of Sulzberger and Garbe was simply nummular dermatitis.

THERAPY Topical corticosteroids are helpful for vesicular and crusted lesions, and oral antibiotics for impetiginized ones.

DEFINITION A keratotic condition of the palms and soles, inherited usually, but sometimes acquired, in which involvement may be diffuse, circumscribed (including striate), or punctate.

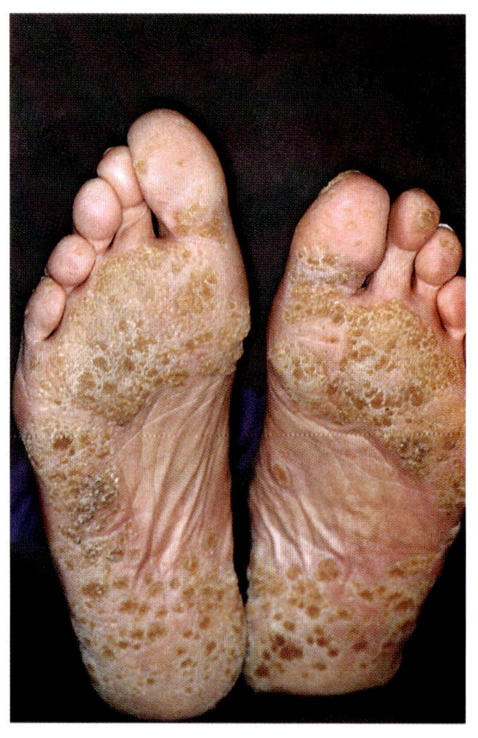

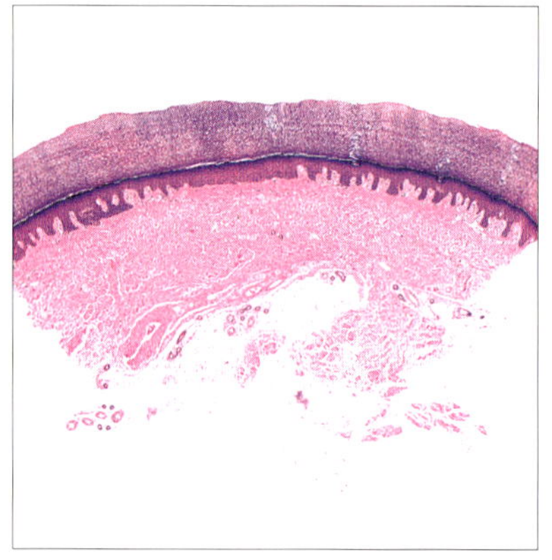

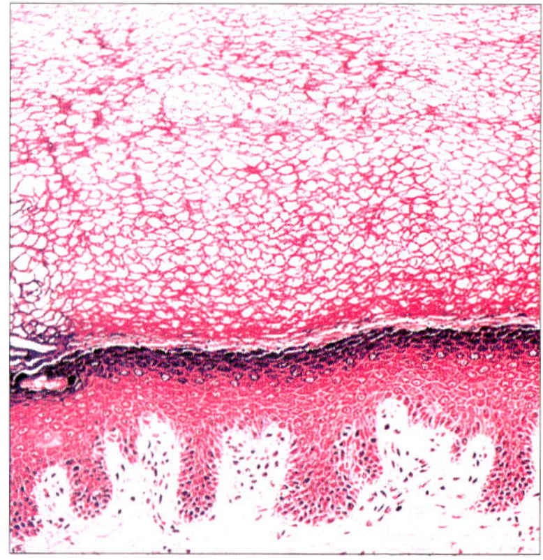

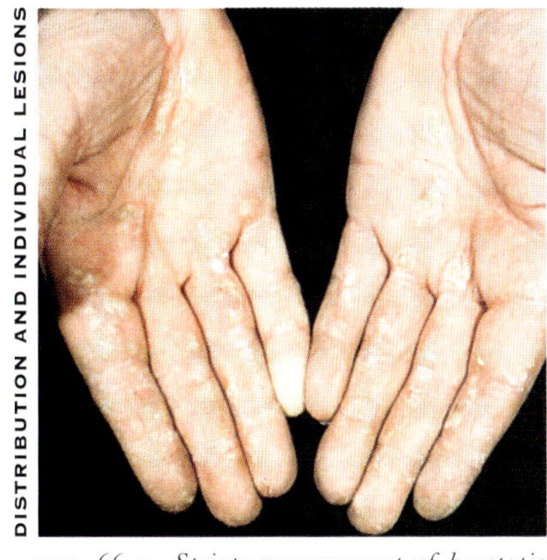

FIG. 66-1 *Striate arrangement of keratotic lesions.*

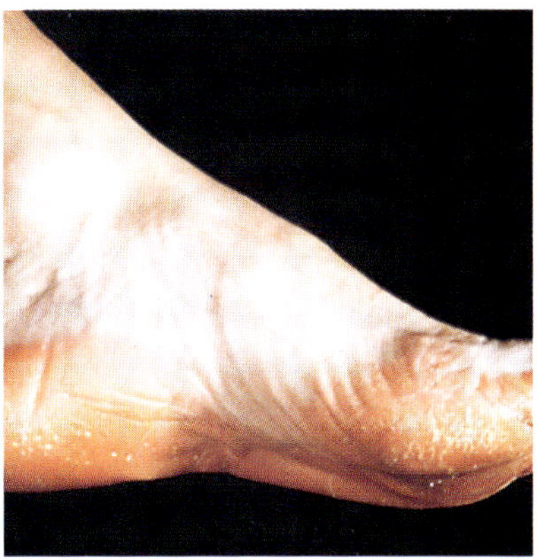

FIG. 66-2 *Diffuse keratoderma.*

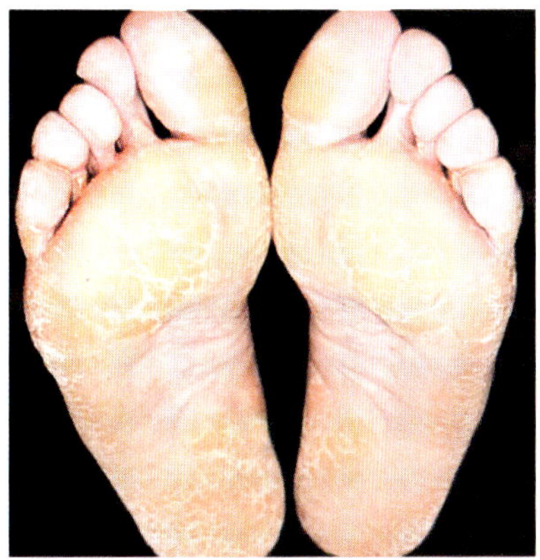

FIG. 66-3 *Circumscribed keratoderma.*

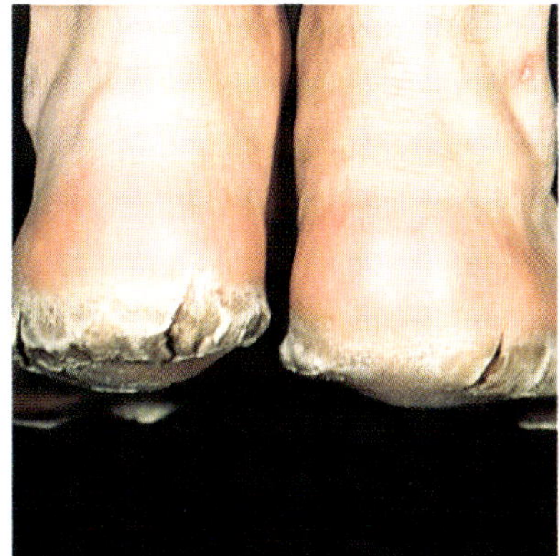

FIG. 66-4 *Circumscribed keratoderma with prominent fissures.*

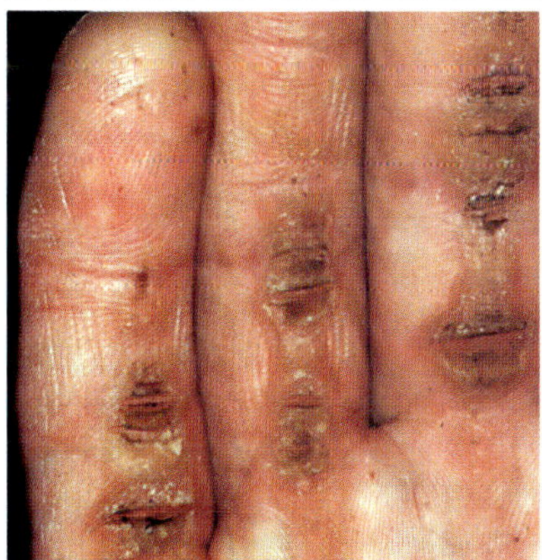

FIG. 66-5 *Circumscribed striate keratoderma.*

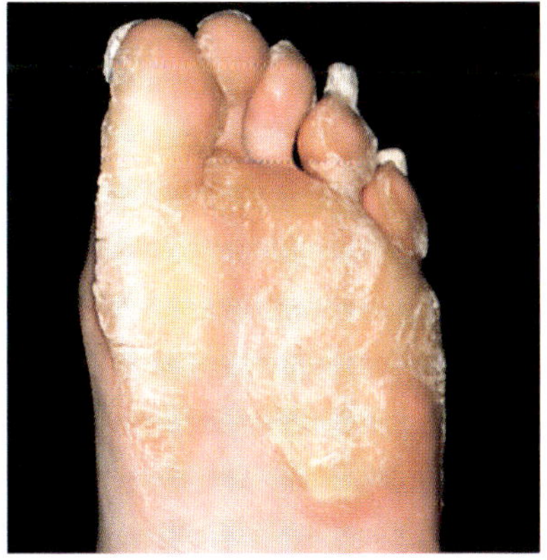

FIG. 66-6 *Circumscribed keratoderma.*

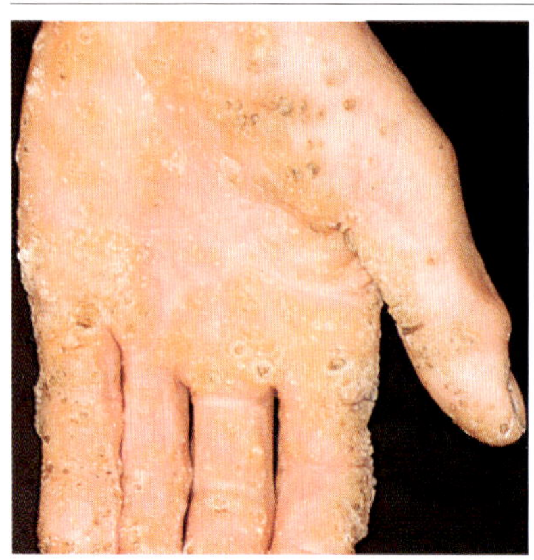

FIG. 66-7 *Keratoderma punctatum.*

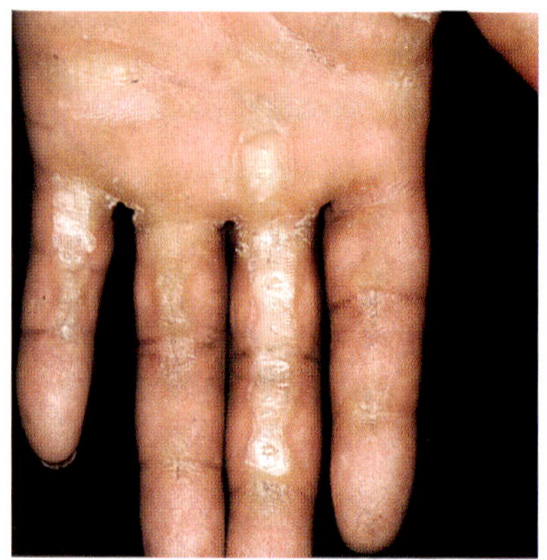

FIG. 66-8 *Keratoderma striatum.*

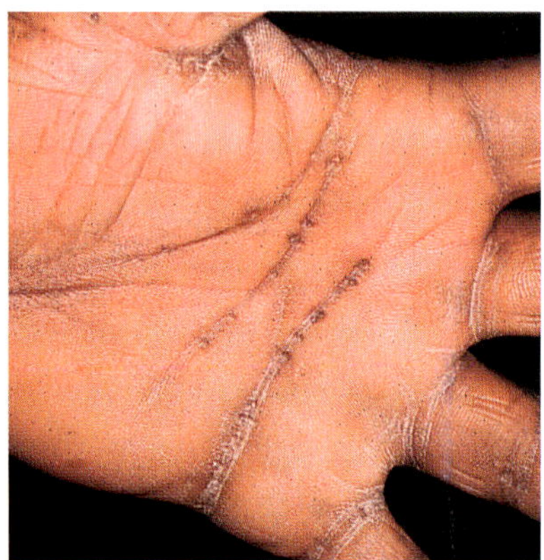

FIG. 66-9 *Localized punctate keratoderma situated in creases of a palm.*

COURSE Once lesions of palmar and plantar keratoderma appear, generally in late childhood or early adulthood, they tend to persist for a lifetime. The lesions, as the title denotes, are keratotic, and may be punctate, striate, or confluent. Each of those types retains its character for the entire course of the process.

INTEGRATION: UNIFYING CONCEPT Palmar and plantar keratoderma is one expression of a basic disorder of cornification analogous to that of so-called epidermal nevi. The latter assume different shapes and have different morphologic appearances, each of which is accompanied by distinctive histopathologic findings. For example, when one type of epidermal nevus is universal, it is called bullous congenital ichthyosiform erythroderma, but when the same type is systematized, it then is termed ichthyosis hystrix; both designations are misnomers. That same type of epidermal nevus, which tends to be digitated and hyperkeratotic clinically and shows signs of epidermolytic hyperkeratosis histopathologically, may involve only palms and soles, and of them completely. On those sites the condition may be considered a palmar and plantar keratoderma, being typified as it is by innumerable digitated keratoses grossly and by epidermolytic hyperkeratosis histopathologically.

An analogy can be drawn between various forms of epidermal nevi and equivalents of them that appear on the palms and soles. First are epidermal nevi that clinically consist of keratotic papules and histopathologically are seen to display signs of focal acantholytic dyskeratosis (like that of Darier's disease), and an equivalent form confined to palms and soles. Second are epidermal nevi that are keratotic clinically and show typical features of cornoid lamellation histopathologically (like that of porokeratosis) and an equivalent form that involves palms and soles by punctate lesions of porokeratosis. Last are epidermal nevi that seem to be digitate hyperkeratotic exaggerations of normal epidermis, i.e., nevus verrucosus, and an equivalent form that involves palms and soles completely. A variety of rare and recondite keratodermas that are determined genetically and go by a host of names, among them, mal de Meleda, also affect palms and soles. They, too, can be conceived of as analogues of epidermal nevi that happen to be restricted to volar skin.

THERAPY Topical treatment consists of so-called keratinolytics, like salicylic acid, and systemic treatment for severe examples of the condition consists of oral retinoids.

DEFINITION A blistering inflammatory disease in which acantholysis occurs in the upper part of the spinous zone or granular zone of the epidermis, the result of the process being flaccid blisters that give way to erosions and crusts accompanied by erythema. When mostly the trunk is affected, the condition is termed "pemphigus foliaceus," when mostly the face and upper part of the chest are involved, it is termed "pemphigus erythematosus." The same malady in Brazil, where it occurs endemically, is designated "fogo selvagem."

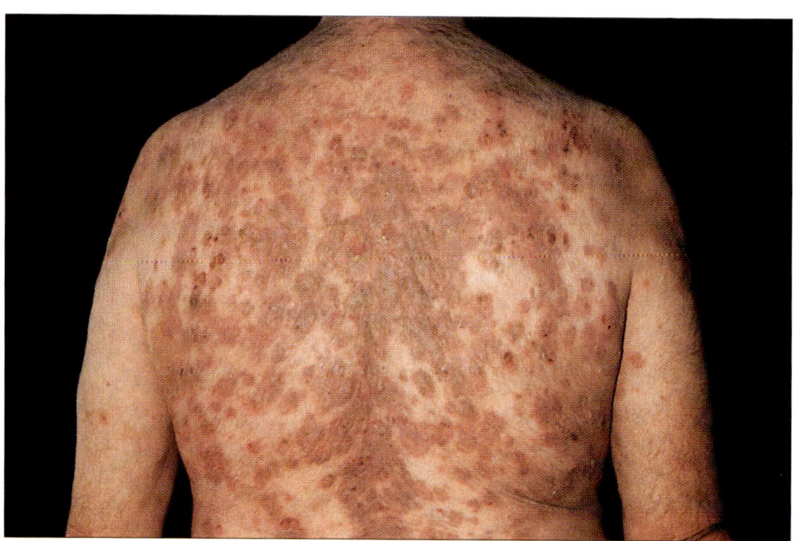

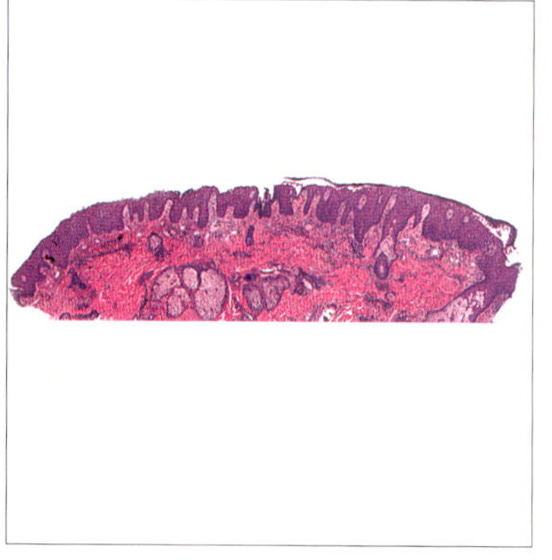

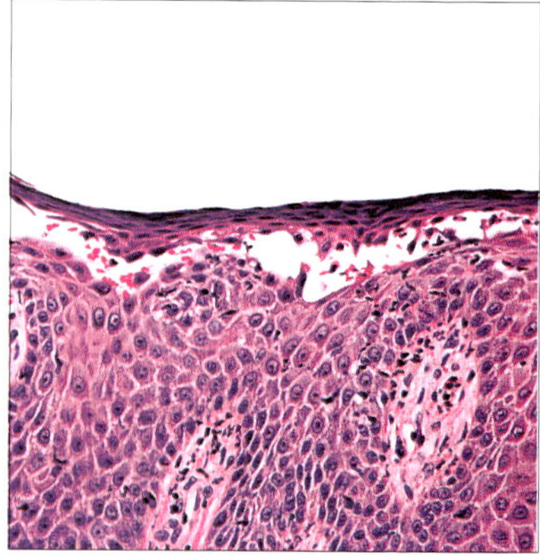

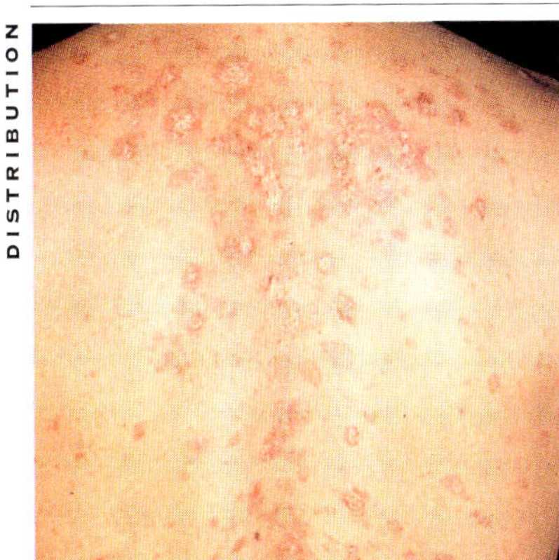

FIG. 67-1 *Numerous erosions and crusts of pemphigus foliaceus.*

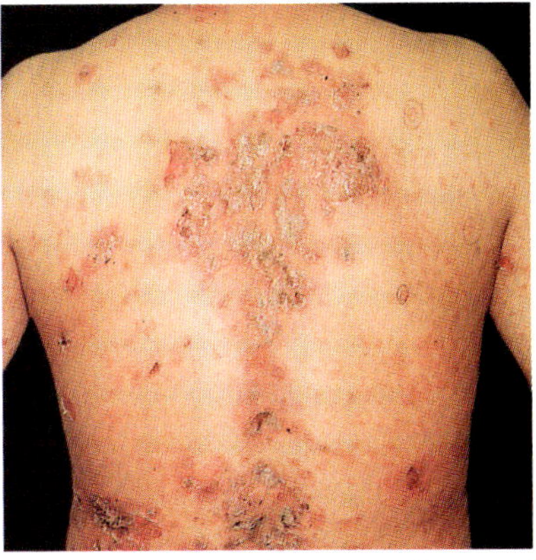

FIG. 67-2 *Widespread erosions and crusts of pemphigus foliaceus.*

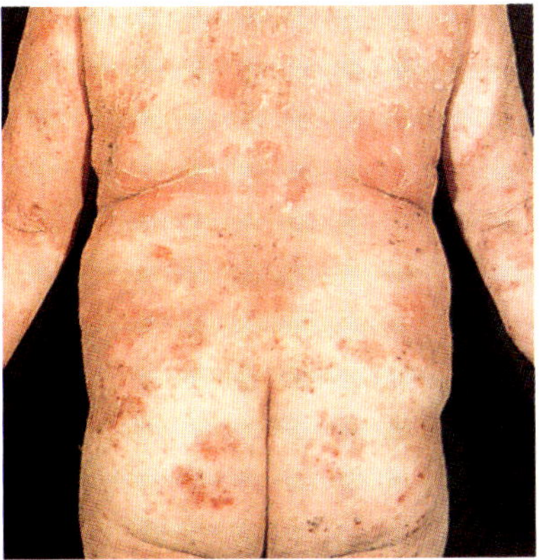

FIG. 67-3 *Widespread erosions, crusts, and scales of pemphigus foliaceus.*

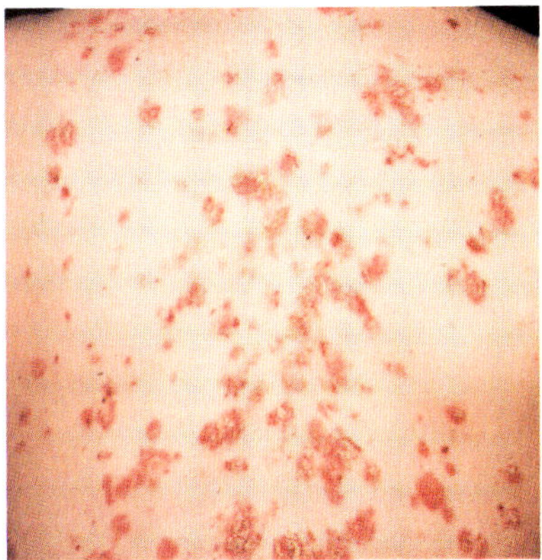

FIG. 67-4 *Erythematous macules, plaques, vesicles, and crusted erosions of pemphigus foliaceus.*

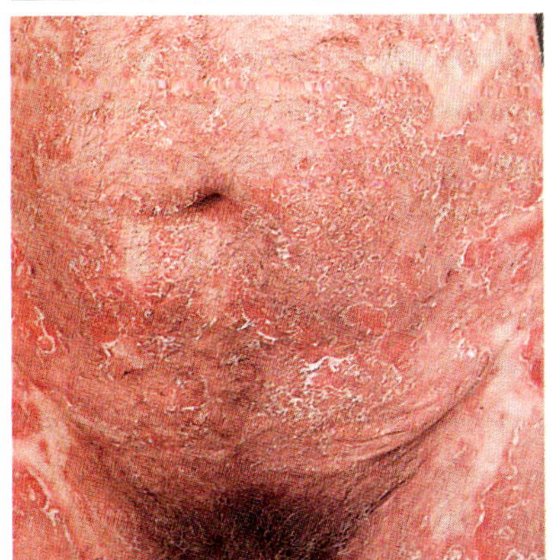

FIG. 67-5 *Confluent erosions and scales of pemphigus foliaceus.*

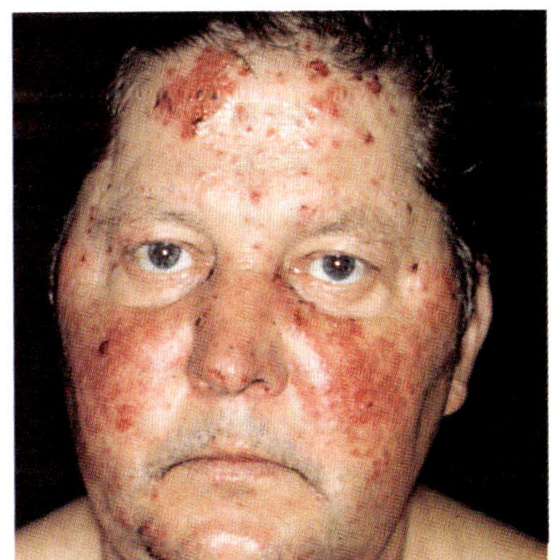

FIG. 67-6 *Erosions and hemorrhagic crusts of pemphigus erythematosus on a cushingoid face.*

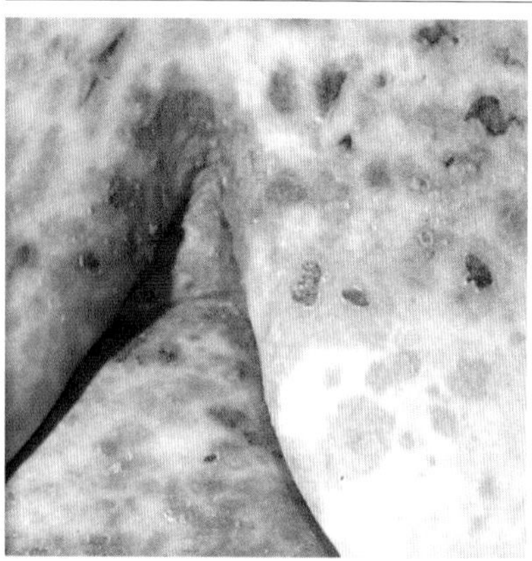

FIG. 67-7 *Erosions and crusts of pemphigus foliaceus on the trunk and breasts.*

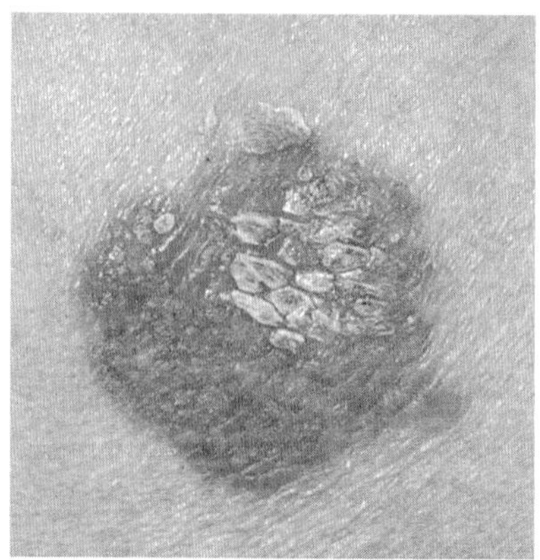

FIG. 67-8 *A re-epithelialized plaque, formerly eroded, covered by scale-crusts represents a healing lesion of pemphigus foliaceus.*

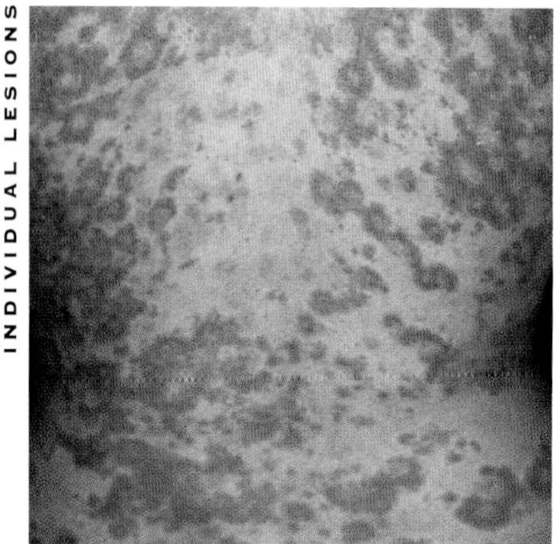

FIG. 67-9 *Eroded papules and plaques of pemphigus foliaceus.*

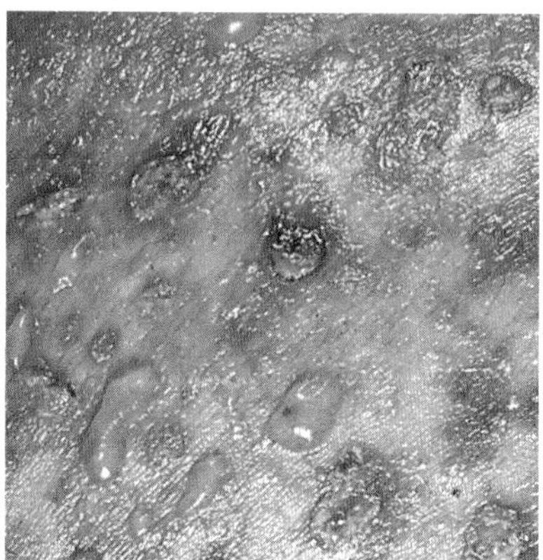

FIG. 67-10 *Vesicles, erosions, and scale-crusts of pemphigus foliaceus.*

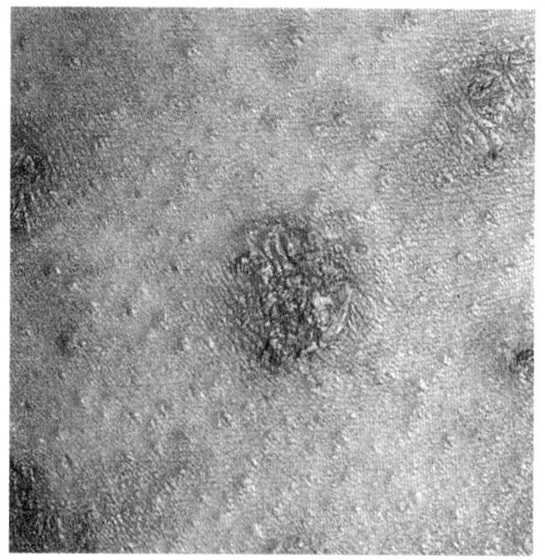

FIG. 67-11 *Crusts, scales, and hyperpigmented macules of pemphigus foliaceus.*

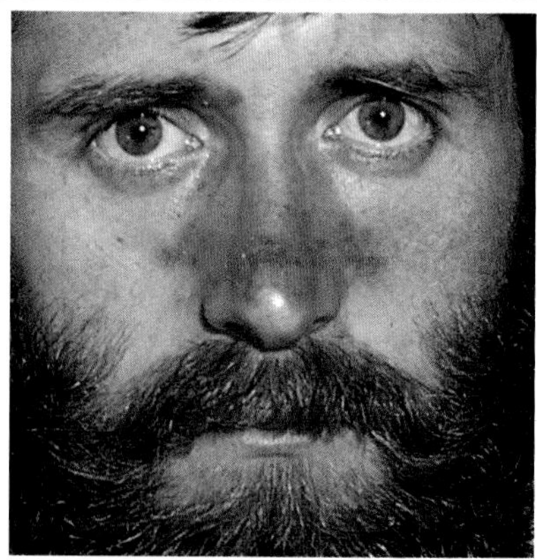

FIG. 67-12 *Erosions in distribution similar to discoid lupus erythematosus; hence the name "pemphigus erythematosus."*

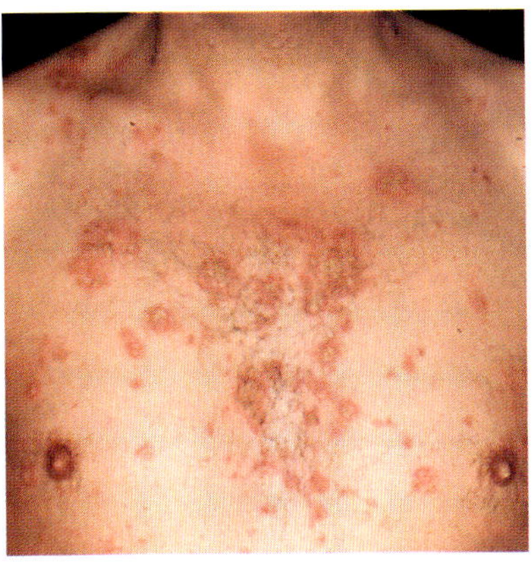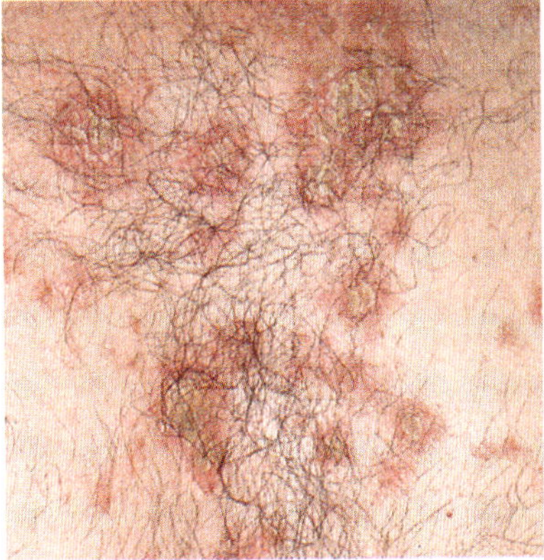

FIG. 67-13 (A, B) *Erosions, crusts, and scales in pemphigus foliaceus.*

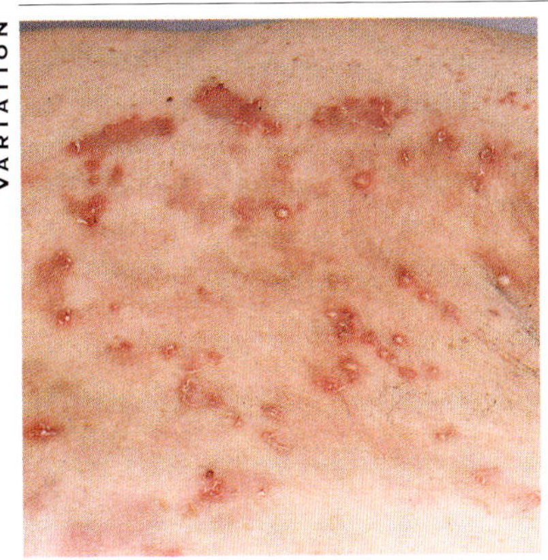

FIG. 67-14 *Pustules in groups and erosions of IgA pemphigus (subcorneal variant).*

ADJUNCTIVE DIAGNOSTIC TEST Immunofluorescence technique on cryostat sections of fresh tissue enable detection of immunoglobulins in intercellular spaces.

COURSE The primary lesion of pemphigus foliaceus is a flaccid blister that may be a vesicle or a bulla. In time, the blister breaks and an erosion comes into being. In time, the erosion is covered by crust and when that is shed, a hyperpigmented macule is residual. The process of pemphigus foliaceus itself lasts for many years and often for a lifetime. The pace of appearance of new lesions is unpredictable, but those lesions resolve in predictable fashion.

INTEGRATION: UNIFYING CONCEPT Pemphigus foliaceus is a distinctive disease in which the blister forms consequent to acantholysis in the upper part of the viable epidermis, namely, the upper part of the spinous zone and the granular zone. Within the blister, acantholytic cells are discernible. Only in ensuing days does the blister come to be situated immediately beneath the stratum corneum, i.e., subcorneally. When lesions of pemphigus foliaceus, which favor the trunk especially, affect the face and the chest in photodistribution, the same condition is known as pemphigus erythematosus (Senear-Usher syndrome). A type of pemphigus foliaceus that occurs endemically in areas of Brazil especially, but also in other parts of South and Central America, and that affects children and adults, is known as fogo selvagem ("wild fire"). The histopathologic findings in pemphigus erythematosus and in fogo selvagem are identical to those in pemphigus foliaceus, all of those conditions seeming to represent a single pathologic process, possibly of different causes.

The term "pemphigus," like "nevus," "id," and "pseudopelade," is confusing because it is used for several different, unrelated conditions. Literally, pemphigus means a blister. Hailey-Hailey disease is a blistering disease wholly unrelated to pemphigus foliaceus, or to any other disease named pemphigus, yet it was originally named "familial benign chronic pemphigus" and often is referred to by that appellation to this day. Pemphigus vulgaris is very different in nearly all respects from pemphigus foliaceus. Even immunopathologically, pemphigus foliaceus differs from pemphigus vulgaris, the antibodies in the former being directed against desmoglein 1 and plakoglobin and those in the latter against desmoglein 3 and plakoglobin. Pemphigus vegetans is simply heaped up, i.e., vegetating, lesions of long-standing pemphigus vulgaris. Pemphigus neonatorum is staphylococcal scalded-skin syndrome, butcher's pemphigus is also a staphylococcal infection, and paraneoplastic pemphigus is not basically a blistering disease, but a dermatitis of the face that develops as a consequence of the effects of a carcinoma or a lymphoma in an internal organ. In sum, all of the diseases known as pemphigus are very different from one another, clinically, histopathologically, and biologically.

THERAPY Systemic corticosteroids are indicated for widespread lesions and in a dosage like that used in treatment of pemphigus vulgaris.

DEFINITION A blistering disease of skin and mucous membranes that presents itself in the skin first as flaccid bullae that soon become eroded, and in mucous membranes as erosions, hemorrhagic crusts, or both. If widespread and untreated, the disease can be fatal.

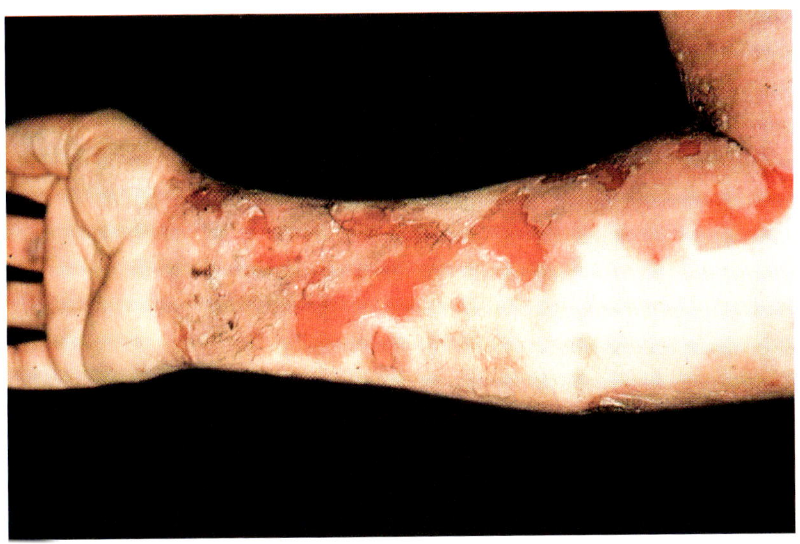

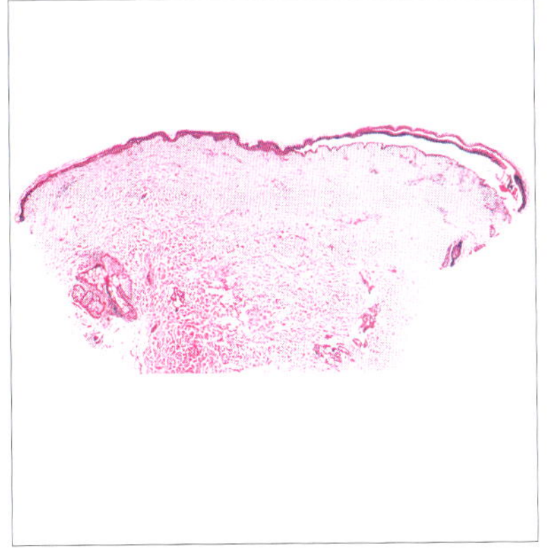

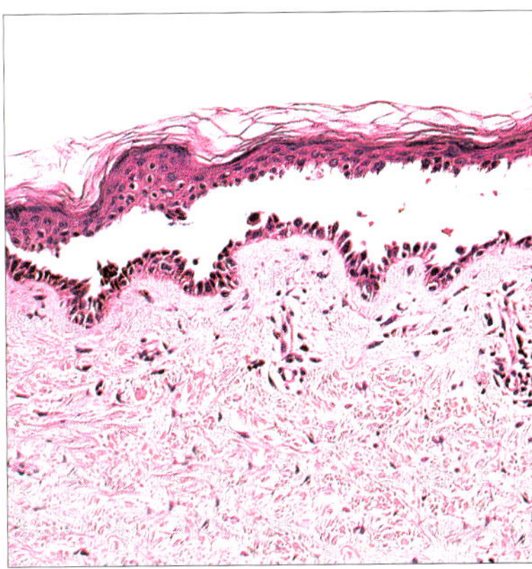

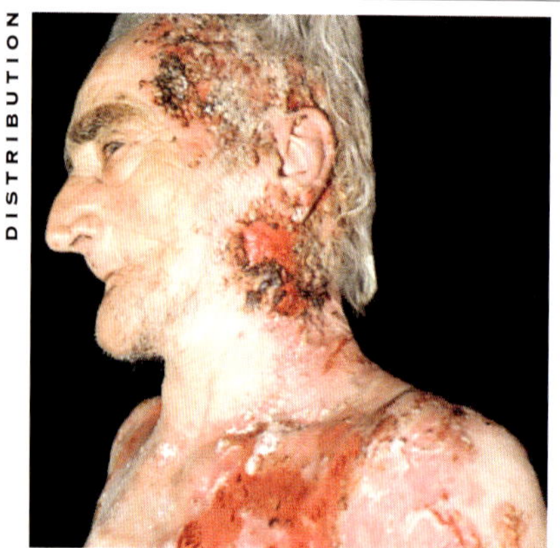

FIG. 68-1 *Widespread erosions and hemorrhagic crusts.*

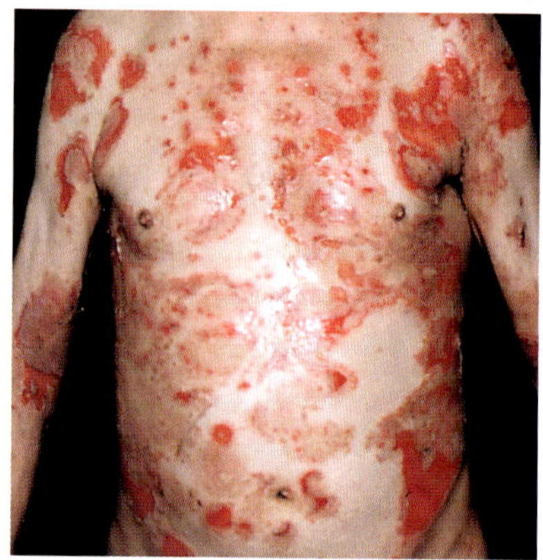

FIG. 68-2 *Scattered tense vesicles and erosions surrounded by the residua of flaccid blisters.*

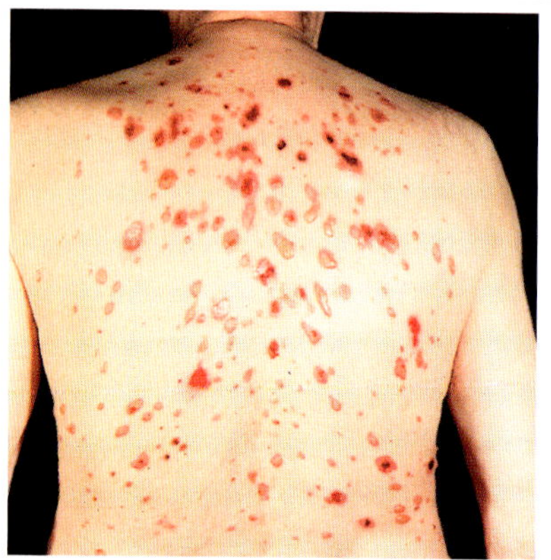

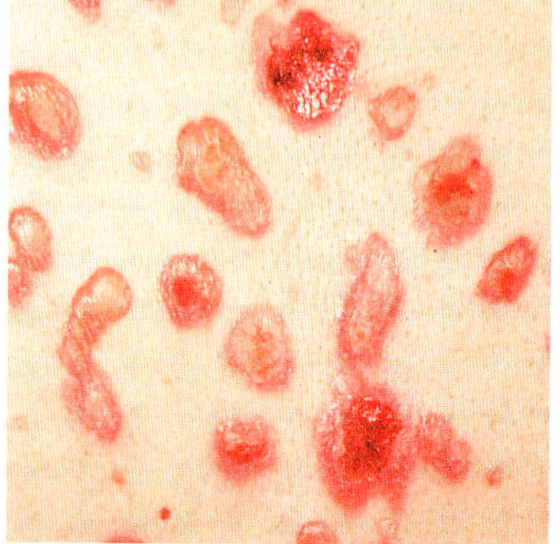

FIG. 68-3 (A, B) *Widespread vesicles, bullae, erosions, and hemorrhagic crusts.*

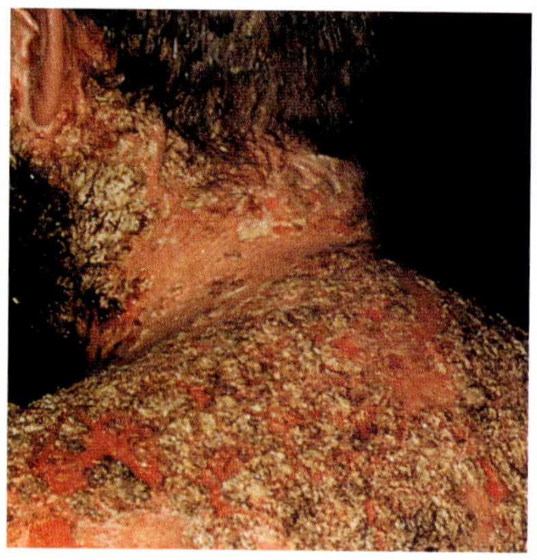

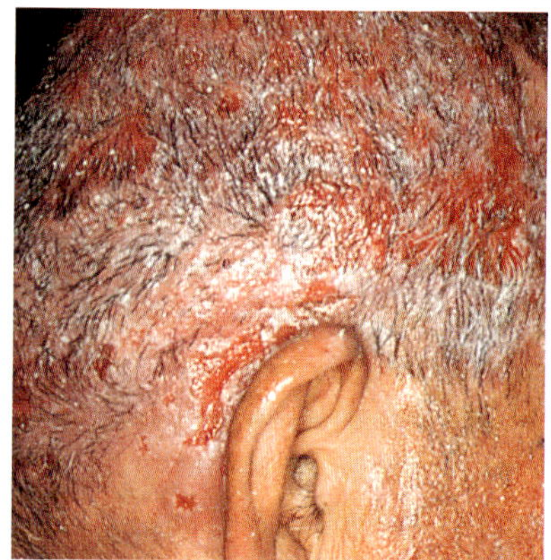

FIG. 68-4 *Widespread erosions and thick scale-crusts.*

FIG. 68-5 *Erosions.*

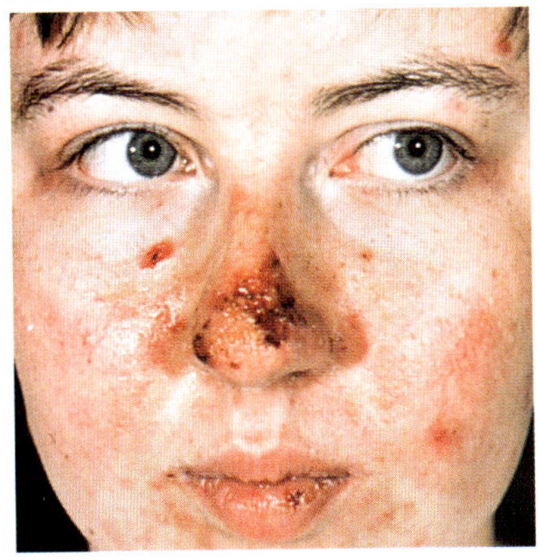

FIG. 68-6 *Erosions and hemorrhagic crusts on the nose and lips.*

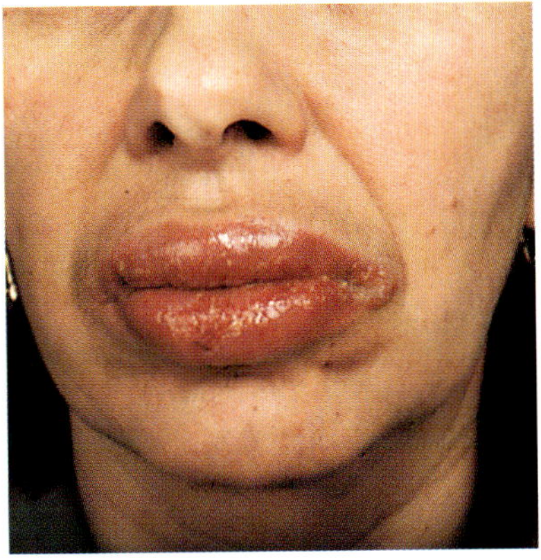

FIG. 68-7 *Erosions and crusts, as well as vegetating lesions.*

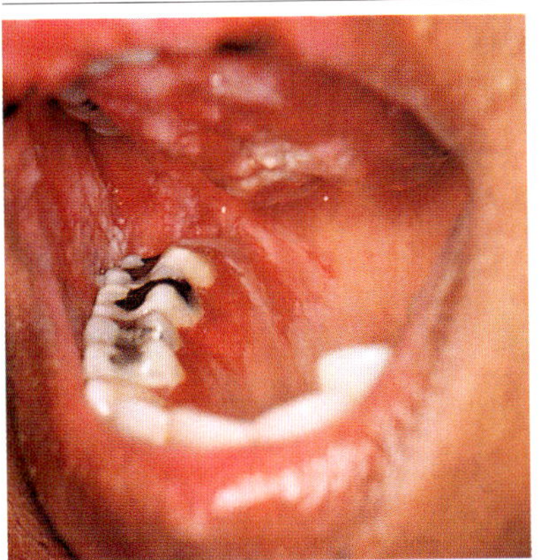

FIG. 68-8 *Erosions and signs of maceration on the buccal mucosa.*

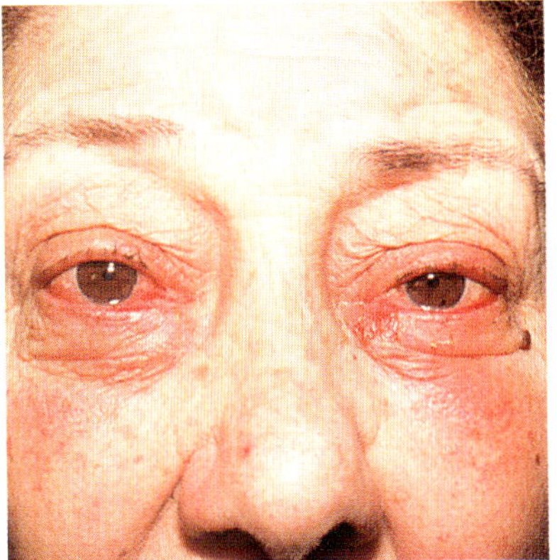

FIG. 68-9 *Erosion on the left eyelid and conjunctivitis bilaterally.*

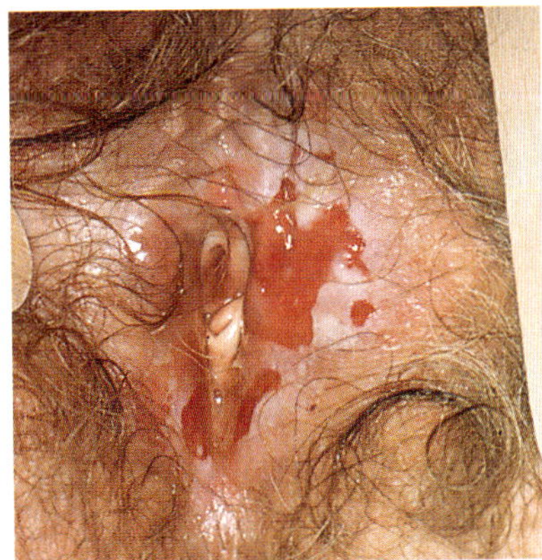

FIG. 68-10 *Erosions and ulcers, in company with maceration, on the vulva.*

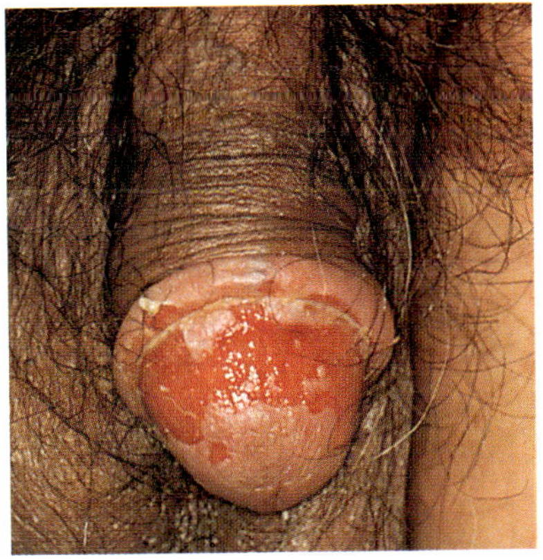

FIG. 68-11 *Erosion with ragged edges.*

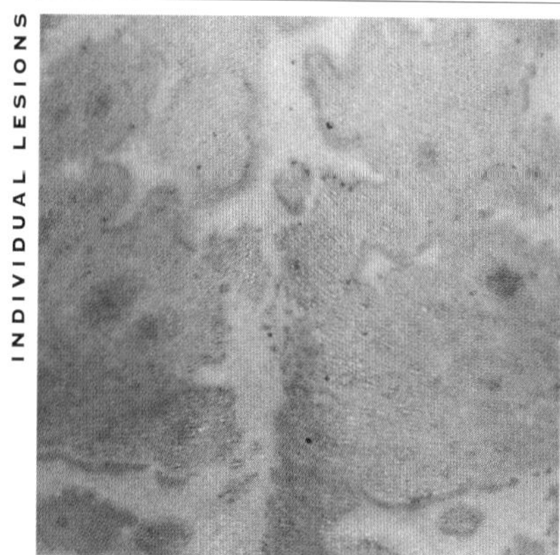

FIG. 68-12 *Hyperpigmented patches at the periphery of which are urticarial papules.*

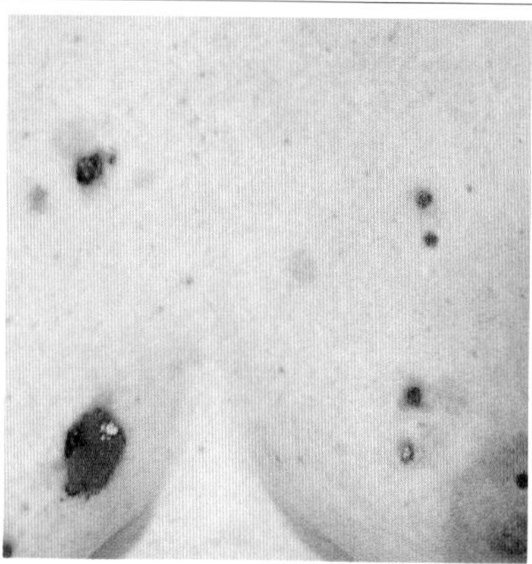

FIG. 68-13 *Erosions and hemorrhagic crusts.*

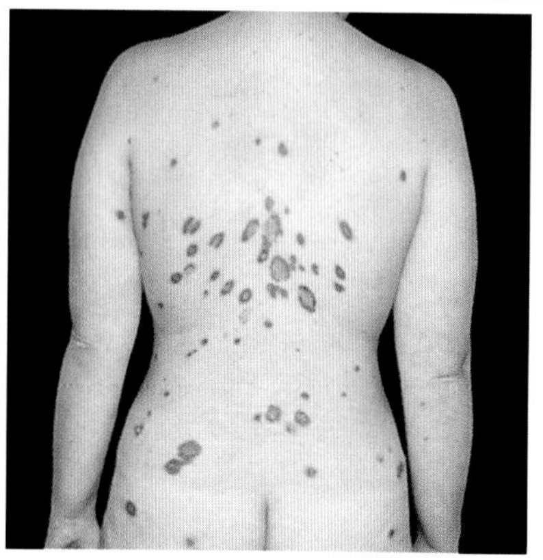

FIG. 68-14 *Eroded plaques, some with annular and arcuate shape.*

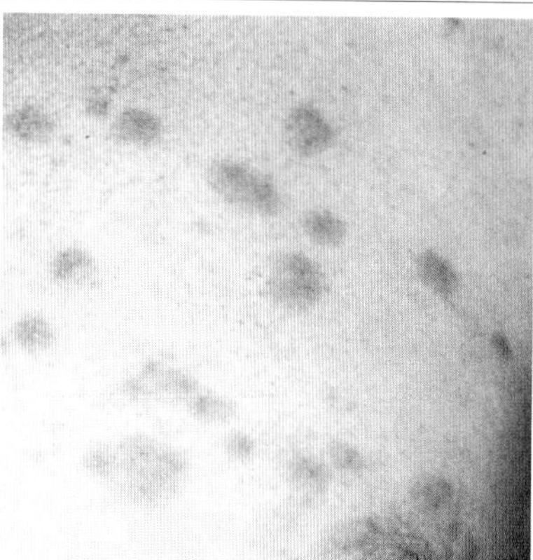

FIG. 68-15 *Urticarial papules and plaques.*

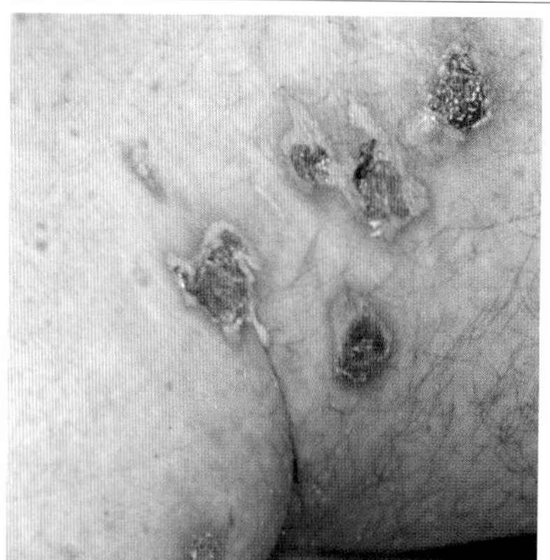

FIG. 68-16 *Flaccid blisters at the margin of erosions and ulcerations that are covered by hemorrhagic crusts.*

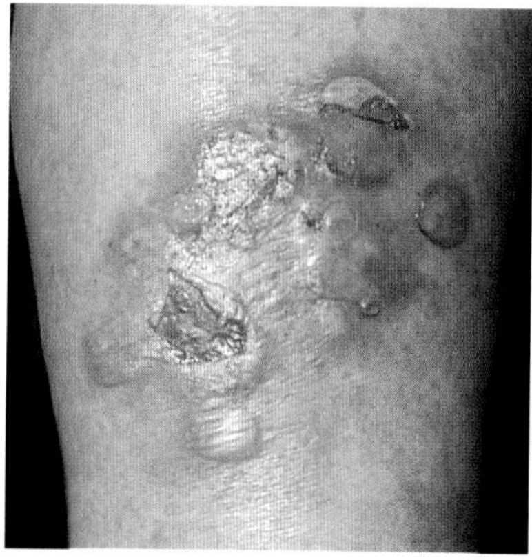

FIG. 68-17 *Vesicle and flaccid bullae in conjunction with erosions.*

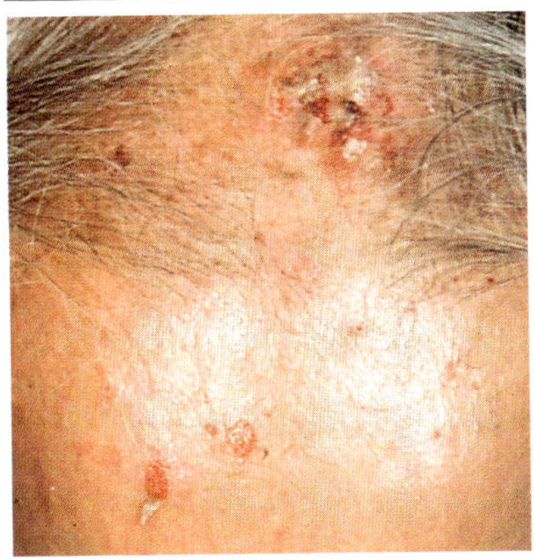

FIG. 68-18 *Erosions and crusts.*

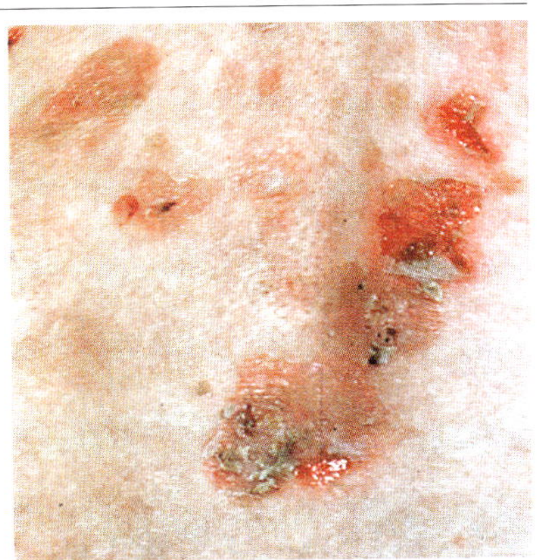

FIG. 68-19 *Flaccid blisters, erosions, and crusts.*

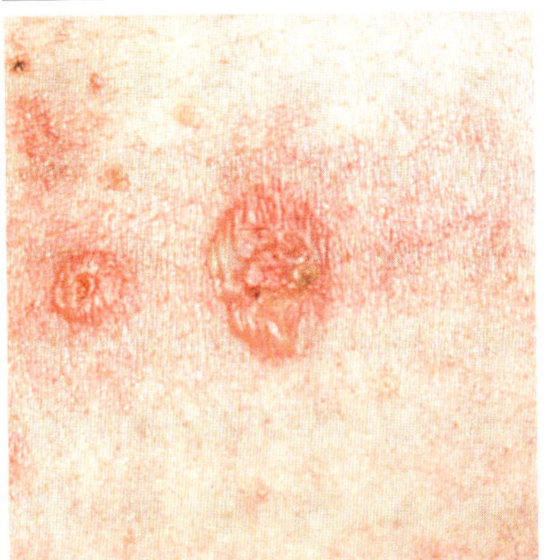

FIG. 68-20 *Flaccid vesicle and bulla.*

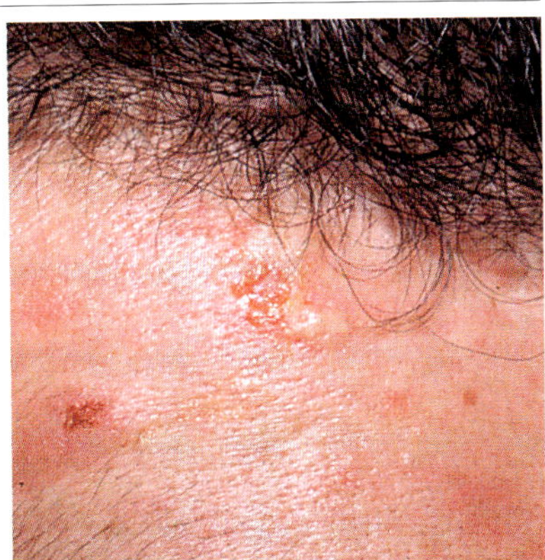

FIG. 68-21 *Flaccid blisters and erosions.*

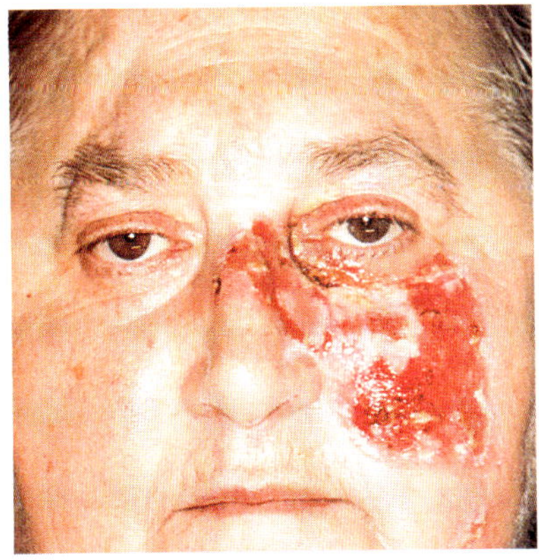

FIG. 68-22 *Large erosion associated with crusts and with signs of re-epithelialization.*

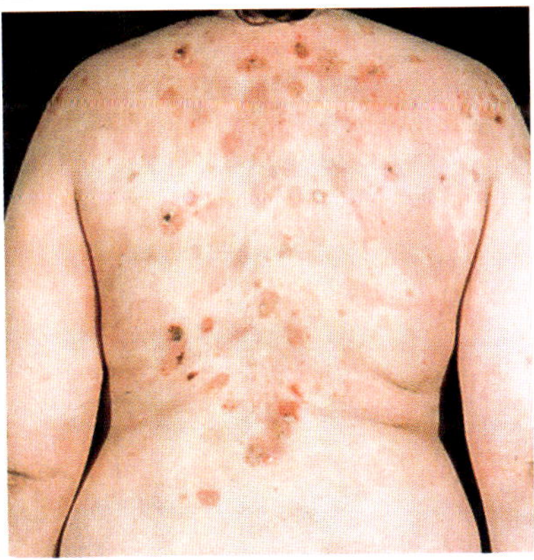

FIG. 68-23 *Flaccid bullae, erosions covered by crusts, and pigmented patches, the latter a sign of lesions having resolved completely.*

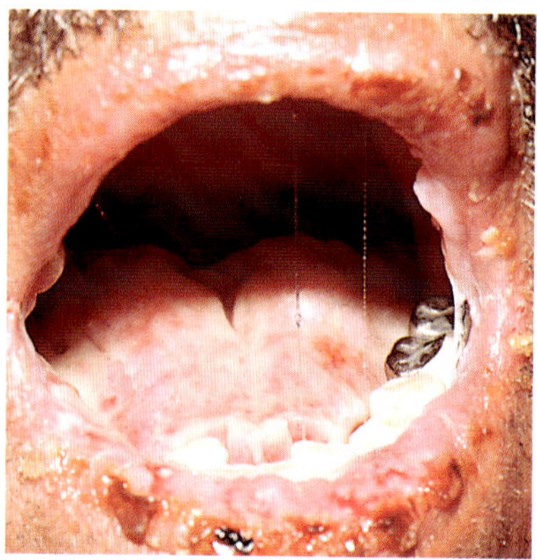

FIG. 68-24 *Erosions and crusts on the lips and buccal mucosa.*

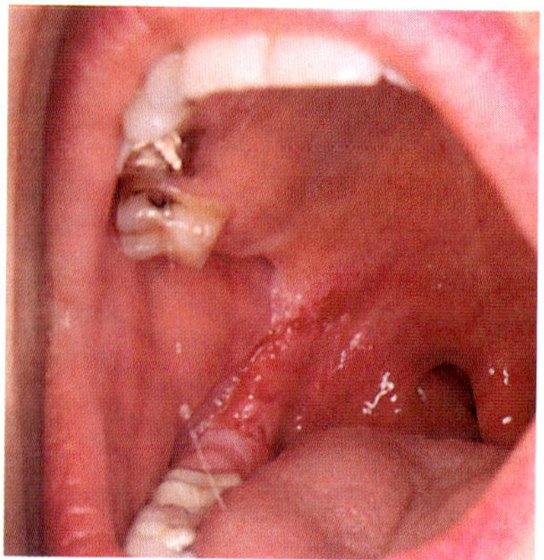

FIG. 68-25 *Ulcerations with jagged outlines on the buccal mucosa and gingival ridge.*

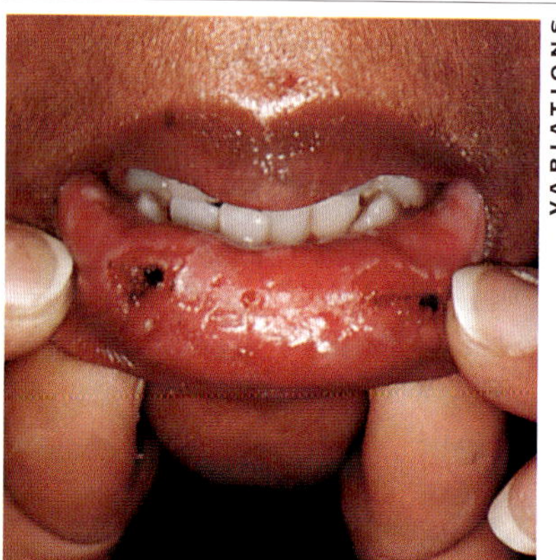

FIG. 68-26 *Erosions and crusts.*

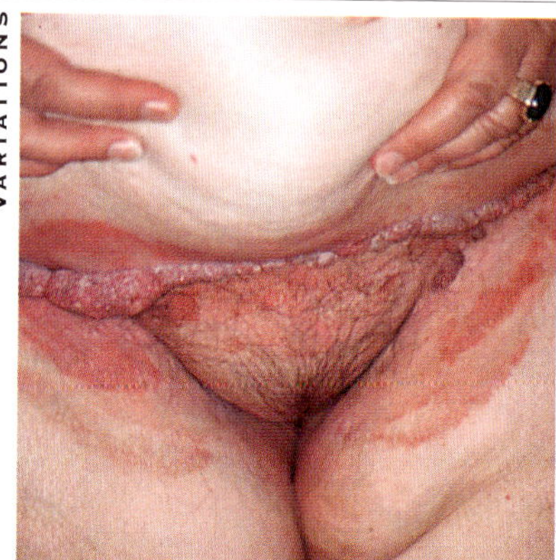

FIG. 68-27 *Vegetations in intertriginous folds (pemphigus vegetans, i.e., vegetating lesions at sites of previous blisters).*

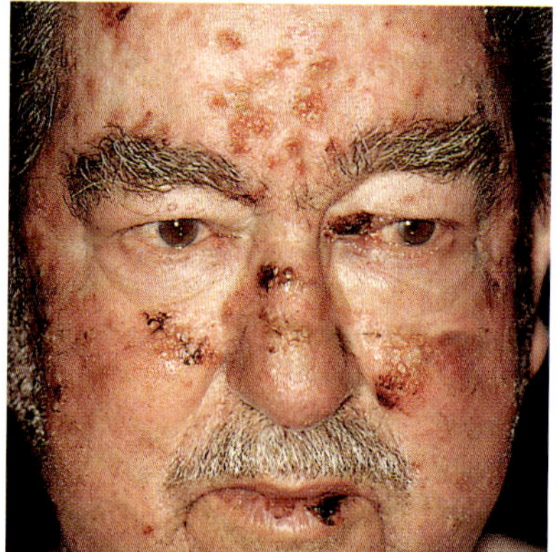

FIG. 68-28 *Erosions and crusts, some hemorrhagic, involving the face and lips.*

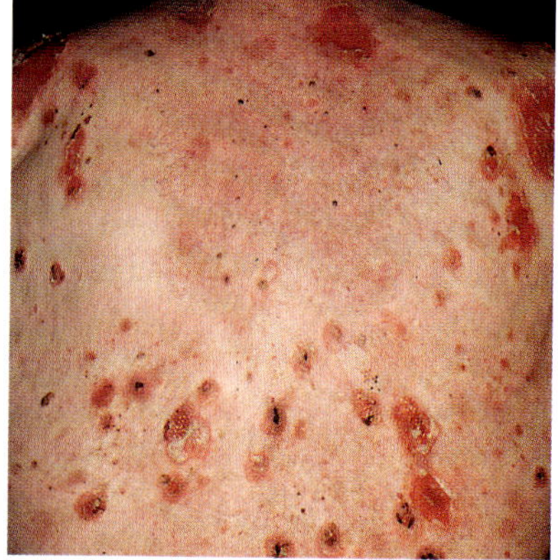

FIG. 68-29 *Flaccid blisters and crusts atop erosions.*

VARIATIONS

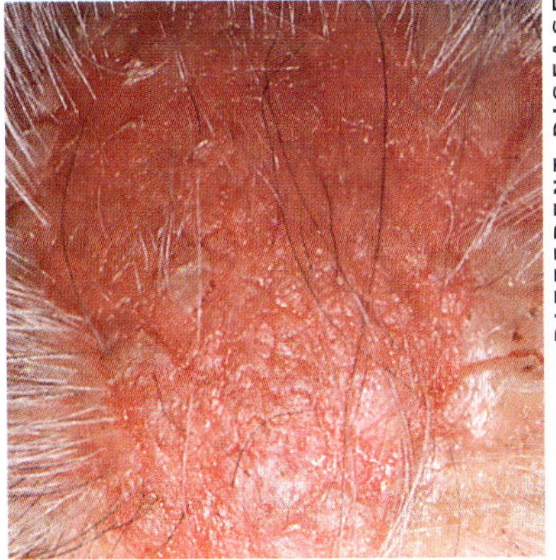

FIG. 68-30 *Alopecia in a plaque whose surface is papillated and crusted.*

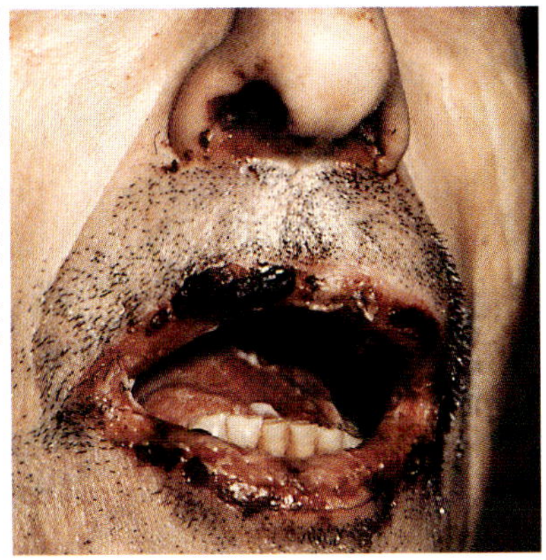

FIG. 68-31 *Erosion and hemorrhagic crusts of paraneoplastic pemphigus.*

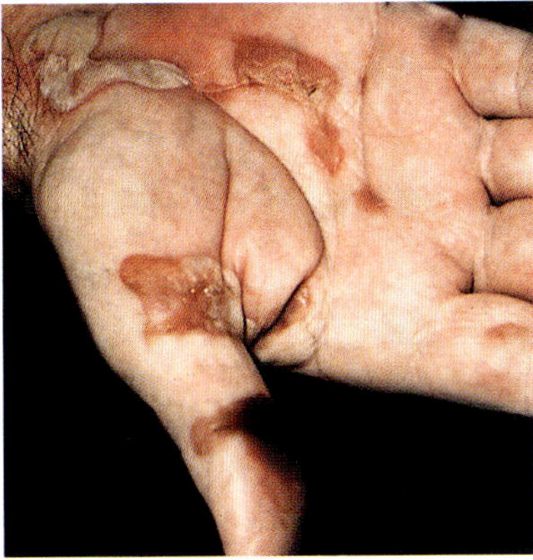

FIG. 68-32 *Bulla and crusts on the palm of a patient with paraneoplastic pemphigus.*

ADJUNCTIVE DIAGNOSTIC TESTS IgG antibodies can be demonstrated against the cell surface of keratinocytes by direct and indirect immunofluorescence techniques.

COURSE Lesions of pemphigus vulgaris present themselves, from the outset, as blisters that usually are flaccid. Individual lesions on the skin generally heal with difficulty and can fester for weeks or months before re-epithelialization occurs. That recalcitrance is even more true for lesions on mucous membranes, especially of the oral cavity, which are subjected to the effects of mastication.

Prior to the advent of parenteral administration of corticosteroids, pemphigus vulgaris was a disease that tended to persist for the course of a lifetime and that often proved fatal. It is not usually fatal today because corticosteroids given systemically are able to control the disease in most patients. The side effects of the corticosteroids themselves may be associated with severe morbidity.

INTEGRATION: UNIFYING CONCEPT The blisters in pemphigus vulgaris, on skin and on mucous membranes as well, result from acantholysis, a process by which epithelial cells separate from one another and then become round. The histopathologic findings, just like the clinical ones, are diagnostic with specificity. The blister occurs above the basal layer and the blister space usually houses only a few acantholytic cells. Most of the epidermis is cohesive and, because the process occurs quickly, there are no alterations of the cornified layer. The acantholytic process involves not only the epidermis, but also epithelial structures of adnexa, sometimes extending along the entire length of follicle and to within lobules of sebaceous glands.

The mechanism of blister formation is thought to be the effects of antibodies to components of desmosomes between keratinocytes in epidermal and adnexal epithelium, and epithelium of mucous membranes. The pemphigus antigens are complexes of desmosomal molecules, organelles that are important in cell-to-cell adhesion. The pemphigus vulgaris antigens are a 130-kD glycoprotein, desmoglein 3, and an 85-kD plaque protein, plakoglobin.

Pemphigus vulgaris is a specific and distinctive pathologic process. It must be differentiated from all other diseases associated with the word pemphigus, such as pemphigus foliaceus (and its variant pemphigus erythematosus), pemphigus neonatorum (which is staphylococcal scalded-skin syndrome), butcher's pemphigus (which was a fulminant pyoderma), and paraneoplastic pemphigus (which is an interface dermatitis associated with very few acantholytic cells). Those four diseases, which carry the word "pemphigus" in their names, are completely unrelated to pemphigus vulgaris.

THERAPY High doses of oral corticosteroids are requisite initially and should be continued until no new blisters form, after which a low dose should be maintained. Immunosuppressive agents, such as azathioprine, may be given in addition to systemic corticosteroids for the purpose of achieving a remission. Alternative methods of treatment include cyclophosphamide, gold, mycophenolate mofetil, plasmapheresis, intravenous immunoglobulins, and a pulse regimen of dexamethasone combined with cyclophosphamide.

Patients with pemphigus vulgaris must be monitored closely and carefully for signs of any ill effects of systemic corticosteroids.

DEFINITION An inflammatory process that involves the acra, in particular fingers and toes, and sometimes the thighs with bluish red papules and nodules which invariably are induced by cold. Chilblain is a synonym for pernio.

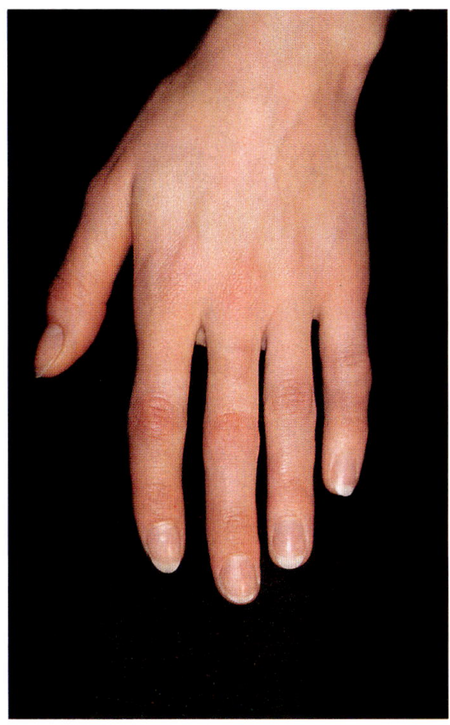

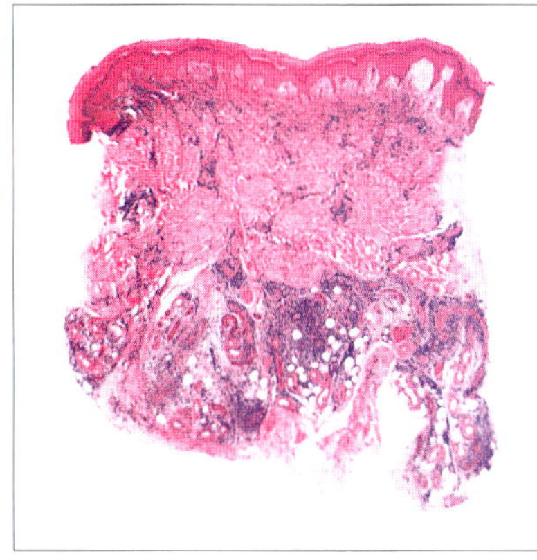

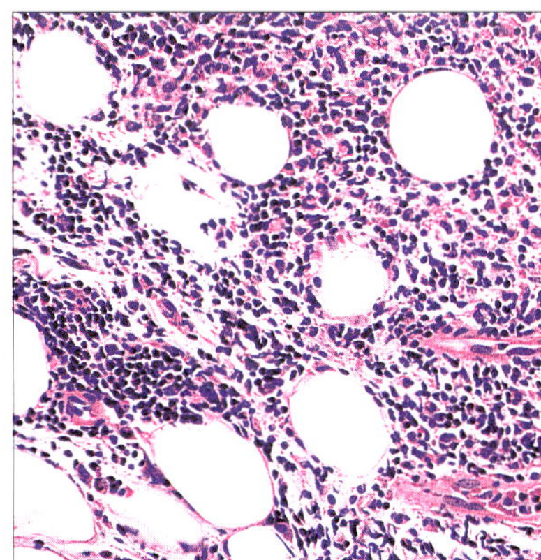

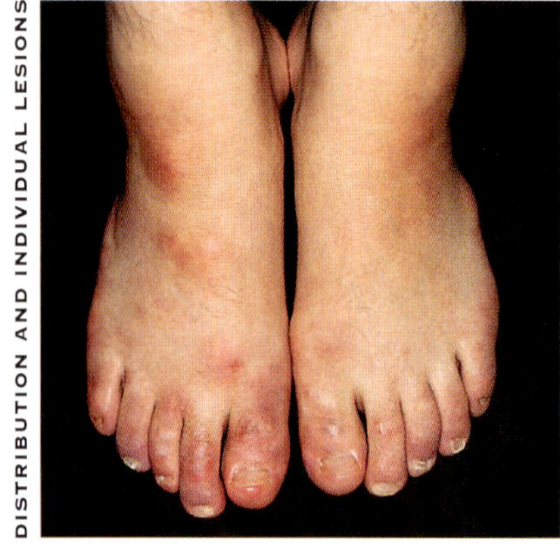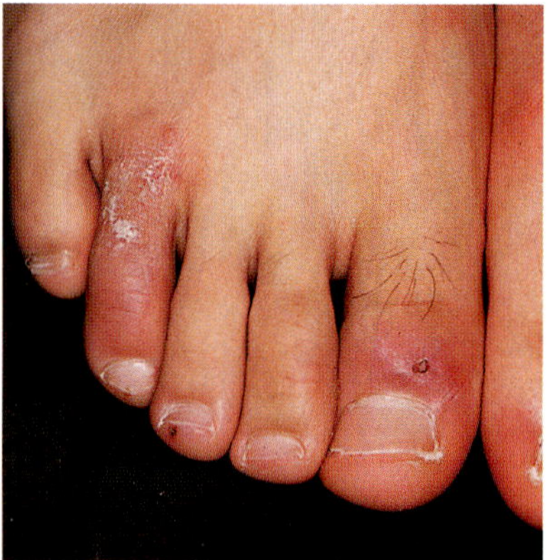

FIG. 69-1 (A, B) *Red papules and nodules of pernio.*

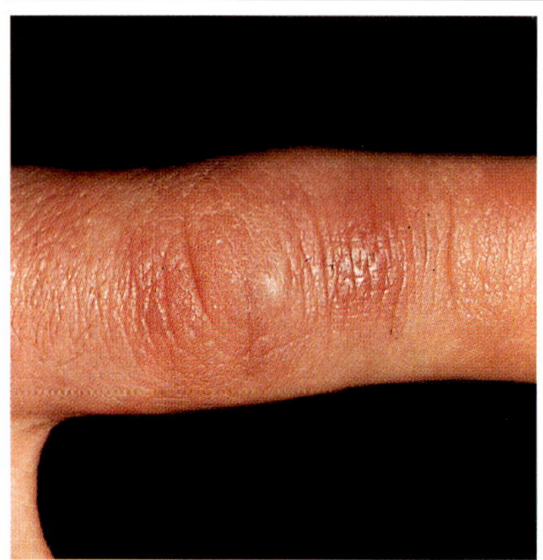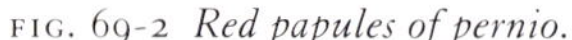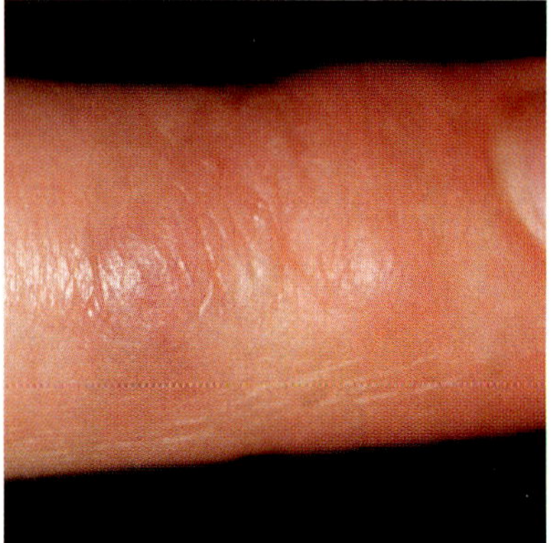

FIG. 69-2 *Red papules of pernio.*   FIG. 69-3 *Pink papules of pernio.*

COURSE The lesions of pernio begin as red macules that may become erythematous or purpuric papules and nodules or purpuric patches and plaques. The inflammatory process is precipitated by cold and once a person with pernio no longer is exposed to cold, the lesions resolve in weeks.

INTEGRATION: UNIFYING CONCEPT Pernio is a dermatitis/panniculitis induced by cold. The histopathologic findings, namely, edema of the papillary dermis, a superficial and deep perivascular infiltrate of lymphocytes, and lymphocytes in patchy array within fat lobules are virtually the same as those encountered in cold panniculitis. In fact, pernio is a type of cold dermatitis/panniculitis that affects young women mostly and often those with actual or latent systemic lupus erythematosus.

Lupus pernio is related neither to pernio nor to lupus erythematosus, but is a particular expression of sarcoidosis.

THERAPY Warm clothing is necessary to protect against the cold and nifedipine, a calcium channel blocker, is indicated when the condition is severe.

DEFINITION An inflammatory process, but not a vasculitis, that involves the legs especially with purpuric macules and subtle papules (Schamberg's disease), lichenoid papules (lichenoid purpura of Gougerot-Blum), and scaly papules (eczematid-like purpura of Doukas and Kapetanakis), all of which seem to be variants of the same basic pathologic process.

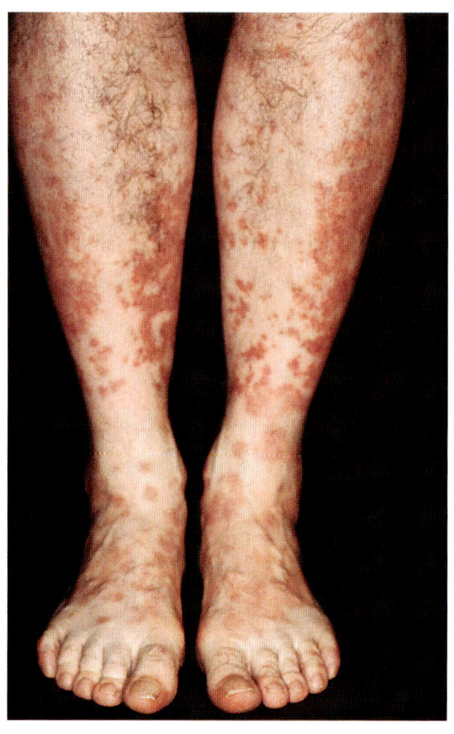

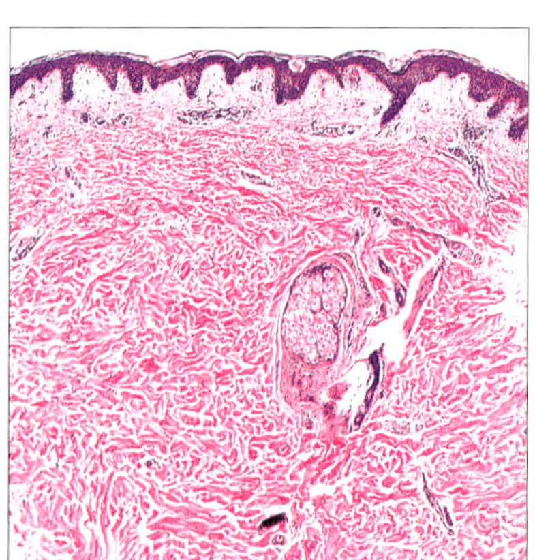

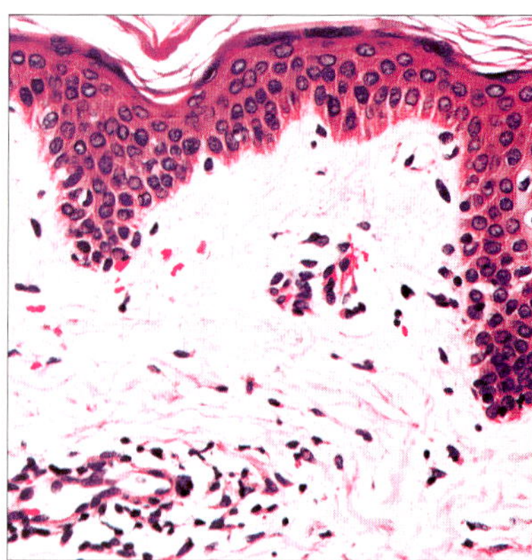

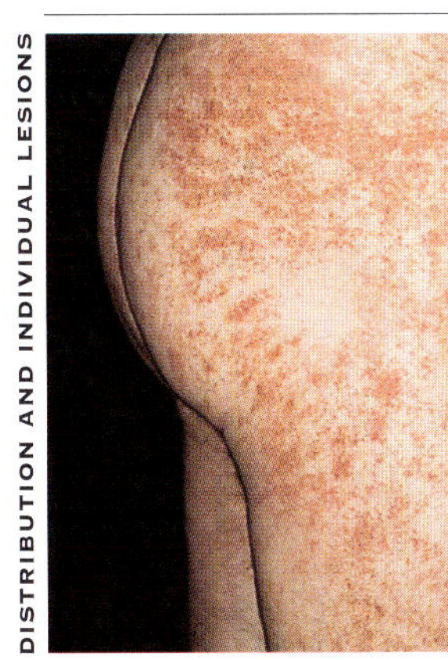
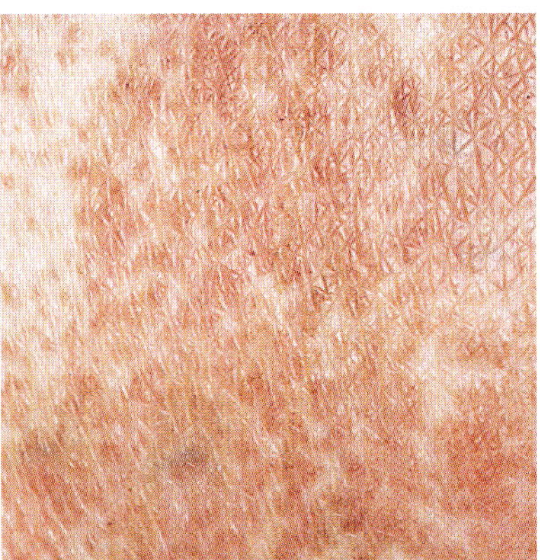

FIG. 70-1 (A, B) *Innumerable purpuric macules and papules that represent an early stage of the process (Schamberg's disease).*

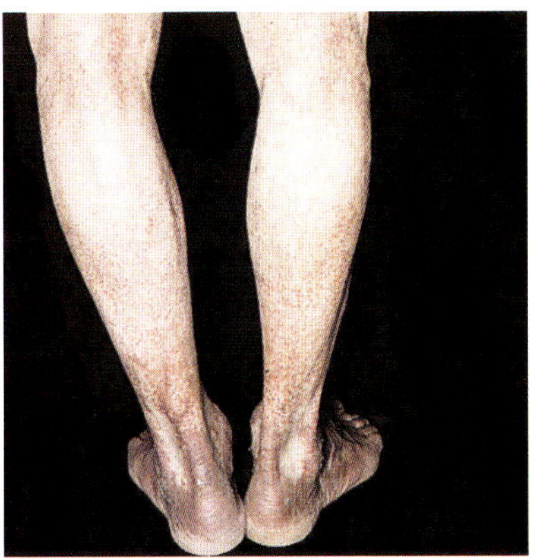

FIG. 70-2 *Pigmented macules that represent a late stage of the process (Schamberg's disease).*

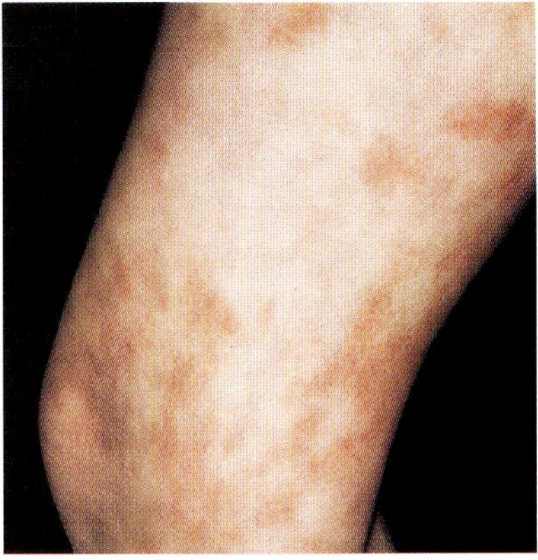

FIG. 70-3 *Pigmented macules, some of which have become confluent to become patches (Schamberg's disease).*

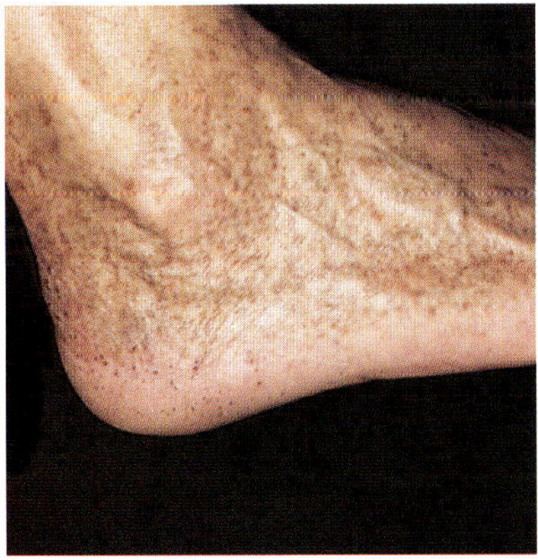
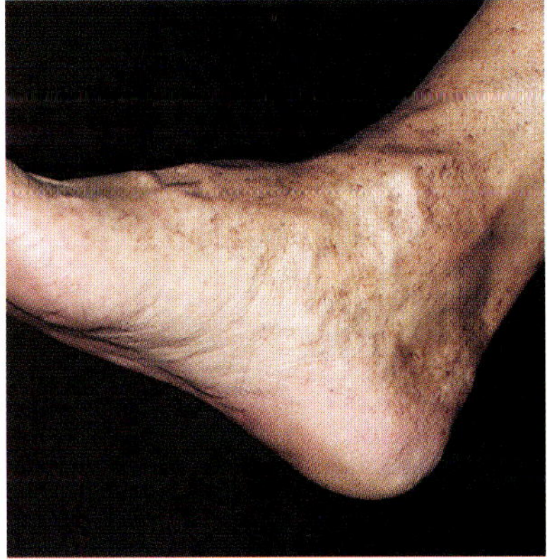

FIG. 70-4 (A, B) *Pigmented macules (Schamberg's disease).*

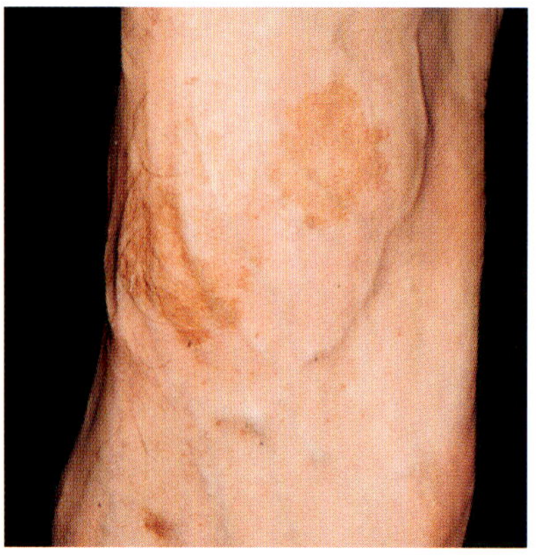

FIG. 70-5 *Pigmented macules and patches (Schamberg's disease).*

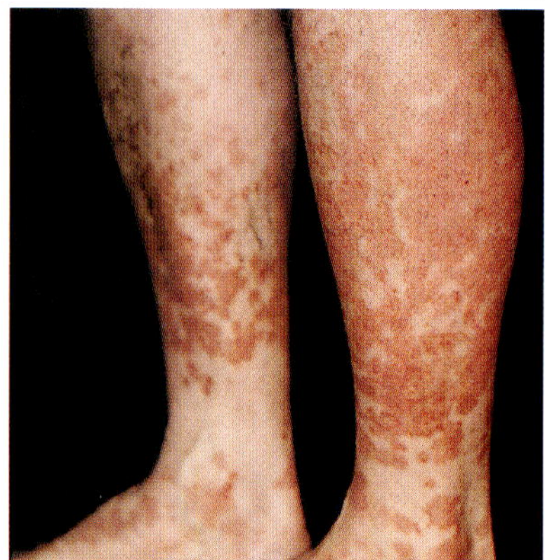

FIG. 70-6 *Lichenoid purpuric papules (Gougerot-Blum).*

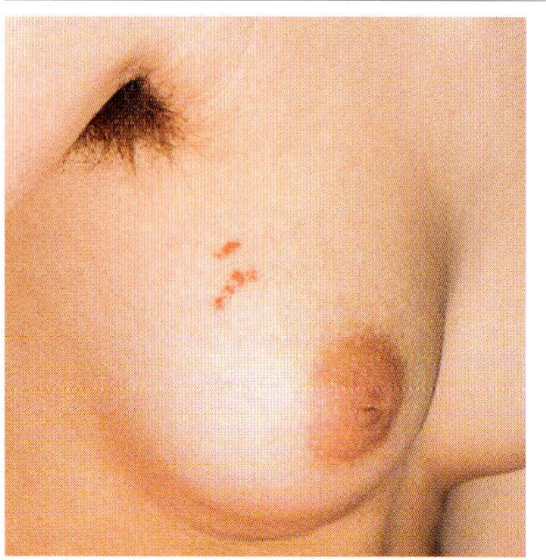

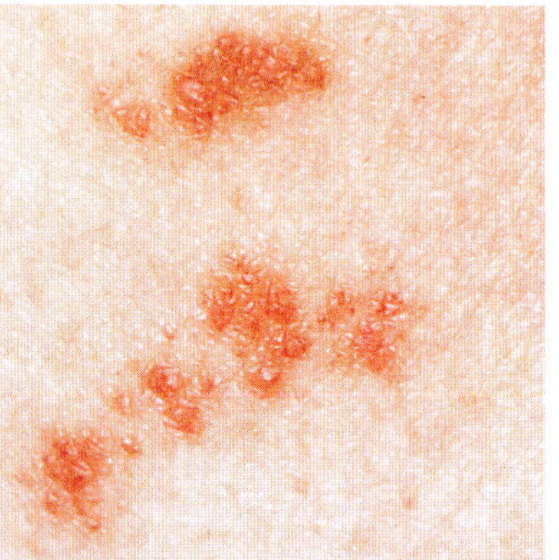

FIG. 70-7 (A, B) *Golden yellow papules, some of them in clusters (lichen aureus).*

COURSE In each of the expressions of persistent pigmented purpuric dermatitis, i.e., Schamberg's, Gougerot-Blum, and Doukas and Kapetanakis, the lesions begin as purpuric macules, and, in the case of Schamberg's disease, they may remain flat. In the other expressions of the process, purpuric macules become purpuric papules. The purpuric papules of the manifestation known for Doukas and Kapetanakis often become slightly scaly. The original purple color of lesions in all three expressions of the process changes in the course of weeks to yellowish and slowly, in months, to brown. New purpuric lesions may develop as older ones fade.

The course of the persistent pigmented purpuric dermatitides is highly variable. In some patients the lesions last for only weeks or months, whereas in others the process persists for decades.

INTEGRATION: UNIFYING CONCEPT The conditions named for Schamberg, Gougerot-Blum, and Doukas and Kapetanakis are morphologic variants of a single pathologic process, namely, persistent pigmented purpuric dermatitis. Those morphologic variants have in common a superficial perivascular and interstitial infiltrate of lymphocytes accompanied by extravasated erythrocytes in the upper part of the dermis. Early lesions of Schamberg's disease have no other histopathologic findings. The clinical variant of Schamberg's disease that consists of annular lesions is known as purpura annularis telangiectodes of Majocchi and it is identical histopathologically to Schamberg's disease.

In evolving lesions of the purpuric dermatitis of Gougerot-Blum, a band-like infiltrate of lymphocytes fills much of the papillary dermis and, at times, obscures the dermoepidermal junction. In the purpuric dermatitis of Doukas and Kapetanakis, there is no lichenoid infiltrate of lymphocytes, but spongiosis is present in foci of an epidermis that is topped by small mounds of parakeratosis. As these expressions of persistent pigmented purpuric dermatitis evolve over months, the number of extravasated erythrocytes decreases and the number of siderophages increases. If siderophages are found in the upper part of the reticular dermis, it is a sign that the process has been present for years. As lesions of this condition fade, their color changes from purple to golden yellow, thus the designation lichen aureus.

Many authors aver that the persistent pigmented purpuric dermatitides are an expression of "capillaritis." In actuality, there is no vasculitis in persistent pigmented purpuric dermatitis. Infiltrates of lymphocytes are present around blood vessels and between bundles of collagen, but there is neither fibrin in the wall of venules nor thrombi within their lumen. Parenthetically, although there are authentic examples of venulitis and arteriolitis in some diseases, capillaritis per se does not exist.

The cause of persistent pigmented purpuric dermatitides is not known.

THERAPY No treatment is really satisfactory, but the lesions wane in time with only pigment as residuum. Systemic corticosteroids have been advocated as helpful in interrupting the process. PUVA also is reported to be beneficial.

PHOTOALLERGIC DERMATITIS

DEFINITION An inflammatory process that results from either topical or systemic sensitization coupled with the effects of ultraviolet light. The lesions, all of which occur in photodistribution, are macules, papules, and blisters that resolve with crusts.

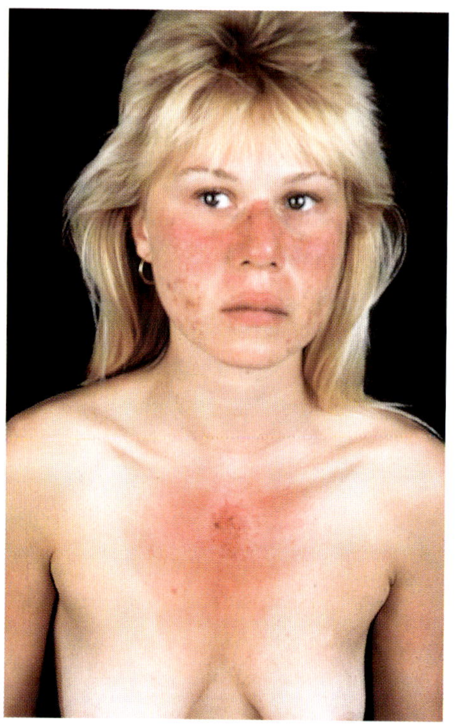

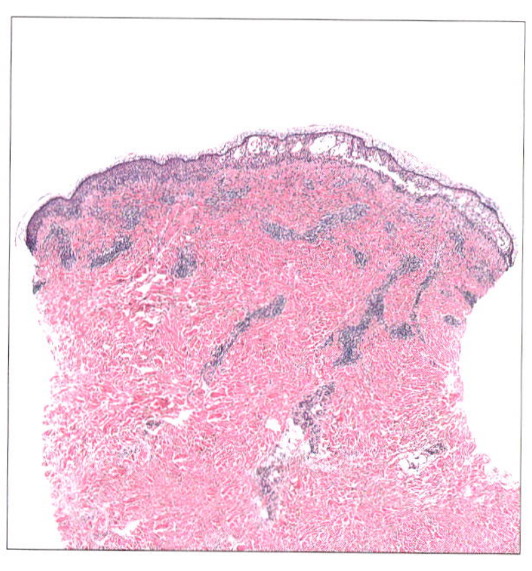

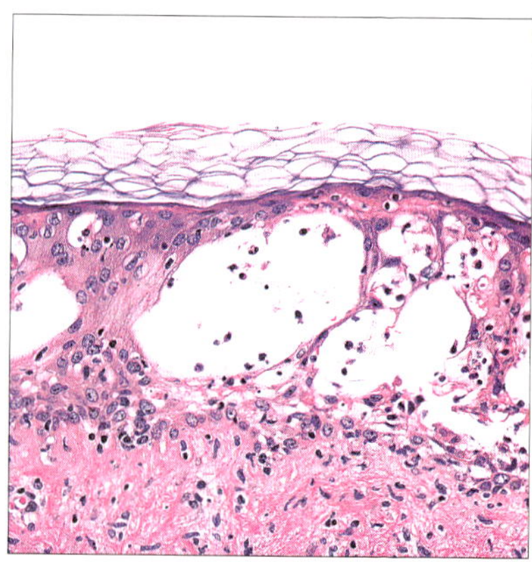

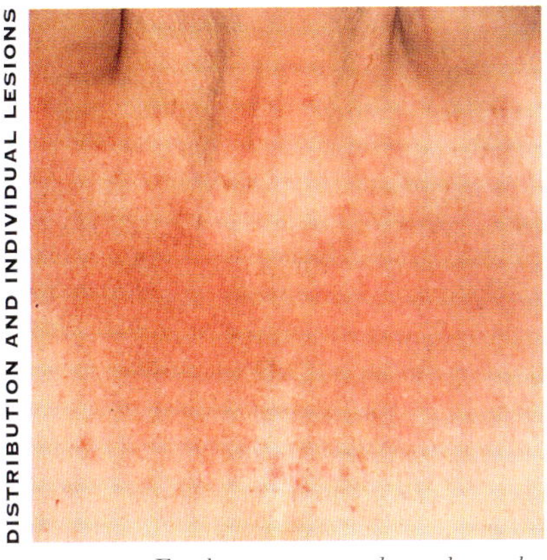

FIG. 71-1 *Erythematous macules and papules in photodistribution.*

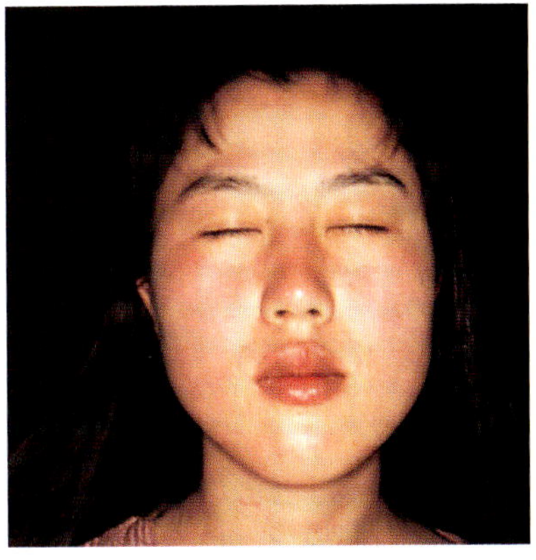

FIG. 71-2 *Erythema and edema of the face and urticarial papules on the neck.*

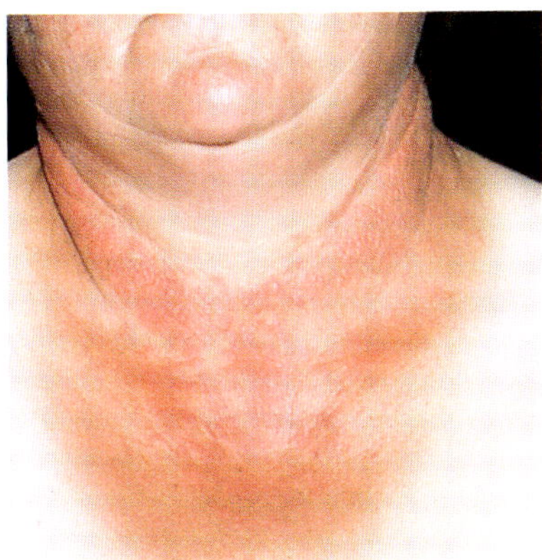

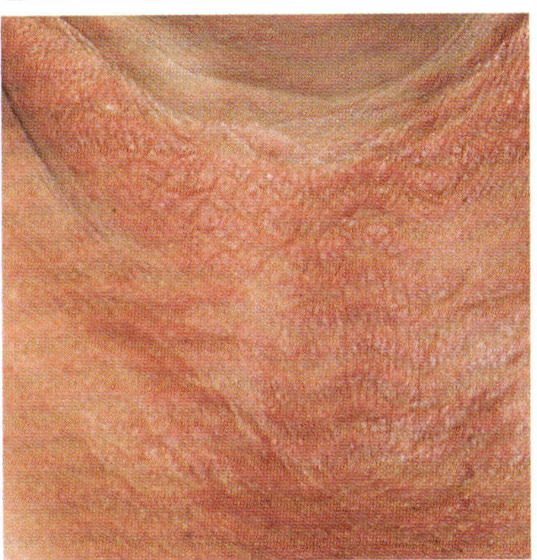

FIG. 71-3 (A, B) *Confluence of papules result in plaques in photodistribution. Sites not exposed directly to ultraviolet light are spared.*

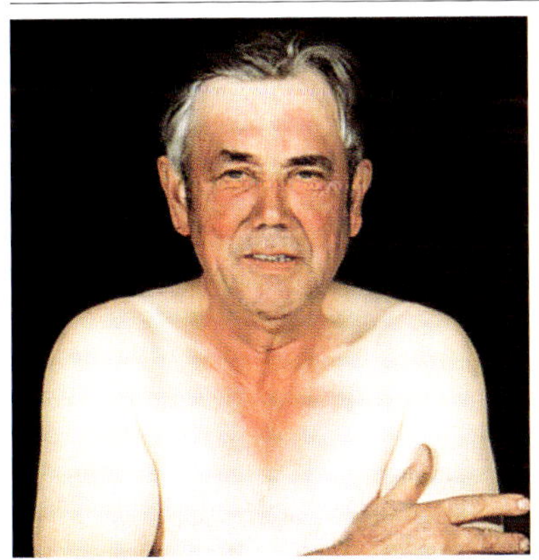

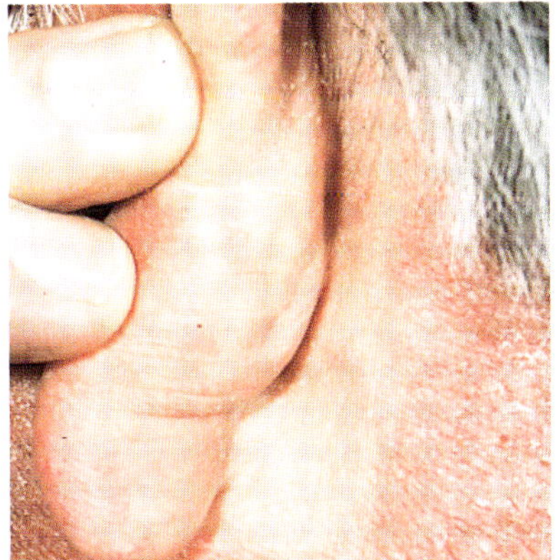

FIG. 71-4 (A, B) *Hyperpigmentation on the face and in the decolletée region. Note that the retroauricular region, protected from the sun's rays by the ear, is spared.*

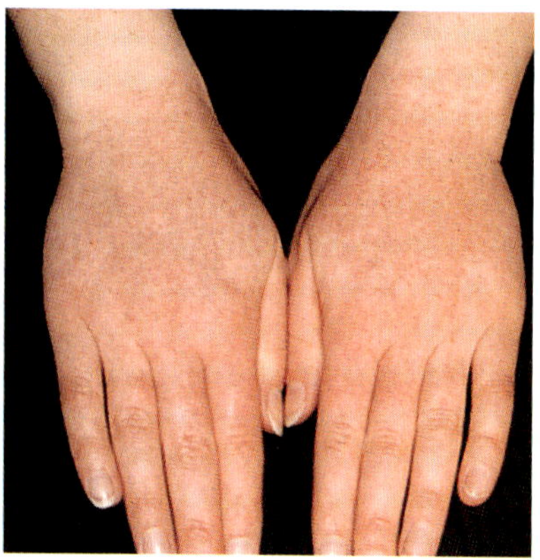

FIG. 71-5 *Innumerable closely-set papules on the dorsa of the hands.*

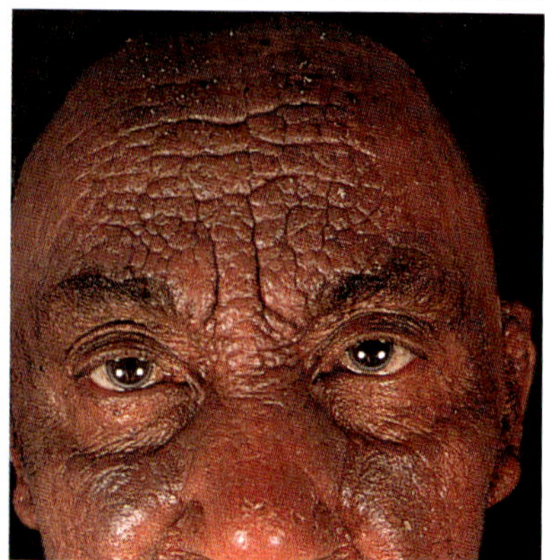

FIG. 71-6 *Severe lichenification secondary to persistent light eruption (actinic reticuloid).*

ADJUNCTIVE DIAGNOSTIC TESTS Phototests and photopatch tests permit identification of the drugs that are responsible for photosensitivity.

COURSE The lesions of photoallergic dermatitis are very much like those of allergic contact dermatitis, and the course of the lesions is similar in both conditions. Papules, papulovesicles, and vesicles develop in response to the combined effects of a sensitizing agent and ultraviolet light. Individual lesions last for days and usually disappear in less than two weeks. The duration of the condition itself turns on the duration of exposure to both the sensitizer and ultraviolet light. New lesions appear if exposure is sustained; the process stops once exposure ceases.

INTEGRATION: UNIFYING CONCEPT Photoallergic dermatitis is analogous to allergic contact dermatitis, the responsible substance being a chemical that is applied topically or administered systemically and that is altered by the effects of ultraviolet light, thereby being transformed into an allergen. The papules, papulovesicles, and vesicles of photoallergic dermatitis represent a continuum of a basically spongiotic dermatitis, the blisters being a consequence of spongiotic vesiculation.

On the basis of morphologic changes of individual lesions alone, namely, clinical and histopathologic features, a photoallergic dermatitis cannot be distinguished from allergic contact dermatitis. Even distribution of lesions is not, in itself, effective in differentiating photoallergic dermatitis from allergic contact dermatitis, because some airborne sensitizers that induce allergic contact

dermatitis cause lesions to appear in the same distribution as those of photoallergic dermatitis. A subtle clue to distinction between the two conditions
clinically is sparing of the skin of the submandibular region in photoallergic
dermatitis and a subtle clue histopathologically is a deep, as well as superficial,
perivascular infiltrate of lymphocytes in photoallergic dermatitis. In the ultimate analysis, photoallergic dermatitis can be differentiated from allergic
contact dermatitis by utilizing phototests, including photopatch tests.

Actinic reticuloid is a particular expression of photoallergic dermatitis,
namely, an extraordinarily long-lasting ("persistent light eruption") and pruritic one, the joint effect of severe photodermatitis and extensive lichen simplex chronicus producing a leonine facies that could be misconstrued as that
of a lymphoma.

PHOTOTOXIC DERMATITIS

DEFINITION An inflammatory process that represents the combined
effects of a toxic substance applied topically or administered systemically in
combination with the effects of ultraviolet light, the result being a caricature
of sunburn. The lesions consist of erythema and blisters, some of which may
be large bullae, and occur on sites exposed directly to ultraviolet light.

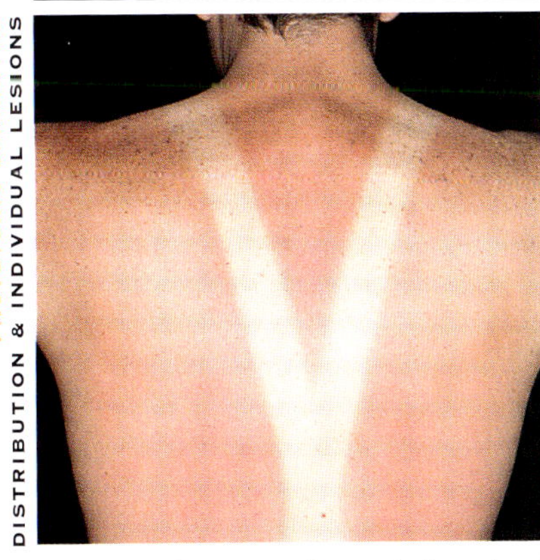

FIG. 71-7 *Intense erythema at sites exposed directly to ultraviolet light.*

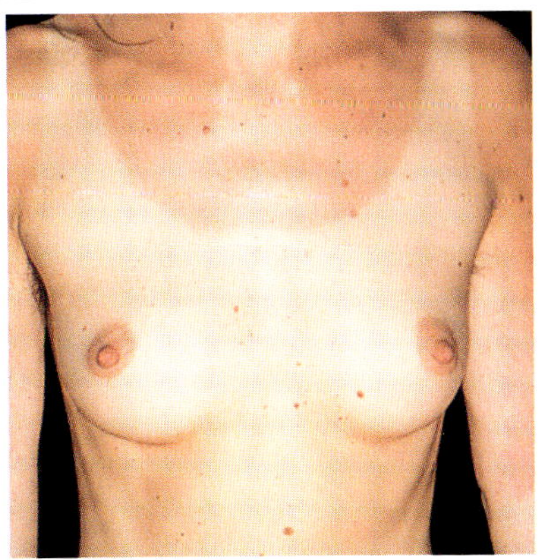

FIG. 71-8 *Postinflammatory hyperpigmentation in photodistribution.*

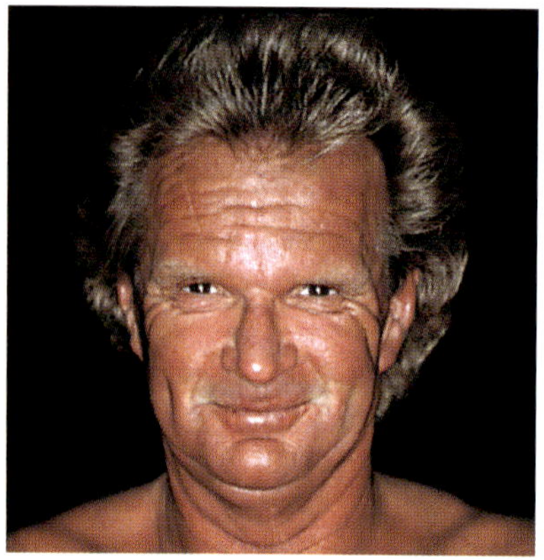

FIG. 71-9 *Erythroderma with sparing of paraoral creases.*

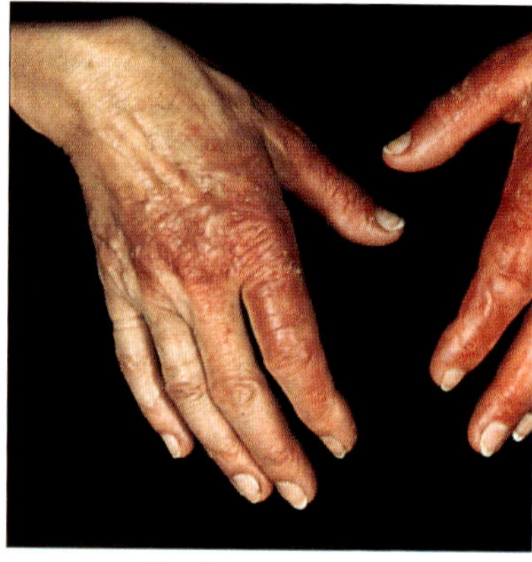

FIG. 71-10 *Erythema, purpura, erosions, and scales on sites most prominently exposed to the effects of sunlight.*

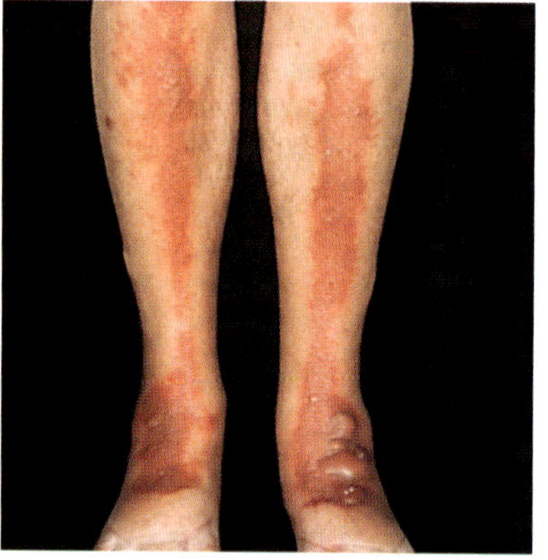

FIG. 71-11 *Redness in linear distribution and bullae of a phytophotodermatitis.*

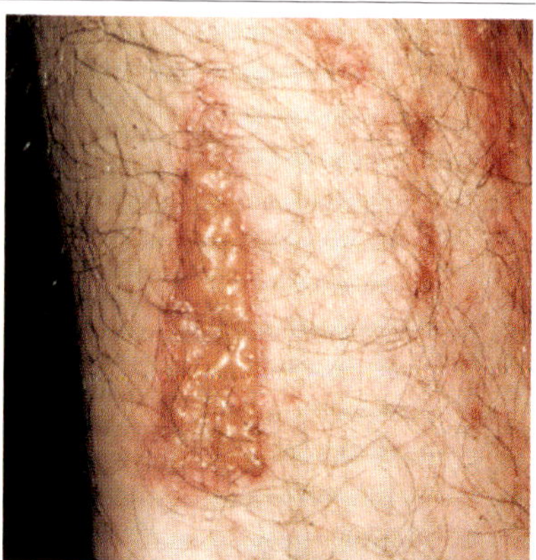

FIG. 71-12 *Vesicles that have become confluent in a lesion that has the shape of an arrowhead.*

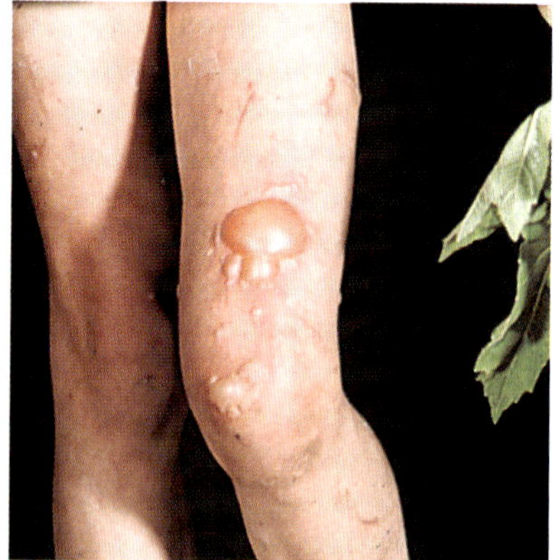

FIG. 71-13 *Vesicles, bullae, and pigmented macules in striate pattern of phytophotodermatitis.*

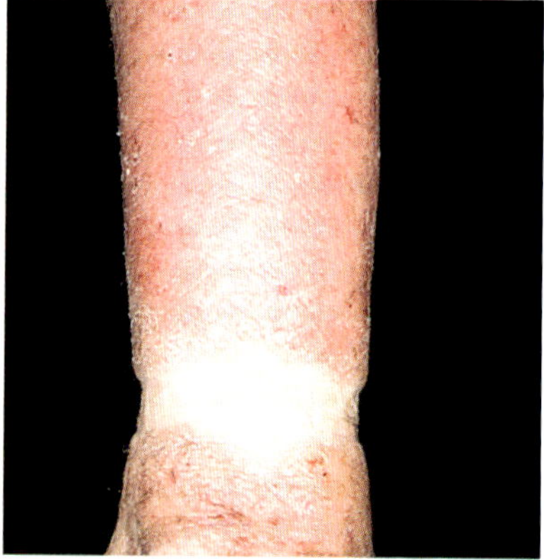

FIG. 71-14 *Erythema, edema, and scales of the arm, except for the region spared by the watchband.*

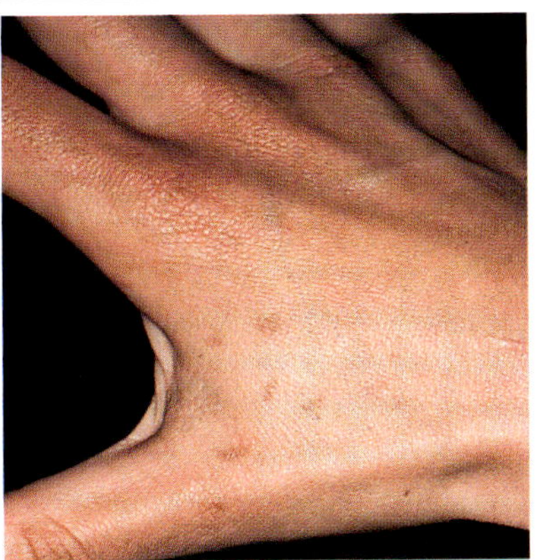

FIG. 71-15 *Pigmented macules of resolving phytophotodermatitis.*

ADJUNCTIVE DIAGNOSTIC TESTS Phototests with assessment of the minimal erythema dose and exposure to ultraviolet light with and without the presence of the toxic substances are confirmatory.

COURSE Phototoxic dermatitis usually is not characterized by discrete papules and vesicles but, depending on the degree of injury, first by patches of redness followed shortly by blisters, many of them large. If there is only a first-degree burn, the lesions disappear in days, but if there is a second-degree burn, with ulceration, it may take weeks before healing is complete.

INTEGRATION: UNIFYING CONCEPT Phototoxic dermatitis is analogous to irritant contact dermatitis; there is no immunologic basis for formation of lesions. The lesions of phototoxic dermatitis, however, tend to be better circumscribed than those of photoallergic dermatitis. In contrast to both photoallergic dermatitis and allergic contact dermatitis, neither of which affects every person exposed to a particular allergen, phototoxic dermatitis and irritant contact dermatitis affect everyone exposed to the responsible agent.

Whereas photoallergic dermatitis and allergic contact dermatitis are spongiotic dermatitides, phototoxic dermatitis and irritant contact dermatitis are ballooning dermatitides. In addition to ballooning that may eventuate in intraepidermal vesiculation, there are also signs of epidermal necrosis, at first as individual necrotic keratinocytes and later as confluent epidermal necrosis. In short, photoallergic dermatitis/allergic contact dermatitis and phototoxic dermatitis/irritant contact dermatitis are fundamentally different pathologic processes, and those differences are expressed clinically, histopathologically, immunopathologically, and biologically.

Phytophotodermatitis refers specifically to that kind of photodermatitis in which the "toxin" is housed in parts of plants, such as parsley, parsnips, figs, meadow grass, limes, and berloque, from which it is transferred to skin.

THERAPY Sun exposure and offending causative agents should be avoided. For mild cases, a topical soothing lotion suffices; if the dermatitis is more severe, a topical corticosteroid cream may be satisfactory, but if it is not, oral corticosteroids for a short course should bring the process to a halt.

DEFINITION An inflammatory process characterized by oval lesions marked at the periphery by collarettes of scale and distributed usually along lines of cleavage on the trunk especially, but in a general range from "the neck to the knees."

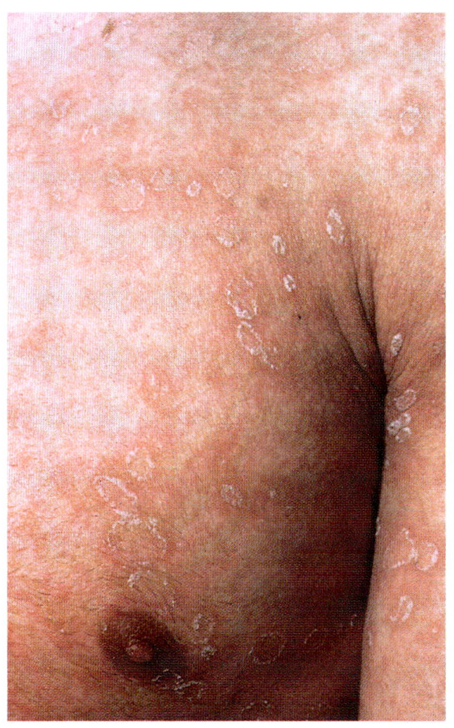

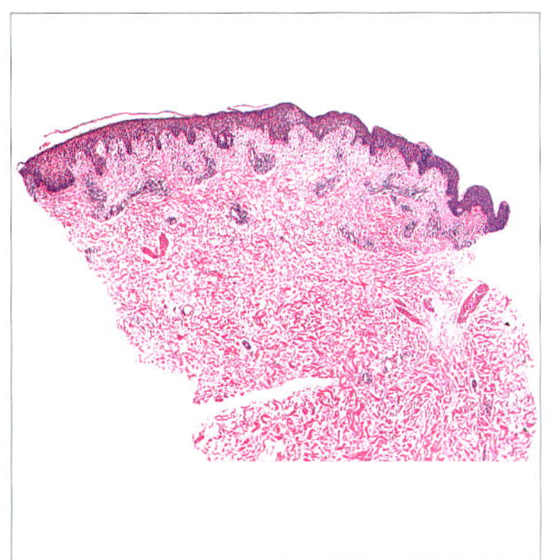

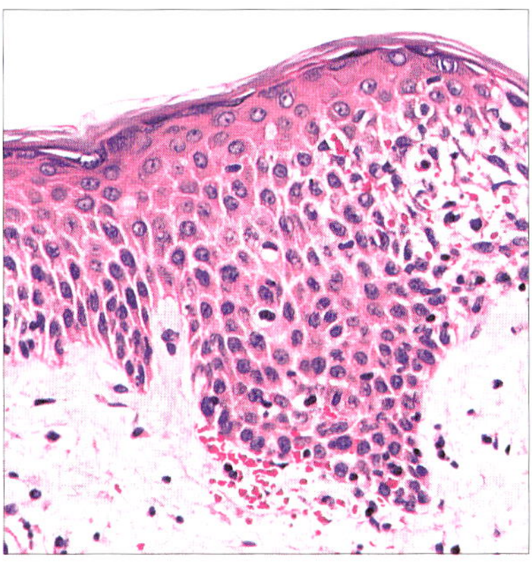

DISTRIBUTION

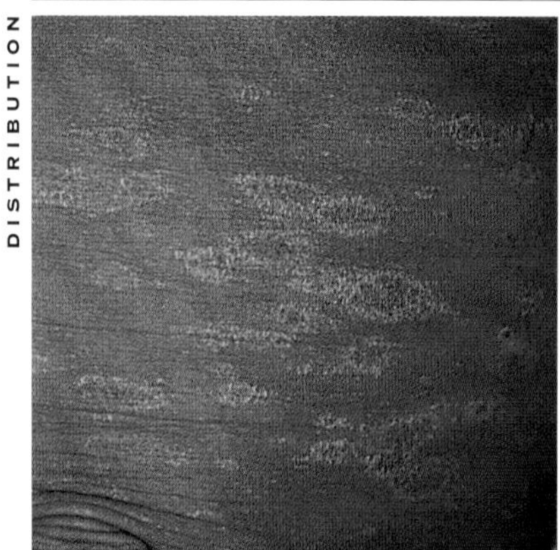

FIG. 72-1 *Collarettes of scales in oval shape along lines of cleavage.*

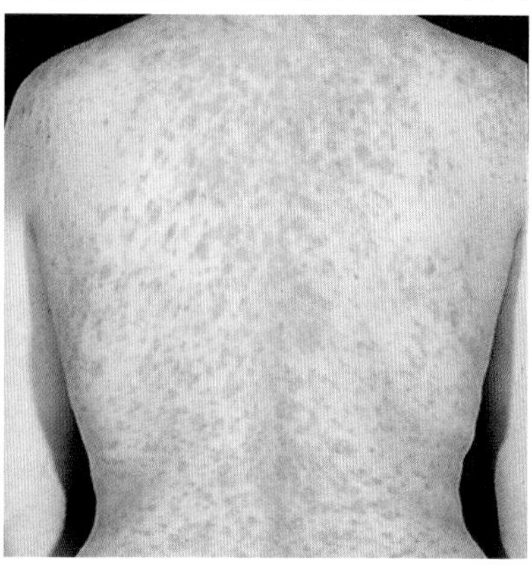

FIG. 72-2 *Oval papules in a distribution on the trunk and sacral region that resembles the branches of an evergreen tree.*

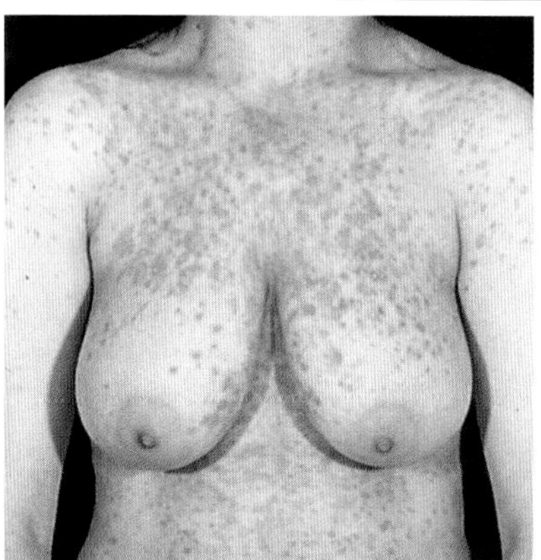

FIG. 72-3 *Oval papules, some of which have become confluent.*

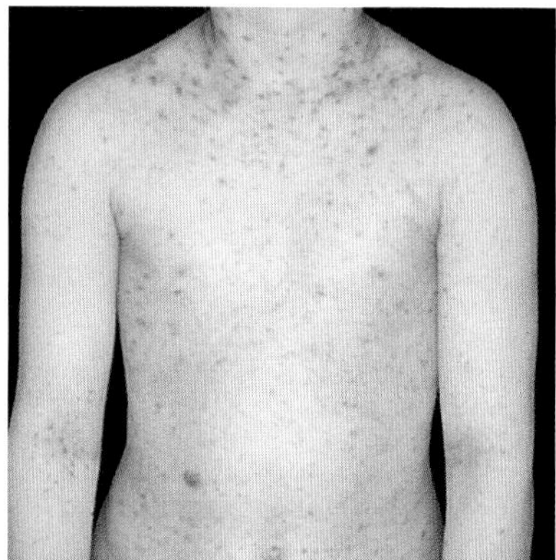

FIG. 72-4 *A "herald" or "mother" patch, which truly is a plaque, in association with smaller daughter lesions.*

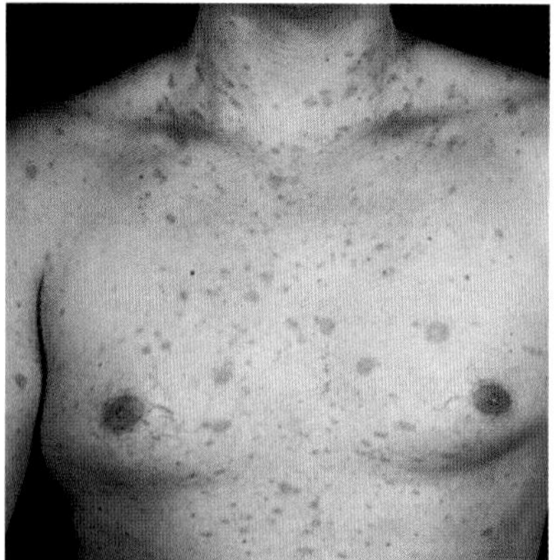

FIG. 72-5 *Oval and round papules, some in annular configuration.*

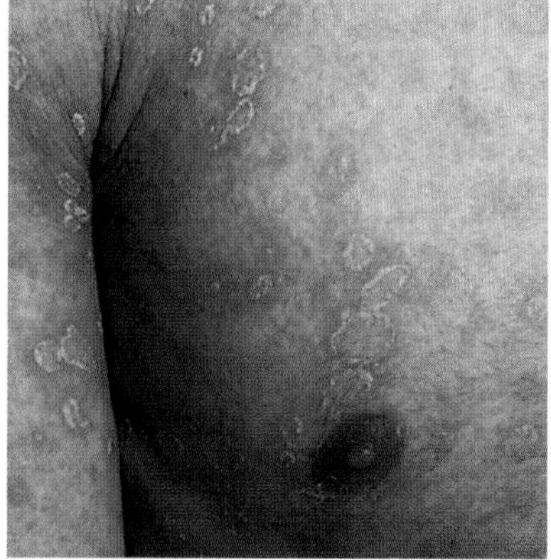

FIG. 72-6 *Patches and subtle plaques characterized by a rim of erythema and collarettes of scale.*

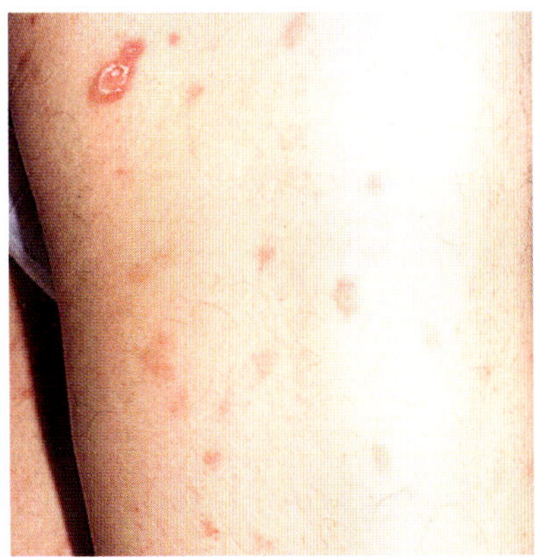

FIG. 72-7 *Macules, papules, and a plaque typified by collarettes of scale on its inner margin.*

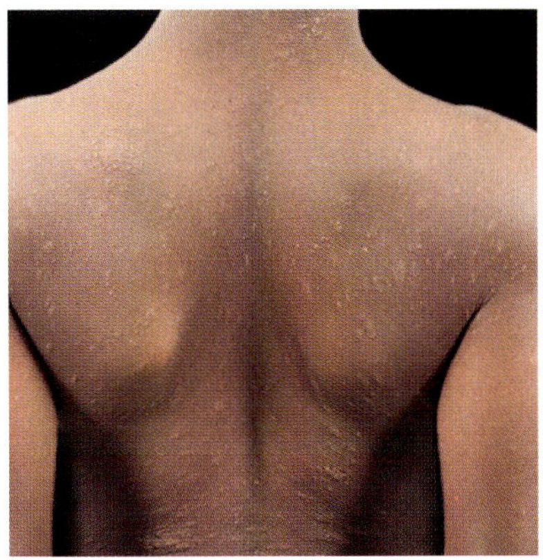

FIG. 72-8 *Papules, some of them clustered to create a fusiform shape.*

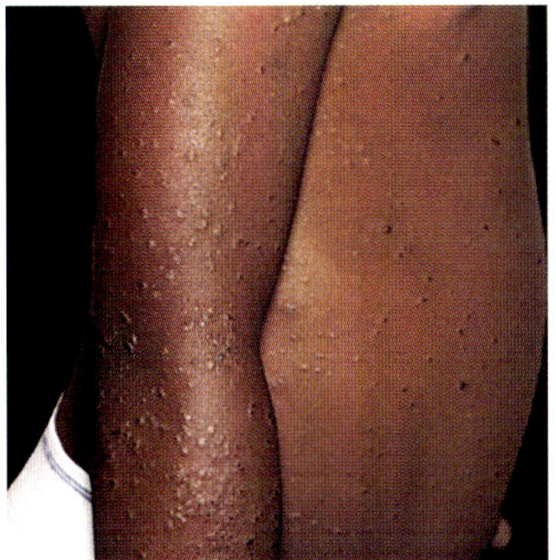

FIG. 72-9 *Papules only.*

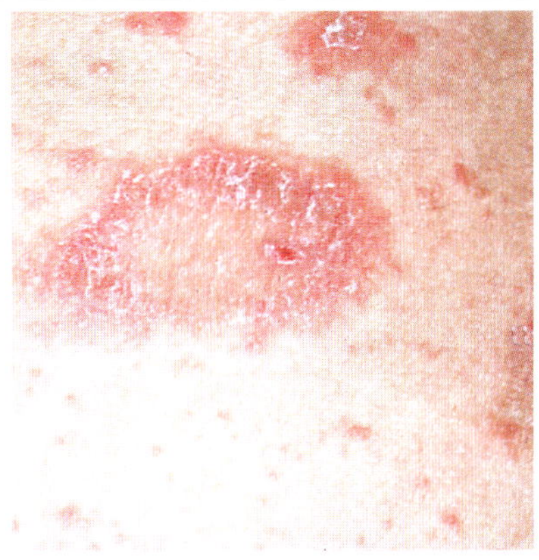

FIG. 72-10 *A "mother" patch, which in reality is a plaque, and "daughter" lesions, which in actuality are papules.*

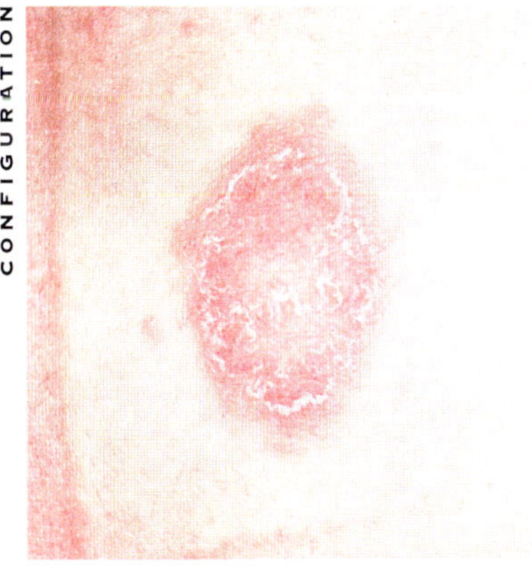

FIG. 72-11 *Coin-shaped lesion associated with a papular rim, the inner margin of which is marked by a collarette of scale.*

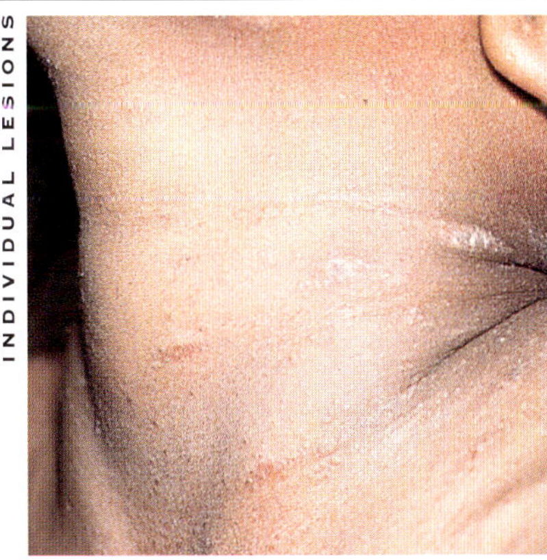

FIG. 72-12 *Scaly and non-scaly papules.*

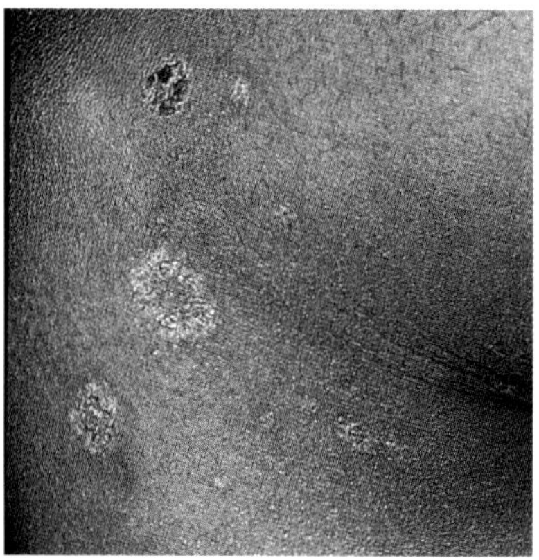

FIG. 72-13 *Scaly and crusted nummular papules and plaques.*

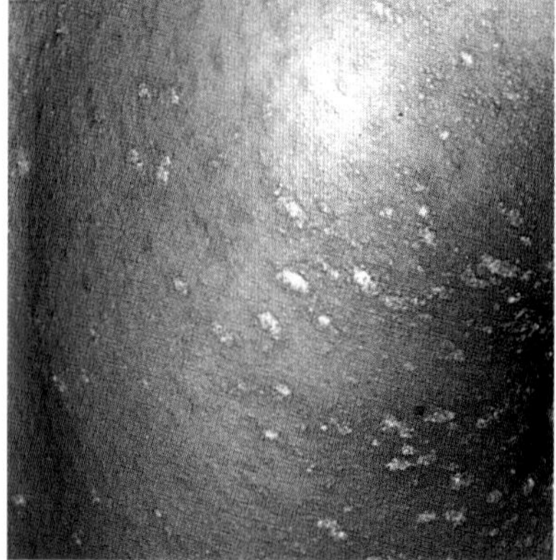

FIG. 72-14 *Scaly ovoid papules.*

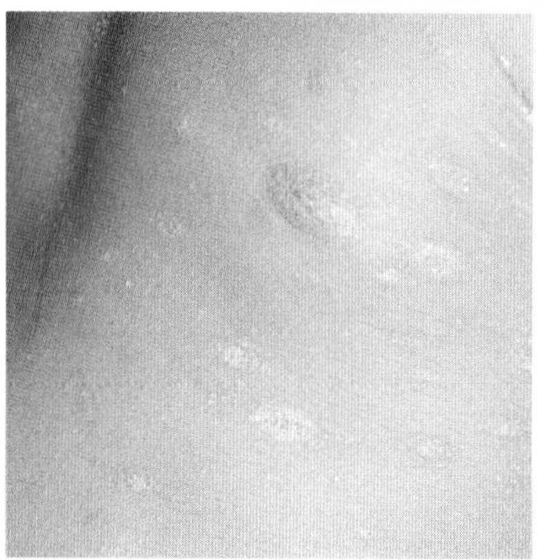

FIG. 72-15 *Papules and plaques with scales in the shape of a collarette at the periphery of them.*

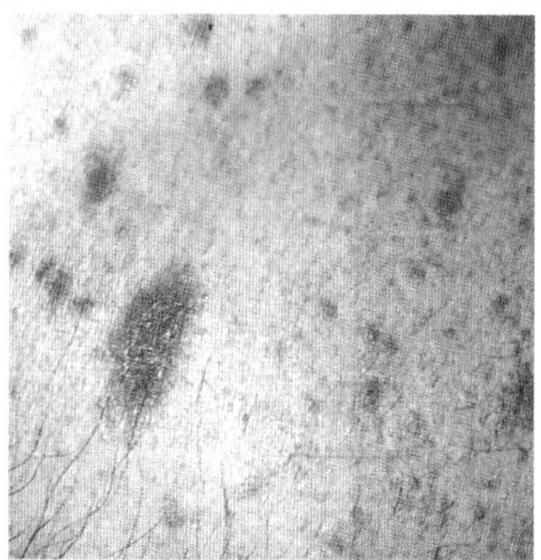

FIG. 72-16 *Papules, some of them covered by subtle crust, and plaque with oval shape and slight scale.*

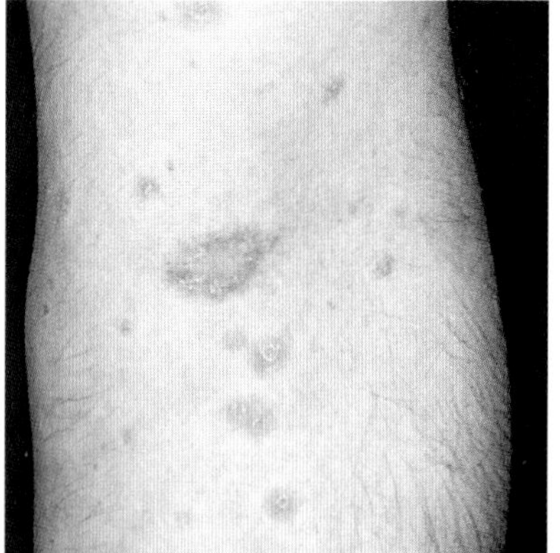

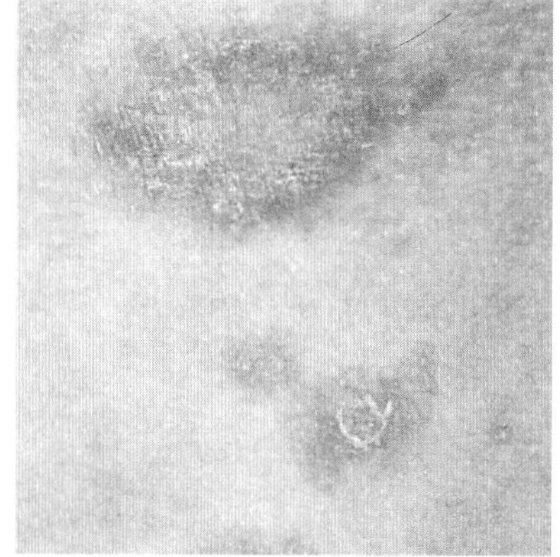

FIG. 72-17 (A, B) *Papules and a plaque marked at its periphery by collarettes of scale.*

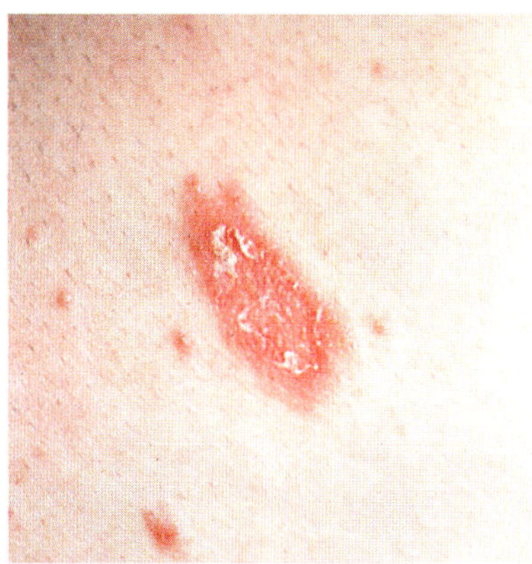

FIG. 72-18 *Papules and a plaque whose surface is covered by collarettes of scale.*

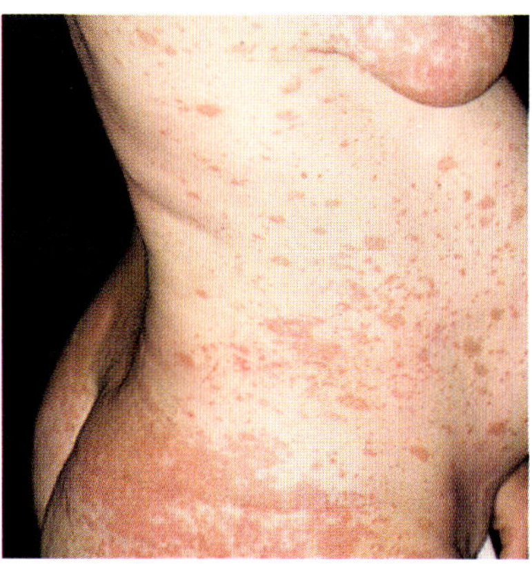

FIG. 72-19 *Oval lesions of pityriasis rosea on a trunk and confluence of those lesions on the breast and buttock.*

COURSE The course of pityriasis rosea is repeatable and predictable; a "herald" or "mother" patch appears, usually on a trunk, followed soon afterward by an eruption of oval scaly macules that become papules that eventuate in subtle plaques. The shower of lesions, which tends to be restricted to the region from the "neck to the knees," ceases after some days and the entire process usually wanes within six weeks. As a rule, there is no residuum.

INTEGRATION: UNIFYING CONCEPT Pityriasis rosea is a distinctive, probably virally-induced disease that has typical morphologic features, clinically and histopathologically. By microscopy, a tissue section of a biopsy specimen from a scaly papule of pityriasis rosea shows a superficial perivascular infiltrate of lymphocytes, variable numbers of extravasated erythrocytes in an edematous papillary dermis, a slightly hyperplastic epidermis that houses foci of spongiosis, and mounds of parakeratosis. The histopathologic findings in pityriasis rosea are indistinguishable from those of erythema annulare centrifugum.

In some black patients with pityriasis rosea, vesicles may develop clinically, and they are seen by conventional microscopy to be the result of extensive spongiosis. As a rule, however, lesions of pityriasis rosea do not vesiculate.

THERAPY Soothing lotions, topical hydrocortisone cream, and ultraviolet light may each ameliorate signs, but they do not hasten the disappearance of lesions, which takes about 6 weeks irrespective of treatment.

DEFINITION An inflammatory process in which lesions present themselves clinically as red macules and subtle scaly papules. They soon become so confluent that there is widespread redness and scaling punctuated by islands of skin that ostensibly are spared and by discrete tiny keratoses positioned equidistant from one another, a consequence of their emanation from ostia of follicles.

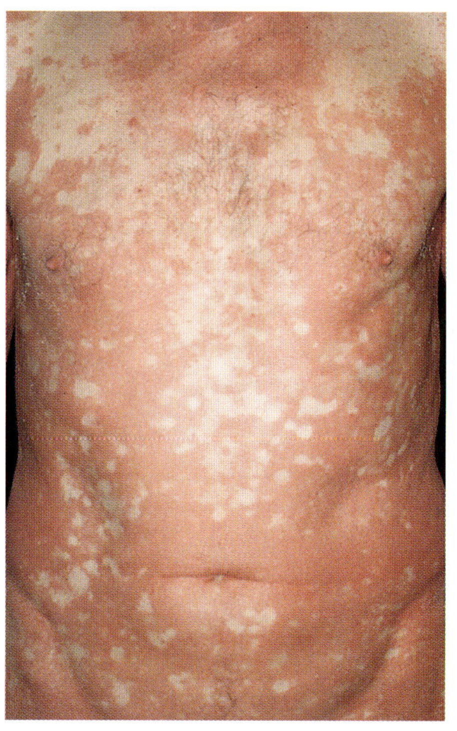

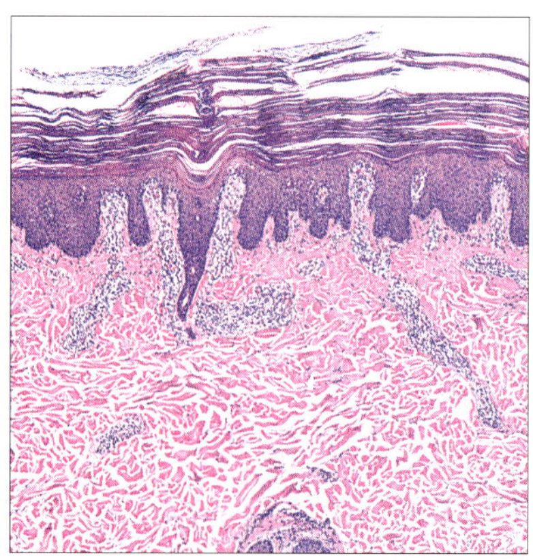

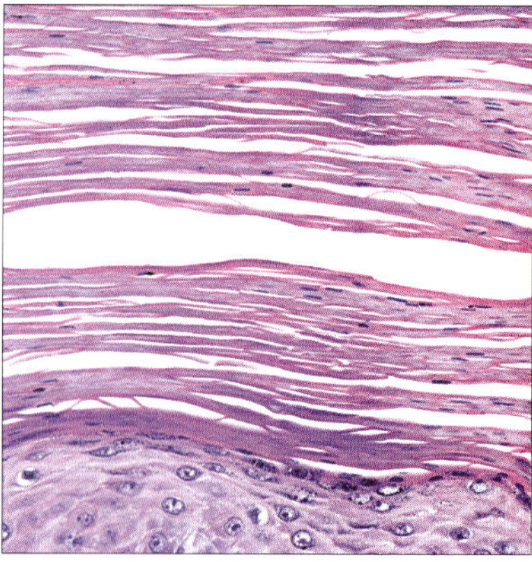

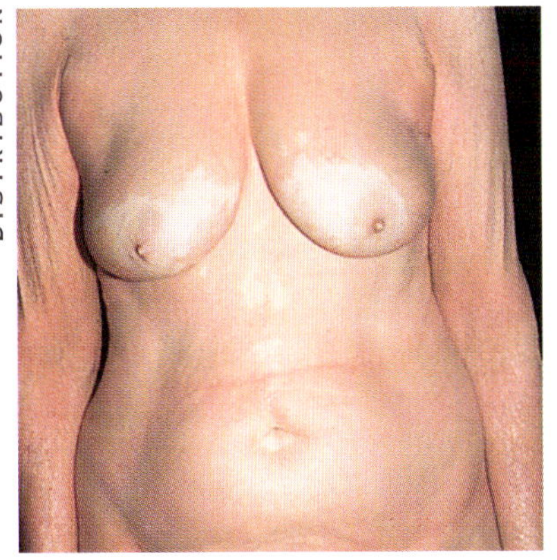

FIG. 73-1 *Erythroderma with sparing of skin in islands.*

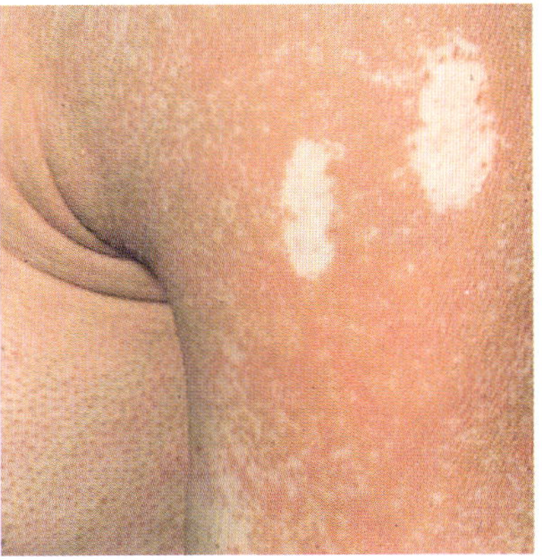

FIG. 73-2 *Erythroderma and keratotic follicular papules, with islands of skin that seem to have been spared by the process.*

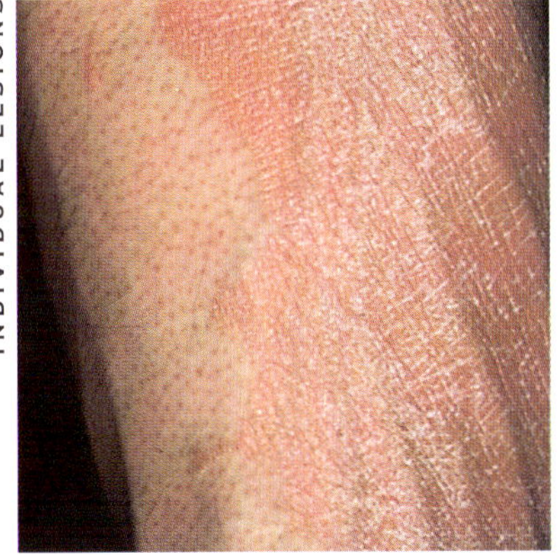

FIG. 73-3 *Sharply circumscribed broad plaque with associated lichenification and scaling, and keratotic follicular papules.*

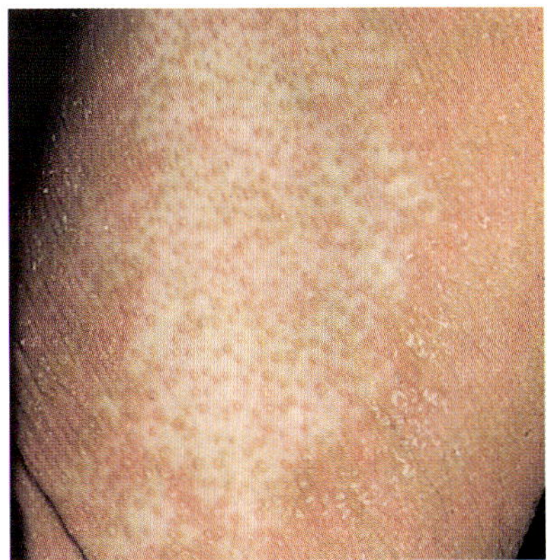

FIG. 73-4 *Keratotic follicular papules equidistant from one another in the midst of exfoliative erythroderma.*

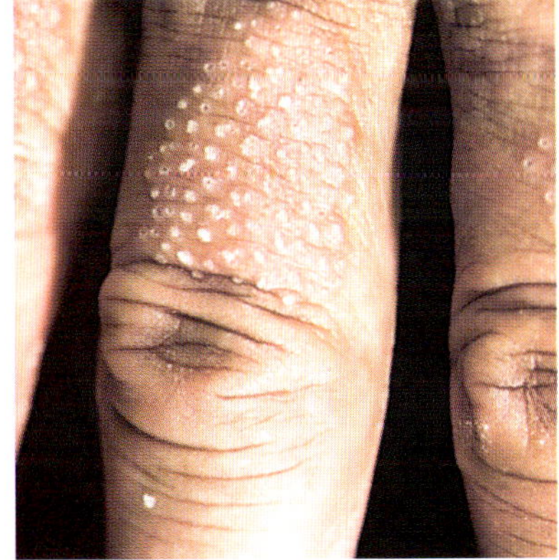

FIG. 73-5 *Keratotic follicular papules equidistant from one another within a plaque.*

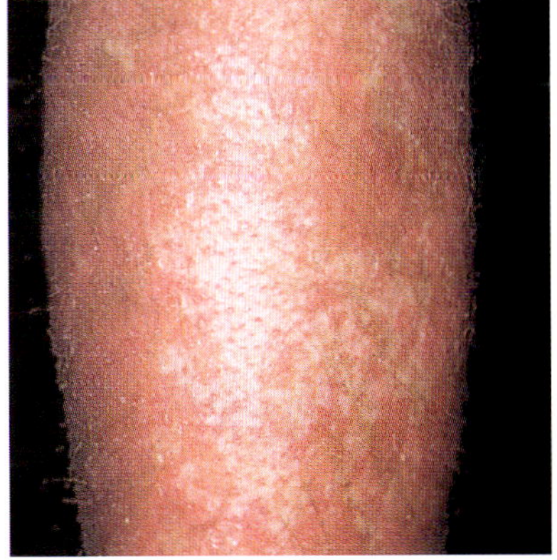

FIG. 73-6 *Follicular papules and erythema in interfollicular zones forming patches.*

COURSE The first lesions of pityriasis rubra pilaris to present themselves are red macules that may become scaly patches, or papules that may become scaly plaques. The disease tends to become progressively widespread and, in time, an erythroderma may result. Characteristically, there are zones within the erythroderma of seemingly unaffected skin ("islands of sparing"). The scaling becomes ever more marked and is expressed most dramatically on the scalp. Palms and soles become hyperkeratotic and have a yellow-orange cast. In addition, ostia of follicles often are seen to be widened and plugged by horny material.

Pityriasis rubra pilaris usually lasts for months, but sometimes for years.

INTEGRATION: UNIFYING CONCEPT Pityriasis rubra pilaris is a distinctive inflammatory process whose morphologic features are unique, clinically and histopathologically. Papules of the condition are characterized by discrete foci of parakeratosis that alternate with orthokeratosis in both vertical and horizontal directions. The granular zone is prominent and the remainder of the epidermis is psoriasiform, rete ridges of the condition being less long and more broad than those of psoriasis. A sparse infiltrate of lymphocytes is present around dilated venules of the superficial plexus. Tissue sections of a biopsy specimen of a horny plug within the ostium of a follicle show a dilated infundibulum filled with corneocytes that are both orthokeratotic and parakeratotic and arranged in a manner similar to that in the altered stratum corneum.

Pityriasis rubra pilaris, especially in its erythroderma expression, could be confused clinically, at first glance, with psoriasis, but the latter disease does not show "islands of sparing," follicular accentuation, or palmar and plantar keratoderma. By contrast to pityriasis rubra pilaris, psoriasis displays histopathologically, in addition to thin rete ridges, thin suprapapillary plates, a mostly absent granular zone, and near confluent parakeratosis that houses some neutrophils. In sum, despite similarities clinically and histopathologically, pityriasis rubra pilaris and psoriasis are very different diseases.

The cause of pityriasis rubra pilaris is not known.

THERAPY Topical corticosteroids are appropriate for localized scaly papules and plaques on the extremities, but PUVA or retinoids given systemically are necessary for treating widespread lesions. Extracorporeal photopheresis and cyclosporine also have been advocated for disease that is widespread.

DEFINITION An inflammatory process that appears on skin exposed to sunlight, especially the face, neck, sternal region, arms, and dorsa of hands, and consists mostly of edematous papules that may become confluent to form plaques, and at times, papulovesicles.

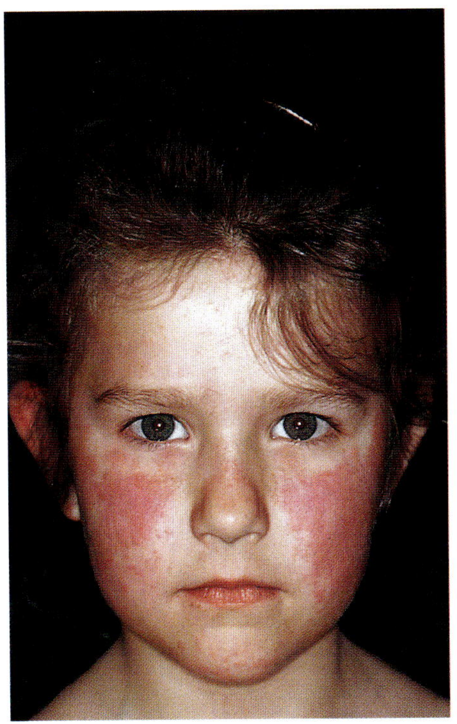

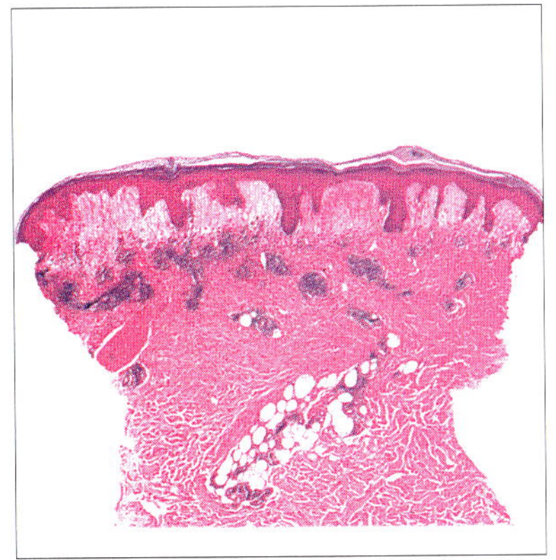

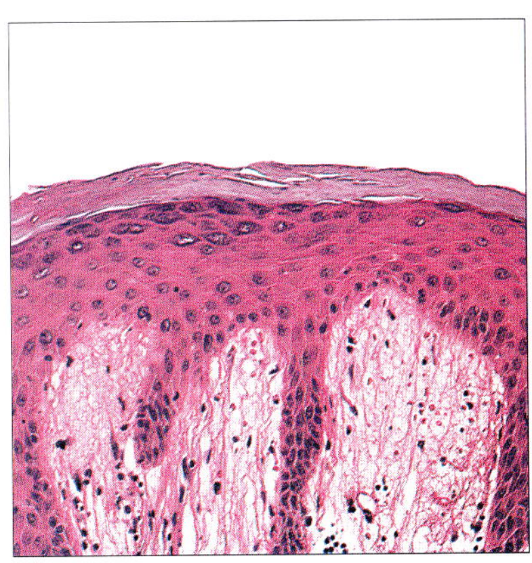

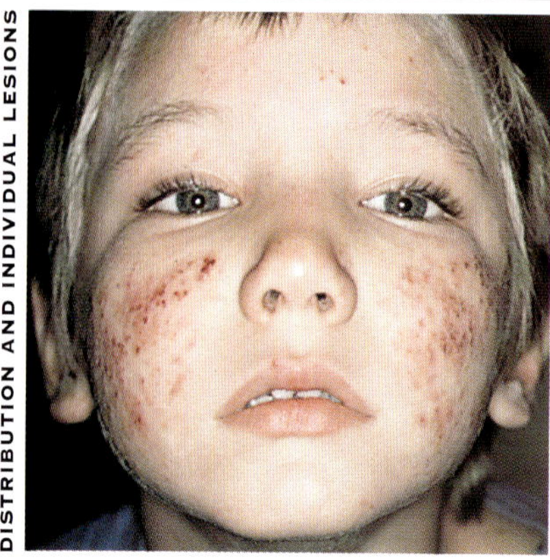

FIG. 74-1 *Macules and eroded papules.*

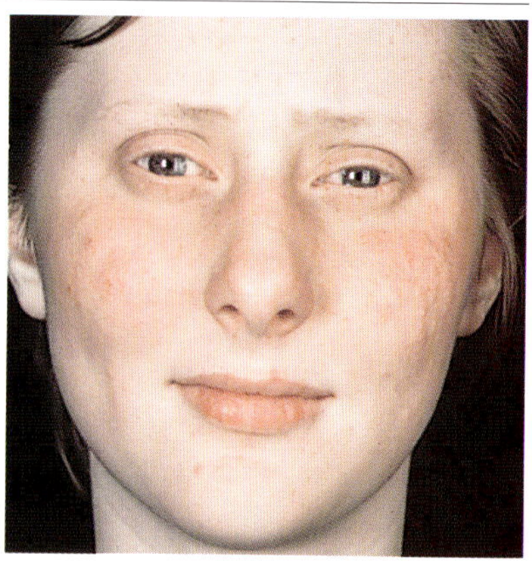

FIG. 74-2 *Papules, some discrete and others confluent, on malar eminences, cheeks, nose, and chin.*

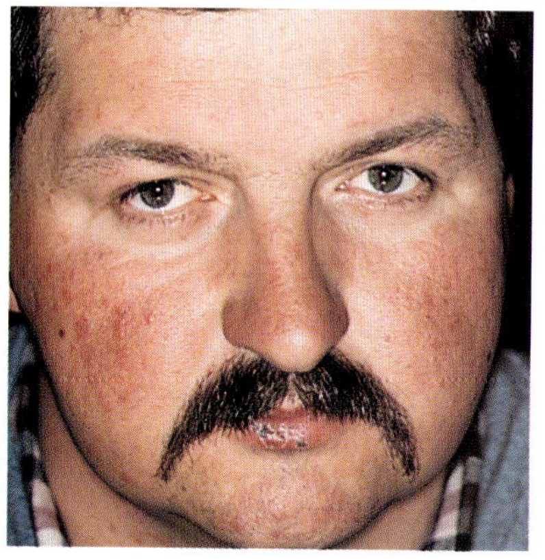

FIG. 74-3 *Papules on the cheeks and nose especially.*

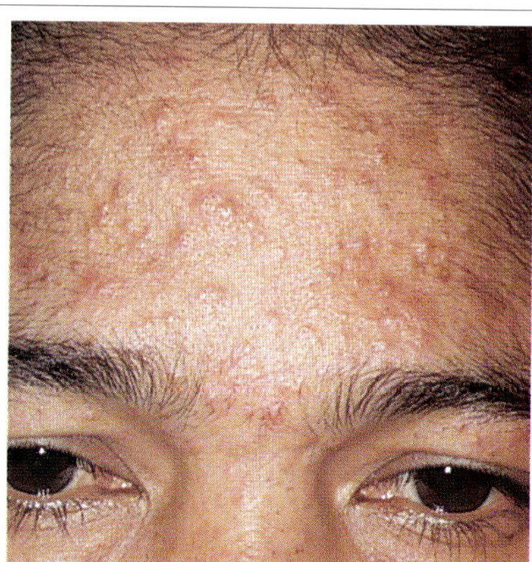

FIG. 74-4 *Discrete papules, some of them in clusters.*

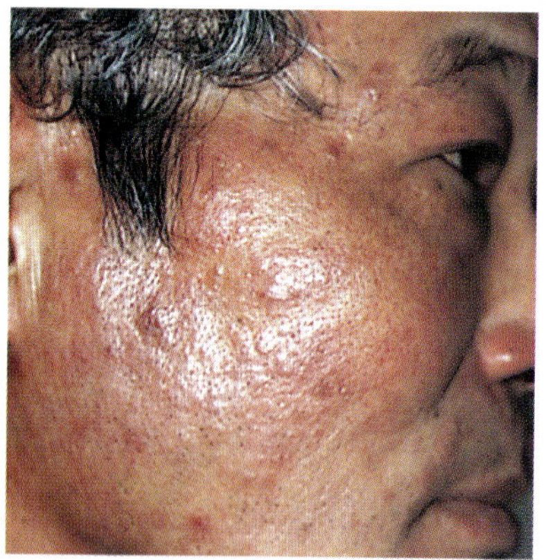

FIG. 74-5 *Edematous papules.*

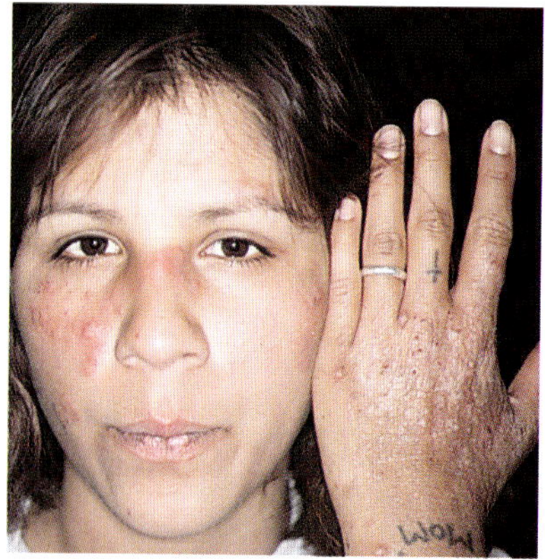

FIG. 74-6 *Papules on the face, and signs of lichen simplex chronicus on the lips and on the dorsum of the hand.*

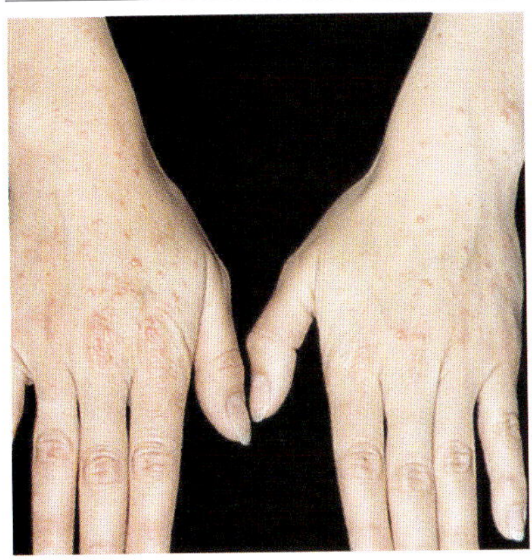 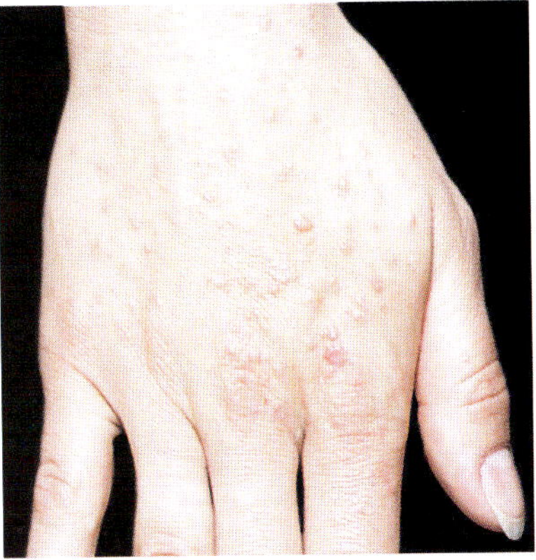

FIG. 74-7 (A, B) *Papules, some of which are edematous.*

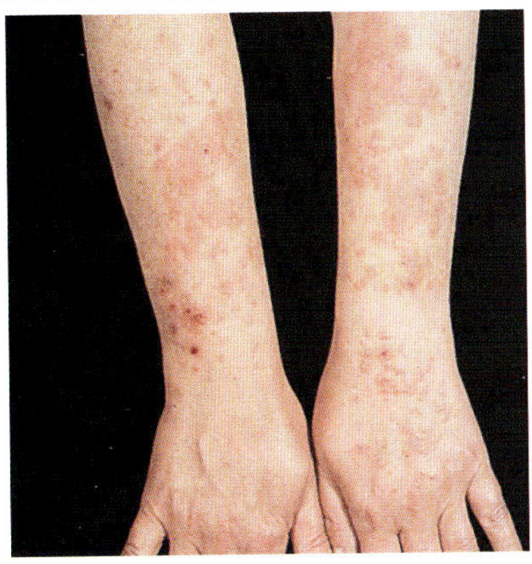 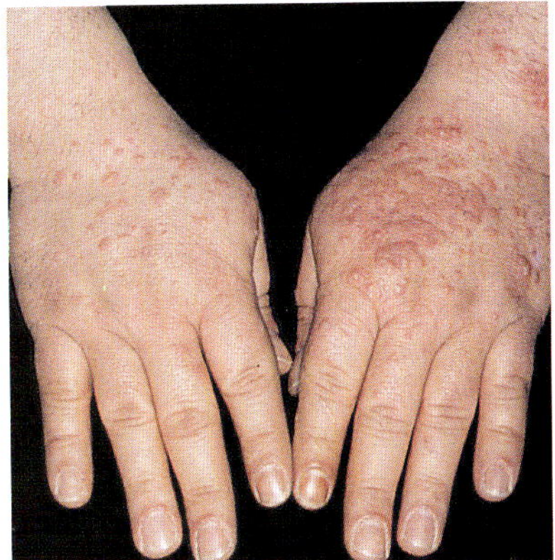

FIG. 74-8 *Papules and plaques, some of them crusted.*

FIG. 74-9 *Papules are markedly edematous and some are in clusters.*

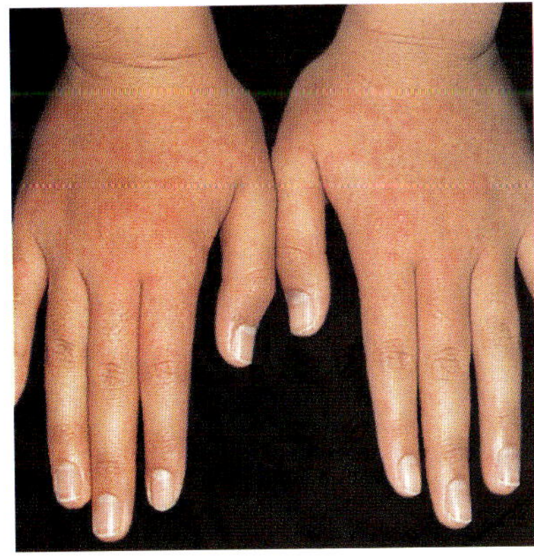 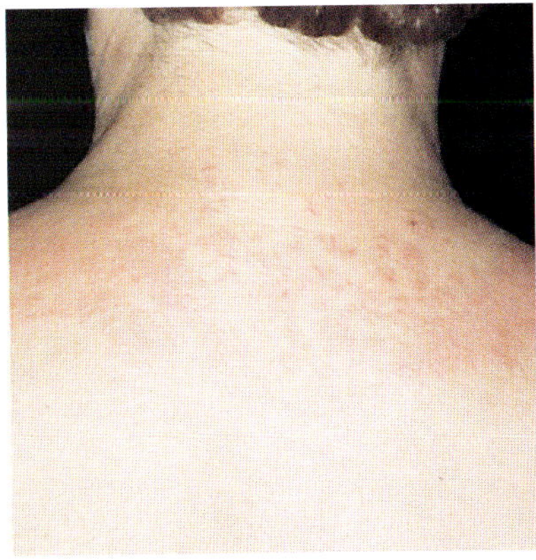

FIG. 74-10 *Edematous papules in clusters.*

FIG. 74-11 *Papules, some of which are discrete, and some of which have become confluent to form plaques.*

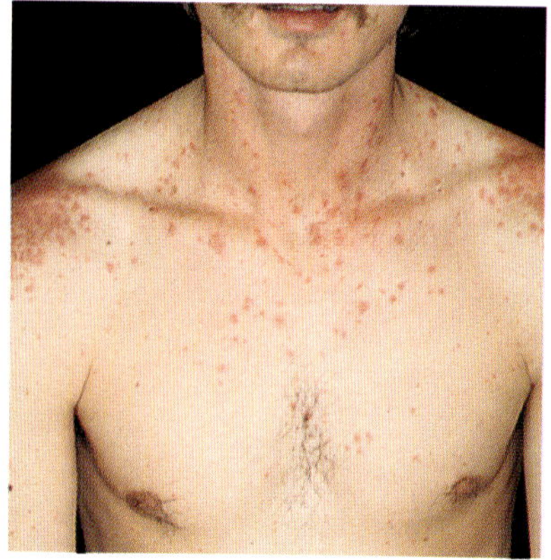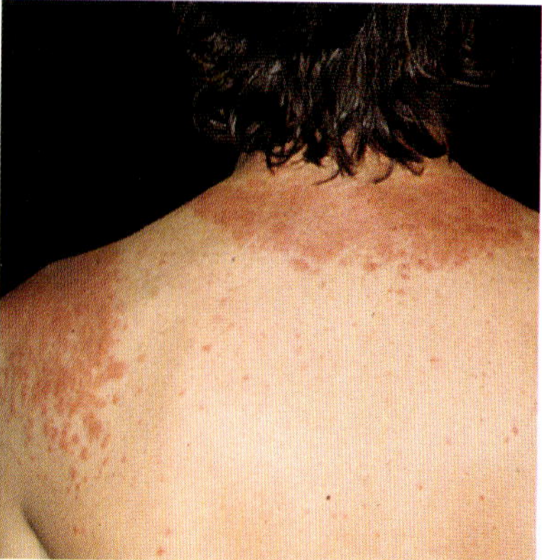

FIG. 74-12 (A, B) *Scattered papules, many of them having become confluent to form plaques.*

ADJUNCTIVE DIAGNOSTIC TESTS A patient's skin, when exposed by phototests to particular wavelengths of ultraviolet light produced by specially designed lamps, responds with lesions typical of polymorphous light eruption.

COURSE Individual papules and papulovesicles of polymorphous light eruption usually last for several days before resolving without residua. The condition itself may persist for as long as the skin is exposed to sunlight.

INTEGRATION: UNIFYING CONCEPT Polymorphous light eruption is a distinctive type of photodermatitis thought to be a consequence of delayed hypersensitivity to a yet undetermined allergen that is either induced or liberated in the skin by the effects of ultraviolet light. Although there are different morphologic expressions of polymorphous light eruption, the most common is edematous papules and plaques. All fully-developed lesions of polymorphous light eruption have in common a superficial and deep perivascular infiltrate of lymphocytes and prominent edema in the papillary dermis. The edema sometimes can be so extensive that it verges on subepidermal vesiculation. Some examples of polymorphous light eruption may display focal spongiosis and scale-crusts.

Polymorphous light eruption can be diagnosed with confidence, clinically and histopathologically, by virtue of repeatable and reliable criteria. It is different, morphologically and mechanistically, from photoallergic dermatitis and phototoxic dermatitis.

THERAPY For prophylaxis, exposure to the sun should be avoided and sun screens should be applied. PUVA may also be employed to "harden" the skin. Corticosteroids may be utilized topically and betacarotene or hydroxychloroquine may be given systemically.

DEFINITION A constellation of conditions that assumes various forms clinically but whose most dependable denominator in common (the exception being the punctate manifestation) is a keratotic ring around a central zone of atrophy, e.g., in a congenital expression that takes the form of a plaque (Mibelli), in a congenital manifestation in which lesions are in linear array (segmental), in an acquired type induced by ultraviolet light (disseminated superficial actinic), and in an acquired form in which lesions are not in photodistribution (disseminated superficial).

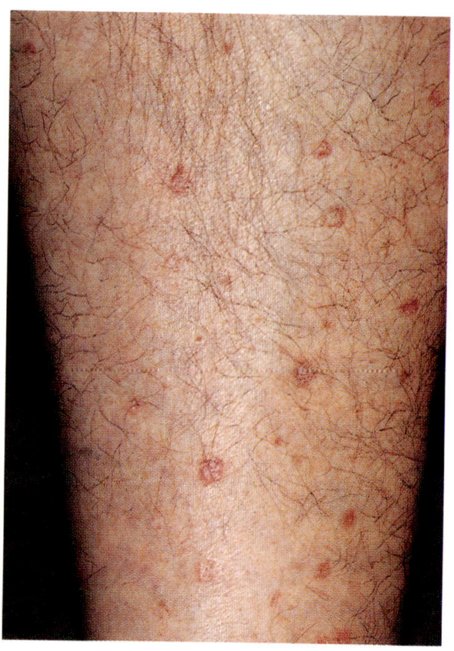

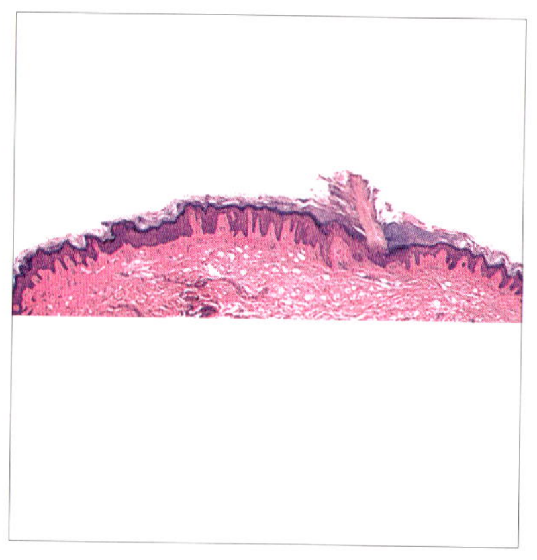

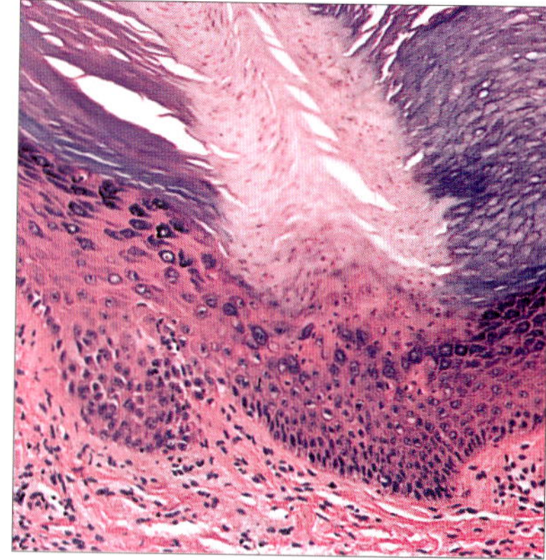

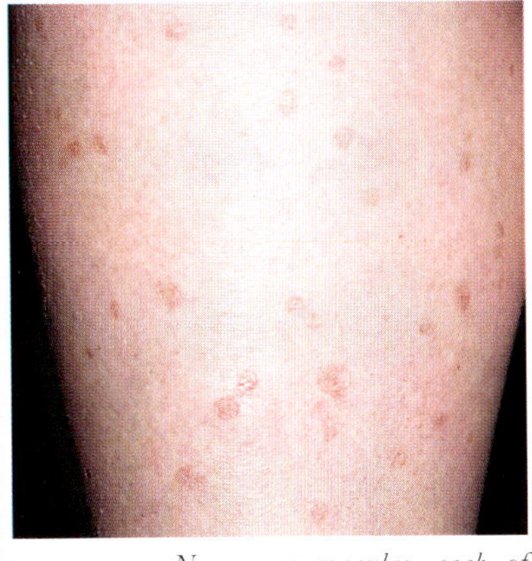

FIG. 75-1 *Numerous macules, each of which is surrounded by a subtle rim of horny material.*

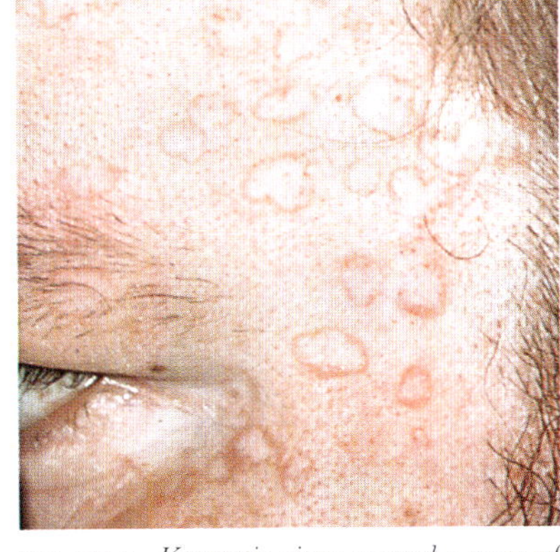

FIG. 75-2 *Keratotic rings around a zone of atrophy.*

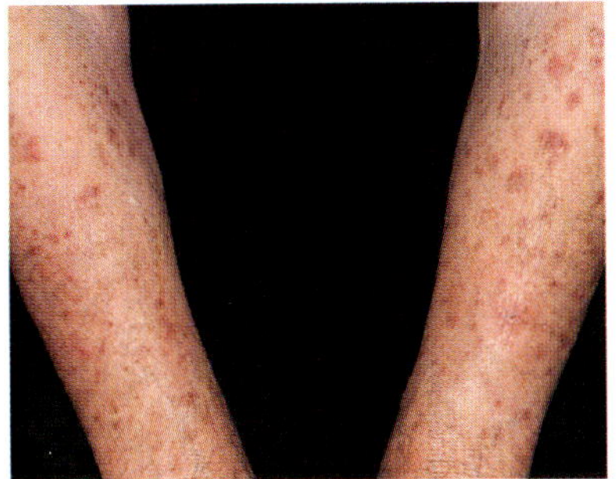

FIG. 75-3 *Widespread papules and small plaques.*

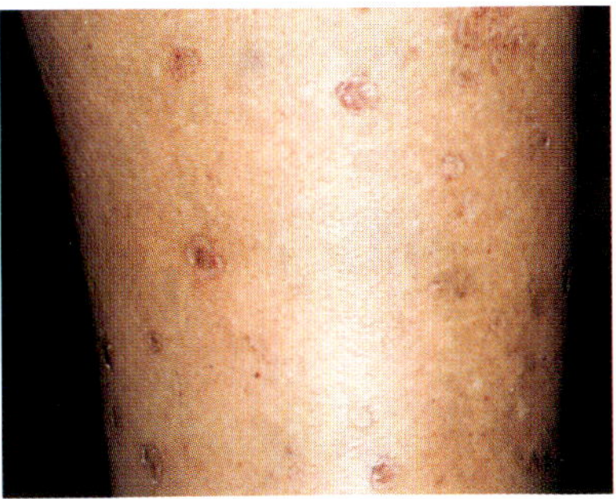

FIG. 75-4 *Annular lesions characterized by a keratotic rim and an atrophic center.*

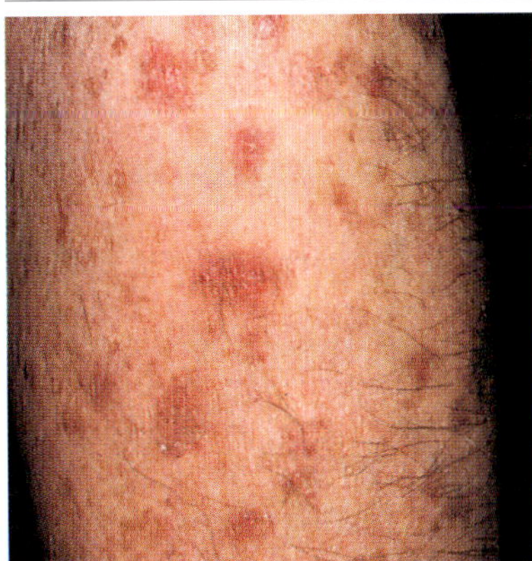

FIG. 75-5 *Keratotic rims around a reddish center. These lesions sometimes are misdiagnosed clinically as solar keratoses.*

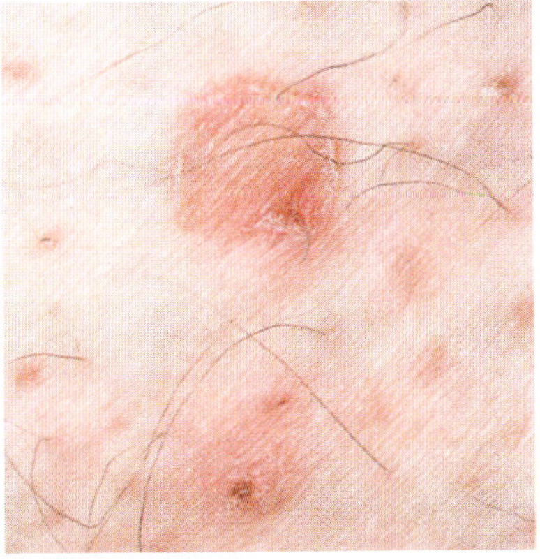

FIG. 75-6 *Erythematous papule with a keratotic rim.*

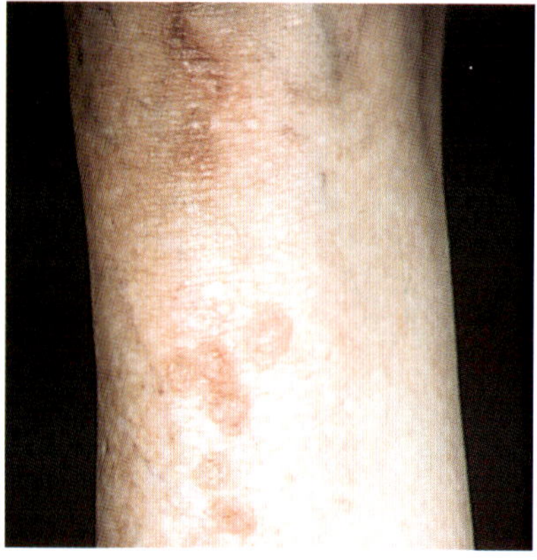

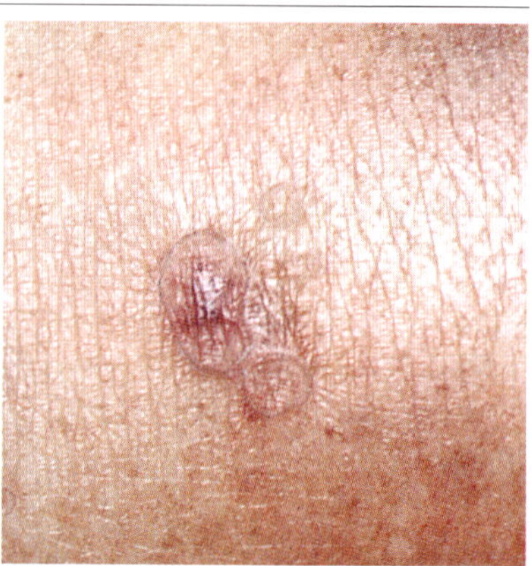

FIG. 75-7 *Tan lesions made up of a keratotic rim and an atrophic center.*

FIG. 75-8 *Papules with a keratotic rim.*

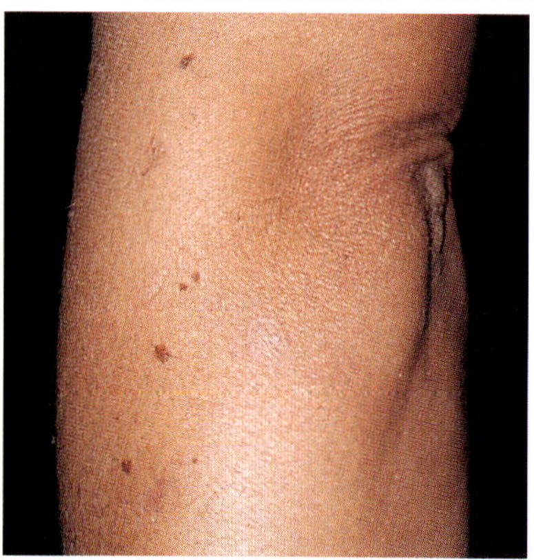

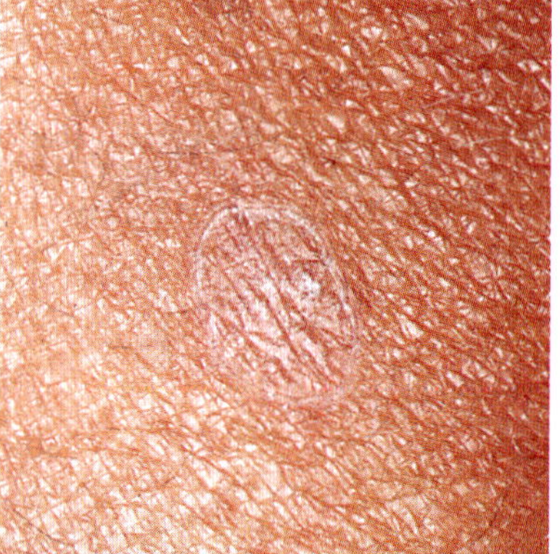

FIG. 75-9 (A, B) *Subtle off-white macules typified by hints of a keratotic rim and an atrophic center. Note also the Clark's nevi.*

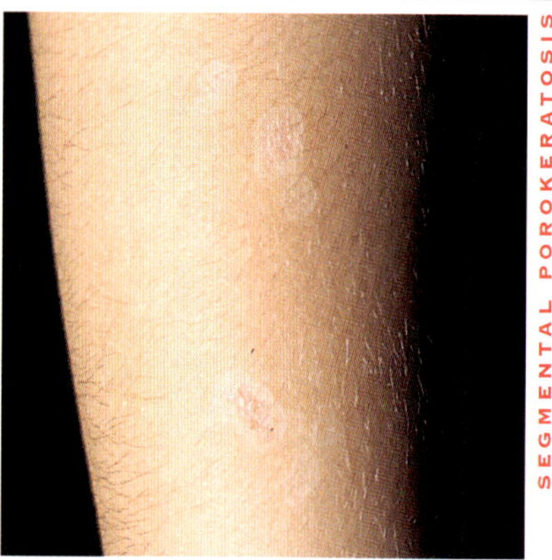

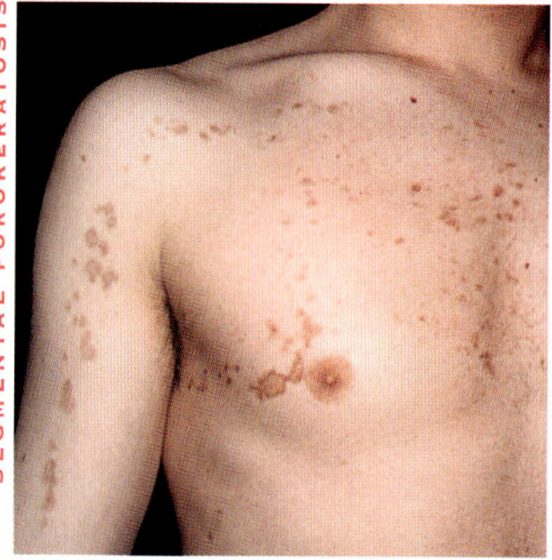

FIG. 75-10 *Subtle off-white macules with a hint of a keratotic rim and an atrophic center.*

FIG. 75-11 *Discrete macules with a keratotic rim and an atrophic center confined to one-half of the body (nevoid type).*

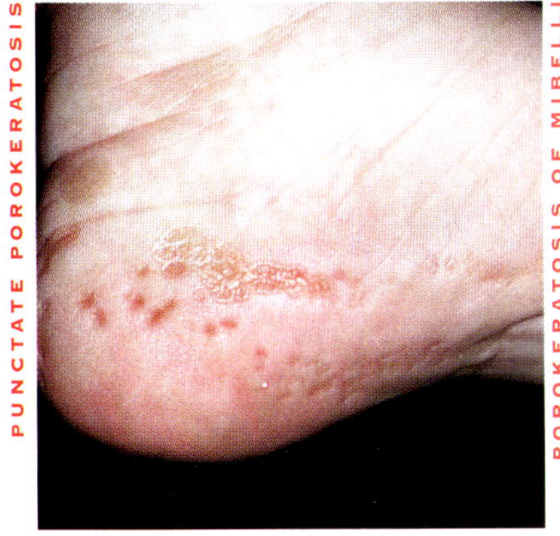

FIG. 75-12 *Discrete depressions with a keratotic rim and in linear arrangement (porokeratosis punctata).*

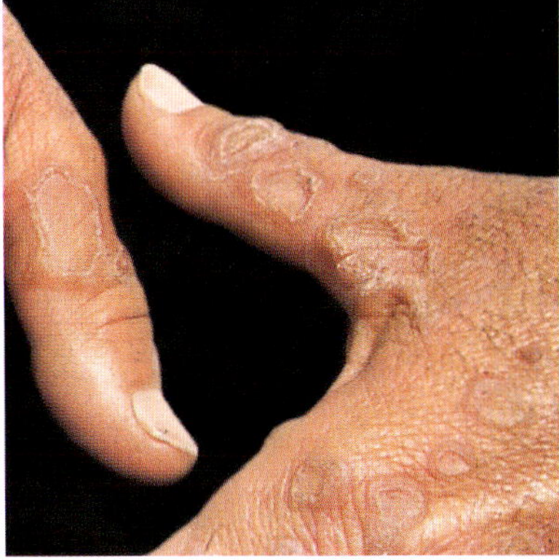

FIG. 75-13 *Prominent keratotic rim around an atrophic center of several lesions.*

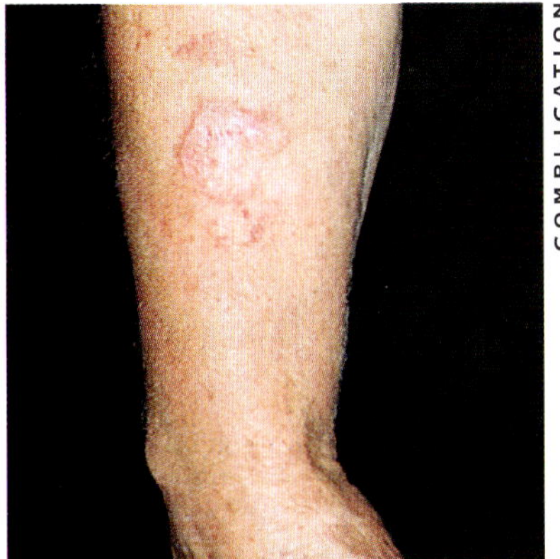

FIG. 75-14 *Patch with keratotic rim.*

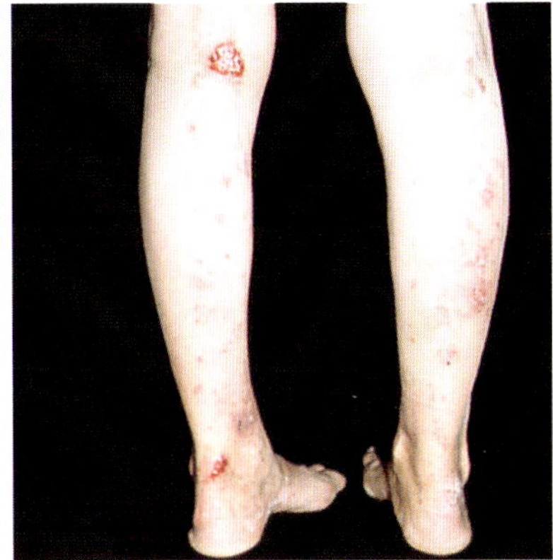

FIG. 75-15 *Lesions with a keratotic rim and an atrophic center in linear array. Two ulcerated plaques are squamous-cell carcinomas.*

COURSE Each of the several different types of porokeratosis, namely, Mibelli, segmental, disseminated superficial actinic, disseminated superficial, and punctate, has a keratotic element associated with it. In the case of all of them, except for punctate, the keratotic aspect takes the form of a rim around a zone that at first is a reddish macule, then a reddish papule, and eventually a hypopigmented atrophic macule. The lesions of porokeratosis characterized by a keratotic rim tend to expand slowly in centrifugal fashion, leaving in their wake a zone of atrophy. At one moment in time, the lesions stop expanding. Punctate keratotic lesions nearly always occur on palms and soles and do not change appreciably over time. Once lesions of porokeratosis have developed, irrespective of type, they tend to last.

A squamous-cell carcinoma may develop rarely in the atrophic center of any type of porokeratosis.

INTEGRATION: UNIFYING CONCEPT The common denominator for all types of porokeratosis is a keratotic dimension clinically and a distinctive column of parakeratosis (a cornoid lamella) that emerges from eccrine ducts, infundibula, and epidermis histopathologically and is the analogue of the keratotic rim seen clinically. Beneath each column of parakeratosis the granular zone is absent and dyskeratotic cells are present in the spinous zone. For practical purposes, the constellation of findings that makes up a "cornoid lamella" signifies porokeratosis. Despite that unifying factor, however, it is likely that the so-called porokeratoses represent different diseases.

Cornoid lamellation represents a histopathologic pattern analogous to epidermolytic hyperkeratosis, focal acantholytic dyskeratosis, pale-cell acanthosis, and follicular mucinosis. Just as cornoid lamellation is an attribute of each of the conditions known as porokeratosis, each different from one another, so too, focal acantholytic dyskeratosis is a denominator common to a variety of conditions known by different names. These conditions include, for example, Darier's disease for a disorder of cornification that is widespread and persistent for a lifetime, a Darier-type of epidermal nevus for a disorder of cornification that is segmental, a Darier-type of keratoderma palmaris et plantaris for a disorder of cornification confined to palms and soles, acantholytic dyskeratotic acanthoma for a solitary papule of a benign neoplasm, and Grover's disease for an inflammatory disease that is either "transient" or "persistent" for a few years.

In sum, cornoid lamellation is common to all types of porokeratosis, each type of which seems to be a very different disease. There is no relationship whatsoever between the Mibelli type of porokeratosis, which represents a genodermatosis, and disseminated superficial actinic porokeratosis, which is a type of photodermatosis. Nor is there any relationship between the segmental epidermal nevus marked by cornoid lamellation and the punctate type of keratoderma on palms and soles that is characterized, too, by cornoid lamellation.

Speculations have been published concerning the mechanism of formation of cornoid lamella, but none of them is compelling, and none has been proven.

THERAPY Cryotherapy, laser surgery, and topical application of 5-fluorouracil or retinoids are effective. When lesions are widespread, systemic retinoids are the treatment of choice.

DEFINITION A disease manifested chiefly in the skin by vesicles and bullae that appear on sites of trauma, especially the face and dorsa of the hands, often in conjunction with macular hyperpigmentation and hypertrichosis of a face and sclerodermoid changes on a chest. The cutaneous manifestations are a consequence of enzymatic defects in porphyrin synthesis.

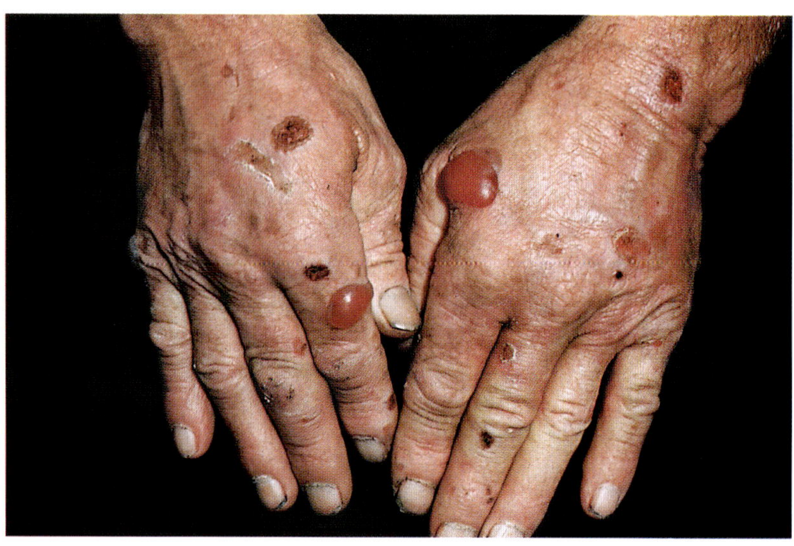

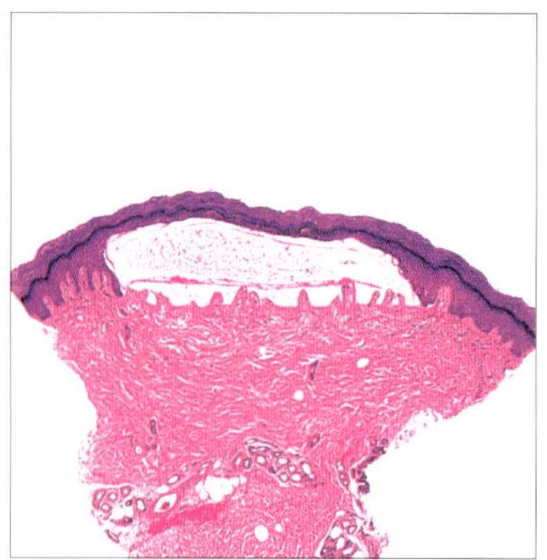

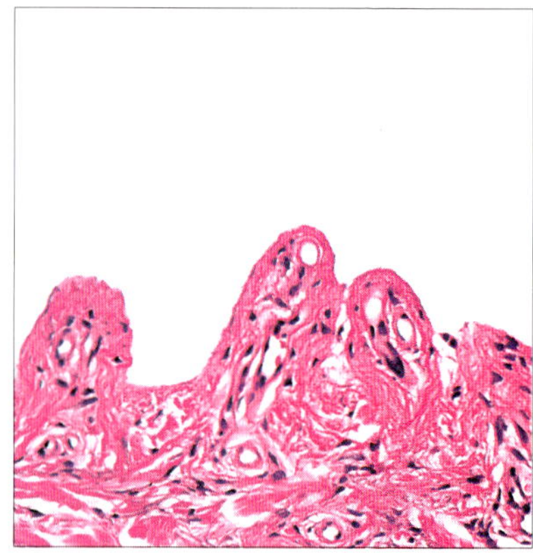

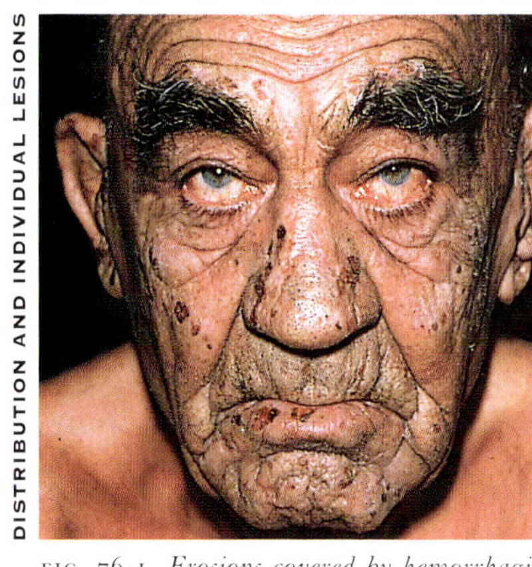

FIG. 76-1 *Erosions covered by hemorrhagic crusts in company with hypertrichosis and hyperpigmentation.*

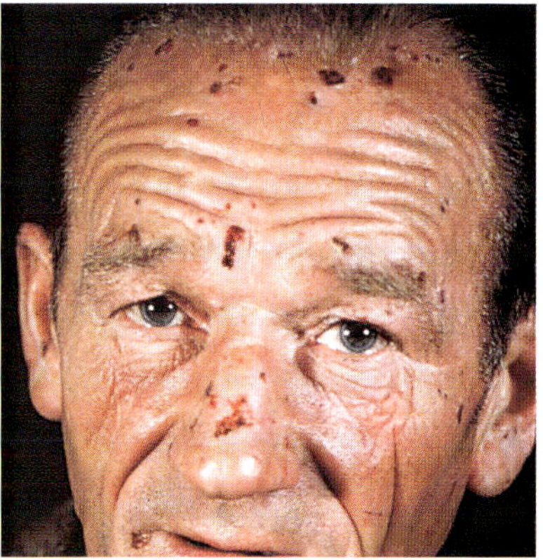

FIG. 76-2 *Hemorrhagic crusts atop erosions.*

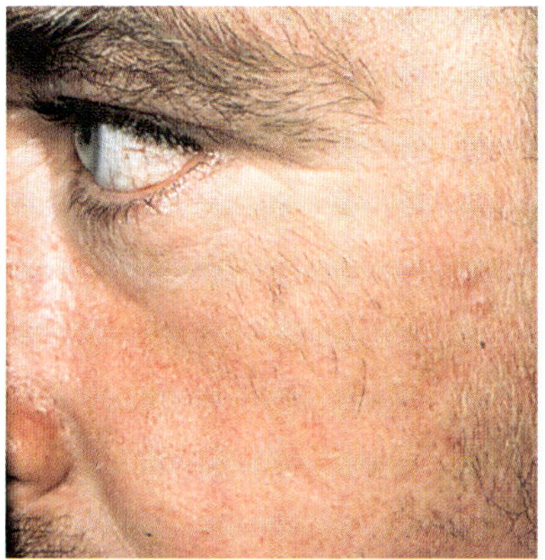

FIG. 76-3 *Hypertrichosis and macular hyperpigmentation.*

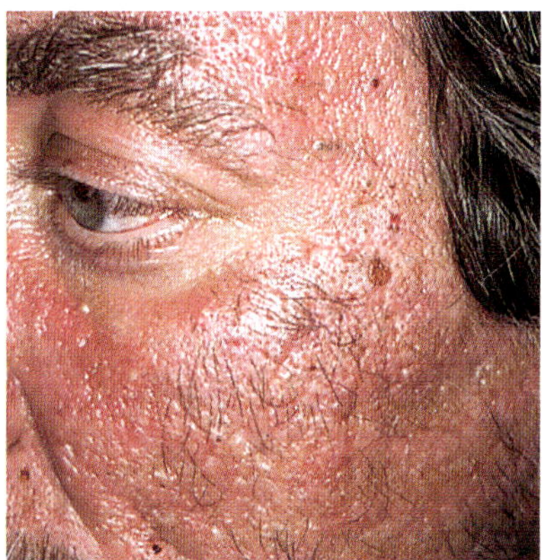

FIG. 76-4 *Hypertrichosis and eroded papules.*

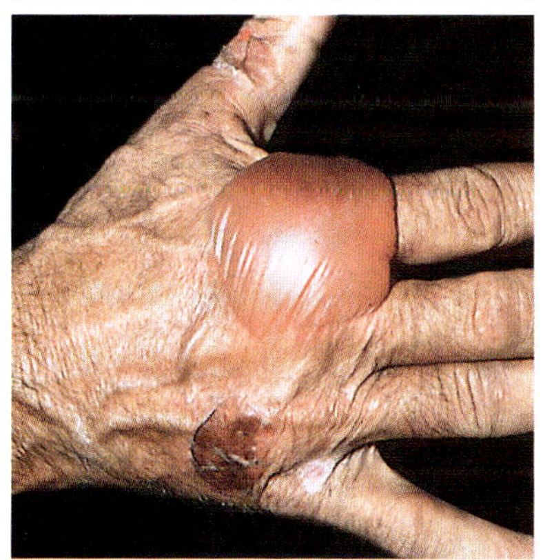

FIG. 76-5 *A bulla, hemorrhagic crusts atop erosions, and an atrophic scar.*

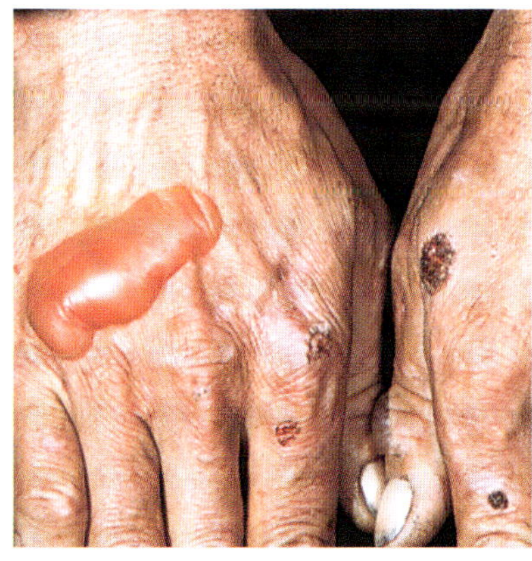

FIG. 76-6 *Vesicles and bullae, hemorrhagic crusts, and scars.*

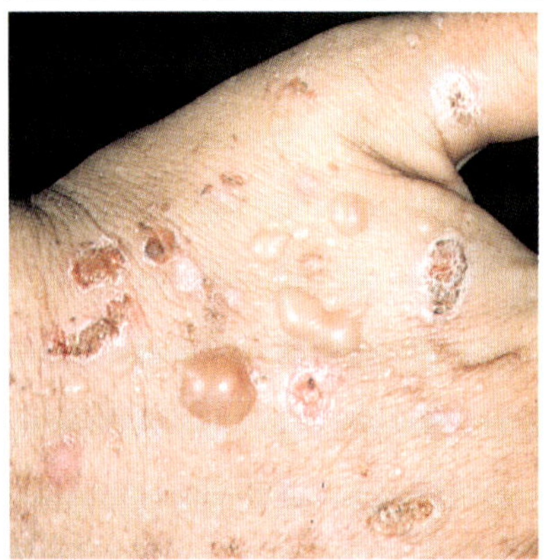

FIG. 76-7 *Large bullae and several blisters that have collapsed and become crusts.*

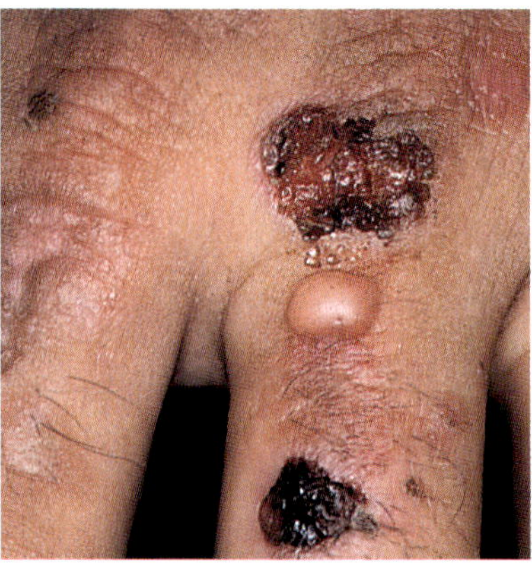

FIG. 76-8 *Erosions, hemorrhagic crusts, and scars. The dome-shaped papule is not a blister, but an infundibular cyst.*

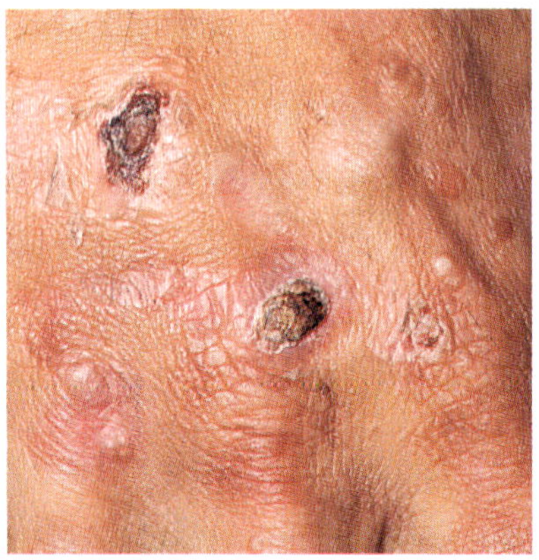

FIG. 76-9 *Vesicles, hemorrhagic crusts atop ulcers, atrophic scars, milia, and postinflammatory hyperpigmentation.*

ADJUNCTIVE DIAGNOSTIC TESTS Assessment should be made of serum iron and ferritin concentrations for evidences of an elevation. Examination of urine with a Wood's lamp should be performed in order to demonstrate pink-red fluorescence. Demonstration of increased quantities of uroporphryin in the urine and increased excretion of isocoproporphyrin infecas are confirmatory.

COURSE The blisters of porphyria cutanea tarda, which usually are vesicles but sometimes are bullae of various sizes, have a characteristic chronologic sequence, which is to break, discharge their fluid contents, and heal within a very few weeks, often with hyper- and hypopigmentation and subtle signs of atrophic scarring. As long as a patient produces abnormal porphyrins, blisters tend to come and go, sometimes for a lifetime.

Types of lesions other than blisters are associated often with porphyria cutanea tarda, among them, hyperpigmentation and hypertrichosis on the face especially, and sclerodermoid changes on the chest in particular. Each of those abnormalities tends to worsen slowly over time, the hyperpigmentation becoming more extensive and more marked, the hypertrichosis becoming ever more apparent, and the peculiar morphea-like changes, in the form usually of a huge butterfly-shaped zone, becoming progressively larger and more yellow. Over the course of many years, the characteristic sclerodermatous changes of porphyria cutanea tarda become less indurated, and the skin becomes more supple.

INTEGRATION: UNIFYING CONCEPT All of the cutaneous manifestations of porphyria cutanea tarda, to wit, blisters, hyperpigmentation, hypertrichosis, and sclerodermatous changes are a reflection of a basic pathologic process that pertains to deficiency of an enzyme crucial to synthesis of porphyrins. The blisters themselves usually are induced by trauma, either mechanical or photochemical. The reasons for the abnormalities of pigmentation, excessive growth of hair, and a morpheiform expression of scleroderma are not known. The pigmentary abnormalities are a consequence of epidermal hyperpigmentation, the hypertrichosis is not reflected in abnormalities of follicles as they are judged histopathologically, and the sclerodermatous changes are seen by conventional microscopy to be just like those of morphea. In regard to the latter, so-called localized scleroderma occurs in very different settings, from porphyria cutanea tarda to tryptophane myalgia syndrome, from en coup de sabre (linear scleroderma on a scalp) to fasciitis with eosinophilia (Shulman's syndrome), from lichen sclerosus et atrophicus limited to genital skin to widespread morphea.

The blisters of porphyria cutanea tarda are subepidermal, and dermal papillae at the base of them tend to be well preserved. That the blistering condition does not qualify as a truly inflammatory one can be told by the absence of infiltrates of inflammatory cells within the dermis. An interesting finding in the upper half of the dermis, however, in addition to extensive solar elastosis, is a rim of homogeneous eosinophilic material around capillaries and venules. The blisters, which result commonly from photosensitivity, are thought to be a consequence of excessive uroporphyrins in the skin. They occur because of the basic deficiency of uroporphyrinogen decarboxylase that follows upon the effects of too much alcohol, estrogen, or iron, or overexposure to hexachlorobenzene or dioxin. Uroporphyrins are induced by UVA to react with other molecules to bring about the morphologic changes typical of the disease.

In sum, porphyria cutanea tarda is but one of several porphyrias, each as different from the other as is each of the sclerodermas, keratoacanthomas, and fibromatoses from the other.

THERAPY Factors that precipitate exacerbations of the disease, such as sunlight, oral contraceptives, and alcohol, should be identified and avoided. Sun screens should be used. Periodic phlebotomy and low doses of an antimalarial, such as chloroquine, taken orally, are very worthwhile.

PRURITIC URTICARIAL PAPULES AND PLAQUES OF PREGNANCY

DEFINITION An inflammatory process in pregnant women near term that consists of urticarial papules and plaques, especially on the trunk and particularly in association with lesions of striae atrophicantes, the lesions disappearing shortly after parturition.

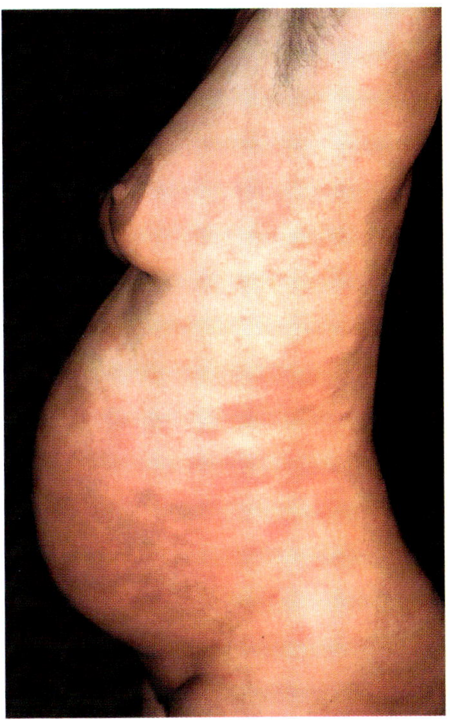

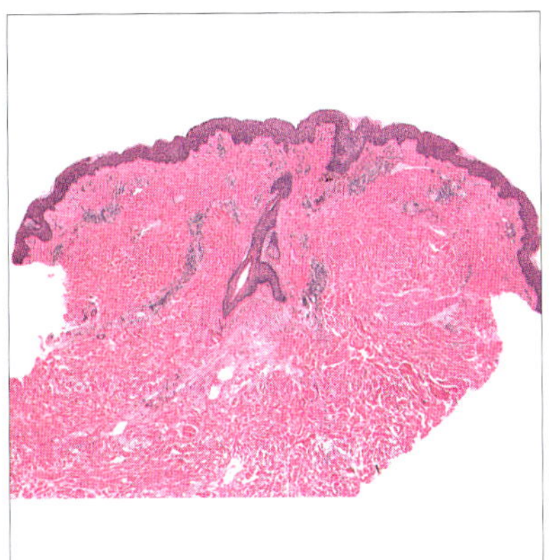

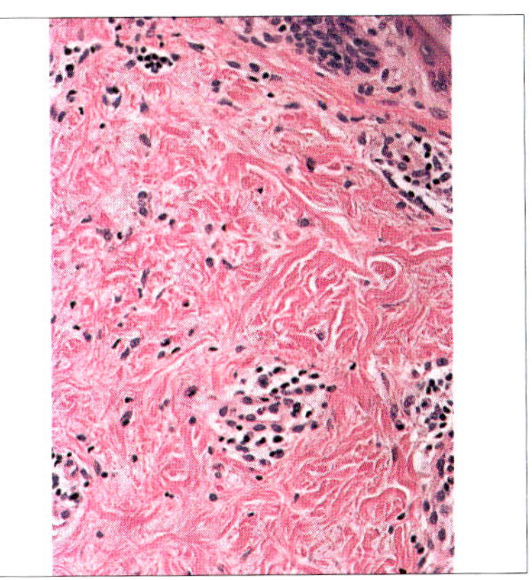

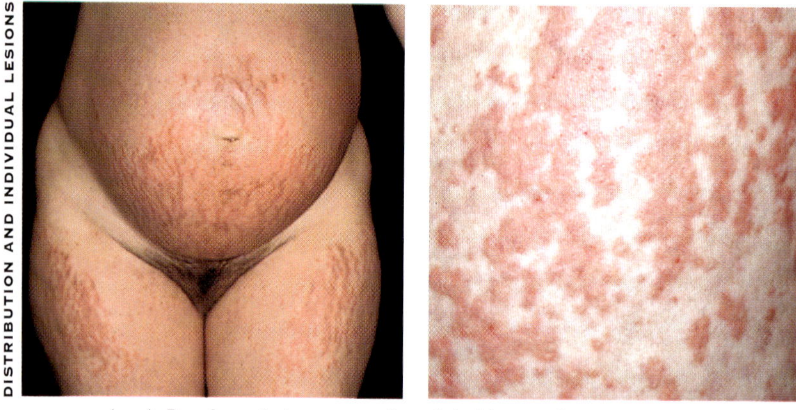

FIG. 77-1 (A, B) *Papules and plaques on a distended abdomen of a woman in the last trimester of pregnancy. The lesions are more prominent in the striae.*

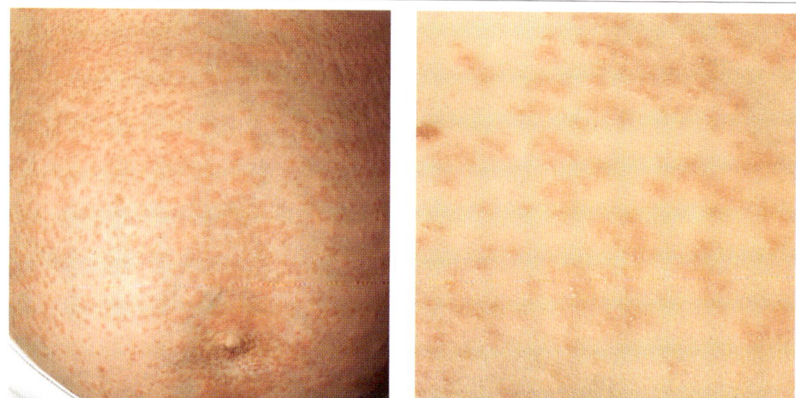

FIG. 77-2 (A, B) *Acuminate papules, some of them isolated and others in clusters.*

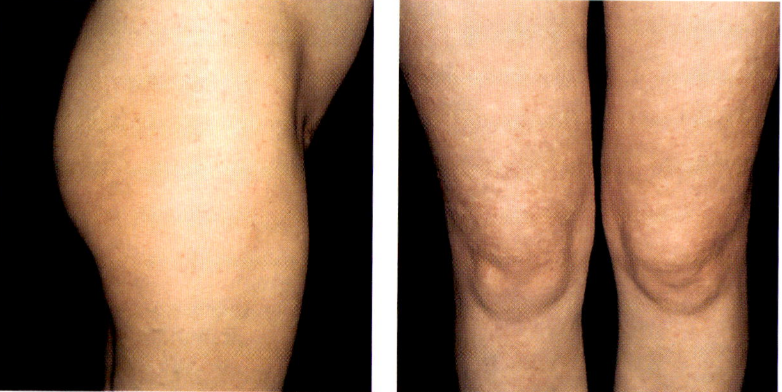

FIG. 77-3 (A, B) *Soon after parturition, papules begin to fade and become skin-colored before disappearing completely.*

COURSE The urticarial papules and plaques that typify this condition of the terminal phase of pregnancy last for many days, but disappear shortly postpartum, as does the condition itself.

INTEGRATION: UNIFYING CONCEPT There are only two major inflammatory diseases of pregnancy, to wit, herpes gestationis and pruritic urticarial papules and plaques of pregnancy. The two diseases are very different from each other, the former being fundamentally a subepidermal blistering disease that bears many morphologic similarities to bullous pemphigoid, whereas the latter is basically a superficial perivascular and interstitial dermatitis that may be associated with spongiosis, which is insufficient to eventuate in vesiculation. Eosinophils are present in extraordinary numbers in herpes gestationis, but usually are only few in pruritic urticarial papules and plaques of pregnancy.

The cause and mechanism of pruritic urticarial papules and plaques of pregnancy is not known, but as the title indicates, the disease is clearly related to events that occur near the end of pregnancy.

THERAPY A topical soothing lotion or hydrocortisone cream helps to alleviate pruritus, but patients with an extensive eruption may require low doses of systemic corticosteroids.

DEFINITION An inflammatory disease of genetic nature that begins with red macules that quickly become nonscaly papules that in turn become scaly papules and plaques. If the process becomes widespread, an erythroderma results, and if it is accelerated, pustules form. The scaly discrete lesions favor extensor surfaces, especially elbows and knees, but any site may be affected, including nail units and, uncommonly, mucous membranes. Approximately 5 percent of patients with psoriasis develop an arthritis that, although it bears similarities to rheumatoid arthritis, seems to be different from it.

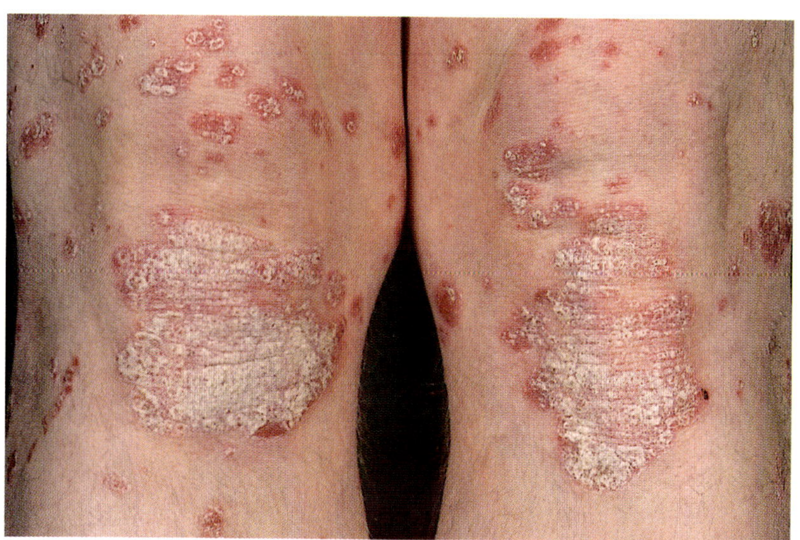

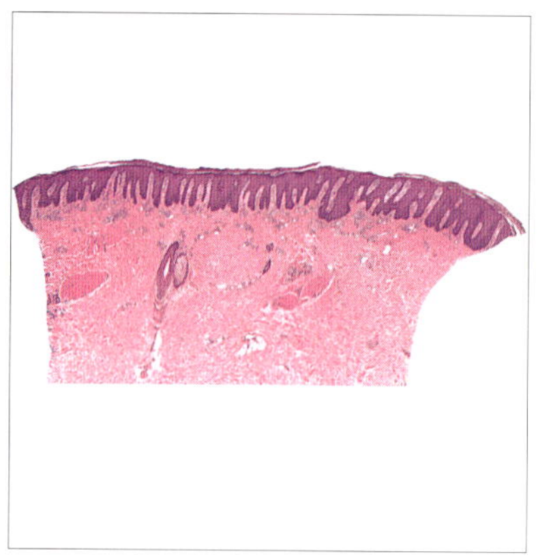

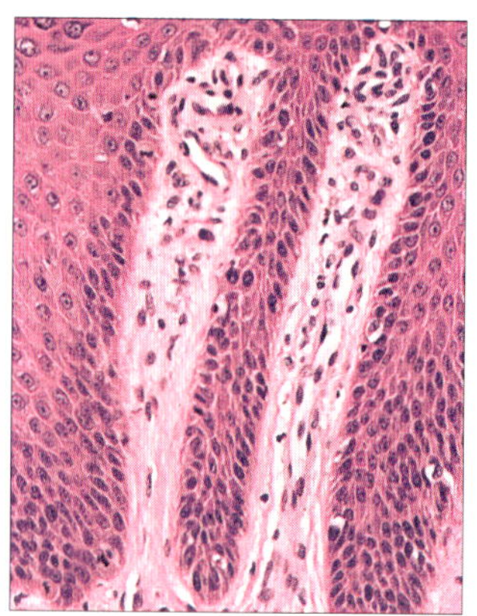

DISTRIBUTION

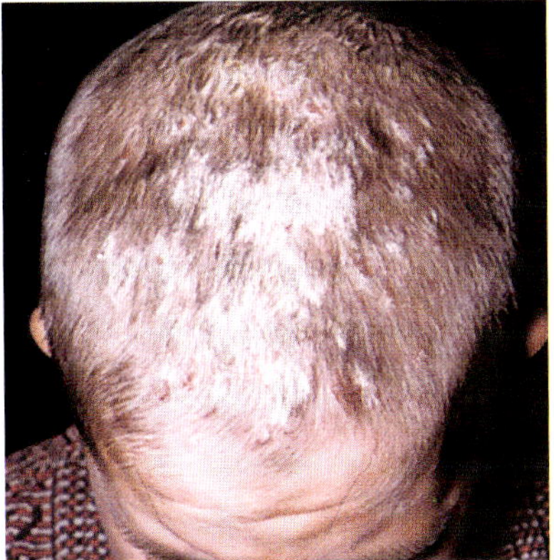

FIG. 78-1 *Scaly papules and keratotic plaques.*

FIG. 78-2 *Plaques that are so keratotic that they have been compared to the appearance of asbestos (tinea amiantacea).*

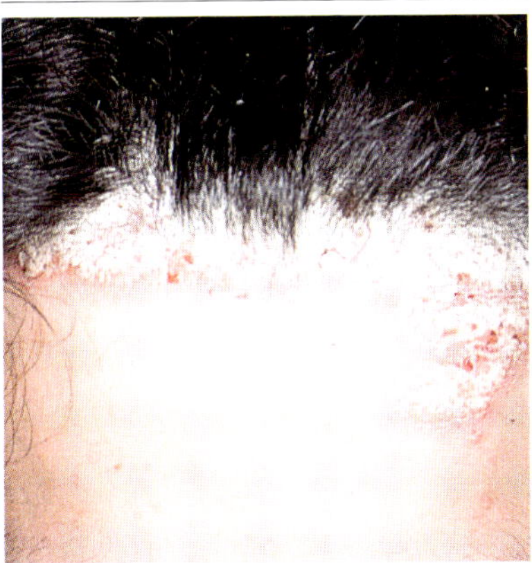

FIG. 78-3 *Plaques along the hairline.*

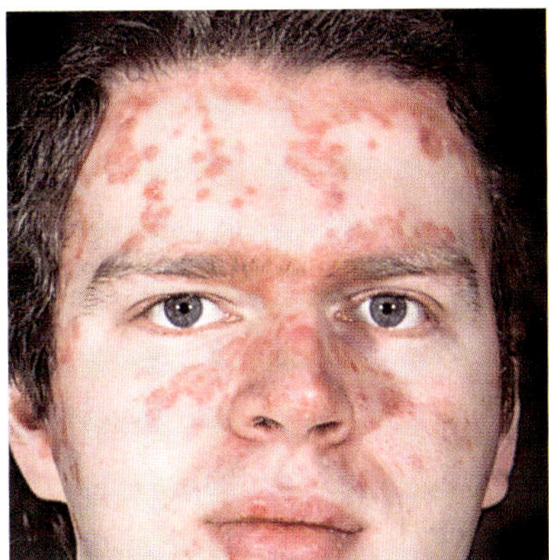

FIG. 78-4 *Lesions on the face and the anterior portion of the scalp.*

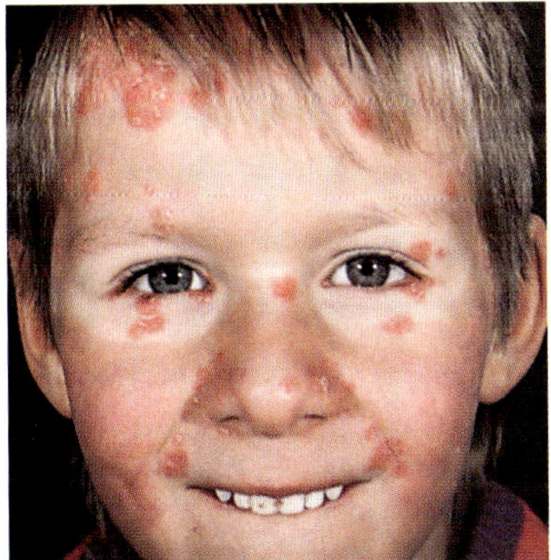

FIG. 78-5 *Papules and plaques on the face and scalp.*

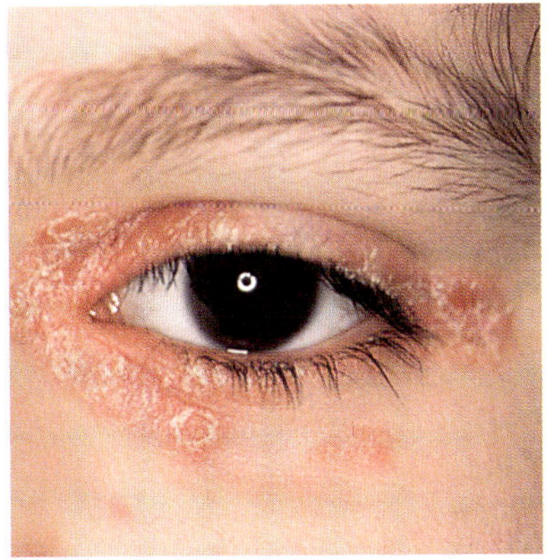

FIG. 78-6 *Scaly papules and plaques on periocular skin.*

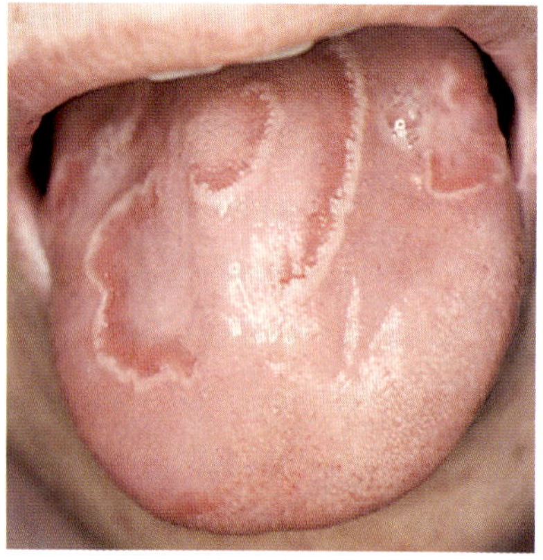

FIG. 78-7 *Figurate lesions (geographic tongue).*

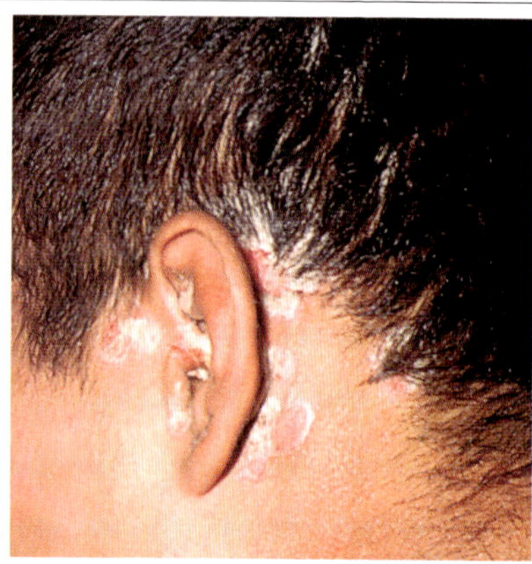

FIG. 78-8 *Scaly plaques.*

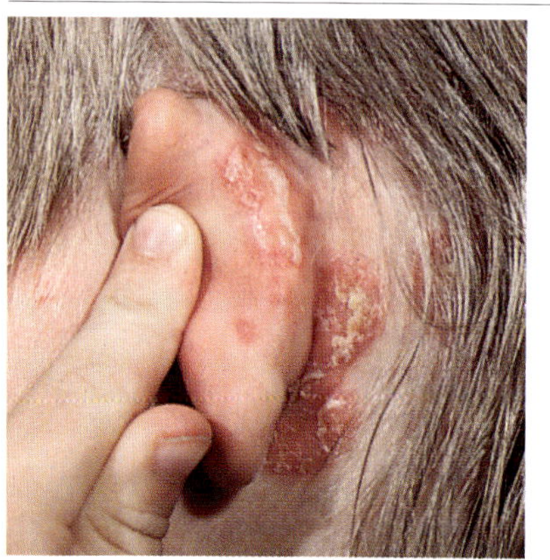

FIG. 78-9 *Scaly plaques.*

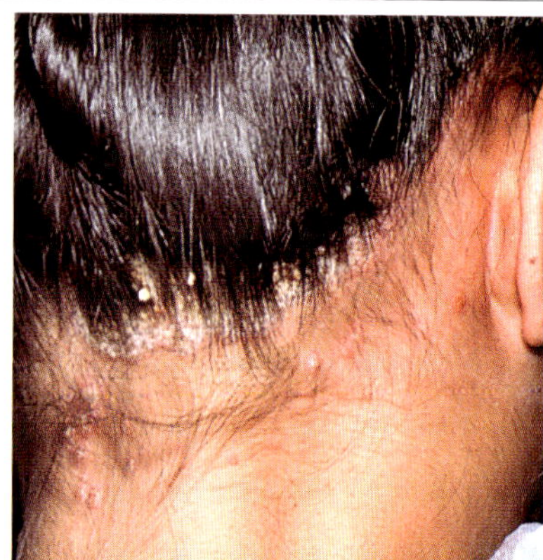

FIG. 78-10 *Scaly papules that have become confluent to form plaques.*

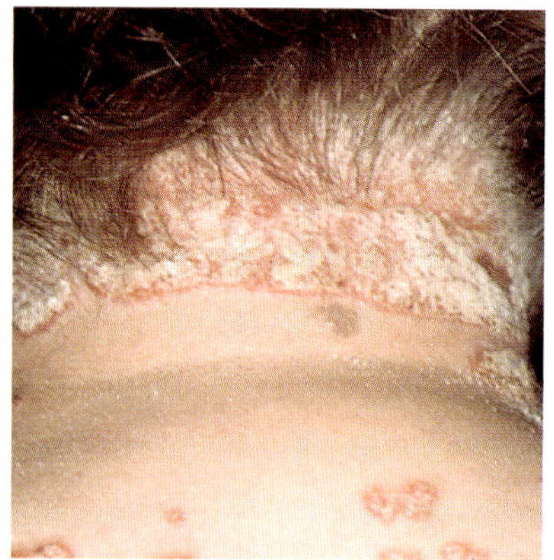

FIG. 78-11 *Scaly papules and plaques.*

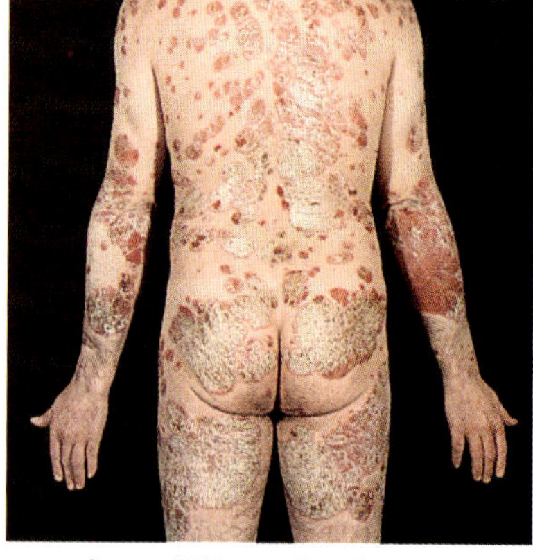

FIG. 78-12 *Widespread scaly papules and plaques.*

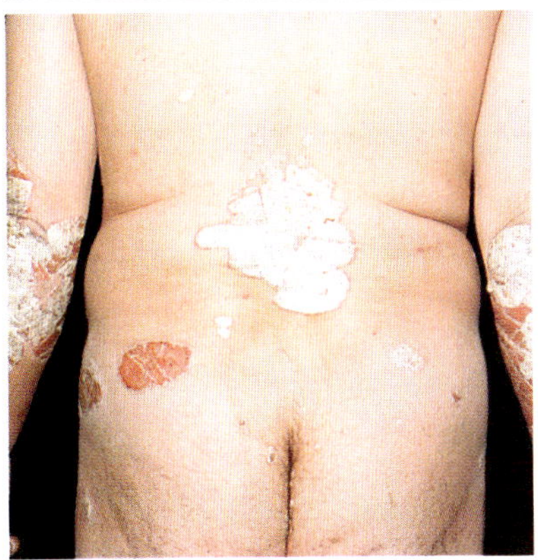

FIG. 78-13 *Scaly papules and plaques.*

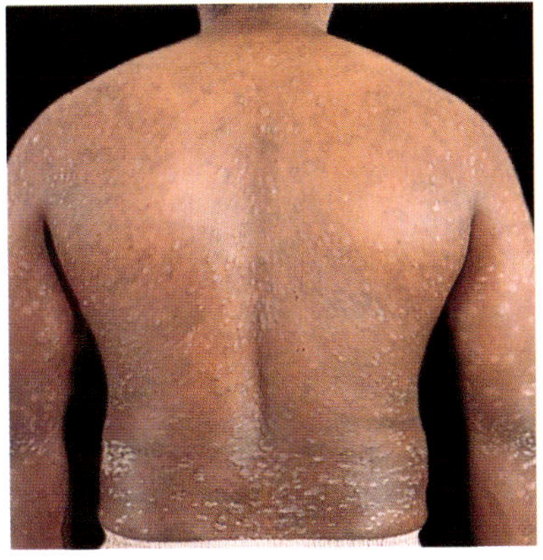

FIG. 78-14 *Widespread nonscaly and scaly papules, some of which have become confluent to form plaques.*

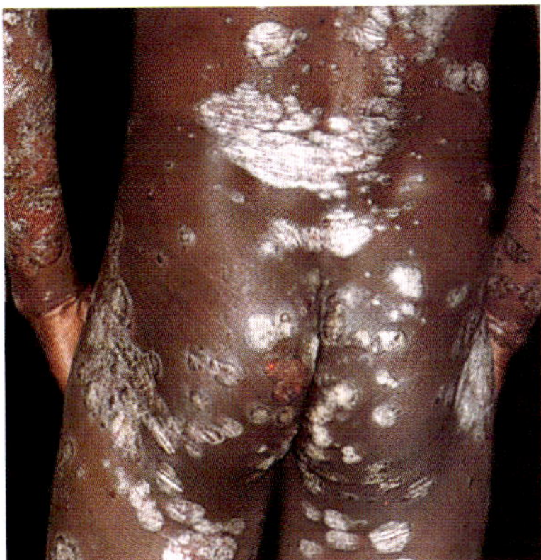

FIG. 78-15 *Scaly papules and plaques.*

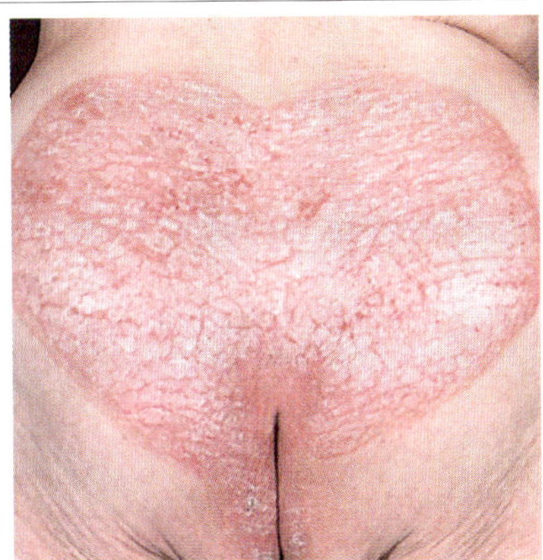

FIG. 78-16 *Broad, scaly plaque.*

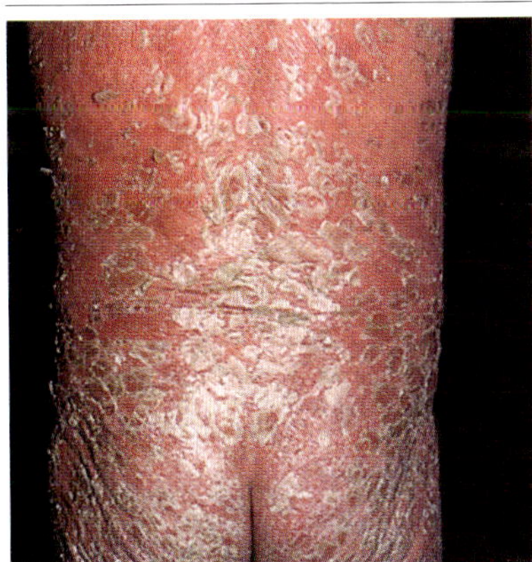

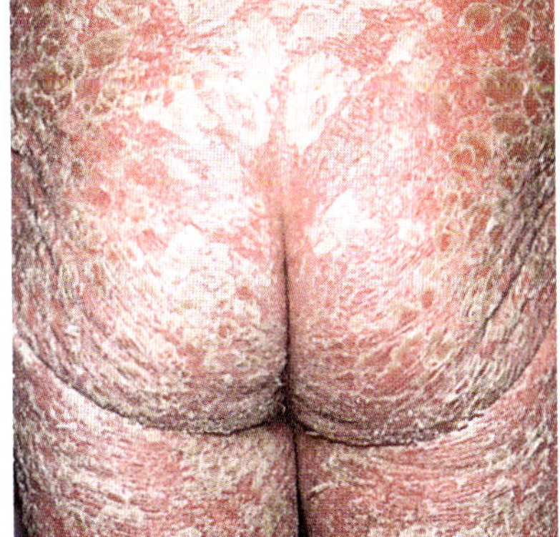

FIG. 78-17 (A, B) *Erythroderma with large gray scales.*

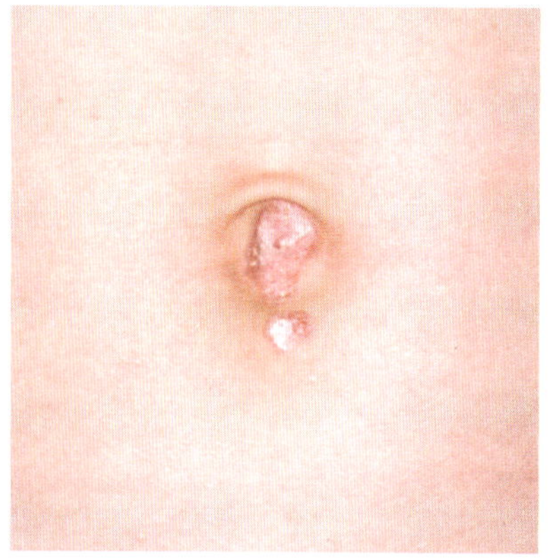

FIG. 78-18 *Scaly papule.*

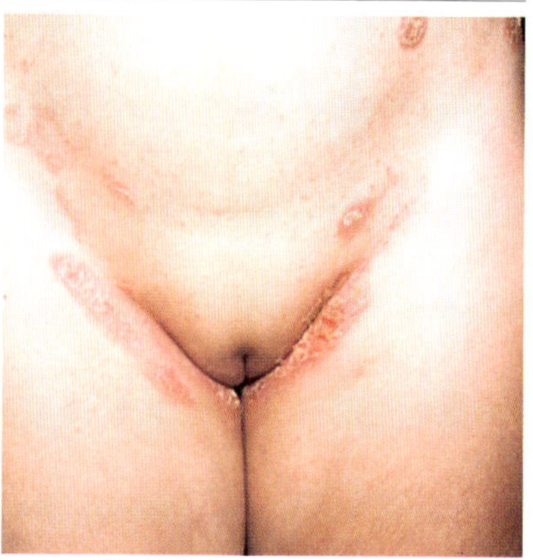

FIG. 78-19 *Scaly plaques.*

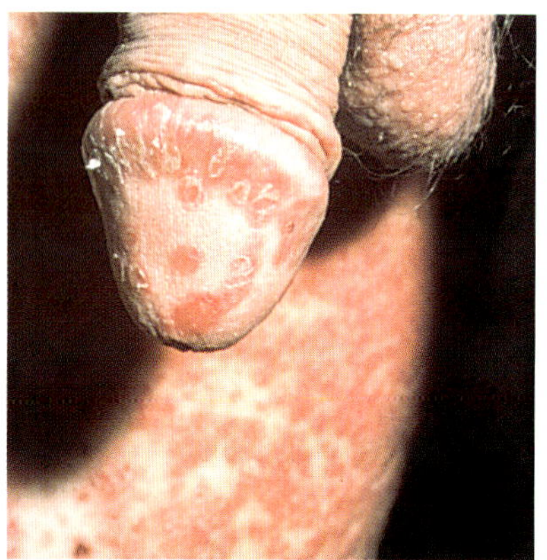

FIG. 78-20 *Scaly papules.*

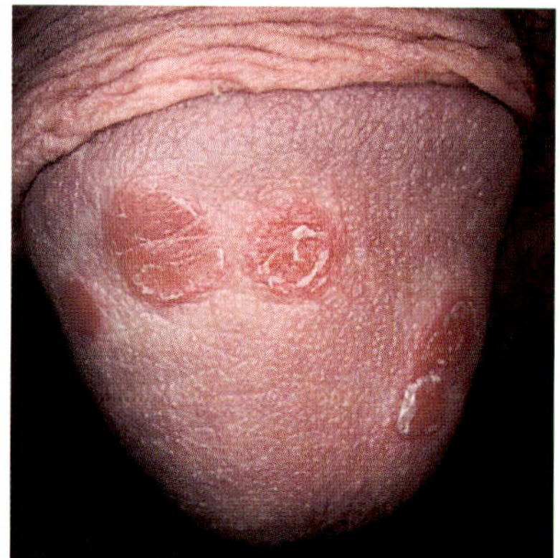

FIG. 78-21 *Scaly guttate papules.*

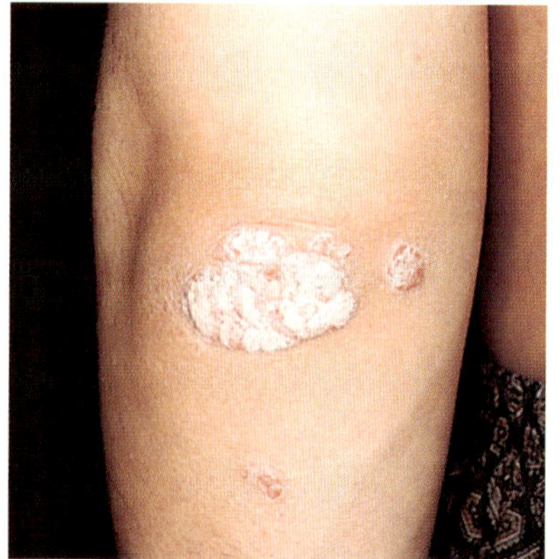

FIG. 78-22 *Scaly plaque on an elbow and two papules in the vicinity of it.*

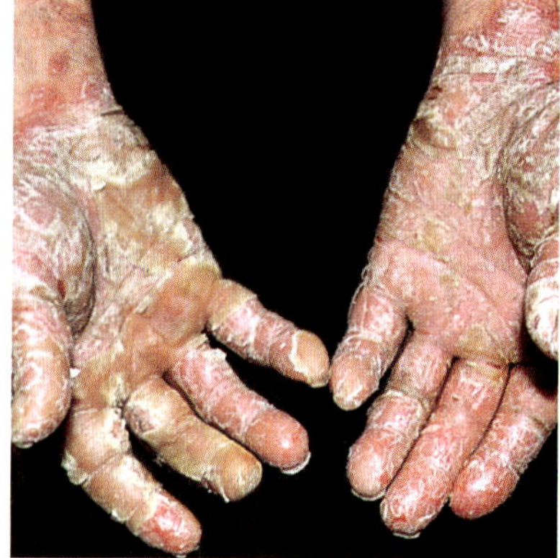

FIG. 78-23 *Scaly plaques.*

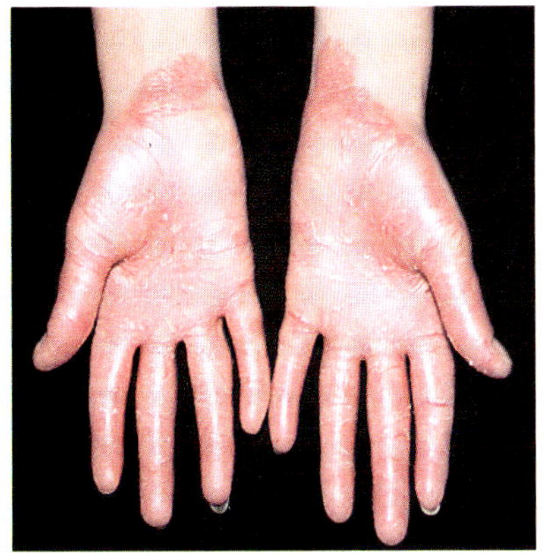

FIG. 78-24 *Diffuse erythema and scaling of atrophic fingers, palms, and wrists.*

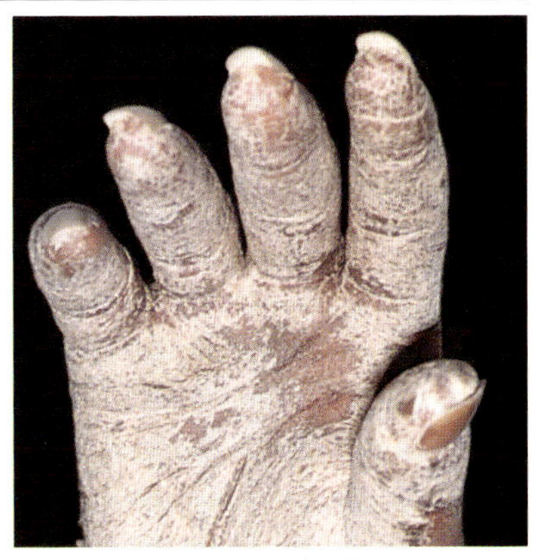

FIG. 78-25 *Extensive scaly plaque.*

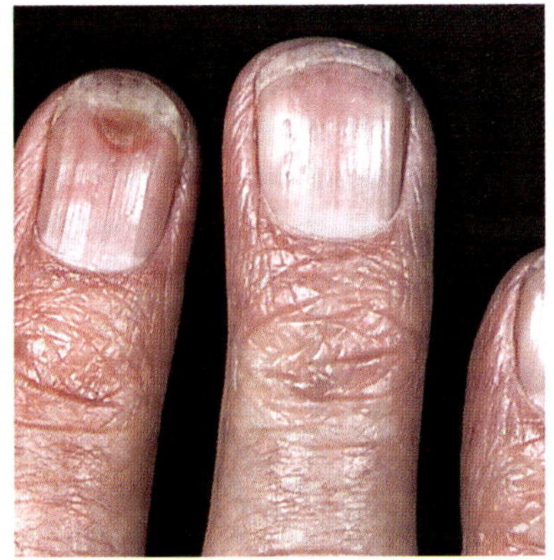

FIG. 78-26 *Prominent pits of the nails and an "oil drop" sign of the nail of the fourth finger.*

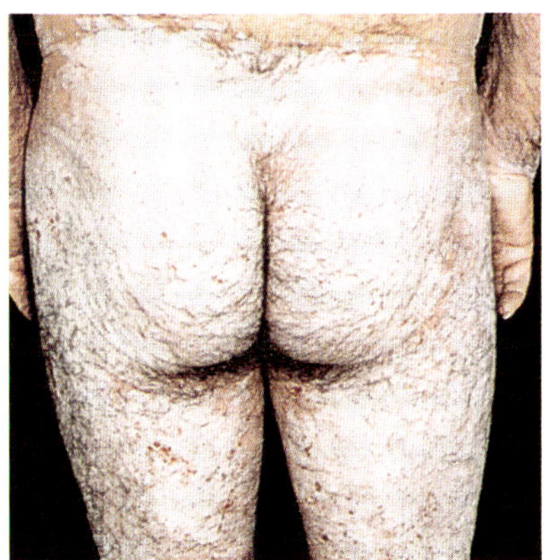

FIG. 78-27 *Diffuse scaly plaque is pruritic as evidenced by excoriations.*

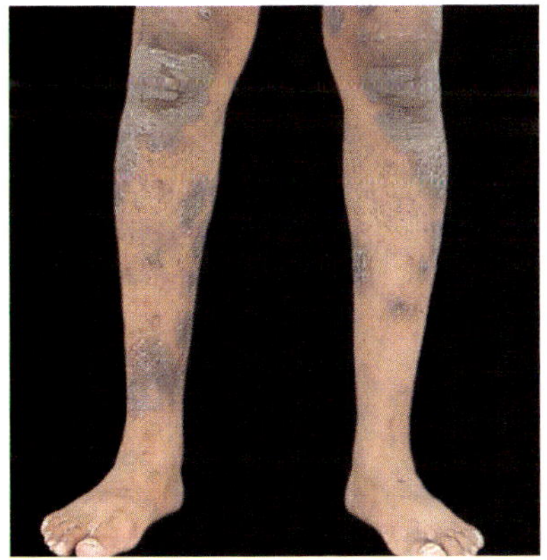

FIG. 78-28 *Scaly plaques.*

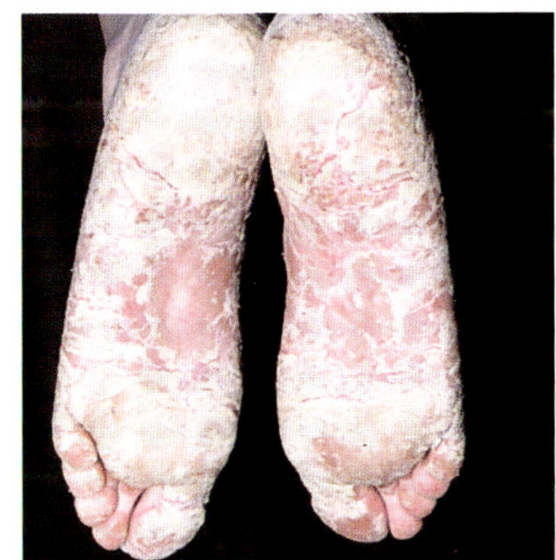

FIG. 78-29 *Scaly plaques on weight-bearing zones especially.*

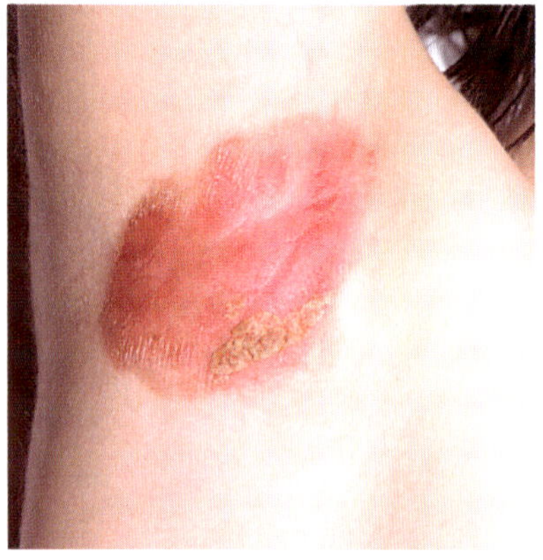

FIG. 78-30 *Eroded crusted plaque in the vault of an axilla (inverse psoriasis).*

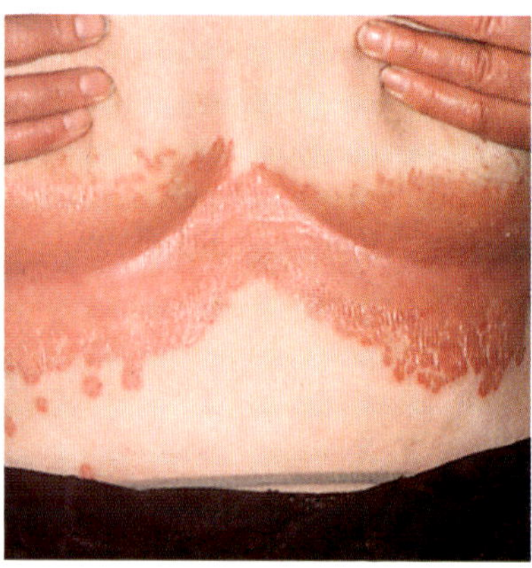

FIG. 78-31 *Broad plaque in the inframammary region.*

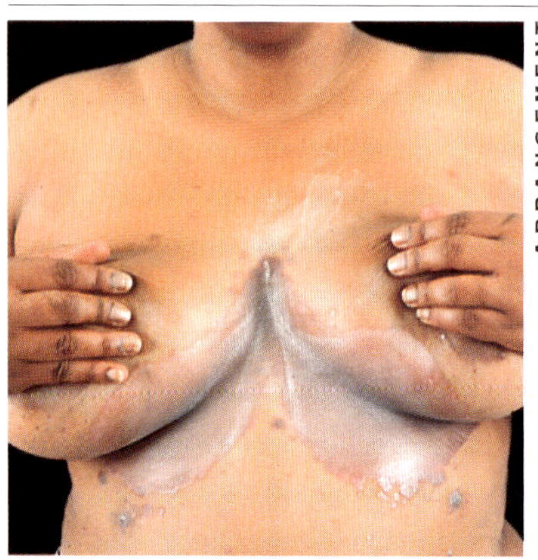

FIG. 78-32 *Broad plaques on the breasts and in the inframammary region.*

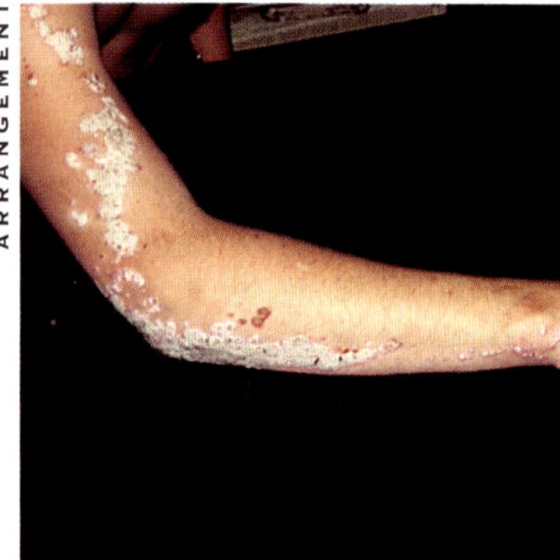

FIG. 78-33 *Scaly papules and plaques in quasilinear "serpentine" array.*

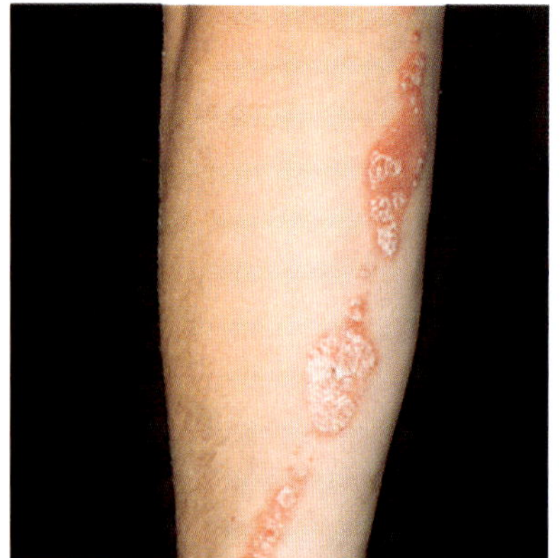

FIG. 78-34 *Scaly papules and plaques in a line.*

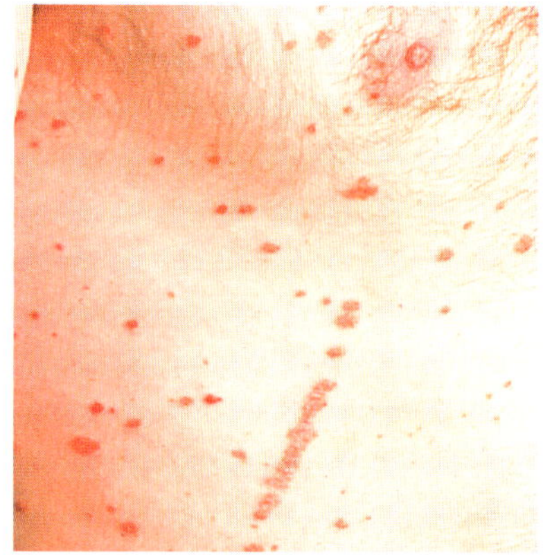

FIG. 78-35 *Slightly scaly papules in striate arrangement ("Koebner") in company with numerous discrete scaly papules and small plaques.*

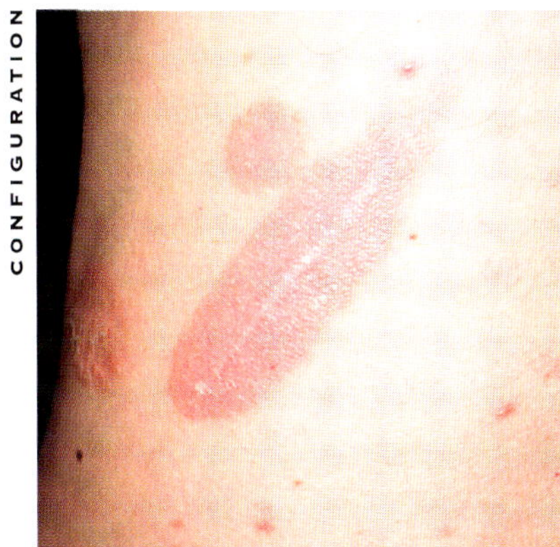

FIG. 78-36 *Linear plaque consequent to external trauma ("Koebner phenomenon") in association with papules and plaques.*

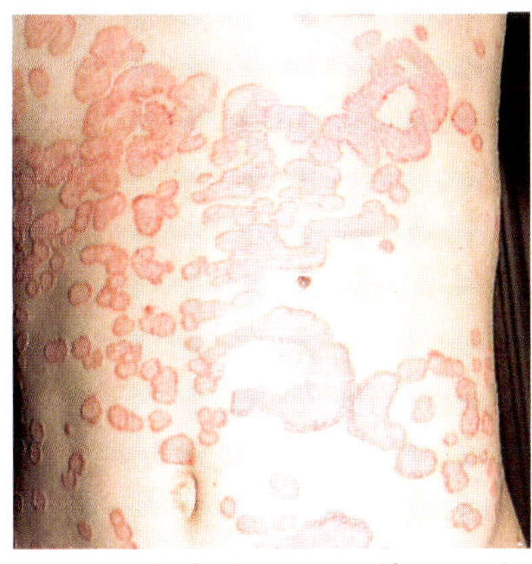

FIG. 78-37 *Scaly plaques in arciform, serpiginous, annular, and nummular shape.*

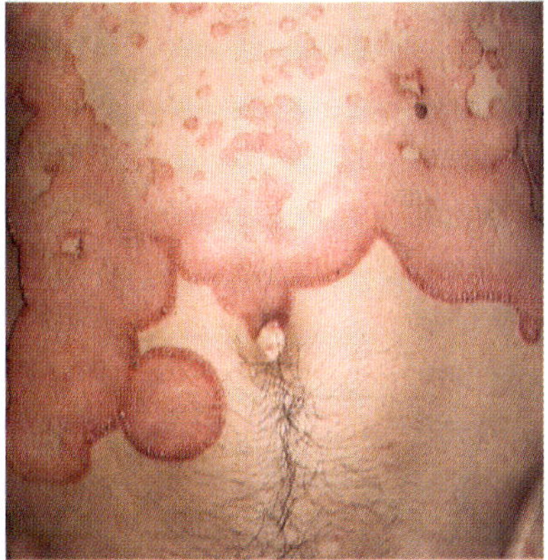

FIG. 78-38 *Sharply circumscribed scaly plaques with polycyclic outlines.*

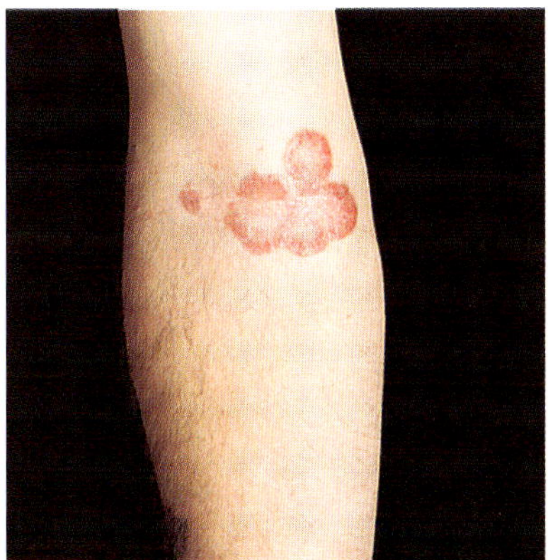

FIG. 78-39 *Polycyclic shape of plaques.*

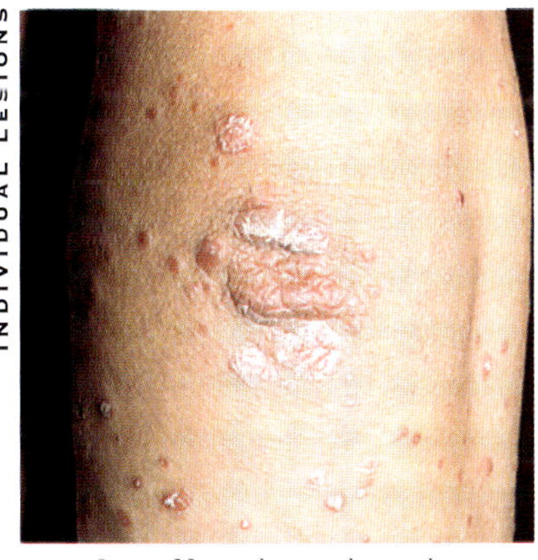

FIG. 78-40 *Nonscaly papules, scaly guttate papules, and scaly plaques illustrate the chronological sequence of lesions.*

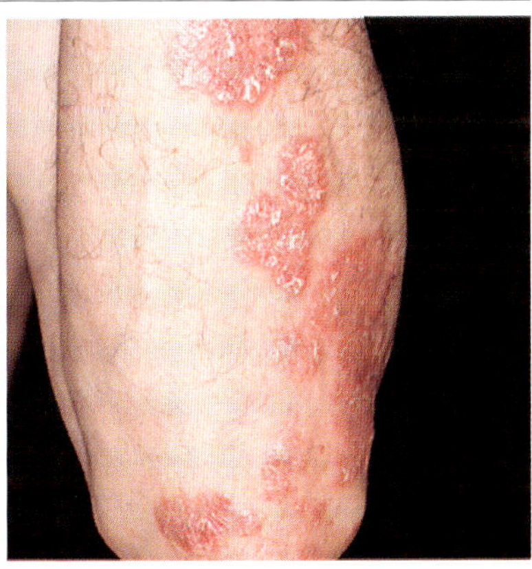

FIG. 78-41 *Scaly papules and plaques of different sizes and shapes.*

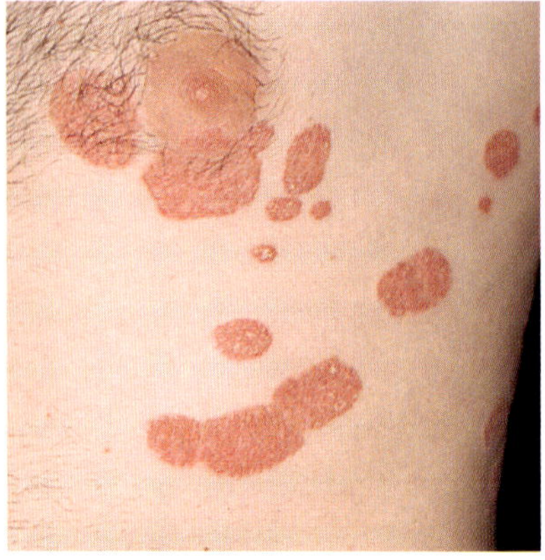 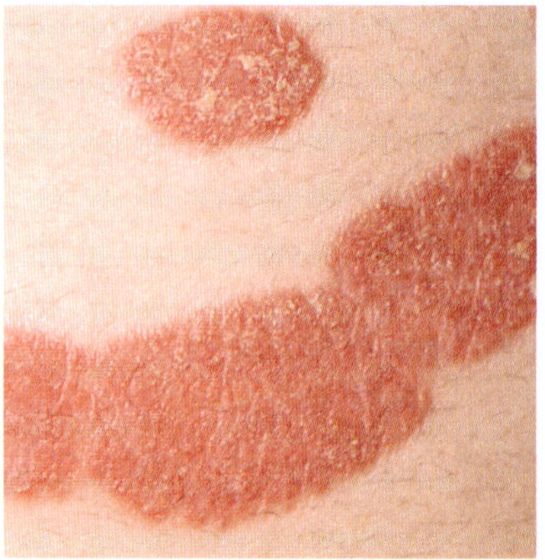

FIG. 78-42 (A, B) *Scaly papules and plaques.*

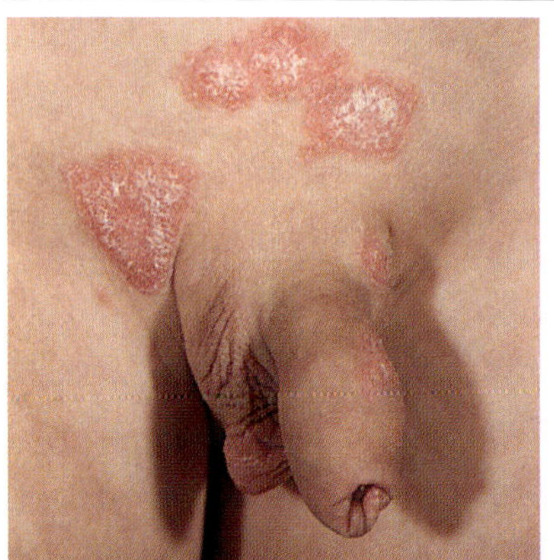 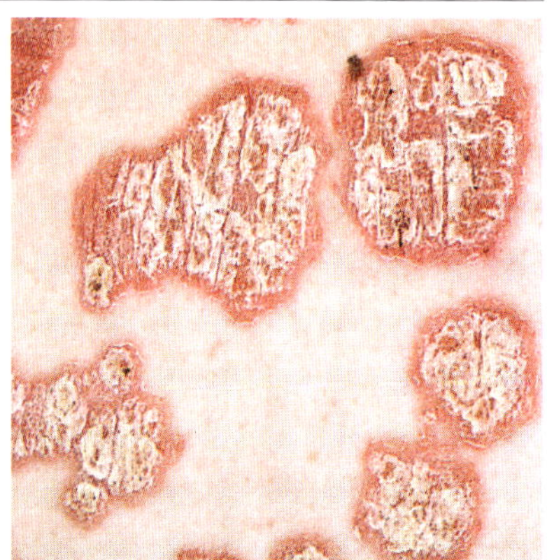

FIG. 78-43 *Scaly papules and plaques.*

FIG. 78-44 *Scaly plaques.*

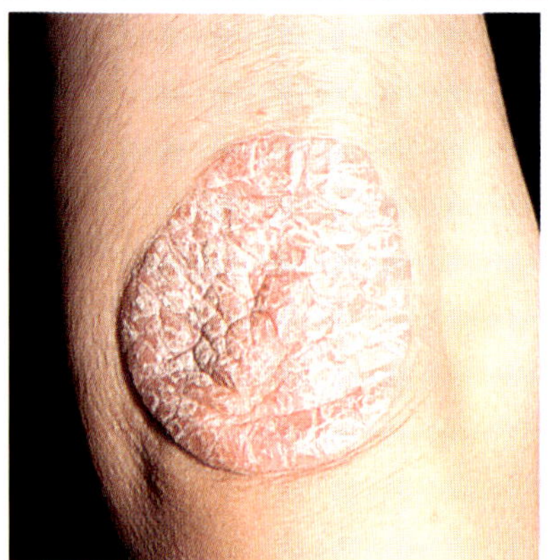 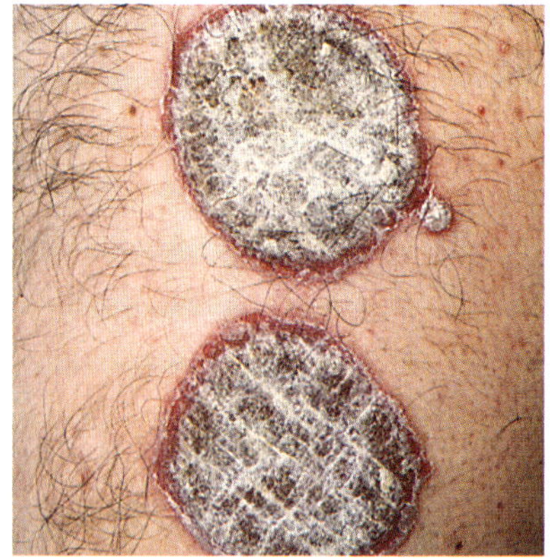

FIG. 78-45 *Sharply circumscribed scaly plaque.*

FIG. 78-46 *Scaly guttate papule and scaly plaques.*

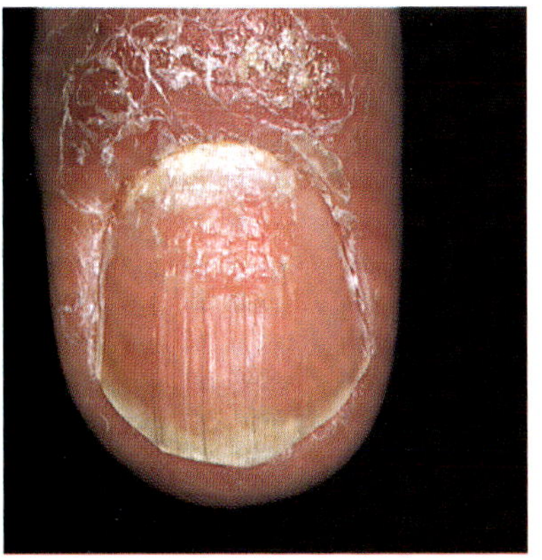

FIG. 78-47 *Scaly plaque of the posterior nail fold (psoriatic paronychia) and onychodystrophy.*

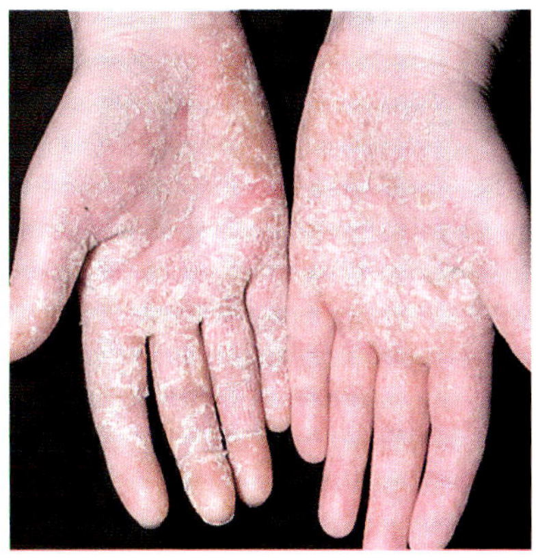

FIG. 78-48 *Diffuse desquamation, many of the scales being in the shape of a collarette.*

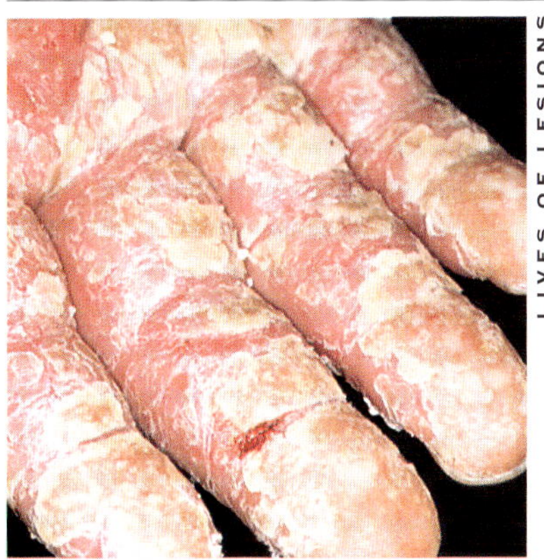

FIG. 78-49 *Diffuse scales and crusts, and a fissure.*

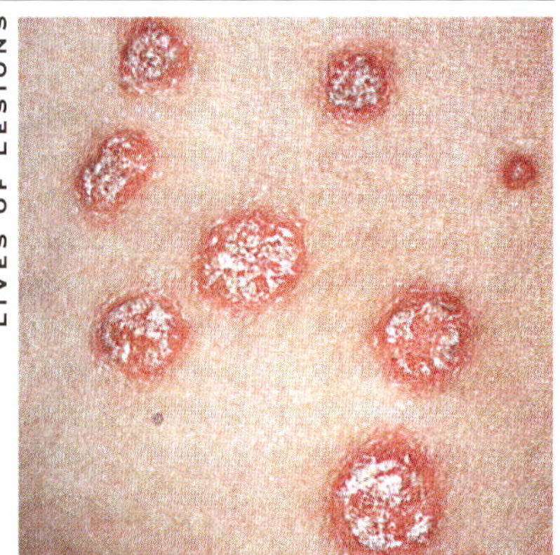

FIG. 78-50 *Discrete scaly papules.*

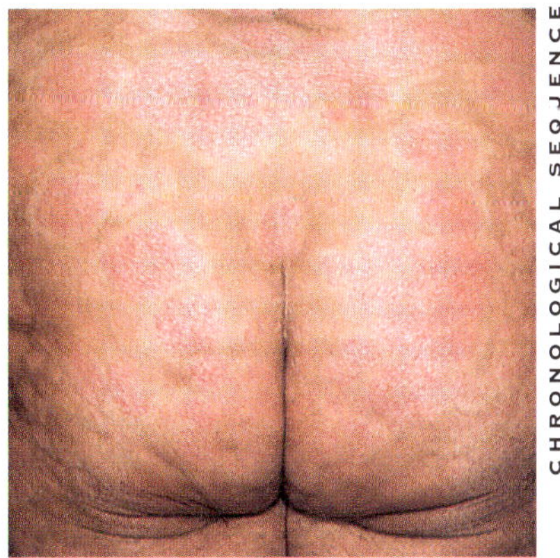

FIG. 78-51 *Subtle scaly reddish plaques surrounded by a white rim (Woronoff's ring), the latter being a sign of regression.*

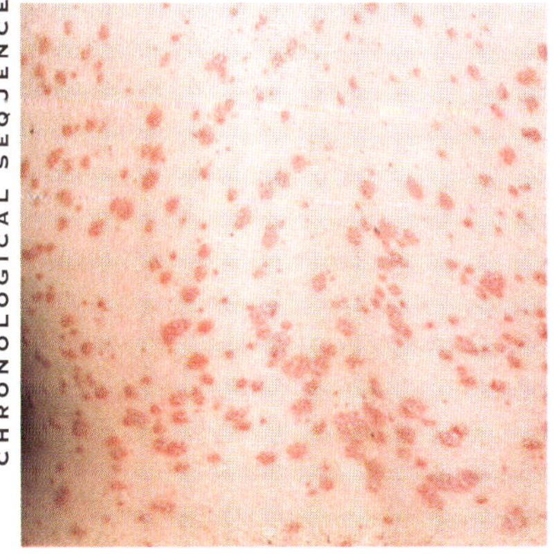

FIG. 78-52 *Slightly scaly guttate (drop-sized) papules, some of which have become confluent to form plaques.*

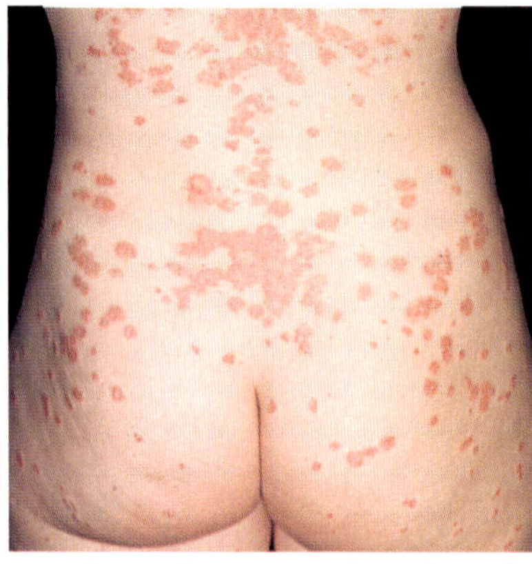

FIG. 78-53 *Guttate macules and papules have become confluent to become plaques.*

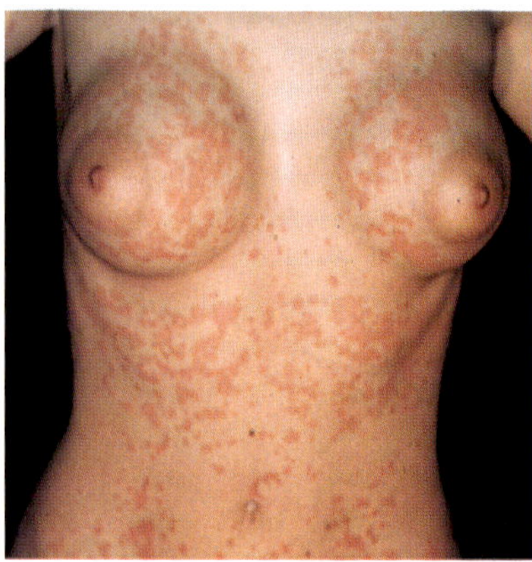

FIG. 78-54 *Papules and plaques of different sizes.*

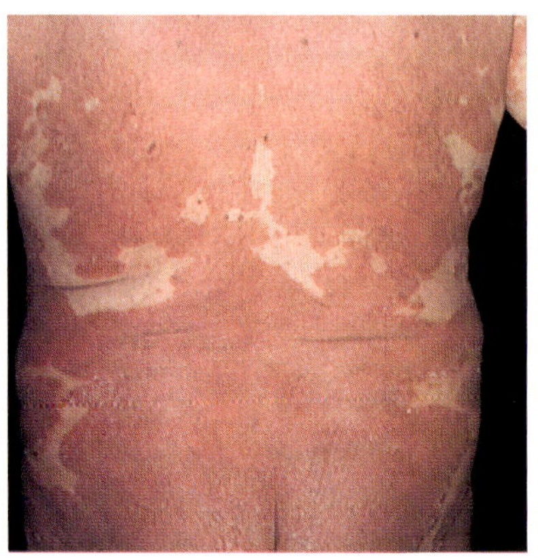

FIG. 78-55 *Extensive confluence of plaques en route to erythroderma.*

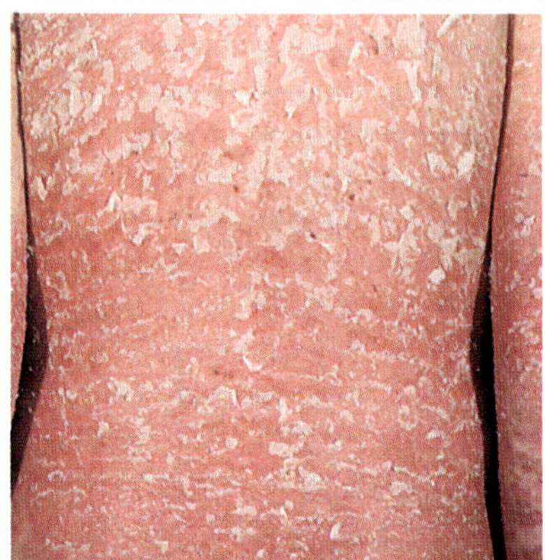

FIG. 78-56 *Erythroderma associated with flake-like scales.*

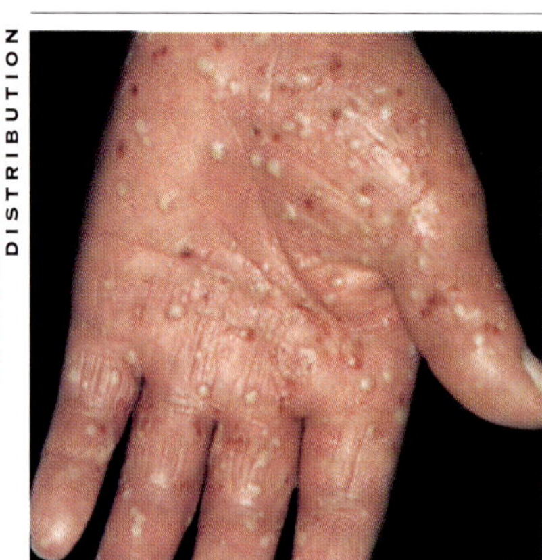

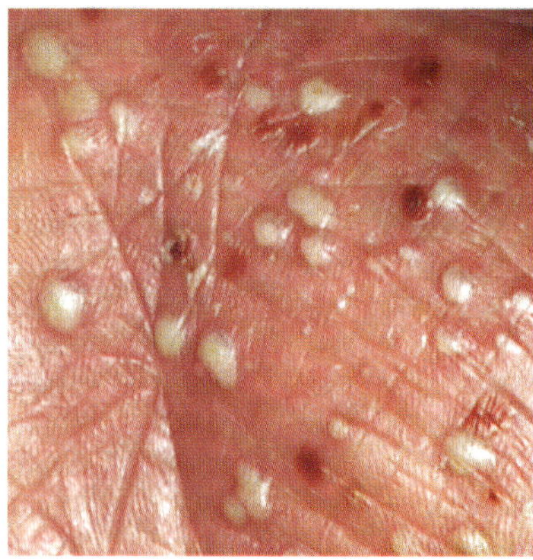

FIG. 78-57 (A, B) *Tiny pustules and larger pustules in company with the residuum of pustules seen here as hemorrhagic crusts.*

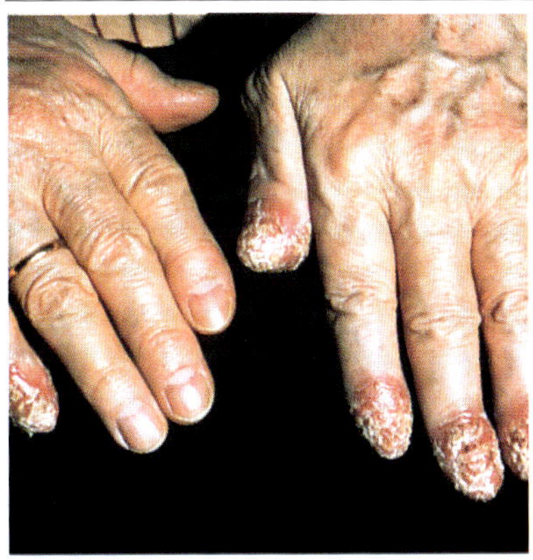

FIG. 78-58 *Crusts on an erythematous base represent the residua of pustules. Nails have been destroyed by the process.*

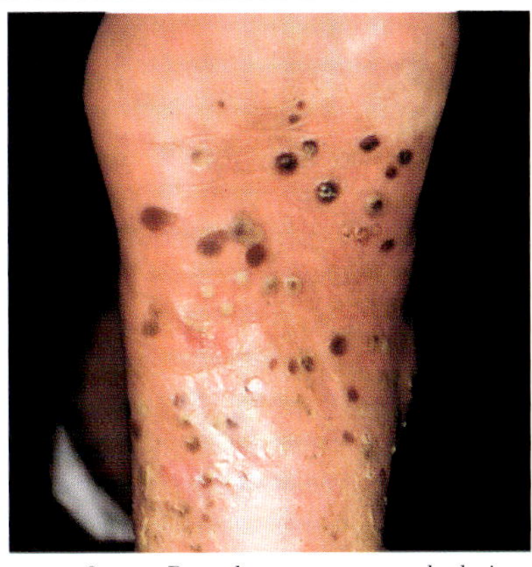

FIG. 78-59 *Pustules represent early lesions and hemorrhagic crusts late ones on a sole.*

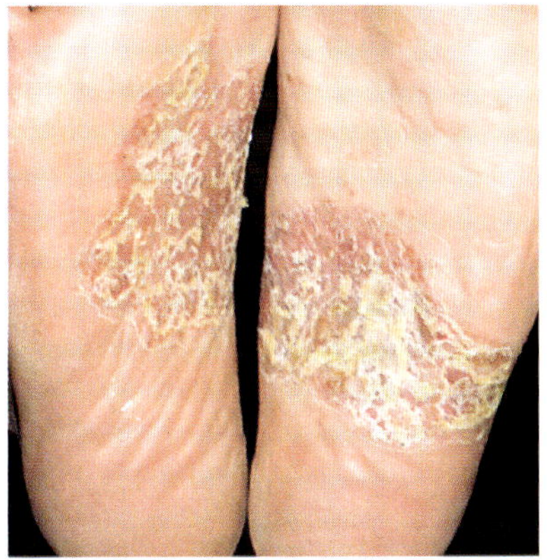

FIG. 78-60 *Plaques covered by scale-crust. The collarettes of scale-crust are indications that intraepidermal pustules were present.*

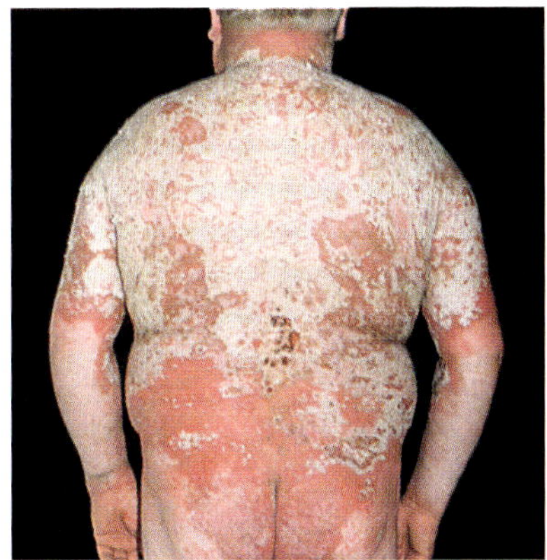

FIG. 78-61 *Widespread, closely-set pustules, crusts, and erythema of the von Zumbusch expression.*

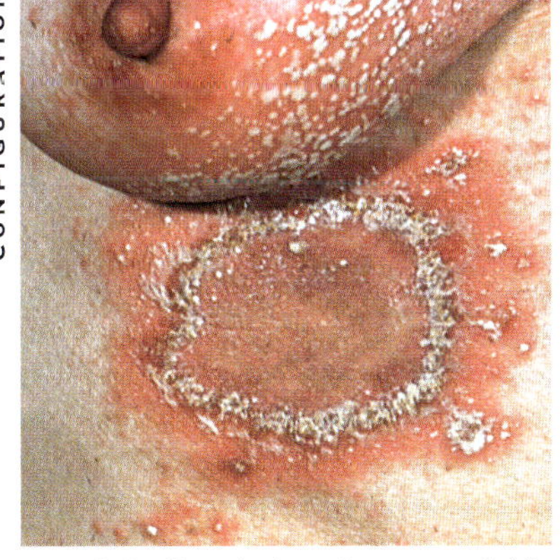

FIG. 78-62 *Pustules in a ring surrounded by erythema. Numerous pustules on a red base are present also on a breast.*

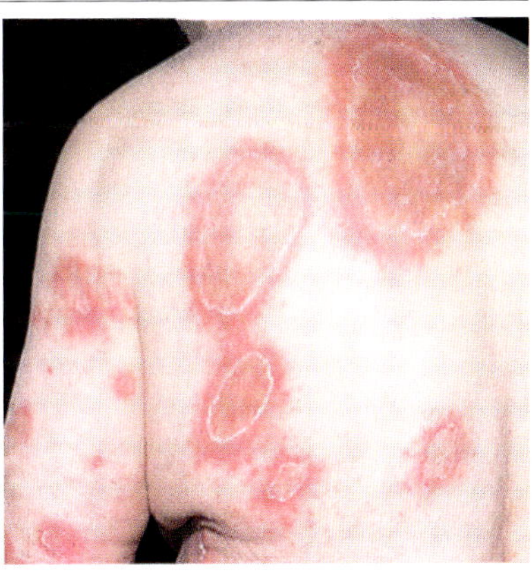

FIG. 78-63 *Annular lesions on whose inner rim are scale-crusts, resembling vaguely erythema annulare centrifugum.*

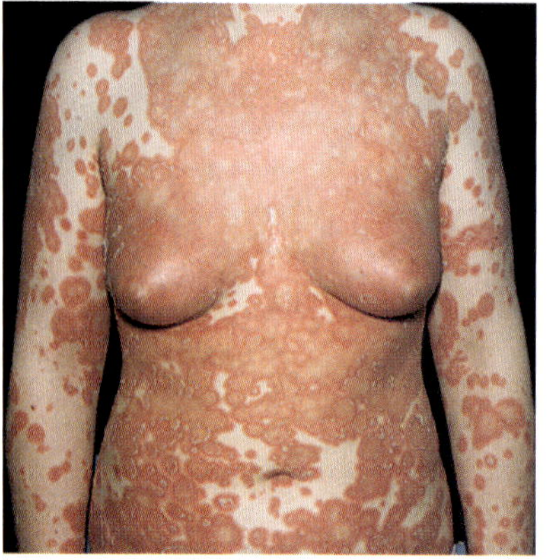

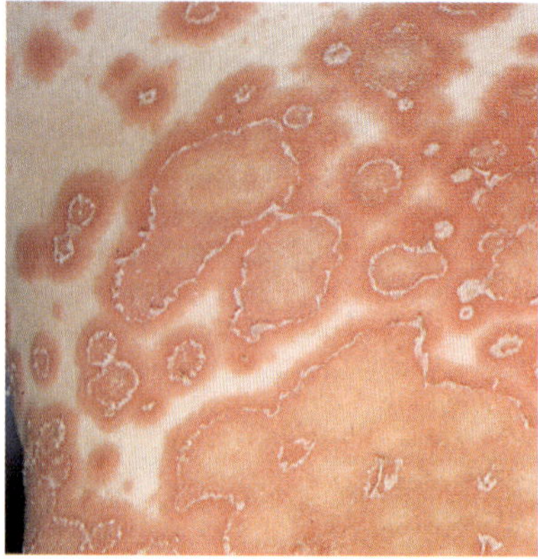

FIG. 78-64 (A, B) *Numerous annular lesions have become confluent to create a polycyclic pattern. On the inner margin of the circles are collarettes of scale-crust, residua of pustules.*

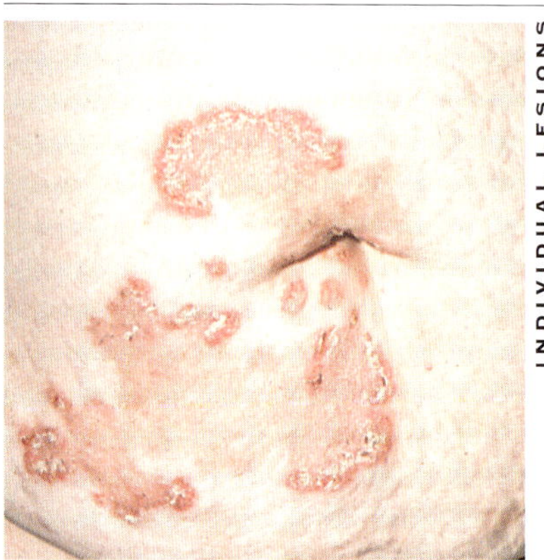

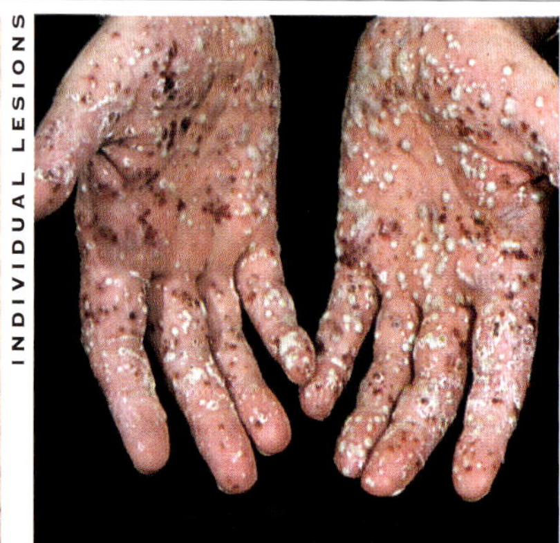

FIG. 78-65 *Arcuate and annular lesions on whose inner border reside scale-crusts. The crusts represent the contents of pustules.*

FIG. 78-66 *Numerous fresh pustules and remnants of old pustules that are seen here as hemorrhagic crusts.*

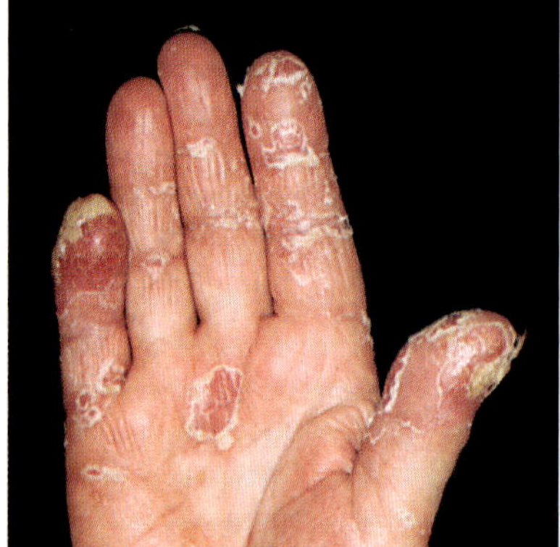

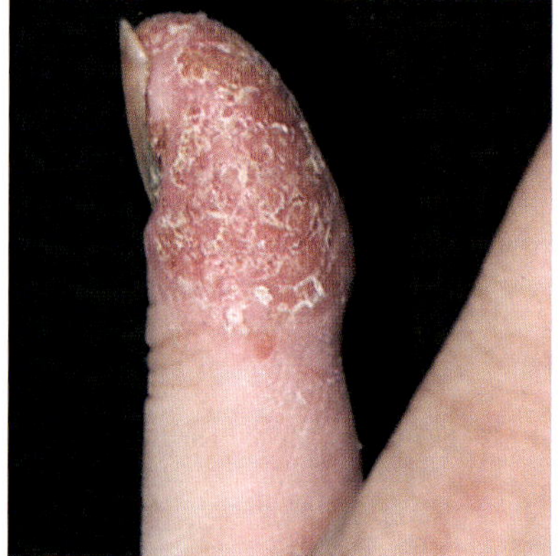

FIG. 78-67 *Collarettes of scale-crust at sites where pustules resided.*

FIG. 78-68 *Scales and crusts atop an erythematous plaque (acrodermatitis continua; dermatitis repens).*

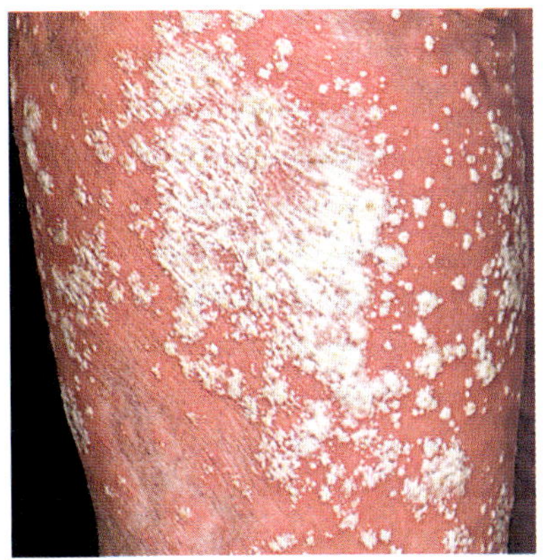

FIG. 78-69 *Many discrete pustules and lakes of pus on an erythematous base on a thigh.*

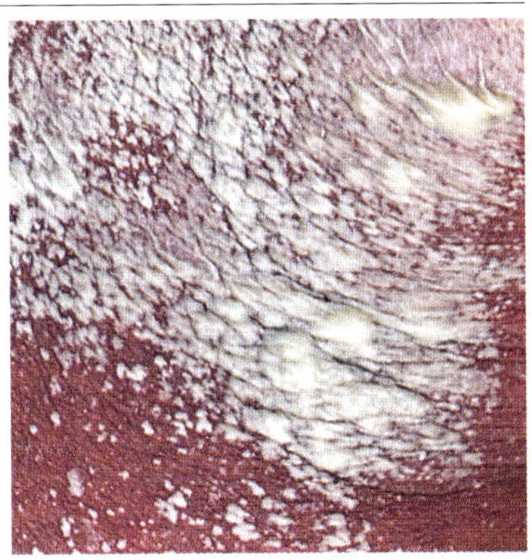

FIG. 78-70 *Tiny discrete pustules and confluence of pustules forming lakes of pus.*

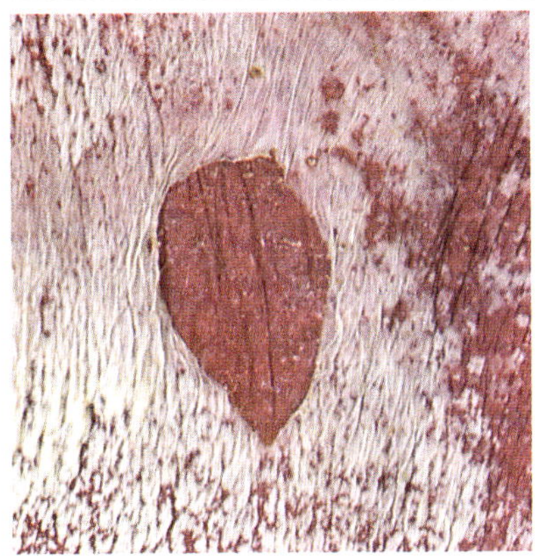

FIG. 78-71 *Individual pustules and lakes of pus. The elliptical zone devoid of pustules is where the stratum corneum was lost.*

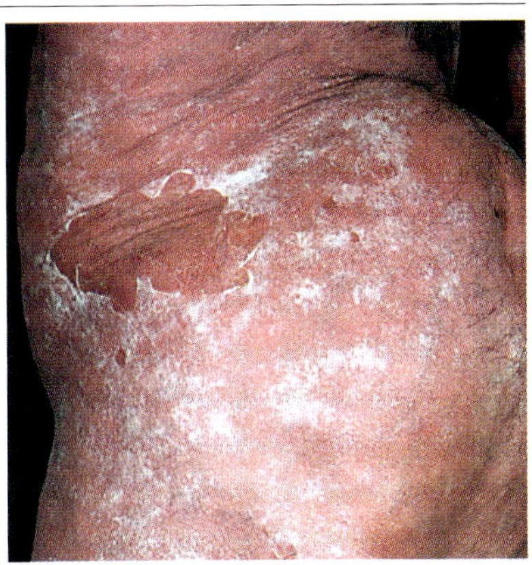

FIG. 78-72 *Countless pustules of the von Zumbusch manifestation.*

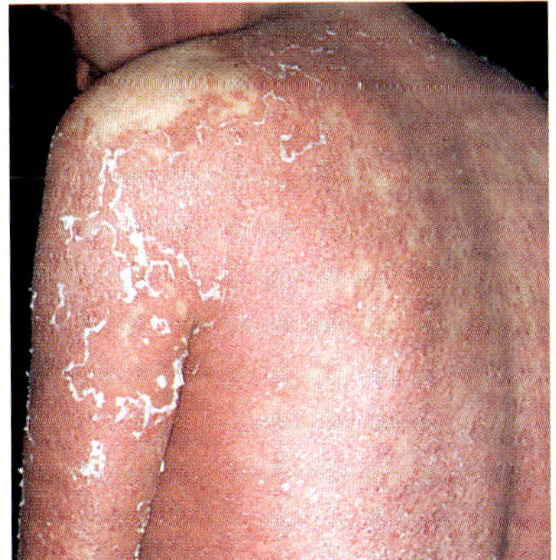

FIG. 78-73 *Collarettes of scale and redness are all that remain of what were myriad pustules at this site.*

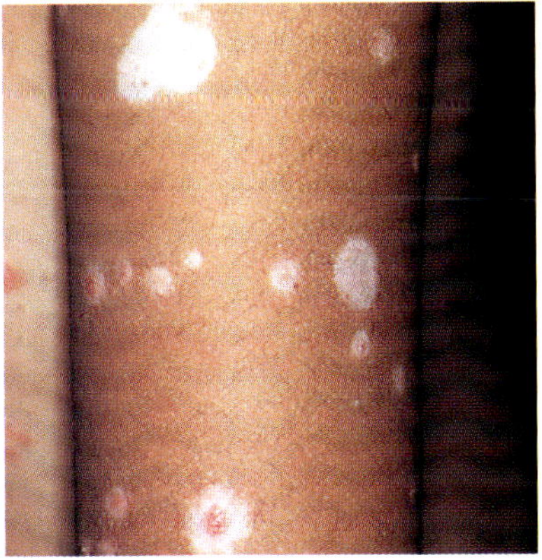

FIG. 78-74 *Scaly papules in company with hypopigmentation and a depigmented patch indicate devolution of lesions.*

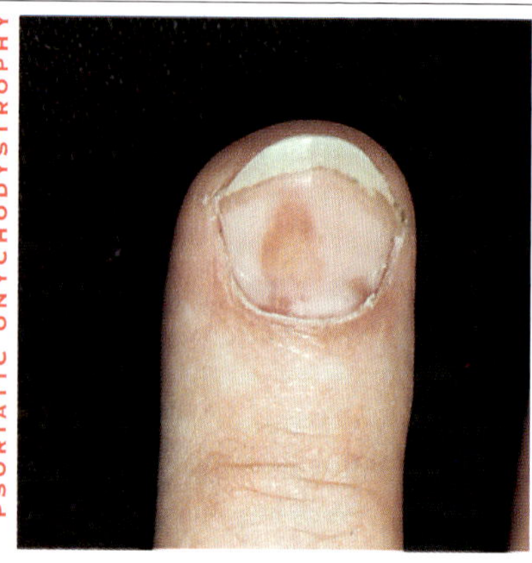

FIG. 78-75 *Arcuate, annular, and serpiginous lesions of geographic tongue, an oral manifestation of psoriasis.*

FIG. 78-76 *The "oil drop" sign indicates involvement of the nail bed by a lesion of psoriasis.*

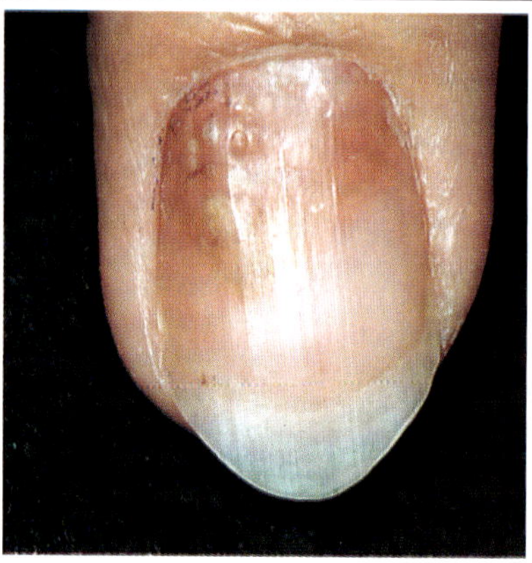

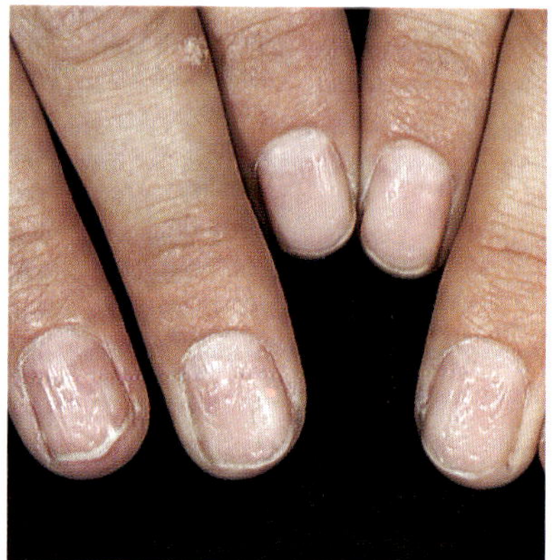

FIG. 78-77 *Combination of pits of the nail plate and an "oil drop" sign.*

FIG. 78-78 *Pits in nails represent the residuum of parakeratotic cells that were lost from the nail plate.*

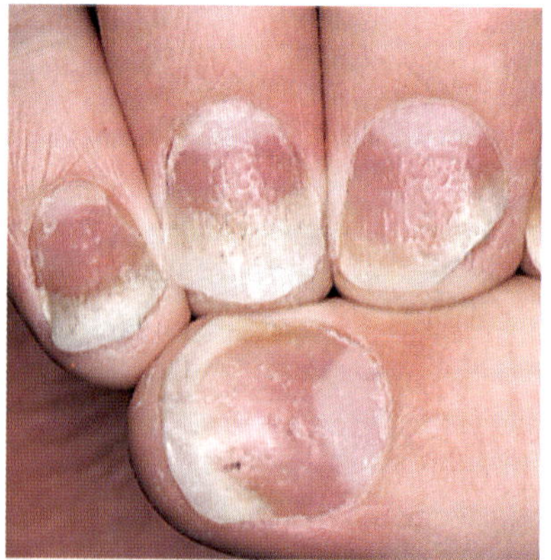

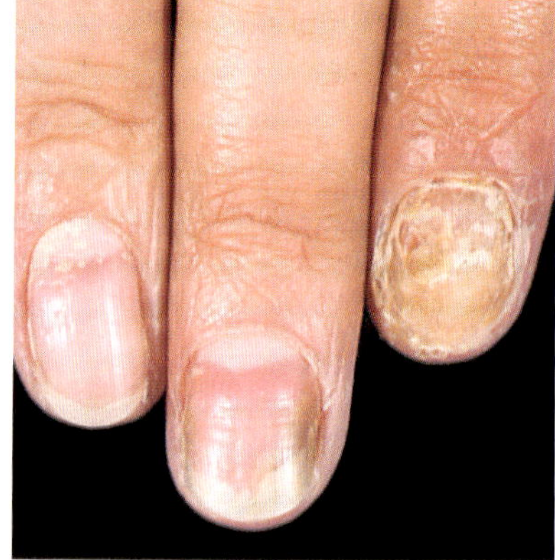

FIG. 78-79 *Pits in the nail plate and discoloration of the nail bed ("oil drop sign").*

FIG. 78-80 *Pits in nails, onycholysis, onychodystrophy, and periungual skin lesions of psoriasis.*

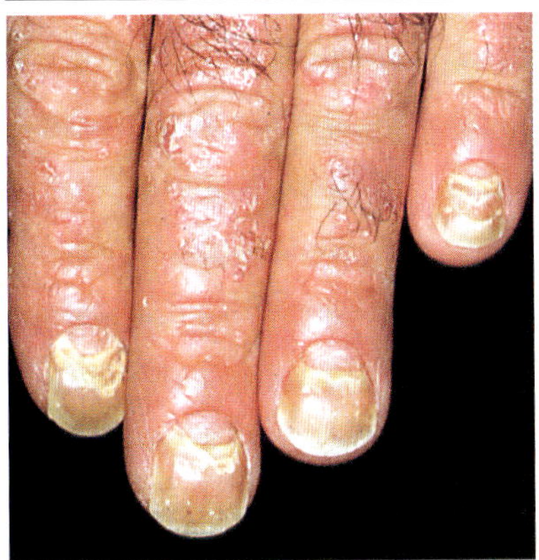

FIG. 78-81 *Severe onychodystrophy and skin lesions of psoriasis.*

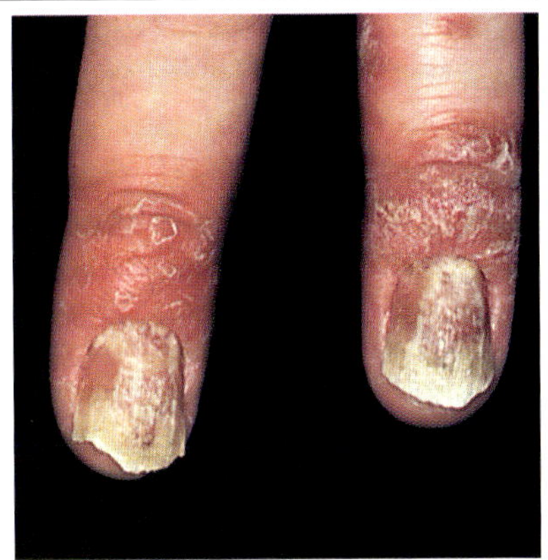

FIG. 78-82 *Severe onychodystrophy and psoriatic paronychia.*

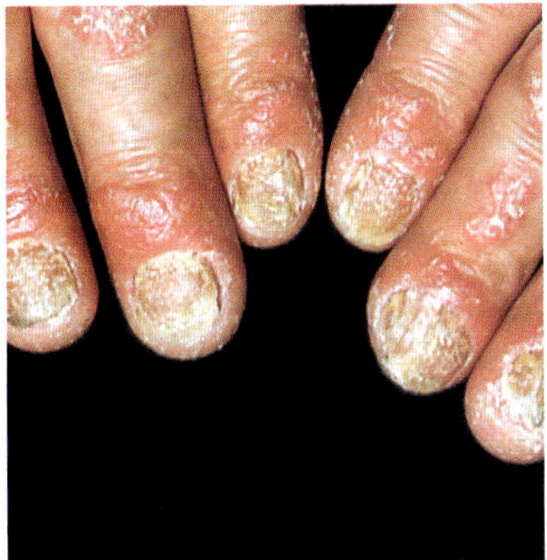

FIG. 78-83 *Severe onychodystrophy and skin lesions of psoriasis.*

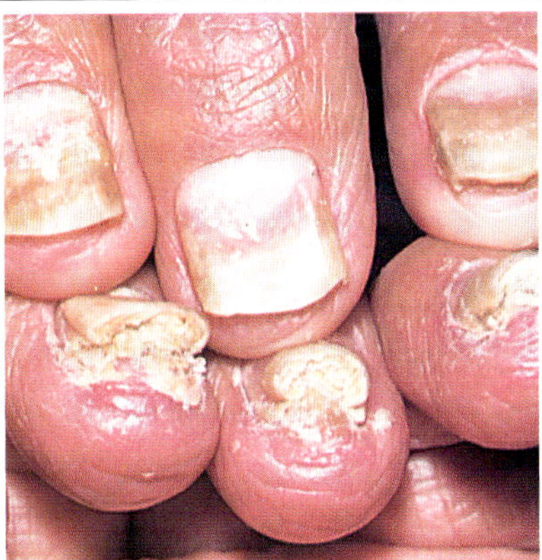

FIG. 78-84 *Severe onychodystrophy, onycholysis, and marked subungual hyperkeratosis.*

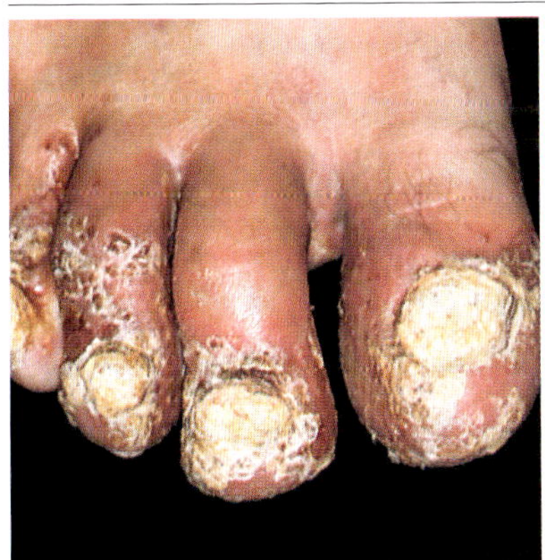

FIG. 78-85 *Ostraceous appearance of dystrophic nail plates and periungual lesions.*

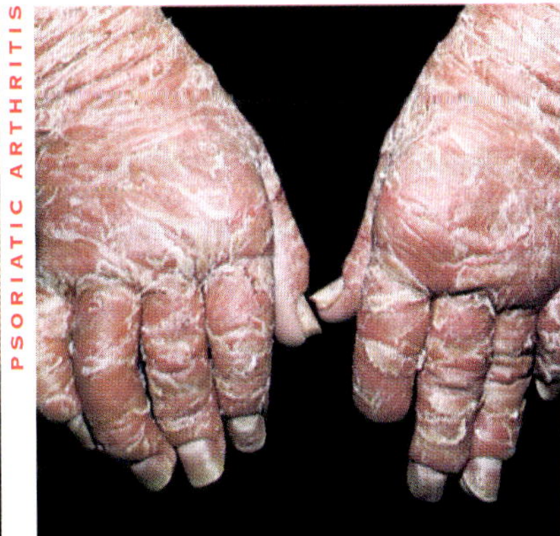

FIG. 78-86 *Mutilating expression of psoriatic arthritis in a patient with psoriatic exfoliative erythroderma.*

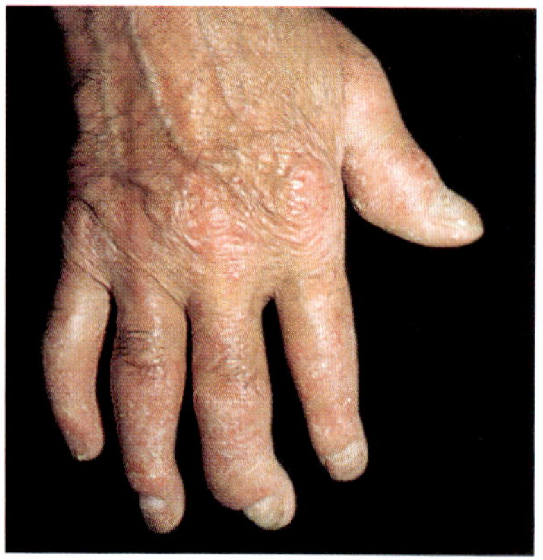

FIG. 78-87 *Psoriatic arthritis in a patient with psoriatic nails and psoriatic skin lesions on fingers and hands.*

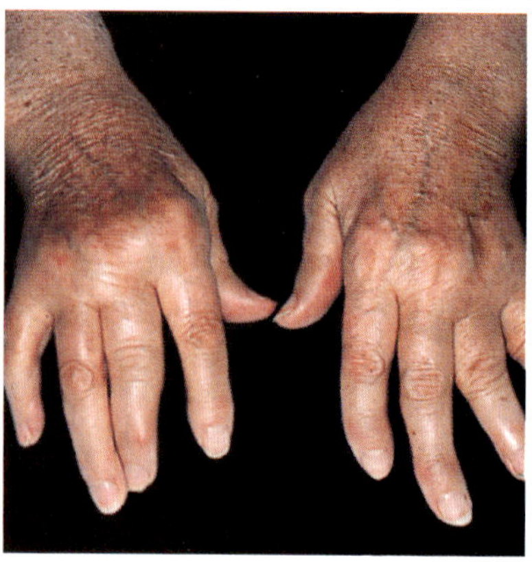

FIG. 78-88 *Typical changes of psoriatic arthritis may resemble those of rheumatoid arthritis.*

COURSE The chronologic sequence of lesions of psoriasis depends on the specific type of lesion. For example, eruptive (guttate) papules of psoriasis may wane and disappear in a matter of weeks, or they may wax to become plaques of psoriasis. Plaques of psoriasis tend to persist and may be confined to sites such as elbows and knees. If plaques are widespread, they may enlarge slowly, become confluent, and eventuate in erythroderma. Remarkably thickened plaques of psoriasis on the scalp, a kind of severe psoriasis totalis known colloquially as tinea amiantacea, tend to persist for decades. The same is true for psoriasis that affects palms and soles. In time, lesions on those latter sites often become fissured.

Pustules that erupt on psoriatic palms or soles come and go in unpredictable fashion. Widespread pustules, a condition known as pustular psoriasis of von Zumbusch, erupt in a shower over the entire integument and, in the course of days or weeks, some pustules heal with crusts at the very same time that new pustules blossom. The course of widespread pustular psoriasis also cannot be predicted; for reasons still inexplicable, the process usually ceases after a matter of weeks, only to return again with equal force when least expected.

INTEGRATION: UNIFYING CONCEPT All manifestations of psoriasis are diagnosable, with surety, clinically and histopathologically. All of those expressions have in common sparse superficial perivascular and interstitial infiltrates of lymphocytes, dilated tortuous capillaries in dermal papillae, and some degree of epidermal hyperplasia. They are usually accompanied by parakeratosis.

Guttate lesions of psoriasis show edema of the papillary dermis, neutrophils within the epidermis in pustules that are given different names according to different organization of neutrophils (e.g., Munro's microabscesses and spongiform pustules of Kogoj) and different sites (e.g., subcorneal and intracorneal pustules), and mounds of parakeratosis that sport neutrophils at their summits and that are staggered throughout the thickened cornified layer. Fully-developed lesions of psoriasis show psoriasiform hyperplasia with thin rete ridges of equal length that alternate with thin dermal papillae. Pallor usually is present in the upper part of the viable epidermis, the granular zone is nearly absent, except at sites of acrosyringia and acrotrichia, and confluent parakeratosis is laced with neutrophils.

Asbestos-like psoriasis on a scalp is typified by all of the changes seen in fully-developed lesions of psoriasis but, in addition, is accompanied by a tremendously thickened parakeratotic layer. Pustular psoriasis is merely an acceleration and exaggeration of the psoriatic process in which neutrophils in large numbers race from capillaries in dermal papillae toward the cornified layer and, en route, form abscesses within the epidermis known by the eponyms previously mentioned. Psoriatic erythroderma exhibits changes of fully-developed psoriasis in which there is only scant parakeratosis because scales are being shed constantly.

In sum, all of the manifestations of psoriasis represent variations on a single pathologic, genetically-conditioned process that seems to be precipitated by different factors, e.g., streptococcal infection, physical trauma, or emotional stress. When that process involves the oral cavity, it is called "geographic tongue." When pustular psoriasis is situated on acral parts, especially on the thumb or fingers, it has gone by names such as acrodermatitis continua of Hallopeau, dermatitis repens of Crocker, and pustular bacterid of Andrews. When pustular psoriasis occurs in someone who is pregnant, the name impetigo herpetiformis has been applied to it. When pustular psoriasis occurs in a patient with Reiter's syndrome, the designation keratoderma blenorrhagicum has been given to it. When pustules of psoriasis are arranged in arcuate, annular, serpiginous, and other figurate patterns, the condition has been called subcorneal pustular dermatosis of Sneddon and Wilkinson. Psoriasis of nail units in the form of pits on nail plates, onycholysis, and subungual hyperkeratosis are all manifestations of the psoriatic process.

That psoriasis is truly a systemic disease can be realized by virtue of involvement by the process not only of the skin and nails, but of mucous membranes, gastrointestinal tract, and joints in the form of an arthritis that may be mutilating.

THERAPY For localized plaques, topical treatment with corticosteroids, anthralin, retinoids, vitamin D3 derivatives, and so-called keratolytics (salicylic acid) is recommended.

For widespread papules and plaques, phototherapy including PUVA, UV-B, and bath-PUVA therapy, as well as the Goeckerman regimen (tar plus UV-B), are advisable.

For nearly universal psoriasis, psoriatic erythroderma, and pustular psoriasis (von Zumbusch), oral retinoids, cyclosporin, or methotrexate in low dose are the treatments of choice.

For psoriatic arthritis, methotrexate or cyclosporin is the best treatment.

For psoriatic nails, injection of posterior nail folds with corticosteroids, albeit painful, is effective.

For tinea amiantacea, solutions of salicylic acid plus corticosteroids are palliative.

DEFINITION An inflammatory process that often begins as a suppurative folliculitis manifested clinically as pustules. It rapidly extends to become ulcers marked at their periphery by boggy tissue. The skin disease is associated commonly with inflammatory bowel disease, especially ulcerative colitis, and sometimes with rheumatoid arthritis, paraproteinemia, and myeloma.

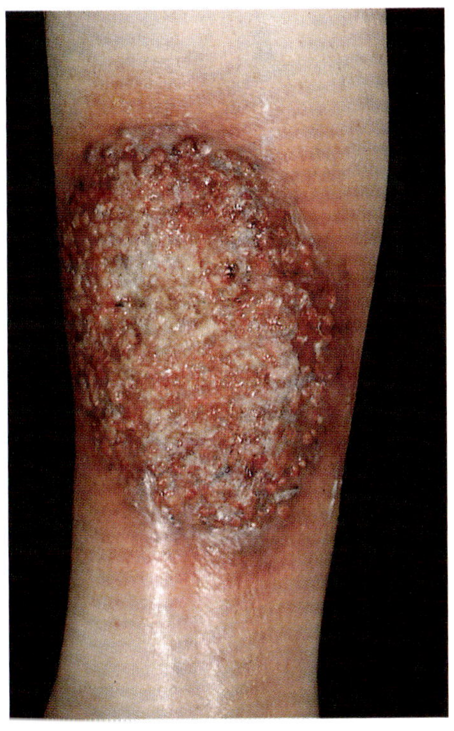

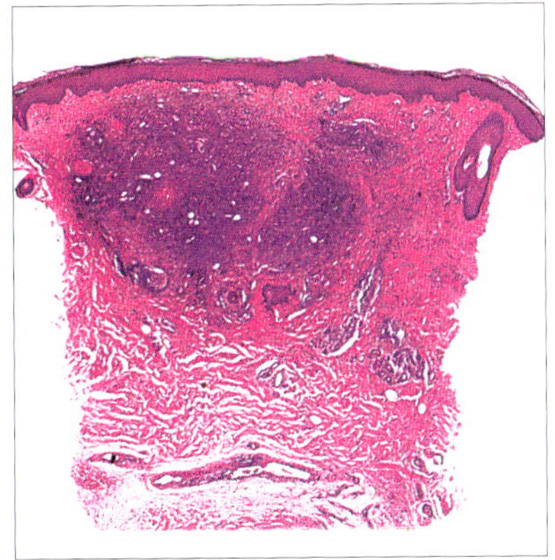

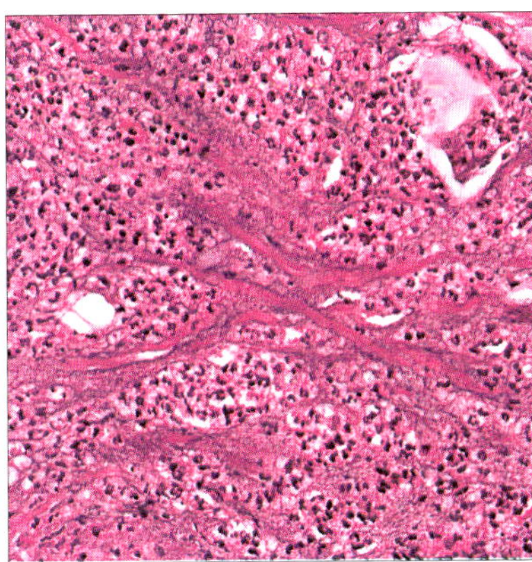

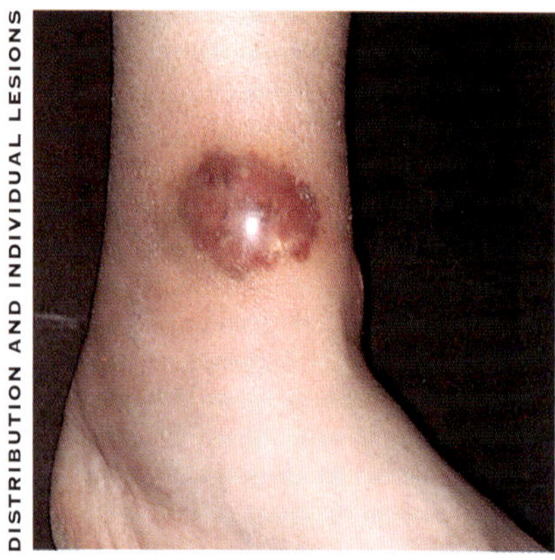

FIG. 79-1 *Hemorrhagic bulla.*

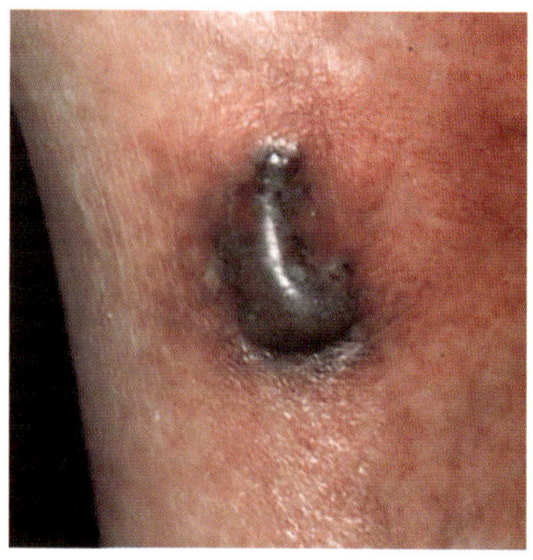

FIG. 79-2 *Hemorrhagic bulla.*

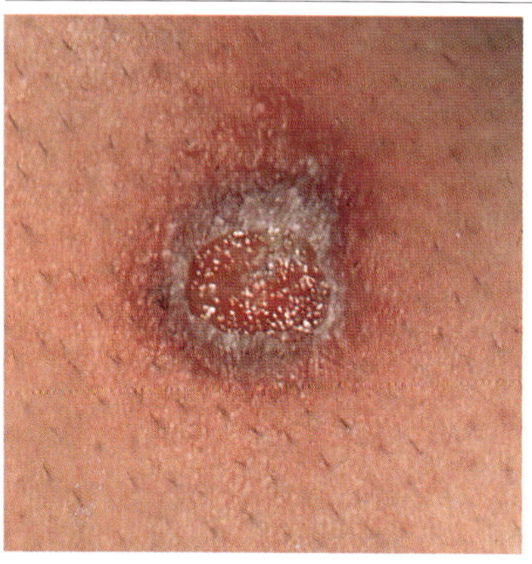

FIG. 79-3 *Ulcer with necrotic overhanging border surrounded by erythema.*

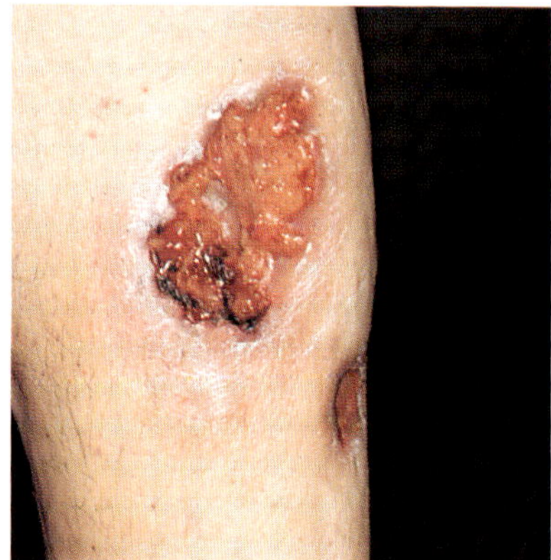

FIG. 79-4 *Deep ulcers with scalloped, overhanging margin.*

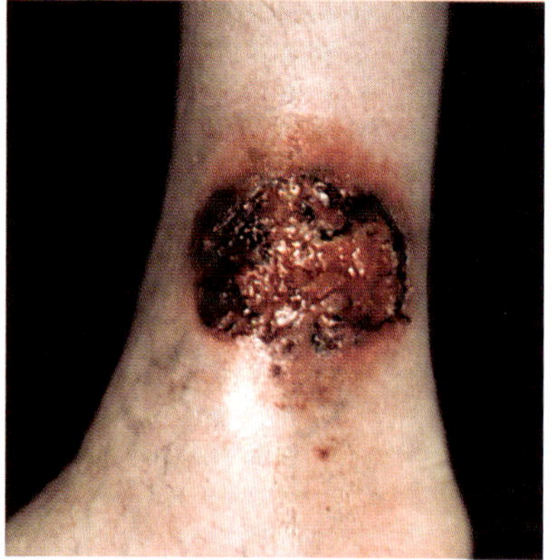

FIG. 79-5 *A large ulcer with a vegetating hemorrhagic surface.*

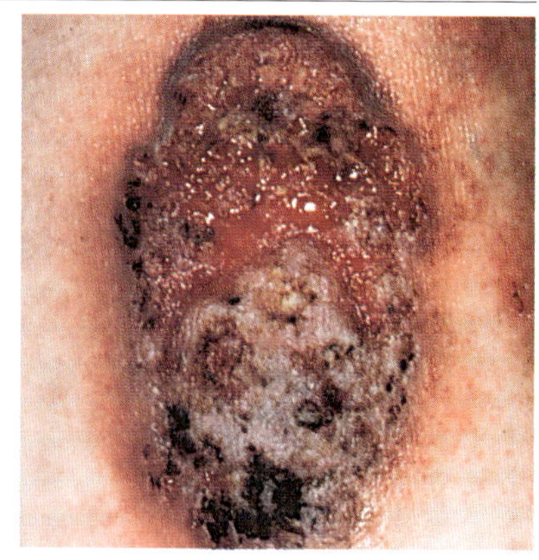

FIG. 79-6 *Ulcer, granulation tissue, hemorrhagic crusts, and gray zones of re-epithelialization.*

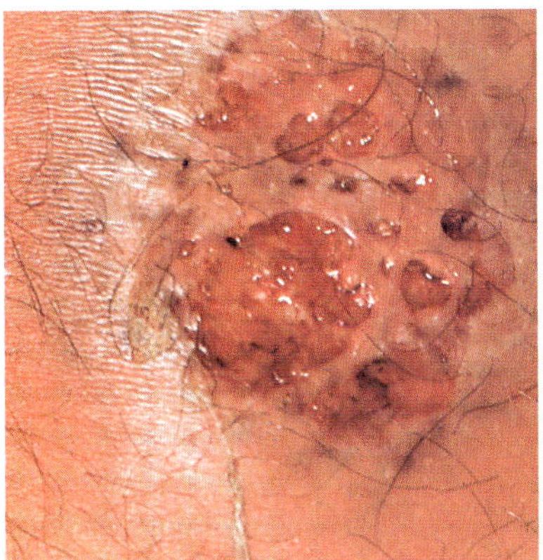

FIG. 79-7 *Cribriform pattern formed by "punched out" ulcers of different sizes and surrounded by a boggy overriding border.*

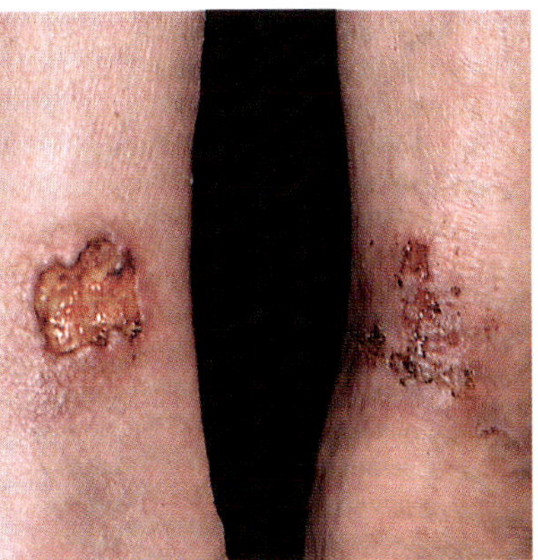

FIG. 79-8 *Deep ulcer with jagged border on the left, and nearly complete healing of what was a similar ulcer on the right.*

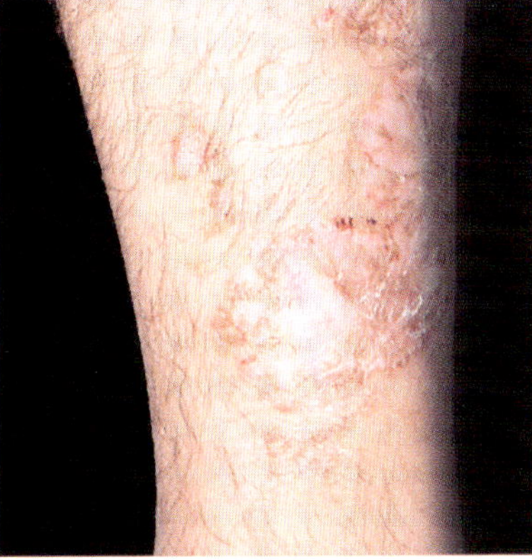

FIG. 79-9 *A large scar with a scalloped border represents the end-stage of pyoderma gangrenosum.*

ADJUNCTIVE DIAGNOTIC TESTS   Search should be undertaken for evidence of systemic disease such as inflammatory bowel disease, arthritis, paraproteinemia, and leukemia.

COURSE The first lesion to appear in pyoderma gangrenosum is a folliculocentric pustule that in a short time ulcerates and becomes surrounded by a boggy undermined inflamed border. That border and the ulcer behind it expand centrifugally, sometimes reaching dimensions of many centimeters. It takes many months, and sometimes years, for the ulcer of pyoderma gangrenosum to heal, the residuum being an atrophic scar that exhibits hypopigmentation and hyperpigmentation.

INTEGRATION: UNIFYING CONCEPT Pyoderma gangrenosum, like Sweet's syndrome, erythema multiforme, erythema nodosum, and allergic vasculitis, is a distinctive morphologic pattern that results from different causes. In the case of pyoderma gangrenosum, the causes may be inflammatory bowel disease, ulcerative colitis in particular, rheumatoid arthritis, paraproteinemia, and chronic active hepatitis. The bullous expression of pyoderma gangrenosum often is a manifestation of a leukemia, and the pyostomatitis vegetans manifestation of pyoderma gangrenosum usually is a reflection of an inflammatory disease of the bowel.

The pustule that heralds the explosive changes that lead to the devastating ulceration of pyoderma gangrenosum is seen histopathologically to be a suppurative folliculitis. When the collection of neutrophils within the infundibulum of a follicle becomes so great that the follicle ruptures, spewing countless neutrophils into the dermis, the stage is set for the phagedenic changes that soon ensue. The contents of extraordinary suppuration in the dermis and subcutaneous fat are discharged to the surface of the severely ulcerated skin. At the periphery of the ulcers, the epidermis is separated from the dermis and appears to "overhang" the edge of the denuded skin. All of the findings just described become progressively more marked over time until, for reasons not understood, the inflammatory process ceases and the lesion heals with scar.

The mechanism whereby pyoderma gangrenosum develops is not known, but the condition seems to be related closely to Sweet's syndrome, the boggy plaques of which also are made up of dense, diffuse infiltrates of neutrophils. Sweet's syndrome, like pyoderma gangrenosum, is secondary to a variety of processes as disparate as ulcerative colitis, rheumatoid arthritis, and acute myeloid leukemia.

THERAPY If an underlying process can be identified, such as ulcerative colitis or rheumatoid arthritis, treatment should be directed toward correcting it. For the ulcers themselves, in addition to local care, systemic treatment with corticosteroids especially, but also of either sulfones or sulfapyridine, is also effective. Chemotherapeutic agents, such as azathioprine and cyclophosphamide, are beneficial in some patients. Newer immunomodulating agents like cyclosporine, mycophenolate mofetil, and tacrolimus (FK506) seem to be of therapeutic value.

DEFINITION   A red, often ulcerated, boggy papule that represents a hyperplasia of small cutaneous vessels which are "fed" by an arteriole in the subcutaneous fat, the lesion resulting consistently from external trauma, usually in the form of a puncture or a yank of a "hang nail." In time, the proliferation of vessels ceases, there is progressive fibroplasia, and the then gray or white papule shrinks and eventually disappears.

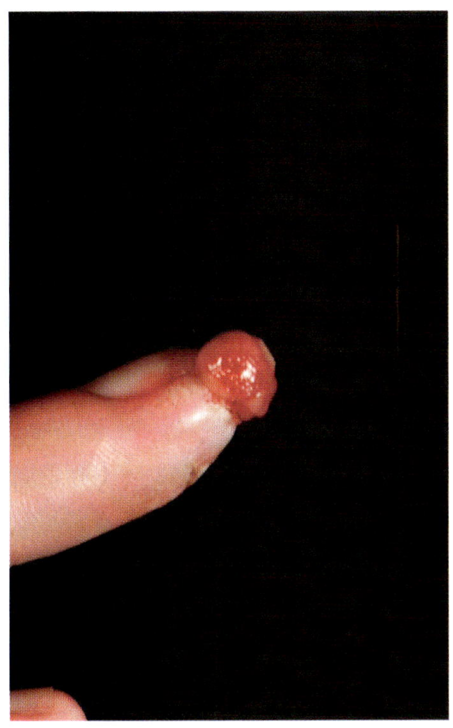

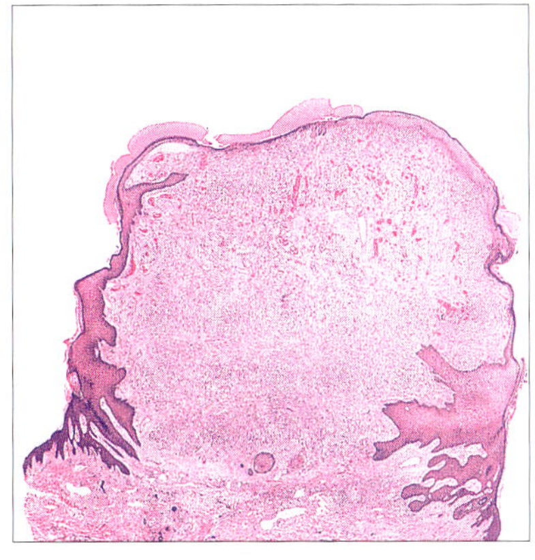

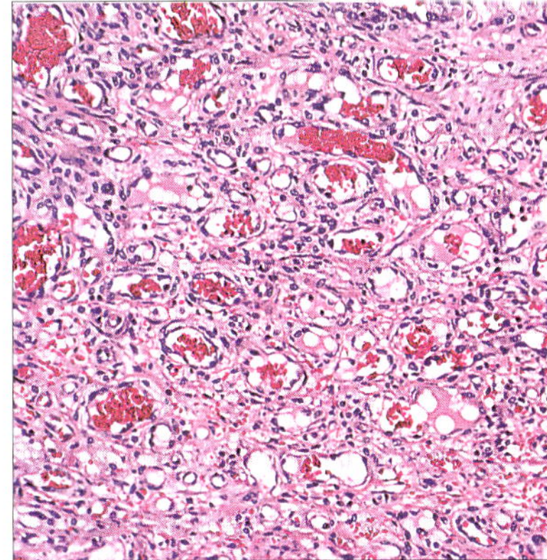

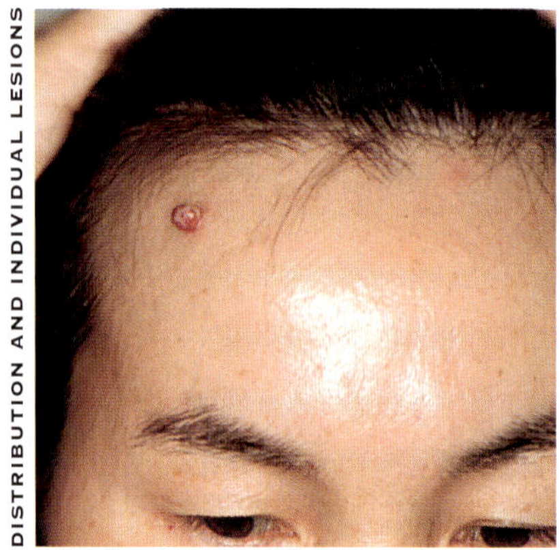
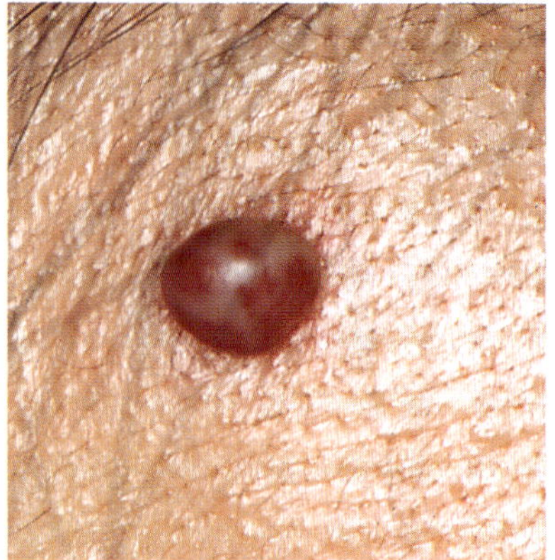

FIG. 80-1 (A, B) *Papule. Resolution with fibrosis as can be told by zones of pallor (B).*

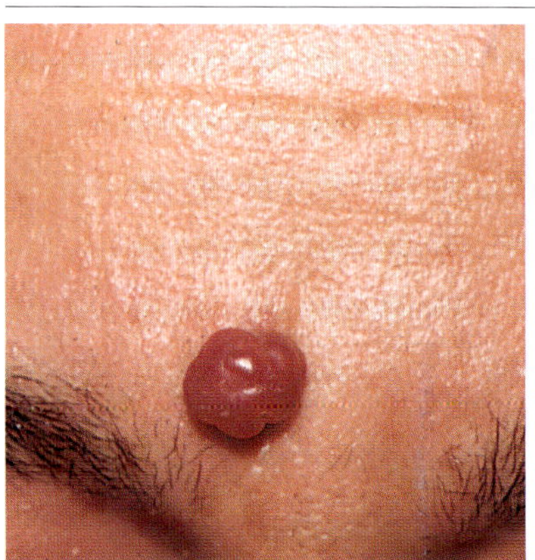

FIG. 80-2 *Multilobate papule.*

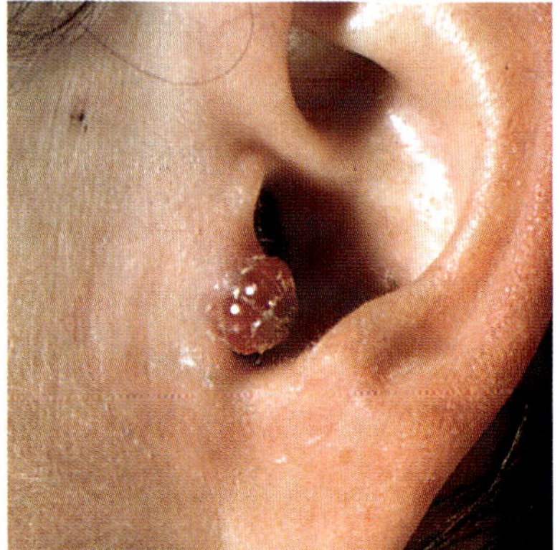

FIG. 80-3 *Multilobulate lesion.*

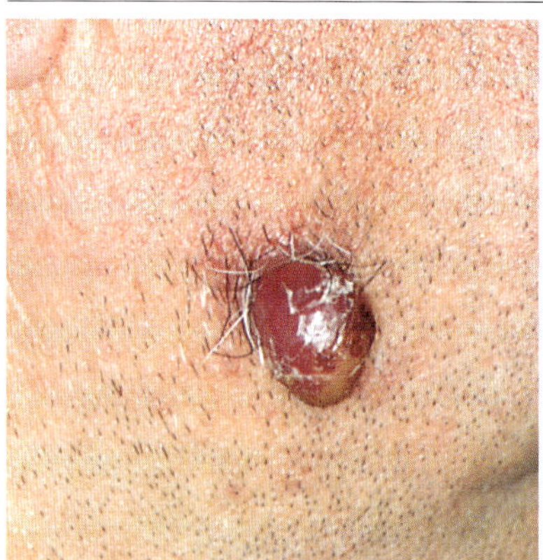

FIG. 80-4 *Ulcerated, partially re-epithelialized lesion covered by scale and crust.*

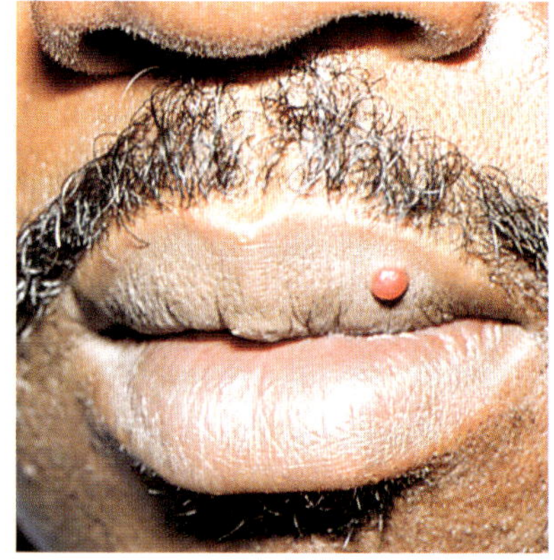

FIG. 80-5 *Smooth-surfaced, domed-shaped papule.*

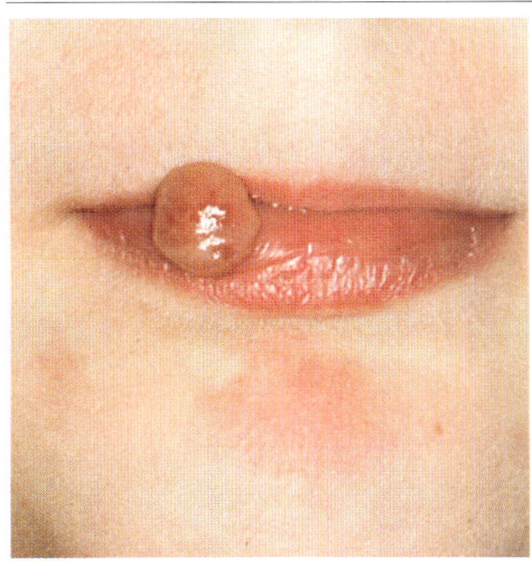

FIG. 80-6 *Shiny eroded polypoid papule.*

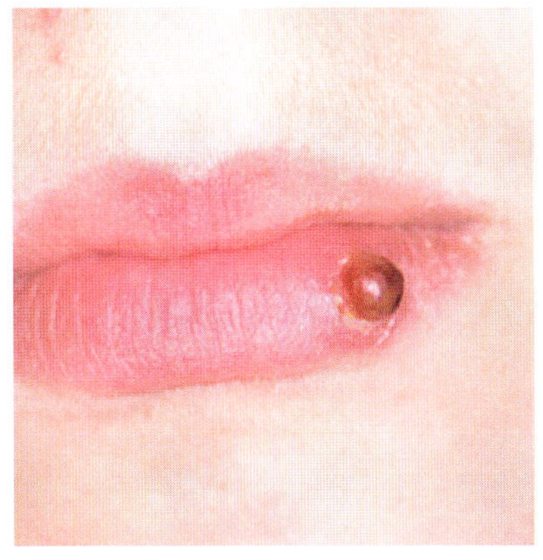

FIG. 80-7 *Globoid smooth-surfaced papule.*

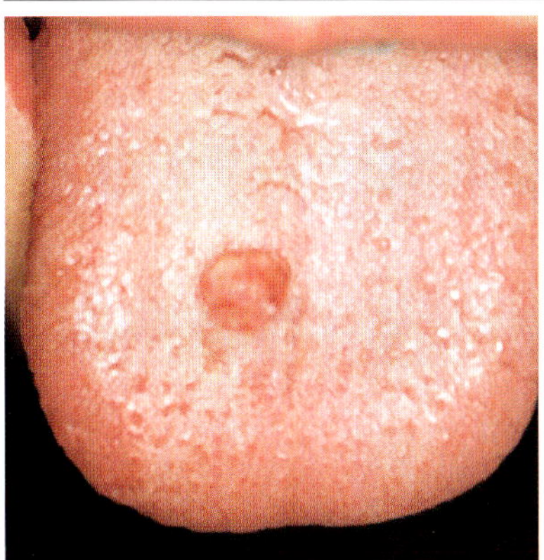

FIG. 80-8 *Rough-surfaced papule.*

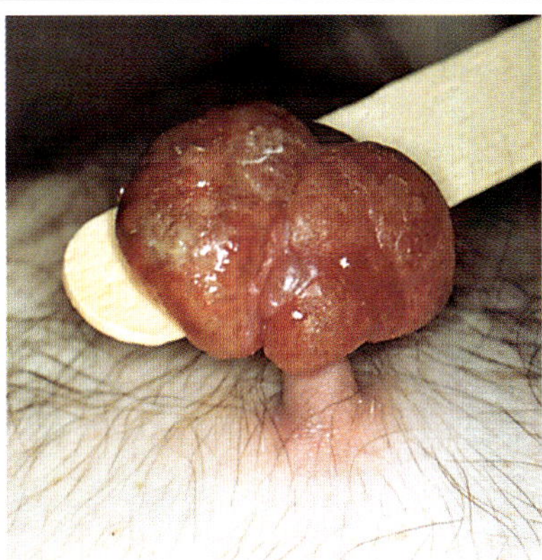

FIG. 80-9 *Mushroom-like, multilobulate, eroded and ulcerated, crusted nodule on a stalk formed by a nipple.*

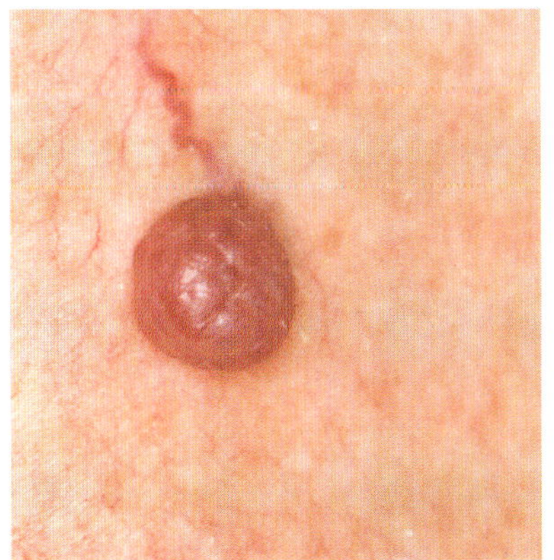

FIG. 80-10 *Typical lesion and its "feeder" arteriole within the subcutaneous fat.*

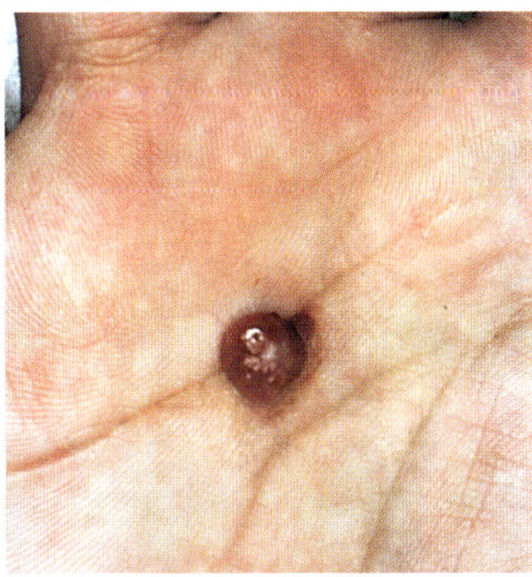

FIG. 80-11 *Ulcerated and partially re-epithelialized lesion.*

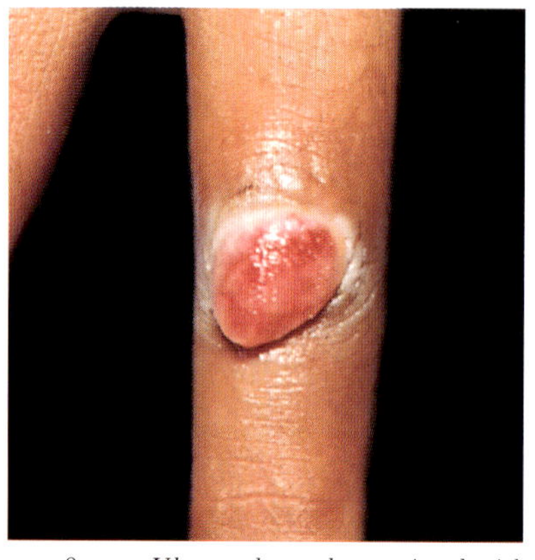

FIG. 80-12 *Ulcerated papule associated with a collarette resembles "proud flesh."*

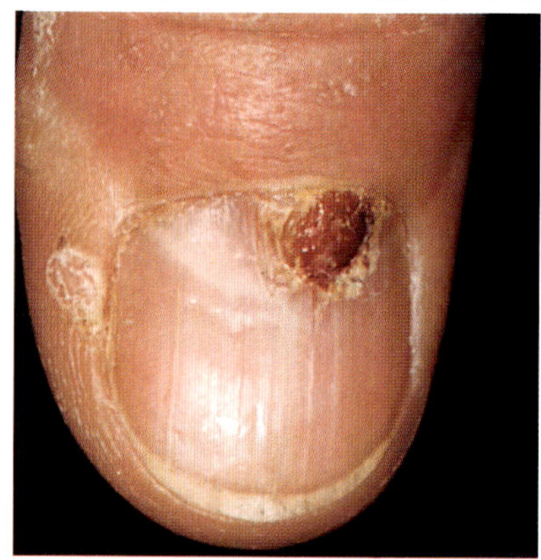

FIG. 80-13 *Ulcerated lesion extending from the nail bed through the nail plate.*

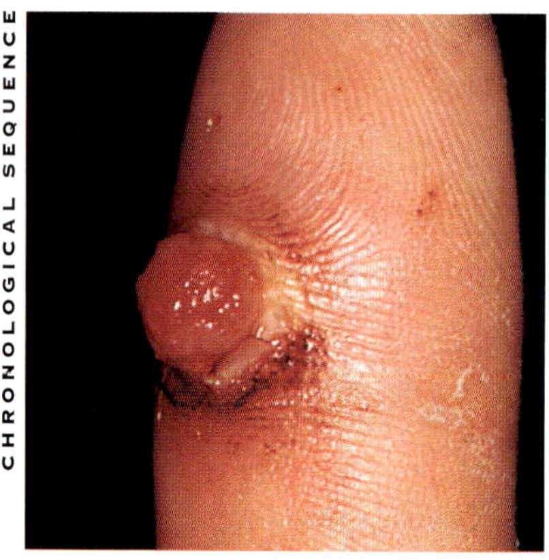

FIG. 80-14 *Ulcerated pyogenic granuloma with a collarette at its base.*

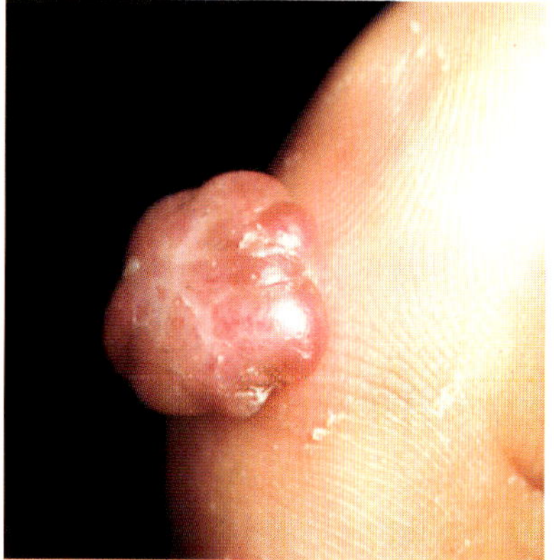

FIG. 80-15 *Multilobate pyogenic granuloma largely re-epithelialized as evidenced by the white surface of much of it.*

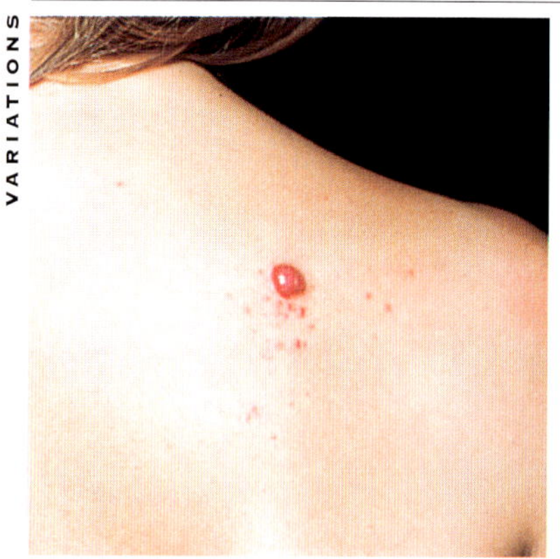

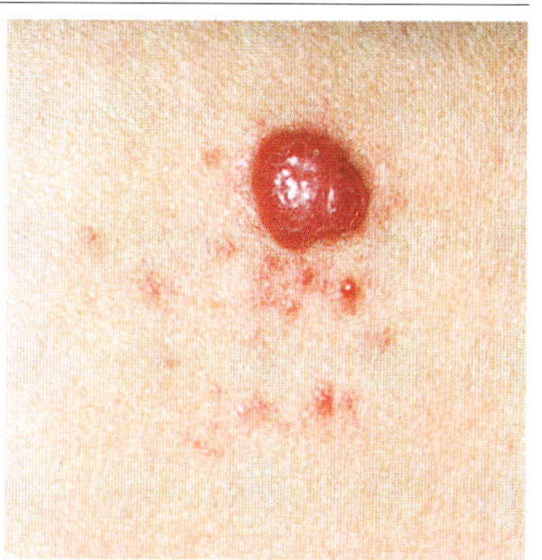

FIG. 80-16 (A, B) *Large pyogenic granuloma with "satellite" smaller pyogenic granulomas.*

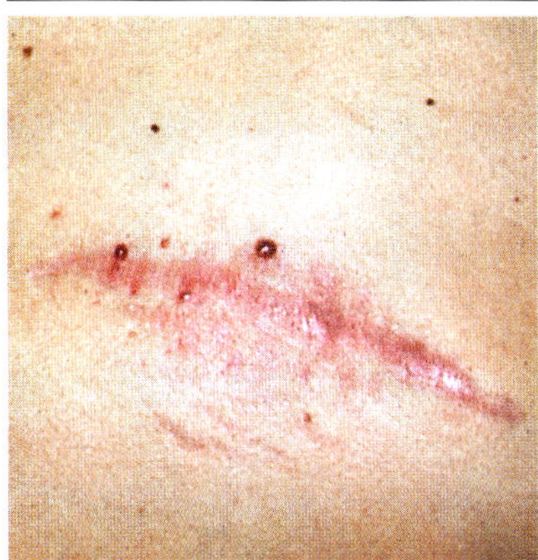

FIG. 80-17 *"Satellite" papules of pyogenic granuloma after excision of a solitary pyogenic granuloma at this site.*

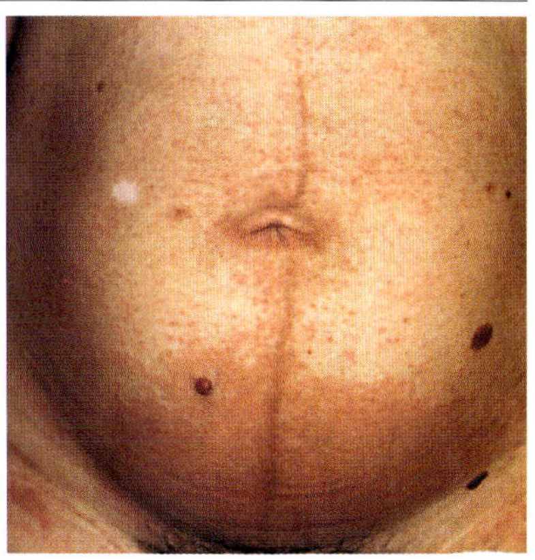

FIG. 80-18 *A red papule of pyogenic granuloma, pruritic urticarial papules and plaques of pregnancy, congenital nevi, and Clark's nevi.*

COURSE The earliest lesions of pyogenic granuloma resemble "proud flesh." The surface is glistening and, in time, comes to resemble a small hemangioma. Over the course of months, the lesion becomes progressively fibrotic, shrinks slowly, and, at last, disappears.

INTEGRATION: UNIFYING CONCEPT Pyogenic granuloma represents a response to trauma to the skin that is sufficiently deep that an arteriole situated in the upper part of the subcutaneous fat has been injured by it. As a consequence of that injury, often by a penetrating wound, but also by "pulling a hangnail," the endothelial cells of the "feeder" vessel become hyperplastic and a structure emerges that clinically resembles "proud flesh" and histopathologically simulates granulation tissue. The surface of the lesion glistens because the denuded granulation tissue is replete with edema and often is covered by fibrin.

In time, the lesion no longer is shiny and comes to resemble a hemangioma because of striking proliferation of small blood vessels in the upper part of the dermis. By the time that multilobulation has occurred consequent to intersection of the proliferation of small blood vessels by fibrous septa, thereby creating distinct lobules of those vessels, the lesion has re-epithelialized completely. In time, a lesion of pyogenic granuloma shrinks steadily consequent to the effects of progressive fibroplasia and finally is lost from the skin.

The term pyogenic granuloma is a misnomer because the lesion is neither pyogenic nor a granuloma. The process is fundamentally a hyperplasia of blood vessels that at first looks like granulation tissue and later a hemangioma, but in actuality is neither.

THERAPY Electrodesiccation destroys the lesion most of the time. Laser ablation and simple surgical excision are alternative methods.

DEFINITION A papular and pustular inflammatory process that is centered in follicles and is distributed mostly in the middle third of the face in both vertical and horizontal directions. Among the varied manifestations of rosacea are innumerable telangiectases, perioral and periocular dermatitis, and rhinophyma. Complications of rosacea include keratitis and conjunctivitis.

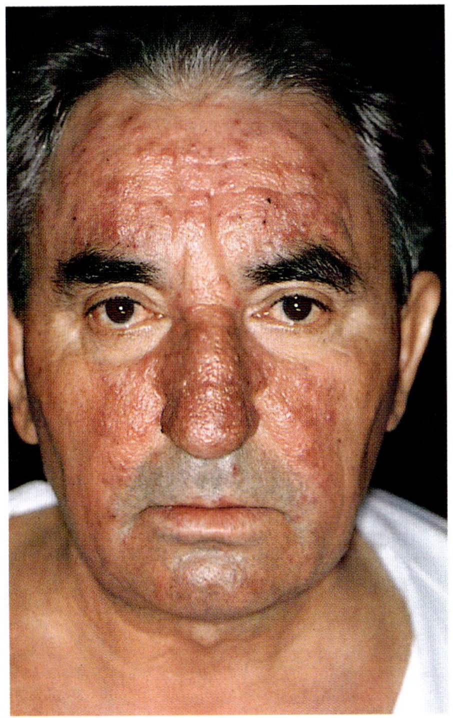

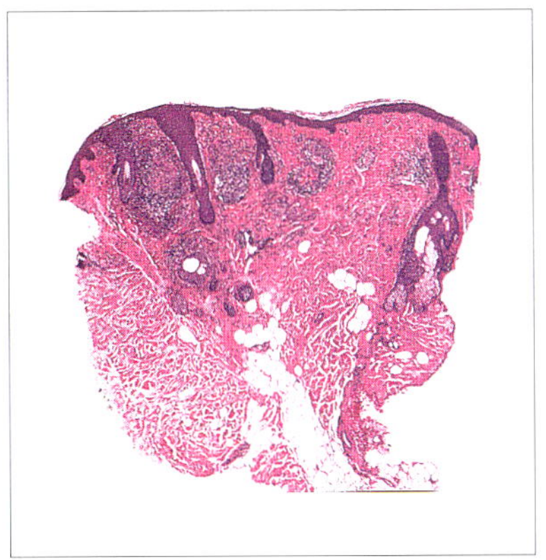

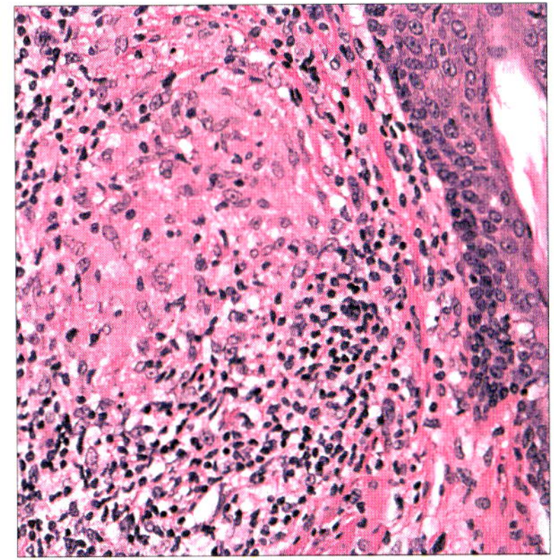

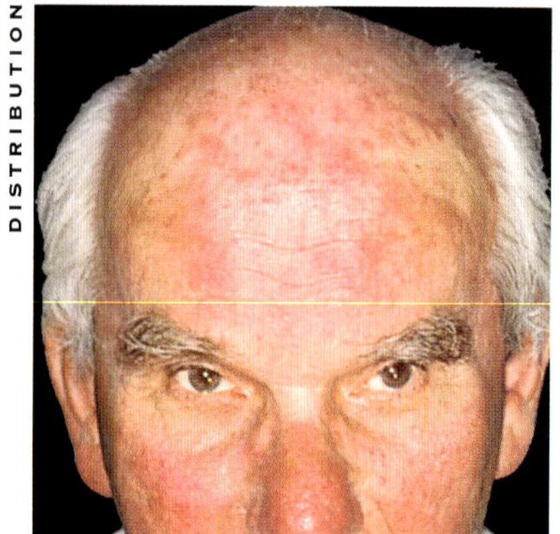

FIG. 81-1 *Telangiectases, papules, and zones of erythema on the scalp, forehead, nose, malar regions, and cheeks.*

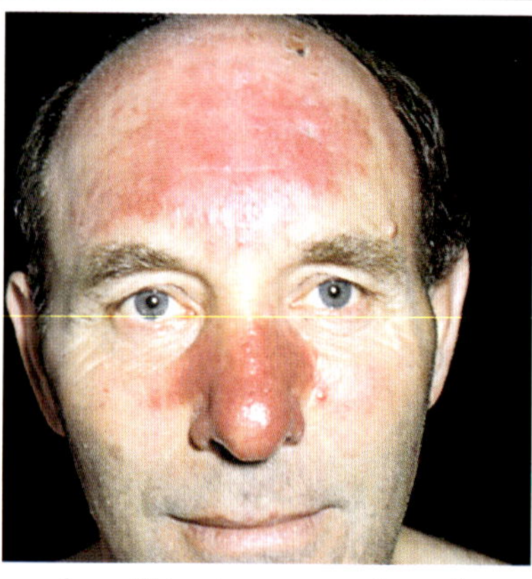

FIG. 81-2 *Telangiectases, papules, and zones of erythema on the forehead, malar regions, and nose especially.*

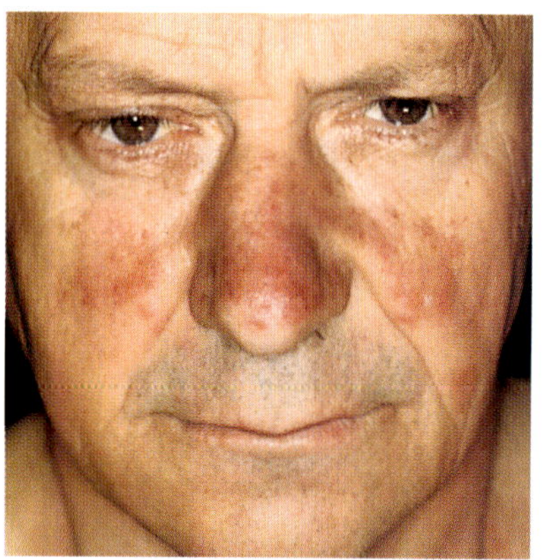

FIG. 81-3 *Telangiectases and papules on the nose, malar eminences, and cheek.*

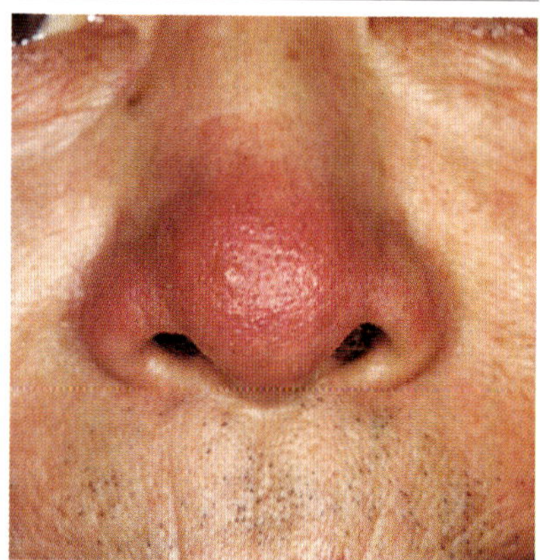

FIG. 81-4 *Erythema and swollen tip of the nose.*

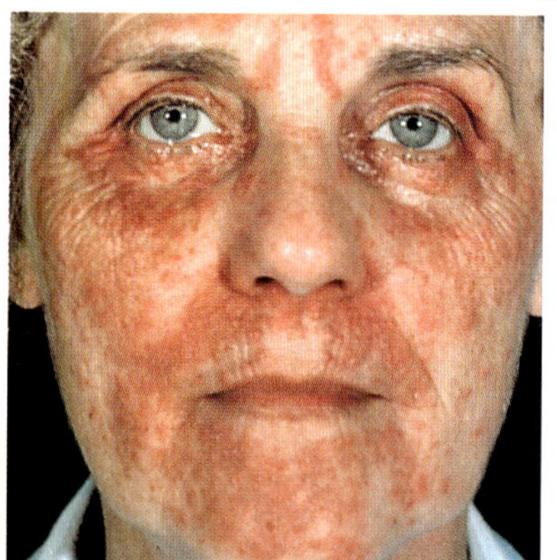

FIG. 81-5 *Papules and pustules of "perioral dermatitis" and of "periocular dermatitis," rosacea both.*

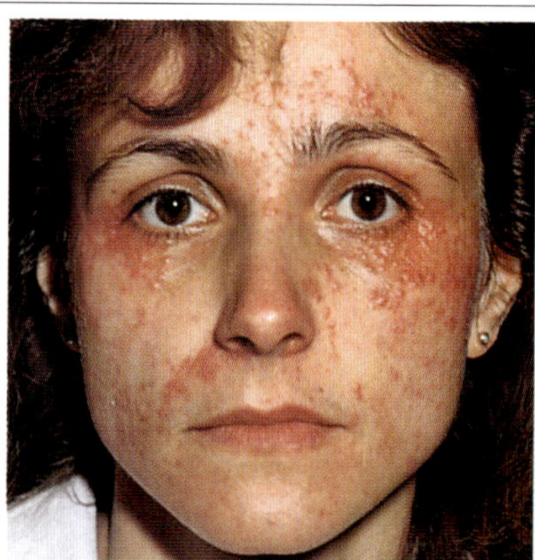

FIG. 81-6 *Papules on the forehead, glabellar region, cheeks, and paranasal and nasolabial regions.*

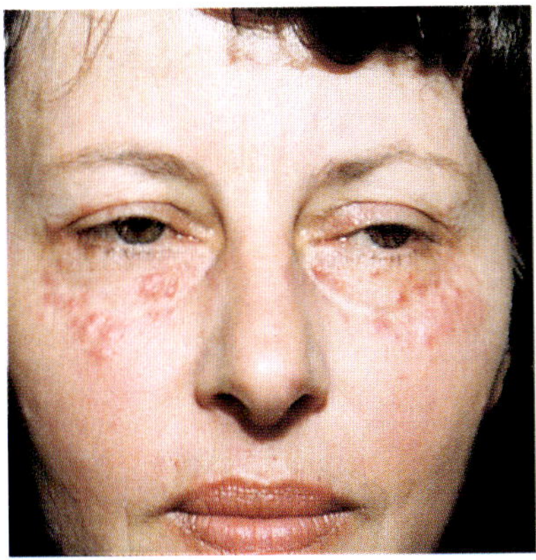

FIG. 81-7 *Papules in the periorbital region (periocular dermatitis).*

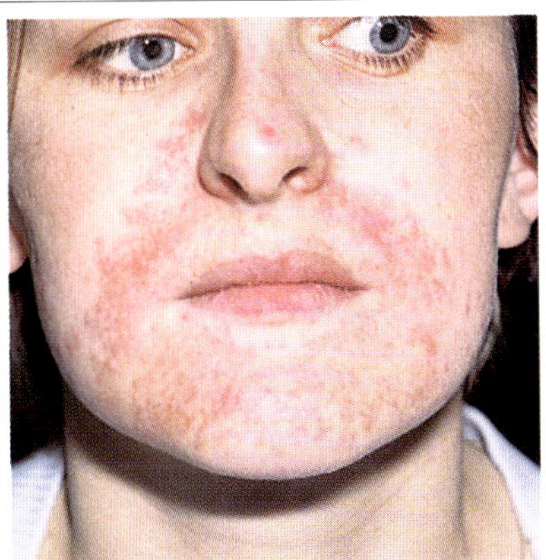

FIG. 81-8 *Papules in the malar region, paranasal region, and chin (perioral dermatitis).*

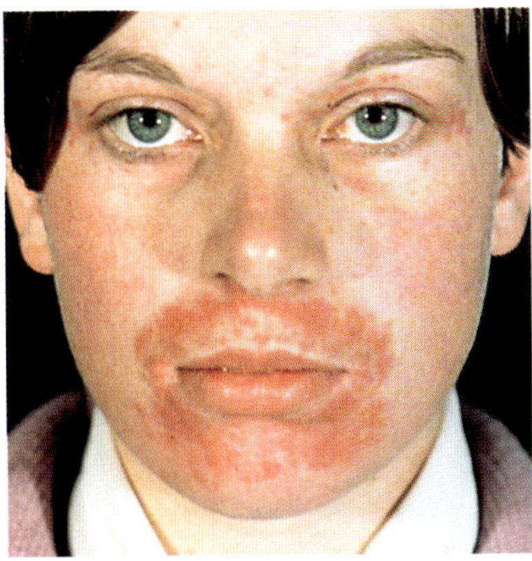

FIG. 81-9 *Papules in periocular and perioral distribution (periocular and perioral dermatitis).*

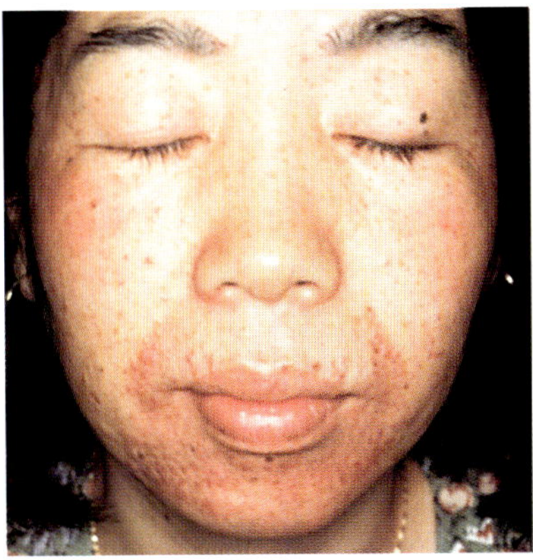

FIG. 81-10 *Papules in the perioral region (perioral dermatitis) and scattered on the malar region, eyelids, and forehead.*

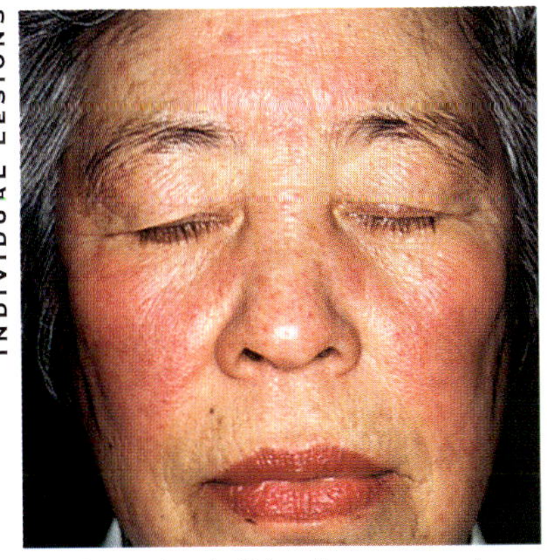

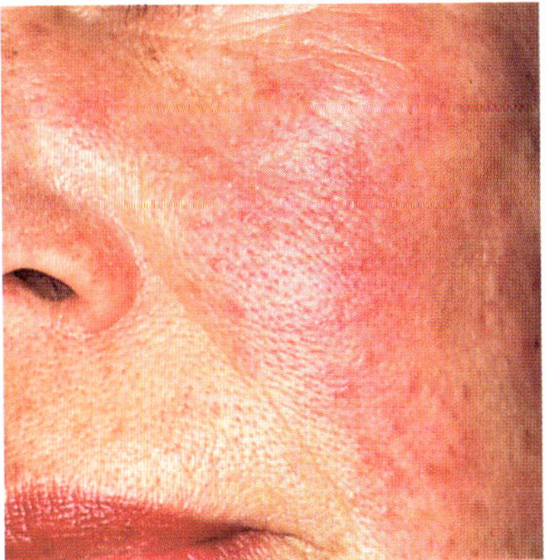

FIG. 81-11 (A, B) *Telangiectases, papules, and diffuse erythema.*

INDIVIDUAL LESIONS

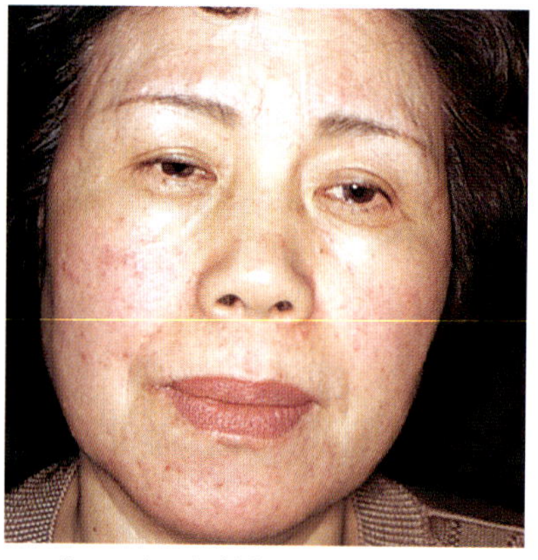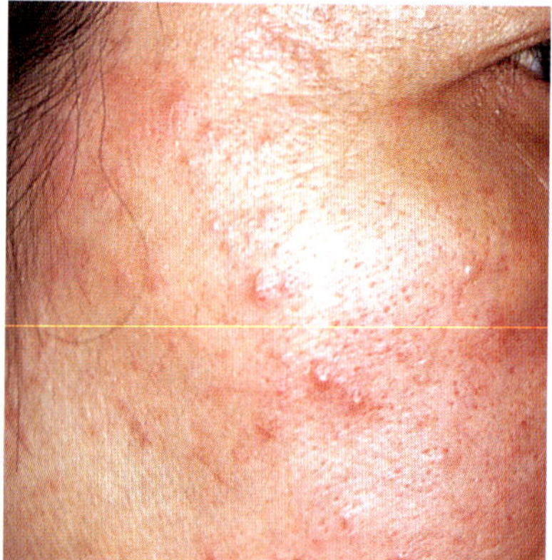

FIG. 81-12 (A, B) *Telangiectases, papules, and diffuse erythema.*

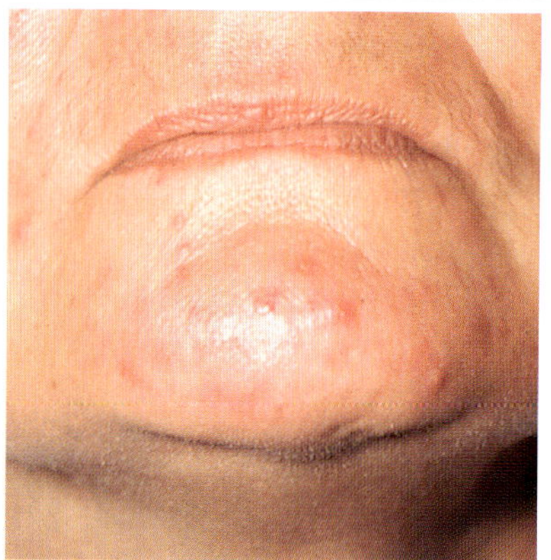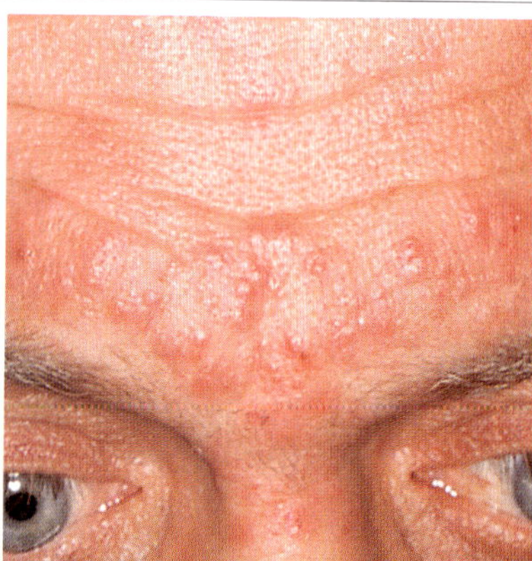

FIG. 81-13 *Papules and papulopustules on an erythematous base.*

FIG. 81-14 *Papules, some of them in clusters.*

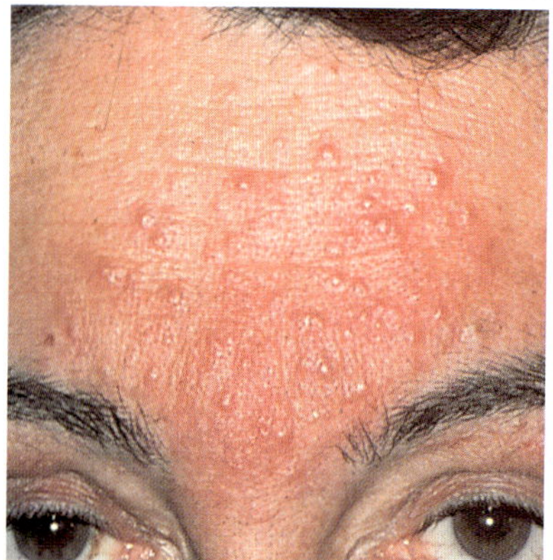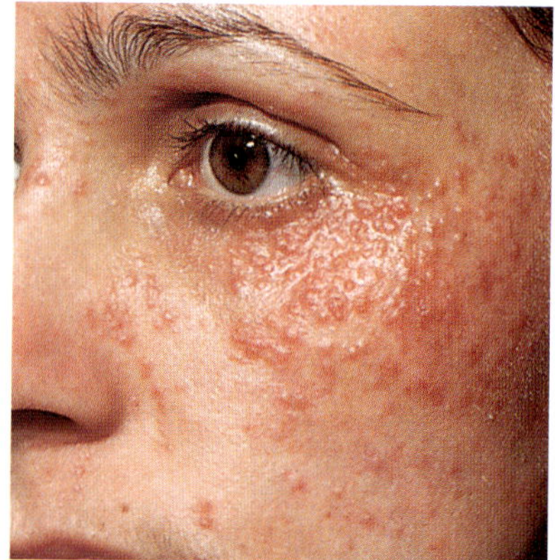

FIG. 81-15 *Papules and papulopustules on an erythematous base.*

FIG. 81-16 *Numerous papules and papulo-pustules.*

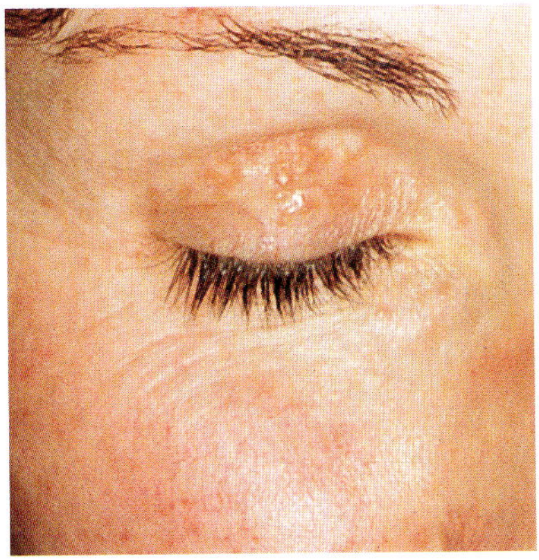

FIG. 81-17 *Cluster of papules.*

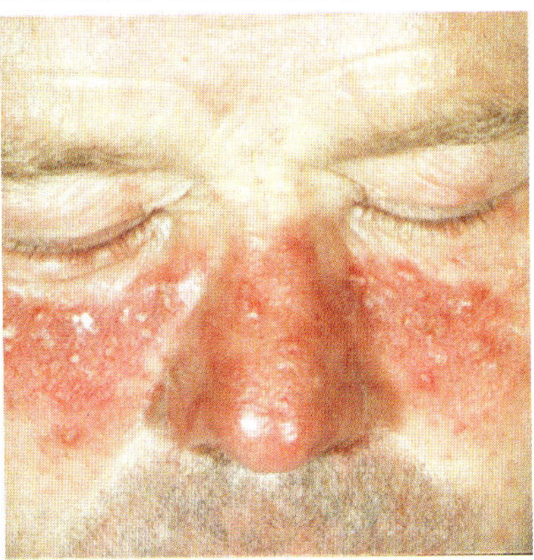

FIG. 81-18 *Papules, papulopustules, scales, and crusts on an erythematous base.*

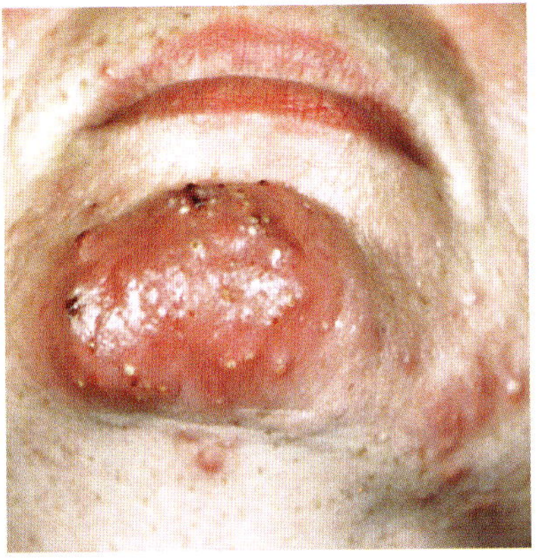

FIG. 81-19 *Papules, papulopustules, pustules, and crusts on a swollen erythematous base (pyoderma faciale, rosacea fulminans).*

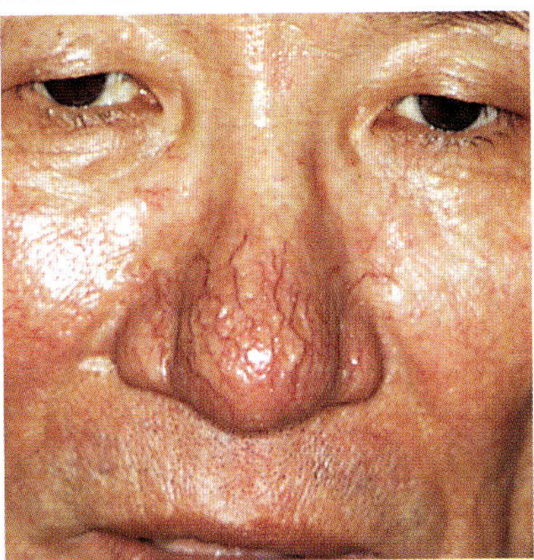

FIG. 81-20 *Varicosities on the nose and telangiectases on the cheeks.*

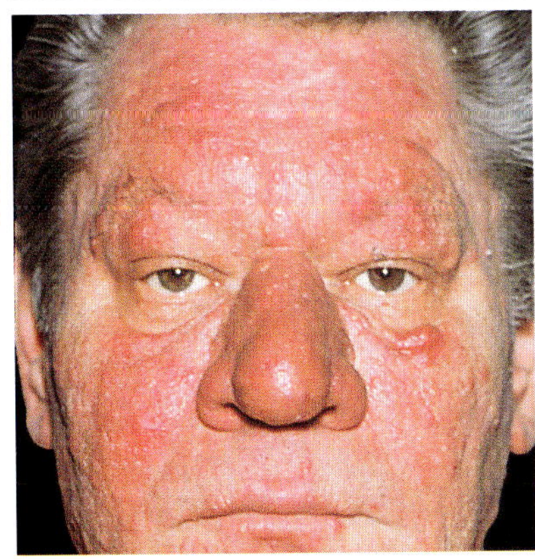

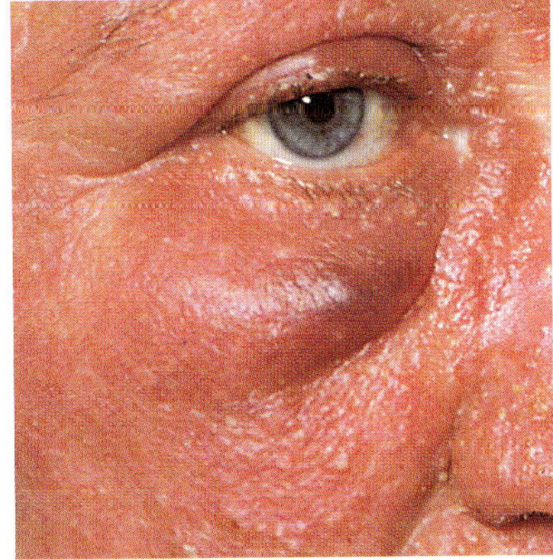

FIG. 81-21 (A, B) *Papules, papulopustules, and nodules on an erythematous base. Periorbital edema is striking (persistent edema of rosacea). In addition to rhinophyma, there are analogous changes on the forehead (metophyma).*

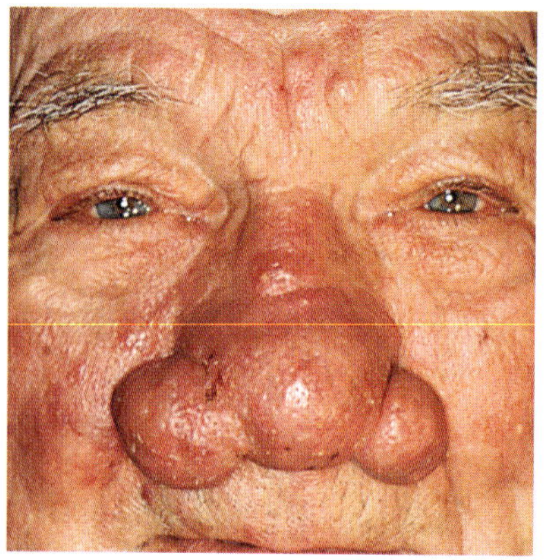

FIG. 81-22 *Rhinophyma and telangiectases, and papules and nodules on the malar region and cheeks.*

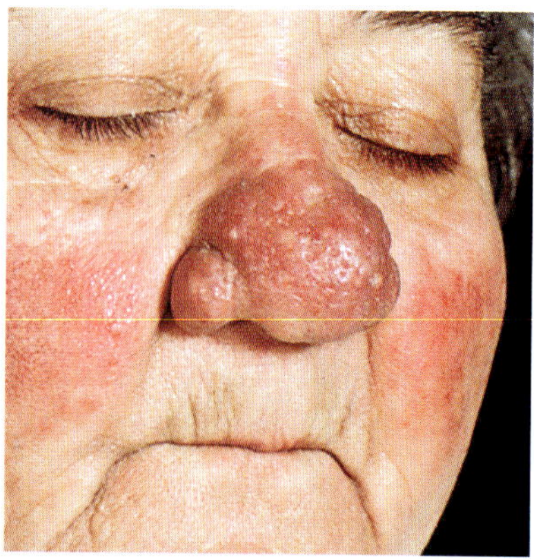

FIG. 81-23 *Rhinophyma and telangiectases, papules, and erythema on the cheeks and chin.*

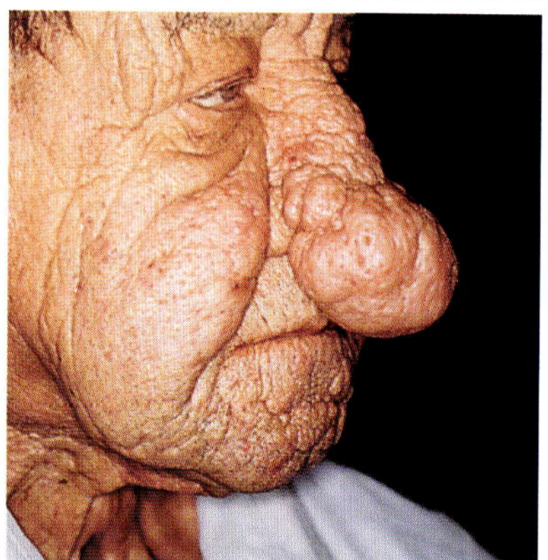

FIG. 81-24 *Rhinophyma.*

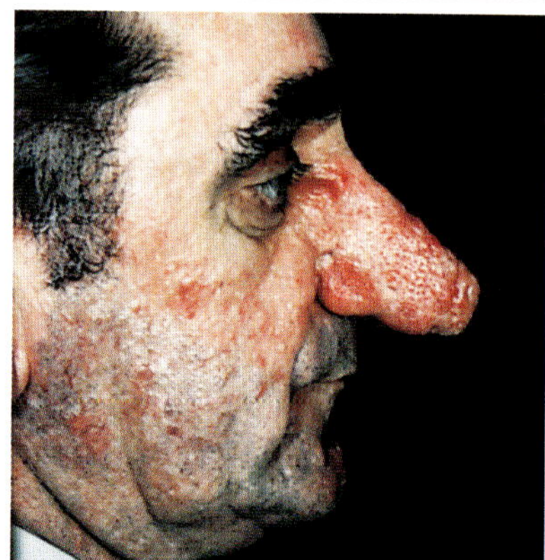

FIG. 81-25 *Cyrano de Bergerac-like nose of rhinophyma. Changes of rosacea are present also on the cheeks and chin.*

CHRONOLOGICAL SEQUENCE

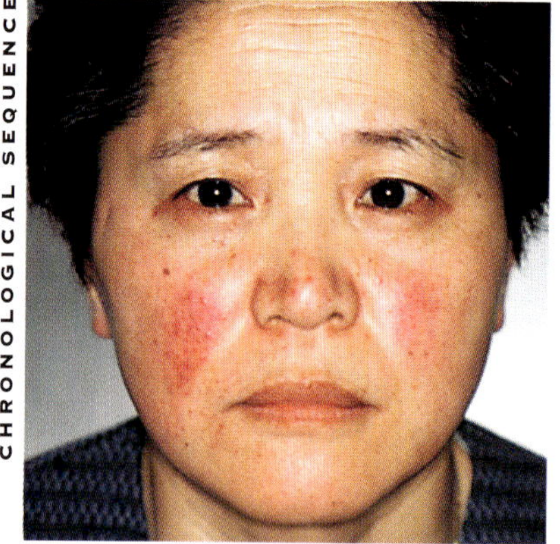

FIG. 81-26 *Telangiectases and papules on an erythematous base.*

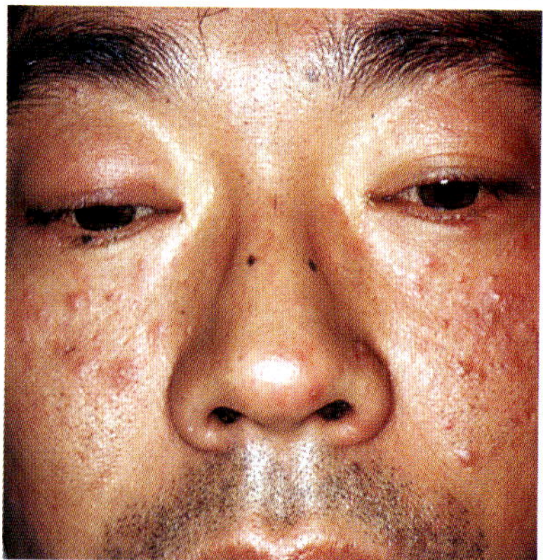

FIG. 81-27 *Papules and papulopustules.*

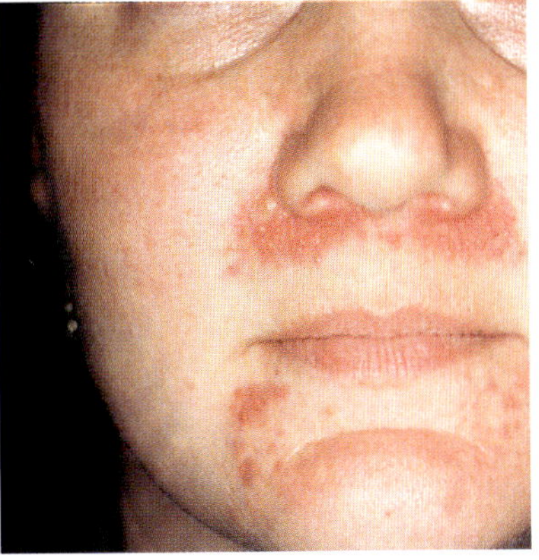

FIG. 81-28   *Pustules on an erythematous base.*

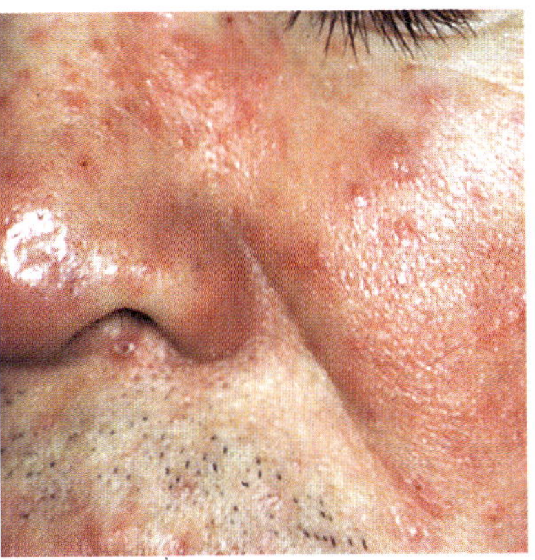

FIG. 81-29 *Papules, papulopustules, and diffuse erythema.*

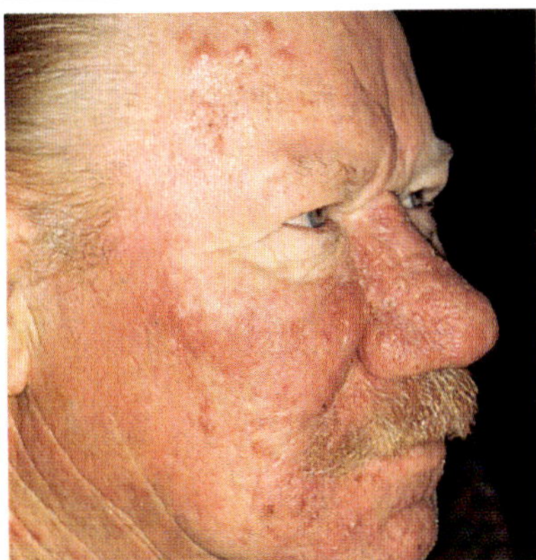

FIG. 81-30 *Telangiectasias, papules, papulopustules, diffuse erythema, and incipient rhinophyma.*

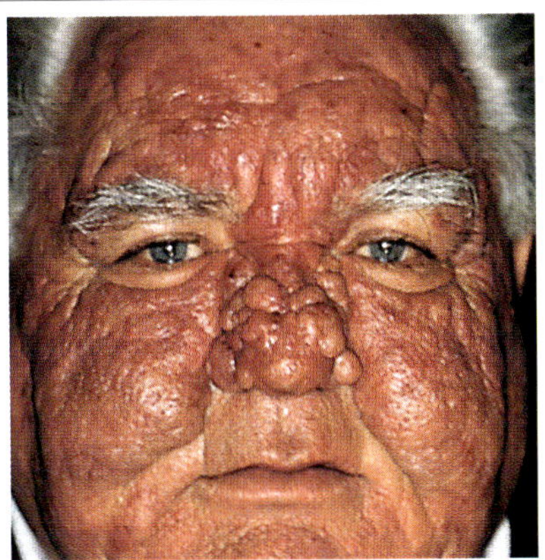

FIG. 81-31   *Nodules and tumors of rhinophyma.*

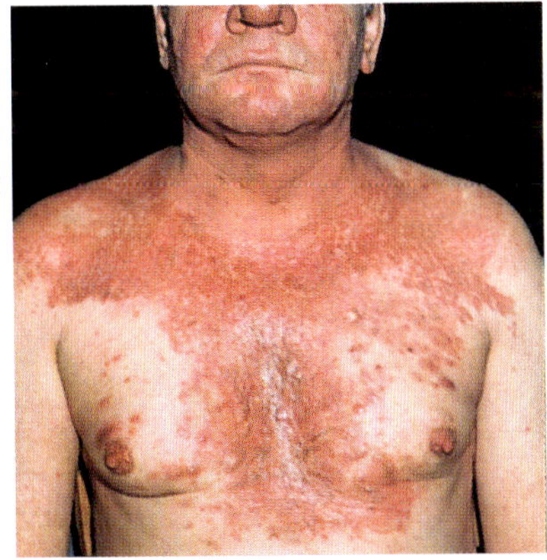

FIG. 81-32   *Extrafacial as well as facial rosacea.*

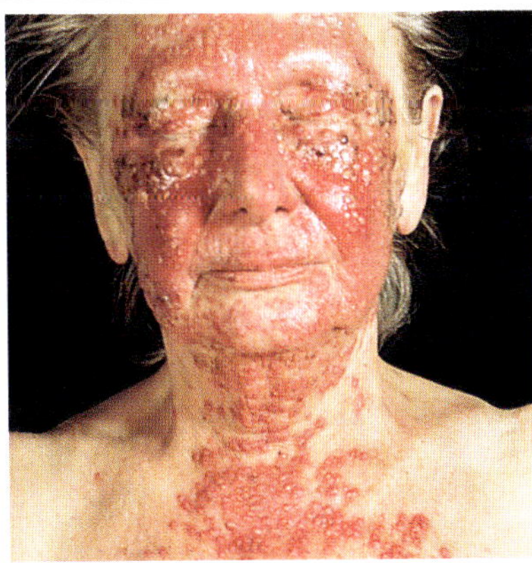

FIG. 81-33   *Facial and extrafacial rosacea with innumerable papules, erosions, ulcers, and crusts (rosacea fulminans).*

COURSE The chronological sequence of lesions of rosacea varies greatly because the lesions themselves vary so greatly. The mostly telangiectatic expression of rosacea simply worsens in time with more telangiectases appearing on the middle third of the face. Papules of rosacea may come and go for years or they may enlarge to become permanent nodules. The rhinophymatous manifestation of rosacea tends to worsen progressively and may be deforming.

In sum, only pustular and papular lesions of rosacea regress, and the latter inconsistently; the telangiectatic and rhinophymatous expressions of rosacea tend to progress and worsen.

INTEGRATION: UNIFYING CONCEPT It is extremely difficult to integrate the various features of rosacea because they are so disparate from one another. How are telangiectases, i.e., dilated end venules, related to papules that consist largely of perifollicular granulomas in company with telangiectases? And how is rhinophyma that represents infundibular cysts that have ruptured and induced suppurative, granulomatous, and fibrosing inflammation combined with prominent sebaceous gland hyperplasia related to keratitis? The answers are not known. Yet another conundrum is posed by the many clinical presentations of the papular expression of rosacea, among them, perioral and periocular dermatitis, rosacea-like tuberculid of Lewandowski, and lupus miliaris disseminatus faciei. In short, rosacea remains an enigma. One issue is clear, namely, that the mite Demodex folliculorum, long claimed to be the etiologic agent of rosacea, is irrelevant to the condition.

A diagnosis can be made of all variants of rosacea clinically, and of papular and rhinophymatous presentations of rosacea histopathologically if attributes of the process pictured in this chapter are identified.

THERAPY Oral tetracyclines modulate the inflammatory response but must be administered for months. Topical metronidazole or topical antibiotics are helpful adjuncts to oral tetracyclines. Dermabrasion or laser ablation is effective for rhinophyma.

DEFINITION An inflammatory (granulomatous) process that involves, among other organs, the lungs, lymph nodes, and skin, and the latter in the form usually of papules, sometimes in arcuate and annular configuration, especially on a face, but also on the extremities, and often in pre-existing scars. In addition to papules, there may be subcutaneous nodules, hypopigmented patches, and ichthyosiform changes.

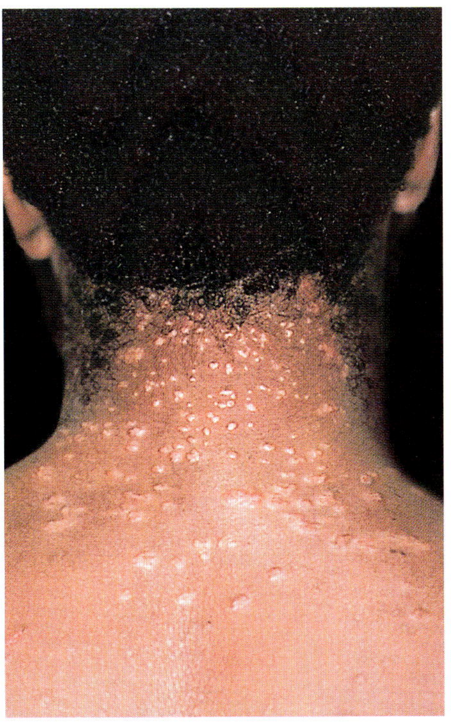

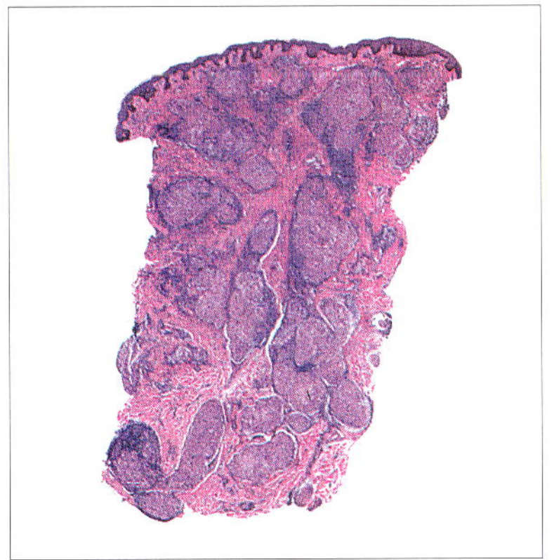

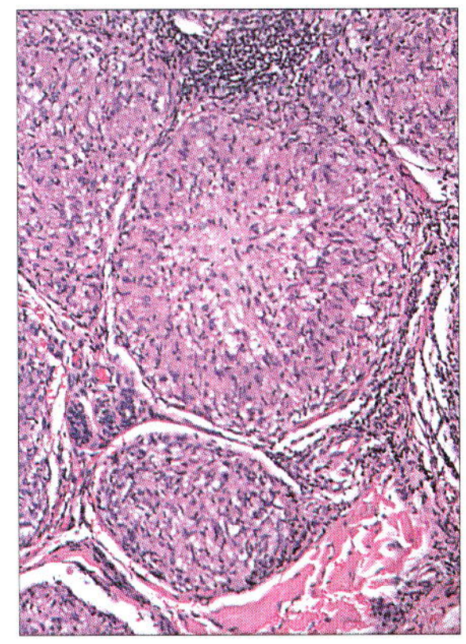

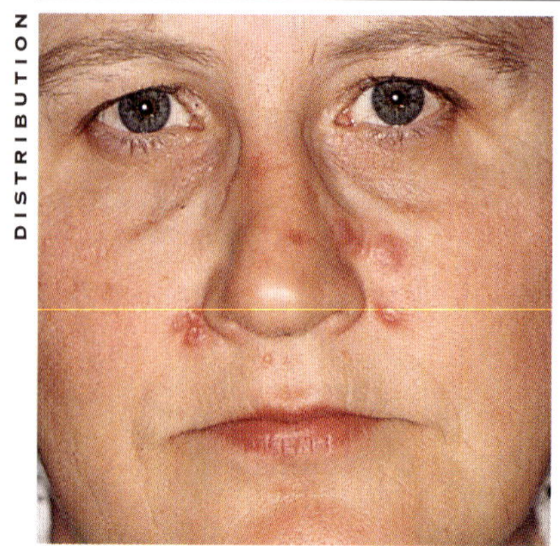

FIG. 82-1 *Papules on and around the nose.*

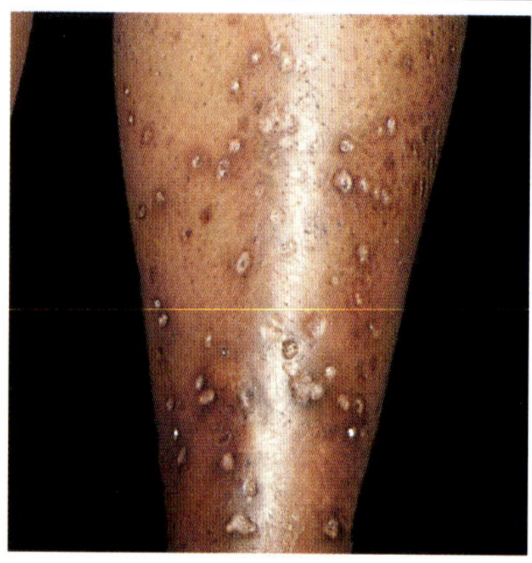

FIG. 82-2 *Ring-like papules, some of them encircling an atrophic center.*

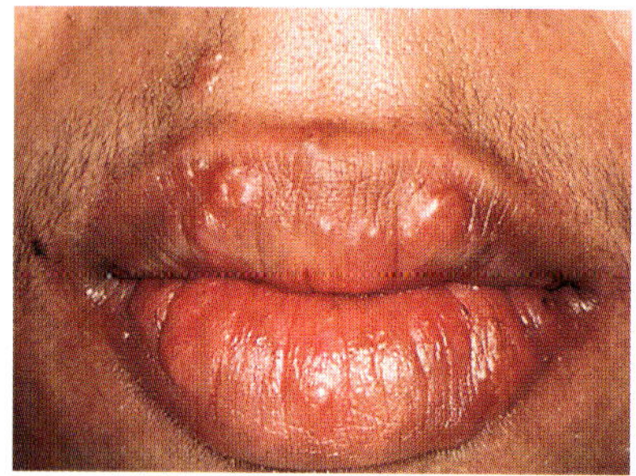

FIG. 82-3 *Papules.*

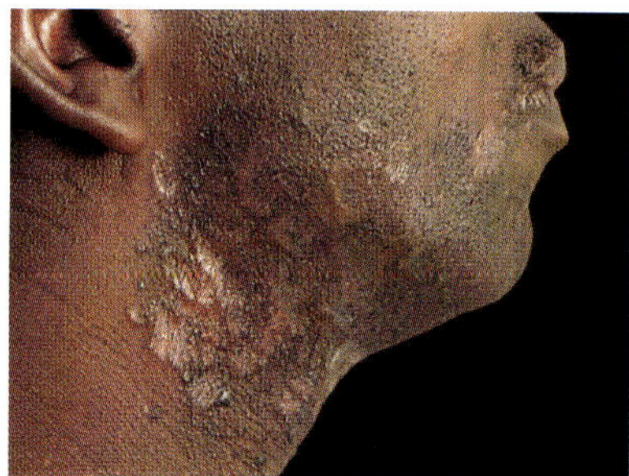

FIG. 82-4 *Dells that represent atrophic scars at sites of former papules of sarcoidosis.*

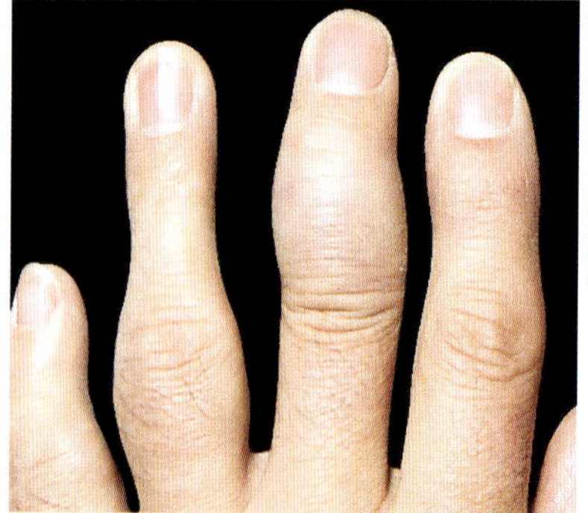

FIG. 82-5 *Fusiform swelling of fingers (osteitis cystica).*

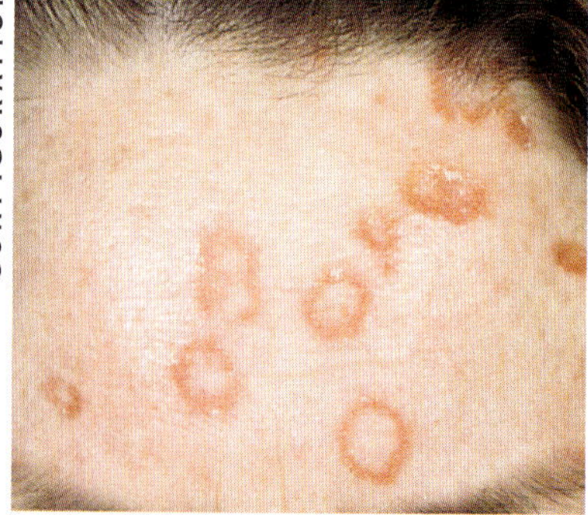

FIG. 82-6 *Annular lesions with a depressed center and a rim made up of tiny, shiny, smooth papules. Some papules are scaly.*

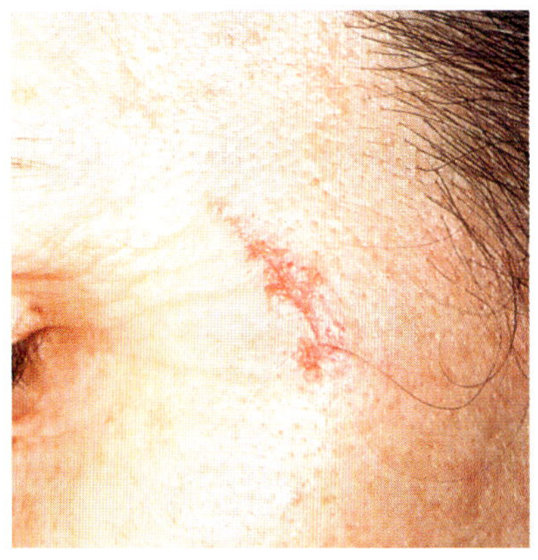

FIG. 82-7 *Papules in and contiguous with a scar.*

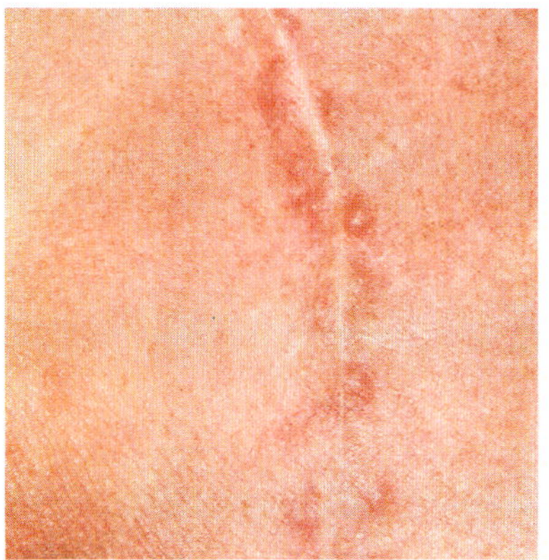

FIG. 82-8 *Papules contiguous with a scar.*

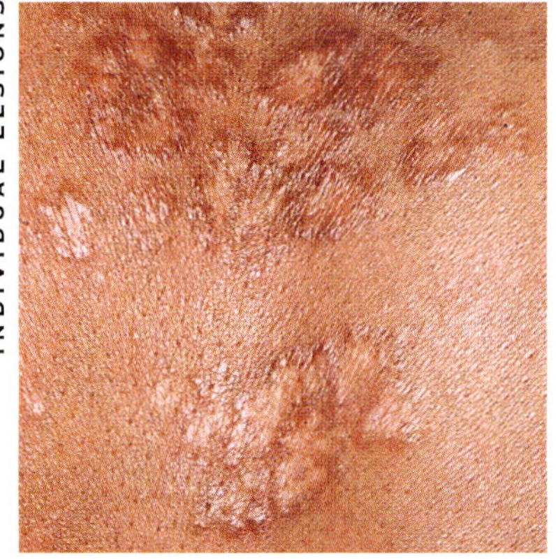

FIG. 82-9 *Papules forming rings.*

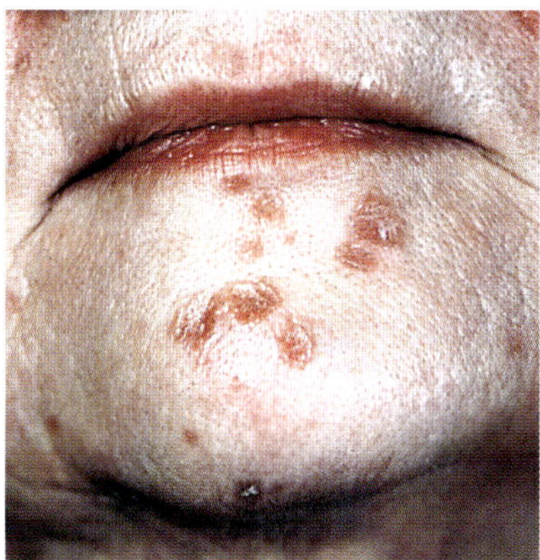

FIG. 82-10 *Atrophic macules surrounded by papules in a ring.*

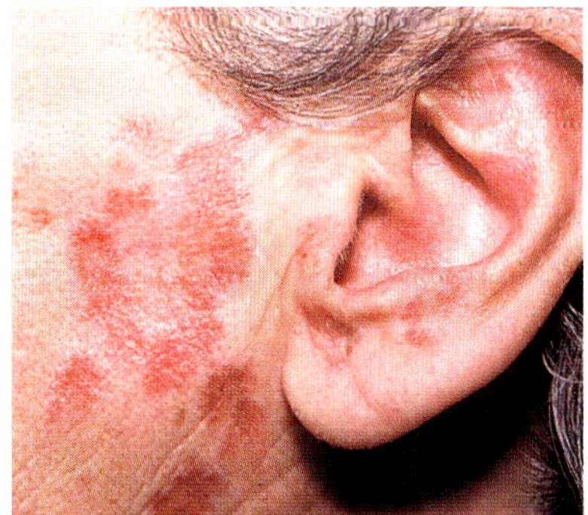

FIG. 82-11 *Plaques with scalloped border and atrophic center.*

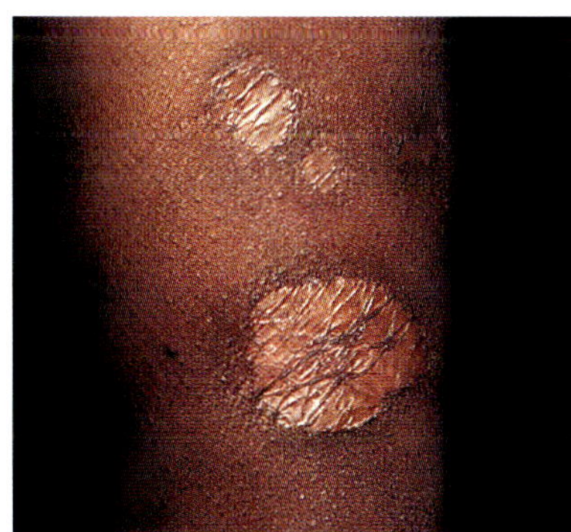

FIG. 82-12 *Atrophic hypopigmented nummular plaques.*

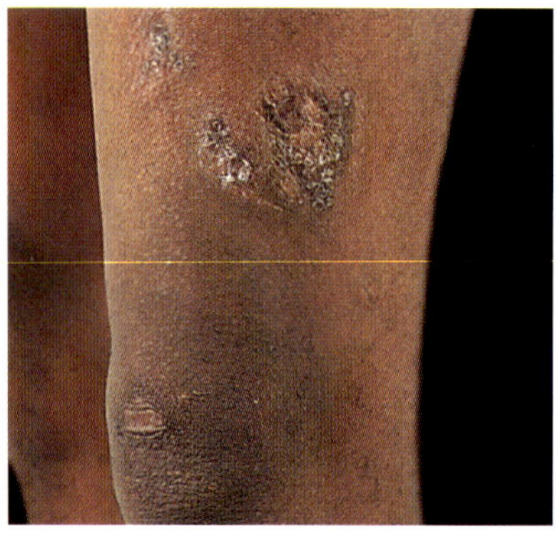

FIG. 82-13 *Scaly hyperpigmented plaques.*

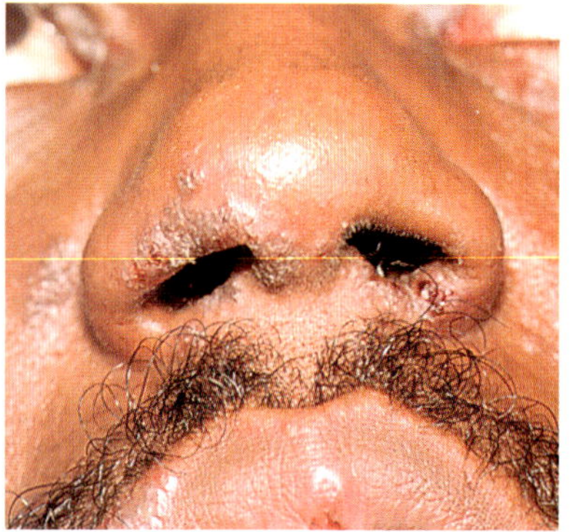

FIG. 82-14 *Papules, some with crusts, on the alae nasae, nasolabial folds, and upper lip.*

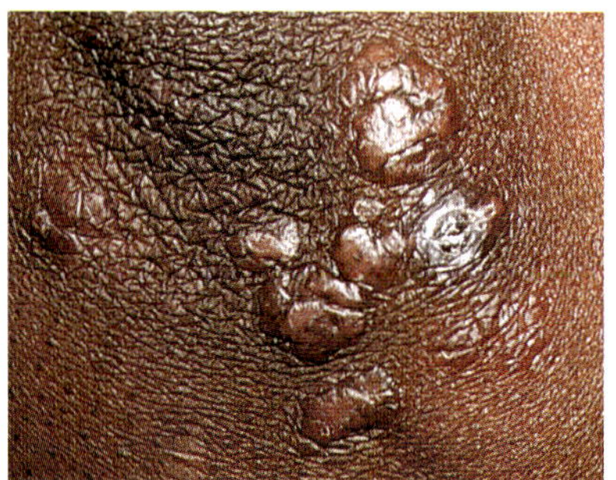

FIG. 82-15 *Smooth-surfaced and scaly papules and plaques.*

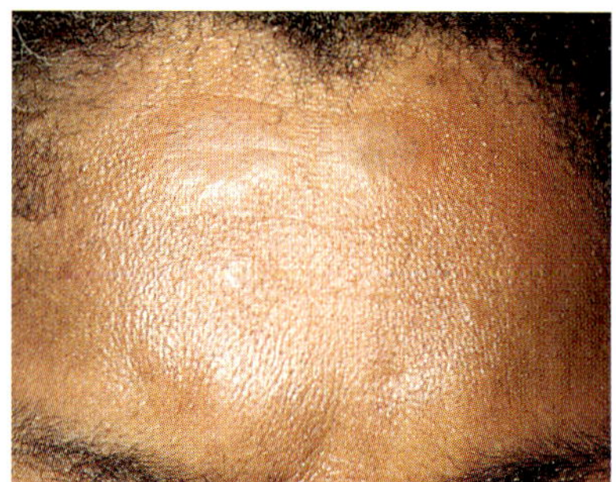

FIG. 82-16 *Smooth-surfaced papules and plaques.*

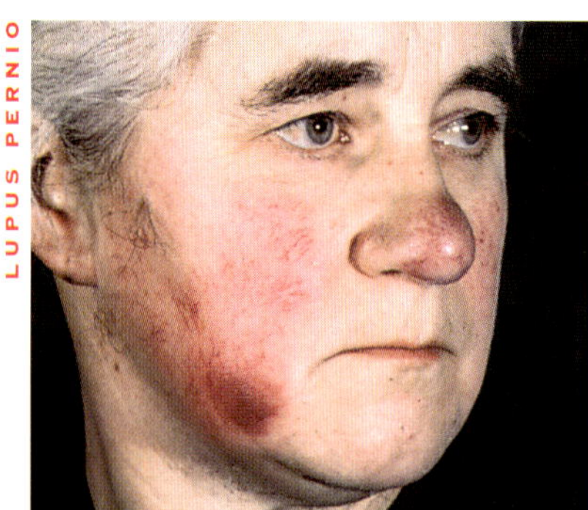

FIG. 82-17 *Nodule on the nose and a plaque on the cheek (lupus pernio).*

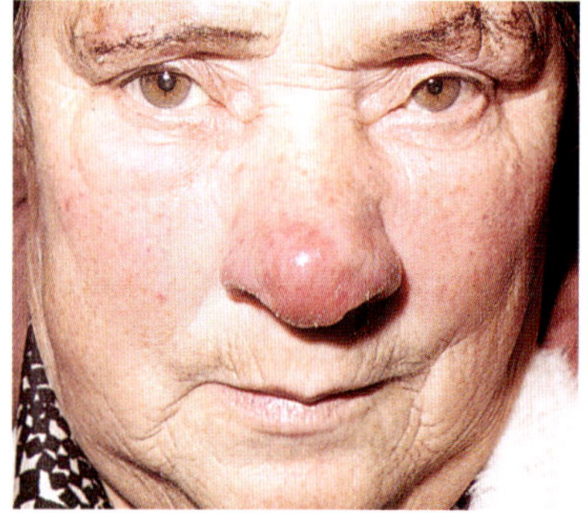

FIG. 82-18 *Nodule on the nose (lupus pernio).*

ADJUNCTIVE DIAGNOSTIC TESTS Chest x-ray is mandatory in order to recognize characteristic manifestations in the lungs, and x-ray of other organs, such as bones, may also be indicated. Calcium levels in the serum should be monitored for signs of hypercalcemia. Serum angiotensin-converting enzyme may be positive in extrathoracic sarcoidosis.

COURSE Tiny papules of sarcoidosis tend to enlarge, but usually do not become nodules. Sometimes those papules are so numerous and set so closely that a plaque results; in other instances the papules may be arranged in an annulus. The papules of sarcoidosis tend to persist, as does the disease itself. New lesions may appear over the course of years, but, as a rule, old lesions do not disappear.

INTEGRATION: UNIFYING CONCEPT The gross and morphologic features of sarcoidosis are distinctive in every organ in which the disease makes itself manifest. In the skin, papules consist of discrete collections of epithelioid histiocytes. Because those collections usually are devoid of encircling dense infiltrates of lymphocytes, they are referred to as "naked tubercles." Plaques of subcutaneous sarcoidosis may involve the dermis in a manner just like that of papules, but, in addition, many granulomas are present within fat lobules and, to a much lesser extent, within septa.

Histopathologic findings like those of sarcoidosis in the skin are seen in lesions of sarcoidosis in organs such as lymph nodes, lung, eye, and bone. In short, sarcoidosis is a systemic granulomatous disease. Involvement of skin by sarcoidosis implies that other organs are also involved by the same pathologic process. The ichthyosiform changes of sarcoidosis usually occur on the legs in the region of the anterior tibiae and, being an expression of "acquired" ichthyosis, they exhibit histopathologic findings indistinguishable from those of ichthyosis vulgaris.

The cause of sarcoidosis is not known, but the histopathologic findings are most consonant with an infectious process.

THERAPY Localized papules and nodules respond to injection of corticosteroids. For widespread papules, which usually signify systemic disease, oral corticosteroids are indicated. An alternative to corticosteroids is an antimalarial like hydroxychloroquine and chloroquine.

SCAR

DEFINITION A type of fibrosing inflammation characterized clinically by lesions that at first are elevated and that do not extend beyond the exact site of injury and that in time tend to shrink, sometimes even becoming atrophic.

KELOID

DEFINITION A fibrosing inflammatory process characterized by papular, plaque-like, nodular, and tumorous lesions that extend well beyond the exact site of injury and that in time tend to shrink somewhat, but never greatly.

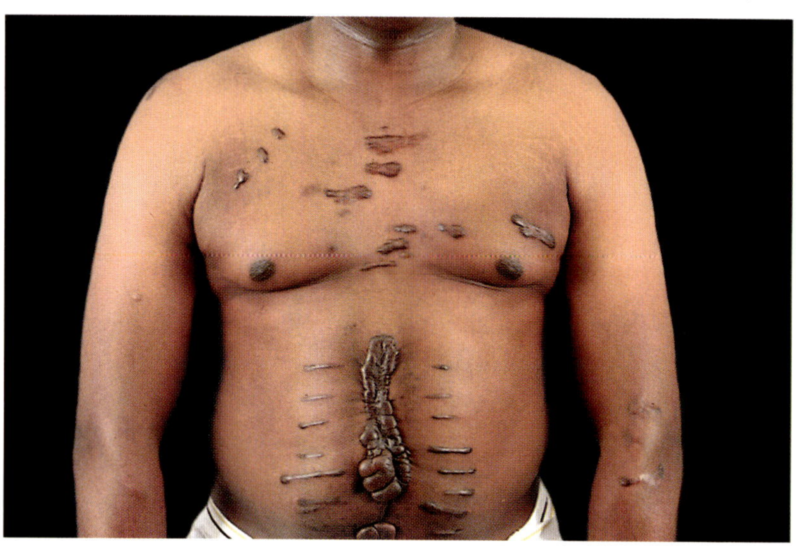

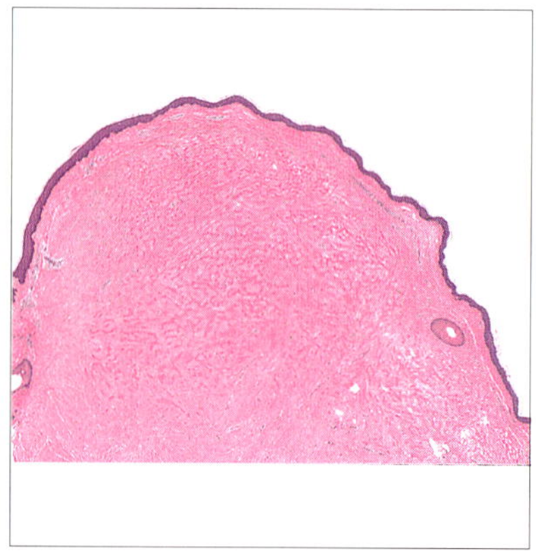

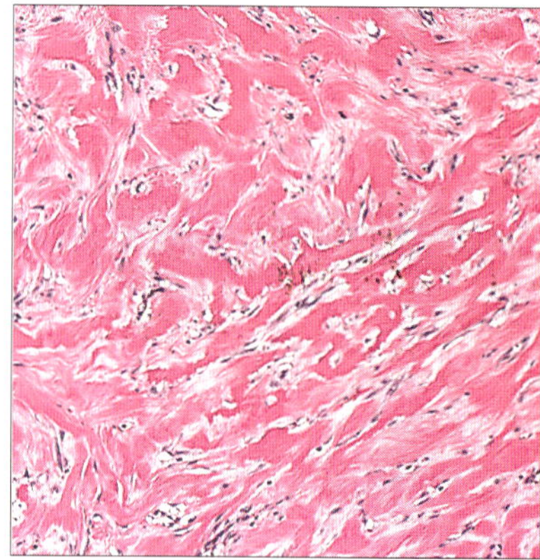

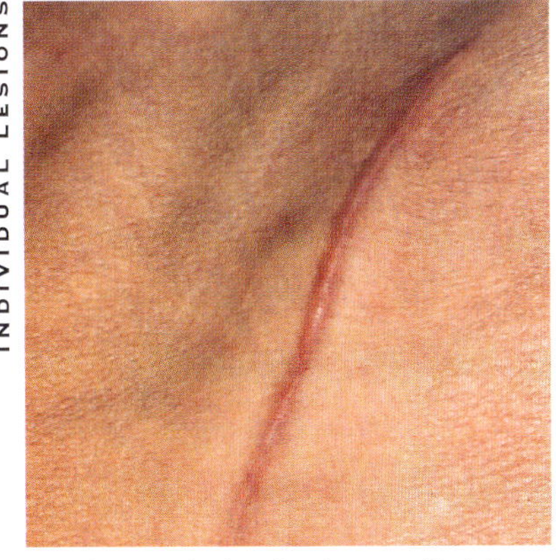

FIG. 83-1 *A sharply circumscribed linear hypertrophic scar.*

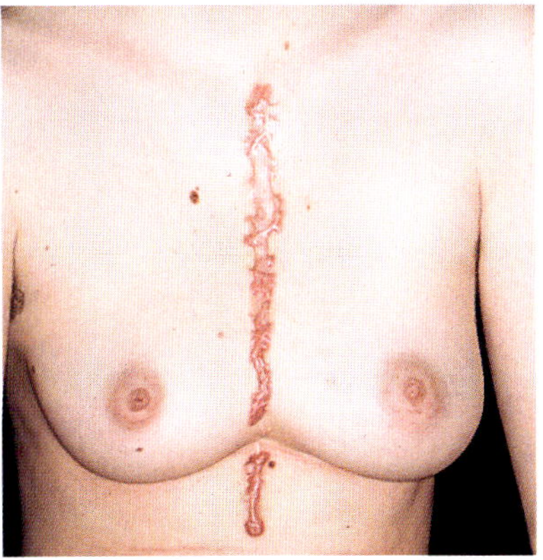

FIG. 83-2 *A poorly circumscribed linear hypertrophic scar.*

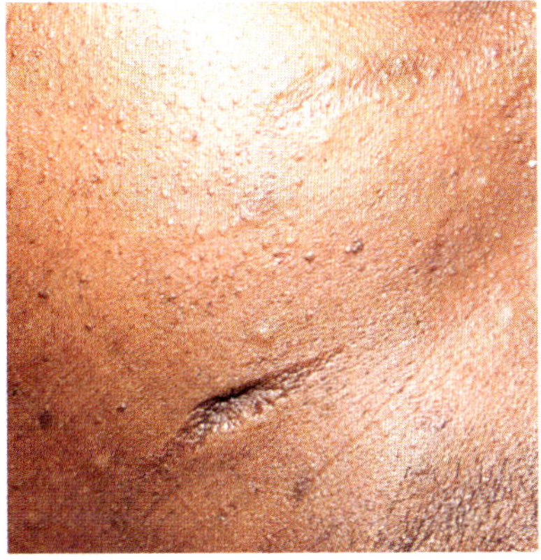

FIG. 83-3 *Two atrophic scars, one of them deep.*

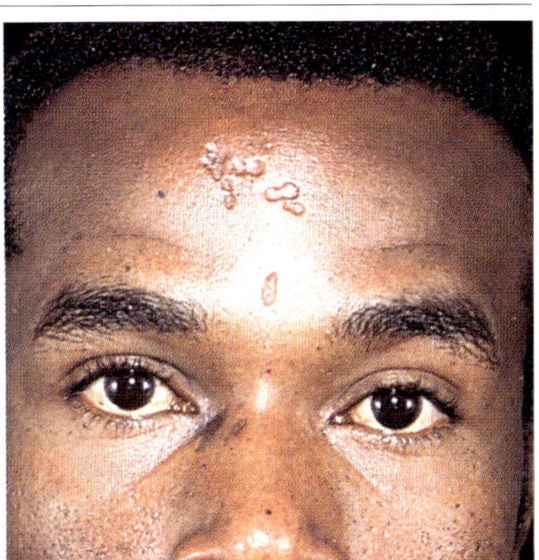

FIG. 83-4 *Atrophic scars.*

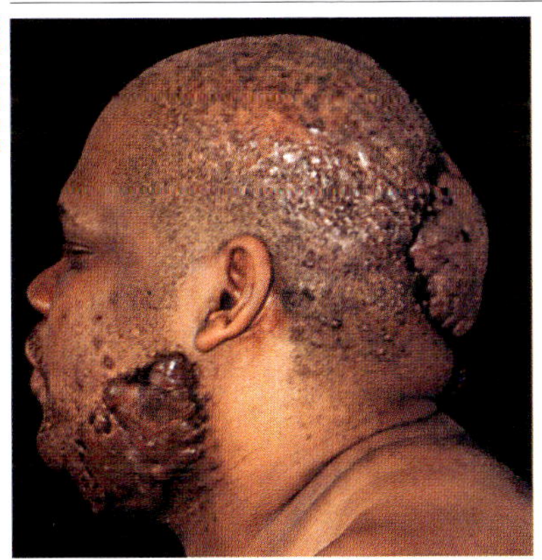

FIG. 83-5 *Huge keloids secondary to suppurative folliculitis so severe that it resulted in formation of sinuses.*

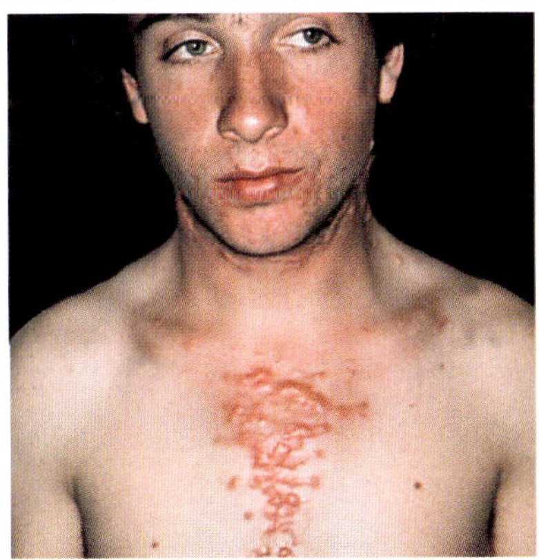

FIG. 83-6 *Keloids, some of them in linear array, secondary to severe acne vulgaris.*

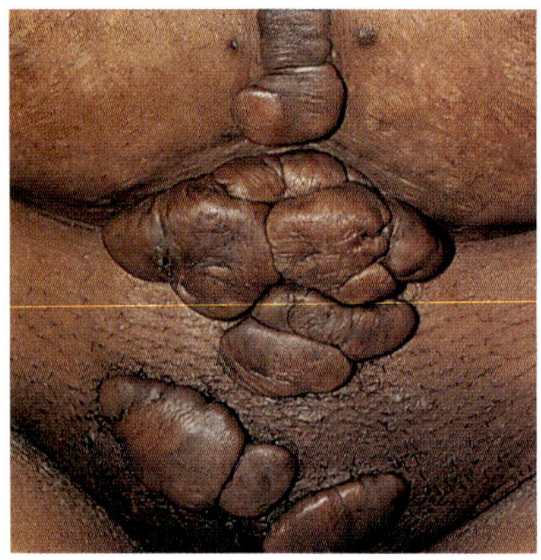

FIG. 83-7 *Keloids that arose secondary to a surgical procedure.*

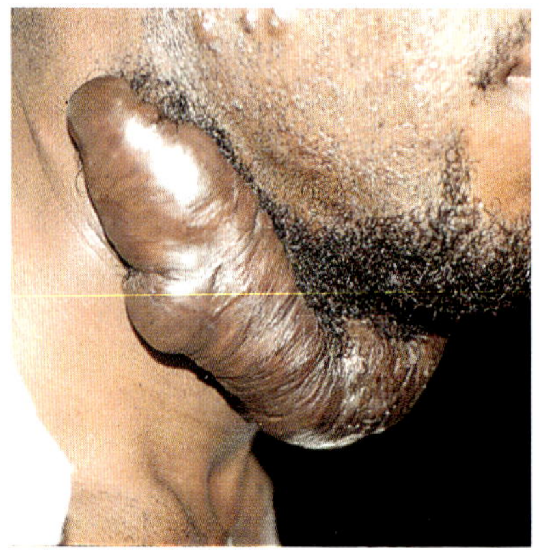

FIG. 83-8 *A sausage-shaped keloid secondary to sycosis barbae.*

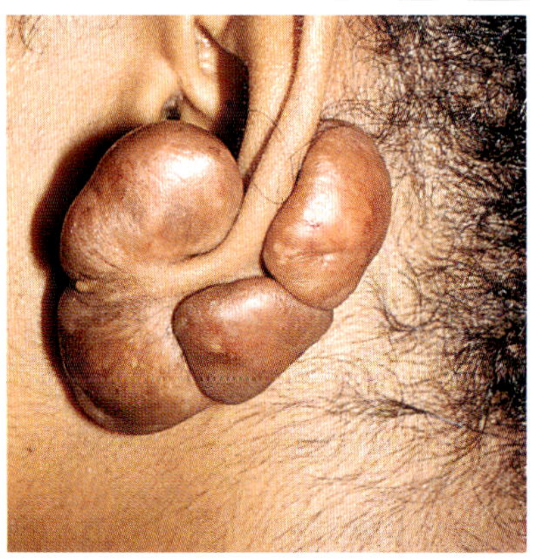

FIG. 83-9 *Keloids secondary to piercing the earlobe.*

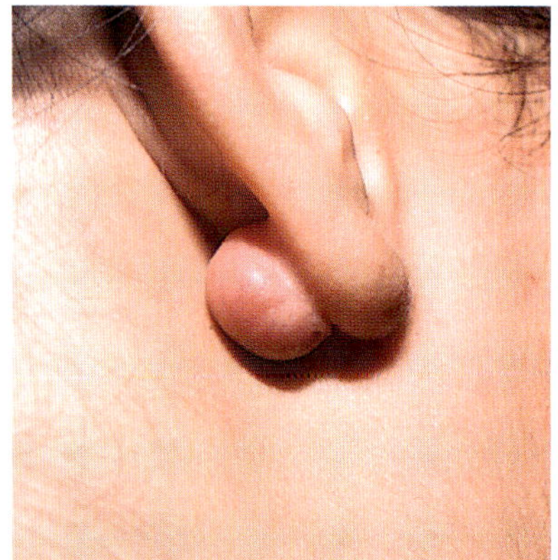

FIG. 83-10 *A keloid on the earlobe secondary to piercing of it.*

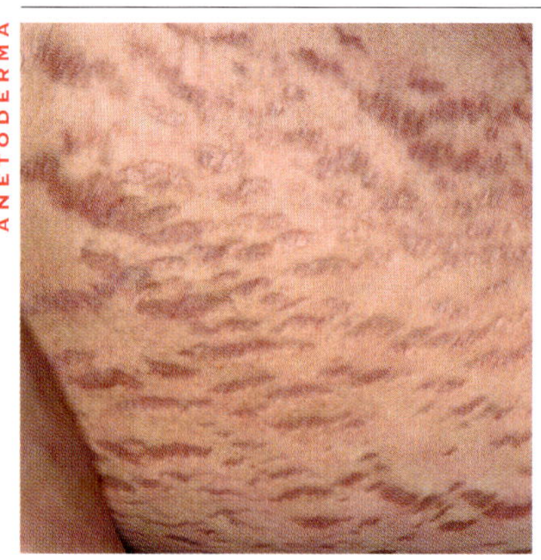

FIG. 83-11 *Atrophic striae.*

ANETODERMA

ANETODERMA

DEFINITION The end-stage of an inflammatory or neoplastic process in which there is loss of collagen and elastic tissue in the mid-reticular dermis with consequent formation of lesions that protrude in dome-like fashion above the skin surface and that can be herniated below the skin surface. The stereotypical expression of a small lesion of anetoderma is "macular atrophy" secondary to destructive changes of acne vulgaris, and of a large lesion of anetoderma is stria atrophicans. Striae are linear lesions that at first are elevated and plethoric (striae distensae) and later, after years, are depressed, atrophic, and white (striae atrophicantes), a result of the combined effects of stretching of the skin and of systemic corticosteroids.

COURSE Scars, keloids, and anetodermas represent the end stage of an inflammatory process that was initiated by trauma of some kind. The earliest change in scars and keloids is granulation tissue that may be present at the surface of an abrasion, at the site of a puncture wound, or as a polyp of "proud flesh." It takes weeks for fibroplasia to replace the granulation tissue and, at that time, the distinctive morphologic characteristics of a scar or keloid may become noticeable. Once a papule, plaque, nodule, or tumor of a scar or keloid is formed fully, it tends to remain more or less that way for years. In time, however, some shrinkage of those fibrosing processes is inevitable. Whereas shrinkage of keloids usually is negligible, some scars may change, over decades, from being hypertrophic to atrophic.

By the time that an atrophoderma, i.e., macular atrophy and other anetodermas, makes itself known, it is already the end stage of a process. Each of those atrophodermas begins as a distinctive inflammatory or neoplastic process, such as acne vulgaris for macular atrophy and a tumor of immunocytoma for anetoderma, but granulation tissue is not a stage of the process. Neither are striae atrophicantes associated with granulation tissue, the earliest changes being those of a subtle inflammatory process as judged histopathologically, but of a not so subtle process as assessed clinically (striae distensae).

INTEGRATION: UNIFYING CONCEPT Scars and keloids are two distinctive types of fibrosing inflammatory processes recognizable for what they are, clinically and histopathologically, by distinctive morphologic findings.

Scars, when fully formed, consist of fibrillary bundles of collagen in conjunction with thin fibrocytes, both of which are aligned parallel to the skin surface, in contrast to adjunctive dilated venules that are oriented perpendicular to the skin surface. A keloid when fully formed, unlike a scar, is made up of markedly thickened bundles of collagen arranged in haphazard fashion. Fibrocytes are aligned along the course of thickened bundles of collagen, and the path of blood vessels parallels that of the bundles of collagen.

By contrast, anetodermas are not truly fibrosing processes, but atrophies that result from loss of collagen and elastic tissue in the midreticular dermis. In every instance, an inflammatory or neoplastic process preceded formation of anetoderma and was responsible for causing destruction of connective tissue elements. Collagen bundles in the midreticular dermis of anetoderma are thinned and widely separated from one another, and elastic fibers are absent. Striae atrophicantes are a specific type of atrophoderma in which loss of collagen and elastic tissue occurs mostly in the upper half of the dermis.

In sum, scars and keloids are fibrosing inflammatory processes, whereas anetodermas represent the atrophic end stage of particular inflammatory or neoplastic processes that resulted in some loss of collagen bundles and total loss of elastic fibers. Striae also are an inflammatory process that ends in atrophy consequent to loss of collagen and elastic tissue.

THERAPY For hypertrophic scars and keloids, intralesional injection of corticosteroids is the mainstay of treatment, but continuous pressure is an important complement to it. Other modalities include cryotherapy, interferon, radiation, laser surgery, and silicone gel dressings.

DEFINITION A generic term for at least two different inflammatory diseases that have in common hardening of the skin by virtue of thickening of bundles of collagen in the dermis and subcutis. One of those diseases manifests itself as localized or widespread patches and plaques (morphea) and by localized linear lesions (linear scleroderma), whereas the other expresses itself diffusely on acral parts of the skin especially, and in internal organs (acrosclerosis, systemic sclerosis).

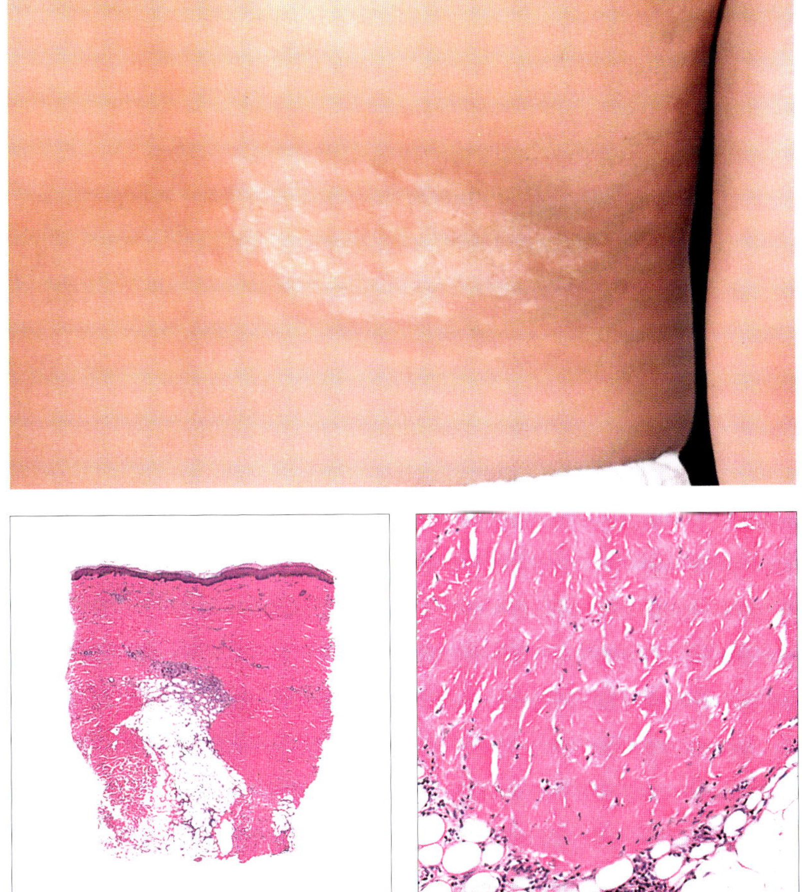

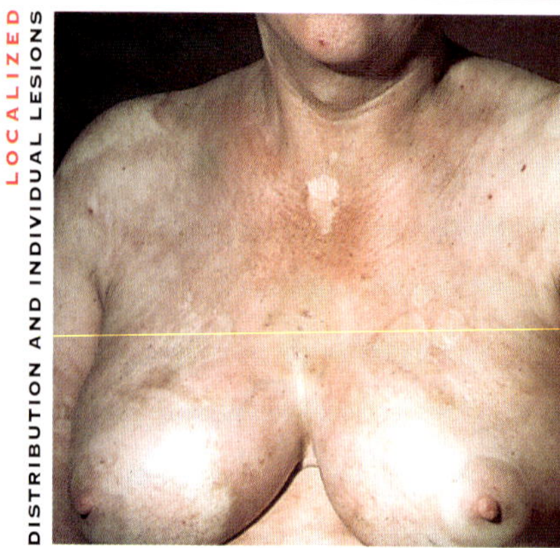

FIG. 84-1 *Widespread morphea manifested as white patches surrounded by a rim of erythema.*

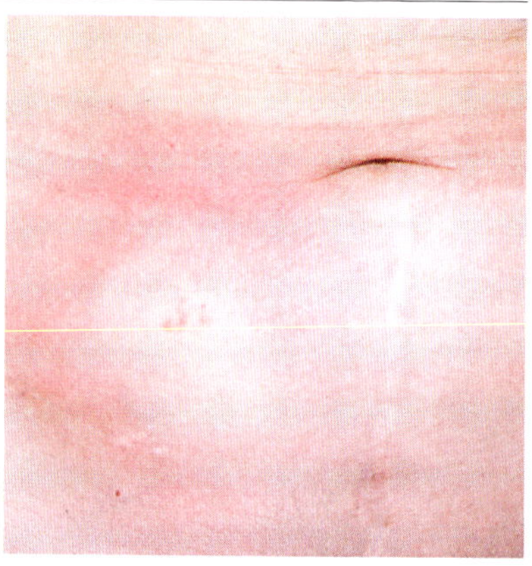

FIG. 84-2 *Lesion of morphea in which a white zone is associated with a diffuse rim of erythema.*

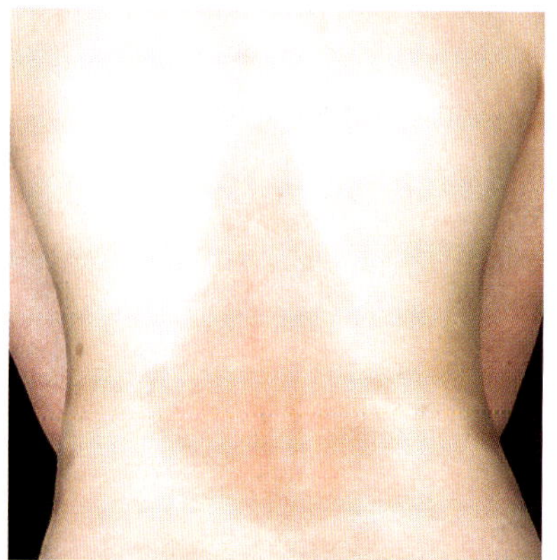

FIG. 84-3 *Atrophic pigmented patch of morphea.*

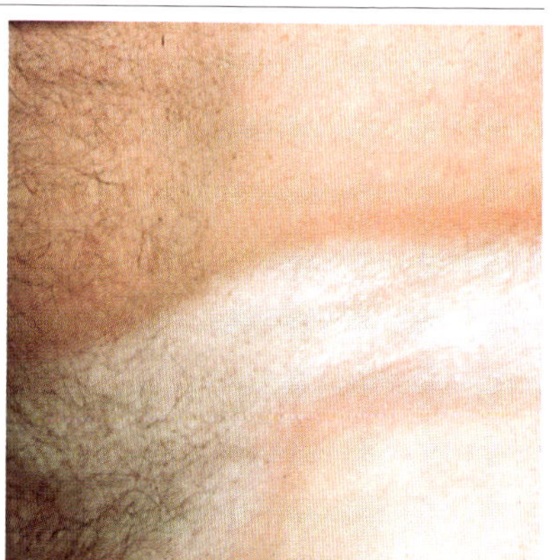

FIG. 84-4 *Atrophic hypopigmented patch with hyperpigmented border of morphea.*

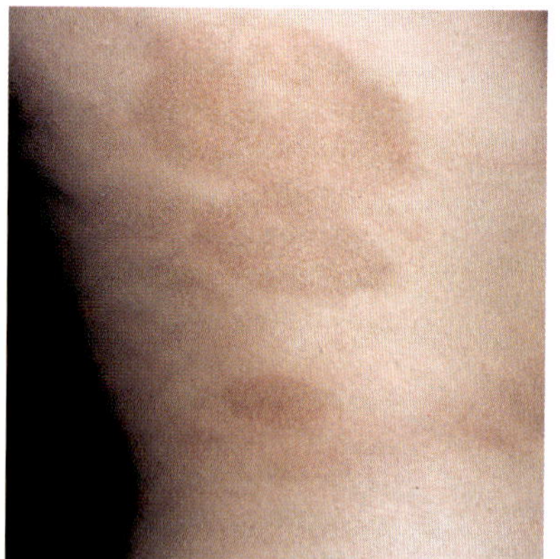

FIG. 84-5 *Hyperpigmented, slightly depressed patches of late lesions of morphea (idiopathic atrophoderma of Pasini and Pierini).*

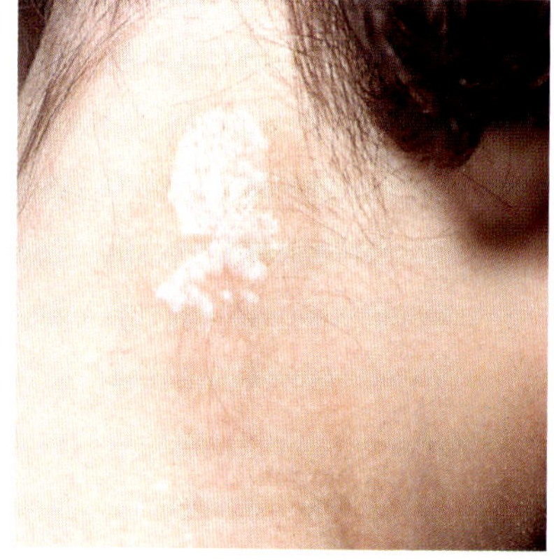

FIG. 84-6 *White papules have become confluent to produce a plaque of lichen sclerosus et atrophicus.*

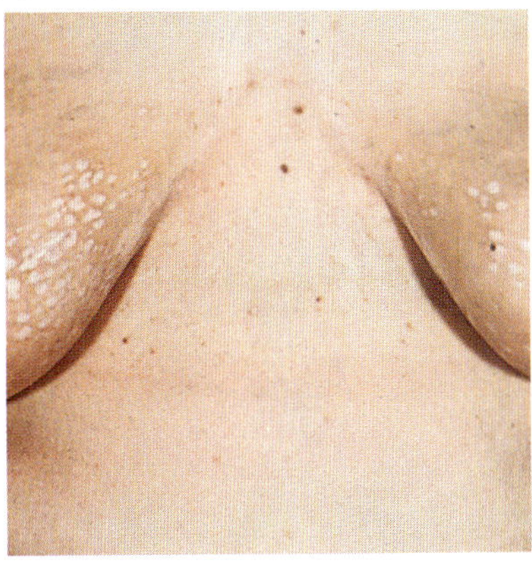

FIG. 84-7 *Hypopigmented papules and atrophic macules and papules of lichen sclerosus et atrophicus.*

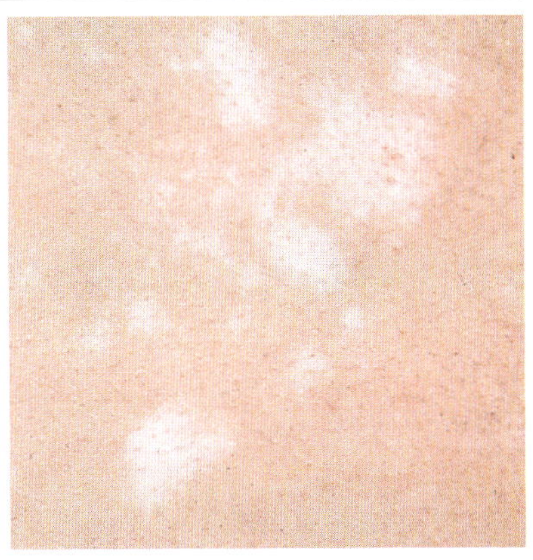

FIG. 84-8 *Hypopigmented atrophic macules, some of which have become confluent, of lichen sclerosus et atrophicus.*

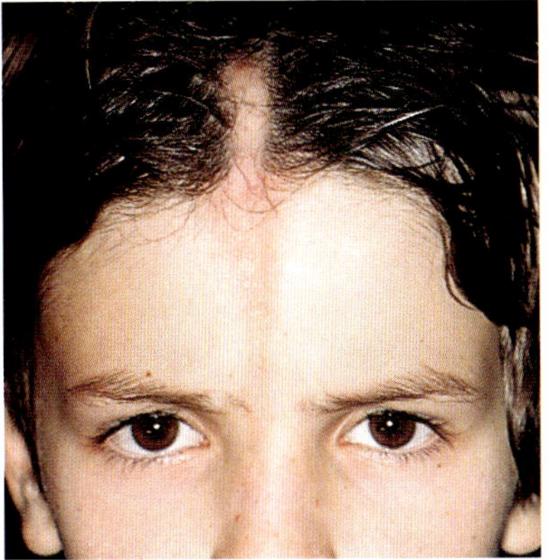

FIG. 84-9 *Linear lesion of scleroderma that extends from the midfrontal part of the scalp to the nose (en coup de sabre).*

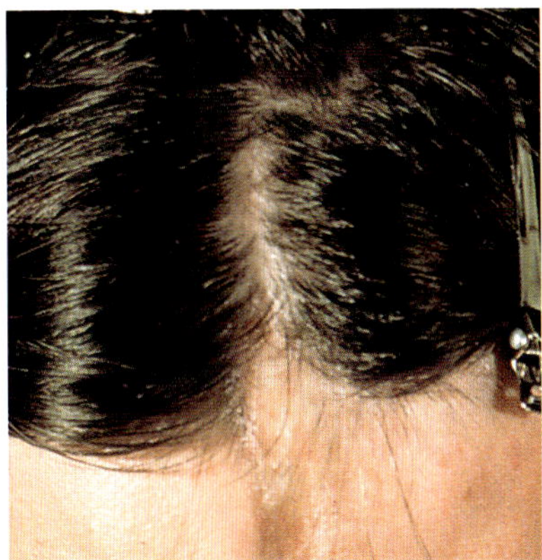

FIG. 84-10 *Linear lesion of scleroderma markedly depressed because of extensive loss of subcutaneous fat.*

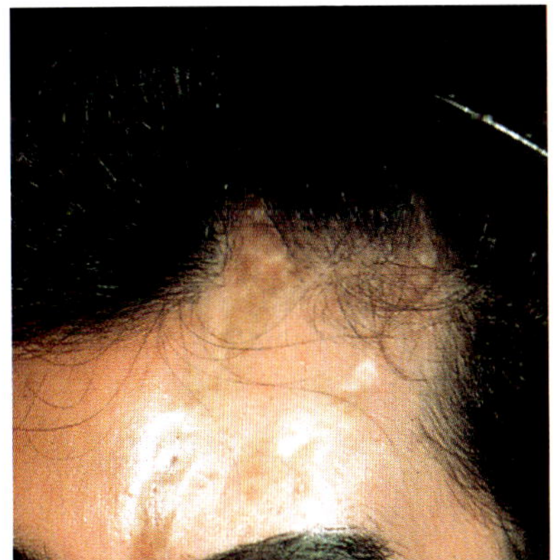

FIG. 84-11 *Linear lesion of scleroderma that has resulted in partial alopecia.*

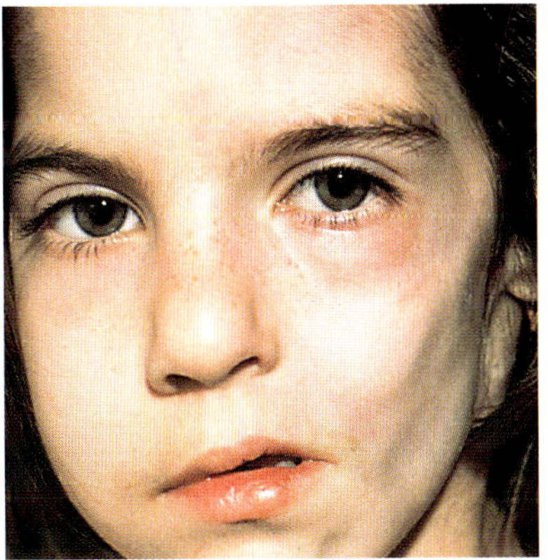

FIG. 84-12 *Involvement of one side of the face by linear scleroderma (hemiatrophy) is distorting physically and emotionally.*

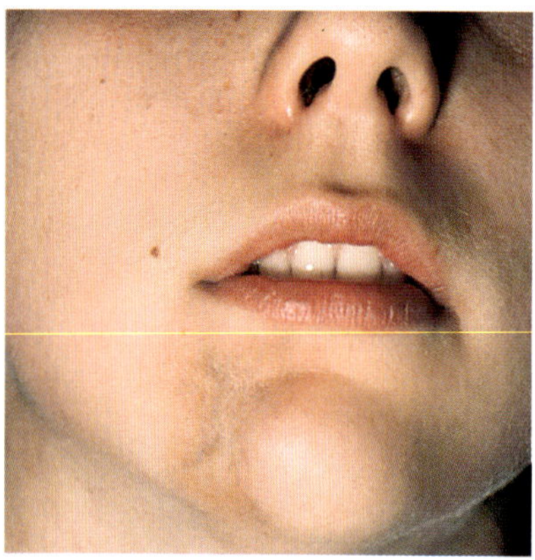

FIG. 84-13 *Deep depression of linear sclero-derma in a band on a chin. Sometimes fascia and skeletal muscle are affected.*

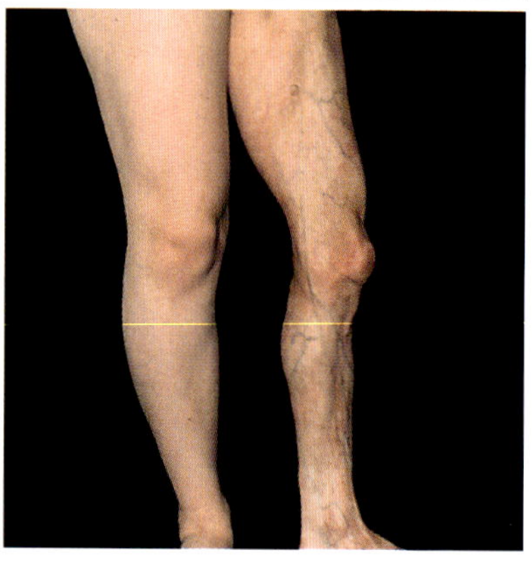

FIG. 84-14 *Markedly shrunken extremity with deep depression in a band of linear scleroderma.*

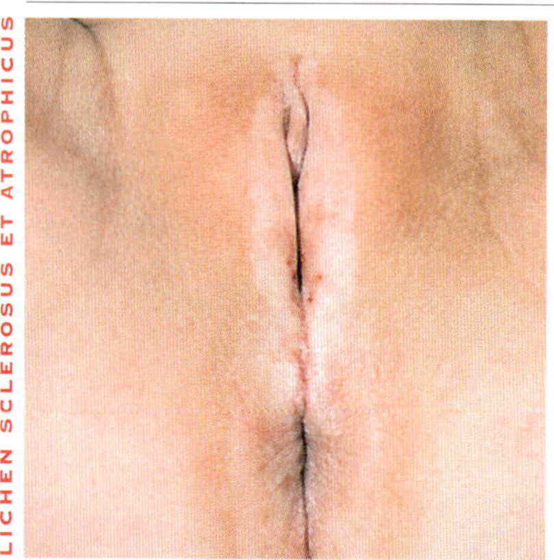

FIG. 84-15 *Atrophic hypopigmented eroded lesions.*

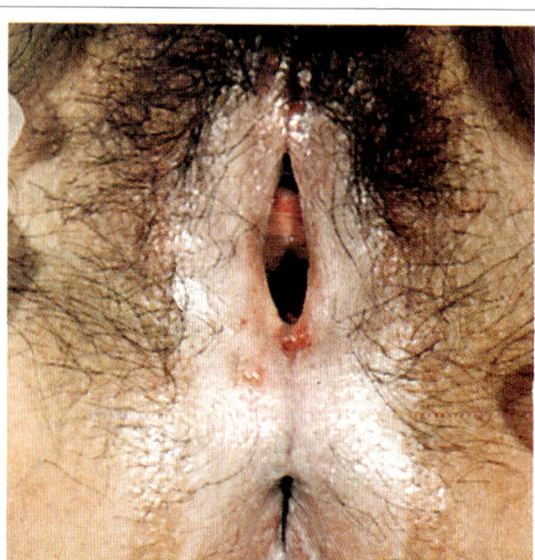

FIG. 84-16 *Hypopigmented papules and plaques.*

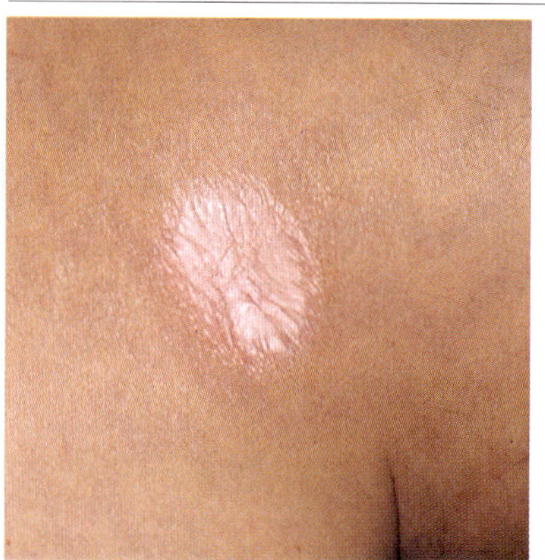

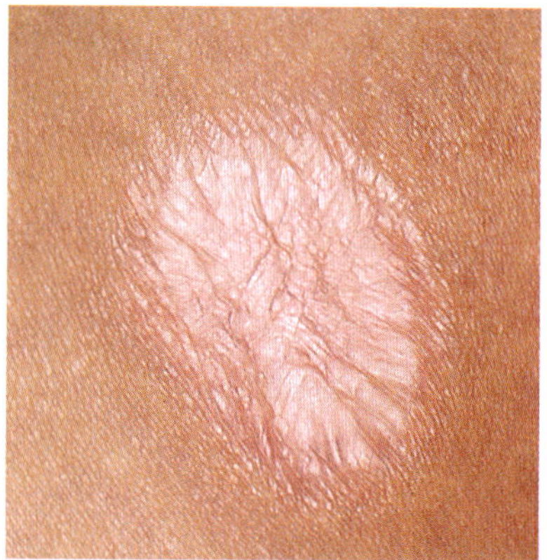

FIG. 84-17 (A, B) *Hypopigmented plaque made up of numerous papules.*

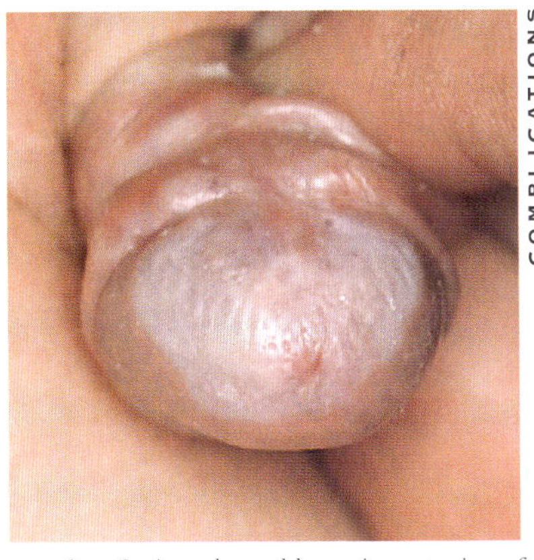

FIG. 84-18 *Atrophy and hypopigmentation of the glans and foreskin (balanitis xerotica obliterans).*

FIG. 84-19 *Phimosis secondary to the effects of lichen sclerosus et atrophicus.*

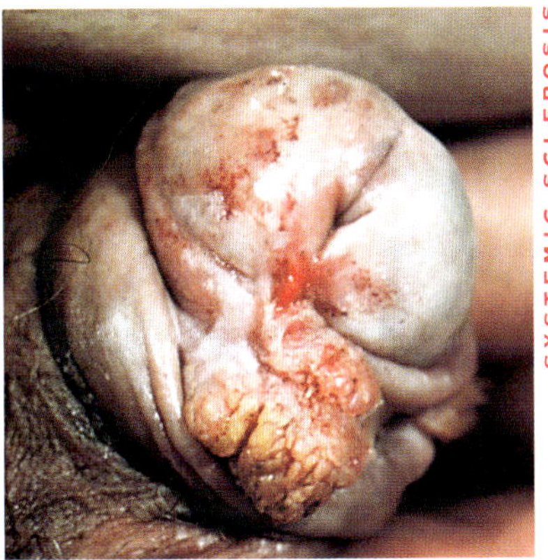

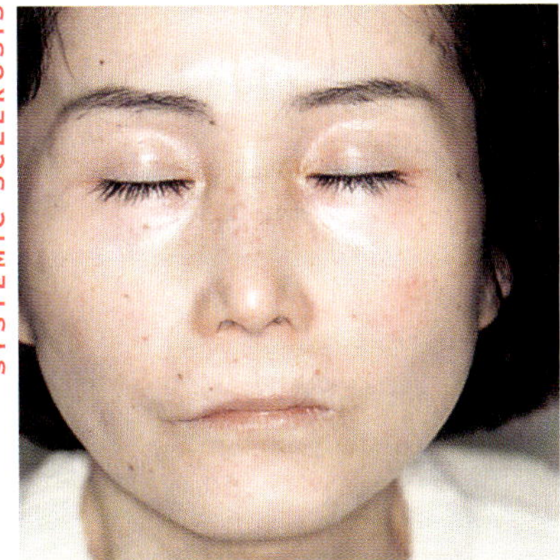

FIG. 84-20 *Squamous-cell carcinoma that developed in a longstanding lesion of lichen sclerosus et atrophicus.*

FIG. 84-21 *A taut, shiny face with pursed lips and numerous telangiectases of acrosclerosis.*

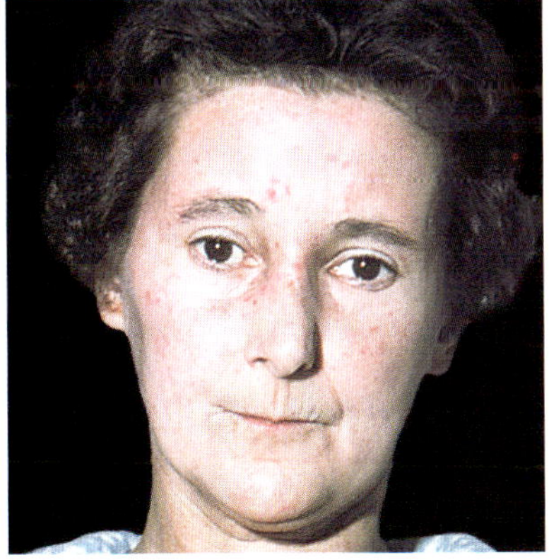

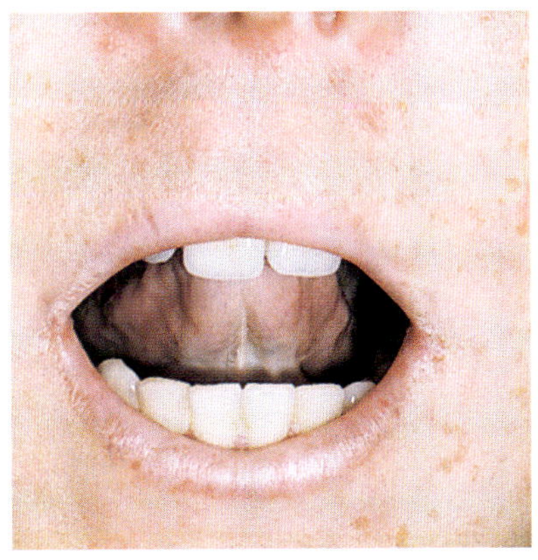

FIG. 84-22 *Pursed lips secondary to tight skin of acrosclerosis.*

FIG. 84-23 *Severe limitation of movement of the mouth due to tight skin of acrosclerosis; the frenulum is shortened.*

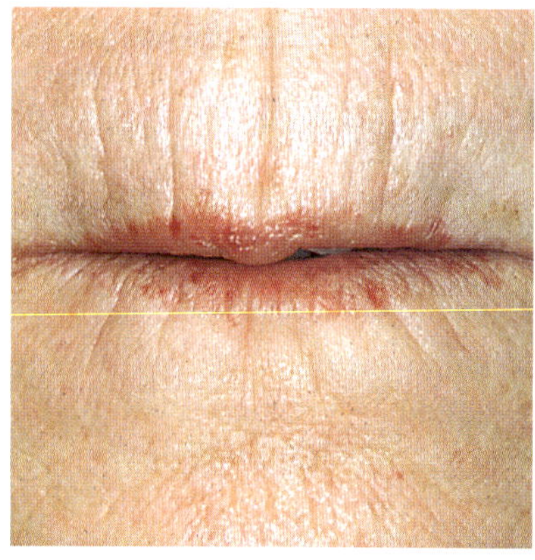

FIG. 84-24 *Pinched mouth associated with pursed lips and matted telangiectases of acrosclerosis.*

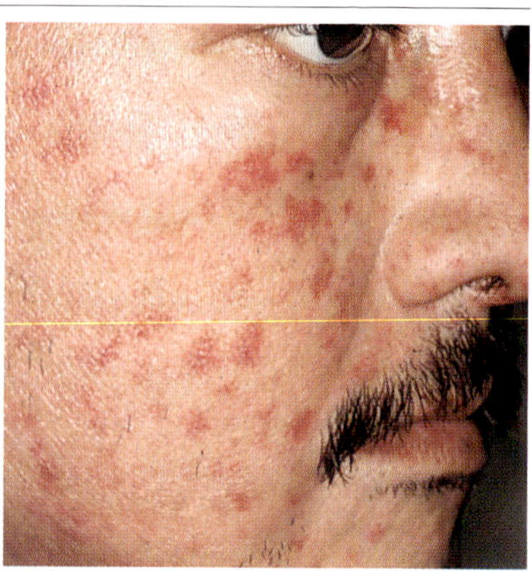

FIG. 84-25 *Mats of telangiectases.*

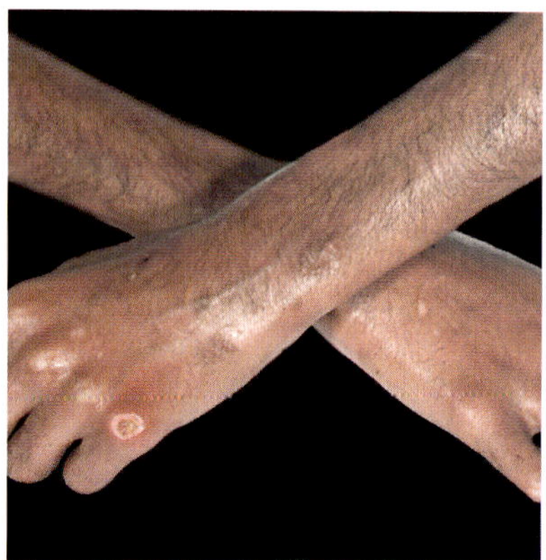

FIG. 84-26 *Tight skin of arms and fingers of acrosclerosis has resulted in flexion contractures and in ulcerations of knuckles.*

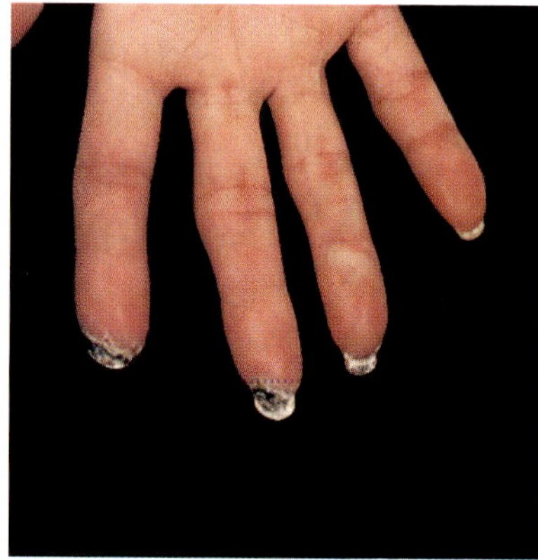

FIG. 84-27 *Patchy redness of fingers, and ulcers covered by eschars at the tips of digits in acrosclerosis.*

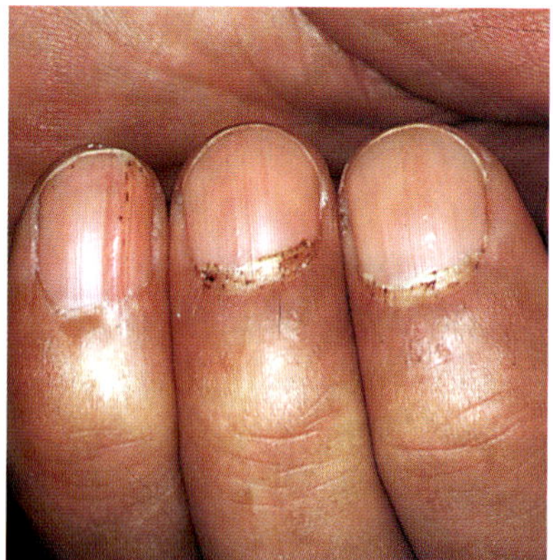

FIG. 84-28 *Petechiae in the cuticle, posterior nail folds, and beneath a nail plate.*

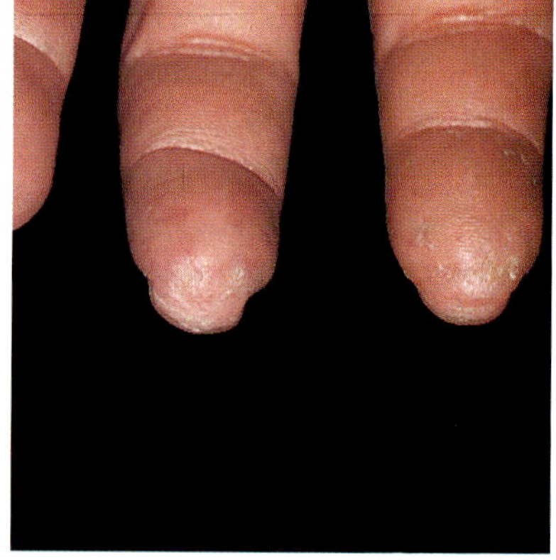

FIG. 84-29 *Depressed scars secondary to infarction, and subsequent necrosis of epithelium and degeneration of collagen.*

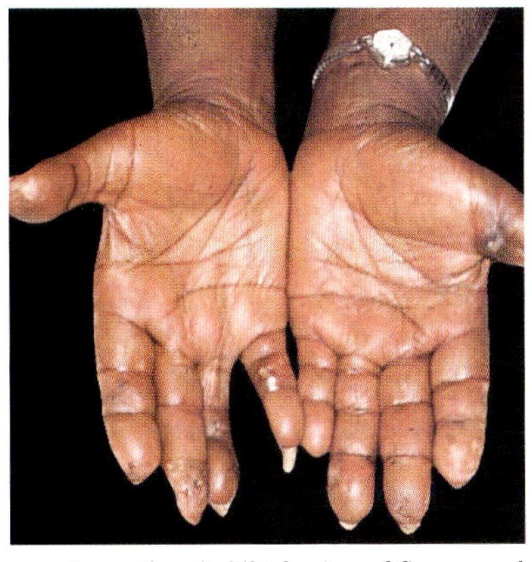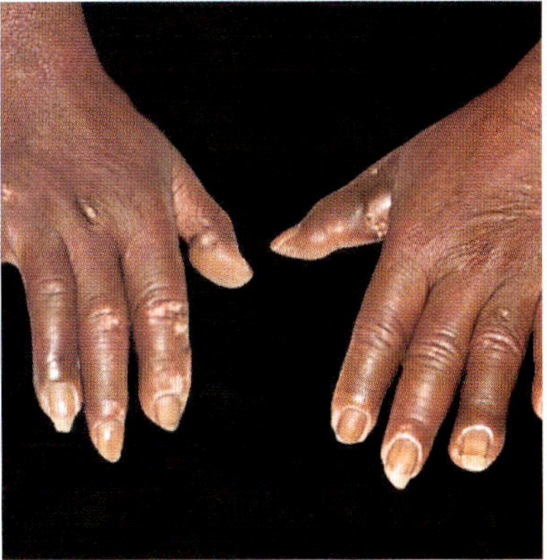

FIG. 84-30 (A, B) *Thickening of fingers and palms, ulcers, depressed scars, and hypopigmentation and hyperpigmentation in acrosclerosis.*

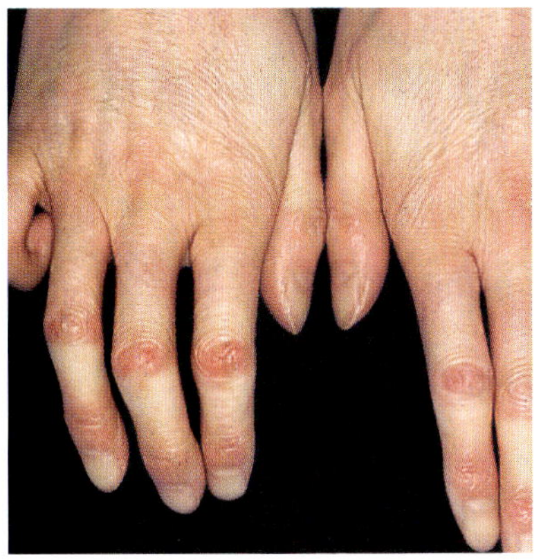

FIG. 84-31 *Raynaud's phenomenon and sclerodactylia.*

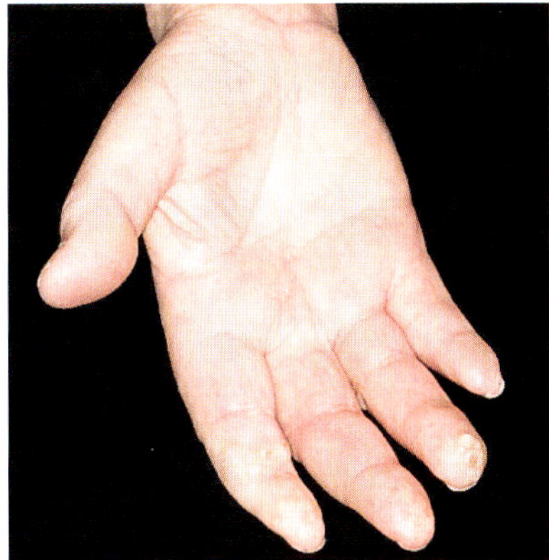

FIG. 84-32 *Deposits of calcium at tips of fingers (CREST syndrome).*

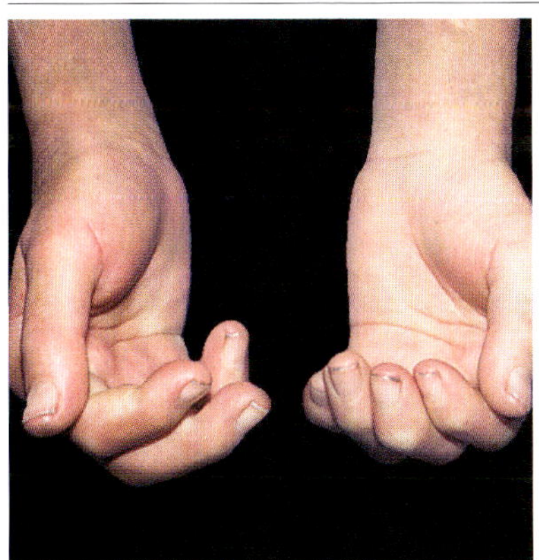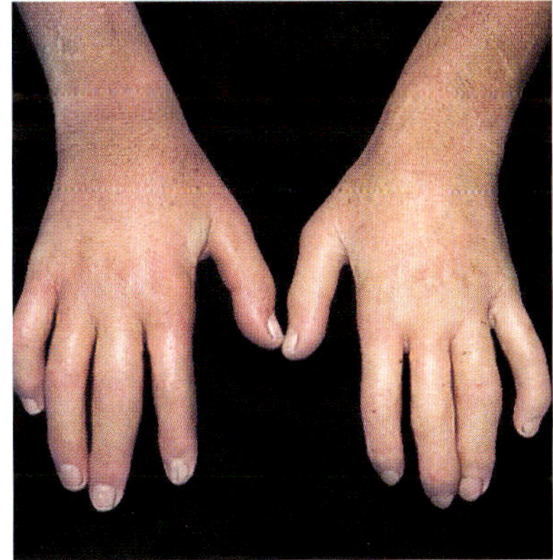

FIG. 84-33 (A, B) *Raynaud's phenomenon and sclerodactylia.*

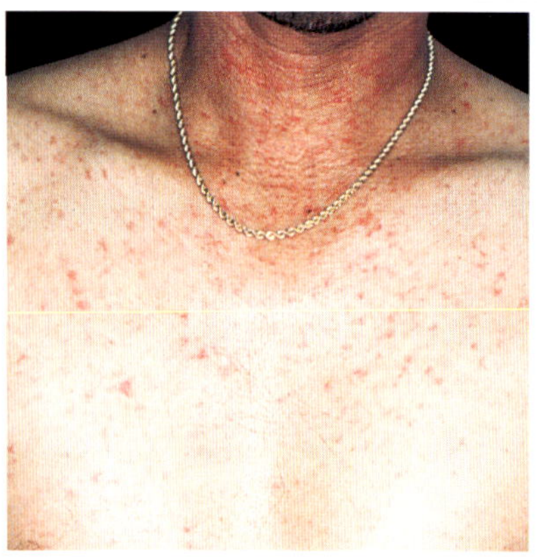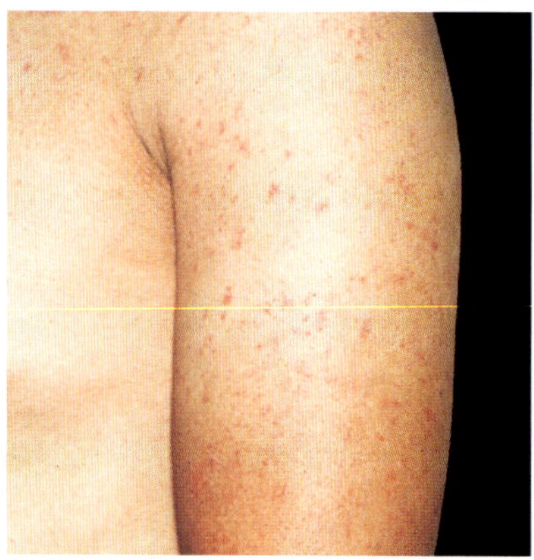

FIG. 84-34 (A, B) *Widespread matted telangiectases.*

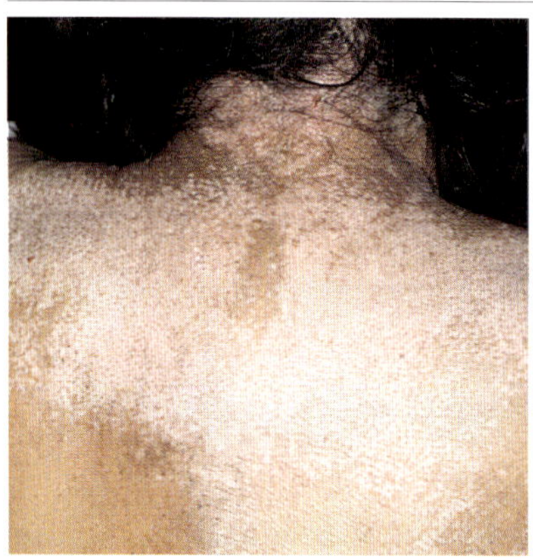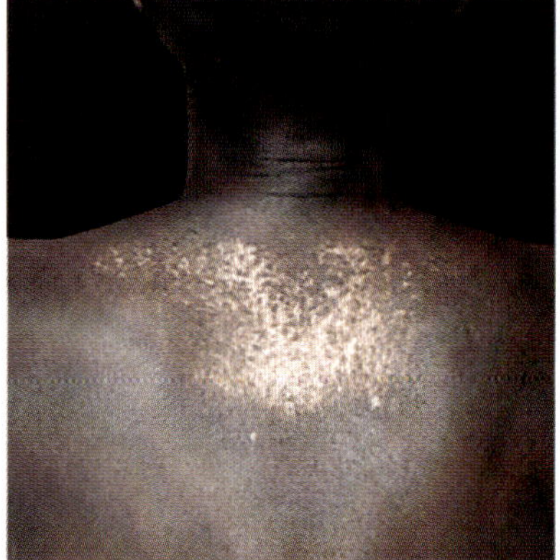

FIG. 84-35 *Macular hypopigmentation in a "salt and pepper" pattern as a consequence of the inflammatory process.*

FIG. 84-36 *"Salt and pepper" pattern on the chest, shoulders, and neck.*

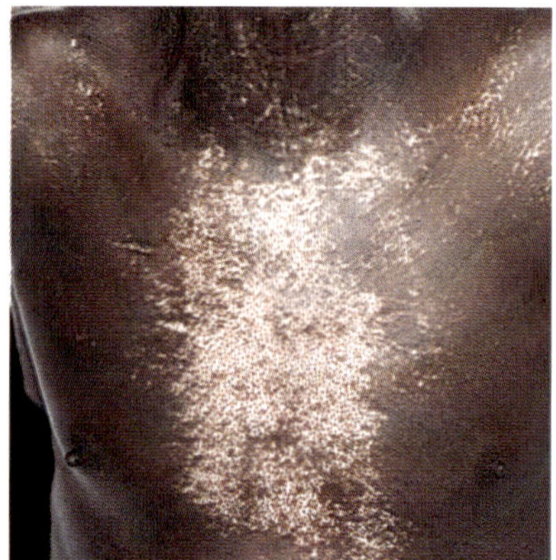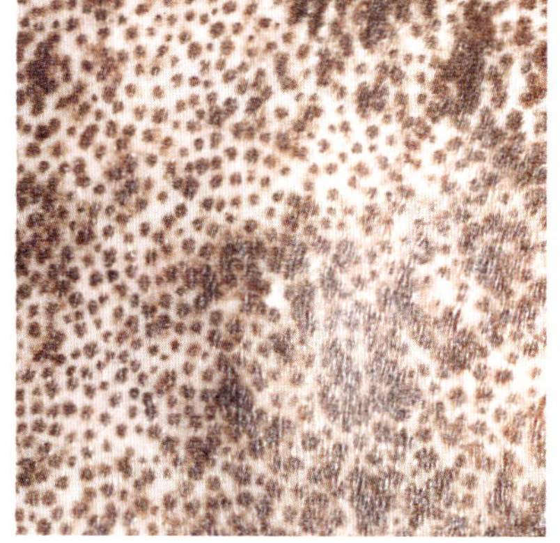

FIG. 84-37 (A, B) *"Salt and pepper pattern" as a consequence of hypopigmentation secondary to the inflammatory process.*

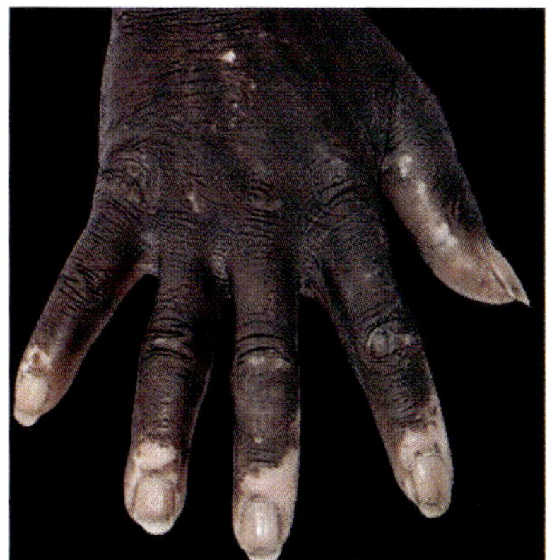

FIG. 84-38 *Depigmented macules and patches in acrosclerosis.*

ADJUNCTIVE DIAGNOSTIC TESTS It is important to assess involvement of internal organs in systemic sclerosis. Demonstration immunopathologically of antinuclear antibodies, including antinucleolar and anticentromere antibodies and of topoisomerase I-antibodies (Scl 70), is confirmatory.

COURSE Localized scleroderma that presents itself as reddish patches of morphea or linear scleroderma progresses, over the course of months, to yellowish plaques rimmed by a patch of violaceous erythema, and, in the course of years, to depressed hyperpigmented patches that are unassociated with erythema. Lichen sclerosus et atrophicus is one of several morphologic expressions of morphea, and it may resolve with atrophic patches or disappear completely without treatment and without residua.

In acrosclerosis, the initial diffuse redness and swelling progress to white or yellow sclerosis associated with marked tightening of skin and, over a period of years, the appearance of numerous telangiectases and ulceration of acral skin that may end with loss of digits.

INTEGRATION: UNIFYING CONCEPT The term "scleroderma" is applied, indiscriminately, to wholly unrelated diseases, to wit, localized scleroderma, i.e., morphea and linear scleroderma, in one case and acrosclerosis, an expression of systemic sclerosis, in another. The situation is analogous to "keratoacanthoma," a term that is applied equally to very disparate neoplasms such as those designated solitary keratoacanthoma, subungual keratoacanthoma, and the familial keratoacanthoma of Ferguson and Smith.

Localized scleroderma is a disease that involves skin and sometimes entire subcutis. The process is an inflammatory one as can be told by biopsy of reddish patches, tissue sections from specimens of which show superficial and deep perivascular and interstitial mixed-cell infiltrates of lymphocytes, plasma cells, and eosinophils around blood vessels. They also show eosinophils, and sometimes neutrophils, within the interstitium of the reticular dermis. Those inflammatory cells also are present within widened septa in the subcutaneous fat. At that stage of the process, there is no detectable alteration in bundles of collagen. At a later stage, localized scleroderma is characterized by superficial and deep perivascular lymphoplasmacytic infiltrates that also are seen as nodules in contiguity with thickened fibrous septa in the subcutaneous fat. Collagen bundles are thickened markedly and are arranged parallel to one another and to the skin surface in the reticular dermis, and parallel to one another and along the long axis of altered septa in the subcutaneous fat.

Late lesions of localized scleroderma are not associated with inflammatory cells, but consist only of markedly thickened bundles of collagen that are crowded and arranged parallel to one another both within the reticular dermis and in the markedly thickened trabeculae of the subcutaneous fat. The idiopathic atrophoderma of Pasini and Pierini represents a "burned out" stage of morphea in which hyperpigmented patches, depressed beneath the skin surface, are made up of thin bundles of collagen that are separated distinctly from one another in the reticular dermis and in fibrous trabeculae of the subcutaneous fat.

Lichen sclerosus et atrophicus is that variant of morphea typified early by violaceous patches and late by white atrophic ones. Early lesions are formed by patchy lichenoid infiltrates of lymphocytes in the upper part of the dermis in company with marked edema there. Late lesions are devoid of infiltrates of inflammatory cells and show sclerosis of a decidedly thickened papillary dermis. Below the sclerosis, collagen bundles in the upper part of the reticular dermis are thickened and crowded in a manner typical of morphea, and above the sclerosis the epidermis is thinned and devoid of rete ridges.

Borrelia burgdorferi has been demonstrated to be the cause of many examples of morphea, especially in Europe. Changes clinically similar and histopathologically identical to those of localized scleroderma are found in circumstances as diverse as in porphyria cutanea tarda, tryptophane-myalgia syndrome, and fasciitis with eosinophilia (Shulman's syndrome).

Acrosclerosis is an inflammatory process that resolves histopathologically in a manner indistinguishable from that of localized scleroderma, to wit, markedly thickened crowded bundles of collagen throughout the reticular dermis and in septa of the subcutaneous fat. Infiltrates of inflammatory cells, in particular, lymphocytes and plasma cells, are known to appear in the dermis and in septa of evolving lesions of acrosclerosis, but the earliest changes seen in that condition have yet to be detailed. On the basis of limited studies, the early histopathologic changes of acrosclerosis seem to be different from those of localized scleroderma.

In sum, it is preferable to write and speak of localized scleroderma and of acrosclerosis, rather than to refer indiscriminately to "scleroderma." In this way it becomes clear that the "sclerodermas" are really different diseases.

THERAPY Topical potent corticosteroids or short-term oral corticosteroids may be effective for morphea in the inflammatory stage of the disease. PUVA-bath photochemotherapy may also be helpful. Oral antibiotics, in particular cephalosporins, are worthwhile in some patients with morphea, presumably by eradicating borrelia that have been implicated as the cause. Local treatment includes administration of emollients and topical corticosteroids, and physical therapy.

Oral corticosteroids, immunosuppressive agents, or PUVA are recommended for systemic sclerosis. D-penicillamine, gamma interferon, or extracorporeal photopheresis is advised for systemic disease that is steadily progressive.

For Raynaud's phenomenon, pentoxyfylline, a calcium channel blocker (nifedipine), and prostacyclines are sometimes beneficial.

Lichen sclerosus et atrophicus may be managed effectively in the inflammatory stage of the process by application of a glucocorticoid or by intralesional injection of corticosteroid. An uncircumsized man with balanitis xerotica obliterans may be aided by circumcision.

DEFINITION An enlargement of normal pre-existing sebaceous lobules on the face, the forehead, cheeks, and nose in particular that results in lesions seen clinically to consist of a rim of yellow papules around a central dell that represents a dilated ostium of a follicle.

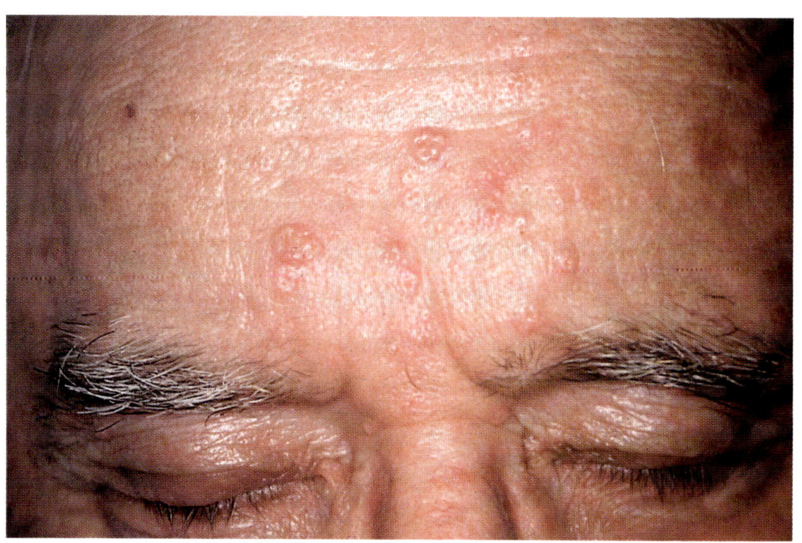

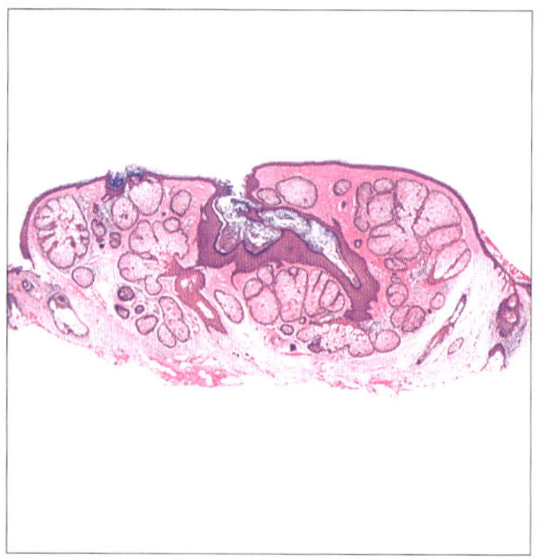

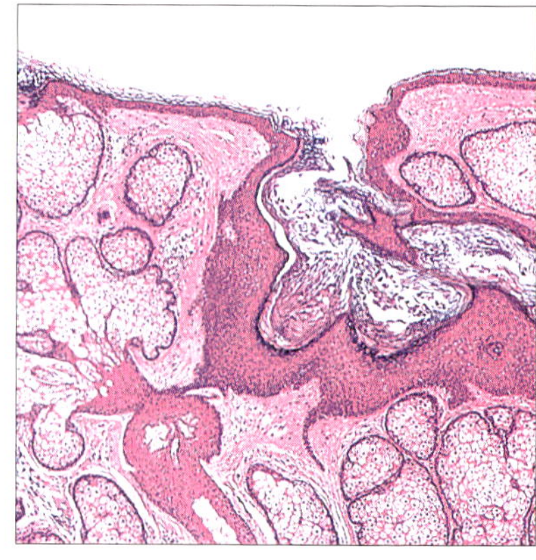

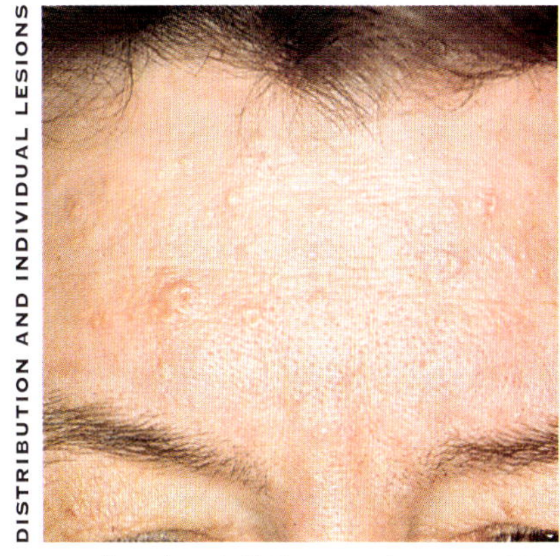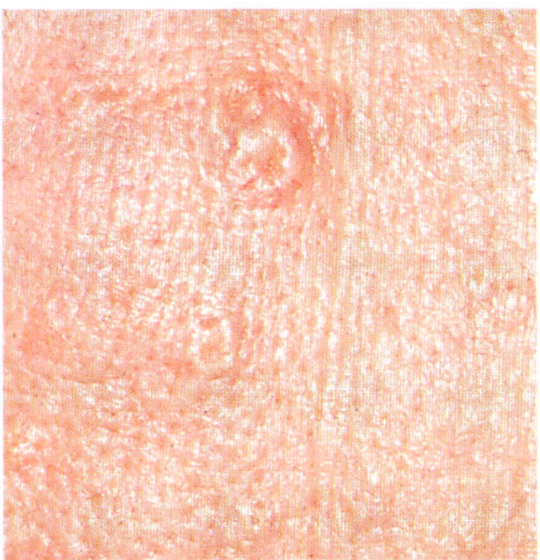

FIG. 85-1 (A, B) *Yellow papules, some of them in a cluster.*

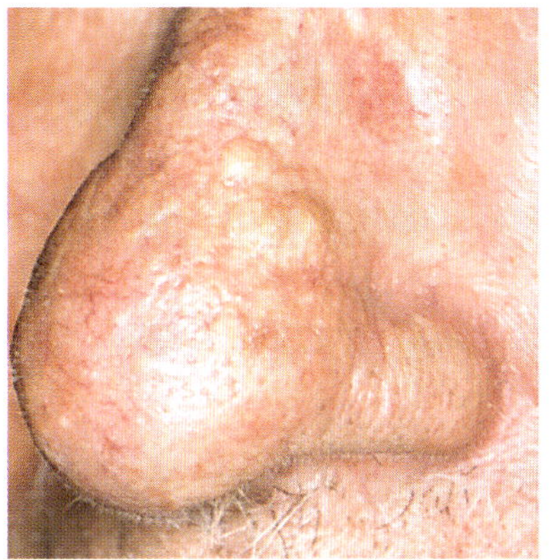

FIG. 85-2 *Yellow papules in a patient with rosacea as evidenced by the bulbous tip of the nose and telangiectases.*

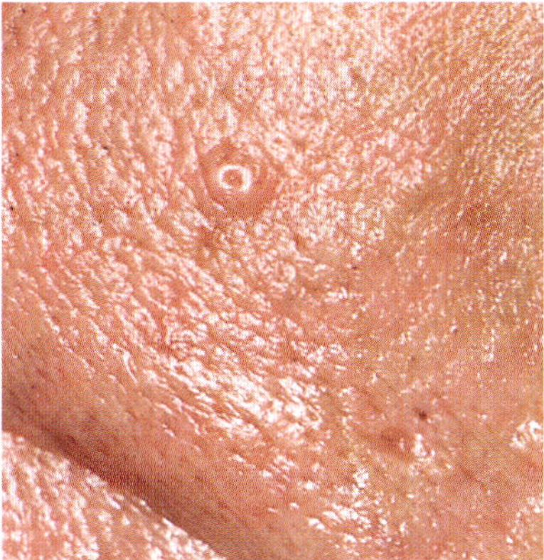

FIG. 85-3 *Doughnut-shaped ever so slightly yellowish papule.*

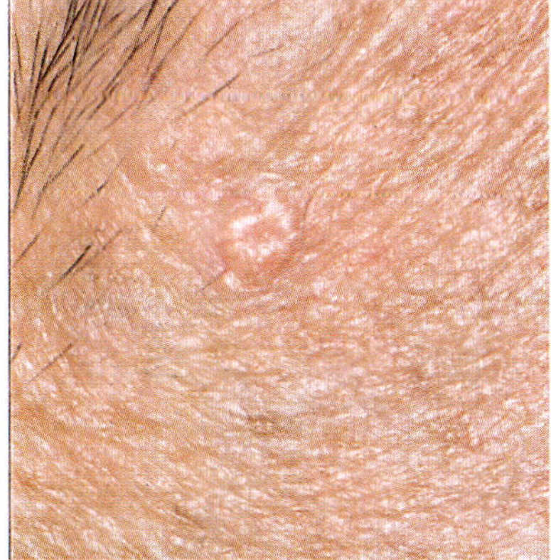

FIG. 85-4 *Yellow papule with central depression.*

COURSE The tiny yellow papules of sebaceous gland hyperplasia at first display a subtle central dell. In time, those ring-shaped papules come to resemble doughnuts with the dell in the center becoming increasingly prominent. Lesions of sebaceous gland hyperplasia tend to persist and to enlarge slowly over time, but some of them actually involute in the absence of treatment. New lesions may appear as some older ones disappear.

INTEGRATION: UNIFYING CONCEPT Sebaceous gland hyperplasia is a true hyperplasia because some of its lesions involute. The yellowish rim of a lesion is made up of large lipid-containing cells of enlarged sebaceous lobules. The central dell is formed by marked dilation of the ostium of a single infundibulum or of several contiguous dilated infundibula.

Sebaceous gland hyperplasia results from the effects of androgens on sebocytes in sebaceous lobules. As the lobules increase in size, a papule forms. Without the flow of androgens to sebocytes by way of blood vessels, hyperplasia of sebocytes could not occur. For this reason, sebaceous gland hyperplasia is much more common in men than women.

In sum, sebaceous gland hyperplasia is a true hyperplasia induced by the effects of androgens, and is very different from a benign neoplasm of sebocytes, i.e., the true adenoma, sebaceoma.

THERAPY Excision, curettage, cryotherapy, and laser surgery are all effective modes of treatment.

DEFINITION An inflammatory process that consists of tiny papules covered by prominent scales and localized typically to the "seborrheic region," namely, scalp, forehead, eyebrows, malar eminences, paranasal and nasolabial folds, and retroauricular zone, and sometimes the chest and axillary vault.

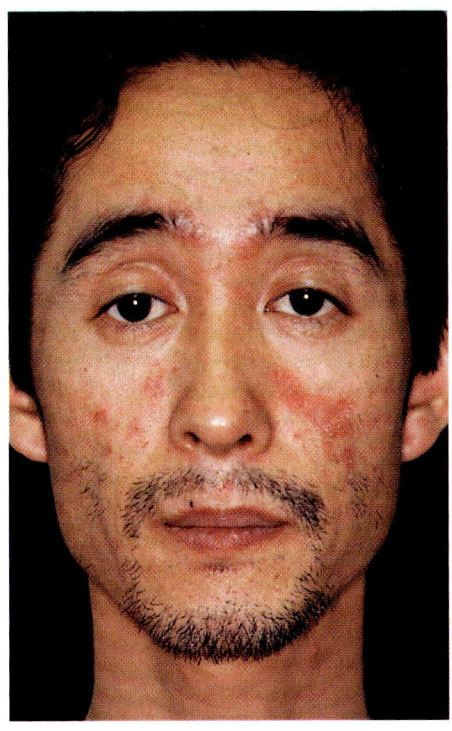

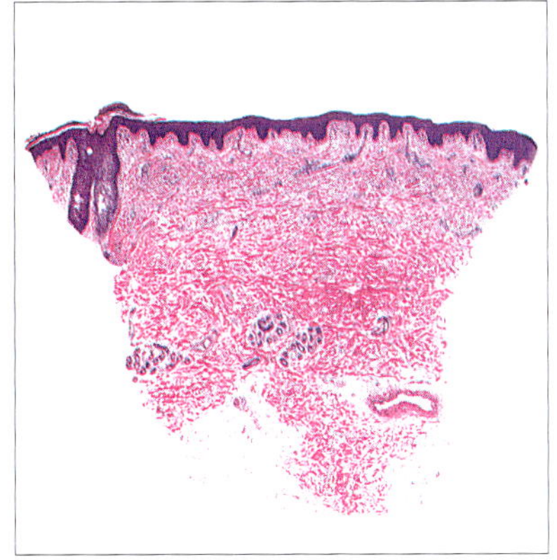

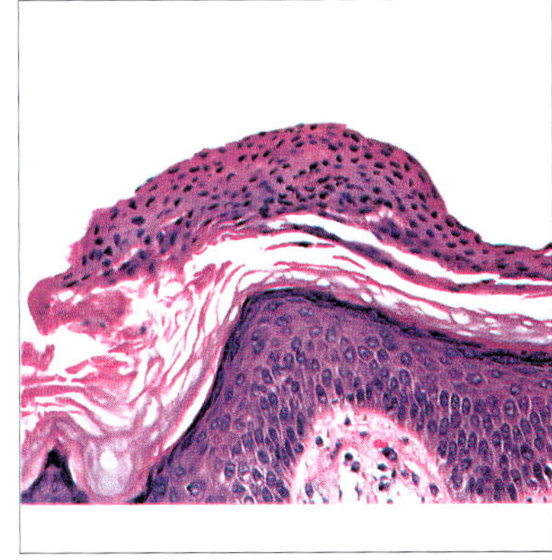

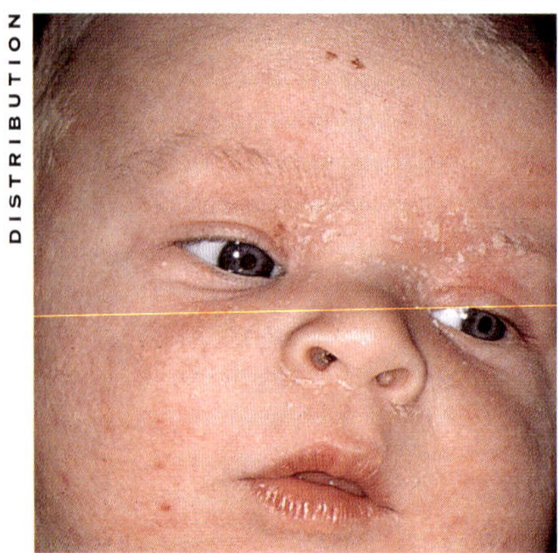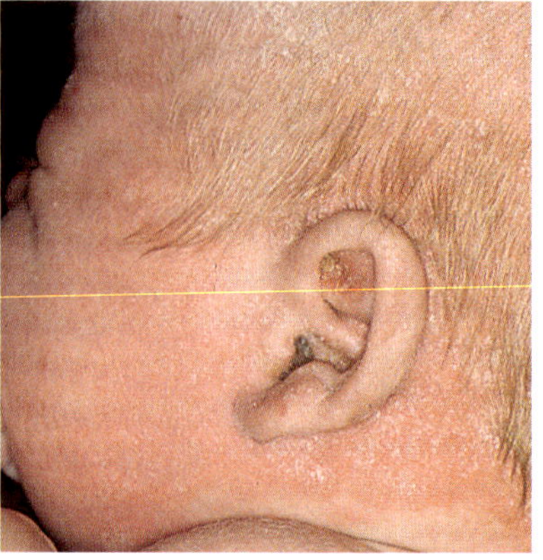

FIG. 86-1 (A, B) *Scaly papules and plaques in characteristic distribution.*

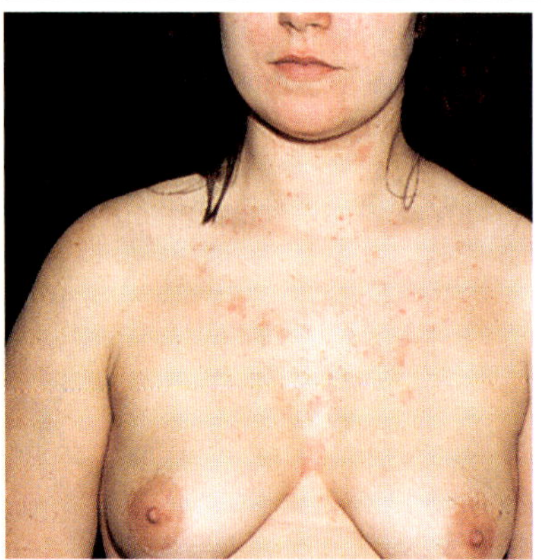

FIG. 86-2 *Widespread papules and plaques in the central third of the face, neck, and chest.*

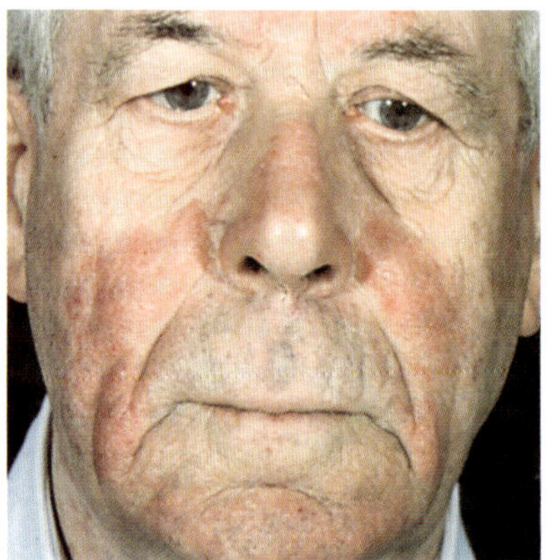

FIG. 86-3 *Scaly, ill-defined plaques on the bridge of the nose, malar region, paranasal region, and chin.*

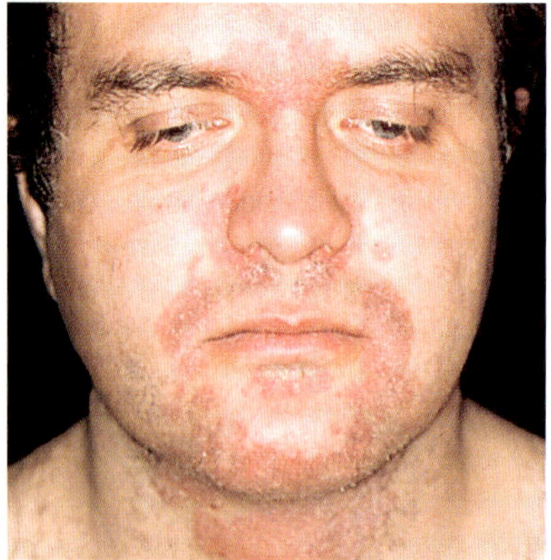

FIG. 86-4 *Scaly red papules and plaques on the face and neck.*

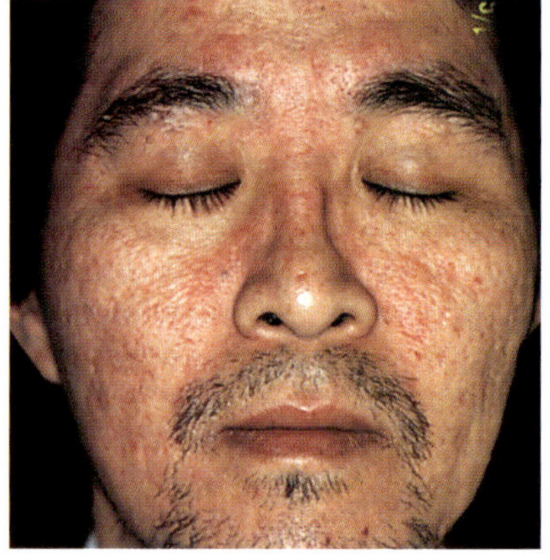

FIG. 86-5 *Blotchy papules and plaques on the forehead, nose, malar regions, cheeks, and chin.*

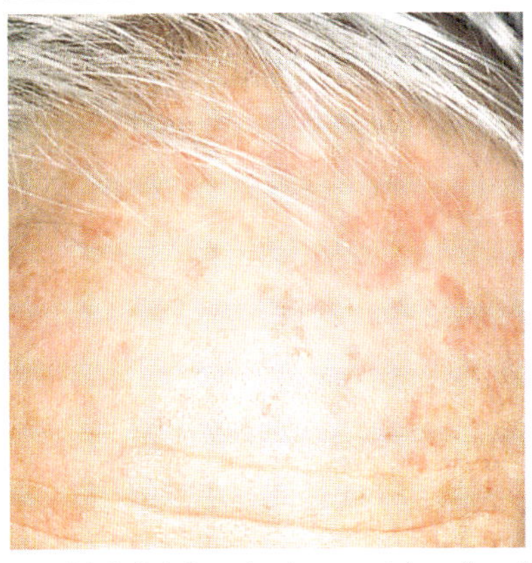

FIG. 86-6 *Subtle scaly plaques with scalloped borders on a scalp and forehead. The numerous tan macules are solar lentigines.*

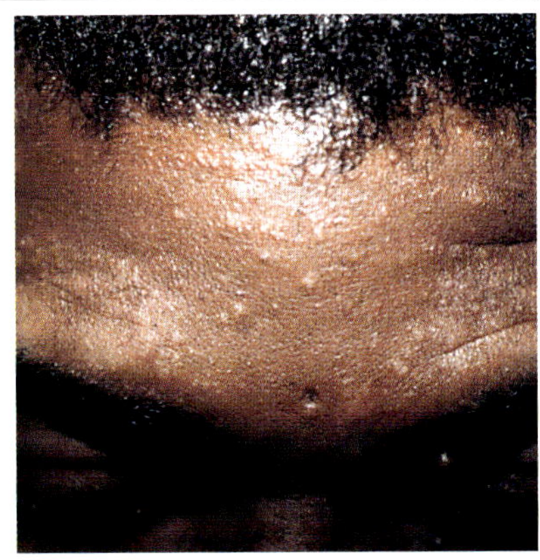

FIG. 86-7 *Hypopigmented scaly papules and patches.*

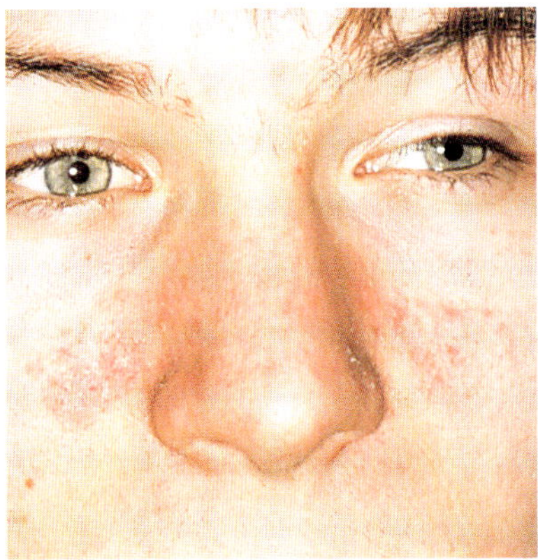

FIG. 86-8 *Scaly papules and plaques on the malar region especially.*

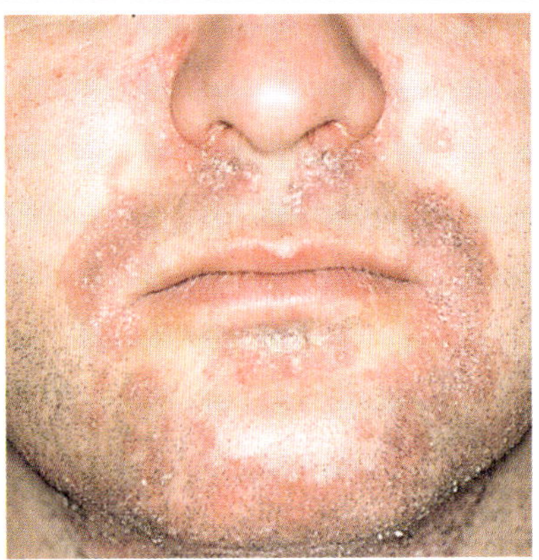

FIG. 86-9 *Scaly macules and plaques, some of them nummular and others with scalloped outlines.*

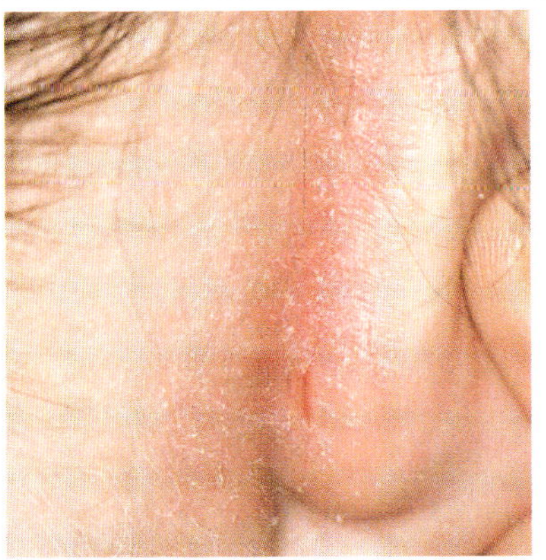

FIG. 86-10 *Scaly patch and fissure.*

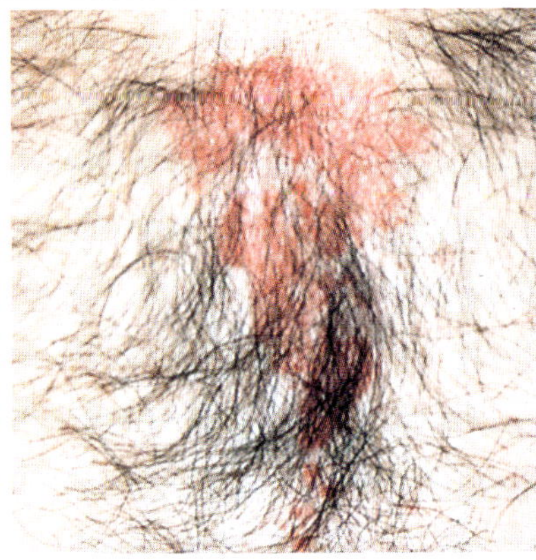

FIG. 86-11 *Scaly patches in the hairy area of the chest have scalloped outlines.*

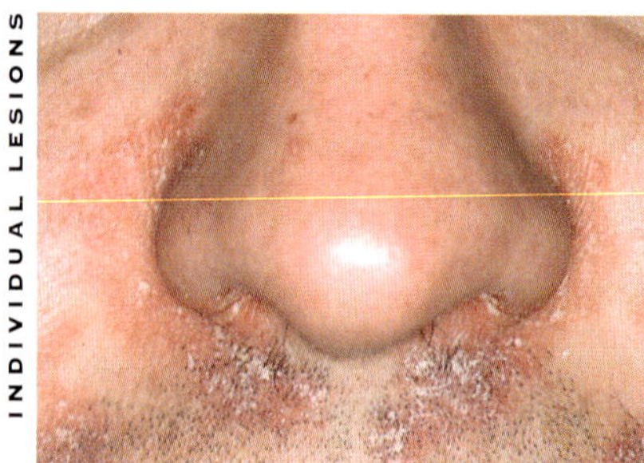

FIG. 86-12 *Scaly papules and plaques.*

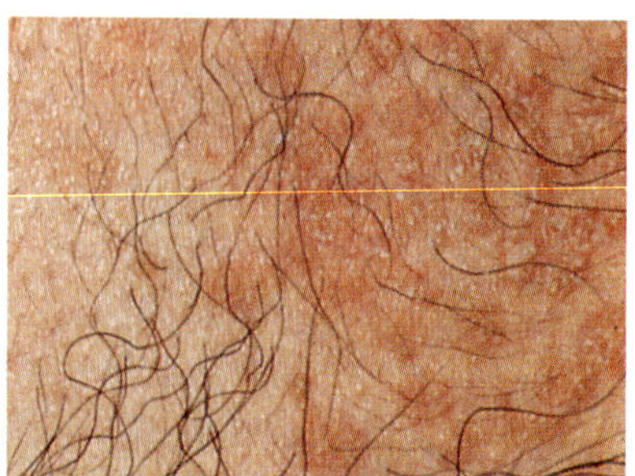

FIG. 86-13 *Scaly patches and subtle plaques, some of which have ill-defined margins.*

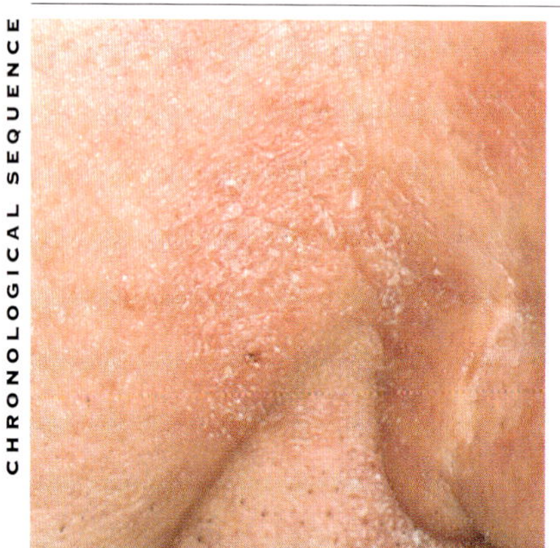

FIG. 86-14 *Pink macules and papules, some of which are covered by delicate scales, in a cluster.*

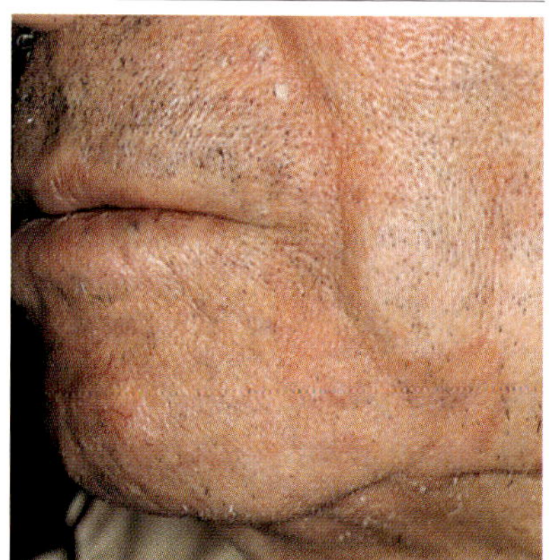

FIG. 86-15 *Scaly papules and plaques.*

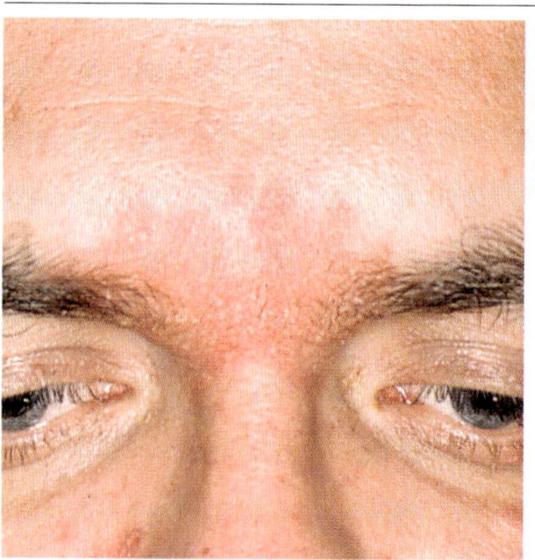

FIG. 86-16 *Scaly plaques.*

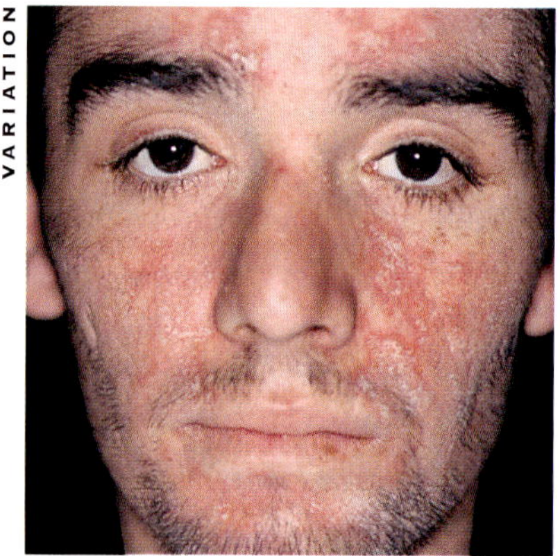

FIG. 86-17 *Extensive seborrheic dermatitis in a patient infected by HIV.*

COURSE Seborrheic dermatitis begins as reddish macules that are covered by subtle scale-crusts. In time, slightly elevated papules come into being and they may be associated with scale-crusts that vary in amount from hardly noticeable to striking. Once lesions of seborrheic dermatitis arise, the tendency is for them to wax and wane, but to persist nonetheless for the life of the person who bears them, expanding ever so slightly but relentlessly. The inflammatory process worsens very slowly, but progressively. First it tends to involve the skin above the nasion near the eyebrows, the malar eminences, and the paranasal folds. Over the course of years it may come to involve most of the forehead, the entire malar region, the paranasal and nasolabial folds, the postauricular regions, and the sternum. How extensive seborrheic dermatitis may become cannot be predicted, but it can be foretold that it will not involute in the absence of therapy.

INTEGRATION: UNIFYING CONCEPT Seborrheic dermatitis is recognizable clinically, not by virtue of study of the individual lesions that compose it, but by virtue of the distribution of those lesions. Sections of tissue of biopsy specimens taken of seborrheic dermatitis, however, show characteristic changes, namely, a superficial perivascular infiltrate of lymphocytes, dilated venules in the upper part of the dermis, slight epidermal hyperplasia, focal spongiosis, and scale-crusts that reside especially at lips of follicular ostia. More longstanding lesions of seborrheic dermatitis, especially those situated over the sternum, show psoriasiform hyperplasia and scant spongiosis, in addition to mounds of scale-crust.

Seborrheic dermatitis is a specific type of inflammatory process, distinct from psoriasis. Lesions referred to as sebopsoriasis or seborrhiasis, implying thereby a combination of two diseases, almost always represent either seborrheic dermatitis or psoriasis, not both of them.

The cause of seborrheic dermatitis is not known.

THERAPY Low-strength topical corticosteroids alone or in combination with topical antimycotics (ketoconazole) are standard treatments, ostensibly to suppress pityrosporum ovale, a saprophyte of the skin that is thought by some students of the subject to play a role in the pathogenesis of seborrheic dermatitis.

DEFINITION A benign neoplasm of keratinocytes that occurs only on skin bearing hair follicles and consists of pigmented macules, papules, and plaques distributed on sun-exposed sites for a solar lentigo and the reticulated type of seborrheic keratosis, which represents a later stage of solar lentigo, and on the trunk mostly for other types of seborrheic keratosis unrelated to solar lentigo.

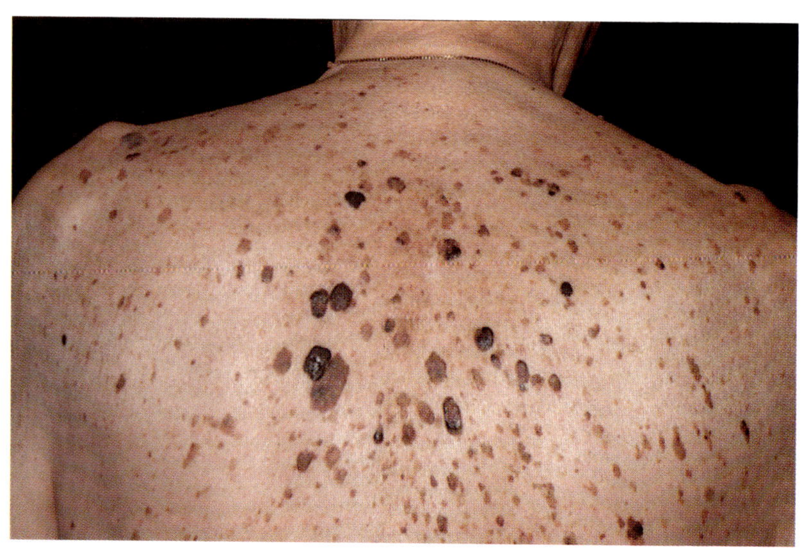

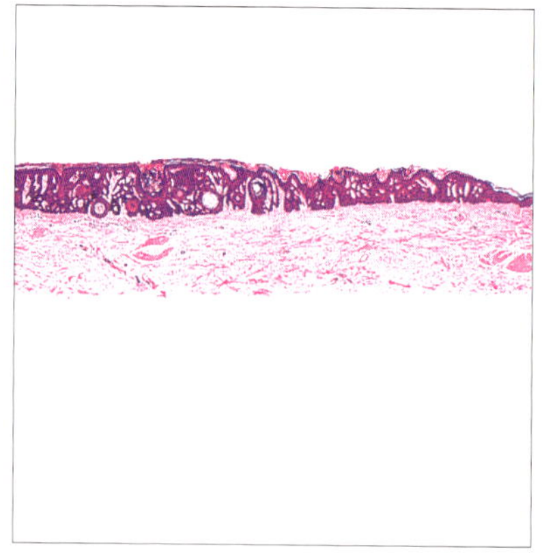

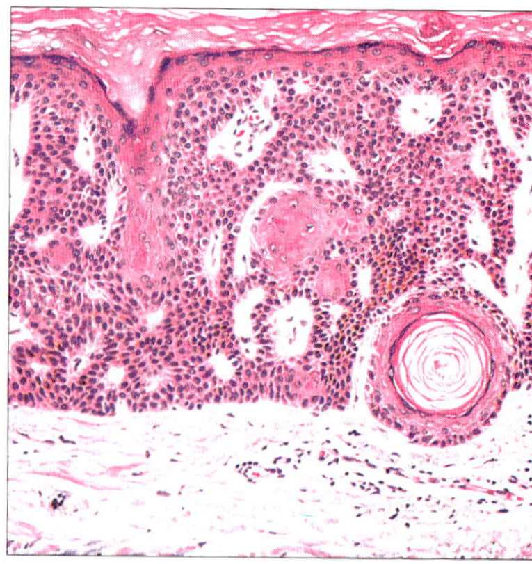

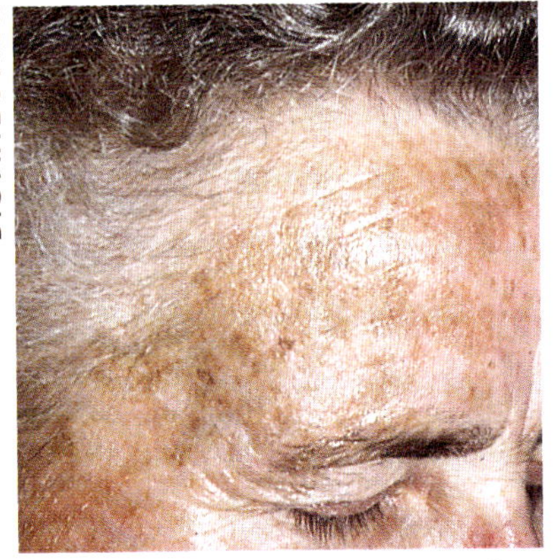
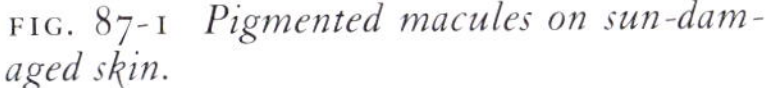

FIG. 87-1 *Pigmented macules on sun-damaged skin.*

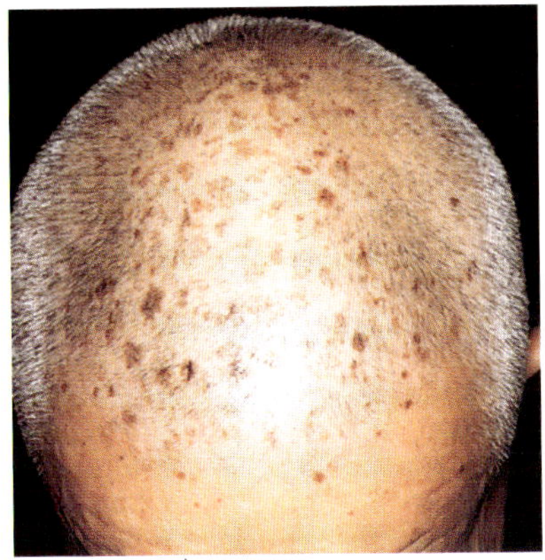

FIG. 87-2 *Pigmented macules of different shades of brown on a bald scalp.*

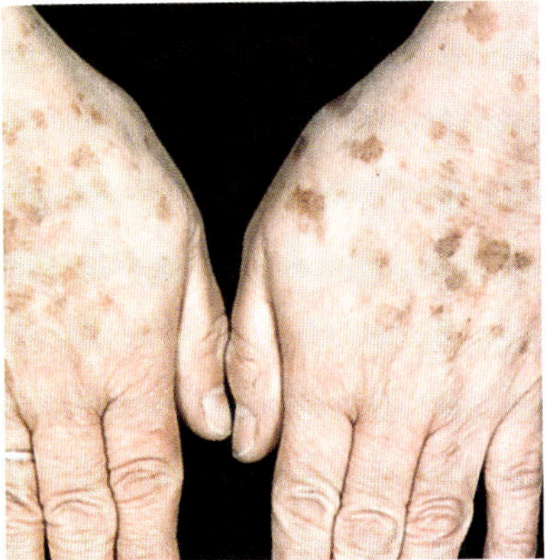

FIG. 87-3 *Pigmented macules and patches, as well as incipient papules and plaques.*

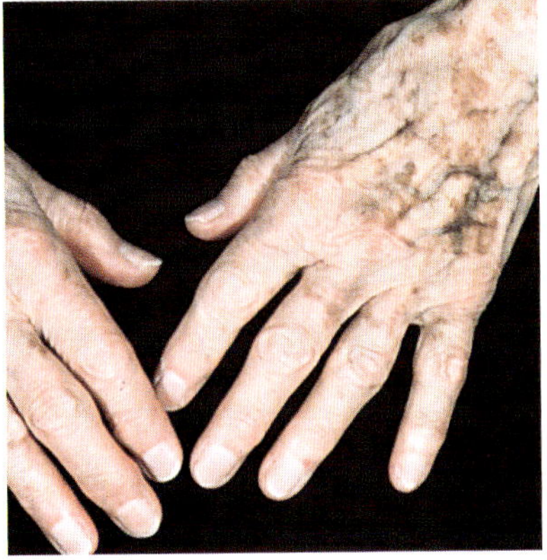

FIG. 87-4 *Pigmented macules and patches on atrophic, sun-damaged skin.*

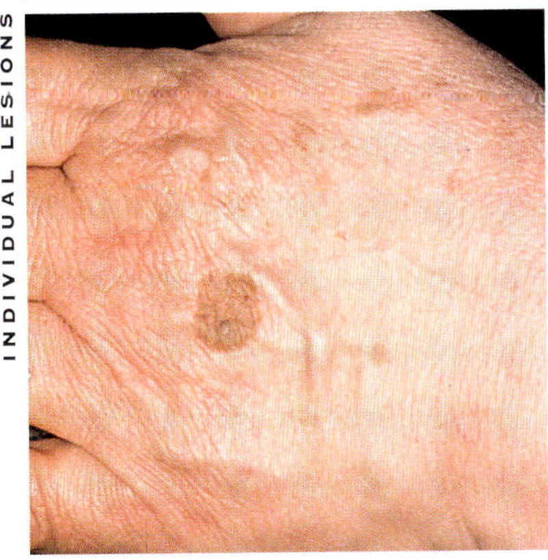

FIG. 87-5 *Pigmented macules and patches of solar lentigo/reticulated seborrheic keratosis, a single pathologic process.*

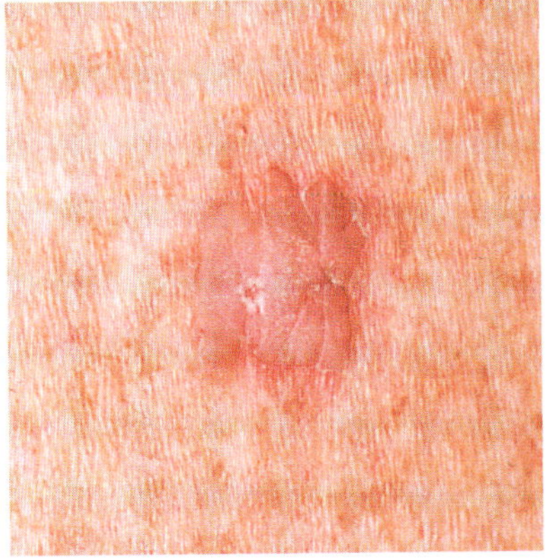

FIG. 87-6 *Keratotic papule with a purplish cast of a resolving lesion of solar lentigo (lichen planus-like keratosis).*

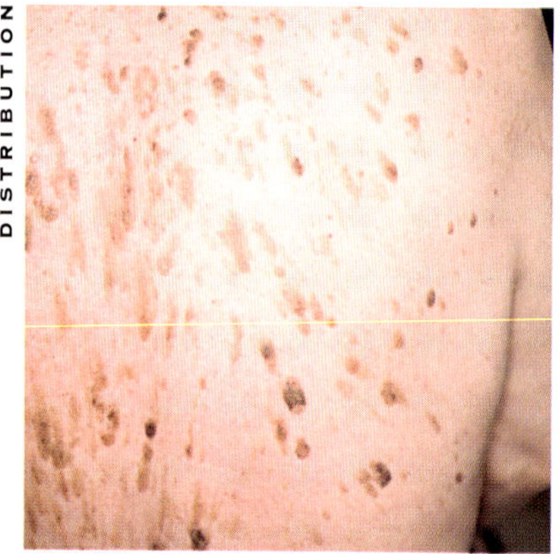

FIG. 87-7 *Innumerable pigmented papules and plaques.*

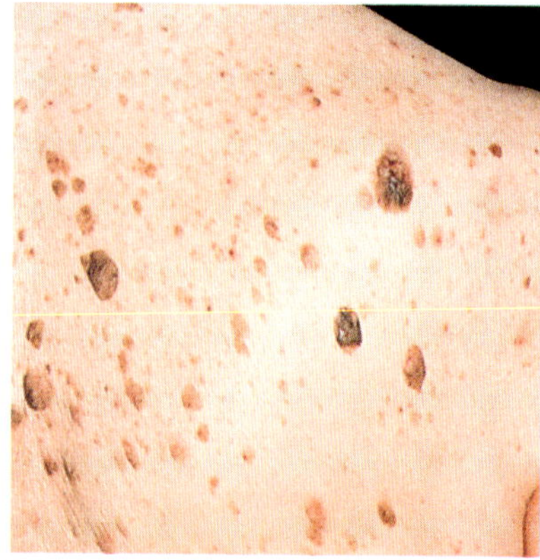

FIG. 87-8 *Pigmented papules and plaques.*

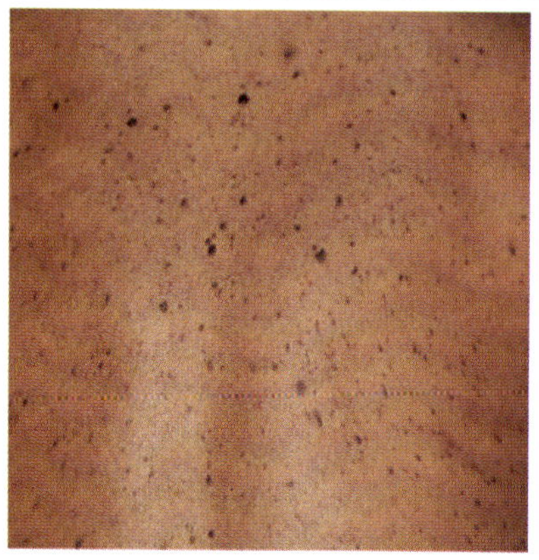

FIG. 87-9 *Pigmented papules, many of them elongated, along lines of cleavage.*

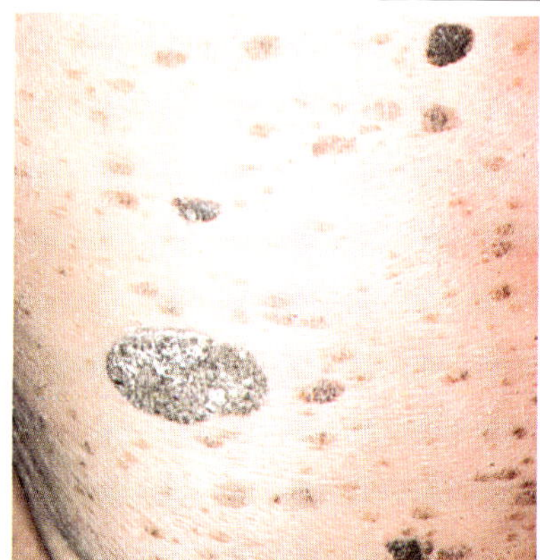

FIG. 87-10 *Pigmented papules and plaques.*

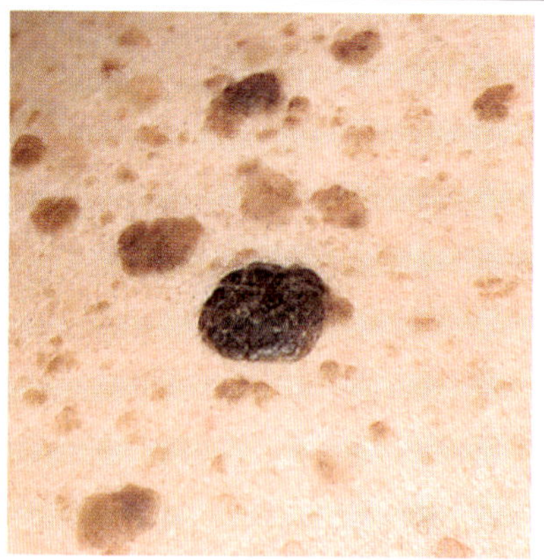

FIG. 87-11 *Pigmented papules and plaques.*

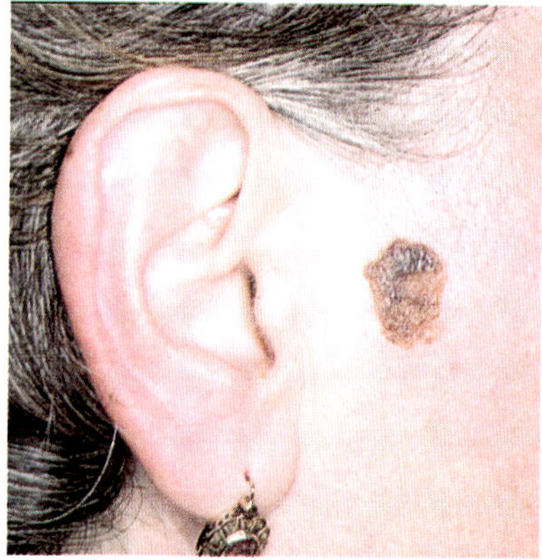

FIG. 87-12 *Pigmented plaque dotted with patulous ostia, unlike the situation in melanoma.*

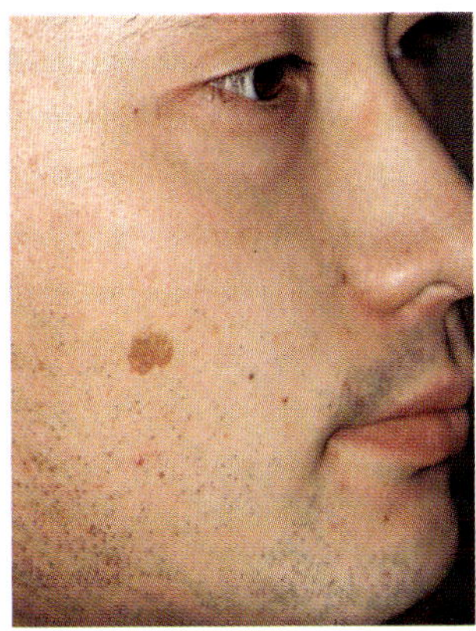

FIG. 87-13 *Small pigmented plaque.*

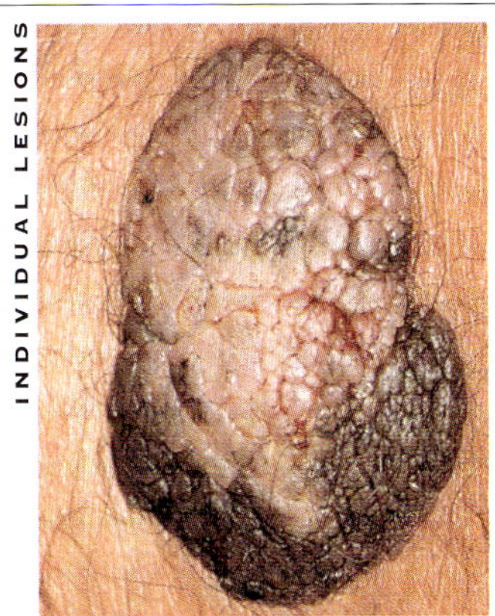

FIG. 87-14 *Pigmented plaque with a multi-lobulated surface.*

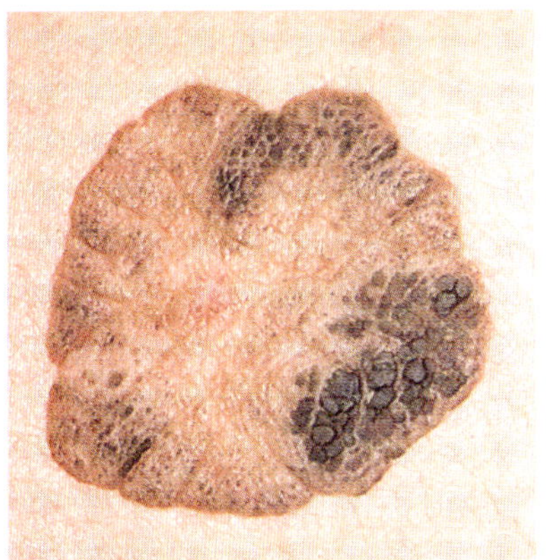

FIG. 87-15 *Sharply circumscribed, scaly, pigmented plaque with plugs of horn within dilated ostia of follicles.*

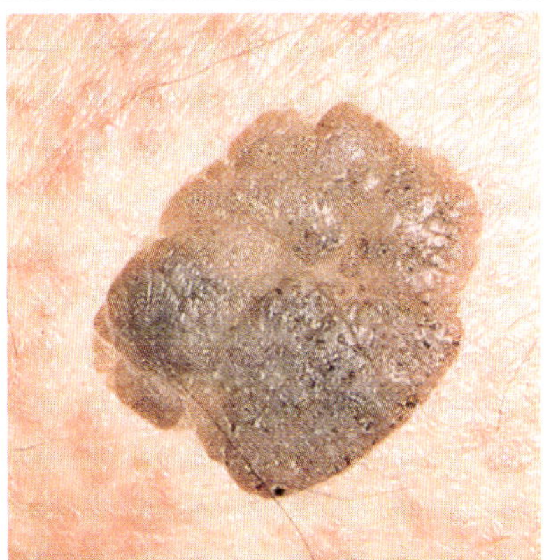

FIG. 87-16 *Sharply circumscribed pigmented plaque with an uneven surface.*

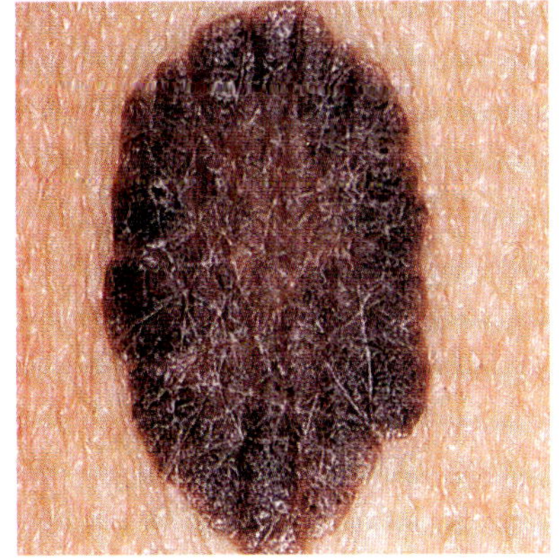

FIG. 87-17 *Sharply circumscribed pigmented plaque.*

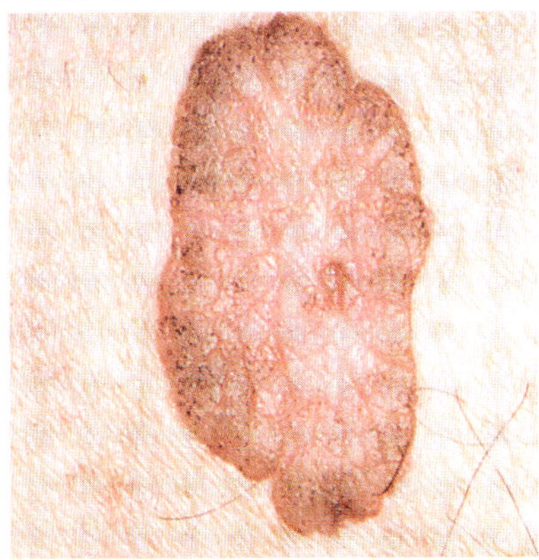

FIG. 87-18 *Sharply circumscribed pigmented plaque with scalloped borders.*

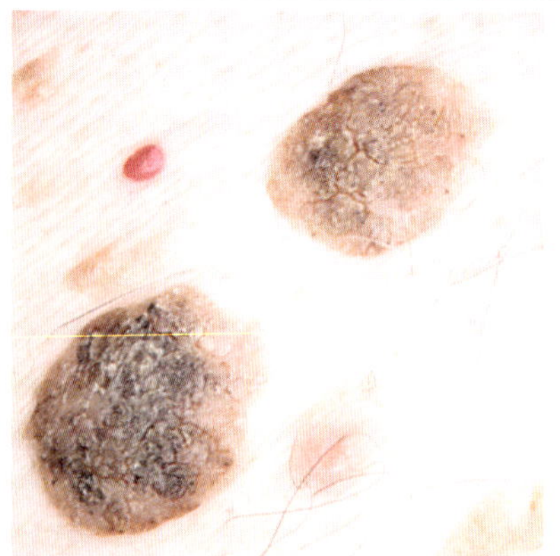

FIG. 87-19 *Pigmented papules and plaques with a keratotic surface. The red papule is a cherry hemangioma.*

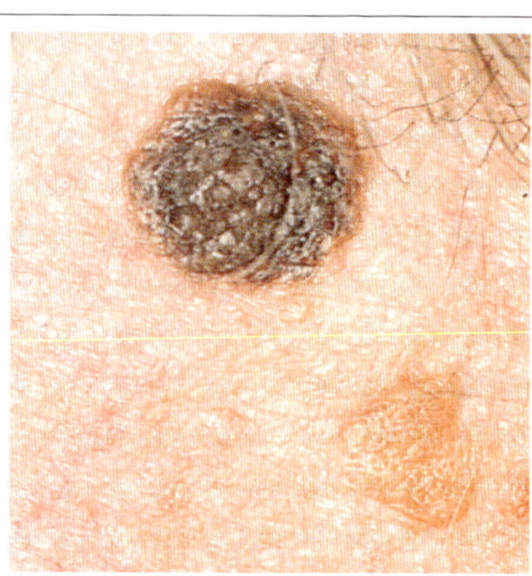

FIG. 87-20 *Keratotic pigmented papule and a keratotic pigmented plaque, the former pigmented lightly and the latter darkly.*

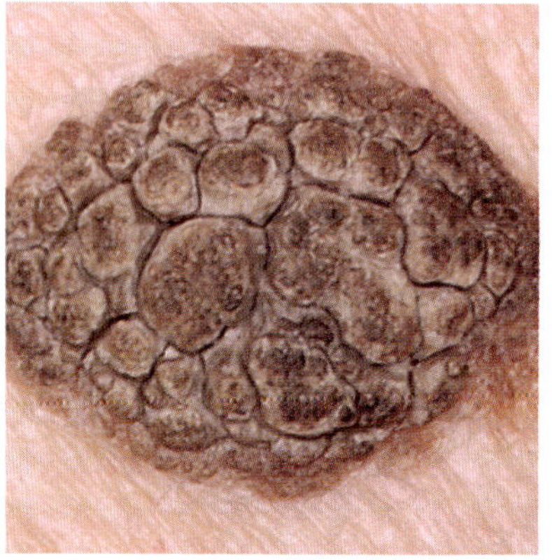

FIG. 87-21 *Pigmented plaque with tortoise shell-like keratotic surface.*

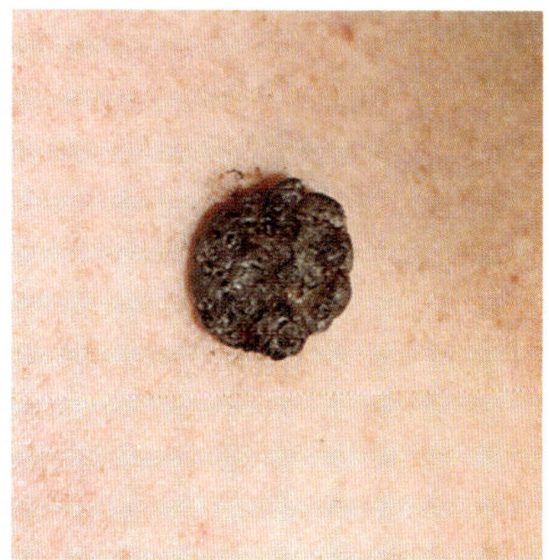

FIG. 87-22 *Sessile papule with a mammillated keratotic surface.*

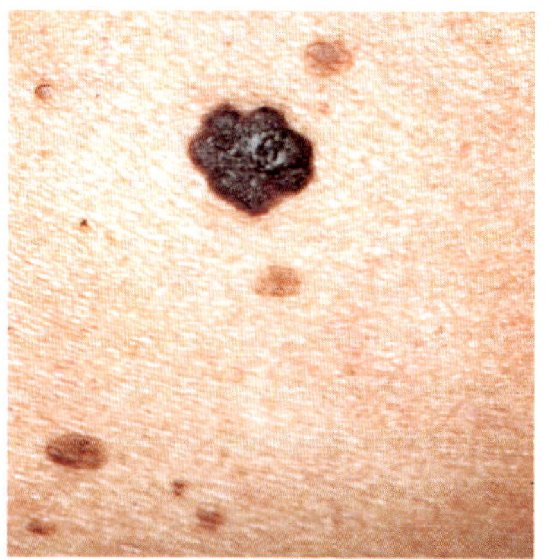

FIG. 87-23 *Papules of different sizes and colors, the largest having a surface punctuated by dilated ostia of follicles.*

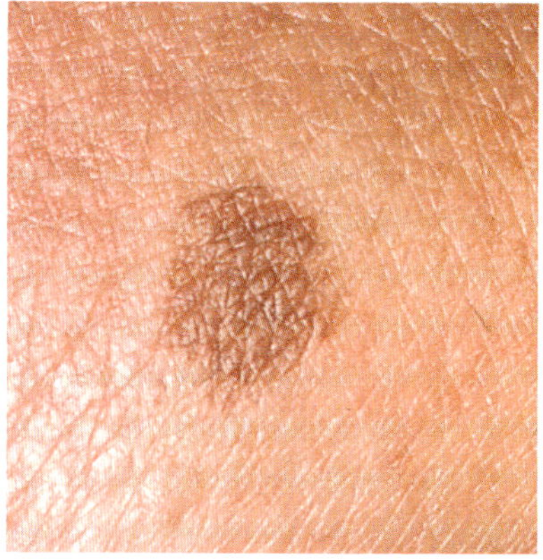

FIG. 87-24 *Pigmented macule. When this solar lentigo thickens it then becomes known as a seborrheic keratosis.*

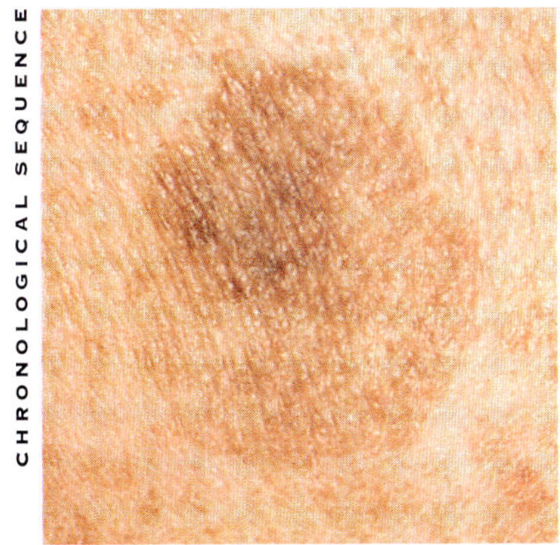

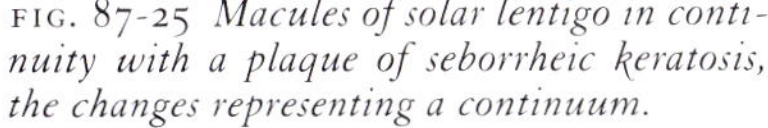

FIG. 87-25 *Macules of solar lentigo in conti-nuity with a plaque of seborrheic keratosis, the changes representing a continuum.*

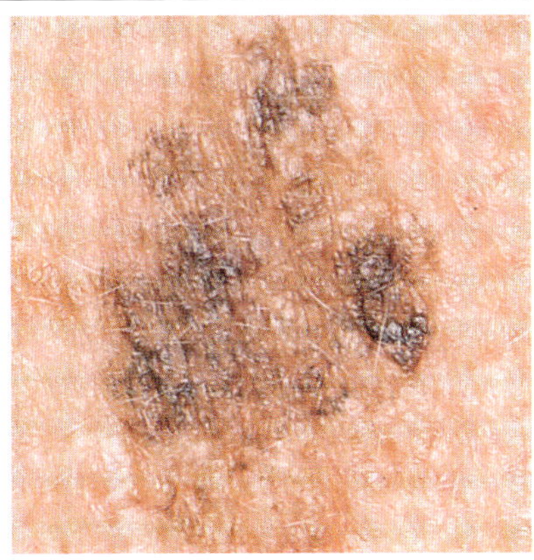

FIG. 87-26 *Elevated keratotic lesions of seborrheic keratosis within a patch of solar lentigo, a continuum.*

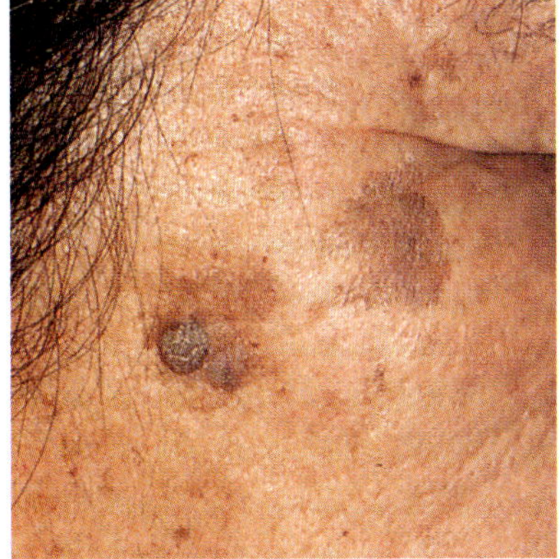

FIG. 87-27 *Numerous solar lentigines with-in one of which are papules of seborrheic ker-atosis, a single process.*

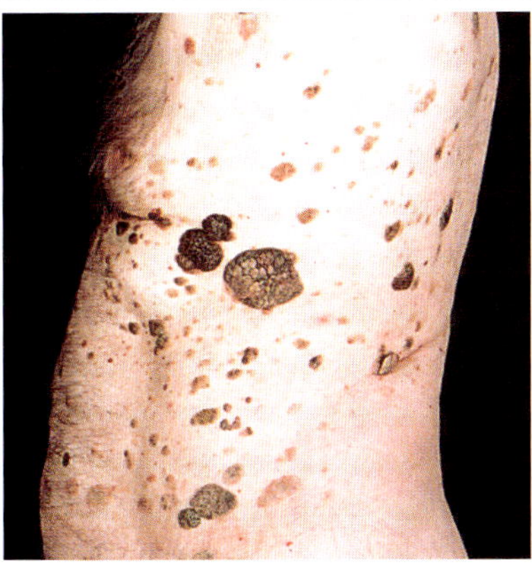

FIG. 87-28 *Seborrheic keratoses at different stages of evolution from macule through papule to plaque and tumor.*

COURSE Solar lentigines appear as pigmented macules on skin injured severely by sunlight, especially the face and the dorsa of hands. Over the course of years, the macules become slightly elevated and darker, and, still later, ever more elevated and even darker papules. The macules are referred to as solar lentigines, the fully developed papules as seborrheic keratoses. Other types of seborrheic keratoses also begin as smooth, pigmented macules that, in time, become pigmented keratotic papules and plaques. Seborrheic keratoses of all types are permanent, except for those (especially of the solar lentigo/reticulated seborrheic keratosis type) that regress completely conse-quent to the effects on them of an onslaught of lymphocytes. Such a seborrheic keratosis in the process of regression, as judged by an associated lichenoid infiltrate of lymphocytes, is known as a "lichen planus-like keratosis."

INTEGRATION: UNIFYING CONCEPT Solar lentigo and reticulated seborrheic keratosis are different names for the same pathologic process at different stages in its chronological course. A tan macule and brown, slightly elevated papule are seen in tissue sections of biopsy specimens to consist of nubbins of pigmented epidermal keratinocytes associated with slight orthokeratosis in which the corneocytes are arranged in laminated fashion. Melanocytes may be increased slightly in number, but they are small and monomorphous, equidistant from one another, and positioned entirely at the dermoepidermal junction. Solar elastosis is present in the upper part of the dermis. Such a lesion is called a solar lentigo.

Over the course of years, the same lesion may become a more elevated brown papule, and when that is biopsied, sections from the specimen show more elongated nubbins of pigmented epidermal keratinocytes that at the base of them make a turn at a right angle to the skin surface. The design thereby created is reticulated and the reticulations are confined to a thickened papillary dermis. In addition, there are tunnels of infundibula that house corneocytes disposed in laminated and basket-woven pattern. Those findings, in toto, are typical of a reticulated seborrheic keratosis. It, like all types of seborrheic keratosis, consists of both "basaloid" and "squamoid" keratinocytes, the squamoid ones being present immediately beneath the stratum corneum and around infundibular tunnels, and the basaloid cells (presumably germinative ones) composing the rest of the neoplasm. In short, solar lentigo/reticulated seborrheic keratosis is a benign pigmented neoplasm composed of both epidermal and infundibular keratinocytes.

There are at least two other types of seborrheic keratosis, namely, an acanthotic type and a verrucous type, both of which are situated mostly on the trunk. The cellular constituents of them are just like those of a reticulated seborrheic keratosis, but the architectural patterns of them are different, the acanthotic type being more solid and endophytic, although always seated above the reticular dermis, and the verrucous type being digitate and residing above the reticular dermis.

That seborrheic keratoses of all kinds consist of follicular as well as epidermal keratinocytes may be inferred not only from the presence of horn-

appear on hair-bearing skin; none occur on palms or soles.

A lichen planus-like keratosis is nothing more than a solar lentigo/reticulated seborrheic keratosis in the throes of regression secondary to the effects of an attack by lymphocytes that are arranged in a band, obscure the junction of the keratosis and the dermis, and induce necrosis of neoplastic keratinocytes, the result of which is disappearance of the lesion.

THERAPY Curettage, cryotherapy, and laser surgery are all efficacious.

DEFINITION A small-vessel vasculitis characterized clinically by vesiculo-pustules on an erythematous base, purpuric macules and papules, and hemorrhagic bullae, and histopathologically by thrombi within venules, a consequence of sepsis.

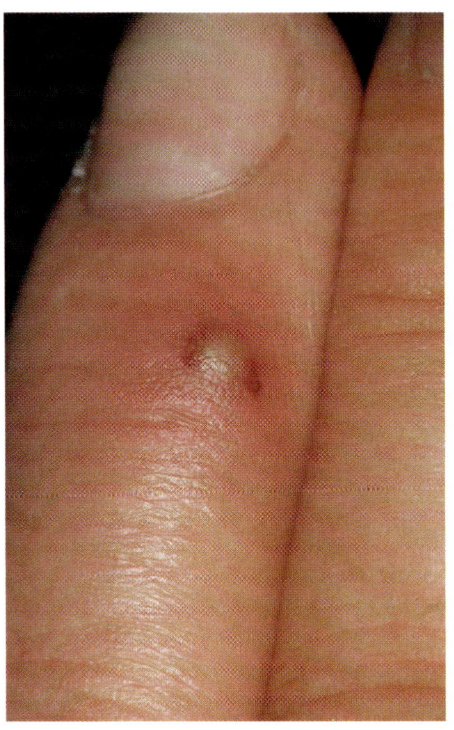

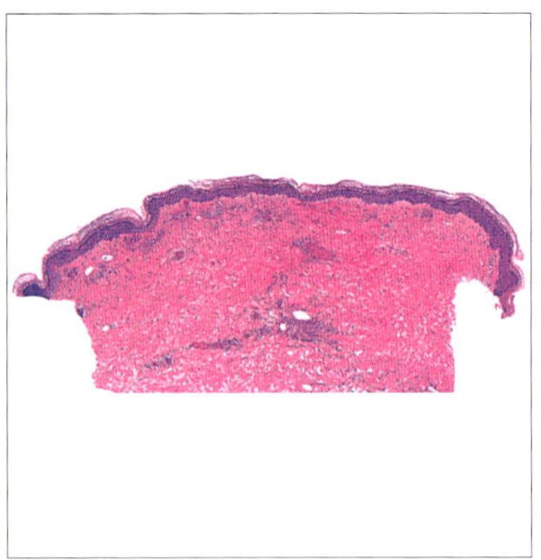

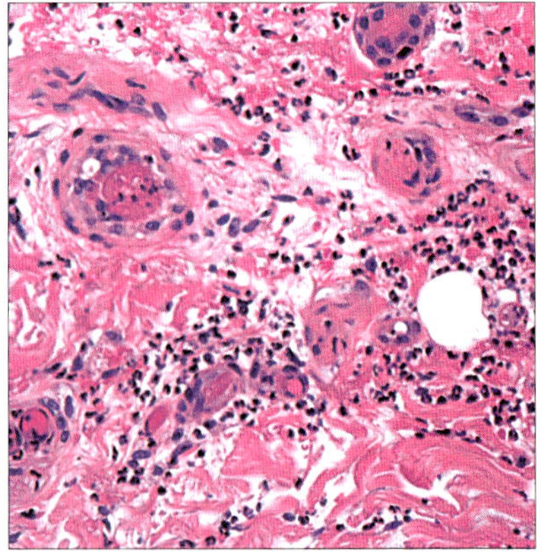

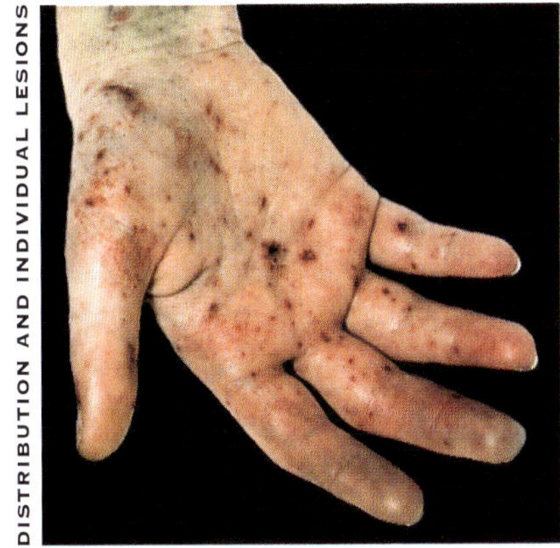

FIG. 88-1 *Purpuric macules and papules of meningococcemia.*

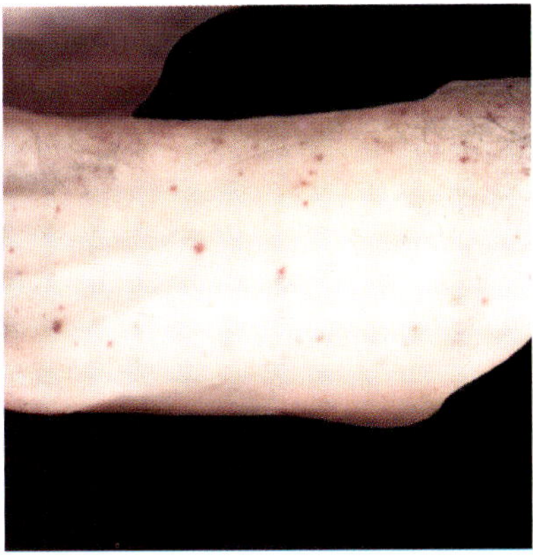

FIG. 88-2 *Purpuric macules and papules of meningococcemia.*

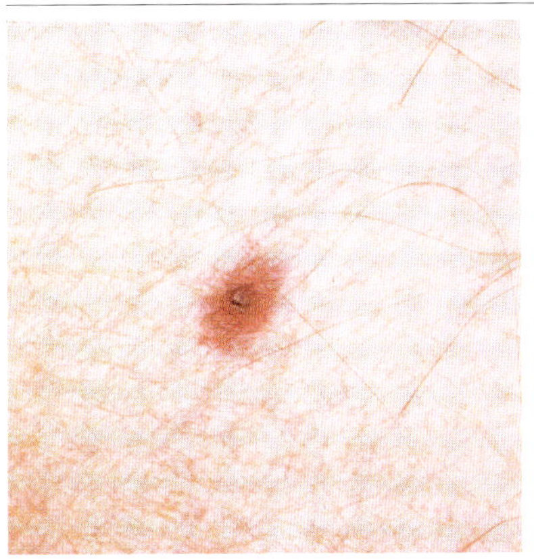

FIG. 88-3 *Purpuric papule with central pustule of disseminated aspergillosis.*

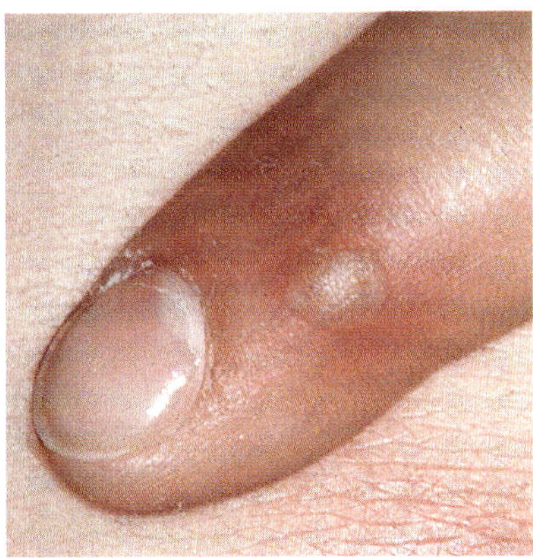

FIG. 88-4 *Pustule of gonococcemia on a red base.*

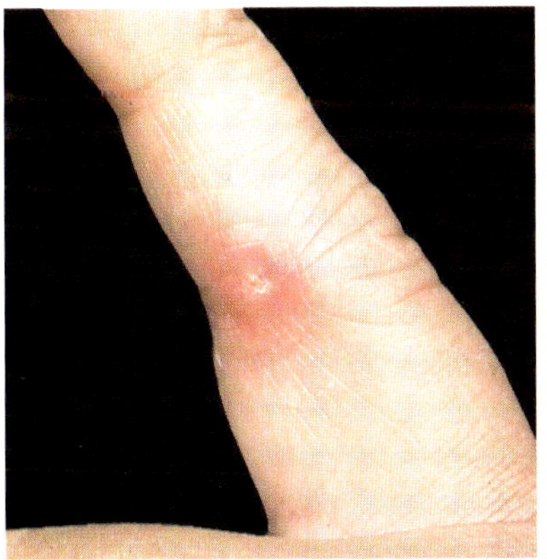

FIG. 88-5 *Vesiculopustule on a broad erythematous areola of gonococcemia.*

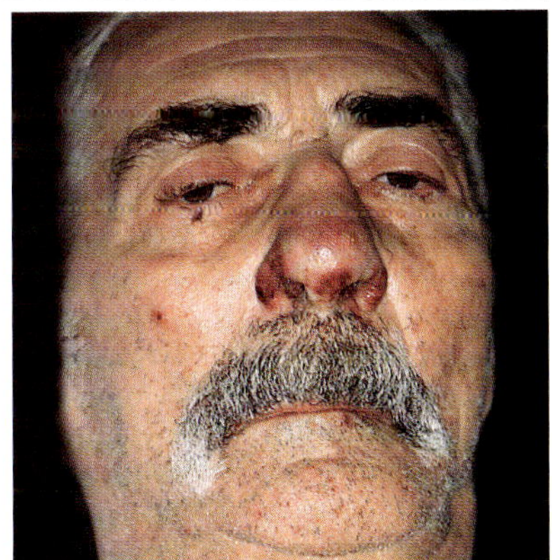

FIG. 88-6 *Purpuric macules and patches of septic vasculitiss in a patient with chronic myelogenous leukemia.*

ADJUNCTIVE DIAGNOSTIC TEST Cultures of blood may be taken in order to promote growth of the causative bacteria.

COURSE The course of septic vasculitides varies enormously, from rapid progression to death in gram-negative septicemia in a person who is immunosuppressed, to remissions and exacerbations over years in a mildly ill patient as in the case of chronic gonococcemia and chronic meningococcemia.

INTEGRATION: UNIFYING CONCEPT The morphologic expressions of septic vasculitis vary markedly, for example, from petechiae, vesiculopustules on a broad erythematous base, and hemorrhagic bullae of chronic gonococcemia and chronic meningococcemia to diffuse purpura in the Waterhouse-Friderichsen syndrome, from hemorrhagic pustules of staphylococcal septicemia to large hemorrhagic bullae that ulcerate in the septicemia caused by pseudomonas (ecthyma gangrenosum).

Irrespective of the morphologic presentation of lesions of septic vasculitis and irrespective of the cause of it, there are certain common denominators, clinically and histopathologically. Clinically, there always is purpura, i.e., a purple hue as a result of extravasation of erythrocytes into at least the upper part of the dermis. Macules, papules, vesicles, bullae, and even pustules are purpuric. Histopathologically, there always are thrombi within the lumen of some venules within the dermis and sometimes in the subcutaneous fat, too. As a result of thrombosis, infarction ensues. It may take the form of simple necrosis of the epidermis, which sloughs to leave behind an erosion or superficial ulcer, or it may be expressed as ballooning intraepidermal vesiculation in conjunction with epidermal necrosis, changes that also soon lead to erosion or ulceration. When thrombi are numerous and infarction extensive, as in the case of ecthyma gangrenosum, hemorrhagic bullae appear, and they are succeeded by deep ulcers.

In sum, septic vasculitis can be caused by many types of gram-positive and gram-negative bacteria, and the morphologic manifestations of that infection result from an interplay between the type of organism on one hand and the capability of the host to respond to it on the other. Irrespective of those considerations, septic vasculitis is characterized by typical clinical and histopathologic findings that permit diagnosis to be made with specificity.

When the process of septic vasculitis is "acute," bacteria can be demonstrated in sections of tissue stained specially for them. When, in contrast, the process is "chronic," as in that particular presentation of gonococcemia and meningococcemia, bacteria can neither be demonstrated in tissue sections nor cultured from lesions, the reason being that they have been ingested by inflammatory cells and have been destroyed.

THERAPY After culture and sensitivity have been performed of skin lesions and blood, intensive treatment with specific antibiotics given intravenously should be instituted post haste.

DEFINITION A malignant neoplasm of keratinocytes that when present as a keratotic macule or papule on skin damaged badly by sunlight is referred to as solar keratosis. When present as a plaque it is termed Bowen's disease, and when present as many papules in the anogenital region it is called bowenoid papulosis. Solar keratosis, Bowen's disease, and bowenoid papulosis, as well as arsenical keratosis and radiation keratosis, are euphemisms for various types of superficial squamous-cell carcinoma. Very episodically, neoplastic cells of those types of squamous-cell carcinoma proliferate wildly, and the primary neoplasm then consists of aggregations that extend throughout the dermis and well into the subcutaneous fat, from which sites they rarely may metastasize.

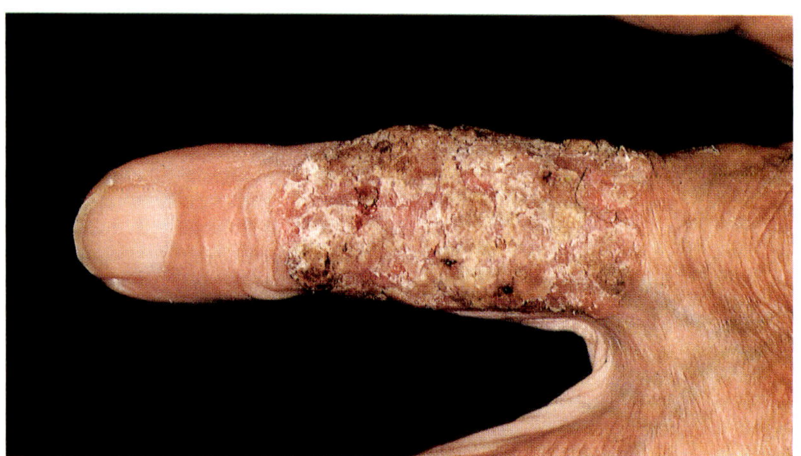

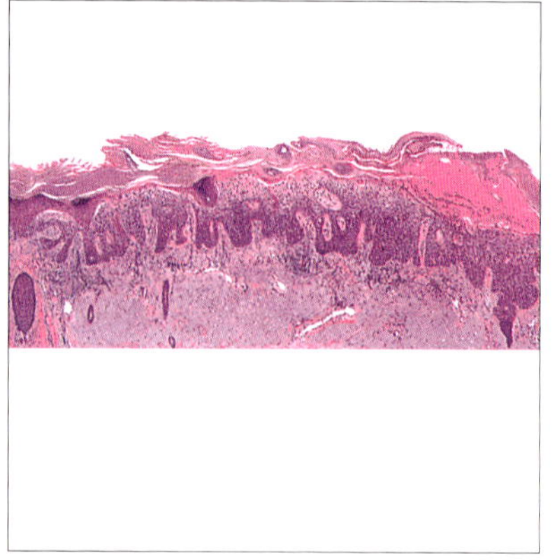

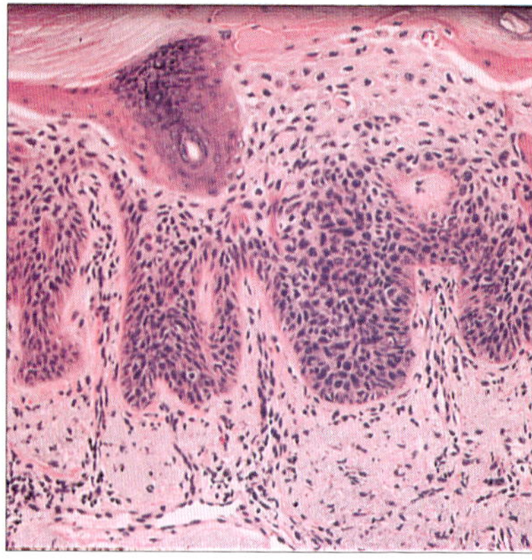

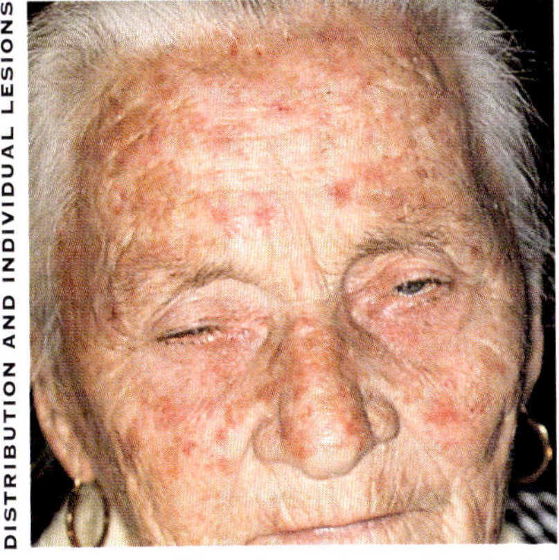

FIG. 89-1   *Many keratotic papules of solar keratosis.*

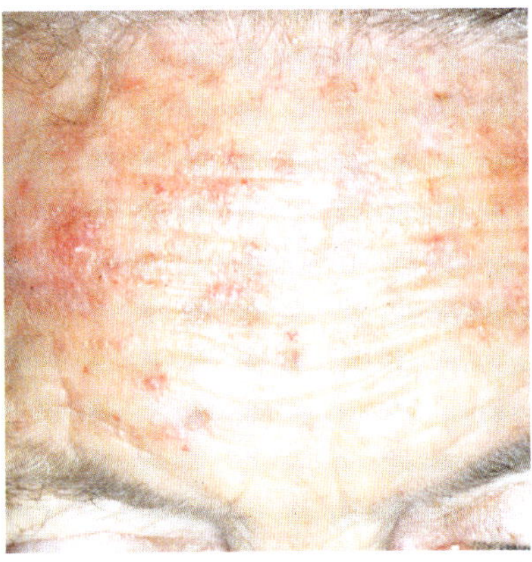

FIG. 89-2   *Numerous closely-set keratotic papules of solar keratosis.*

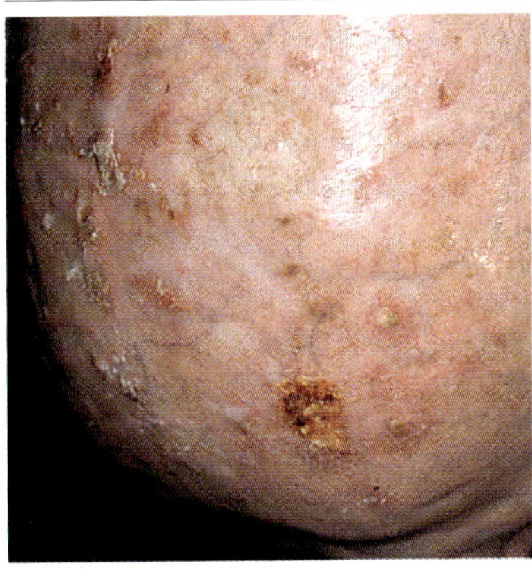

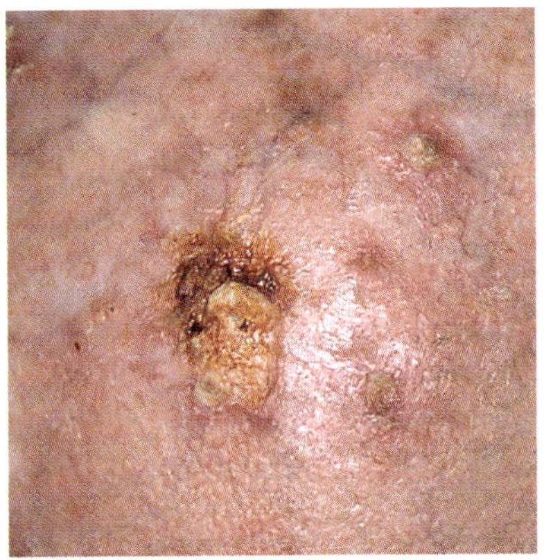

FIG. 89-3 (A, B)   *Numerous closely-set and confluent papules of solar keratosis, superficial squamous-cell carcinomas all.*

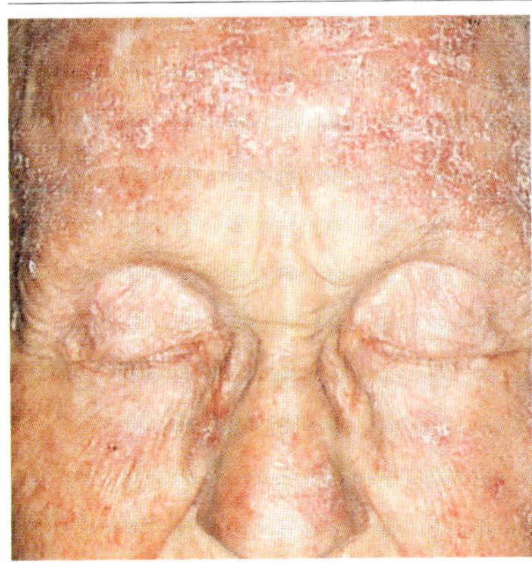

FIG. 89-4   *Confluence of keratotic lesions of solar keratosis.*

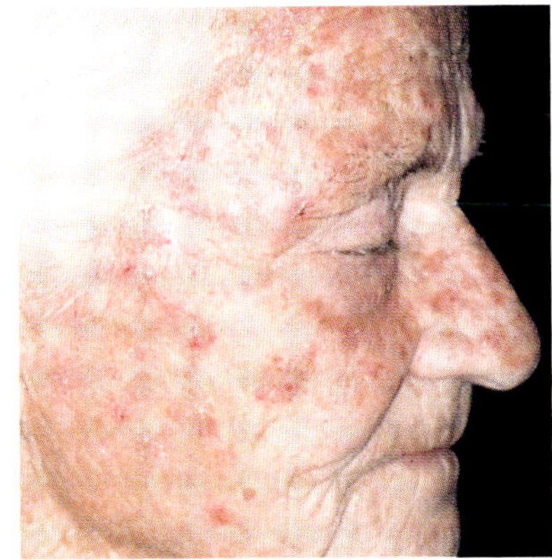

FIG. 89-5   *Solar keratoses and solar lentigines (the brown macules).*

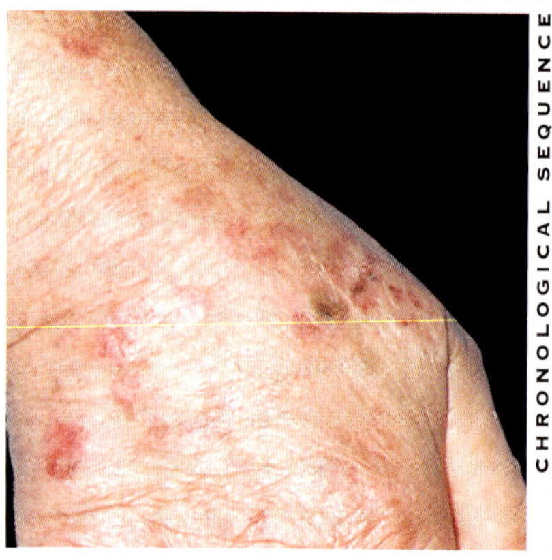

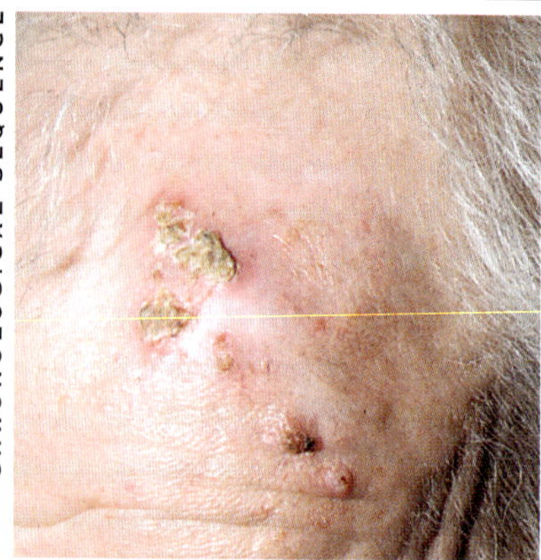

FIG. 89-6 *Solar keratoses and solar lentigines (the brown macules).*

FIG. 89-7 *Squamous-cell carcinomas at stages of evolution from keratotic macules of solar keratosis to keratotic papules.*

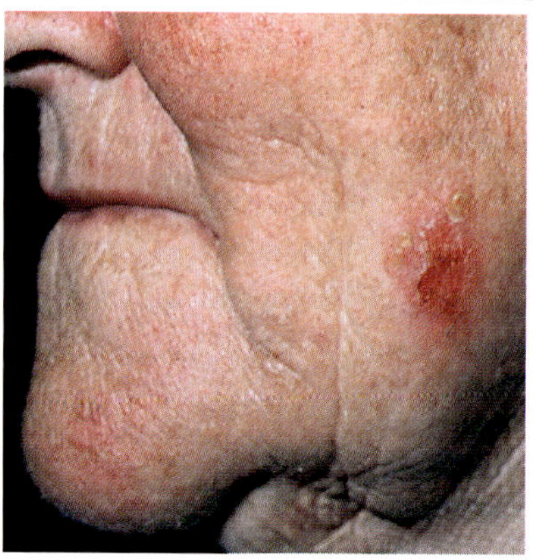

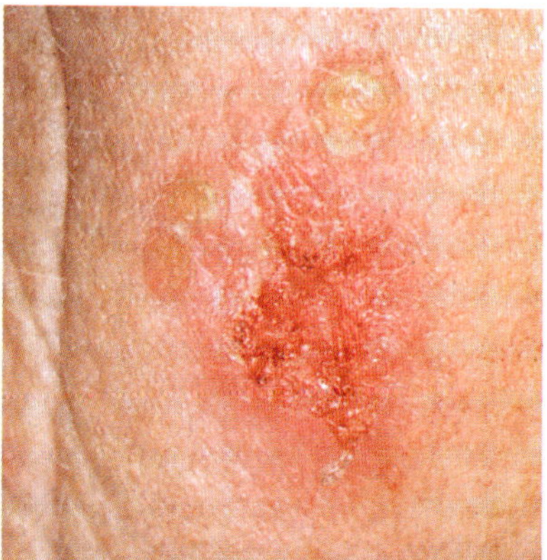

FIG. 89-8 (A, B) *Scaly lesions represent superficial squamous-cell carcinomas (solar keratoses), whereas eroded lesions are deeper squamous-cell carcinomas (solar keratotic type).*

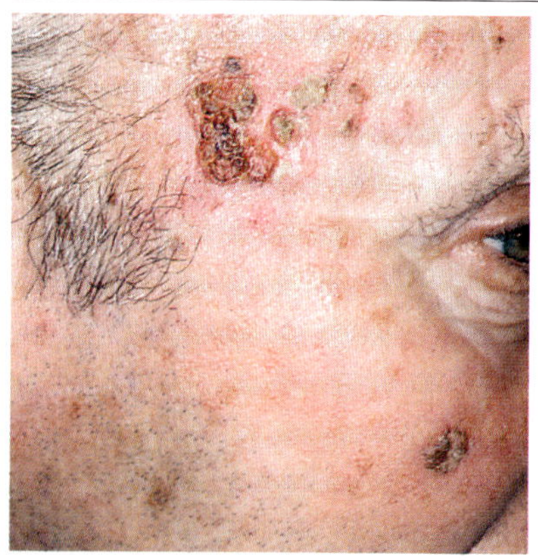

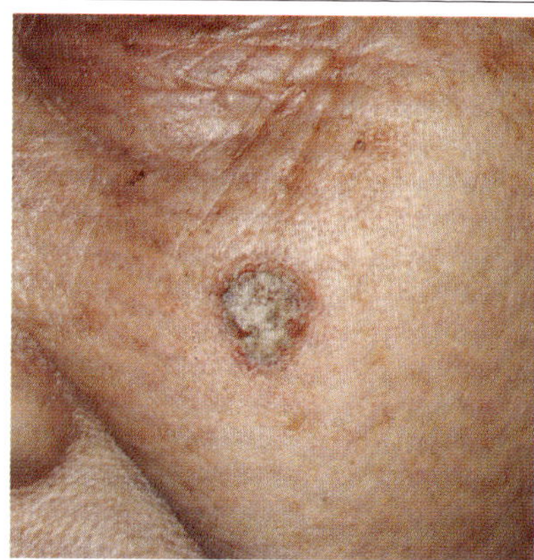

FIG. 89-9 *Spectrum of lesions of squamous-cell carcinoma from keratotic macules of solar keratosis to keratotic plaques.*

FIG. 89-10 *A keratotic plaque is a thick squamous-cell carcinoma, and keratotic papules (solar keratoses) are thin carcinomas.*

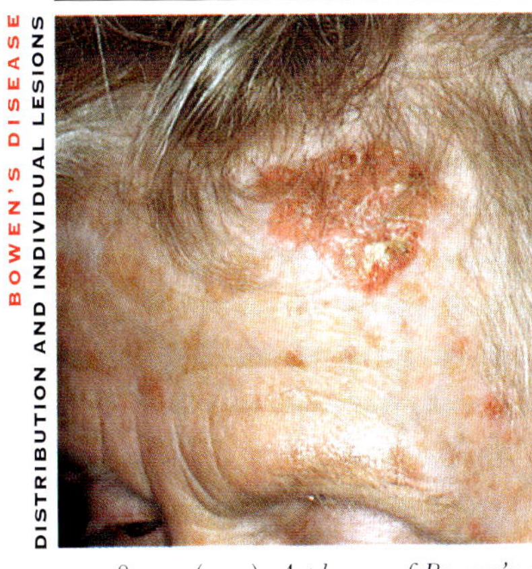
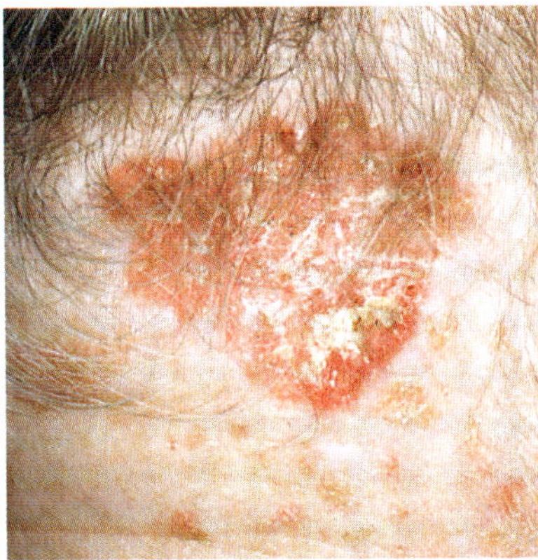

FIG. 89-11 (A, B) *A plaque of Bowen's disease and papules of solar keratosis, all superficial squamous-cell carcinomas.*

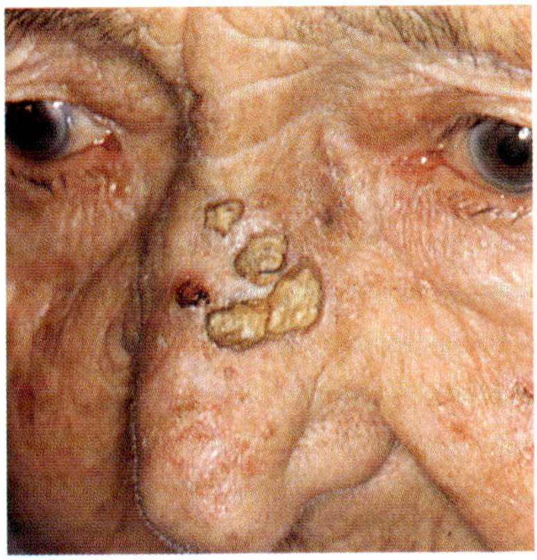

FIG. 89-12 *Keratotic plaques of Bowen's disease in company with papules of solar keratosis.*

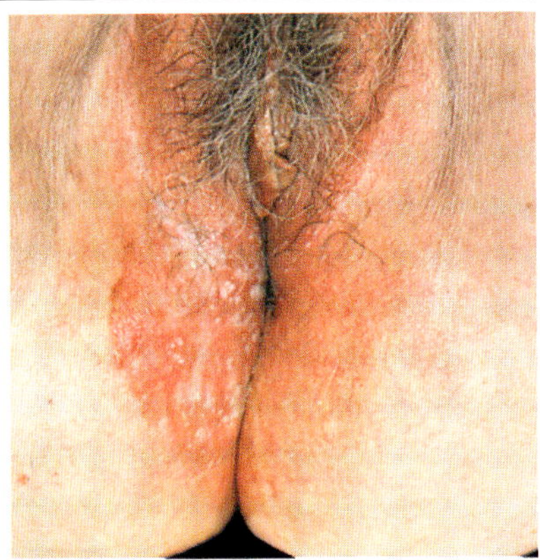

FIG. 89-13 *Eroded scaly plaque of Bowen's disease.*

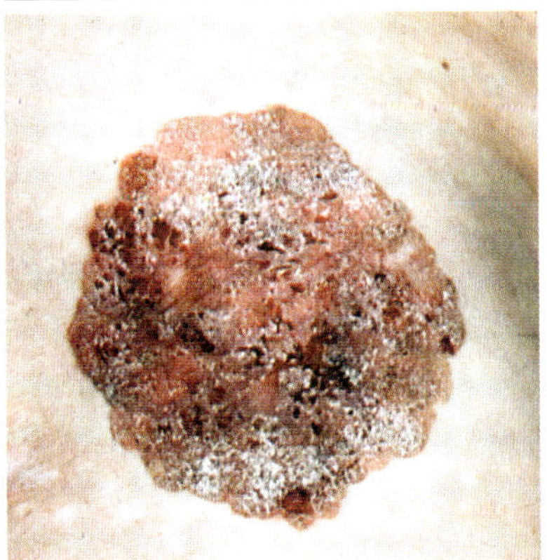

FIG. 89-14 *Scaly plaque of Bowen's disease with various shades of brown.*

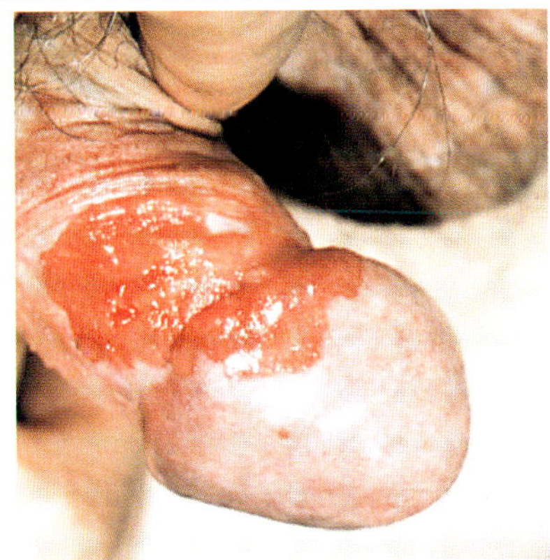

FIG. 89-15 *Ulcerated plaque of squamous-cell carcinoma (erythroplasia of Queyrat). The findings are the same as Bowen's disease.*

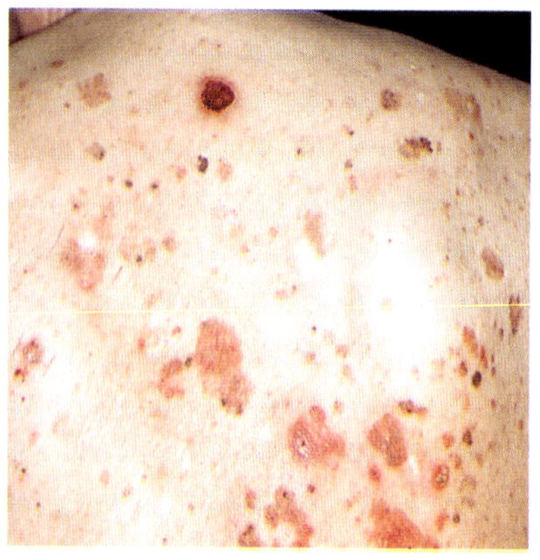

FIG. 89-16 *Numerous reddish brown plaques of Bowen's disease and an ulcerated squamous-cell carcinoma, Bowen's type.*

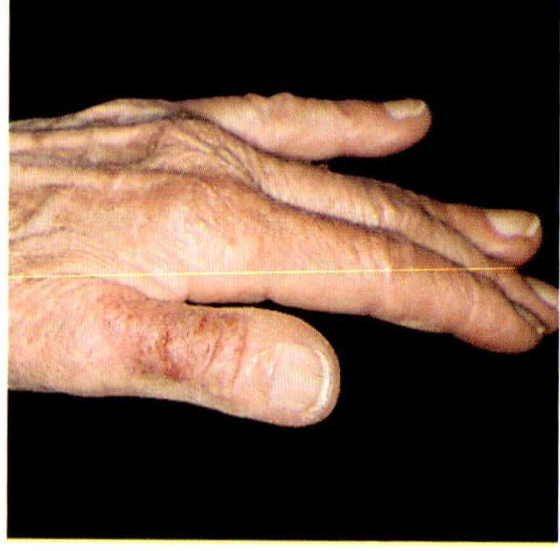

FIG. 89-17 *Scaly crusted plaque of Bowen's disease.*

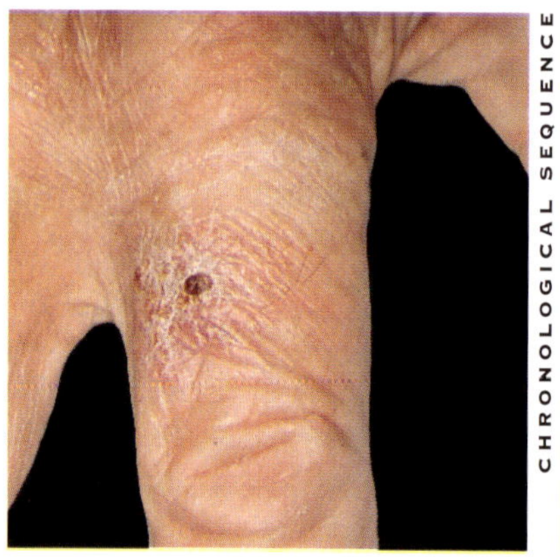

FIG. 89-18 *Scaly crusted plaque.*

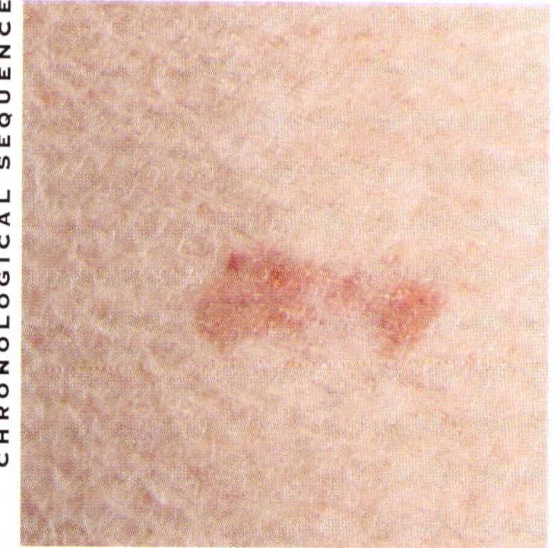

FIG. 89-19 *Scaly crusted plaque.*

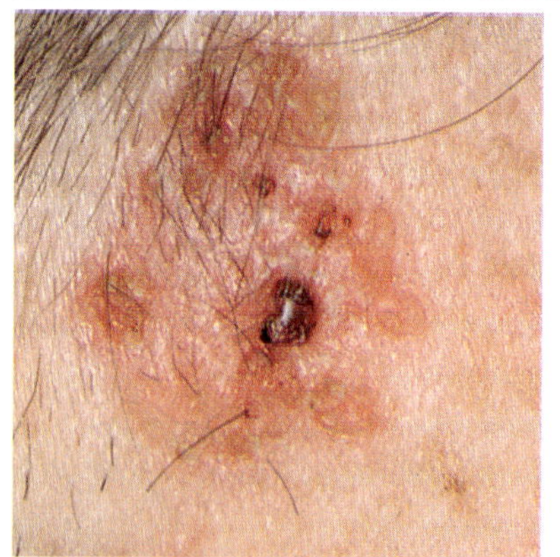

FIG. 89-20 *Scaly crusted plaque.*

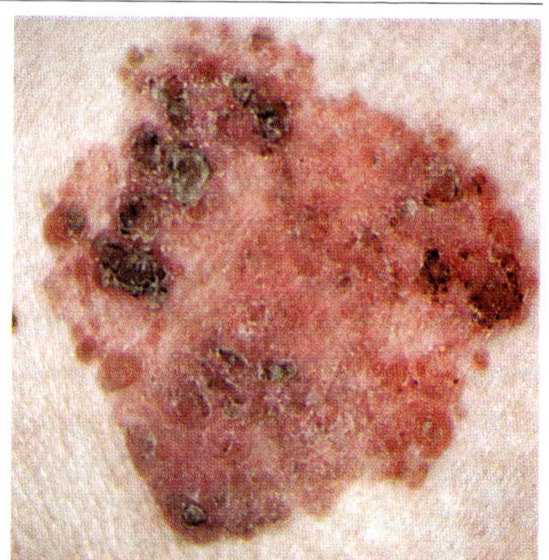

FIG. 89-21 *Large scaly crusted plaque.*

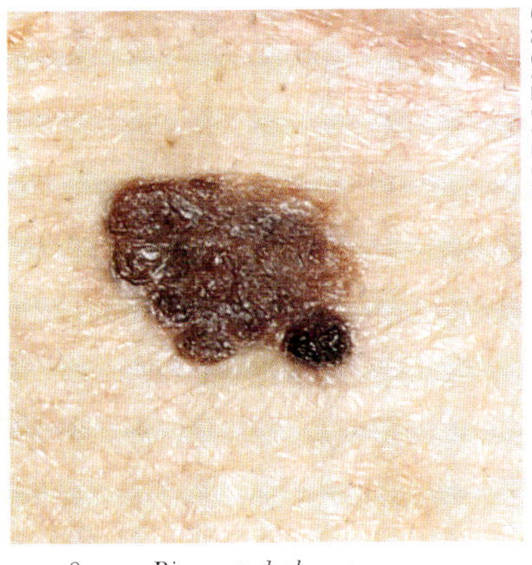

FIG. 89-22 *Pigmented plaque.*

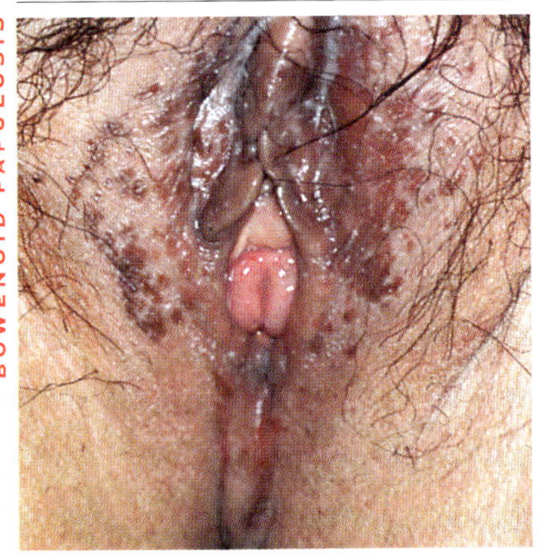

FIG. 89-23 *Pigmented plaques.*

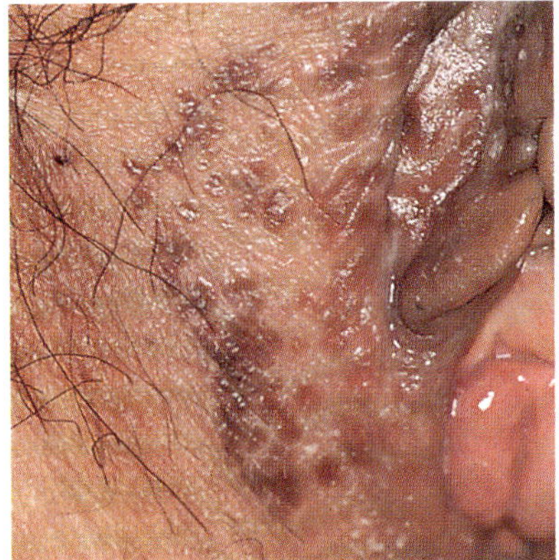

FIG. 89-24 (A, B) *Pigmented papules and plaques.*

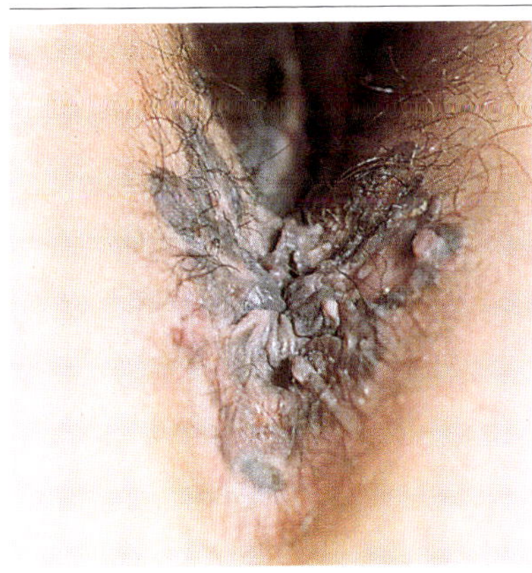

FIG. 89-25 *Perianal plaques.*

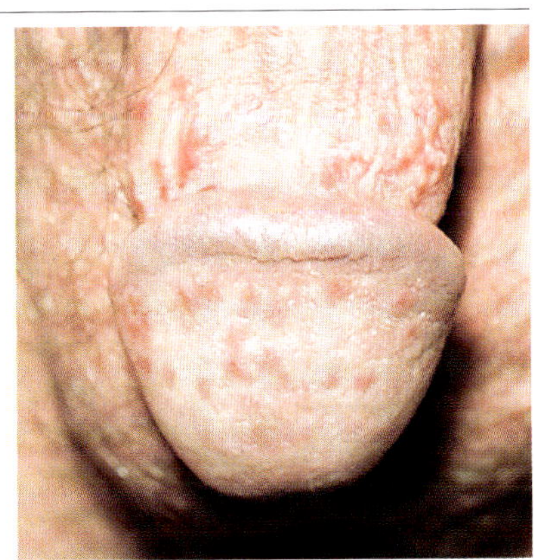

FIG. 89-26 *Papules of bowenoid papulosis.*

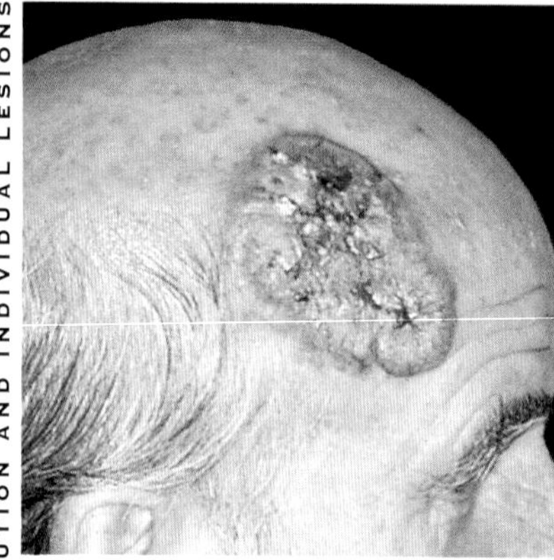

FIG. 89-27 *Ulcerated, crusted plaque/tumor.*

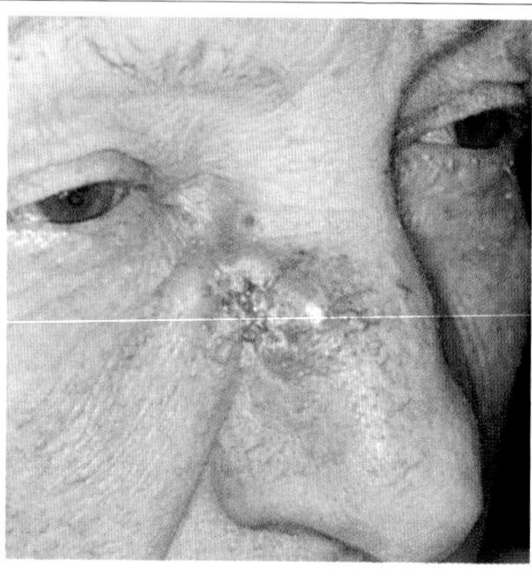

FIG. 89-28 *Ulcerated crusted squamous-cell carcinoma surrounded by numerous telangiectases.*

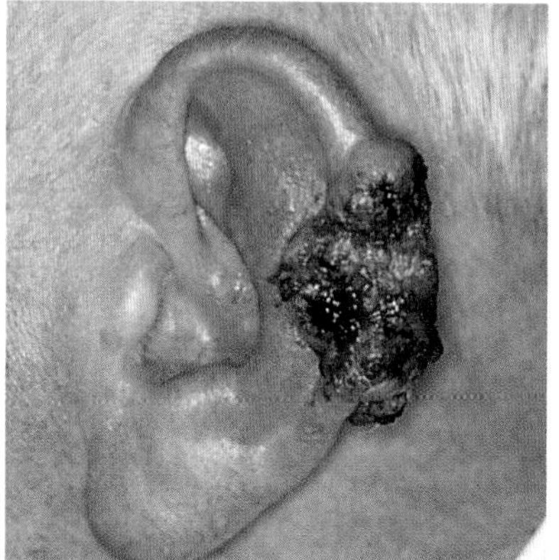

FIG. 89-29 *Ulcerated squamous-cell carcinoma covered by hemorrhagic crusts.*

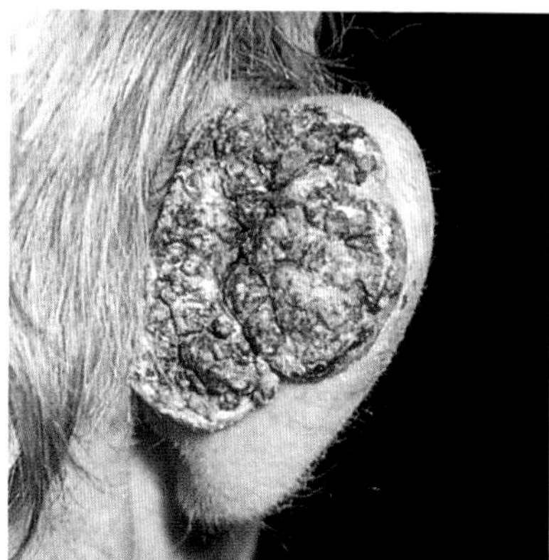

FIG. 89-30 *Markedly keratotic ulcerated plaque.*

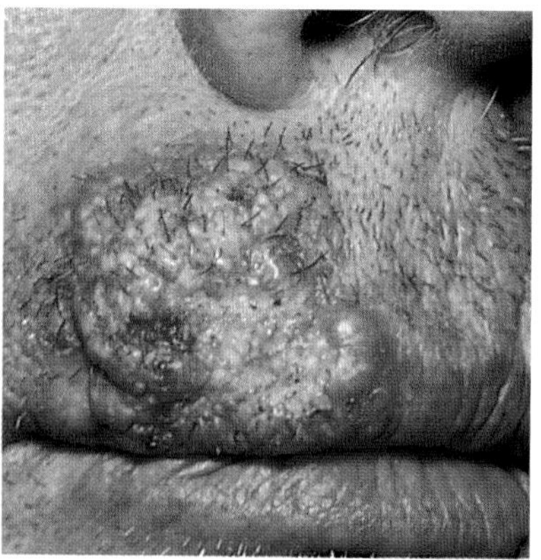

FIG. 89-31 *Ulcerated plaque with a mammillated center.*

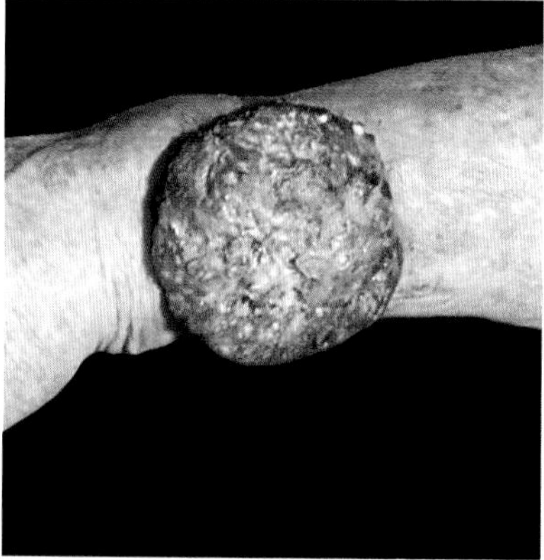

FIG. 89-32 *Sessile, ulcerated, crusted tumor.*

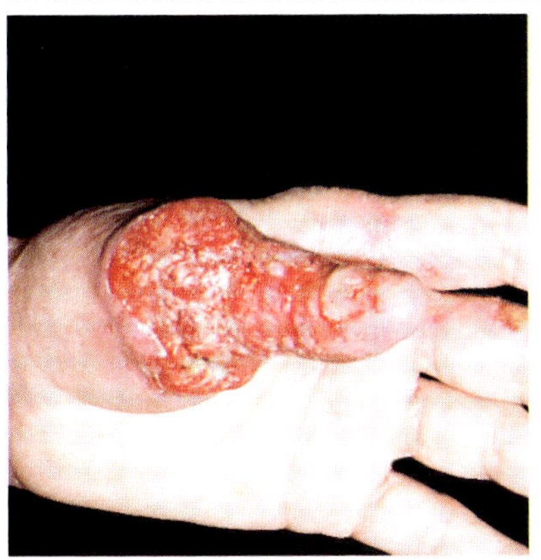

FIG. 89-33 *Ulcerated squamous-cell carcinoma in company with several solar keratoses on the fingers.*

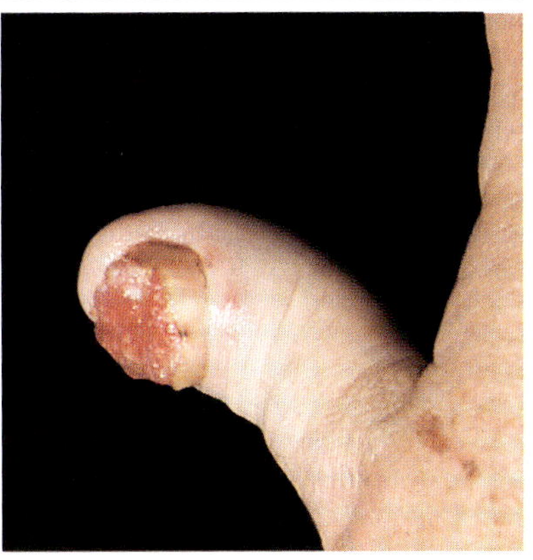

FIG. 89-34 *Ulcerated subungual squamous-cell carcinoma and a solar lentigo on the dorsum of a hand.*

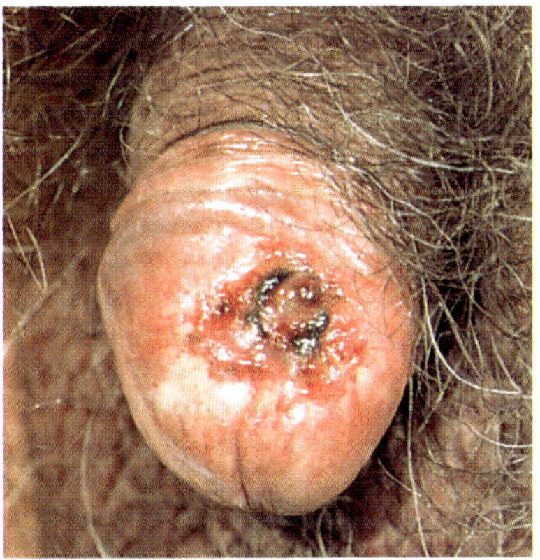

FIG. 89-35 *Ulcerated squamous-cell carcinoma with an elevated, smooth-surfaced, papillated rim.*

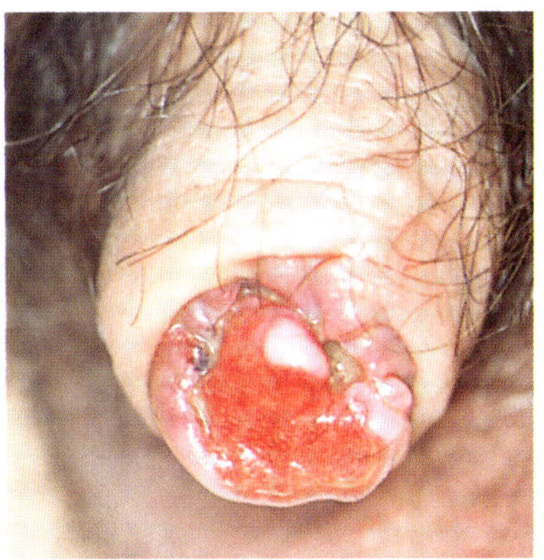

FIG. 89-36 *Papules forming a plaque with a central ulcer.*

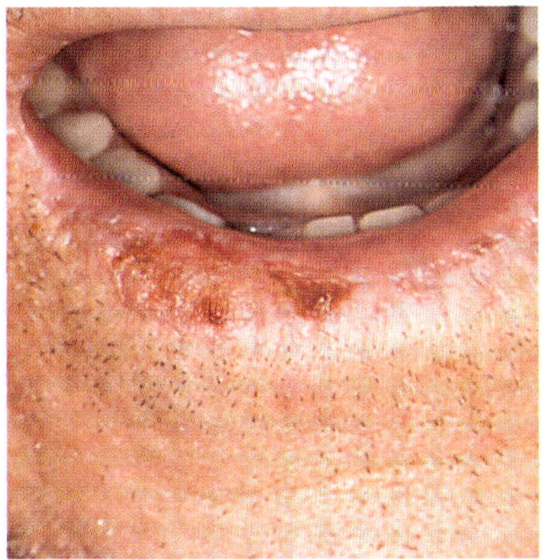

FIG. 89-37 *Incipient squamous-cell carcinoma manifested by whiteness, erosions, and crusts ("actinic cheilitis").*

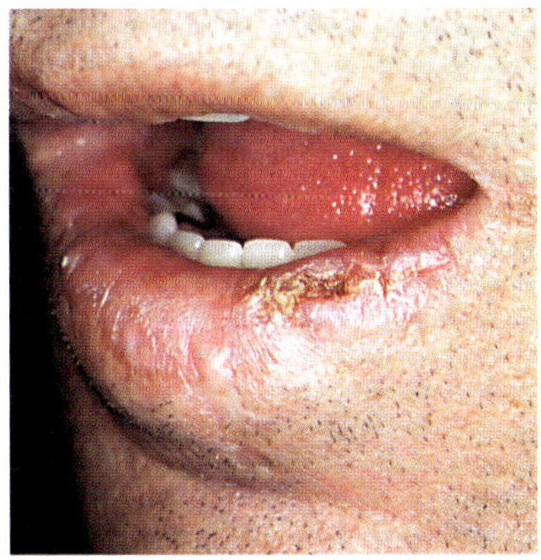

FIG. 89-38 *Keratotic ulcerated plaque of squamous-cell carcinoma on the lip.*

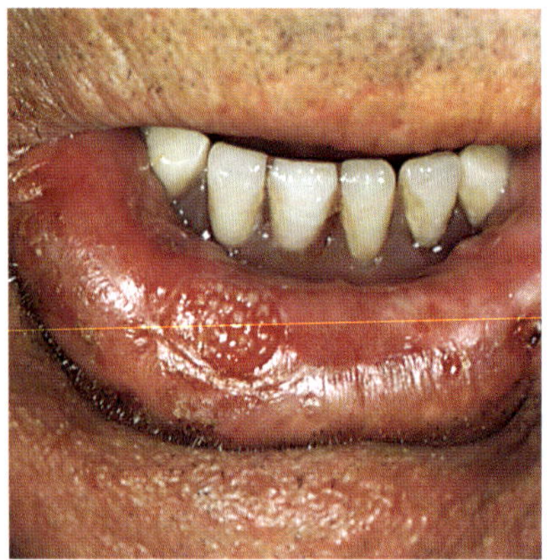

FIG. 89-39 *Squamous-cell carcinoma evidenced by whiteness, crusts, and deep ulcers.*

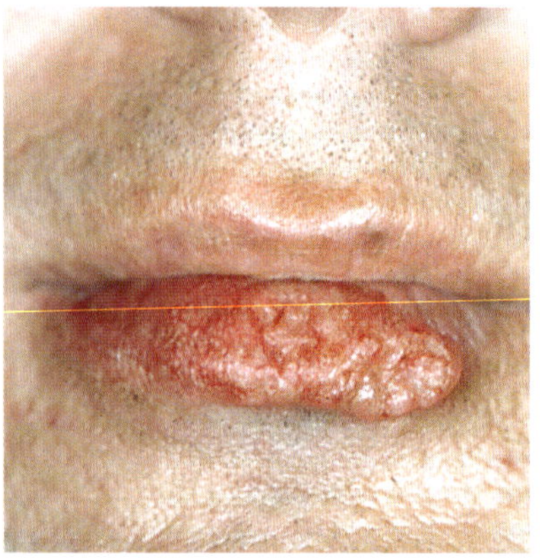

FIG. 89-40 *A plaque of squamous-cell carcinoma characterized by a markedly keratotic surface and by fissures.*

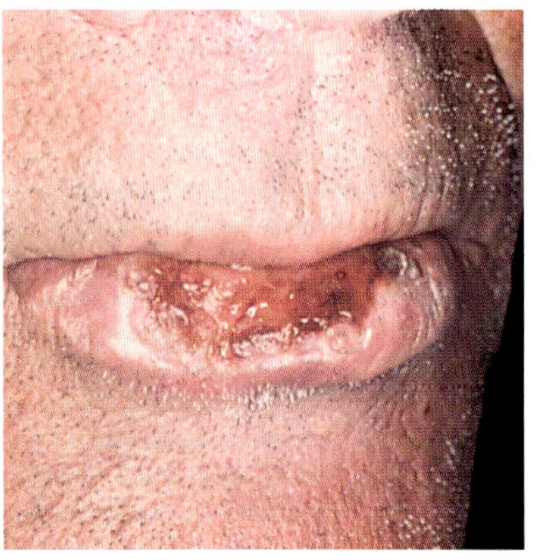

FIG. 89-41 *An ulcerated crusted squamous-cell carcinoma.*

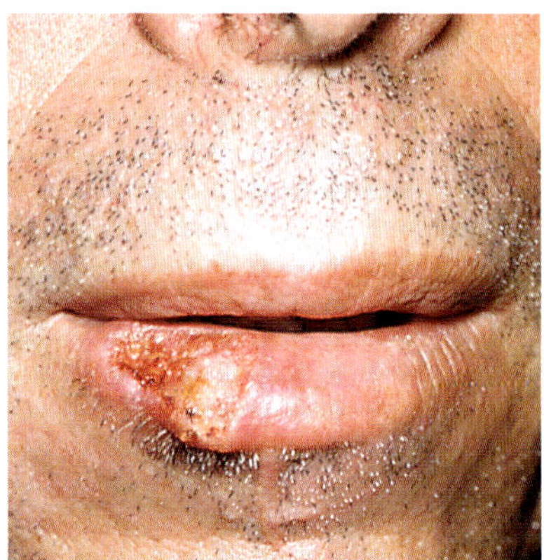

FIG. 89-42 *An ulcerated, crusted, keratotic squamous-cell carcinoma.*

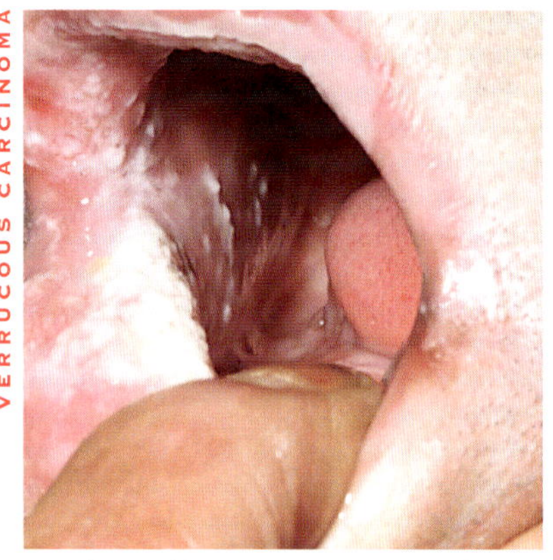

FIG. 89-43 *Verrucous carcinoma of the buccal mucosa (oral florid papillomatosis) at different stages.*

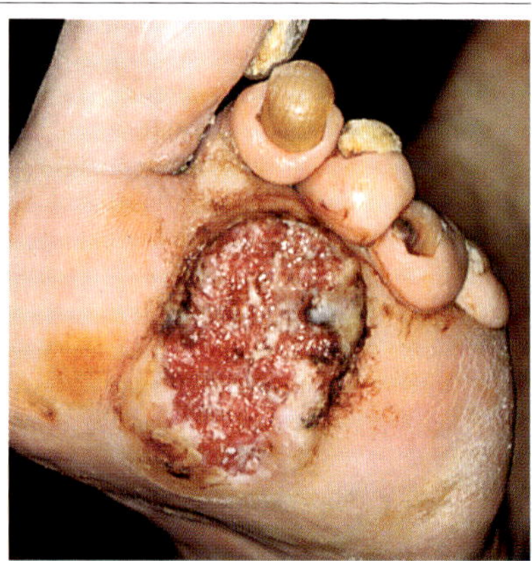

FIG. 89-44 *An ulcerated, crusted, papillated verrucous carcinoma on the sole (carcinoma cuniculatum).*

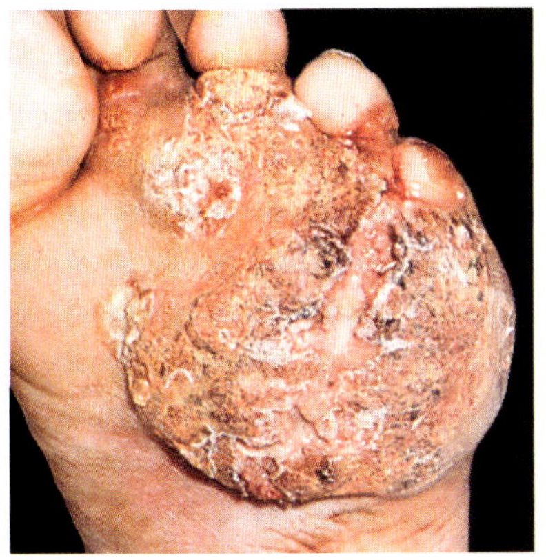

FIG. 89-45   *A verrucous carcinoma on the sole (carcinoma cuniculatum).*

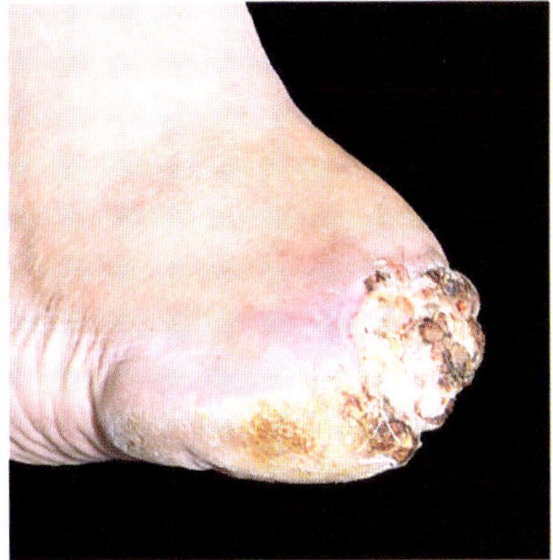

FIG. 89-46   *An ulcerated crusted tumor on a stump (verrucous carcinoma).*

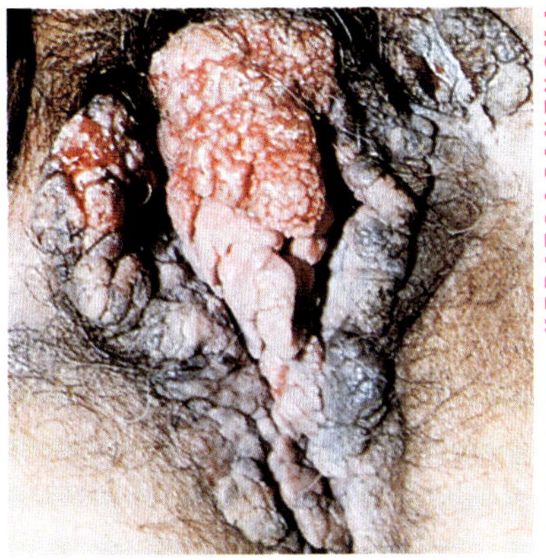

FIG. 89-47   *Cauliflower-like mass of verrucous carcinoma on the vulva and perianal region (giant condyloma).*

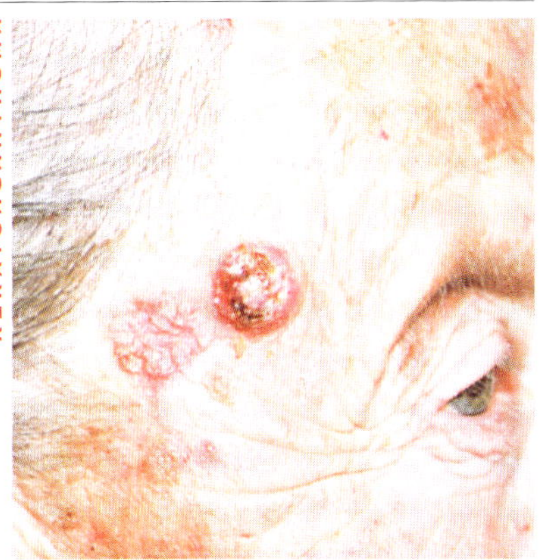

FIG. 89-48   *The tumor with a keratotic center is a keratoacanthoma. At its left is a plaque of Bowen's disease.*

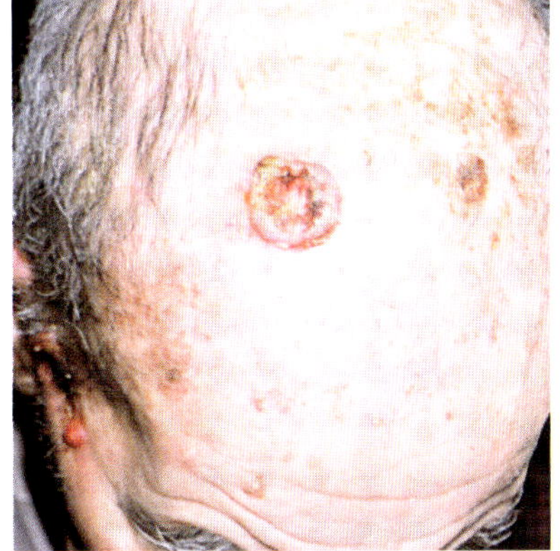

FIG. 89-49   *A tumor of keratoacanthoma with a central crater devoid of a keratotic plug is surrounded by solar keratoses.*

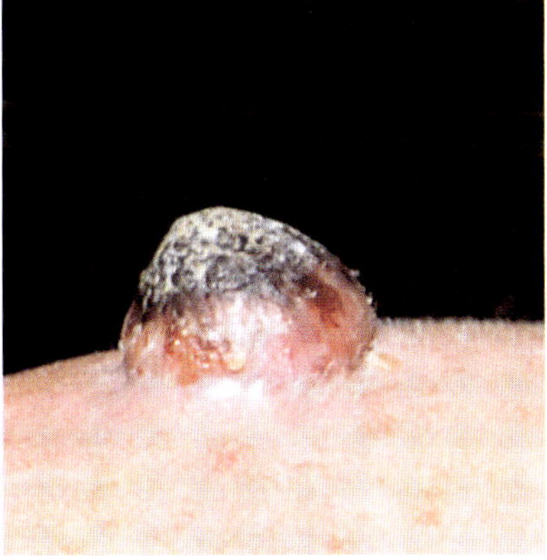

FIG. 89-50   *Rising from the center of the keratoacanthoma is a dome-shaped keratotic mass.*

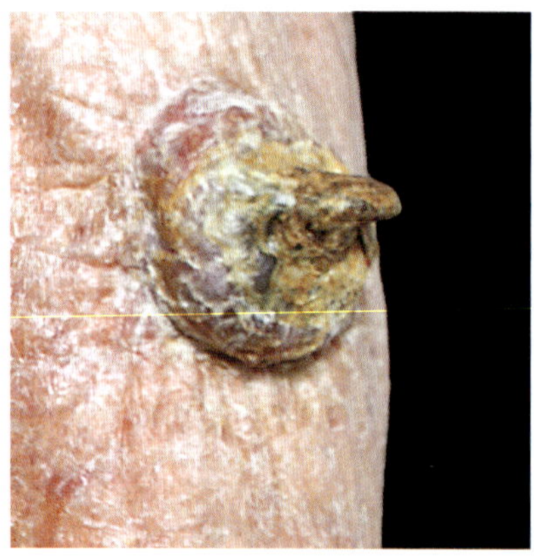

FIG. 89-51 *A keratoacanthoma surrounded by solar keratoses; two different types of squamous-cell carcinoma.*

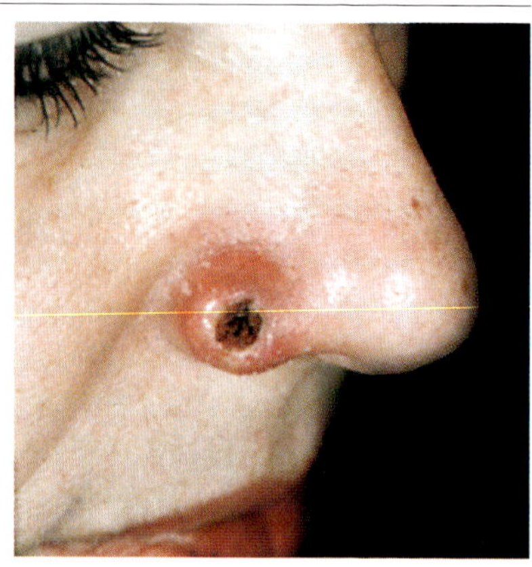

FIG. 89-52 *Dome-shaped nodule of keratoacanthomatous squamous-cell carcinoma with a central horn-filled crater.*

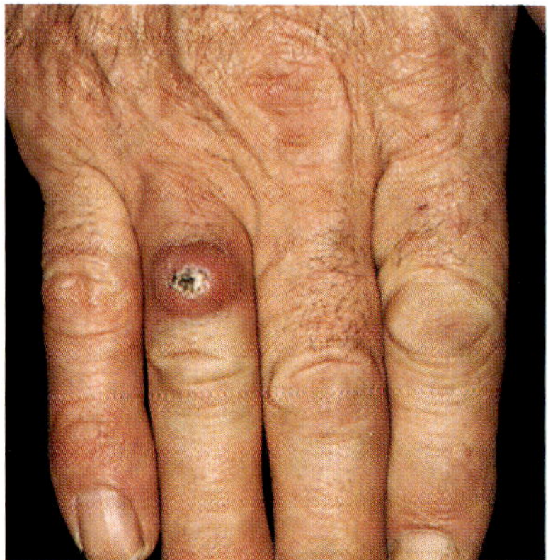

FIG. 89-53 *Dome-shaped keratoacanthoma with a central crater filled with horny material.*

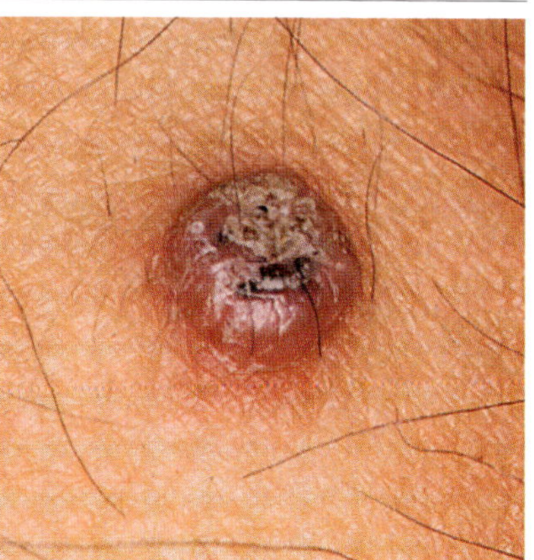

FIG. 89-54 *Dome-shaped keratoacanthoma punctuated by a central crater plugged with horny material.*

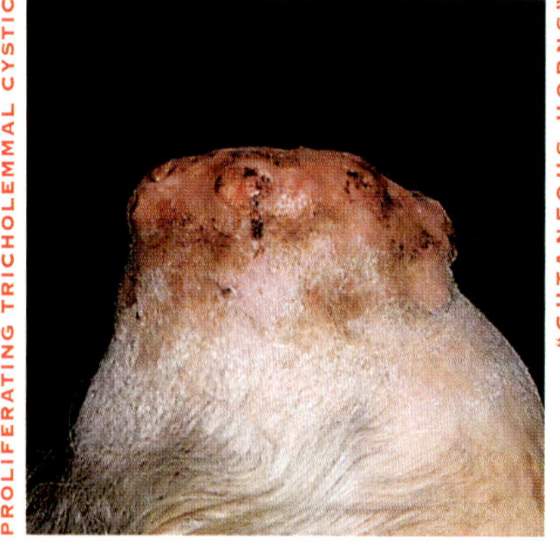

FIG. 89-55 *Fungating ulcerated example of proliferating tricholemmal cystic squamous-cell carcinoma.*

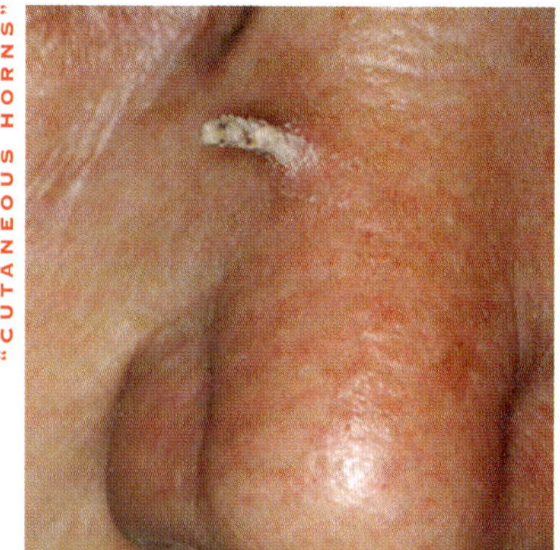

FIG. 89-56 *A superficial squamous-cell carcinoma (solar keratosis) produced the column of horn.*

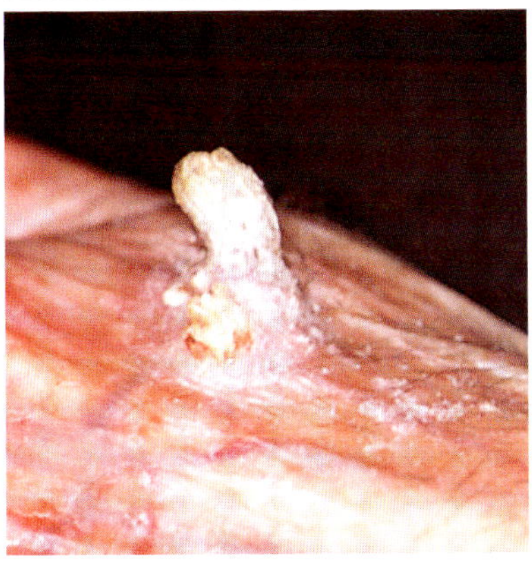

FIG. 89-57 *A squamous-cell carcinoma, solar keratotic type, manufactured the column of horn.*

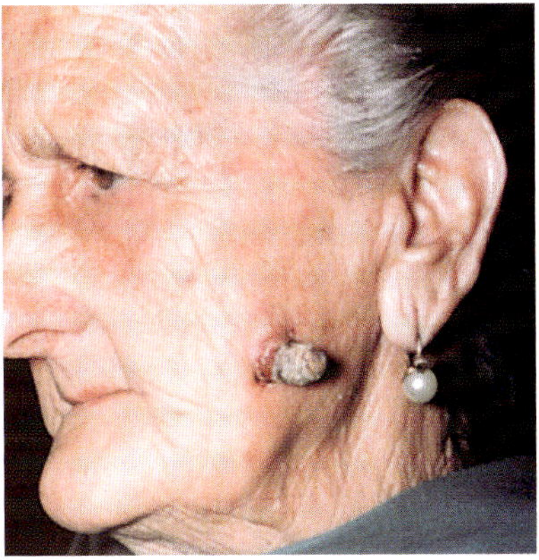

FIG. 89-58 *A column of horn represents the product of maturation of abnormal keratinocytes of a squamous-cell carcinoma.*

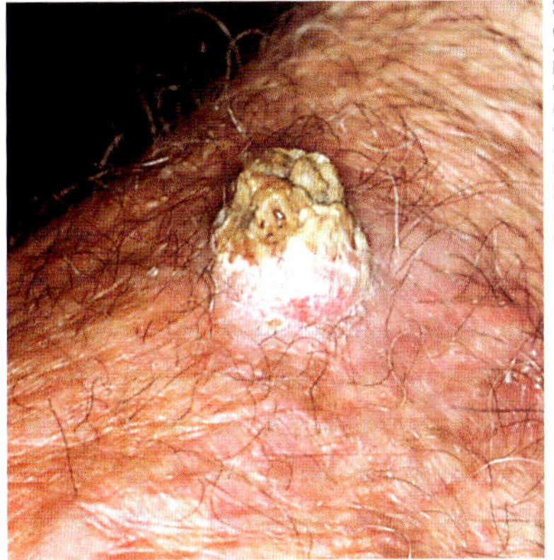

FIG. 89-59 *A stubby column of horn sits atop the rest of a squamous-cell carcinoma, presumably solar keratotic type.*

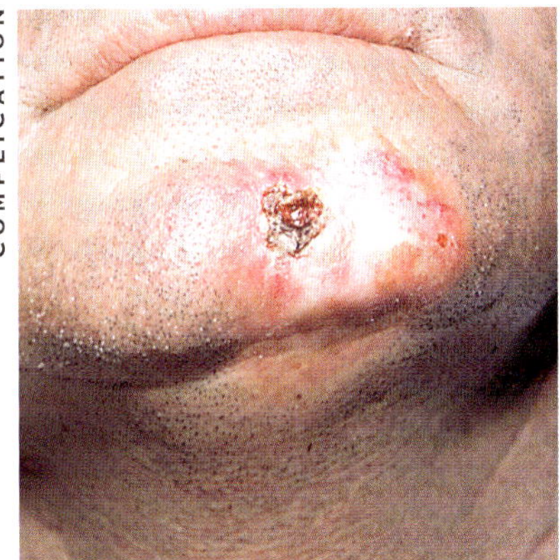

FIG. 89-60 *Squamous-cell carcinoma that developed in an atrophic scar caused by radiation therapy.*

COURSE There are different types of squamous-cell carcinoma in skin, but each of them (except for the proliferating tricholemmal cystic type) is recognized first as a small keratotic macule or papule that usually is keratotic. In time it becomes a larger keratotic papule and, sometimes, a keratotic plaque, keratotic nodule, or keratotic tumor. Very large lesions may ulcerate. The vast majority of squamous-cell carcinomas in skin are solar keratoses, and those keratotic papules tend to remain a very superficial squamous-cell carcinoma for the lifetime of the person who bears them. Sometimes, however, and unpredictably, a solar keratosis or Bowen's disease becomes vastly thicker and metastasizes.

INTEGRATION: UNIFYING CONCEPT The most common type of cutaneous squamous-cell carcinoma is solar keratosis, analogues of which are radiation keratosis, arsenical keratosis, and actinic "cheilitis." Another type of squamous-cell carcinoma in skin is Bowen's disease, and its analogue is bowenoid papulosis. Erythroplasia of Queyrat is merely Bowen's disease on a mucous membrane or a mucocutaneous surface. Each of the conditions just mentioned is an authentic squamous-cell carcinoma, akin to superficial basal-cell carcinoma. All clinicians and histopathologists acknowledge that superficial basal-cell carcinoma is a true basal-cell carcinoma (the name tells that!), but few clinicians and histopathologists are prepared to accept the fact that solar keratosis is just as much a squamous-cell carcinoma as Bowen's disease is. The latter neoplasm is understood to be a squamous-cell carcinoma because the synonym for it is "squamous-cell carcinoma in situ."

The term "solar keratosis" neither connotes nor denotes squamous-cell carcinoma, but that neoplasm, nonetheless, is a squamous-cell carcinoma, albeit a superficial one. Solar keratosis is not a premalignancy and does not "convert" or "transform" into squamous-cell carcinoma; it is a squamous-cell carcinoma from the outset. If left to its own devices, solar keratosis may extend progressively deeper into the dermis and when that happens, all pathologists, universally, then designate it squamous-cell carcinoma. No boundary exists between solar keratosis and squamous-cell carcinoma because solar keratosis *is* a squamous-cell carcinoma.

What has just been written for solar keratosis applies equally to radiation keratosis, arsenical keratosis, Bowen's disease, and bowenoid papulosis. The last enumerated is simply a condyloma acuminatum in which the hyperplasia induced by papillomavirus has progressed to malignant neoplasia, to wit, squamous-cell carcinoma in situ. Bowenoid papulosis has the silhouette of a condyloma and the cytologic features of squamous-cell carcinoma.

The cytologic attributes of squamous-cell carcinoma are nuclei of keratinocytes that are crowded, large, and pleomorphic, individual keratinocytes that are cornified abnormally (dyskeratotic), and groups of keratinocytes that mature abnormally in the form of either parakeratosis in foci in the stratum corneum or as "horn pearls" within dermal aggregations of the neoplasm. Using these criteria, solar keratosis, radiation keratosis, arsenical keratosis, actinic "cheilitis," Bowen's disease, and bowenoid papulosis fulfill requirements for diagnosis of squamous-cell carcinoma.

In addition to the types of squamous-cell carcinoma already mentioned, there are other cutaneous expressions of squamous-cell carcinoma, to wit, verrucous carcinomas, keratoacanthomas, and proliferating tricholemmal cystic squamous-cell carcinomas. The clinical expressions of verrucous carcinoma are giant condyloma of Buschke and Löwenstein in the anogenital region, carcinoma cuniculatum on the sole or palm, and florid oral papillomatosis in the oral cavity or on other mucous membranes. They are merely different names for the same process on different sites. Each of those neoplasms is exo-endophytic, and the endophytic component is bulbous. The cytologic features at the periphery of bulbous aggregations are typical of squamous-cell carcinoma.

Keratoacanthomas are a special type of squamous-cell carcinoma. The type called "solitary" (but which may be multiple) occurs on skin injured by the effects of sunlight and is characterized by rapid growth and often by involution in months in the absence of therapy. It has a characteristic crateriform appearance as a consequence of dilation of contiguous infundibula that are filled with corneocytes. The squamous-cell carcinoma seems to derive from infundibular keratinocytes. The "solitary" kind of keratoacanthoma is a squamous-cell carcinoma, not only for reasons that pertain to architectural and cytologic characteristics, but because, rarely, the neoplasm metastasizes (especially in persons who are immunosuppressed).

Subungual keratoacanthoma is wholly unrelated to "solitary" keratoacanthoma, being unassociated as it is with follicles. It also has a crateriform appearance and it burrows, slowly but surely, through the subungual soft tissues and often into bone of the distal phalanx. Other types of keratoacanthoma are the eruptive, the familial, and the gigantic.

What for decades has been called proliferating tricholemmal cyst is not a cyst or a benign neoplasm, but a type of squamous-cell carcinoma (proliferating tricholemmal cystic squamous-cell carcinoma). Not surprisingly, that distinctive type of squamous-cell carcinoma has capability for metastasis, which it sometimes exercises.

In sum, there are several different types of cutaneous squamous-cell carcinoma, and each has its own diagnostic features, clinically and histopathologically, and biologic characteristics. Each can be identified for what it is by those particular features. When squamous-cell carcinoma no longer is superficial, it often loses its peculiar character and then may be designated "squamous-cell carcinoma," unmodified. Had such a squamous-cell carcinoma been examined histopathologically at an earlier stage, its specificity could have been recognized, for example, solar keratotic type, Bowen's type, or verrucous type. The overwhelming majority of squamous-cell carcinomas are solar keratotic type, that is, they begin as what is trivialized as solar keratosis.

THERAPY Topical 5-fluorouracil, curettage, cryosurgery, laser ablation, or photodynamic therapy are satisfactory for solar keratosis, Bowen's disease, and bowenoid papulosis, and complete surgical excision, including Mohs' micrographic surgery, are indicated for nodular and tumorous expressions of squamous-cell carcinoma. In older persons, radiotherapy may be given for nodules and tumors.

DEFINITION Alterations in the skin and subcutaneous fat, such as pigmentation and induration, secondary to the effects of long-term stasis, and ulcers that occur on the lower part of the legs as a consequence of the effects, combined, of incompetent valves of veins and thrombosis within veins situated deep.

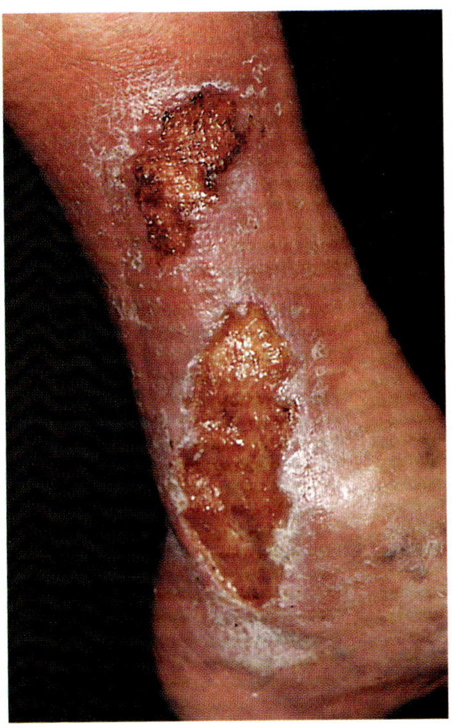

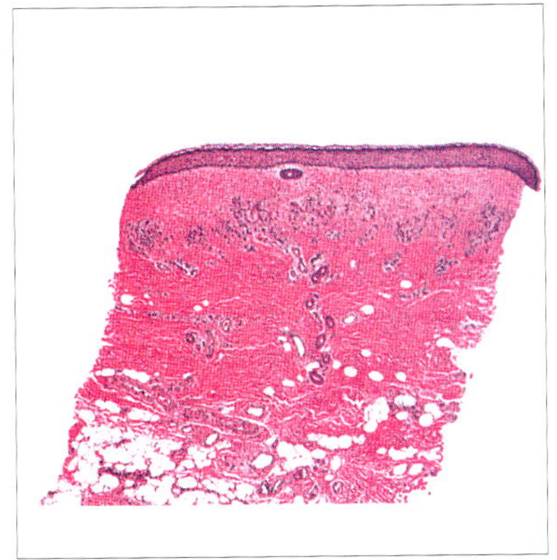

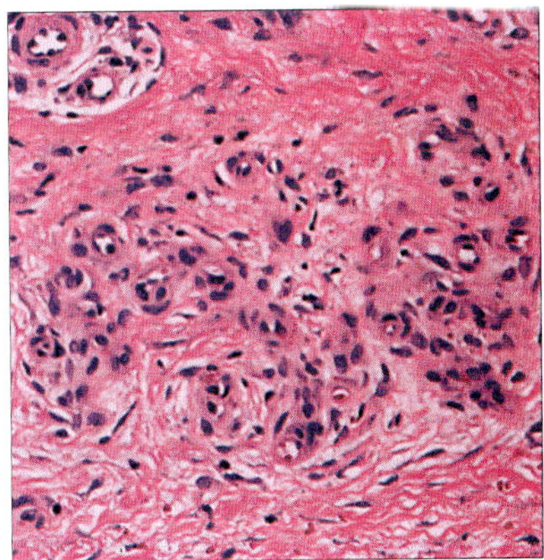

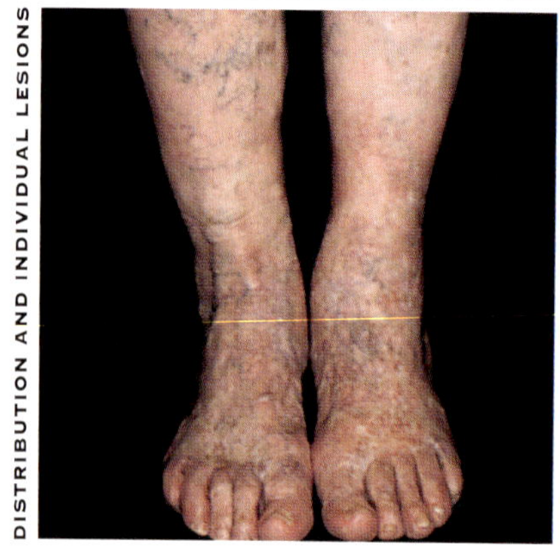
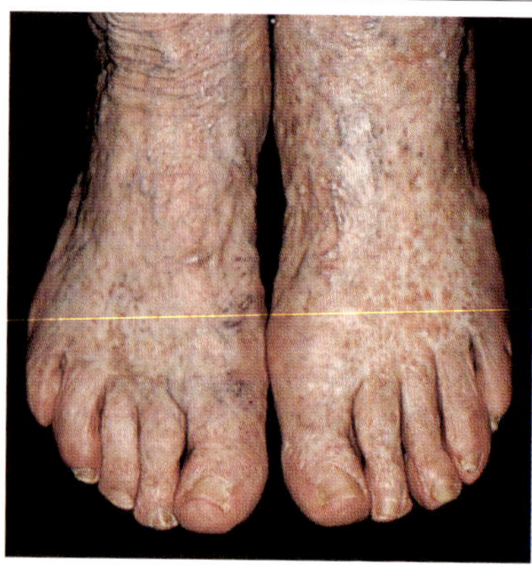

FIG. 90-1 (A, B) *Varicosities, mottled pigmentation, and numerous stellate-shaped white scars.*

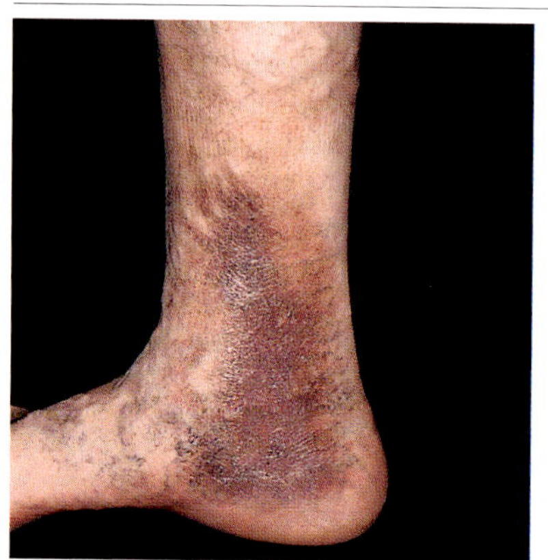
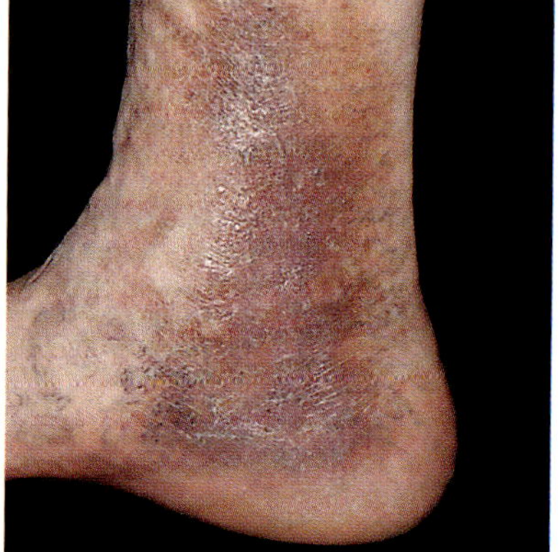

FIG. 90-2 (A, B) *Mottled pigmentation and off-white scars.*

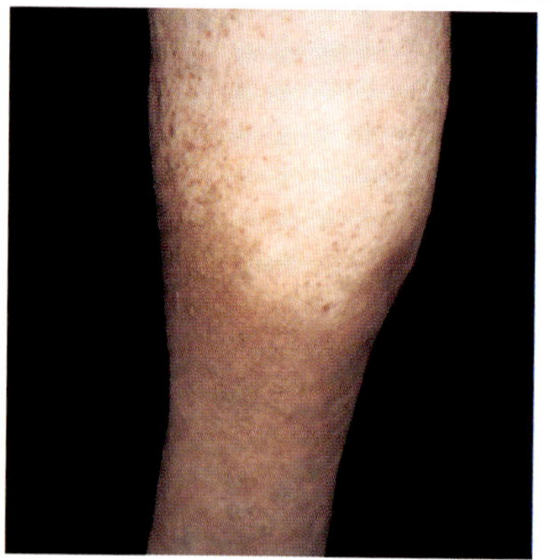
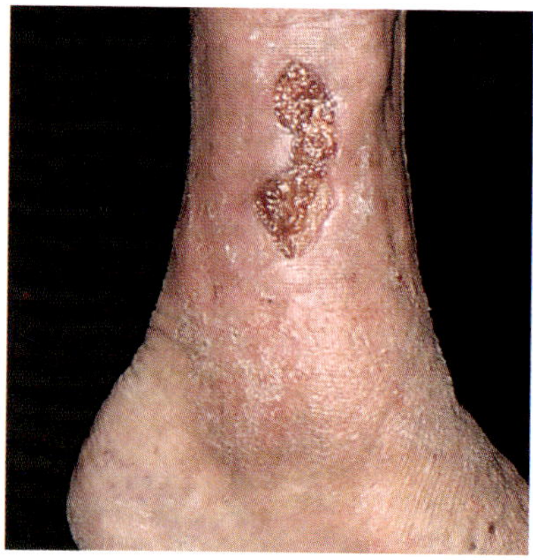

FIG. 90-3 *Diffuse pigmentation and induration (hypodermitis sclerodermiformis; lipodermatosclerosis).*

FIG. 90-4 *Stasis changes and an ulcer surrounded by induration.*

COURSE The first evidence of changes in the skin secondary to the effects of stasis are seen in the region of malleoli. At first there are purpuric macules that, over time, undergo characteristic changes in color, from purple to yellow to brown. As compromise in venous return continues and steadily worsens, more and more mottled pigmented lesions appear on the leg, first in the immediate vicinity of malleoli, and then progressively upward, sometimes extending to near the knee. After many years, pigmentation is extensive. When insufficiency of veins is sufficiently great, ulcers appear, and, in time, those defects usually heal with scars.

INTEGRATION: UNIFYING CONCEPT Because of the posture of human beings, namely, upright on two legs, it is inevitable that in the course of decades veins in the legs become progressively compromised and are unable to fulfill optimally their role in helping to return blood to the heart. As a consequence of that decline, erythrocytes leak into the dermis and, at first, the changes are manifested as mere purpuric macules. As damage to veins increases, more and more erythrocytes are lost into the dermis. Purpuric macules are joined by pigmentary abnormalities that assume a reticulated and mottled appearance. If, in time, veins are altered further by progressive incompetence of valves and by thromboses, ulcers in the skin are inevitable. Those defects heal with difficulty and with scars. Bacterial infection of the skin in the immediate vicinity of the ulcers may produce recurrent cellulitic changes that, in the course of years, resolve as brawny induration.

Unless the compromise of deep veins is corrected surgically, changes of stasis progress to involve much of the leg, and venous ulcers become more numerous and more refractory to healing. Some fail to heal.

The photomicrographs shown at the beginning of this chapter display signs of severe changes of stasis, namely, a markedly increased number of thick-walled venules lined by endothelial cells with a plump nucleus. The section of tissue comes from a biopsy specimen taken at some distance from the ulcers.

THERAPY Reduction of edema is accomplished by compression of the leg. Occlusive permeable biosynthetic wound dressings are helpful. Antiseptics or antibiotics may be used topically if there are signs of infection. If necessary, grafts (punch or meshed) should be applied.

DEFINITION An inflammatory process expressed clinically by markedly edematous acuminate papules and edematous plaques situated mostly on the face, upper part of the trunk, and arms, especially the hands, and often accompanied by fever and leukocytosis. It may be idiopathic or a manifestation of a systemic disorder, such as acute myelogenous leukemia.

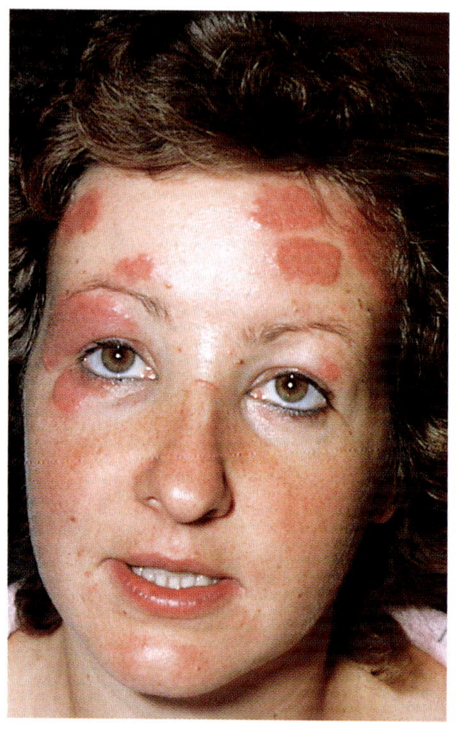

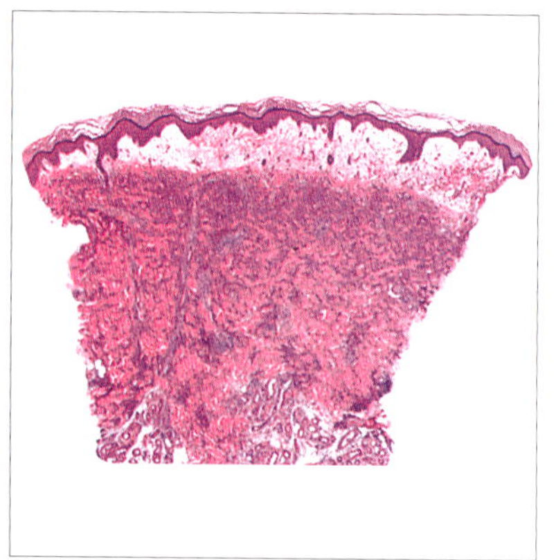

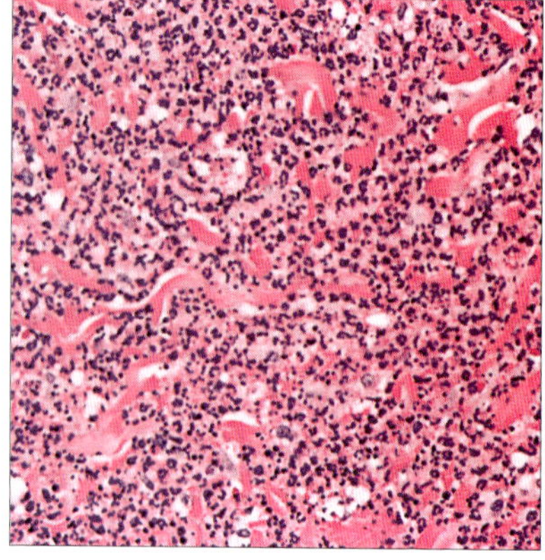

DISTRIBUTION

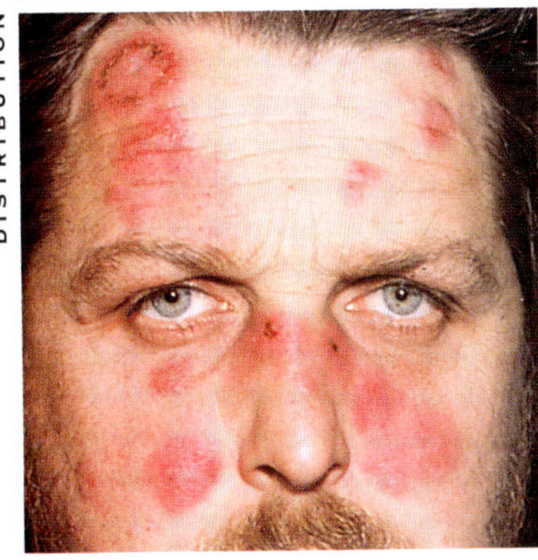

FIG. 91-1 *Papules and plaques, some of which are crusted.*

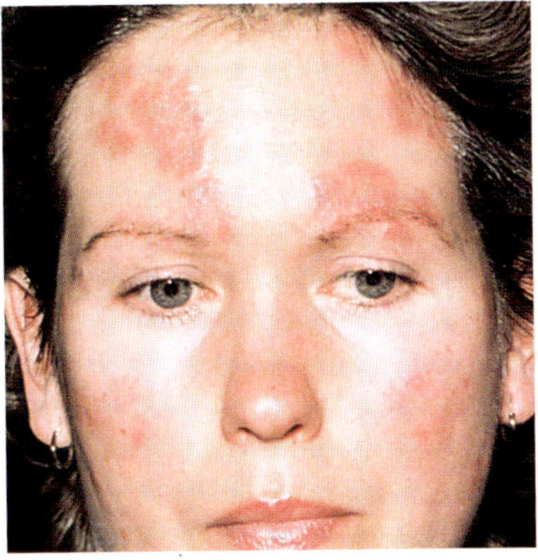

FIG. 91-2 *Macules, papules, and plaques with an elevated border.*

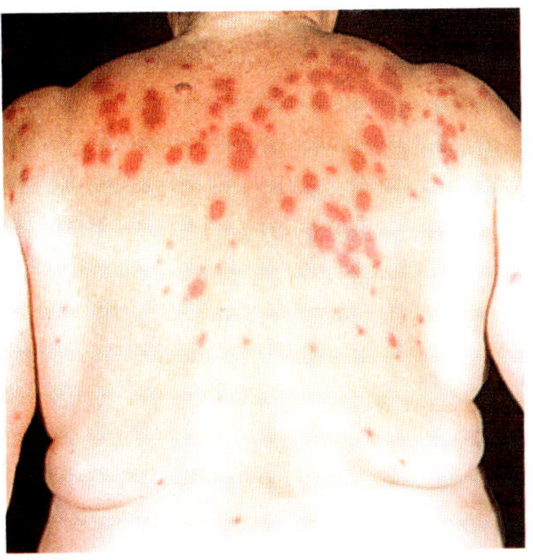

FIG. 91-3 *Papules and plaques, some of which have become confluent.*

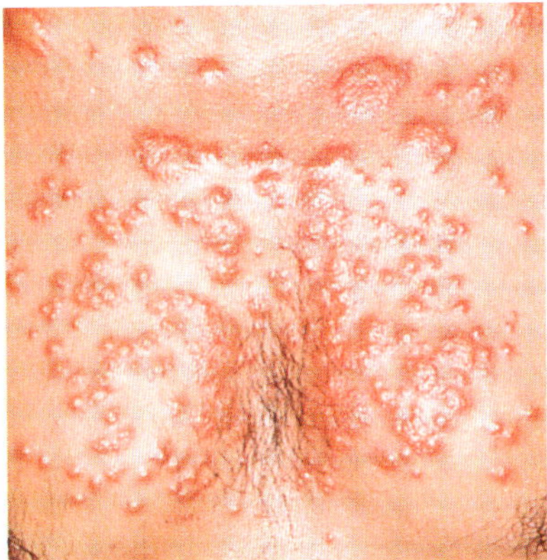

FIG. 91-4 *Markedly edematous acuminate papules and edematous plaques.*

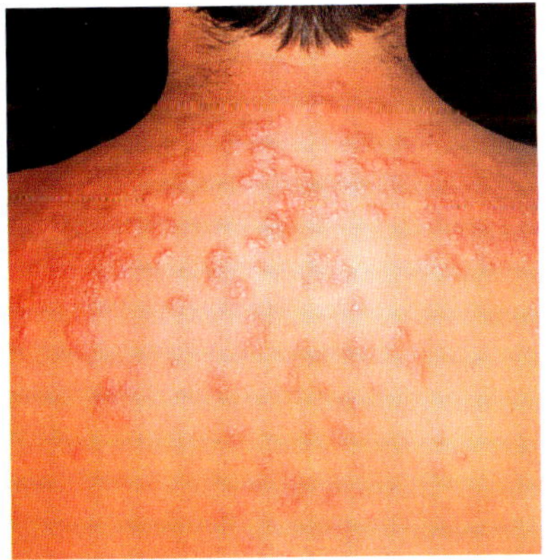

FIG. 91-5 *Papules and plaques made up of numerous closely-set papules; some plaques have become confluent.*

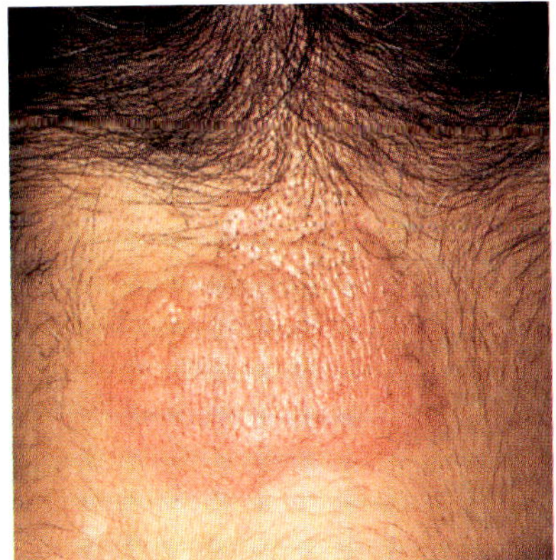

FIG. 91-6 *Plaque with a slightly scalloped border in a patient with acute myelogenous leukemia.*

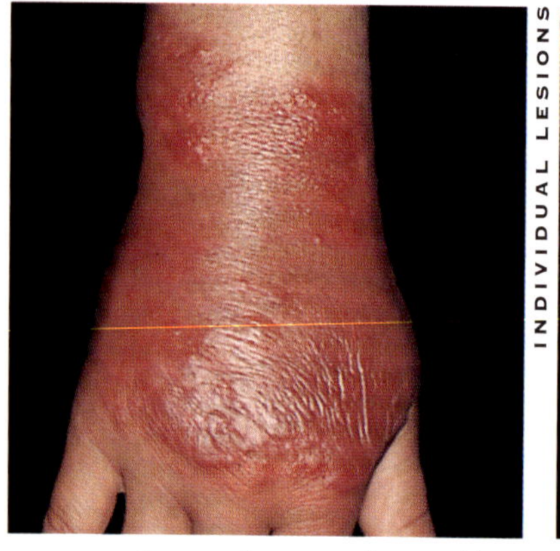

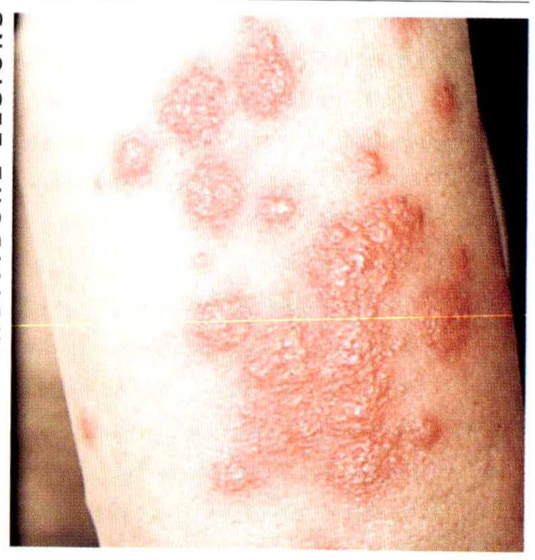

FIG. 91-7 *Large, edematous plaque with an incipient blister and, at the periphery, discrete papules.*

FIG. 91-8 *Markedly edematous well-circumscribed papules and plaques.*

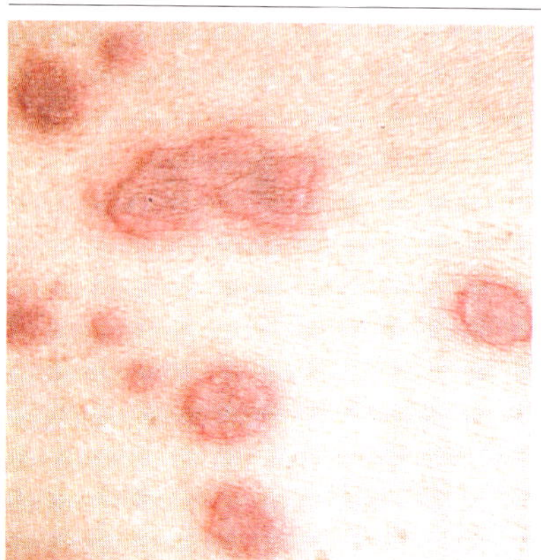

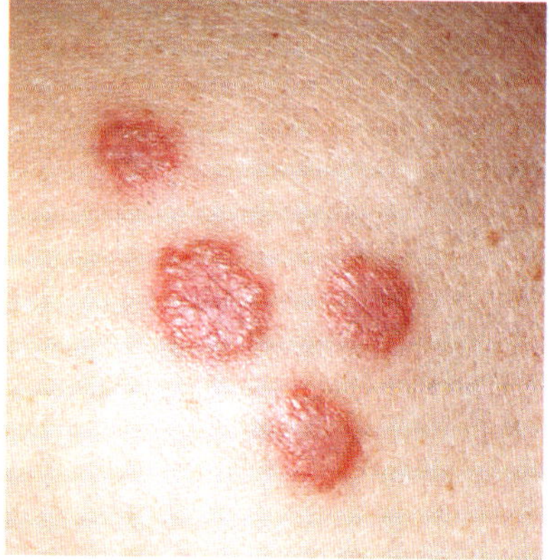

FIG. 91-9 (A, B) *Edematous papules and plaques, the latter sporting an elevated border. The surface of some papules is mammillated.*

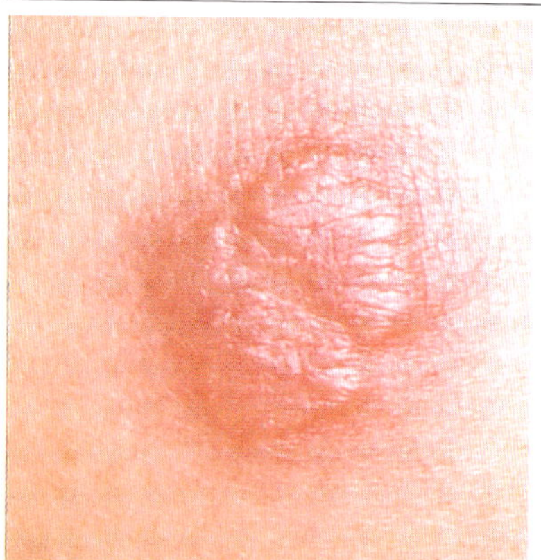

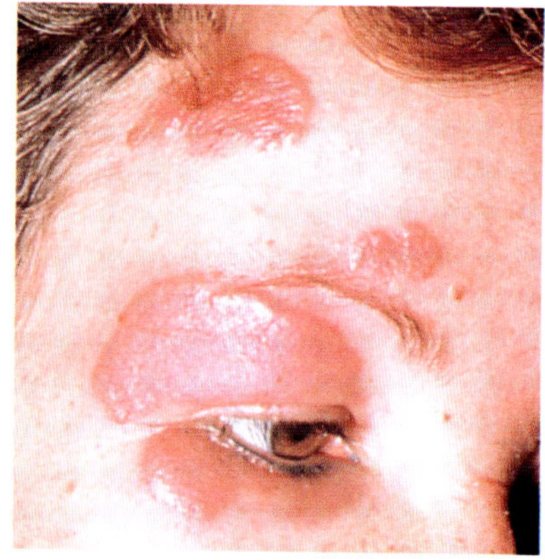

FIG. 91-10 *Edematous plaque composed of confluent papules.*

FIG. 91-11 *Sharply circumscribed edematous plaques.*

ADJUNCTIVE DIAGNOSTIC TESTS Hematologic investigations are worthwhile in order to rule out an associated blood disorder.

COURSE After an evanescent macular stage, erythematous papules come into being and they tend to eventuate in erythematous edematous plaques. The plaques are formed by marked edema in the upper part of the dermis and by nodular and diffuse infiltrates of neutrophils in at least the upper half of the reticular dermis. Extensive nuclear "dust" of neutrophils usually is present concurrently. The histopathologic findings in a plaque of Sweet's syndrome are more or less the same, irrespective of the cause of it. An exception, however, is certain lesions of the syndrome that occur as a consequence of acute myelogenous leukemia. In those lesions, in addition to innumerable neutrophils, there are also abnormal myeloblasts. Plaques of Sweet's syndrome slowly become less edematous, begin to wane in weeks, and disappear completely in months.

INTEGRATION: UNIFYING CONCEPT Sweet's syndrome, like pyoderma gangrenosum, erythema multiforme, erythema nodosum, and allergic vasculitis, is a distinctive morphologic pattern, clinically and histopathologically, and one that nearly always signifies the existence of a process that underlies it, such as ulcerative colitis, rheumatoid arthritis, acute myelogenous leukemia, and, episodically, lymphoma. Just as a clinician or histopathologist cannot look at lesions of erythema multiforme or allergic vasculitis and, on the basis of the morphologic changes alone, infer the cause of them, so too it is for Sweet's syndrome. Only in those lesions that are accompanied by myeloblasts of acute myelogenous leukemia can a cause be identified by morphologic changes alone, that is, by conventional microscopy.

THERAPY Systemic corticosteroids are the treatment of choice, but dapsone, indomethacin, and aspirin are also effective in some patients.

DEFINITION An inflammatory process, caused by the spirochete Treponema pallidum, that tends to evolve through three stages, namely, primary (typified usually by a solitary chancre), secondary (characterized by widespread macules and papules on skin and mucous membranes in conjunction with signs and symptoms of systemic disease), and tertiary (manifested by gummas in the skin and destructive lesions also in the bones, eyes, brain, and elsewhere, resulting in debilitation and often death).

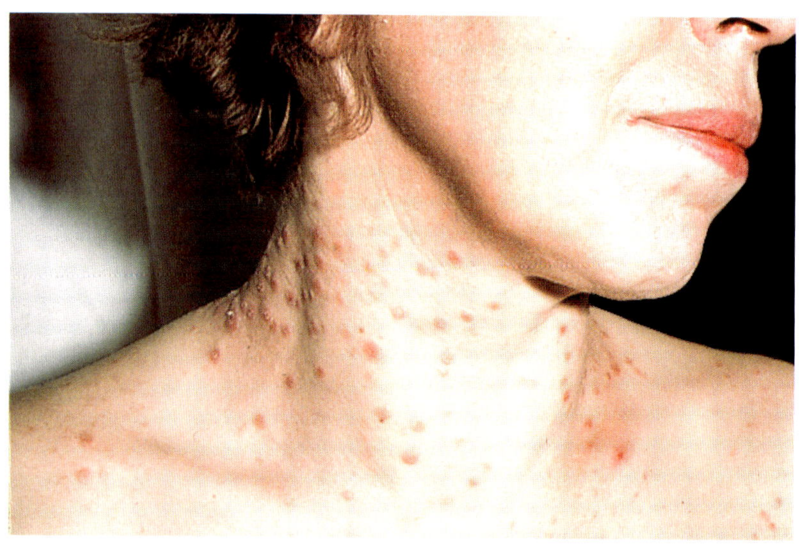

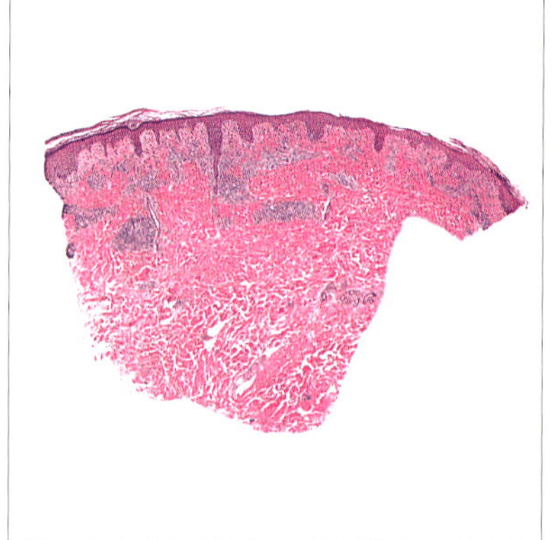

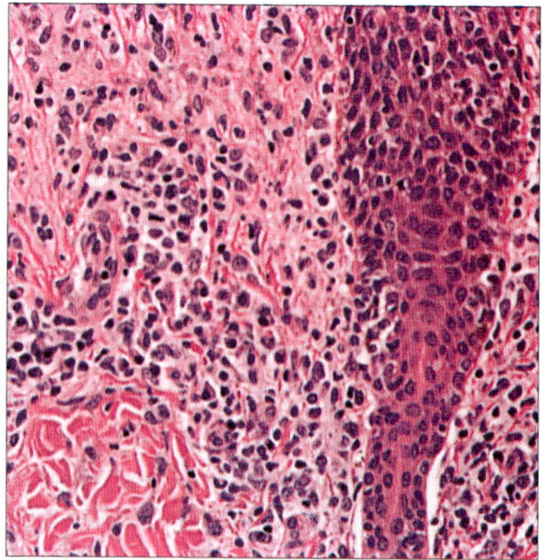

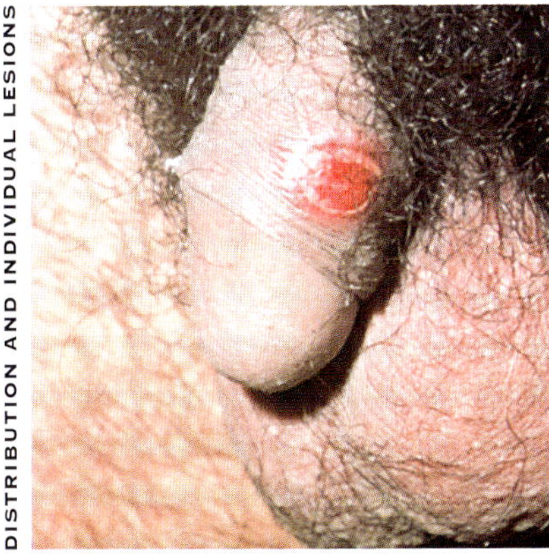

FIG. 92-1 *Chancre.*

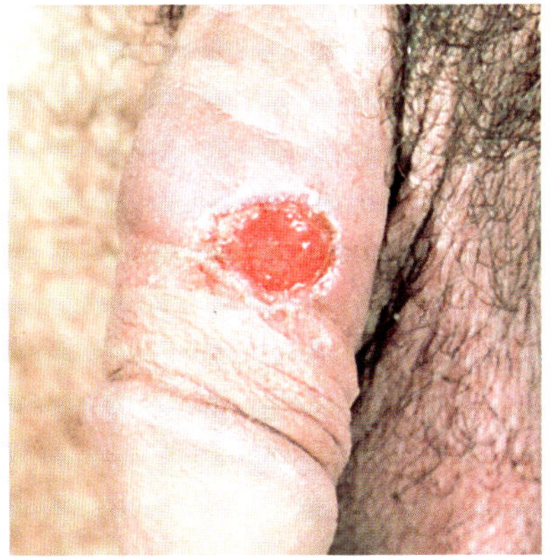

FIG. 92-2 *Chancre.*

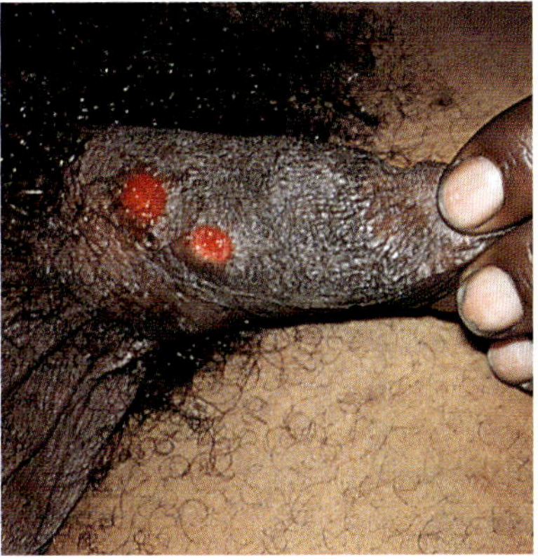

FIG. 92-3 *Multiple chancres.*

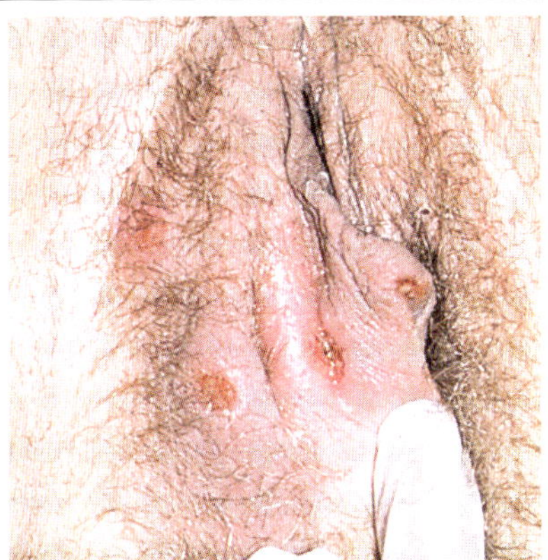

FIG. 92-4 *Several chancres.*

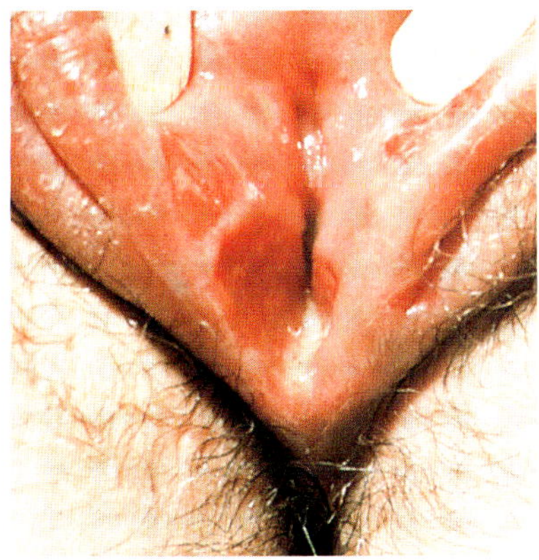

FIG. 92-5 *"Kissing" chancres.*

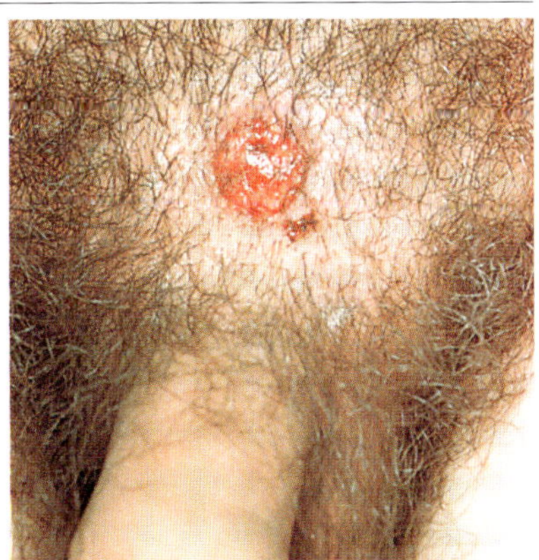

FIG. 92-6 *Chancre.*

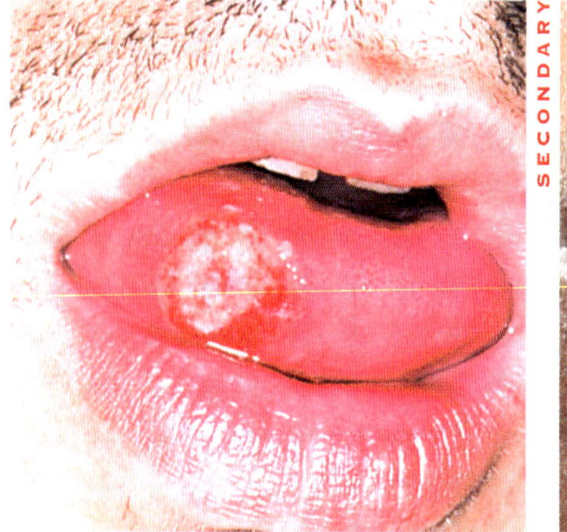

FIG. 92-7 *Chancre on the tongue.*

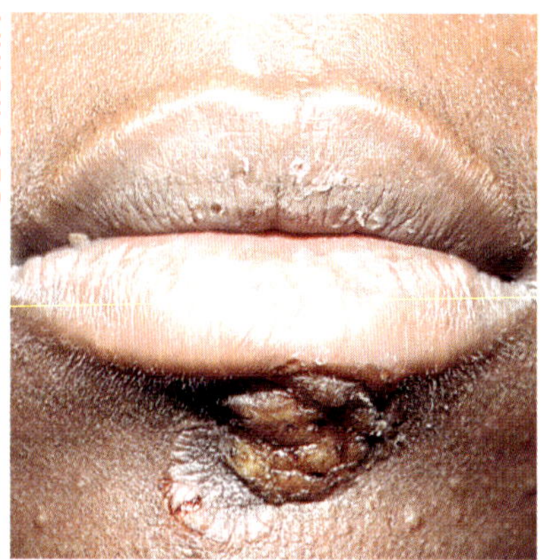

FIG. 92-8 *Smooth-surfaced papules, some in the form of a ring and some in clusters in a multilobulate nodule.*

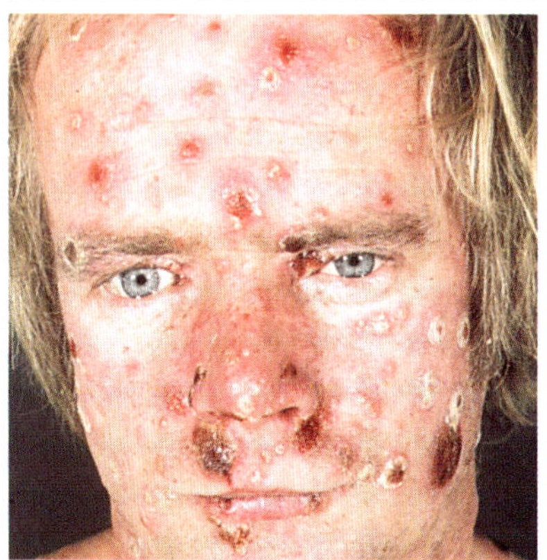

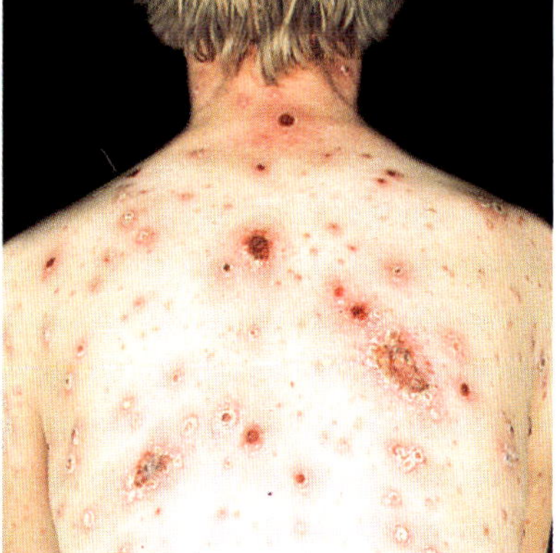

FIG. 92-9 (A, B) *Scaly and crusted papules and plaques.*

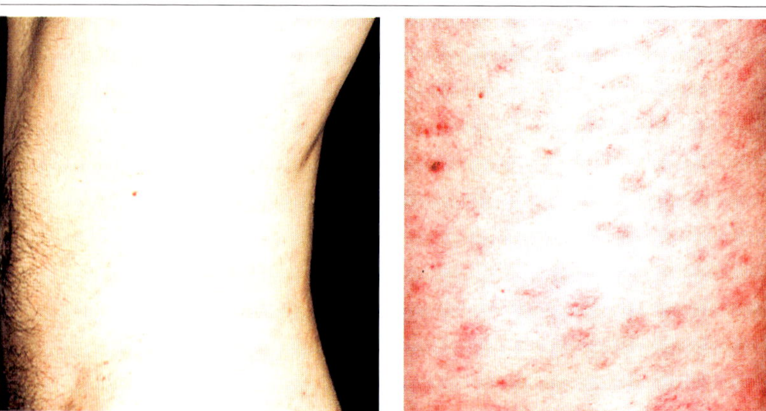

FIG. 92-10 (A, B) *Widespread macules and papules.*

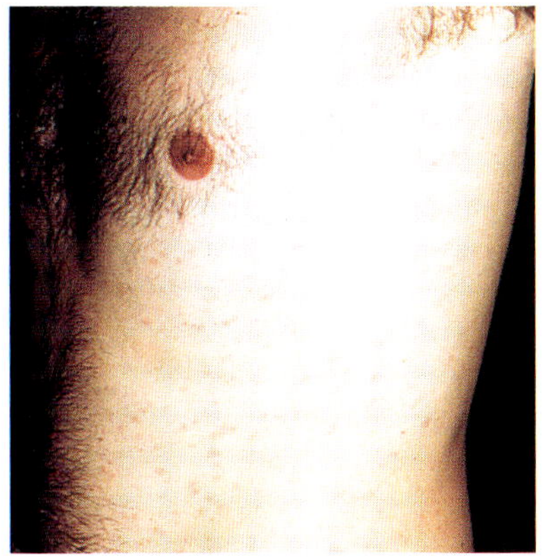

FIG. 92-11 *Widespread subtle macules and papules.*

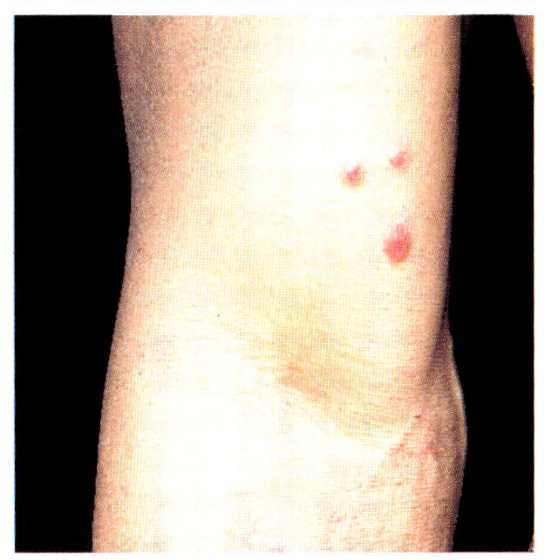

FIG. 92-12 *Discrete papules.*

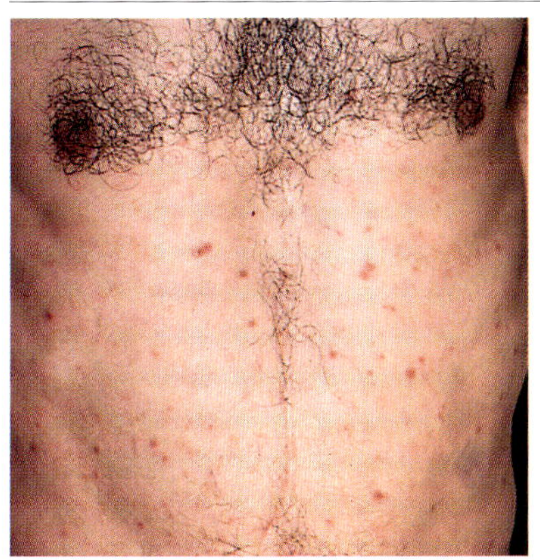

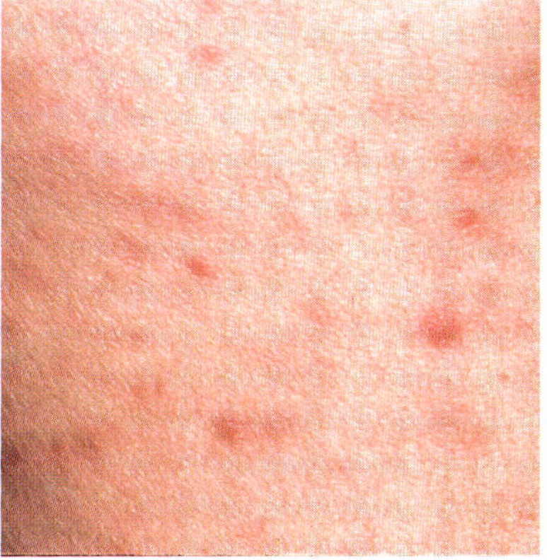

FIG. 92-13 (A, B) *Smooth and scaly papules of late secondary syphilis.*

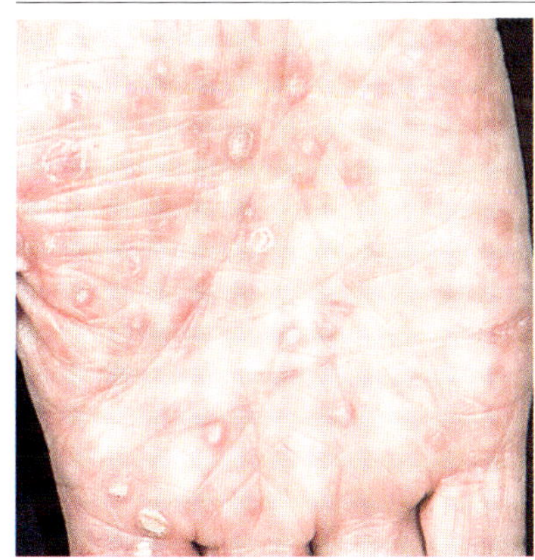

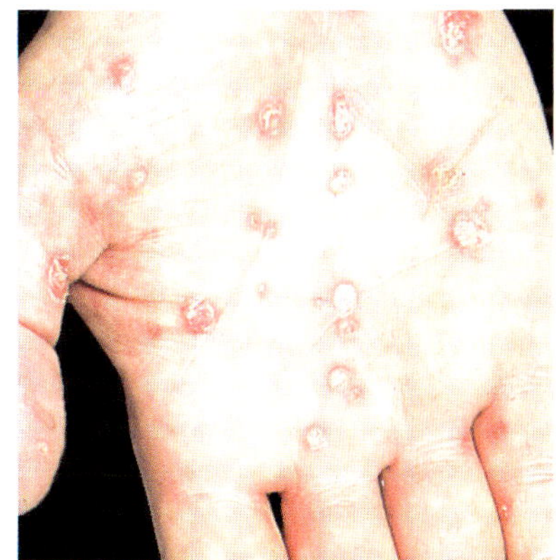

FIG. 92-14 *Macules and both smooth and scaly papules. Some of the scales are in the shape of a collarette.*

FIG. 92-15 *Scaly papules typical of secondary syphilis.*

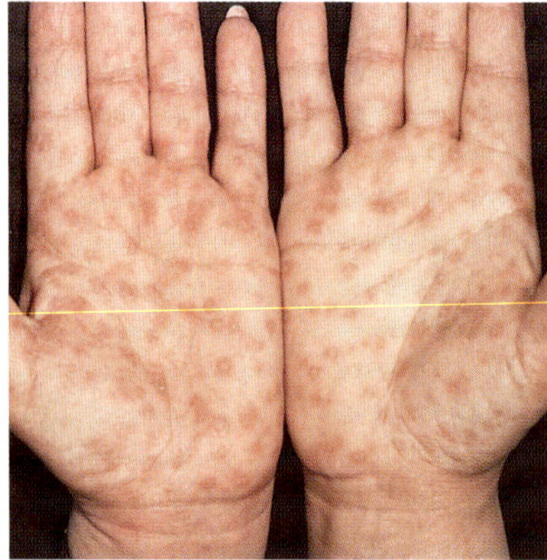

FIG. 92-16 *Discrete scaly papules distributed symmetrically on the palms (and soles).*

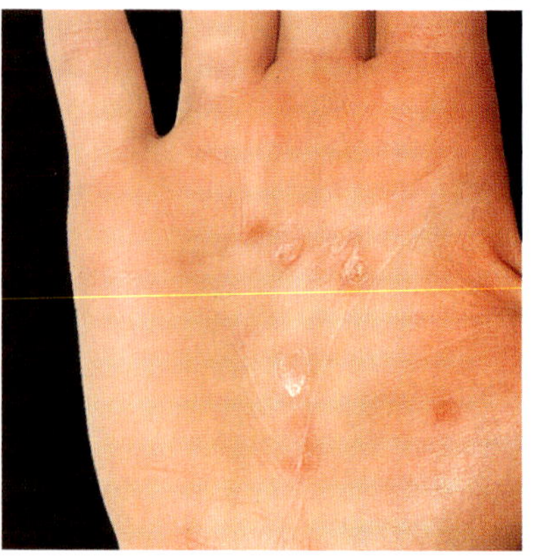

FIG. 92-17 *Lichenoid scaly papules.*

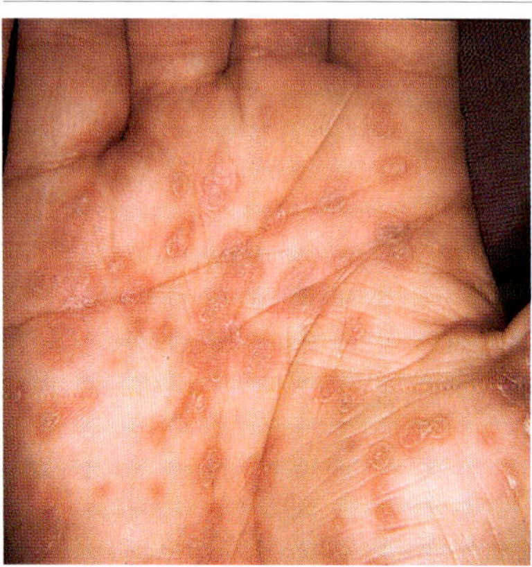

FIG. 92-18 *Scaly papules.*

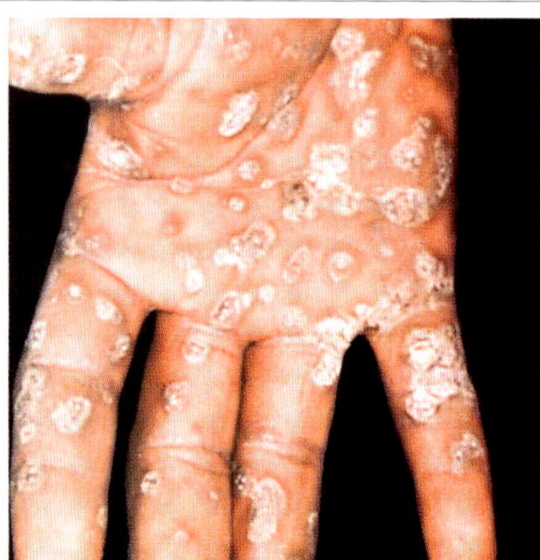

FIG. 92-19 *Keratotic papules and plaques.*

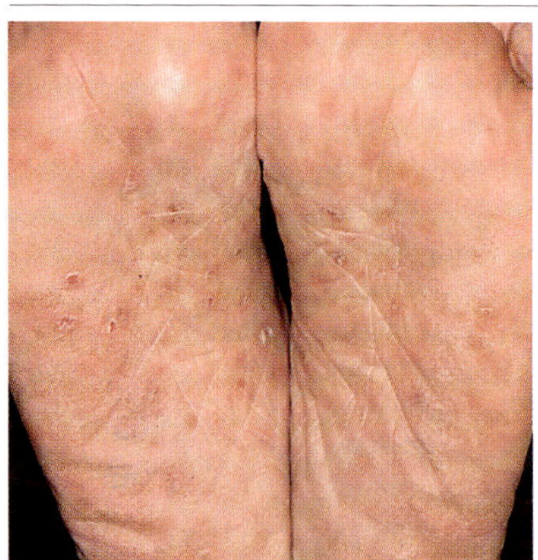

FIG. 92-20 *Smooth-surfaced papules in company with scaly papules.*

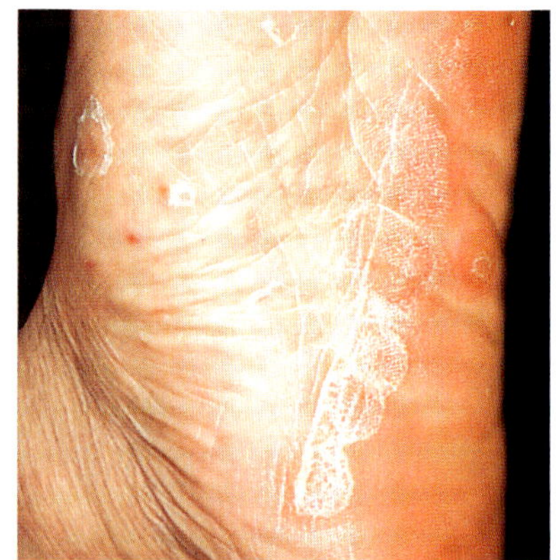

FIG. 92-21 *Scaly papules and plaques in annular configuration.*

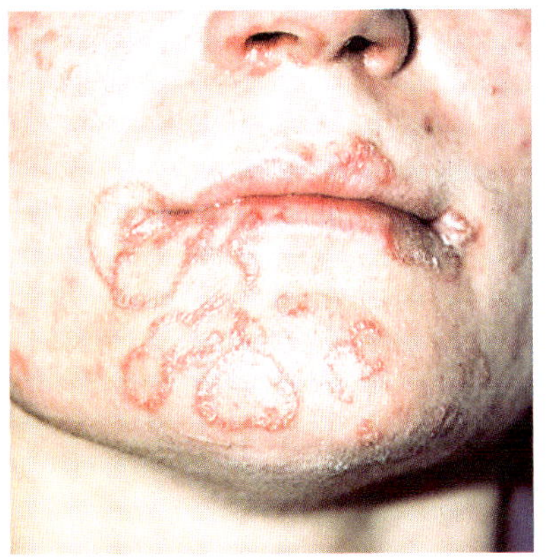

FIG. 92-22 *Scaly and crusted papules and plaques in the shape of a ring.*

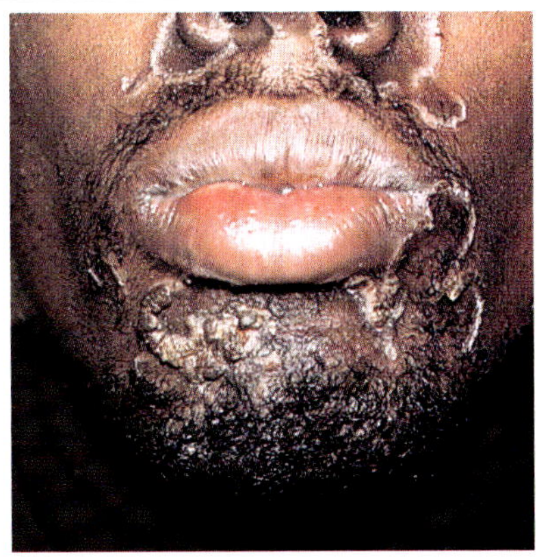

FIG. 92-23 *Scaly papules and plaques in an annulus.*

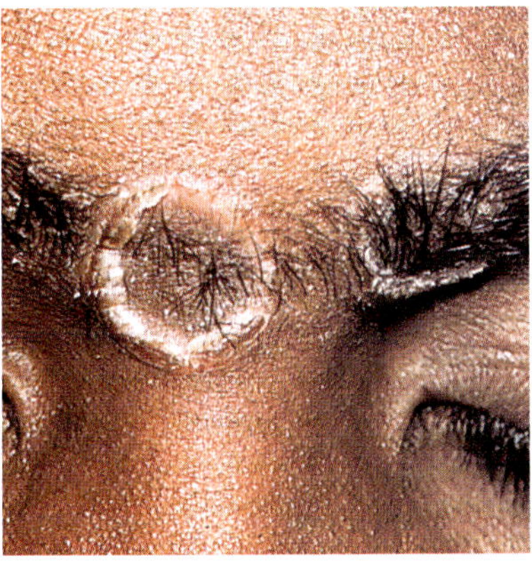

FIG. 92-24 *Annular papules.*

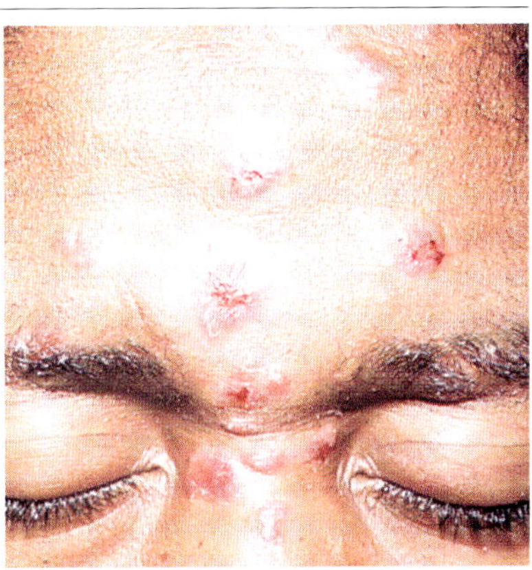

FIG. 92-25 *Eroded and ulcerated papules.*

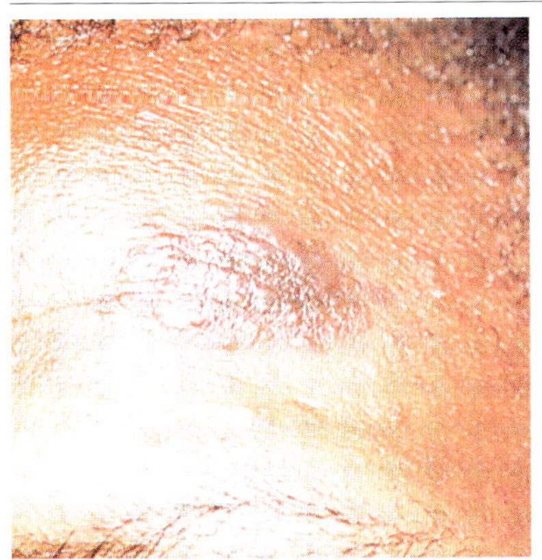

FIG. 92-26 *Hyperpigmented plaque.*

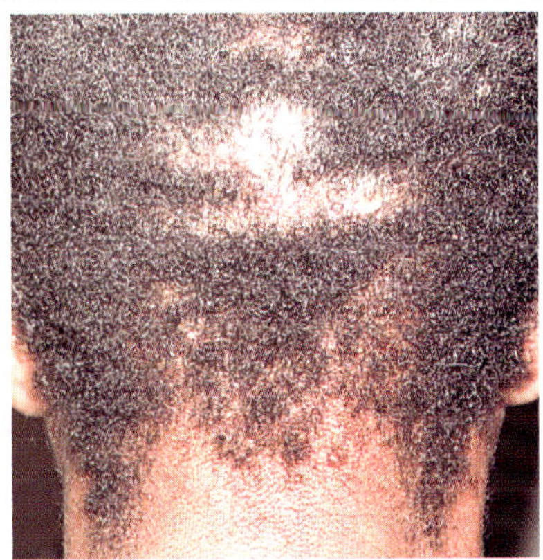

FIG. 92-27 *"Moth-eaten" alopecia.*

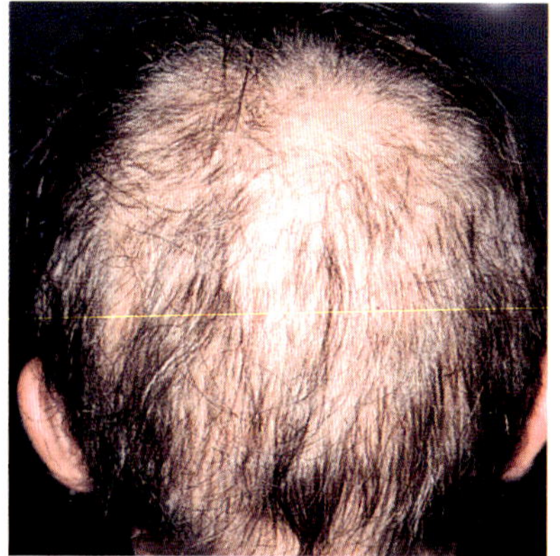

FIG. 92-28 *Patchy alopecia.*

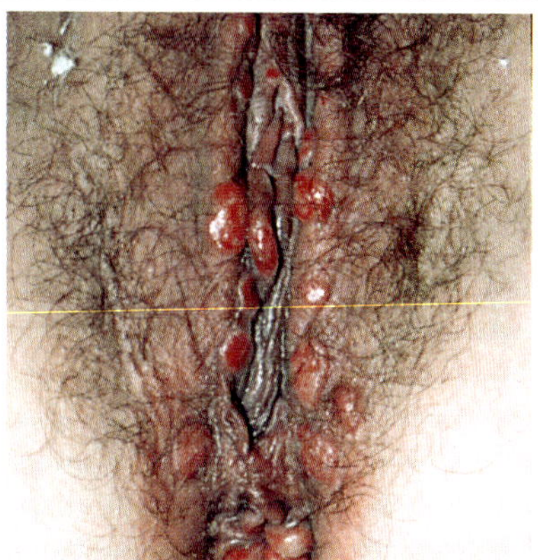

FIG. 92-29 *Papules of condylomata lata.*

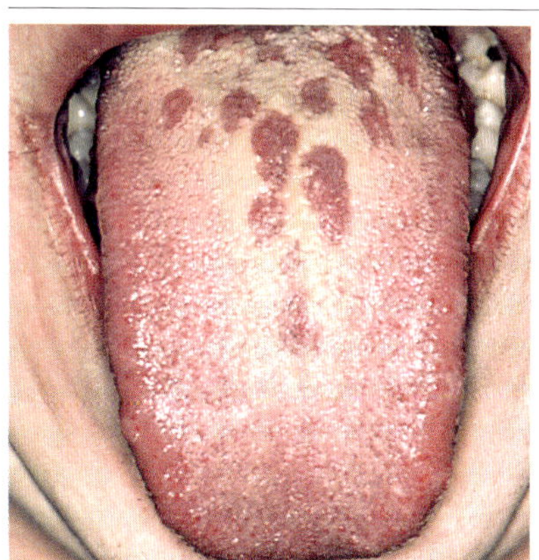

FIG. 92-30 *Mucous "patches."*

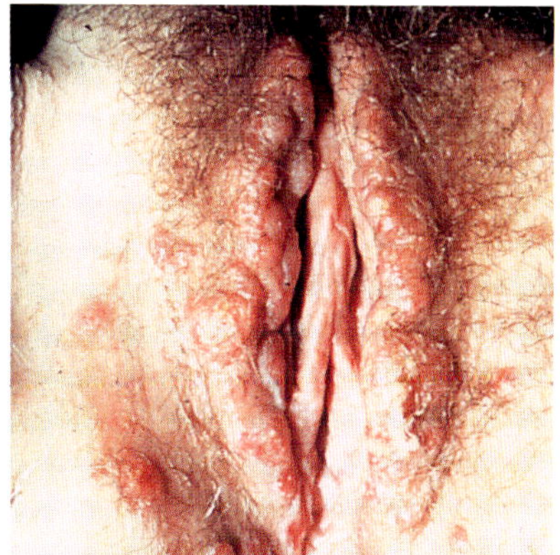

FIG. 92-31 *Papules, some of them eroded, of condylomata lata.*

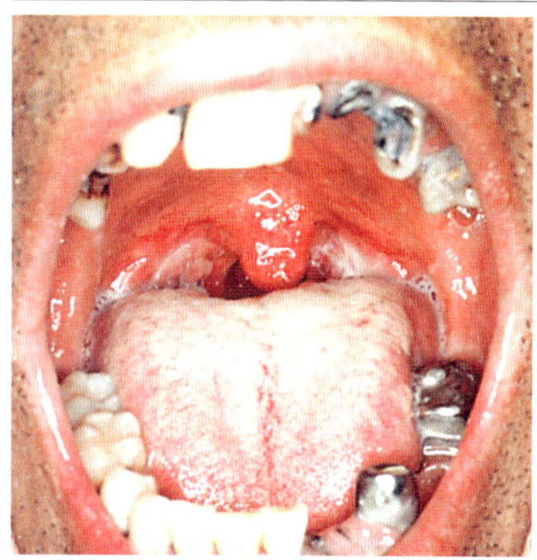

FIG. 92-32 *Mucous "patches" on the soft palate.*

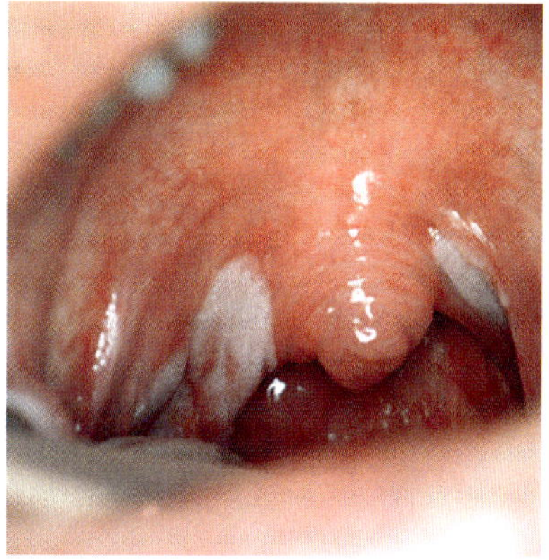

FIG. 92-33 *Mucous "patches" on the soft palate and on a tonsil.*

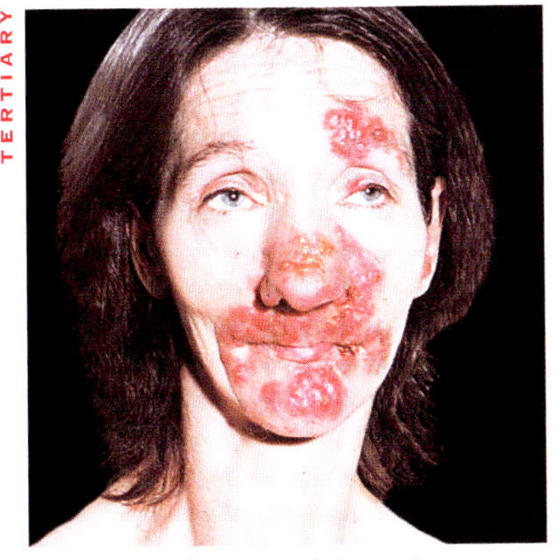

FIG. 92-34 *Plaques, nodules, and tumors.*

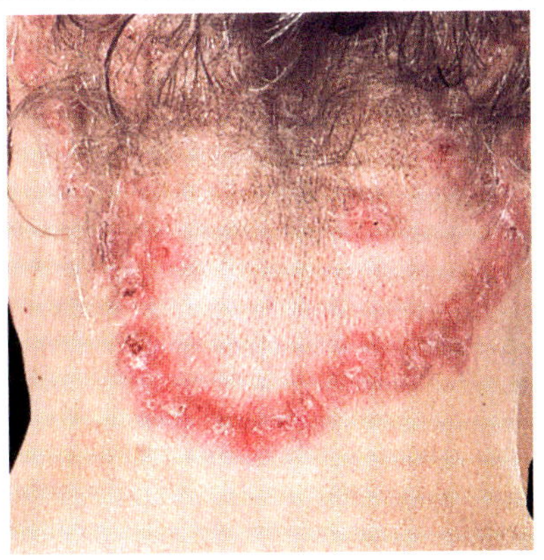

FIG. 92-35 *Scaly papules in a ring.*

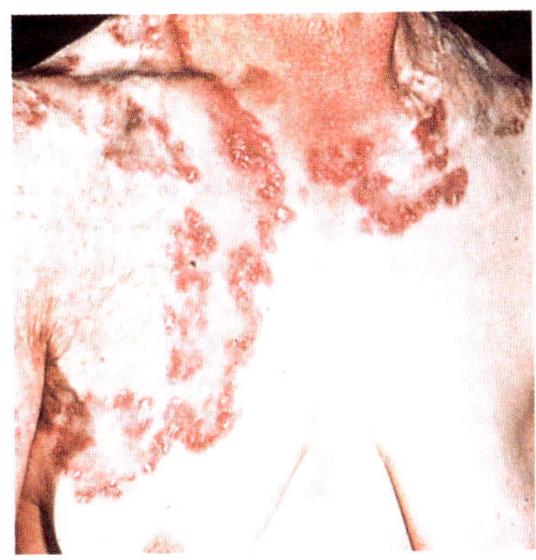

FIG. 92-36 *Scaly and crusted papules, plaques with a scalloped border, and zones of atrophy.*

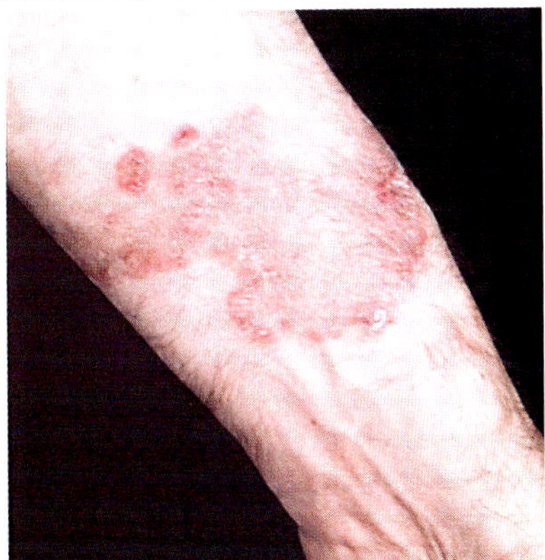

FIG. 92-37 *Scaly plaque with a scalloped border.*

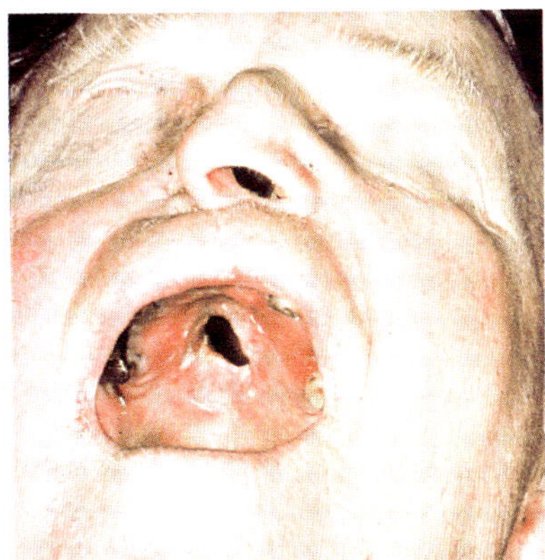

FIG. 92-38 *Perforation of a palate and of the nasal septum.*

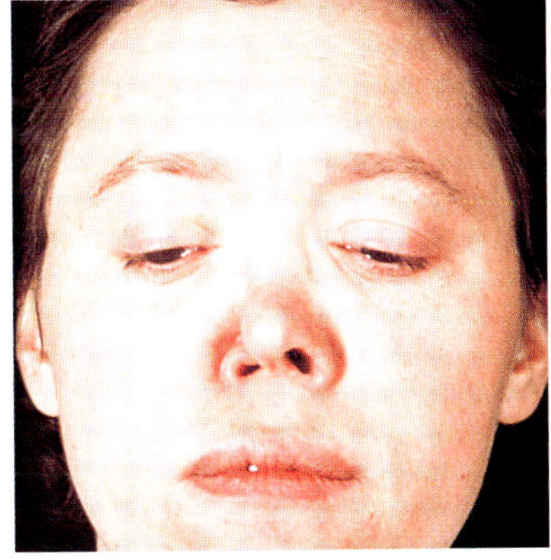

FIG. 92-39 *Depression of the bridge of the nose consequent to destruction of cartilage ("saddle nose").*

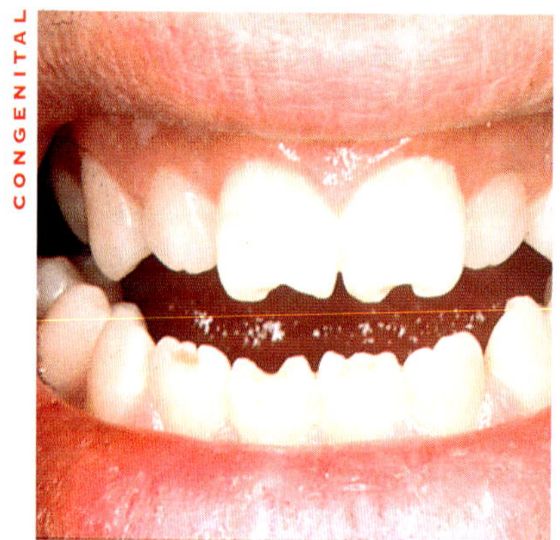

FIG. 92-40 *Hutchinson's teeth.*

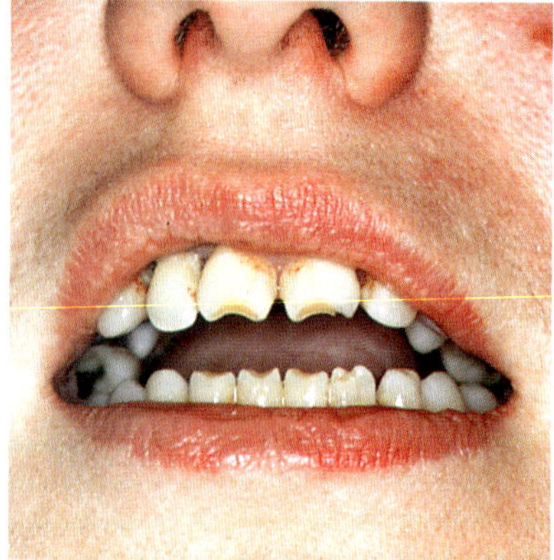

FIG. 92-41 *Hutchinson's teeth.*

ADJUNCTIVE DIAGNOSTIC TESTS Demonstration by darkfield microscopy of spirochetes in the exudate of a lesion. Serologic tests for syphilis, including the VDRL-test, FTA-ABS-test, TPHA-test, IgM-solid phase hemadsorption assay, and ELISA-methods are confirmatory.

COURSE Individual lesions of secondary syphilis have different names depending on the stage of the disease. The chancre of primary syphilis usually presents itself as an ulcerated papule or nodule that heals in weeks. The papules of secondary syphilis often are scaly and widespread, and may last for weeks or even months before they disappear. A gumma of tertiary syphilis usually is an ulcerated plaque in the center of which may be an atrophic scar. Only gummas are permanent, although a chancre may heal with a scar and some lesions of secondary syphilis with macular atrophy.

INTEGRATION: UNIFYING CONCEPT All of the findings in the skin in syphilis are a direct consequence of the effects of spirochetes of Treponema pallidum and the immunologic response of the host to them. A chancre teems with spirochetes, as do early lesions of secondary syphilis on mucous membranes, especially condylomata lata. Early lesions of secondary syphilis in the skin are replete with spirochetes, whereas late lesions of secondary syphilis contain few or none of them. In a gumma, spirochetes may be present, but they are detected with extraordinary difficulty. Although spirochetes may be found in the dermis of a chancre or in a papule of secondary syphilis, they are seen best in an epidermis that has been exposed to an immunoperoxidase stain specific for Treponema pallidum. The spirochetes also can be demonstrated readily with specialized silver stains such as those named eponymically for Warthin and Starry, for Steiner, and for Levaditi.

When sections of tissue of a chancre are studied by conventional microscopy, an ulcer is seen and beneath it is a dense, somewhat diffuse, mixed infiltrate of inflammatory cells in which plasma cells abound. In papules of secondary syphilis, there is a superficial and deep perivascular infiltrate composed mostly of histiocytes and plasma cells, and those cells often are arranged also in lichenoid pattern beneath a pallid psoriasiform epidermis. Neutrophils present within the epidermis of secondary syphilis are an indication that that surface epithelium houses innumerable spirochetes.

As the process of secondary syphilis evolves, neutrophils disappear from lesions and epithelioid histiocytes appear in ever greater numbers, eventually forming collections (granulomas). At that granulomatous stage, spirochetes no longer can be found. A gumma, as its name denotes, is characterized by gummatous inflammation in which necrosis of inflammatory cells and degeneration of collagen is extensive, that debris being surrounded in turn by granulomatous inflammation joined by a lymphoplasmacytic infiltrate and by fibroplasia.

Syphilis has traditionally been regarded by clinicians to be a "great mimicker"; the same can be said by histopathologists.

THERAPY Penicillin is the drug of choice at all stages. In primary, secondary, and early latent syphilis, intramuscular benzathine penicillin (2.4 million units) as a single dose, or tetracycline or erythromycin for 14 days, and, in late syphilis, excluding neurosyphilis, intramuscular benzathine penicillin or oral tetracyclines for 21 days.

DEFINITION A benign neoplasm of apocrine ductal nature within the upper half of the dermis that manifests itself clinically as tiny, smooth, skin-colored, round or oblong papules that usually are situated in periorbital skin, but may be seen on other sites, such as the neck or genitalia, or even be widespread.

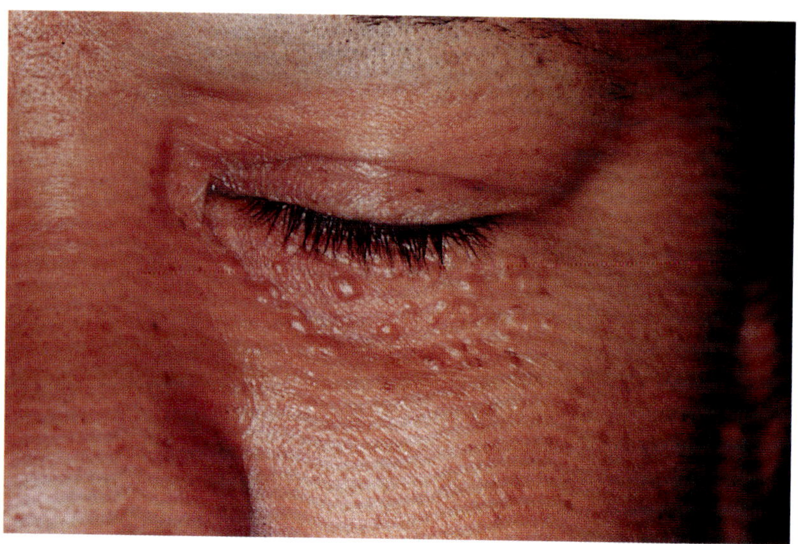

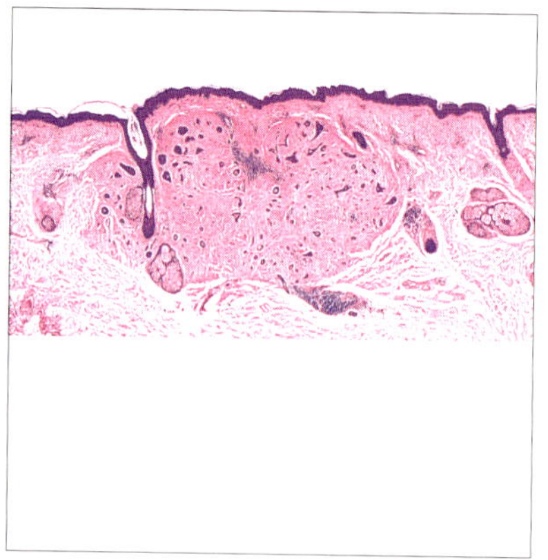

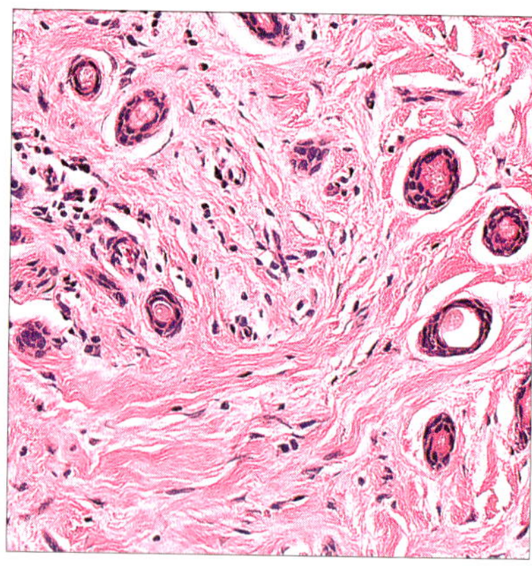

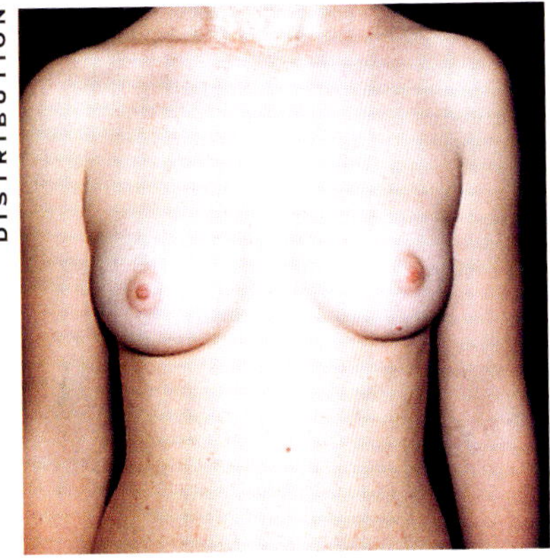

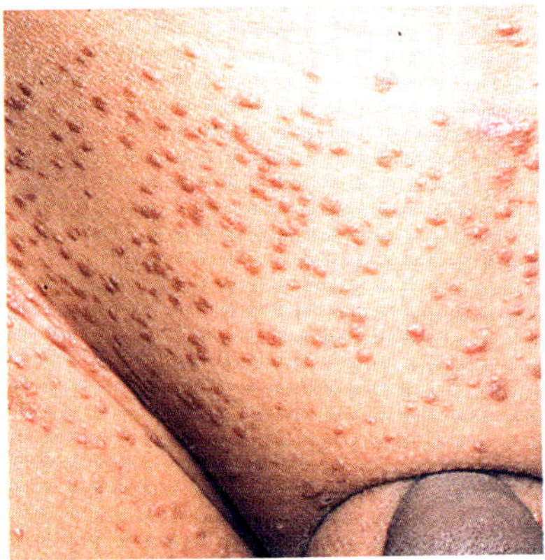

FIG. 93-1   *Tiny papules are present on every site pictured here.*

FIG. 93-2   *In addition to round papules, there are oblong ones.*

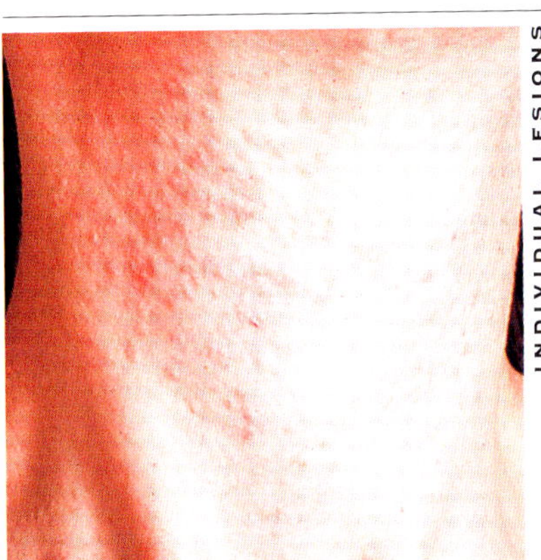

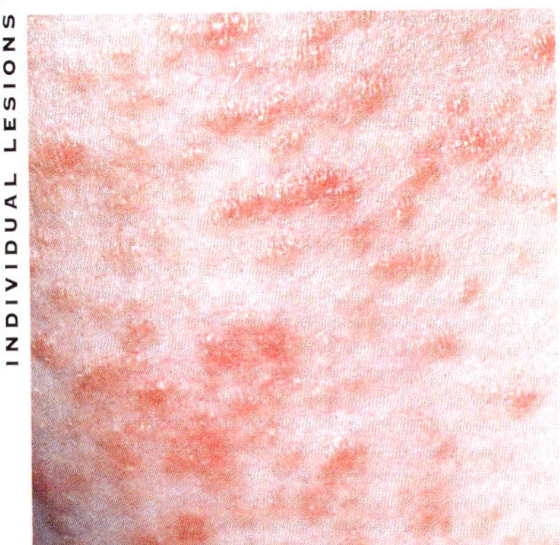

FIG. 93-3   *Papules have become confluent in foci.*

FIG. 93-4   *Some smooth papules have become confluent to form lesions with geometric shapes, among them, linear.*

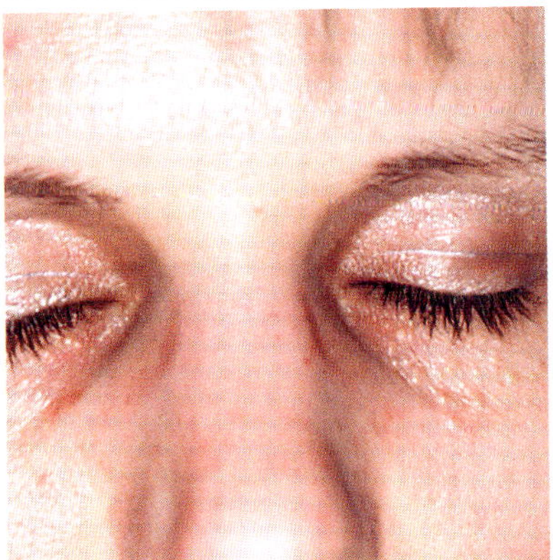

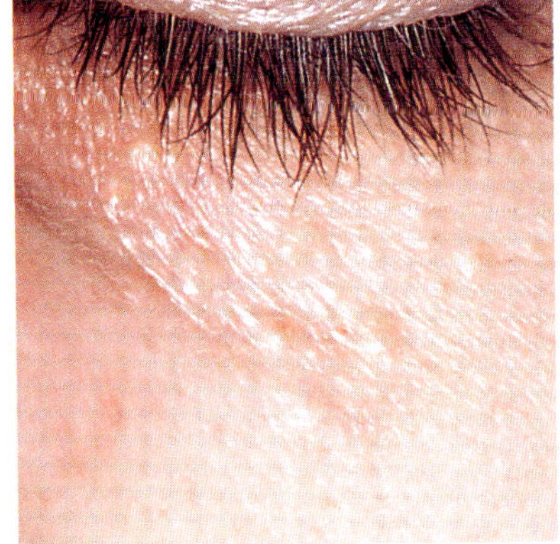

FIG. 93-5 (A, B)   *Discrete smooth papules are distributed symmetrically.*

COURSE Once papules of syringoma come into being, which usually is after puberty, they remain as they are for a lifetime, changing hardly at all over the course of decades.

INTEGRATION: UNIFYING CONCEPT Syringomas are benign neoplasms, presumably with apocrine ductal differentiation. A clue to apocrine character is found in clear-cell syringomas, a manifestation of the diabetic state, in which the proliferation of clear cells is indistinguishable in foci from findings in clear-cell (apocrine) hidradenomas.

Each papule consists of both epithelium and stroma. The epithelial component presents itself in two forms, namely, solid and tubular. The stroma, which is scant, consists of crowded bundles of collagen.

Syringomas usually are numerous, being situated as a rule on and around eyelids, but sometimes they are widespread, involving particularly the skin of genitalia. If a solitary plaque, especially one situated on an upper lip, is biopsied superficially by punch technique, and if the biopsy report reads "syringoma," a clinician should be alert to the likelihood that the lesion is not really a syringoma, but either a syringomatous carcinoma or a microcystic adnexal carcinoma. Syringoma does not occur as a solitary lesion on the lip and, not uncommonly, those carcinomas are misinterpreted as syringoma, especially in biopsy specimens that fail to sample the neoplasm adequately.

THERAPY For reasons of cosmesis, laser surgery, shave (saucerization) removal, and electrocautery are satisfactory modalities, but not ideal because they cannot destroy the lesion without leaving a noticeable scar.

DEFINITION An inflammatory disease caused by the fungus *Malassezia furfur*, the organisms of which proliferate in a slightly thickened stratum corneum. It manifests clinically as white or light brown macules that may be discrete or confluent, on the trunk especially.

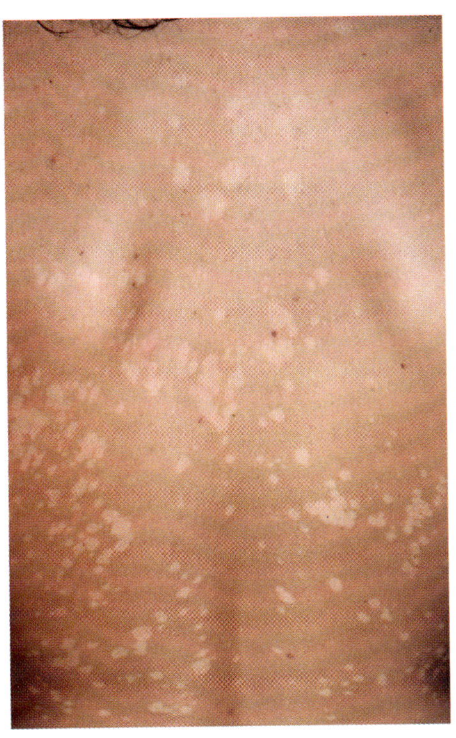

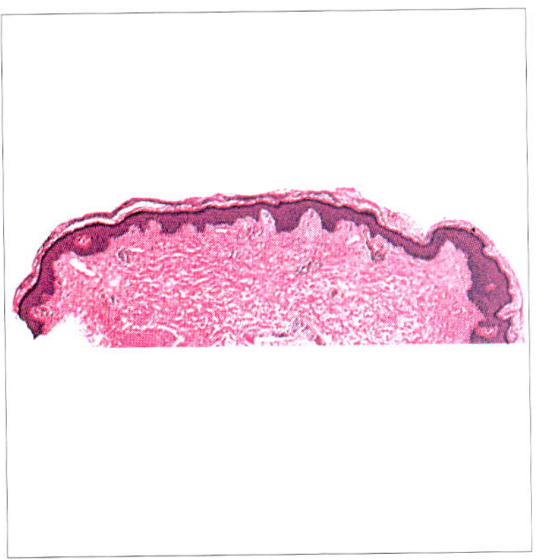

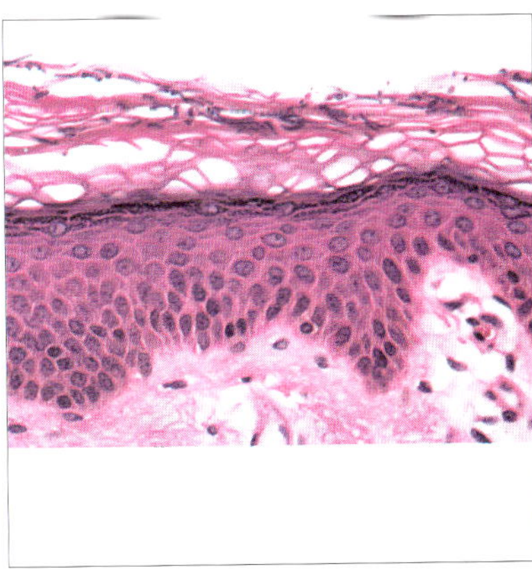

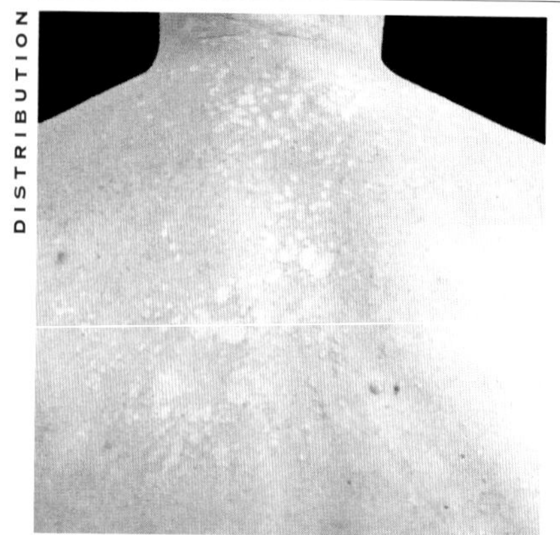

FIG. 94-1 *Off-white and pink macules and papules. The polypoid, skin-colored lesion is an Unna's type of melanocytic nevus.*

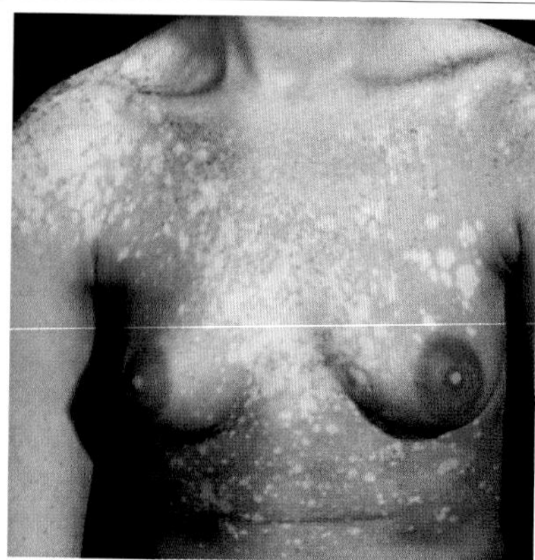

FIG. 94-2 *Hypopigmented macules and patches.*

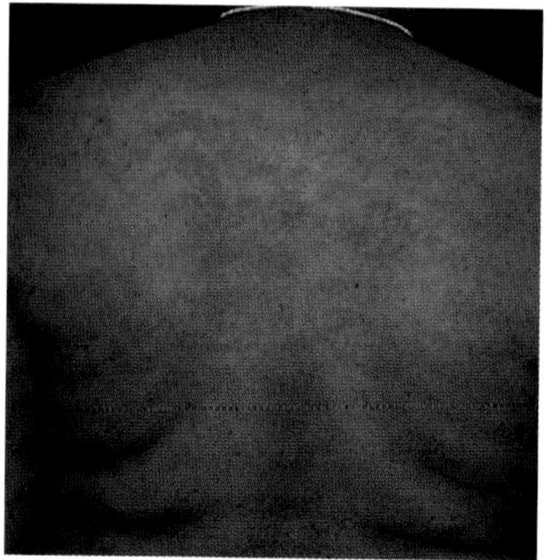

FIG. 94-3 *Off-white macules and patches.*

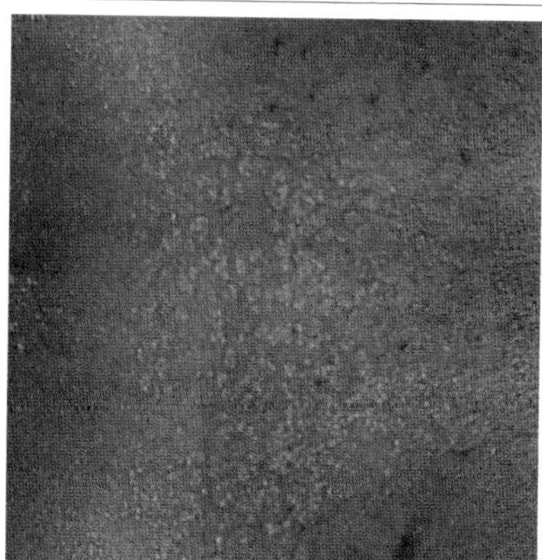

FIG. 94-4 *Off-white macules and papules.*

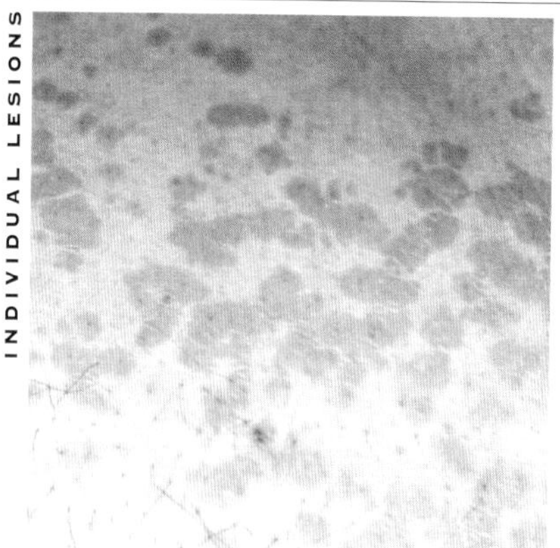

FIG. 94-5 *Fawn-colored macules covered by fine scale. Some lesions have become confluent.*

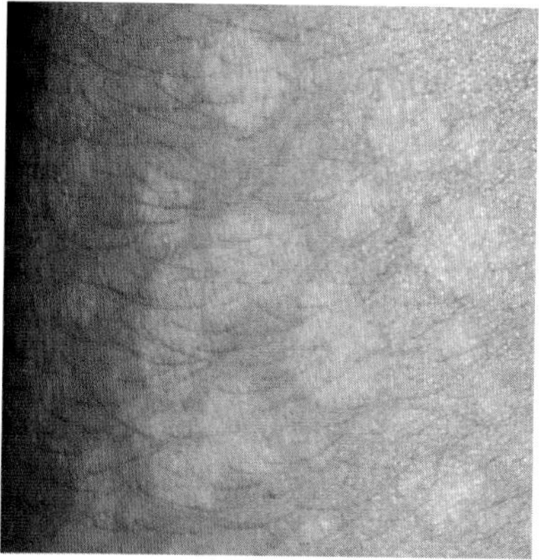

FIG. 94-6 *Scaly pink macules.*

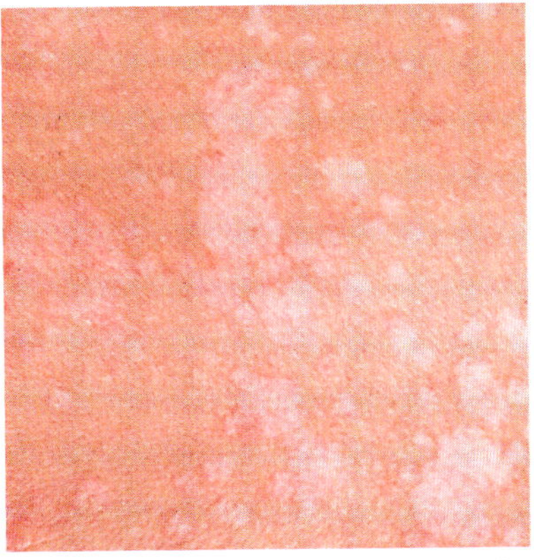

FIG. 94-7 *Pink macules and papules, patches and plaques.*

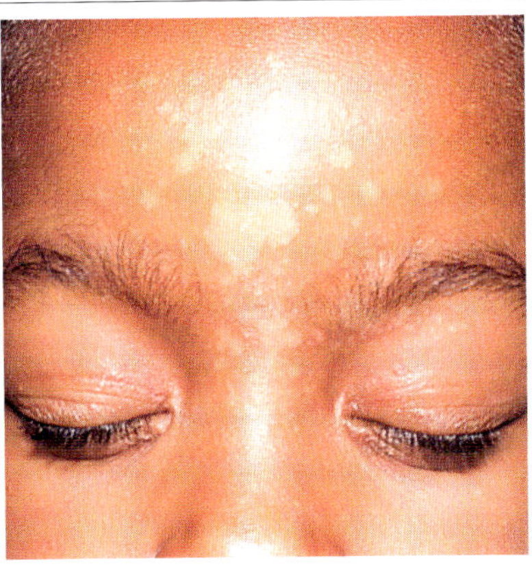

FIG. 94-8 *Off-white macules and patches*

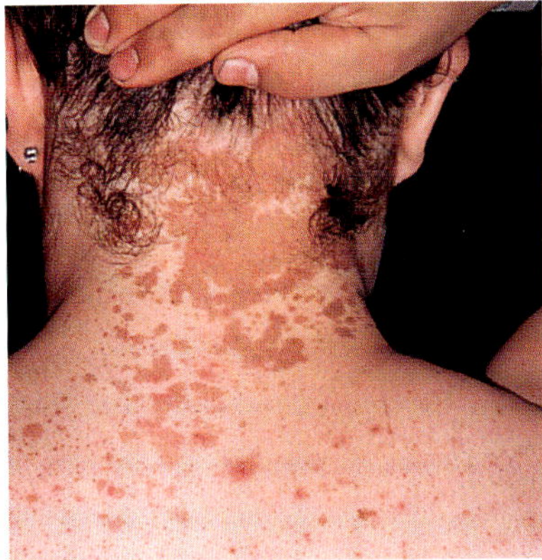

FIG. 94-9 *Hyperpigmented macules and patches.*

ADJUNCTIVE DIAGNOSTIC TEST Scales scraped from lesions and placed in KOH may be scrutinized by conventional microscopy for spores and hyphae of Malassezia furfur.

COURSE Macules with delicate scales of tinea versicolor often become confluent in the course of months to become patches. Depending upon the immunologic status of the host, those macules and patches may sometimes persist for years.

INTEGRATION: UNIFYING CONCEPT Tinea versicolor is caused by the fungus Malassezia furfur. The organisms, pityrosporum ovale and orbiculare, are confined to the stratum corneum of skin on the upper half of the trunk especially. Sections of tissue of a lesion of tinea versicolor show a mostly basket-woven stratum corneum in which short stubby hyphae and round spores abound. The organisms usually induce only a scant infiltrate of inflammatory cells, to wit, a few lymphocytes around venules of the superficial plexus. Because those vessels are ever so slightly dilated, the lesions are never seen to be brightly erythematous clinically, at most being only pink in light-skinned Caucasians.

Lesions of tinea versicolor assume different colors in people of different color and at different times of the year. It is for this reason that the condition is named "versicolor." In dark-skinned persons, the lesions with fine scales seem white by contrast with the background color of normal skin, whereas in light-skinned persons the same lesions, by contrast, often have a brown hue. In summer months, if the skin of Caucasians is tan, lesions of tinea versicolor appear pale by comparison, yet during winter months, when the tan has faded, they seem to be darker. It has been hypothesized that hypopigmentation of lesions following exposure to sunlight may result from production by the fungus of a substance that protects the skin from ultraviolet light.

THERAPY For localized disease, administration of topical antimycotics, such as azoles, or selenium sulfide in a shampoo eliminates the causative organisms; for widespread lesions, oral ketoconazole, itraconazole, or fluconazole is curative.

DEFINITION An inflammatory process caused by Mycobacterium tuberculosis. In the skin, it may be primary as a consequence of direct inoculation (tuberculosis verrucosa cutis) or secondary to a focus of tuberculosis in another organ (the lung for lupus vulgaris, and bones, as well as lymph nodes, for scrofuloderma).

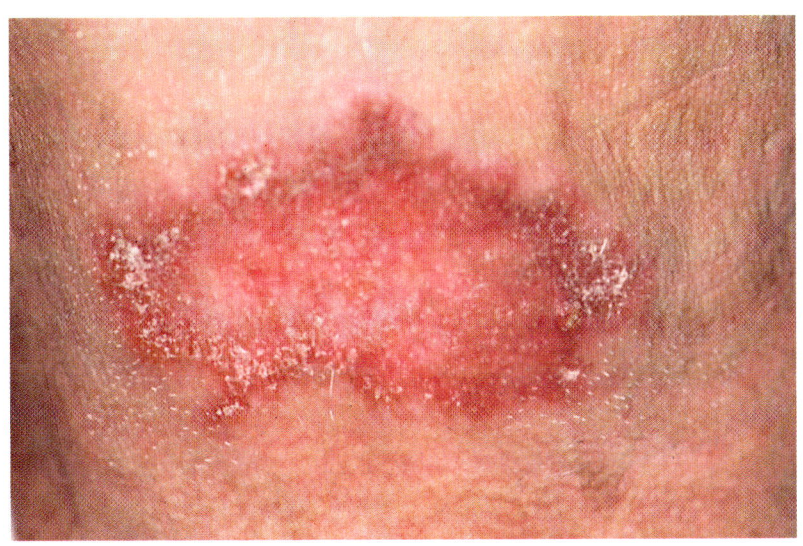

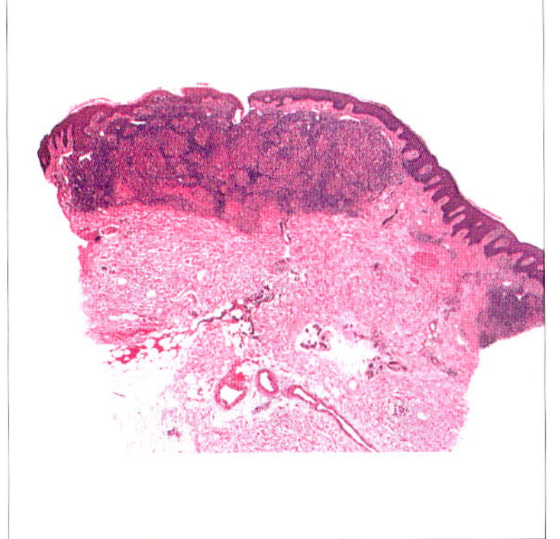

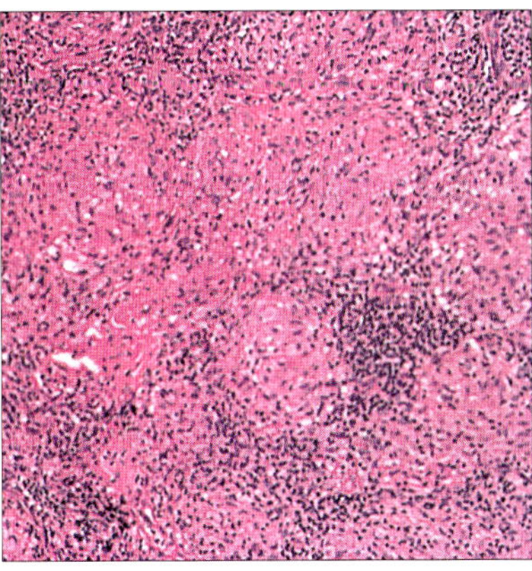

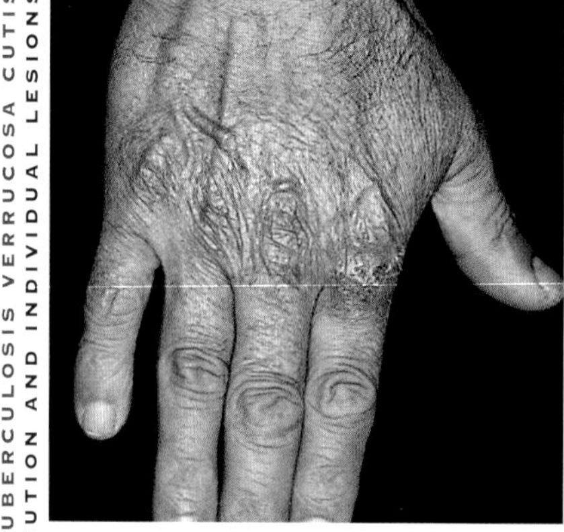
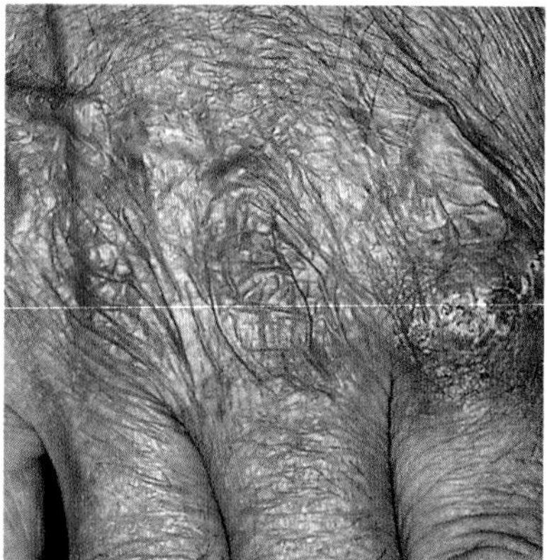

FIG. 95-1 (A, B) *Plaques with scales and crusts.*

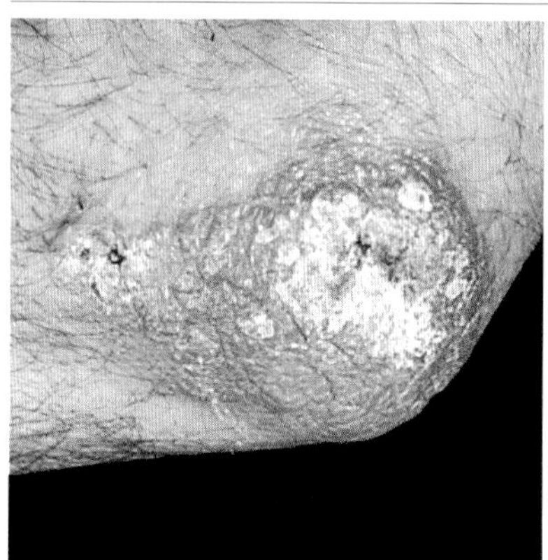

FIG. 95-2 *A keratotic plaque.*

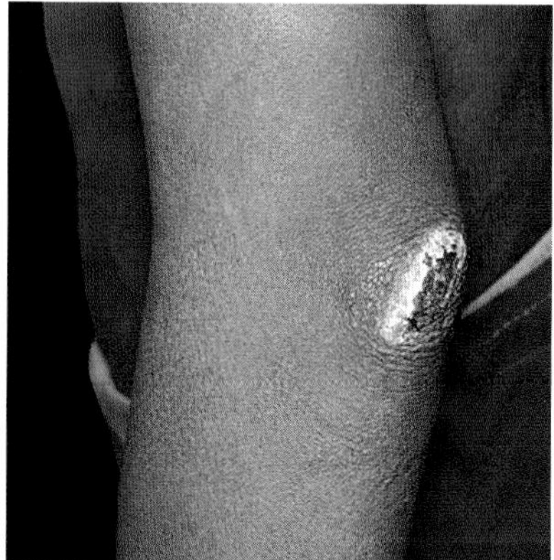

FIG. 95-3 *A verrucous keratotic plaque in annular configuration.*

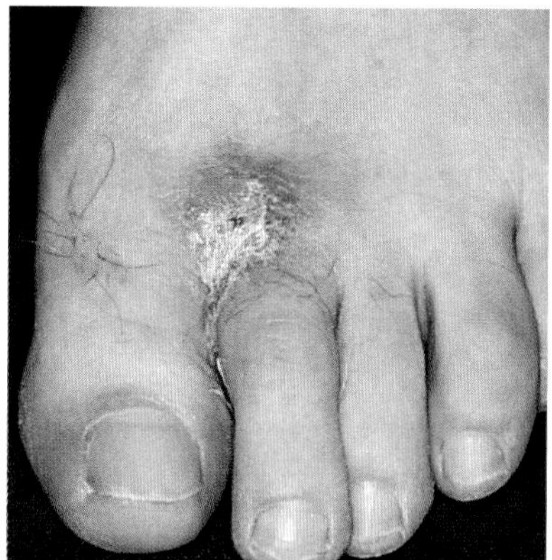
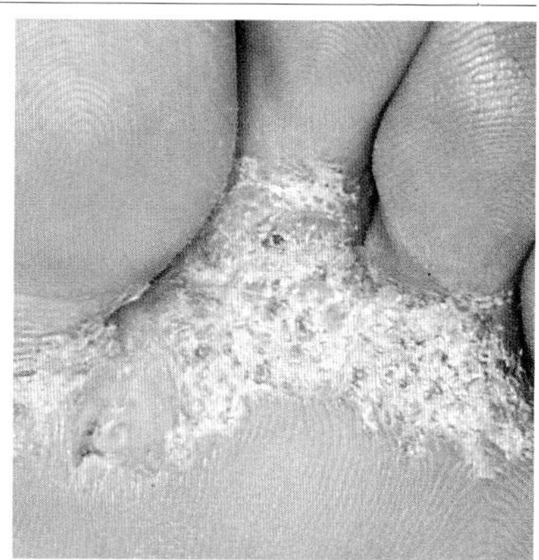

FIG. 95-4 (A, B) *Crusted and scaly plaque.*

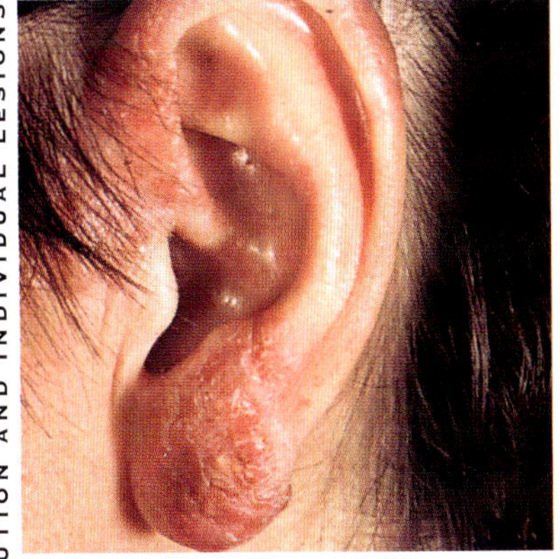

FIG. 95-5 *Slightly scaly orange papules that have become confluent to form plaques.*

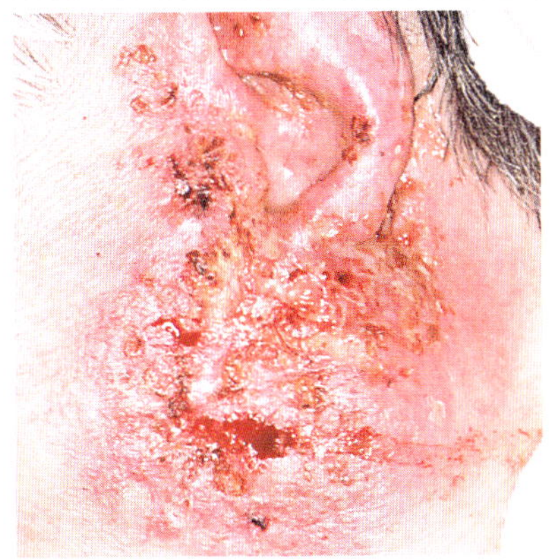

FIG. 95-6 *Ulcerated mass with partial destruction of an ear.*

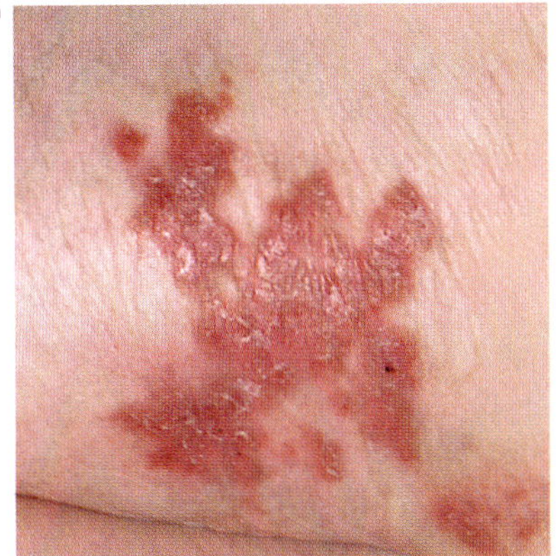

FIG. 95-7 *Violaceous plaque with a scalloped border.*

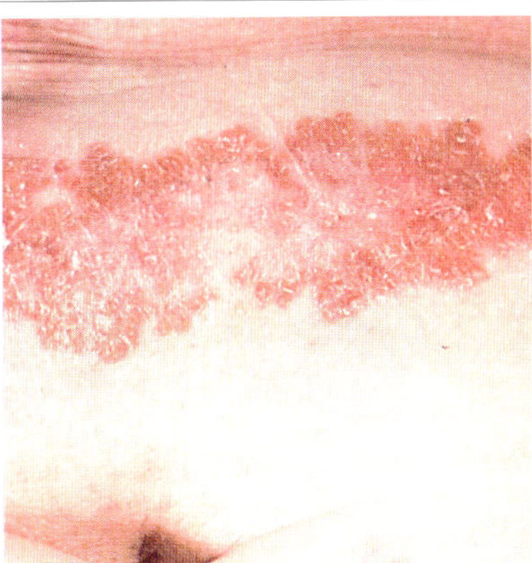

FIG. 95-8 *A large plaque with a scalloped border and scars, in foci, in the center.*

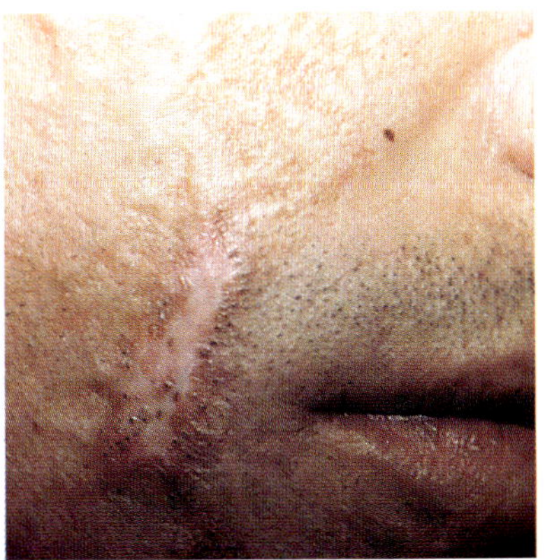

FIG. 95-9 *Brown papules around an extensive hypopigmented scar.*

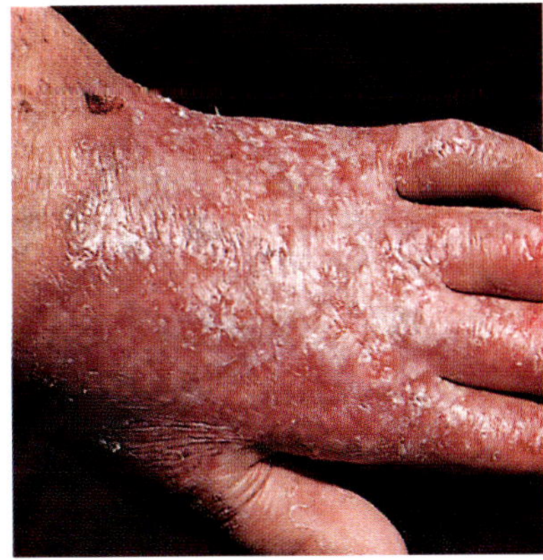

FIG. 95-10 *A large erythematous plaque associated with white scales.*

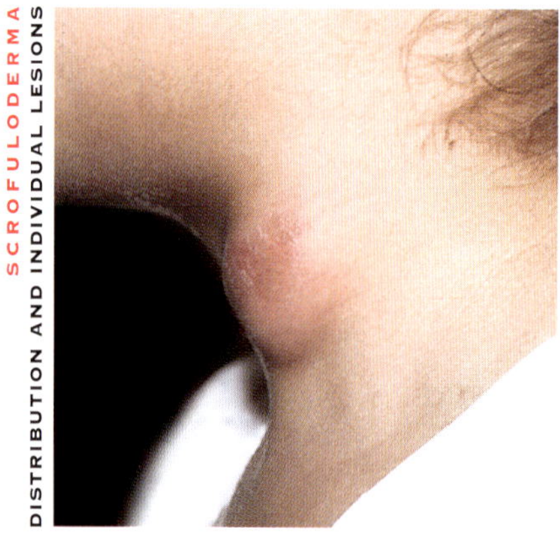

FIG. 95-11 *A tumor with a smooth surface.*

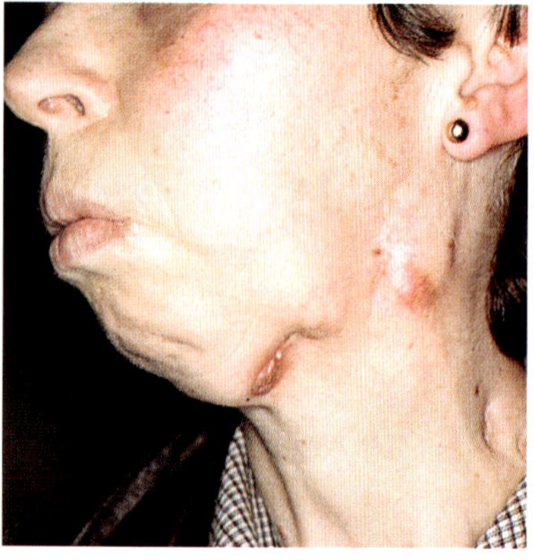

FIG. 95-12 *Granulation tissue at sites of draining sinuses, and a still active nodule.*

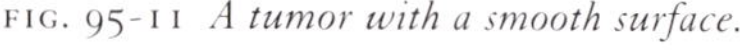

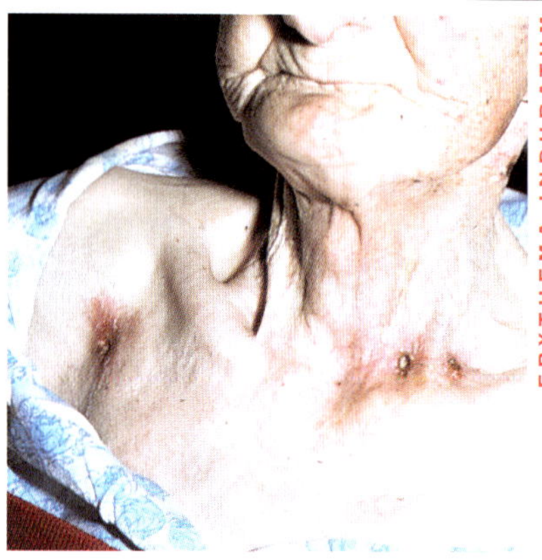

FIG. 95-13 *Ostia that represent openings of draining sinuses.*

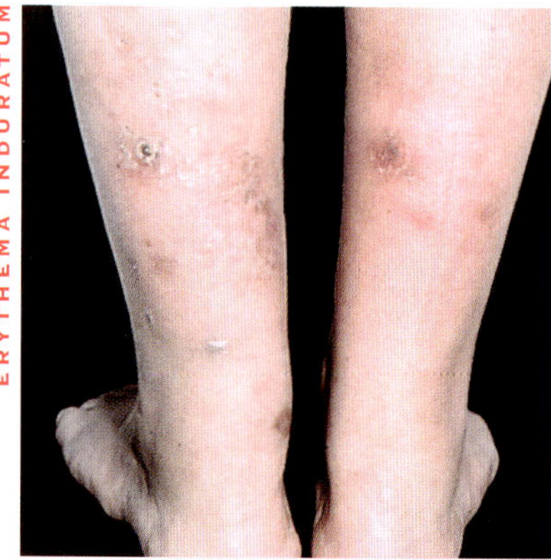

FIG. 95-14 *Crusted nodules and depressed scars mostly on the calves.*

ADJUNCTIVE DIAGNOSTIC TESTS Tuberculin skin test (tine test; Mantoux) induces a papule at the site of injection in a person who has developed delayed hypersensitivity to M. tuberculosis. Acid-fast organisms can be demonstrated in smears from ulcers. Culture of tissue from biopsy specimens of skin may verify the diagnosis. Polymerase chain reaction is effective in demonstrating mycobacterial DNA in tissue sections of skin biopsy specimens.

COURSE Each of the several types of lesions induced by Mycobacterium tuberculosis has a different course. For example, tuberculosis verrucosa cutis, known also by the picturesque term "prosector's wart" that in times past characterized the condition accurately, presents itself as a papule that becomes keratotic and in a few years involutes by scarring. In contrast, lupus vulgaris also presents itself as one or more papules that in time expand centrifugally, becoming increasingly hyperkeratotic or crusted, an ulcer often forming in the center of the lesion. After decades, a lesion of lupus vulgaris may attain a size of many centimeters, with scaly crusted papules at its periphery and an atrophic scar in its center. Such a lesion persists indefinitely and continues at a petty pace to extend outward. Lesions of scrofuloderma, from nearly the outset, consist of draining sinuses that, in time, are joined by granulation tissue and later still by scar. As some lesions heal with scar, new draining sinuses may appear. The nodule or tumor of erythema induratum ulcerates and heals with a scar. Lichen scrofulosorum consists of grouped papules that involute by scarring. Papulonecrotic tuberculid is made up of ulcerated papules and nodules that also resolve by scarring.

The "tuberculids," erythema induratum, lichen scrofulosorum, and papulonecrotic tuberculid, all begin as papules and end as scars. In reality, there is no justification for the concept of tuberculids; the notion is spurious.

INTEGRATION: UNIFYING CONCEPT Common to all of the kinds of lesions of cutaneous tuberculosis are granulomas composed of epithelioid histiocytes surrounded by moderately dense infiltrates of lymphocytes. Moreover, each of the clinical variants of tuberculosis has its own distinctive histopathologic features, such as pseudocarcinomatous hyperplasia with marked hyperkeratosis for tuberculosis verrucosa cutis, suppuration within sinuses in scrofuloderma, and necrosis accompanied by suppuration, granulomatous inflammation, and fibroplasia in lobules in the subcutaneous fat of erythema induratum.

Primary inoculation tuberculosis (tuberculous chancre) results from direct inoculation of tubercle bacilli into the skin of a person who has never before been exposed to the organism. In contrast, tuberculosis verrucosa cutis develops in a person who has immunity to the tubercle bacillus as a consequence of exposure to it previously. Lupus vulgaris occurs in people who have pulmonary tuberculosis and from which site bacilli travel through the bloodstream to the skin, usually of the face. The tuberculous process in people with scrofuloderma usually is seated in lymph nodes and involves the skin secondarily, the mycobacteria being transported to and through the skin by way of sinuses. Miliary tuberculosis develops as a consequence of large numbers of tubercle bacilli being disseminated through the bloodstream of a person who is immunosuppressed; it signifies impending death.

In sum, all of the cutaneous manifestations of tuberculosis can be explained on the basis of immunological mechanisms, just as is the case for cutaneous manifestations of leprosy and leishmaniasis, and many other infectious diseases of the skin.

THERAPY The same treatment is appropriate for cutaneous tuberculosis as is given for pulmonary tuberculosis, namely, a combination of isoniazid, rifampicin, pyrazinamide, and ethambutol. Lesions of tuberculosis verrucosa cutis lend themselves to local excision in toto.

DEFINITION An inflammatory process that consists of transient, slightly erythematous, edematous papules and plaques characterized by a pseudopod-like border. They may be of either allergic or non-allergic cause, among the former being ingestants, injectants, inhalants, and infestations, and among the latter physical phenomena such as pressure, heat, and cold.

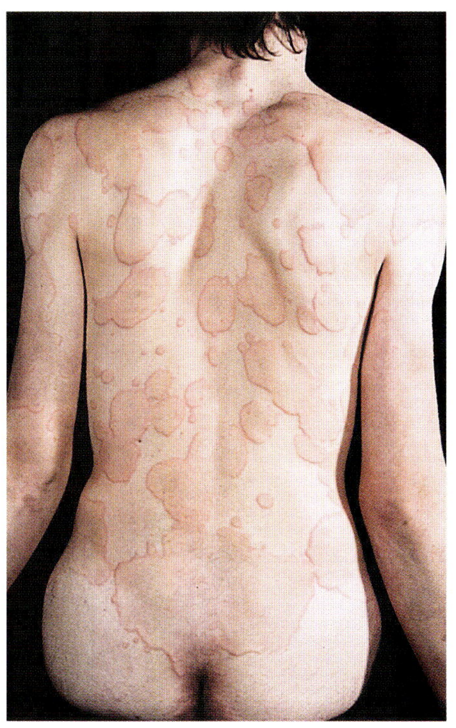

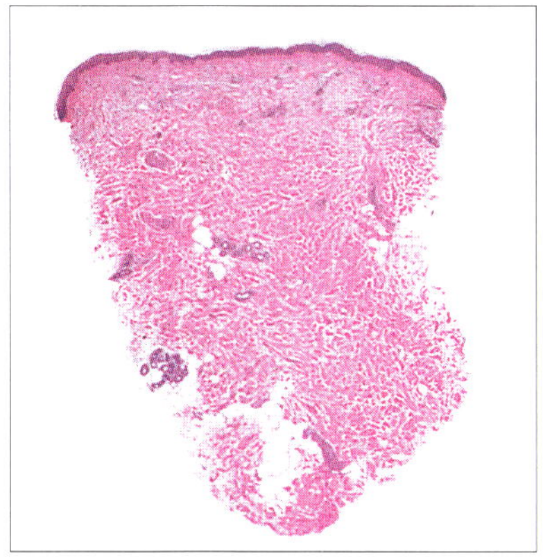

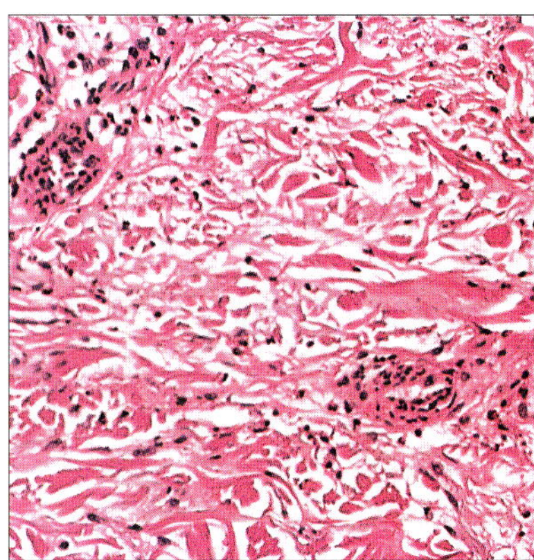

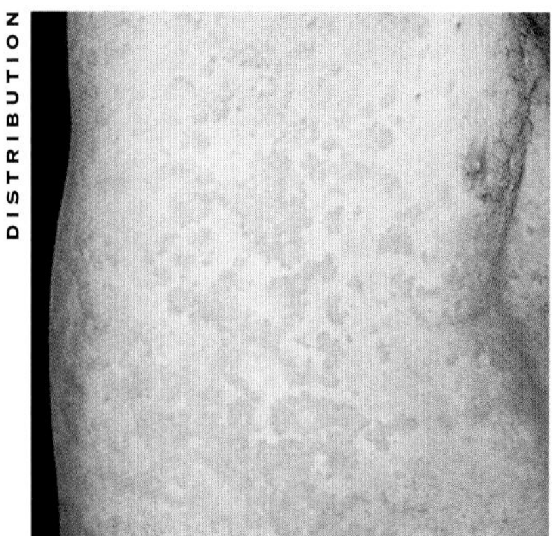

FIG. 96-1 *Papules and plaques.*

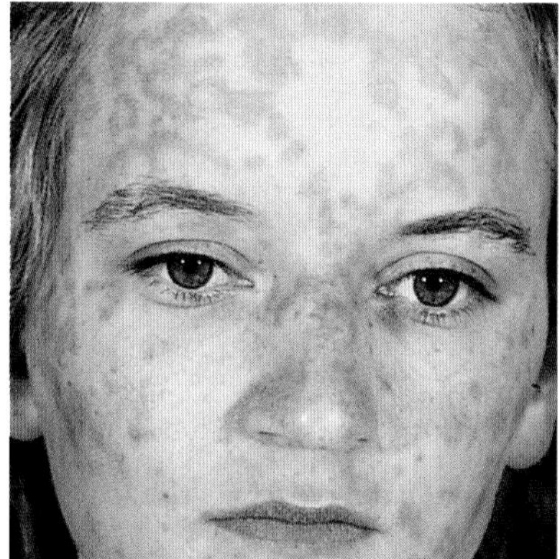

FIG. 96-2 *Papules and plaques.*

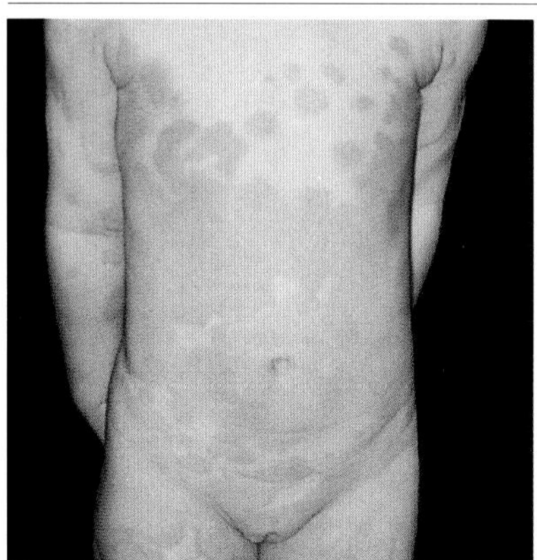

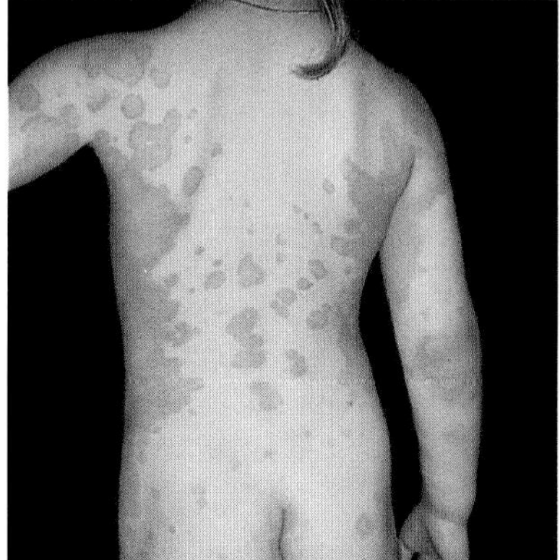

FIG. 96-3 (A, B) *Papules and plaques have become confluent.*

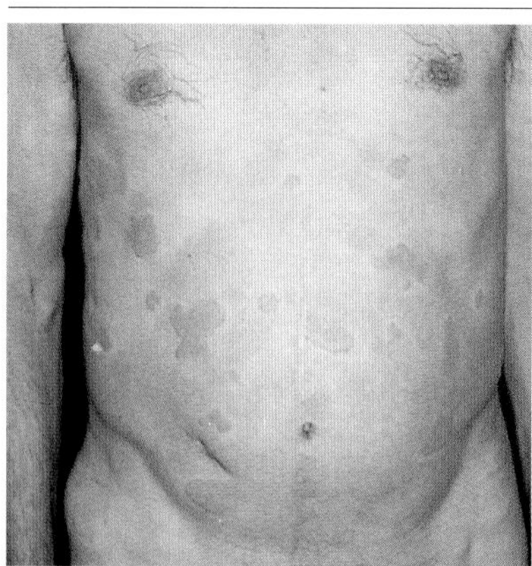

FIG. 96-4 *Plaques mostly, but also some papules.*

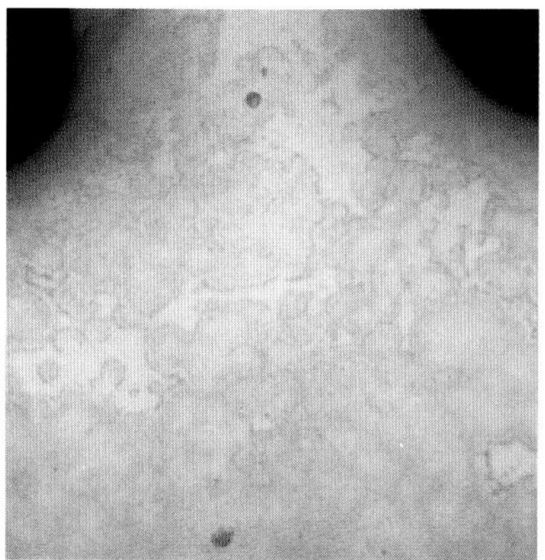

FIG. 96-5 *Arcuate, annular, and serpiginous outlines of lesions. Note two melanocytic nevi of Unna's type.*

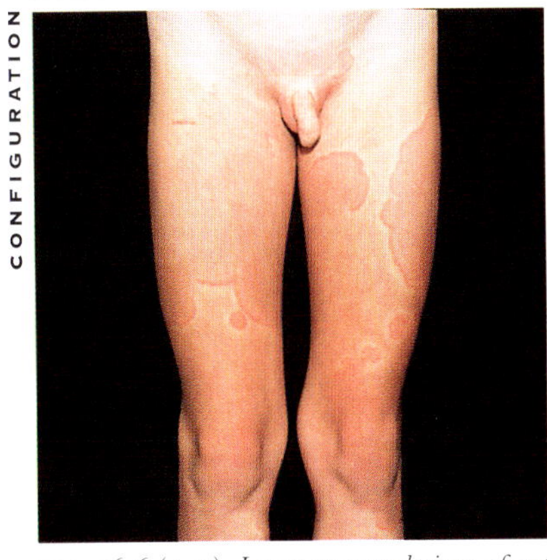 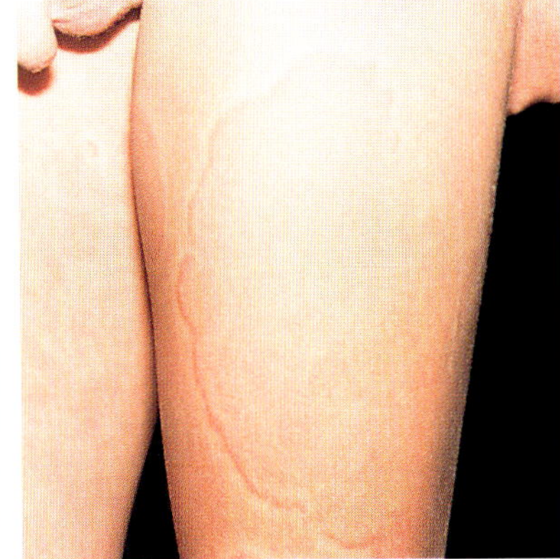

FIG. 96-6 (A, B) *Large arcuate lesions of urticaria.*

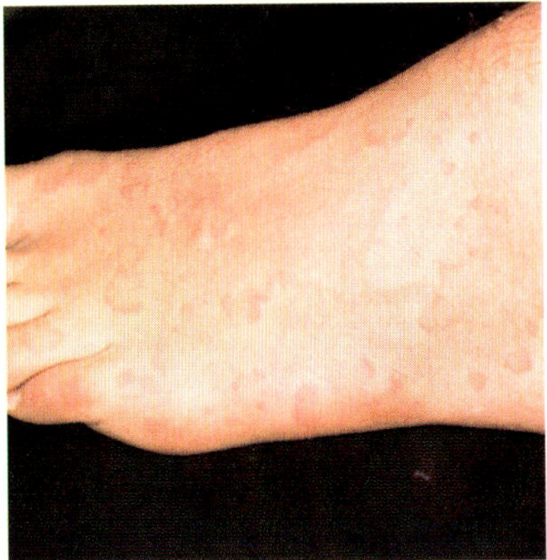

FIG. 96-7 *Papules, some of them in arcuate configuration.*

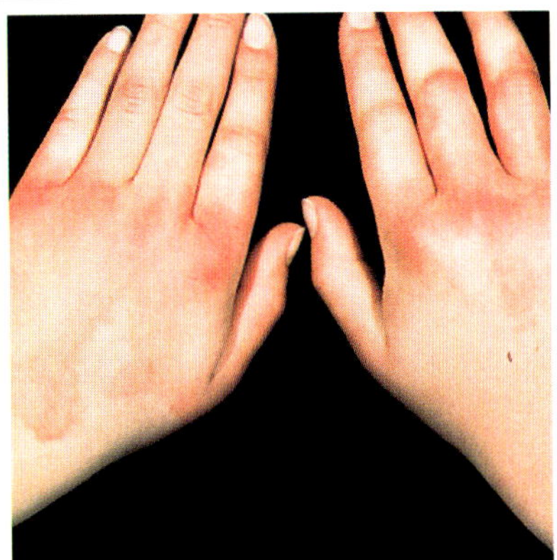

FIG. 96-8 *Papules and plaques have become confluent.*

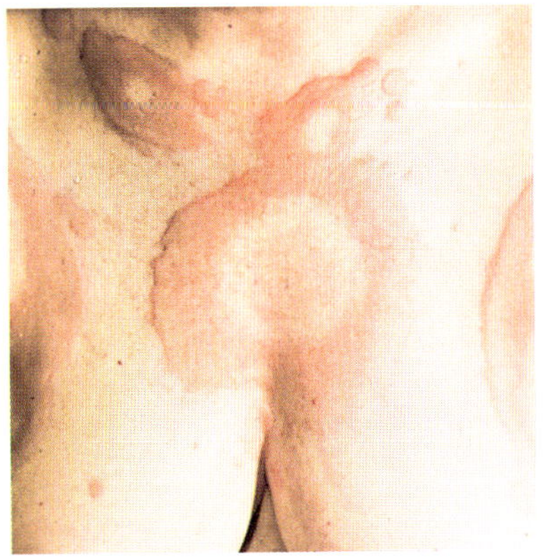

FIG. 96-9 *Large annular plaques in company with small and large papules, and with small plaques.*

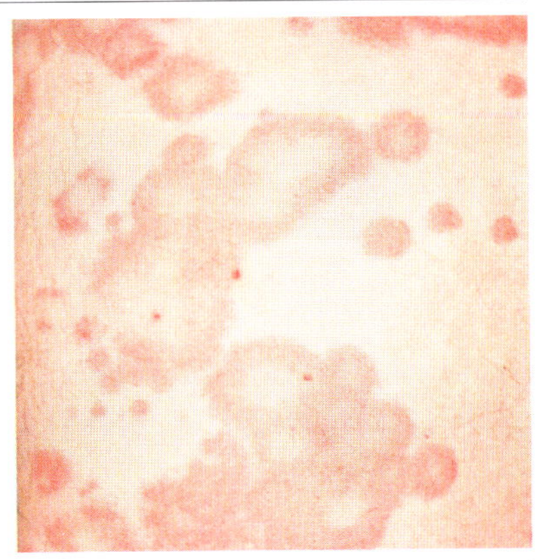

FIG. 96-10 *Papules and plaques, some of them annular.*

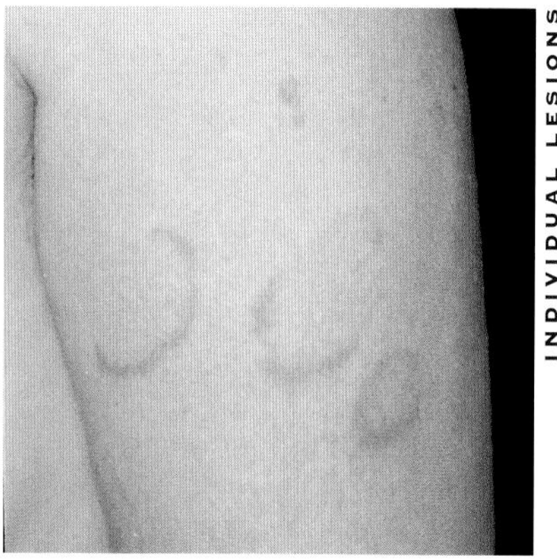

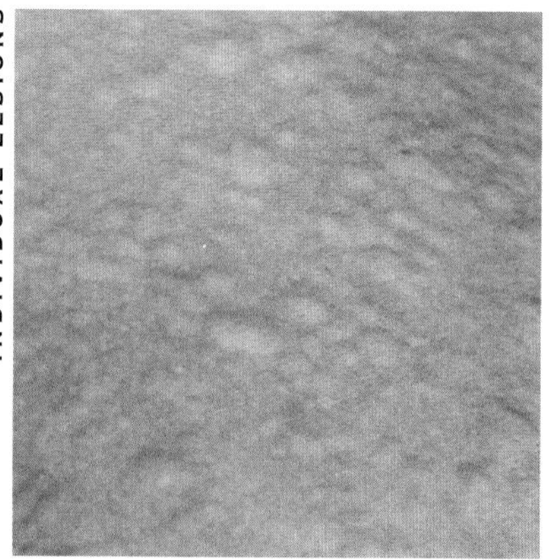

FIG. 96-11 *Small arcuate lesions of urticaria.*

FIG. 96-12 *Markedly edematous papules surrounded by subtle erythema.*

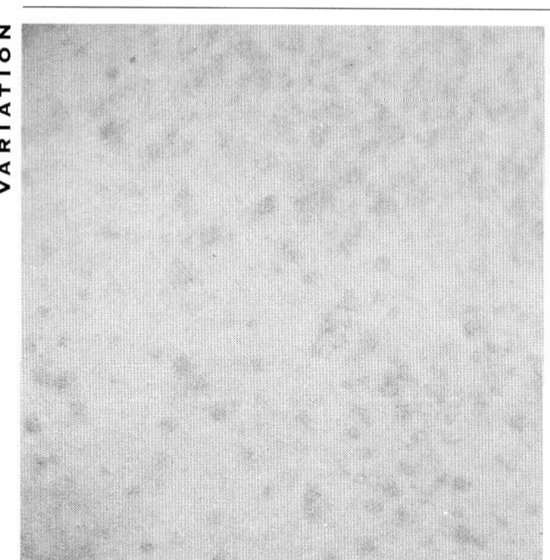

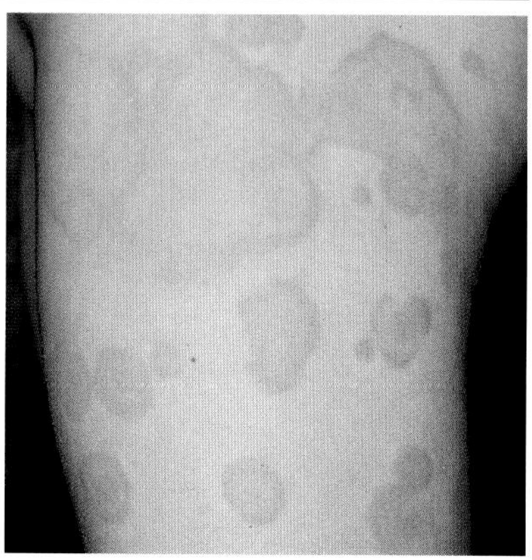

FIG. 96-13 *Small, edematous papules are not discrete (so-called cholinergic urticaria).*

FIG. 96-14 *Papules and plaques, some of them with a scalloped border, and some which have become confluent.*

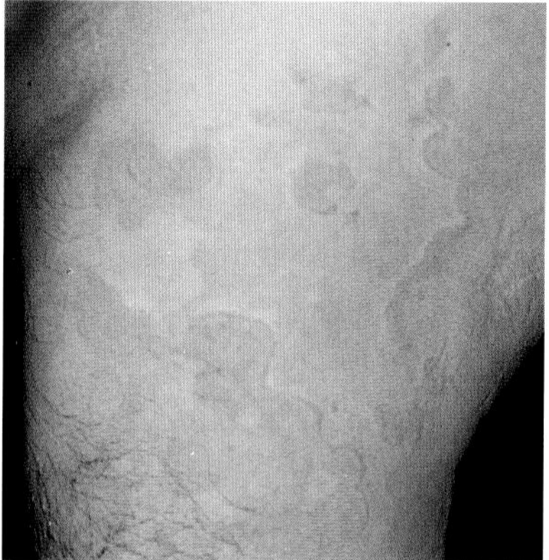

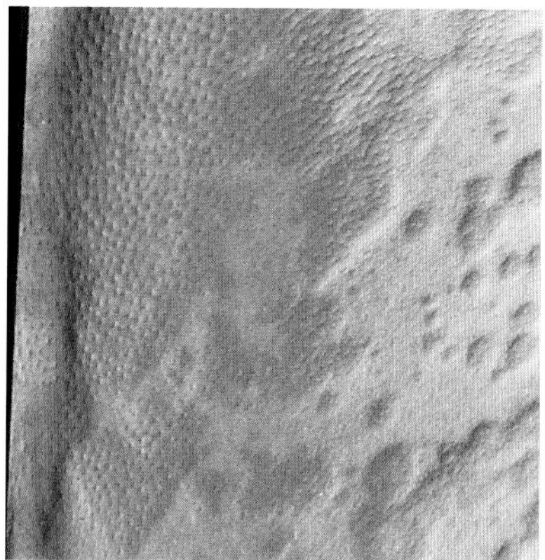

FIG. 96-15 *Papules and plaques, some of them with an arcuate outline and a scalloped border.*

FIG. 96-16 *Small and large edematous papules and plaques that have become confluent.*

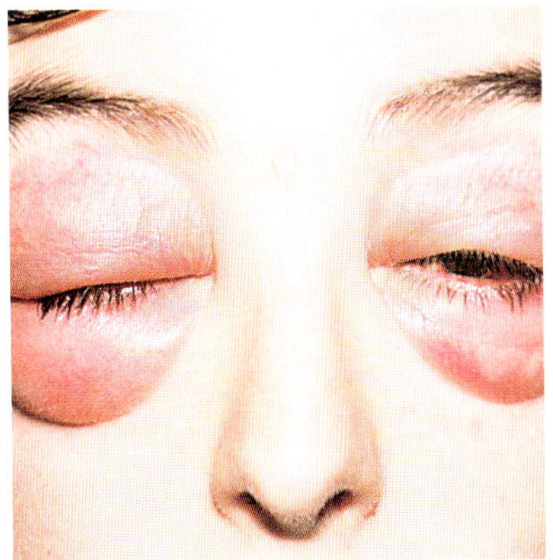

FIG. 96-17 *Extensive swelling of both eyelids secondary to massive edema (angioedema).*

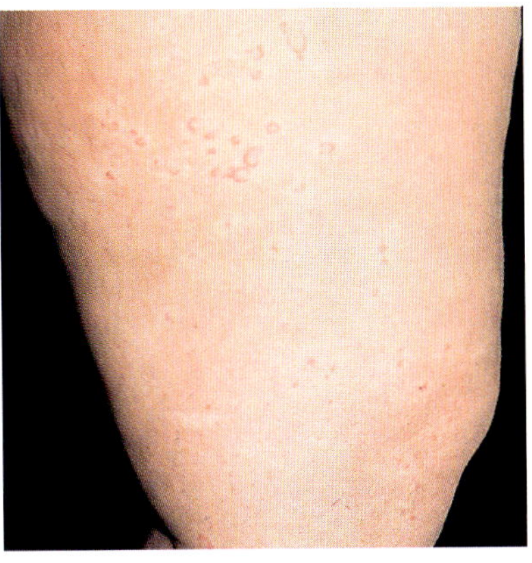

FIG. 96-18 *Tiny papules, some of them arcuate. Pallor around the lesions is a result of vasoconstriction.*

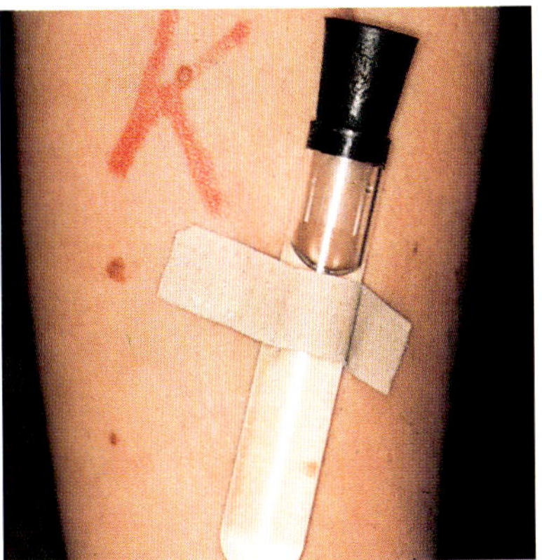

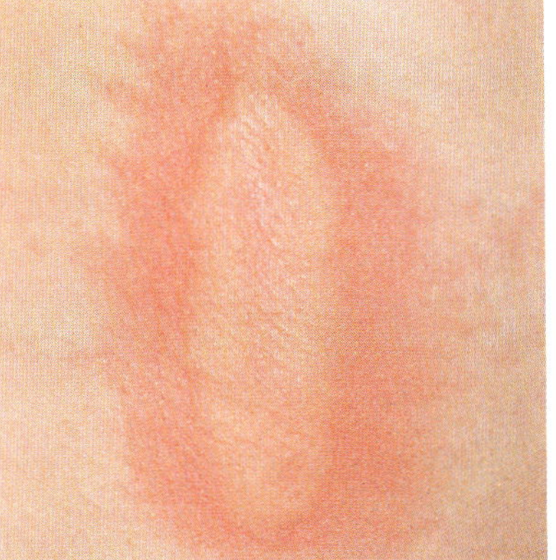

FIG. 96-19 (A, B) *This elongated wheal surrounded by a rim of erythema developed 10 minutes after application of ice to the skin (cold urticaria). The numerous melanocytic nevi are of Clark's type.*

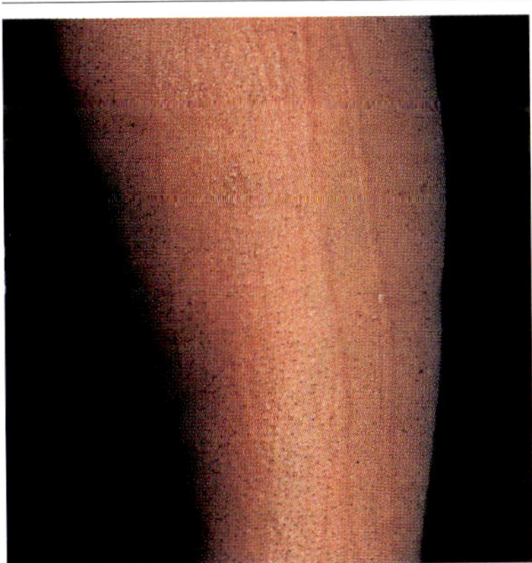

FIG. 96-20 *Urticarial dermographism.*

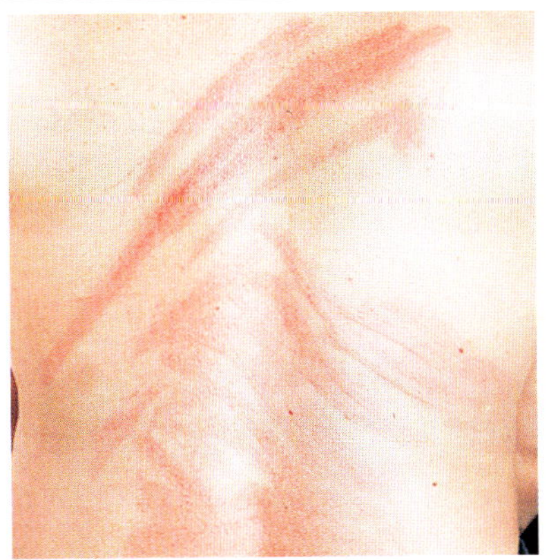

FIG. 96-21 *Urticarial dermographism.*

ADJUNCTIVE DIAGNOSTIC TESTS There are many ways to verify the cause of urticaria, depending on the type of it, e.g., allergic, cold, pressure, and so on. The patient may be exposed to the putative responsible factor, for example, an ice cube, and if a hive develops at the site the suspicion of cold as cause is confirmed.

COURSE An individual lesion of urticaria has a very short life, usually only a few hours. A patient who has urticaria, however, may suffer for years from hives that themselves come and go quickly. In most instances, the course of urticaria itself is short lived, particularly when it is a response to an allergen such as a food or drug. That condition, termed conventionally "acute urticaria," usually lasts for less than 24 hours but sometimes for a few days. If hives come and go for more than that period of time, it is likely that the process is "chronic" in the sense that lesions of urtica will come and go for many months and even years. No cause is usually found for "chronic urticaria." An exception to that general rule is when an allergen resides for a long time in a person, such as the product of parasites housed within the gastrointestinal tract. When those parasites are identified and destroyed by therapy specific for them, hives cease to appear.

INTEGRATION: UNIFYING CONCEPT Hives, irrespective of cause and irrespective of duration of the process, are similar morphologically, that is, clinically and histopathologically. A hive is an evanescent edematous papule, and biopsy of it shows a sparse to moderately dense superficial and deep perivascular and interstitial mixed-cell infiltrate of lymphocytes, neutrophils, and eosinophils around venules, and neutrophils and eosinophils in the interstitium of the reticular dermis. No inflammatory cells are present in the papillary dermis or the epidermis. When lesions of urticaria affect sites where the skin is remarkably extensible, the result is angioedema. Hives never vesiculate.

In sum, even though urticaria has many causes, among them, allergic, physical, and chemical, morphologic expressions of them are the same. The cause of hives that come and then go once and for all almost always is allergic, and the offender is usually identified precisely, often by the patient. The cause of hives that come and go for years, however, usually cannot be determined and is thought to be due to a mechanism other than an immunologic one.

THERAPY Treatment must be directed at the cause of urticaria, at least when the cause is identifiable. When no cause can be found, antagonists to H-1 antihistamine receptors are effective, but a combination of H-1 and a stabilizer of mast cells (Ketotifen) also may be employed. Oral and parenteral corticosteroids are indicated in acute cases that are severe and may be life threatening.

DEFINITION A benign neoplastic process of mast cells. In children the condition manifests itself as papules, nodules, and tumors that urticate upon rubbing, and as blisters; in adults it expresses itself as macules and papules accompanied by telangiectases (telangiectasia macularis eruptiva perstans). In adults the lesions increase steadily in number and do not go away. The lesions in children tend to regress and disappear within months.

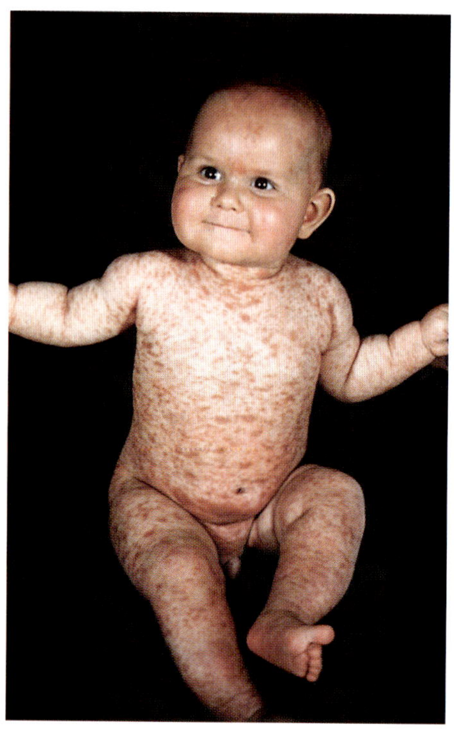

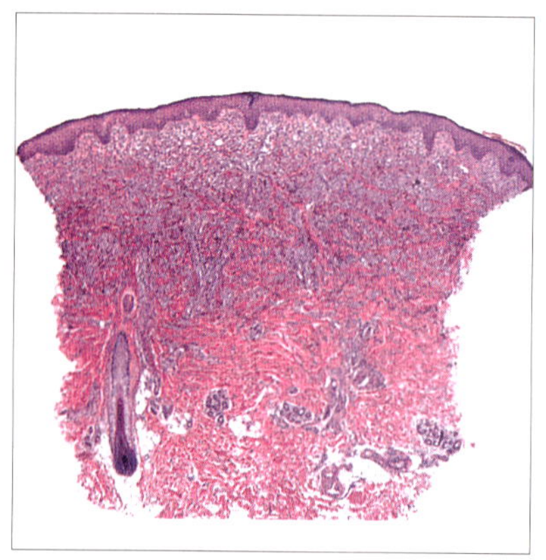

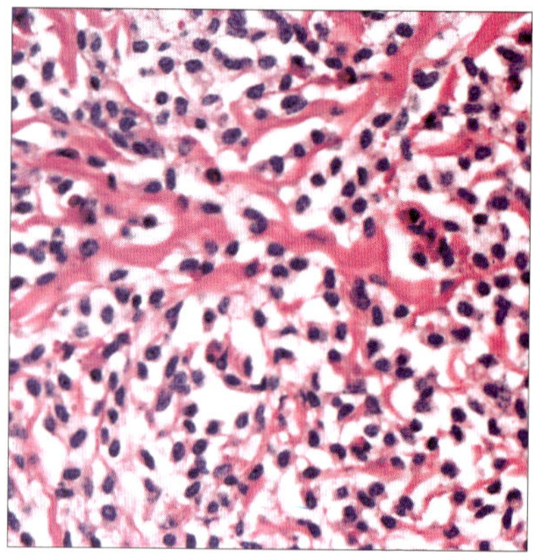

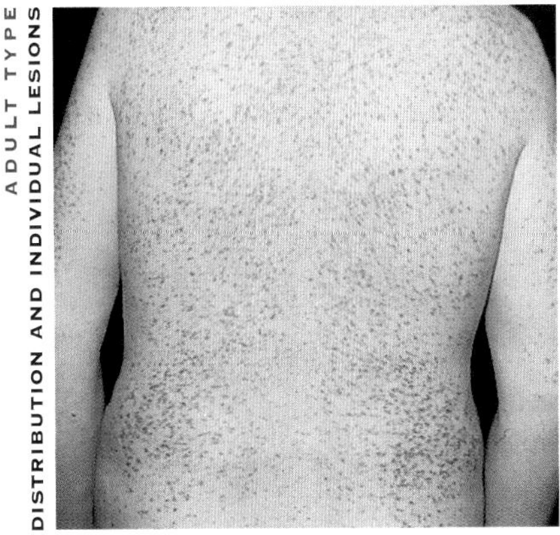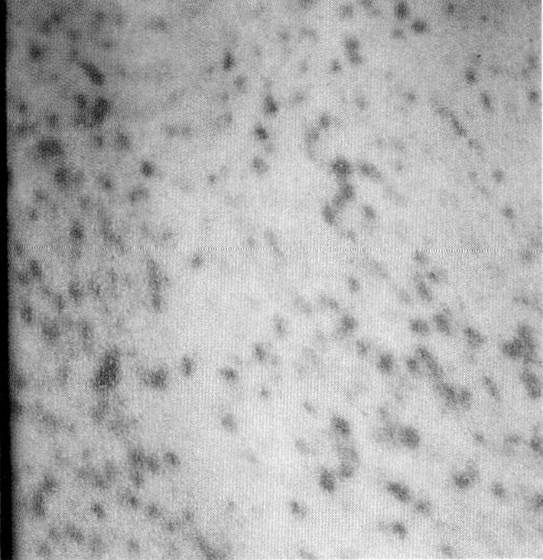

FIG. 97-1 (A, B) *Widespread red-purple macules and papules.*

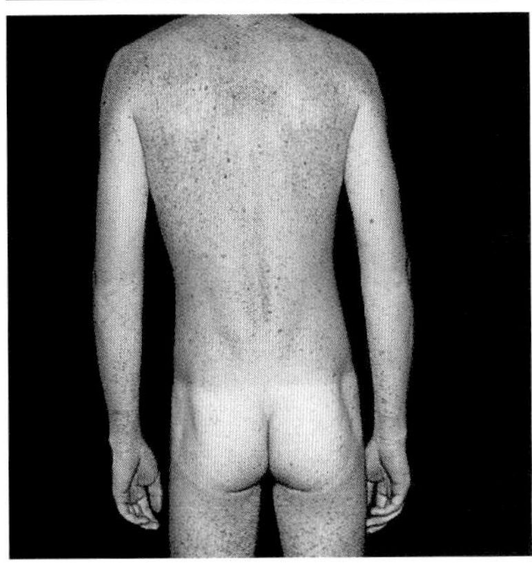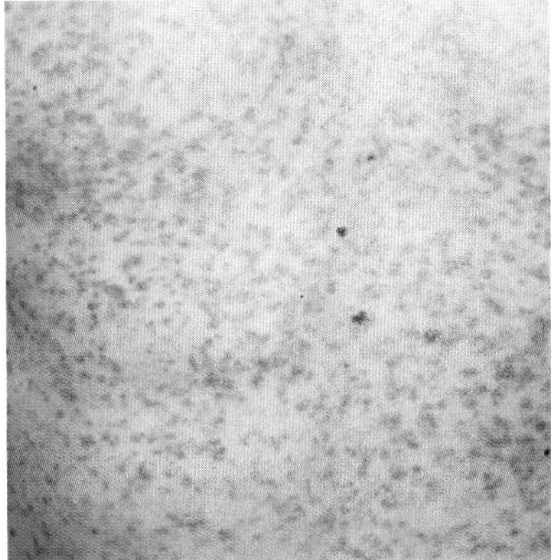

FIG. 97-2 (A, B) *Widespread closely-set macules and papules.*

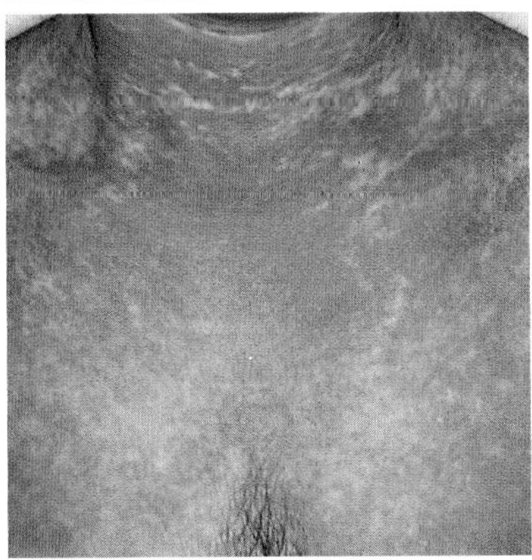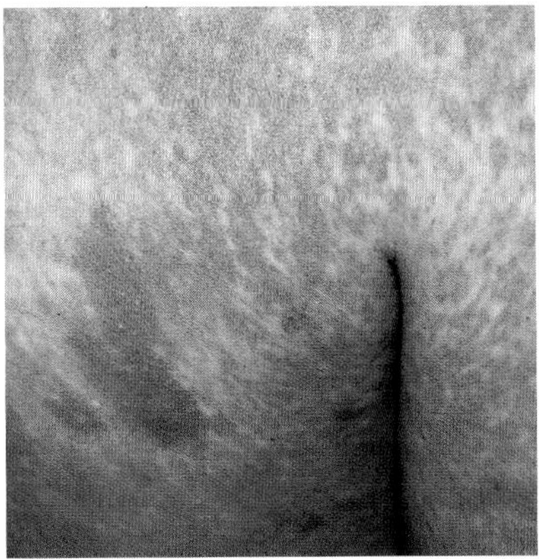

FIG. 97-3 (A, B) *Dusky erythematous macules and papules, most of which have become confluent to form an ill-defined but extensive plaque.*

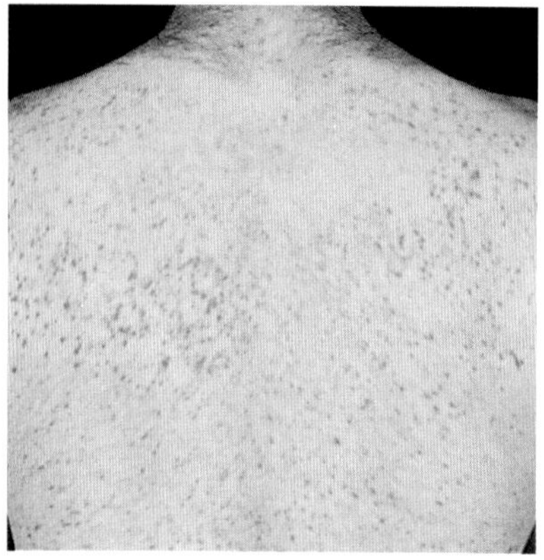

FIG. 97-4 *Widespread reddish brown papules.*

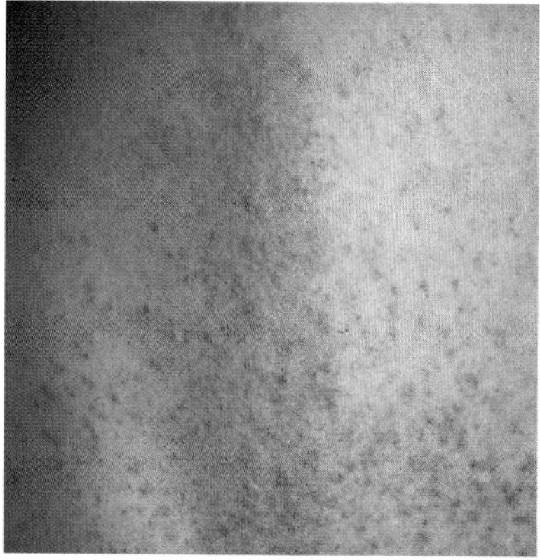

FIG. 97-5 *Darier's sign (urtication of lesions upon trauma).*

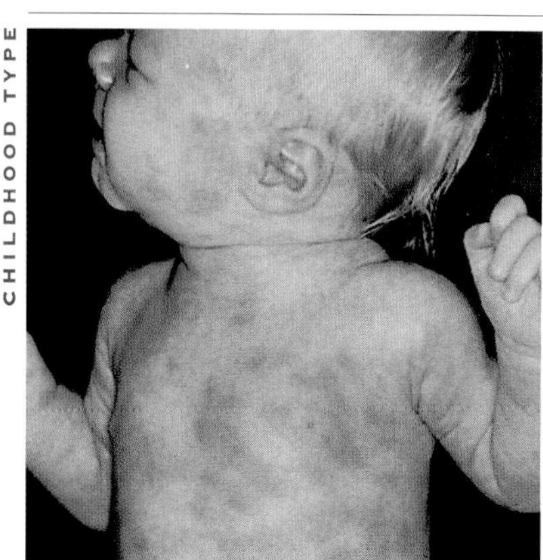

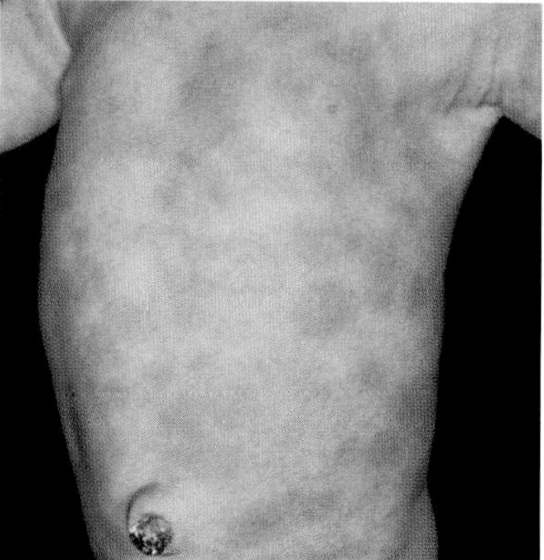

FIG. 97-6 (A, B) *Macules, patches, papules, and plaques.*

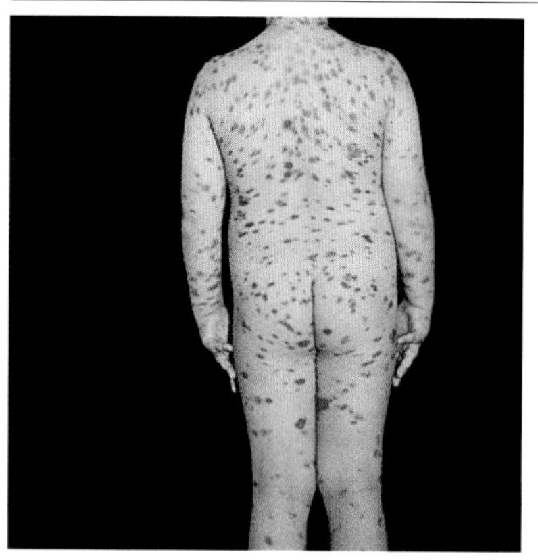

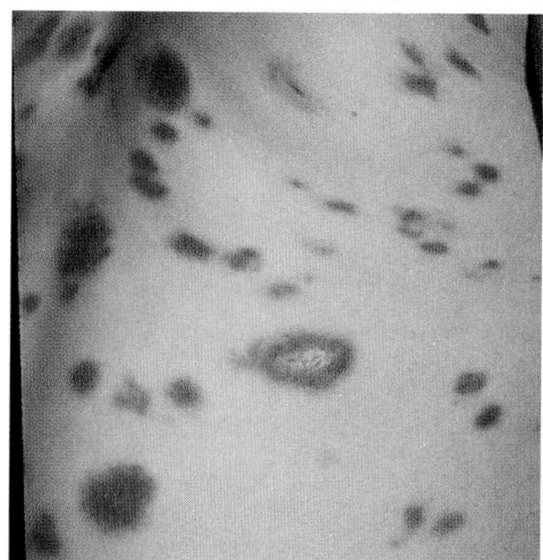

FIG. 97-7 (A, B) *Macules, papules, plaques, and nodules.*

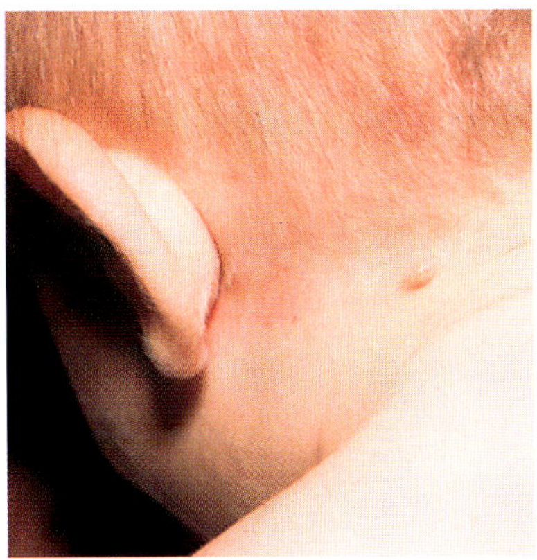

FIG. 97-8 *Papule.*

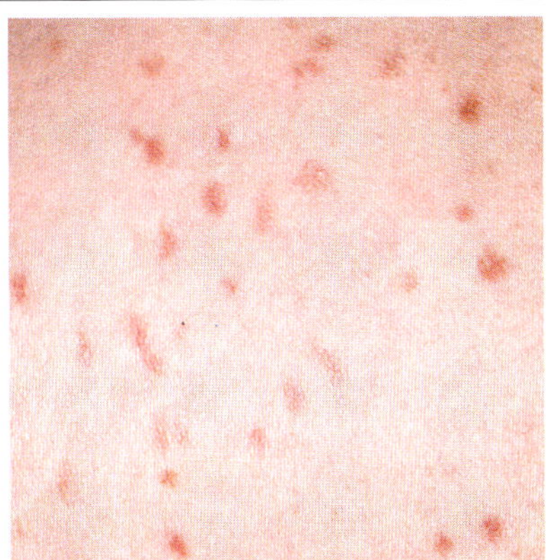

FIG. 97-9 *Numerous papules.*

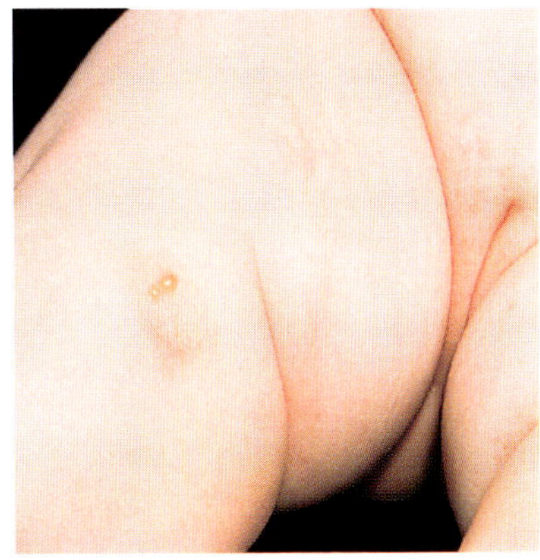

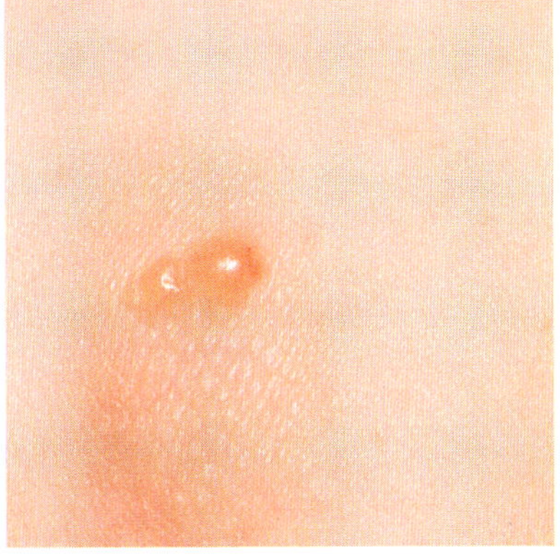

FIG. 97-10 (A, B) *Vesicles on a plaque whose surface is mammillated.*

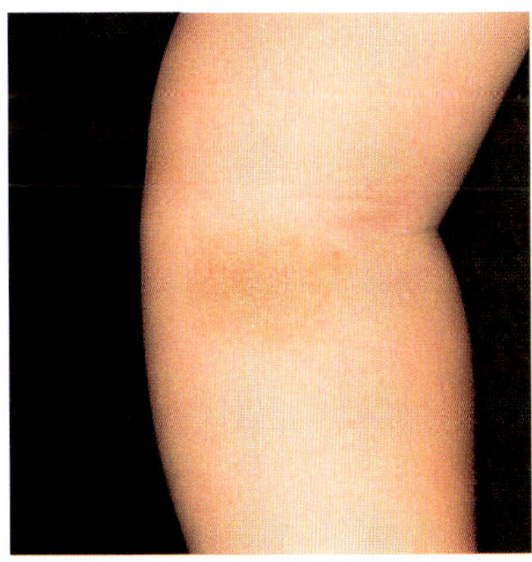

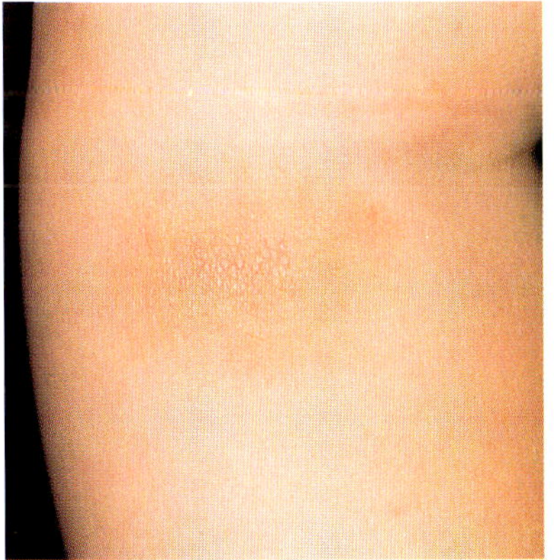

FIG. 97-11 (A, B) *Patch on which there are agminated papules.*

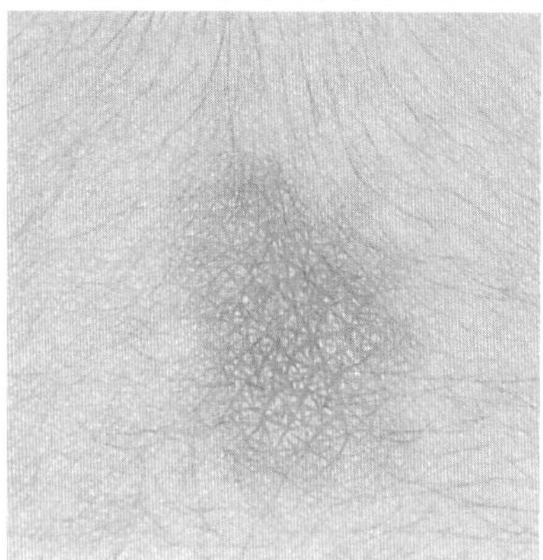

FIG. 97-12 *Yellow plaque with ill-defined borders made up of closely-set papules. Skin markings are accentuated.*

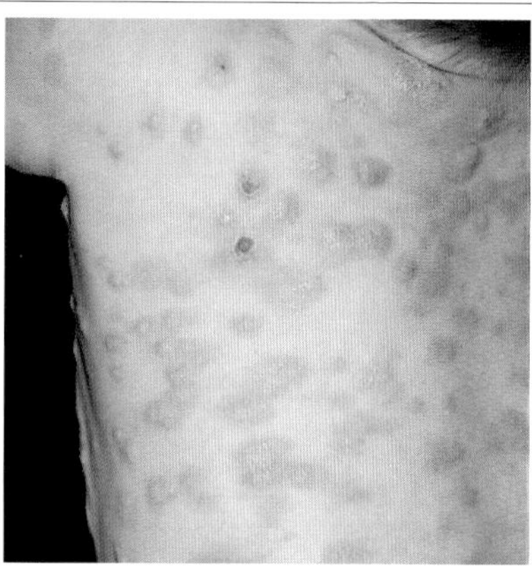

FIG. 97-13 *Widespread patches, papules, plaques, vesicles, and bullae.*

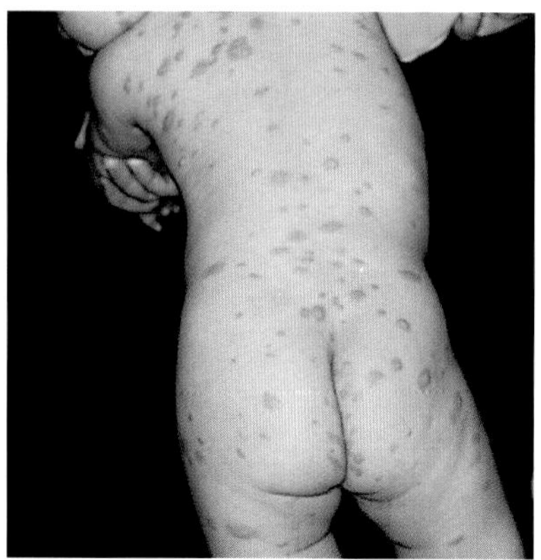

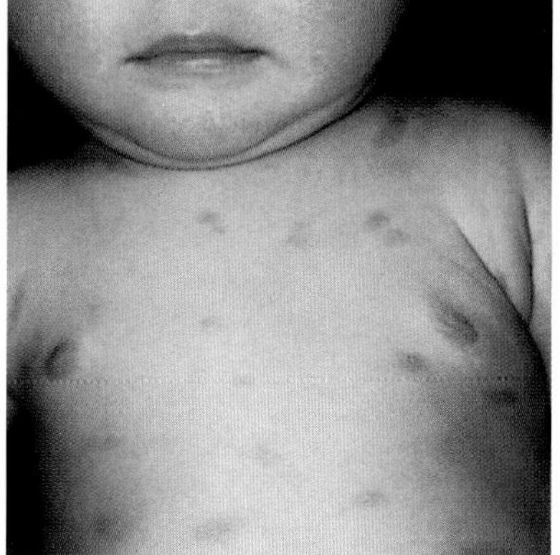

FIG. 97-14 (A, B) *Widespread macules, papules, plaques, and nodules.*

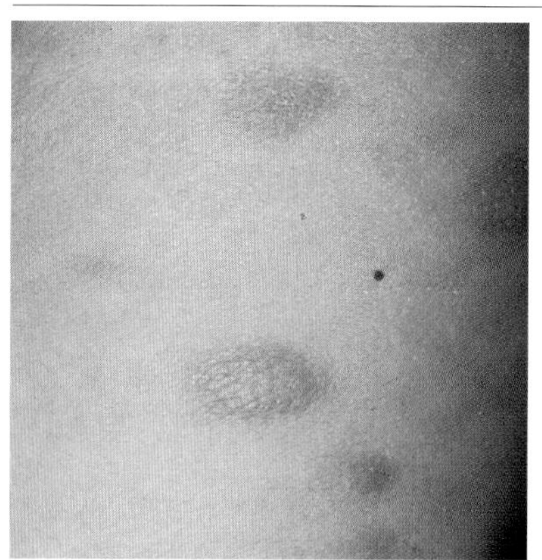

FIG. 97-14 (C) *Mammillated papules.*

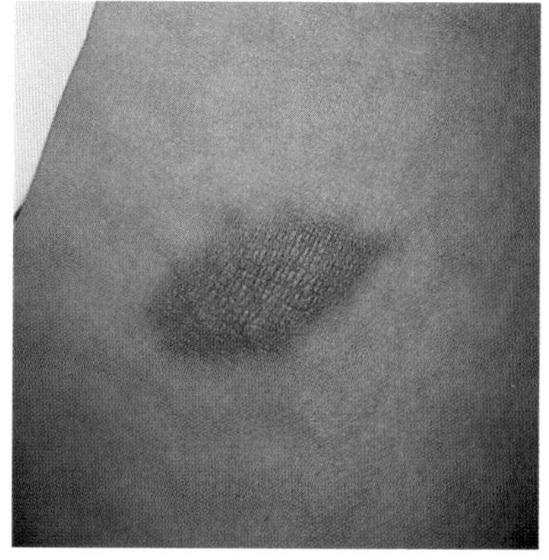

FIG. 97-15 *Ellipsoid red-brown plaque, the skin markings of which are accentuated.*

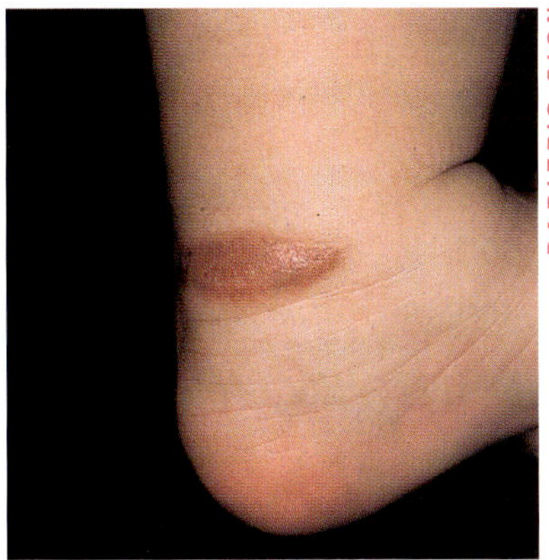

FIG. 97-16 *Fusiform plaque.*

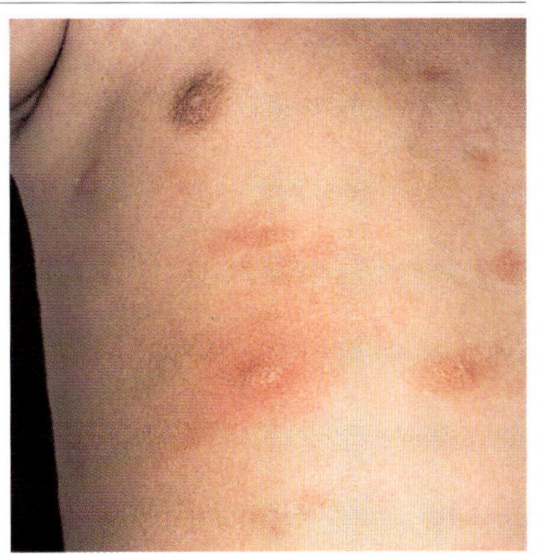

FIG. 97-17 *Urtication of a papule surrounded by a flare of erythema within minutes of rubbing of it firmly.*

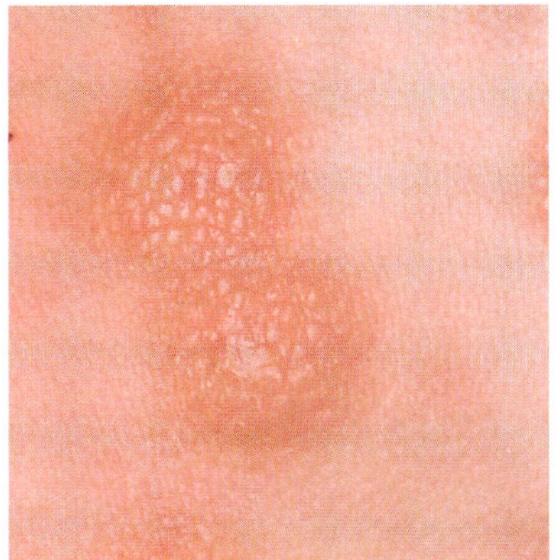

FIG. 97-18 *Papules with a mammillated surface and a surrounding flare of erythema following vigorous rubbing.*

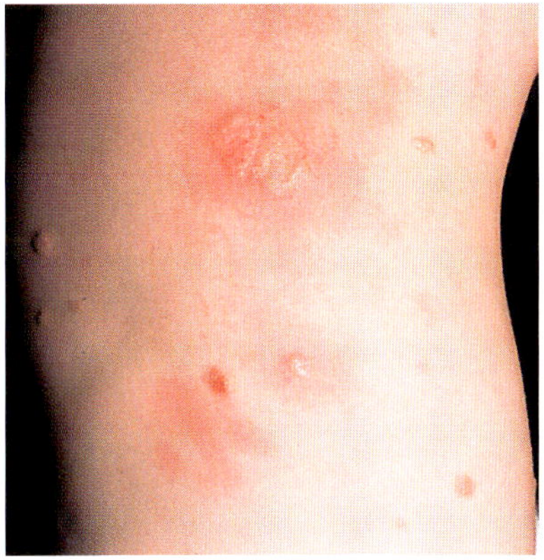

FIG. 97-19 *Blisters that have been induced in a child by vigorous external trauma. A flare surrounds the blisters.*

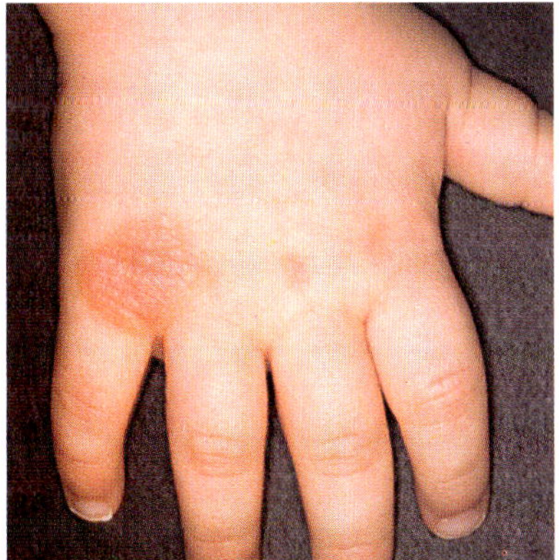

FIG. 97-20 *Nodule with "peau d'orange" appearance.*

ADJUNCTIVE DIAGNOSTIC TESTS Specialized stains for mast cells should be applied to sections of tissue from specimens of skin, the Leder stain being the most dramatic, coloring mast cells brisk red. If clinically there is evidence of disease of internal organs, search should be undertaken for it—bone scan, for example, and aspiration biopsy of bone marrow.

COURSE The course of lesions of urticaria pigmentosa depends on the type(s) of lesions that constitute it. Papules, nodules, and blisters in children usually wane in weeks. By contrast, macules and papules in adults, called telangiectasia macularis eruptiva perstans, not only persist, but become progressively more numerous and widespread.

INTEGRATION: UNIFYING CONCEPT Urticaria pigmentosa, irrespective of the patient's age at onset or its morphologic presentation, is a benign neoplasm composed of mast cells. Nodules of urticaria pigmentosa in children are characterized histopathologically by dense, diffuse infiltrates of mast cells. If such lesions have been rubbed prior to biopsy, the mast cells will be seen by conventional microscopy to have been joined by innumerable eosinophils, a consequence of sudden release from mast cells of pre-packaged (in cytoplasmic granules) eosinophilic chemotactic factor. Bullous lesions of urticaria pigmentosa in children show a subepidermal blister in addition to the same features in the dermis that are present in nodules of the condition.

In adults, macular and papular lesions of telangiectasia macularis eruptiva perstans are characterized by sparse superficial perivascular infiltrates of mast cells around widely dilated venules of the superficial plexus, and those cells also are scattered in the interstitium of the upper part of the reticular dermis. Mast cells usually are not found in the papillary dermis of the macular and papular expression of urticaria pigmentosa, and never are they present within the epidermis.

Although there are clear morphologic differences in types of urticaria pigmentosa as they present themselves in children and in adults, the process is fundamentally a benign neoplastic one of mast cells.

THERAPY For widespread macules and papules, antihistamines (H-1 and H-2 receptor antagonists) are valuable in alleviating pruritus. Orally administered cromolyn sodium and PUVA also may be useful.

For discrete persistent nodules and tumors, surgical excision is appropriate.

DEFINITION Papules on skin and mucous membranes that result from infection of keratinocytes by different types of papillomavirus and classified according to their silhouettes, to wit, papillated (verrucae vulgares on different sites such as volar skin, i.e., verrucae palmares et plantares, and near or on mucous membranes, i.e., condylomata acuminata) and flat (verrucae planae), and by the type of inciting papillomavirus, HPV 6 and 11 for condylomata acuminata, for example, and HPV 5 and 8 for epidermodysplasia verruciformis.

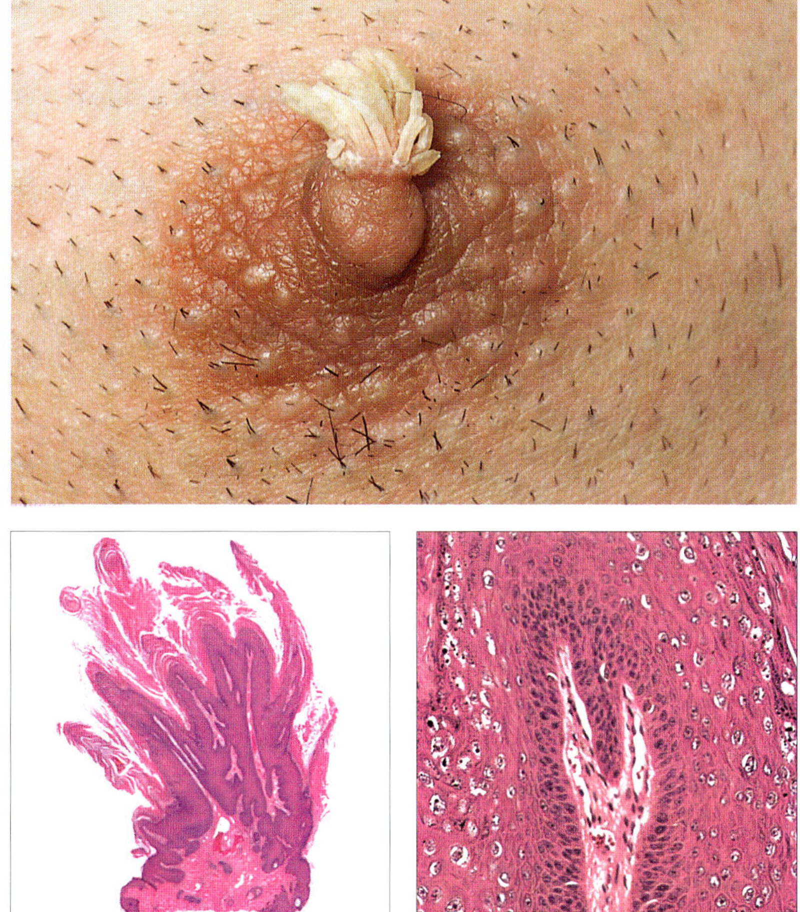

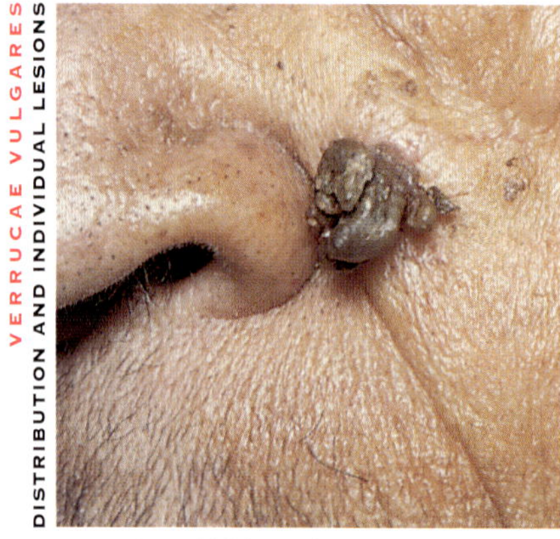

FIG. 98-1   *Filiform keratotic papules in a cluster.*

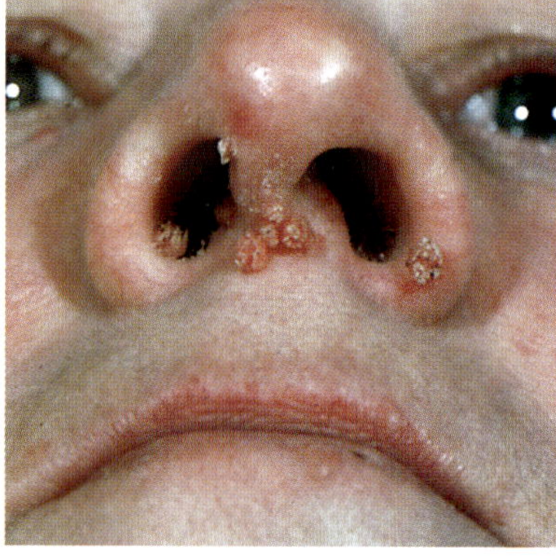

FIG. 98-2   *Filiform keratotic papules.*

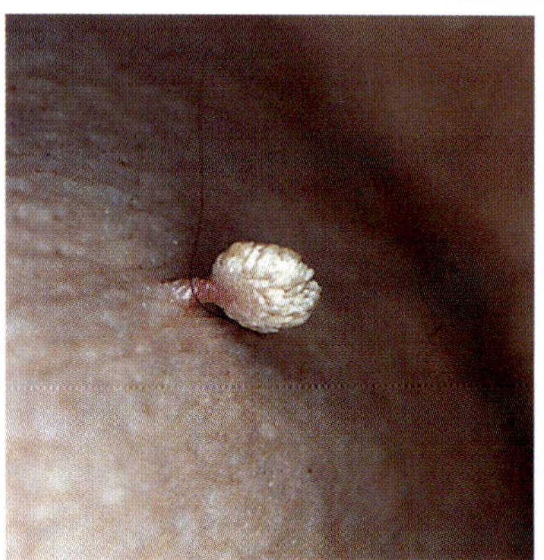

FIG. 98-3   *Pedunculated filiform papule.*

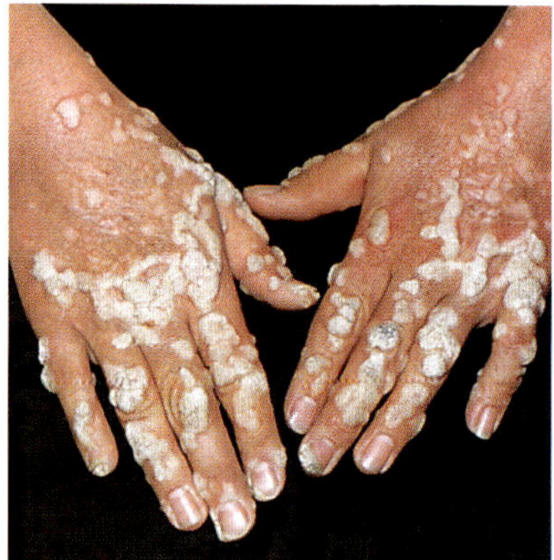

FIG. 98-4   *Numerous keratotic papules, some of them periungual.*

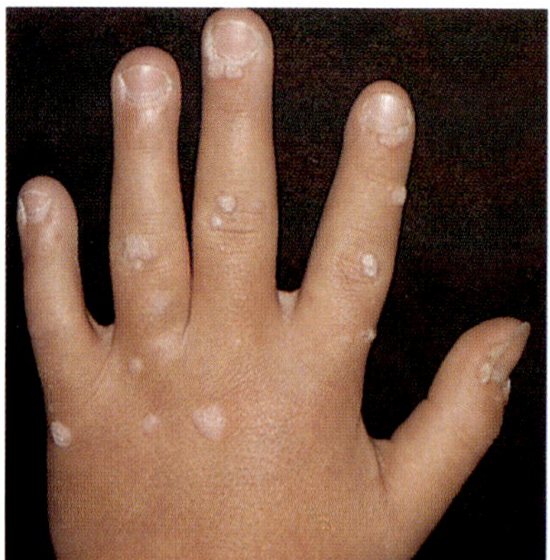

FIG. 98-5   *Scattered keratotic papules, some of them periungual.*

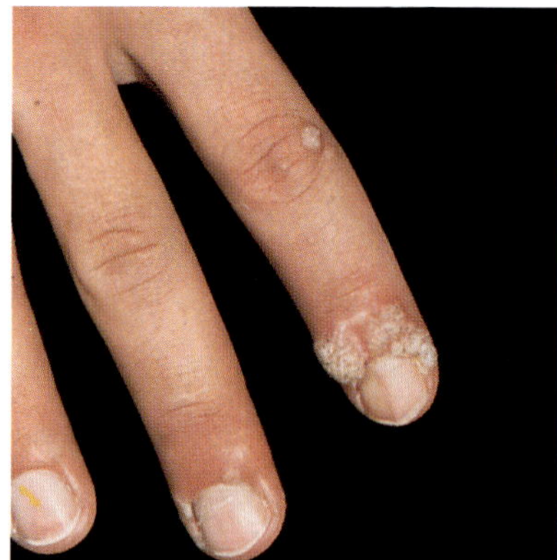

FIG. 98-6   *Periungual keratotic papules and a discrete keratotic papule over a knuckle.*

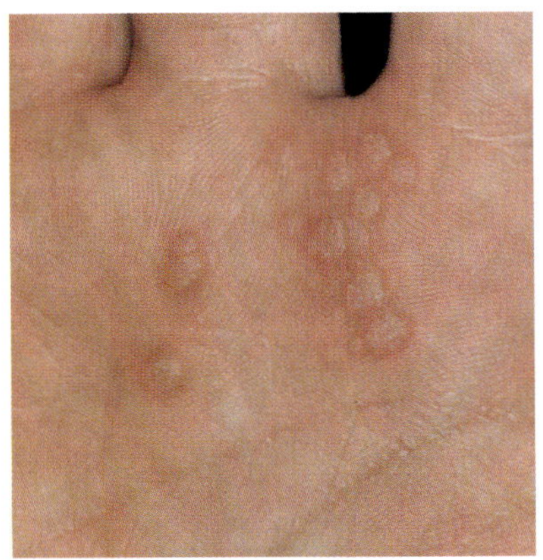

FIG. 98-7 *Keratotic papules, some of them in a line.*

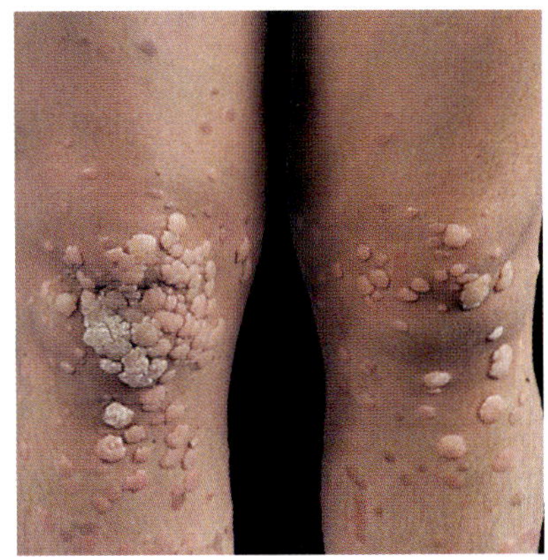

FIG. 98-8 *Keratotic papules, many of which are set closely.*

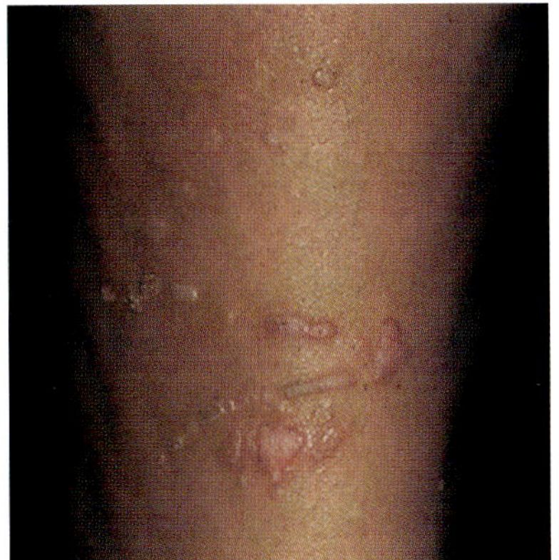

FIG. 98-9 *Keratotic papules, some in linear array (autoinoculation).*

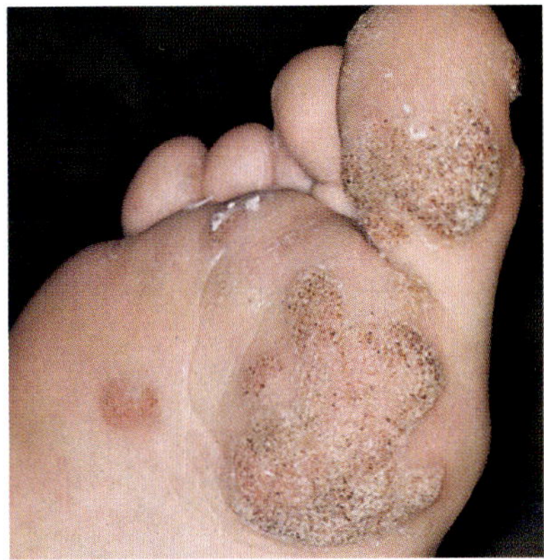

FIG. 98-10 *Keratotic papules and plaques (mosaic warts).*

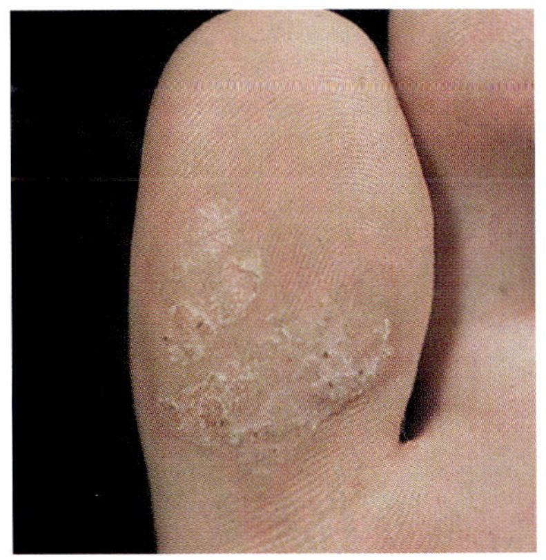

FIG. 98-11 *Keratotic plaque (mosaic wart).*

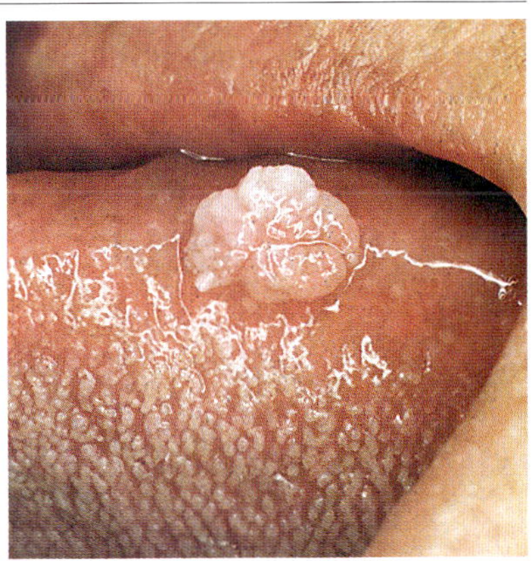

FIG. 98-12 *Macerated keratotic papule.*

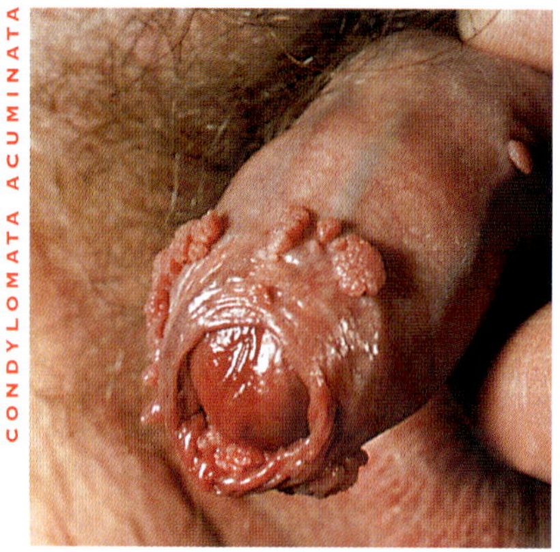

FIG. 98-13 *Papules with a mammillated surface.*

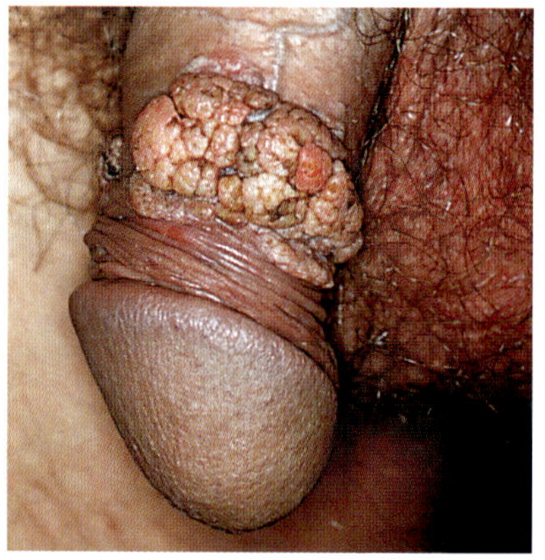

FIG. 98-14 *Plaque composed of verrucous papules.*

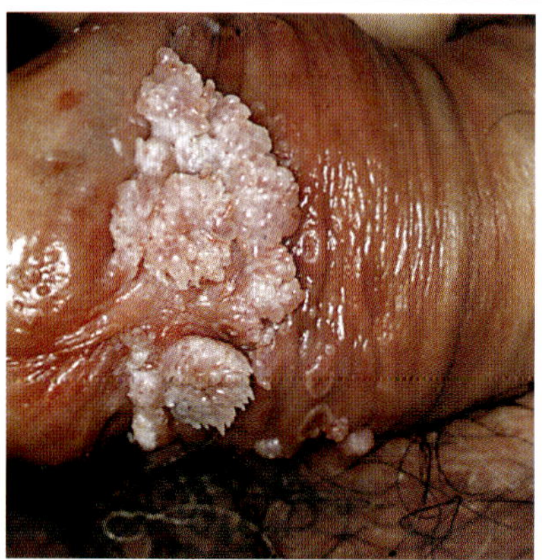

FIG. 98-15 *Plaque made up of verrucous papules.*

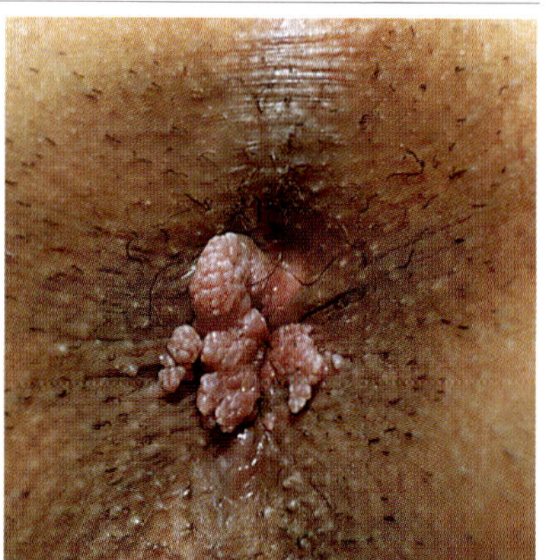

FIG. 98-16 *Sessile keratotic papules.*

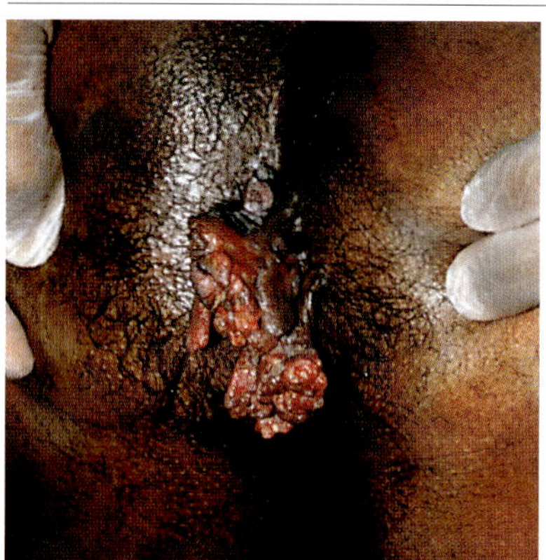

FIG. 98-17 *Verrucous nodules.*

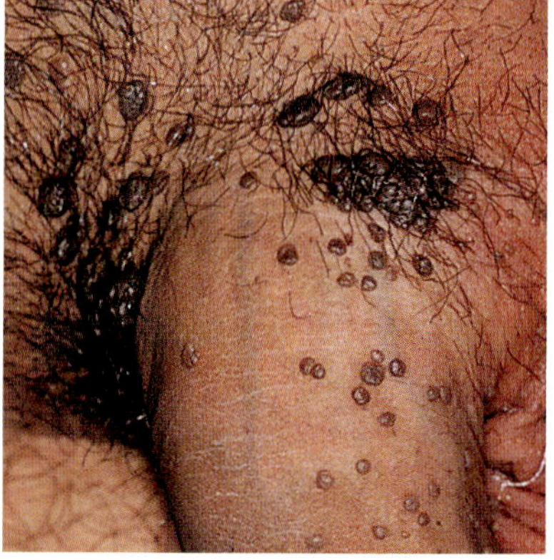

FIG. 98-18 *Pigmented papules, some of them having become confluent to form a plaque.*

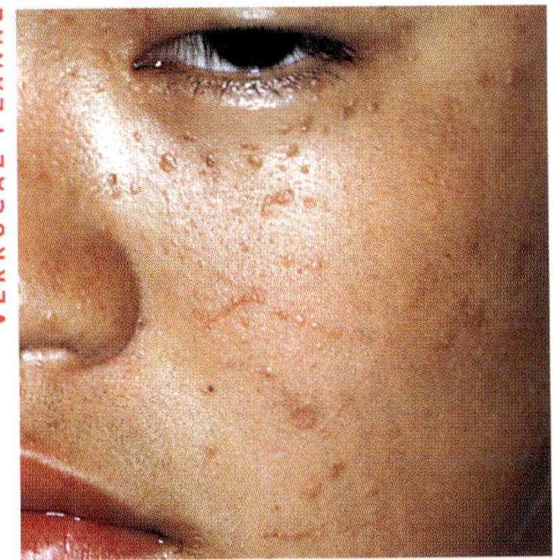

FIG. 98-19 *Tiny papules of flat warts.*

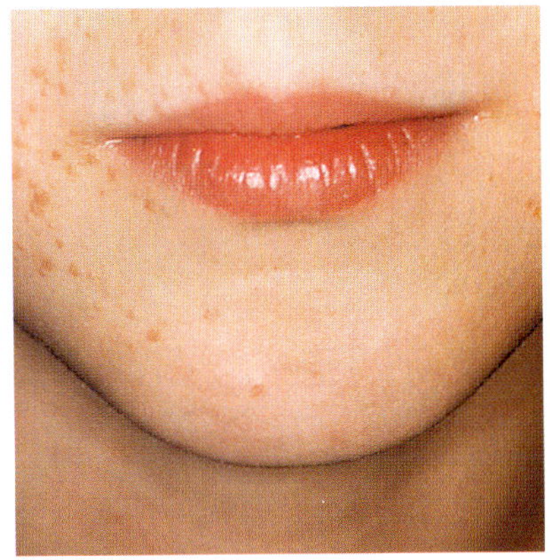

FIG. 98-20 *Papules of verruca planae.*

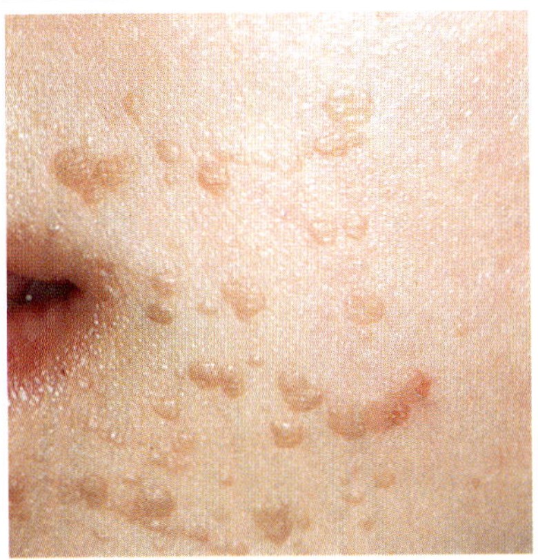

FIG. 98-21 *Tan flat-topped papules, some of which are arranged in a line.*

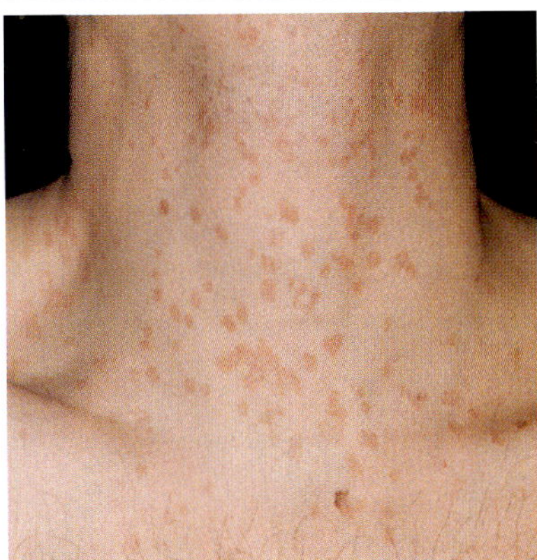

FIG. 98-22 *Papules, some in linear arrangement.*

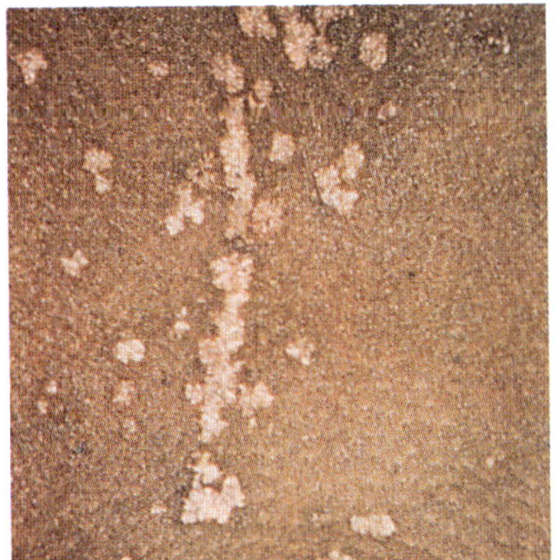

FIG. 98-23 *Flat-surfaced papules of verrucae planae (epidermodysplasia verruciformis), many of them in a line (autoinoculation).*

COURSE There are different types of verrucae vulgares, among them, those that appear on palms and soles, where they are called verrucae palmares et plantares, and on genital skin, where they are termed condylomata acuminata. In contrast to verrucae vulgares are verrucae planae, known also as flat warts. Individual verrucae of both kinds usually have a limited life span; in most instances, their lives are played out in months. Sometimes, however, warts on different anatomic sites may last for longer periods of time, i.e., years, and, in those instances, the people who bear them usually are immunosuppressed.

INTEGRATION: UNIFYING CONCEPT Verrucae are classified conventionally as vulgares, palmar-plantar, condylomata acuminata, and plane. Warts on glabrous skin, on palms and soles, and in the anogenital region may be thought of as examples of verrucae vulgares that look different because of the peculiarities of those different anatomic sites and possibly because of the specific type of papillomavirus responsible for them. In contrast to papillated warts are those that are only ever so slightly mammillated and for practical purposes have a somewhat flat surface, namely, those of verrucae planae. All warts, irrespective of morphologic appearance, are caused by papillomavirus, and warts on certain anatomic sites seem to be caused by certain types of that virus. The relationship between anatomic site of warts and specific type of papillomavirus, however, is not invariable.

Evolving lesions of verrucae vulgares are exo-endophytic lesions whose corneocytes in the stratum corneum house large, round nuclei that are jammed with virions of papillomavirus. The granular zone is markedly thickened by plate-like clumps of keratohyaline. The epidermis is hyperplastic and digitated. Within dermal papillae, dilated capillaries spiral to just beneath the base of the epidermis. At a later stage, verrucae vulgares show parakeratosis at the tips of digitations, prominent hypergranulosis but without large aggregations of keratohyaline, and digitated epidermal hyperplasia above dilated tortuous capillaries in thin dermal papillae. Late lesions of verrucae vulgares are largely endophytic and on the face may be associated with tricholemmal differentiation of hyperplastic infundibula ("tricholemmoma"), with "squamous eddies" within hyperplastic infundibula ("inverted follicular keratosis"), and even with signs of sebaceous or apocrine differentiation, or both of them together. On palms and soles, verrucae sometimes resolve as angiofibromas that are positioned in a discrete focus in the upper part of the dermis.

Papillomavirus has the capability to induce keratinocytes to first become hyperplastic and then malignantly neoplastic. One example of such transformation is bowenoid papulosis, which begins as condyloma acuminatum and eventuates in squamous-cell carcinoma in situ. Another example is epidermodysplasia verruciformis, consisting of plane warts that may then become squamous-cell carcinoma in situ and sometimes even "invasive" carcinoma. It has been shown that some verrucous carcinomas on different anatomic sites begin as an infection by papillomavirus. That association may be demonstrated one day, too, for "solitary" and subungual keratoacanthoma and perhaps even for proliferating tricholemmal cystic squamous-cell carcinoma.

THERAPY For warts, application of solutions or lotions that contain salicylic acid is judicious, as is cryotherapy. Electrocautery and laser coagulation are also effective.

For condylomata, podophyllin, electrocautery, cryotherapy, intralesional interferon, and laser surgery are all beneficial. Aldara cream that enhances an immunologic response is said to be worthwhile.

DEFINITION An inflammatory process manifested by a transient, usually widespread eruption, made up typically of macules and papules, and episodically of vesicles and pustules. It is caused by a virus disseminated hematogenously.

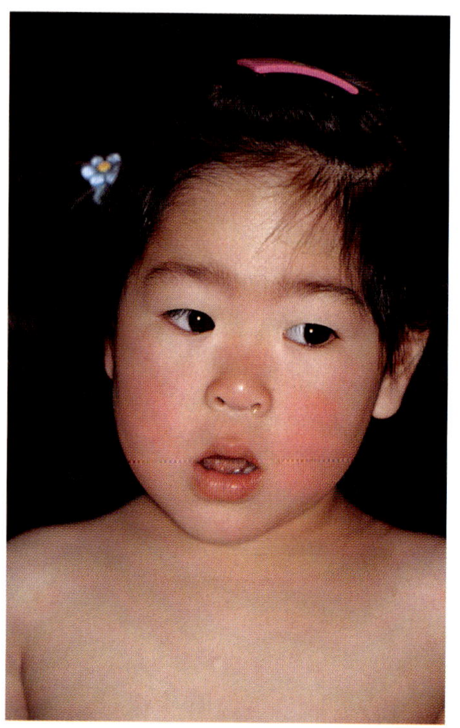

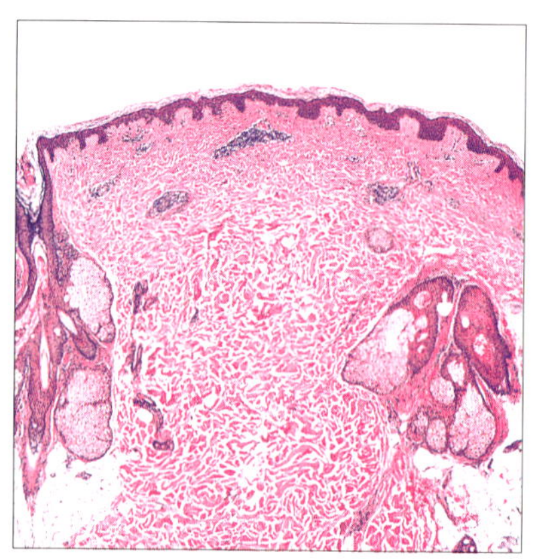

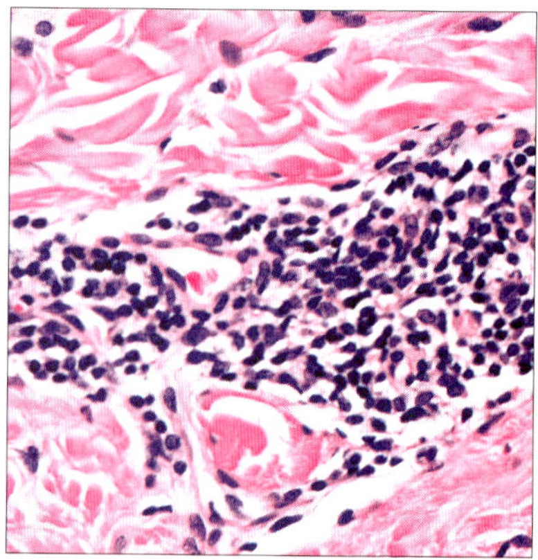

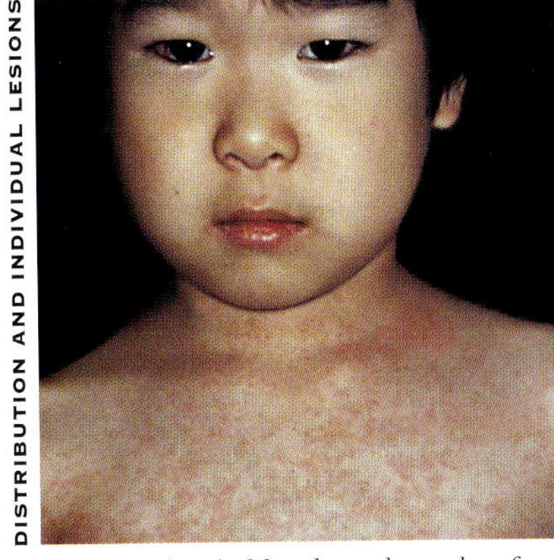
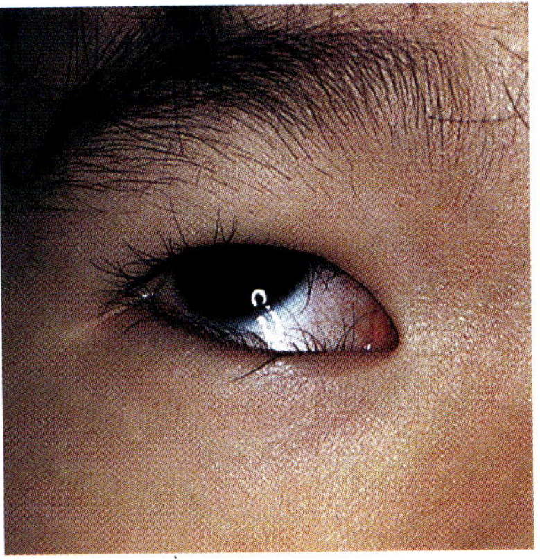

FIG. 99-1 (A, B) *Macules and papules of measles with associated conjunctivitis.*

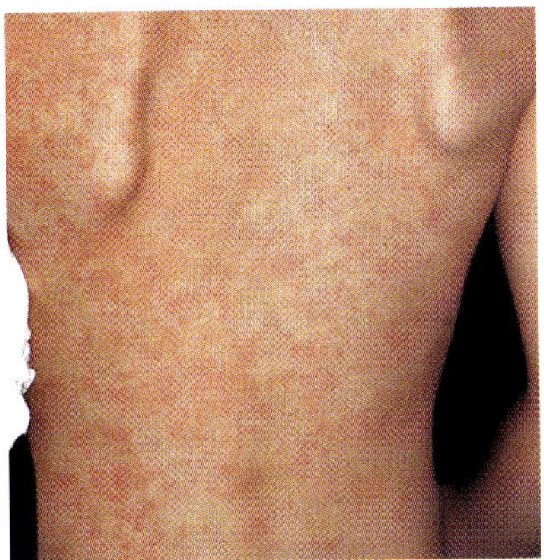
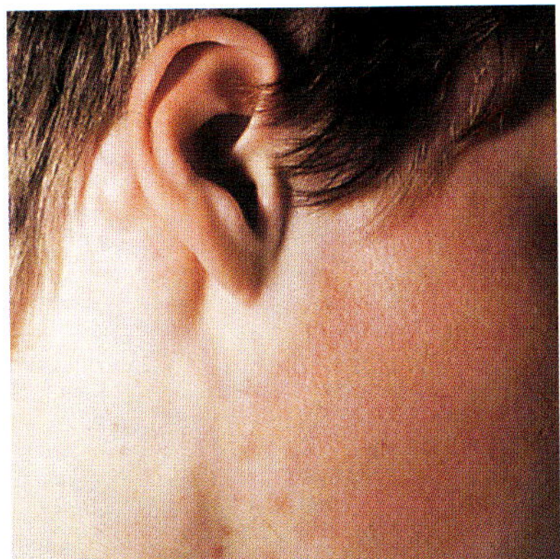

FIG. 99-1 (C) *Macules and papules of measles.*

FIG. 99-2 *Lymphadenopathy in a youngster with German measles.*

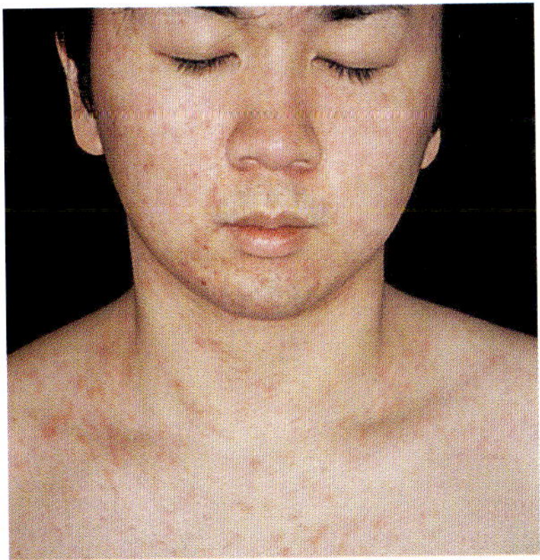
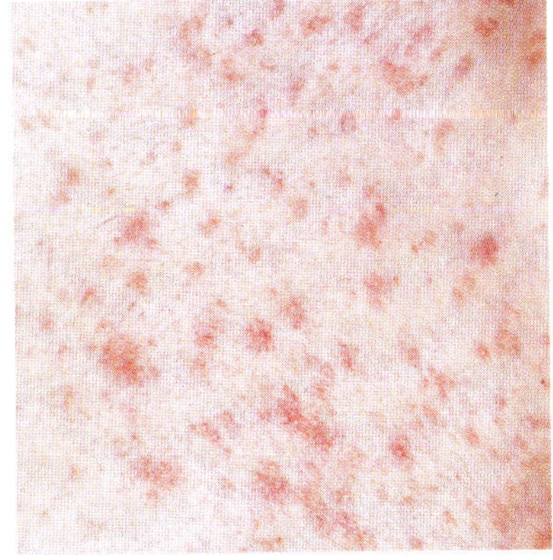

FIG. 99-3 (A, B) *Macules and papules in confluence of measles.*

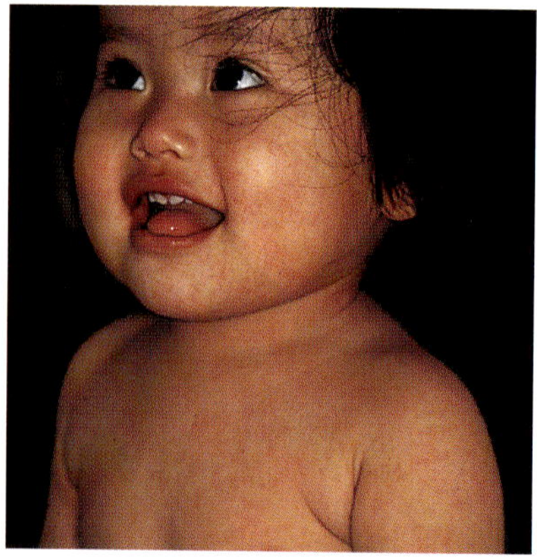
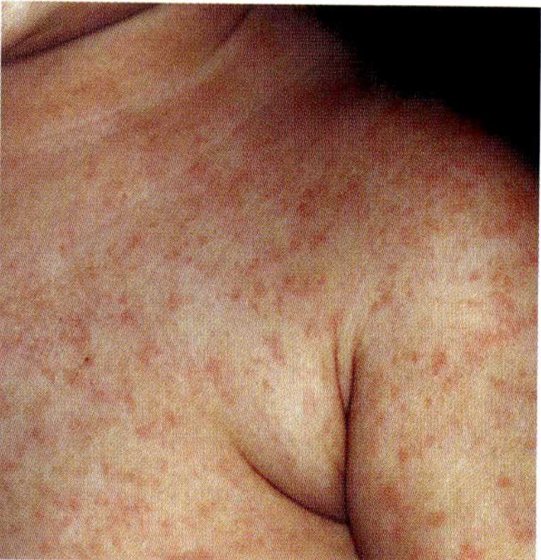

FIG. 99-4 (A, B) *Macules and papules in confluence of German measles (rubella).*

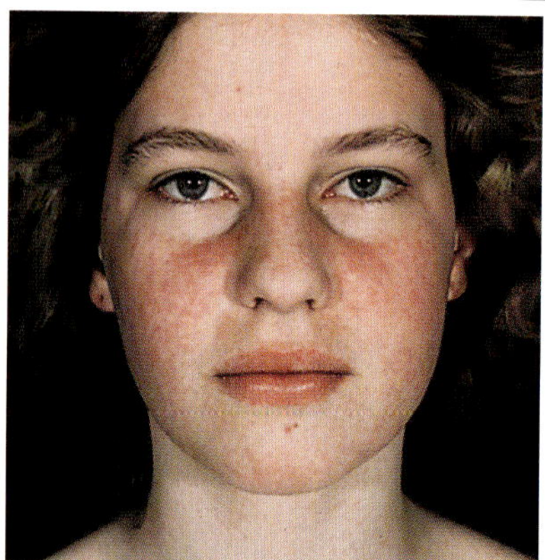
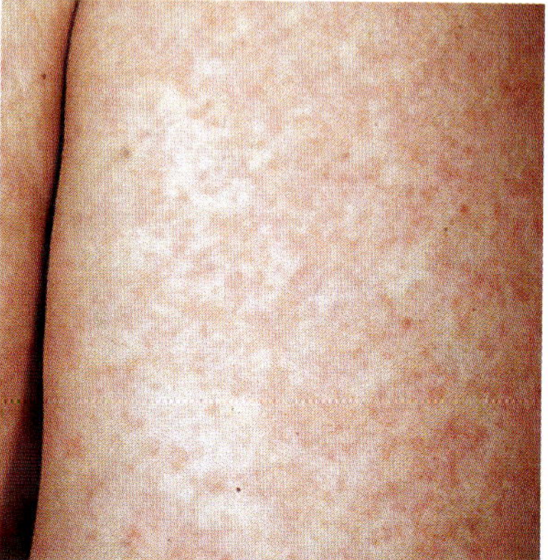

FIG. 99-5 (A, B) *Macules and papules in confluence of German measles.*

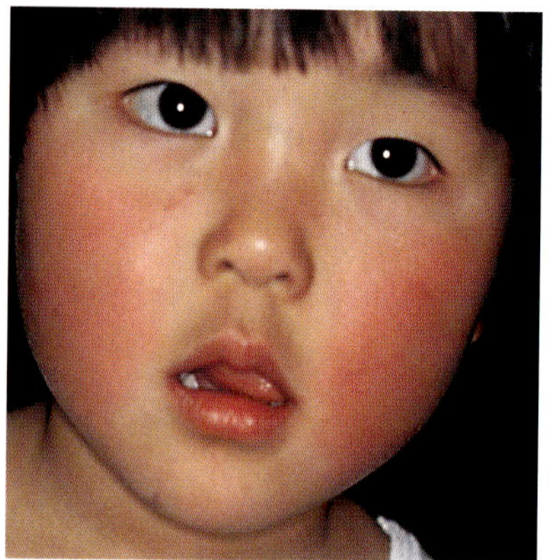
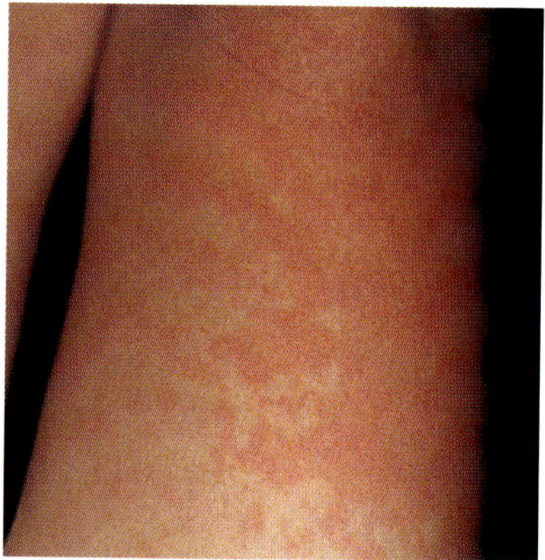

FIG. 99-6 (A, B) *Macules and papules in confluence ("slapped skin" appearance) of Fifth disease (erythema infectiosum), and as discrete macules and papules.*

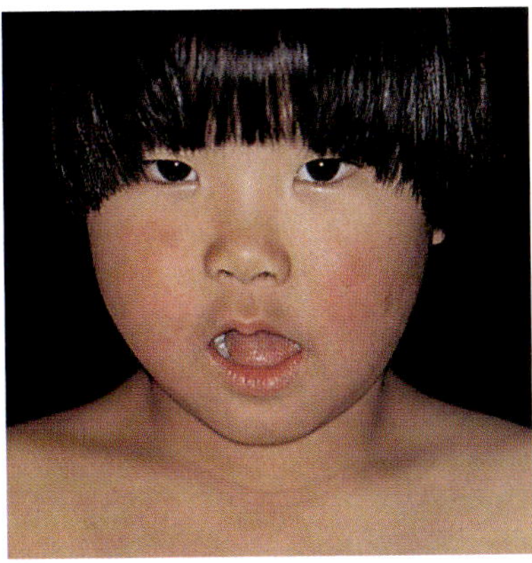
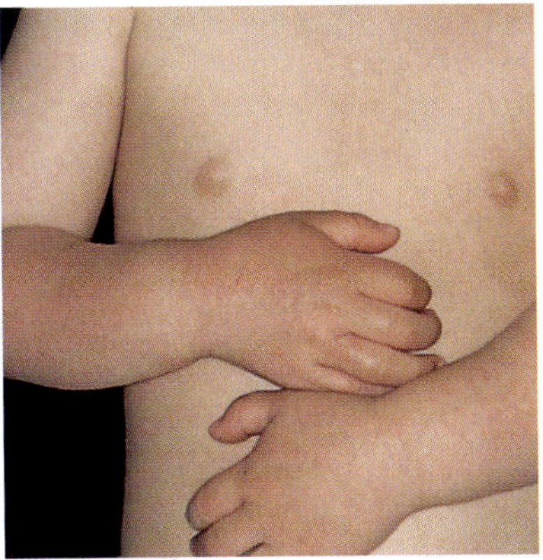

FIG. 99-7 (A, B) *"Slapped cheeks," and macules and papules in confluence on swollen hands and arms of a child with Fifth disease (erythema infectiosum).*

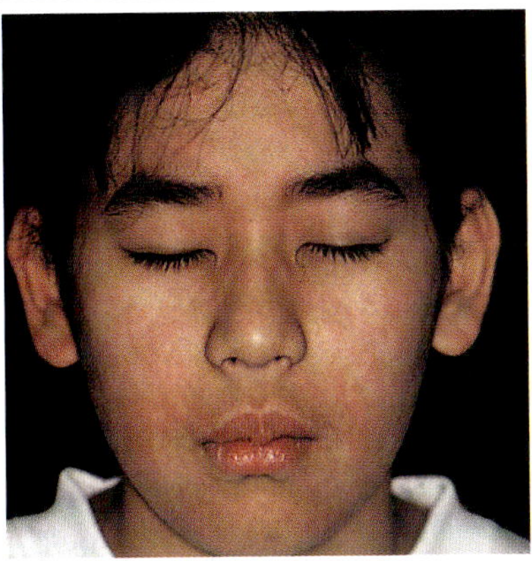
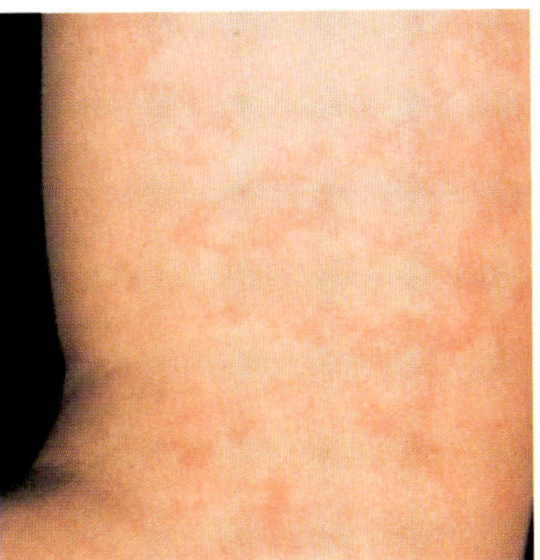

FIG. 99-8 *Macules and papules of Fifth disease.*

FIG. 99-9 *Arcuate and annular lesions in Fifth disease.*

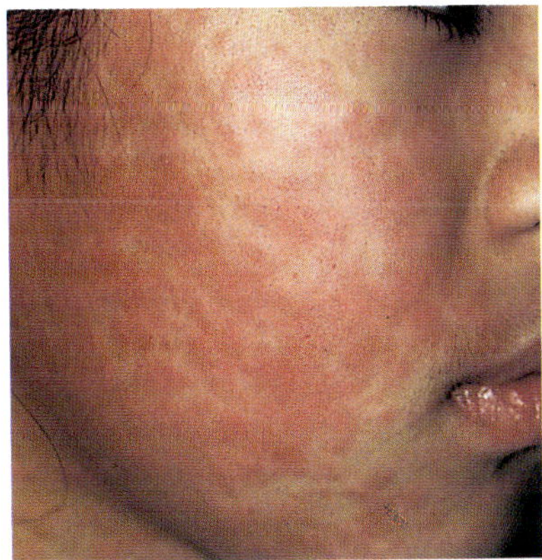
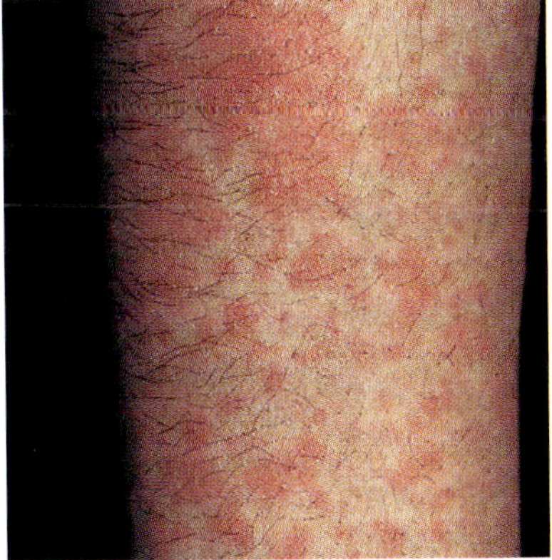

FIG. 99-10 (A, B) *Macules and papules of Fifth disease.*

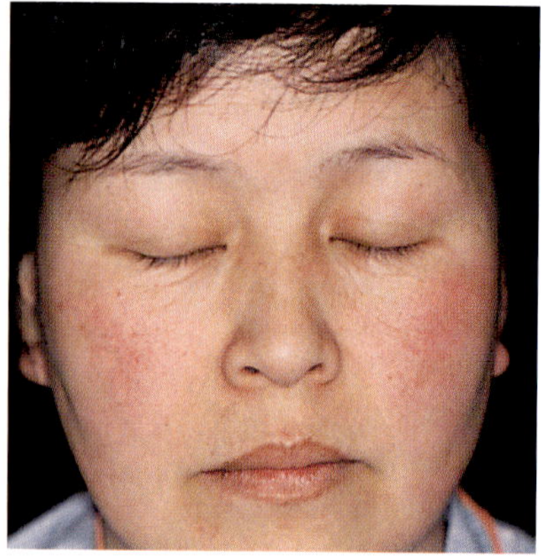

FIG. 99-11 *"Slapped cheeks" of Fifth disease.*

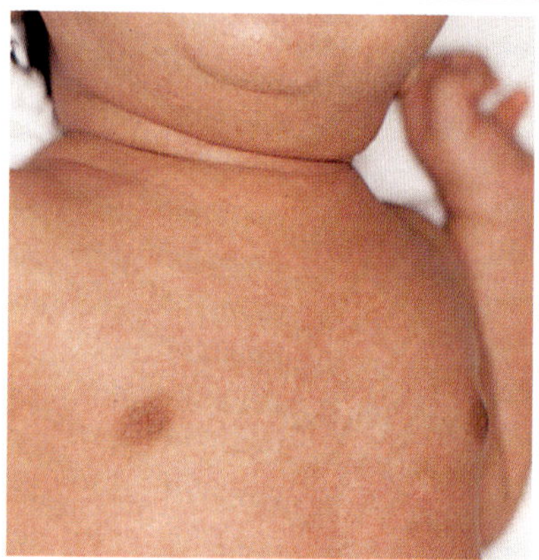

FIG. 99-12 *Widespread macules and papules of Sixth disease (exanthema subitum).*

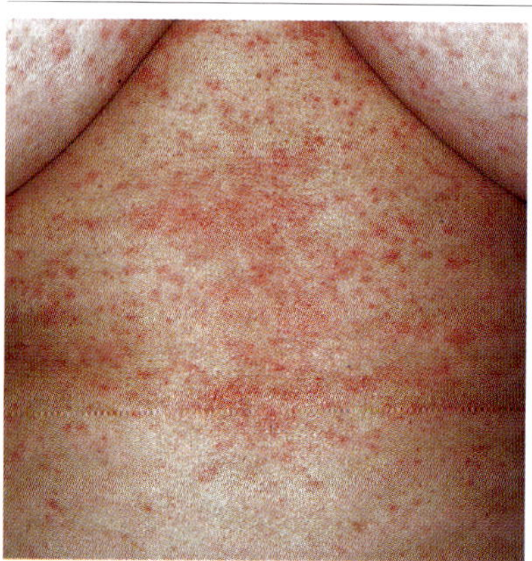

FIG. 99-13 *Widespread macules and papules of exanthema subitum.*

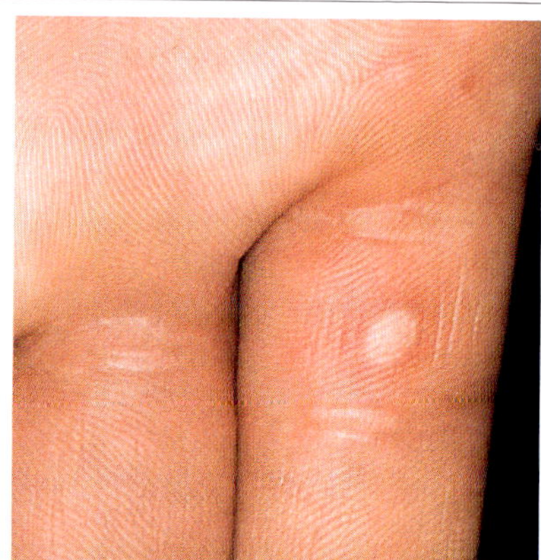

FIG. 99-14 *Oblong gray-roofed vesicles surrounded by a rim of erythema of hand, foot, and mouth disease.*

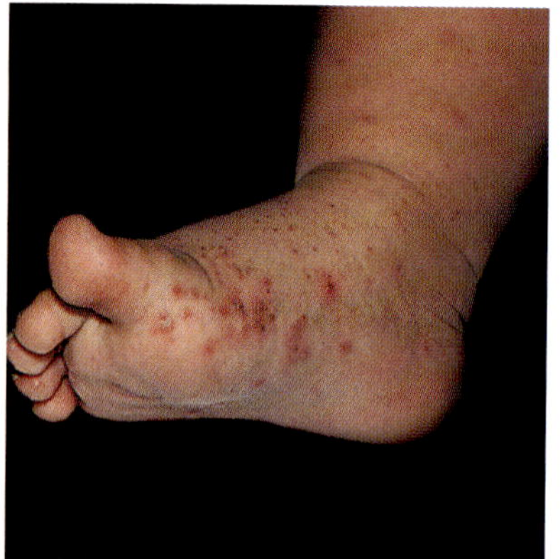

FIG. 99-15 *Papules and papulovesicles in hand, foot, and mouth disease.*

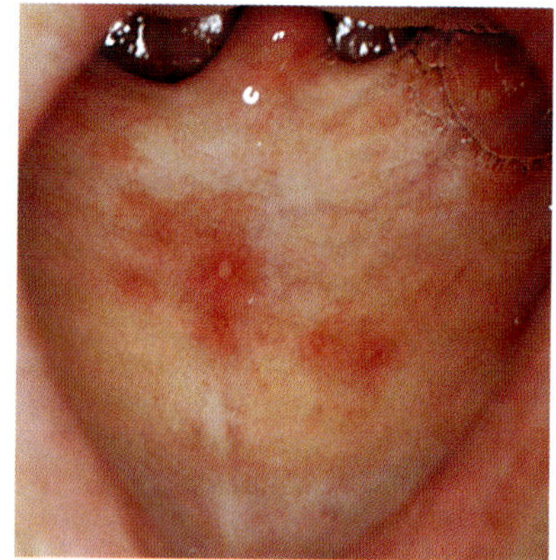

FIG. 99-16 *Papules and vesicles on the hard palate in hand, foot, and mouth disease.*

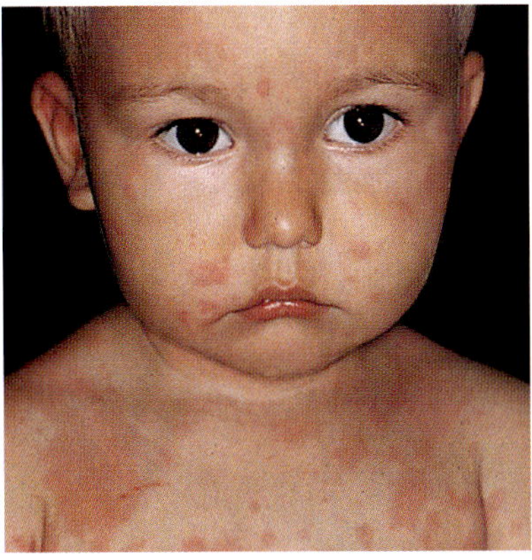 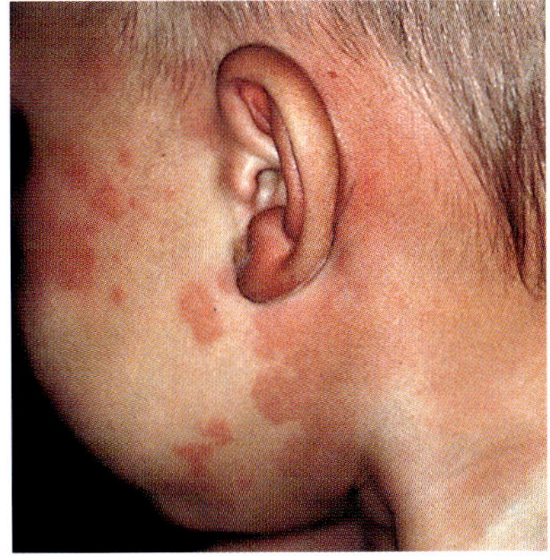

FIG. 99-17 (A, B) *Erythematous patches, papules, and plaques of viral cause, presumably Coxsackie.*

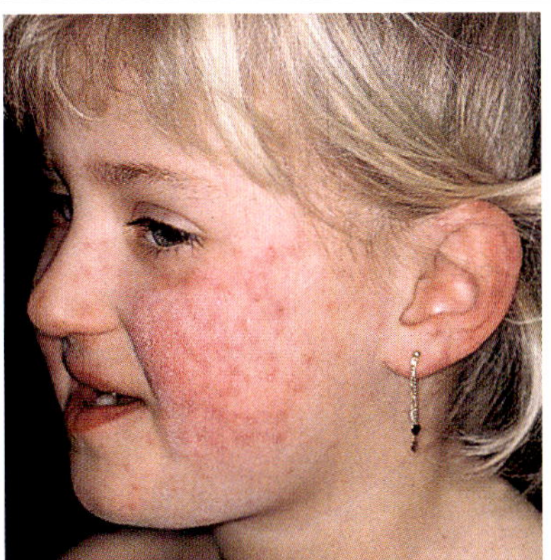 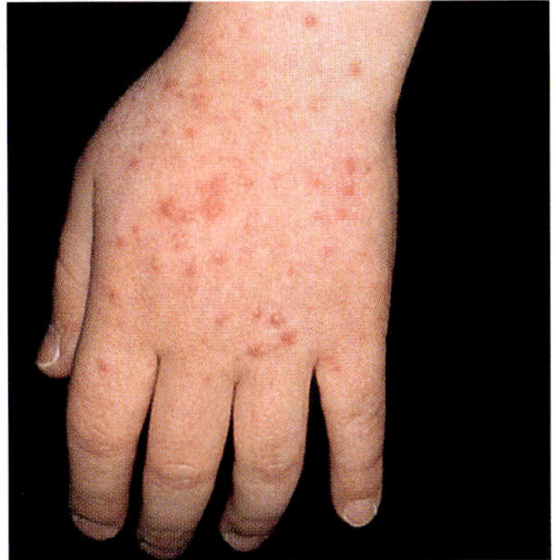

FIG. 99-18 (A, B) *The tiny red papules of Gianotti-Crosti syndrome favor the cheeks and the extremities.*

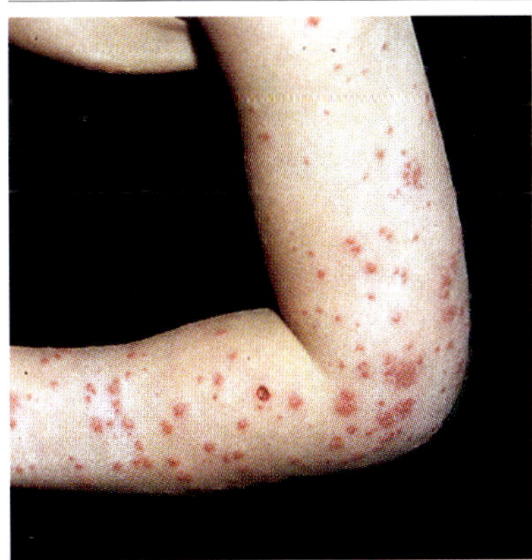

FIG. 99-19 *Papules of Gianotti-Crosti syndrome.*

ADJUNCTIVE DIAGNOSTIC TESTS Cultures, polymerase chain reaction, and specific serologic examination may be performed in an effort to identify the virus.

COURSE There are many types of viral exanthems, most of them composed of macules and papules, but some of vesicles and even pustules. As a rule, the macules and papules disappear completely in several days without residuum, whereas vesicles and pustules resolve as crusts and may at times leave behind slightly atrophic scars.

INTEGRATION: UNIFYING CONCEPT Most viral exanthems are readily diagnosable clinically because each is so distinctive—for example, "slapped cheek disease" (Fifth disease or erythema infectiosum) and "hand-foot-mouth disease" caused by Coxsackie A 5, 10, and 16. Diagnosis of viral exanthems on the basis of histopathologic findings alone is more recondite; it often is impossible to diagnose with specificity a viral exanthem only on the basis of histopathologic findings, there being just a superficial perivascular infiltrate of lymphocytes. In measles, one may be fortunate to see in the epidermis multinucleate epithelial cells that are the analogue of Warthin-Finkeldey cells in tonsils. Unless a marker such as those is seen, a diagnosis of viral exanthem with specificity by conventional microscopy may be impossible.

THERAPY No specific treatment is available.

DEFINITION An inflammatory process that is idiopathic and results in depigmentation of the skin consequent to loss of melanocytes from the epidermis, and in whitening of hair that follows loss of melanocytes from the bulb of follicles.

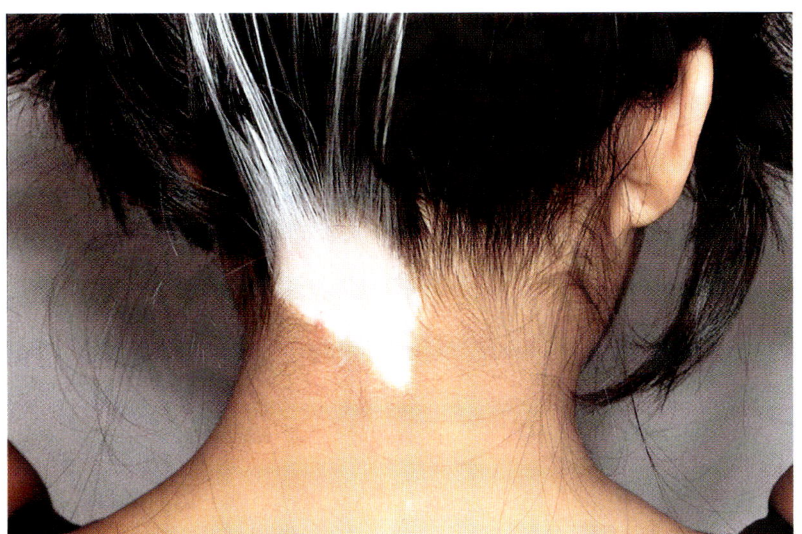

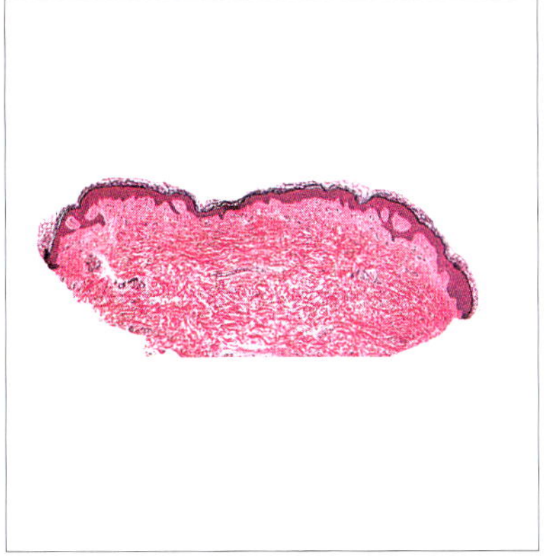

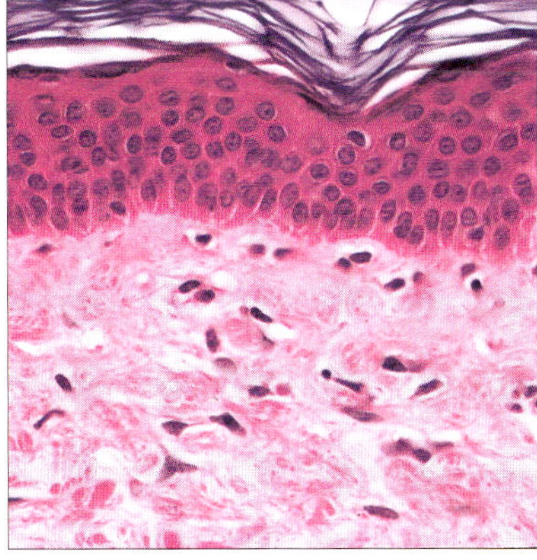

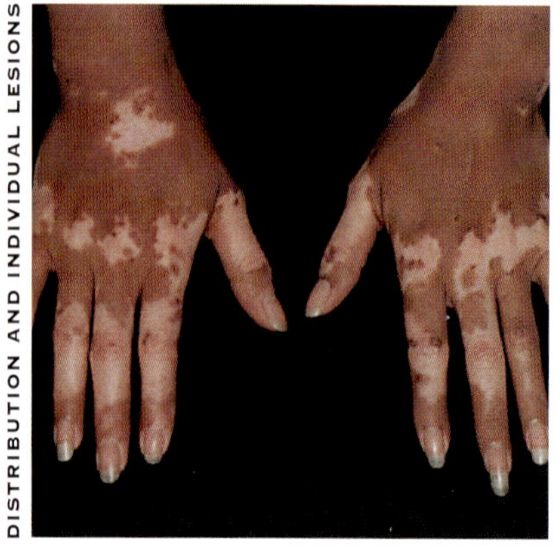

FIG. 100-1   *Bilateral, nearly symmetrical patches.*

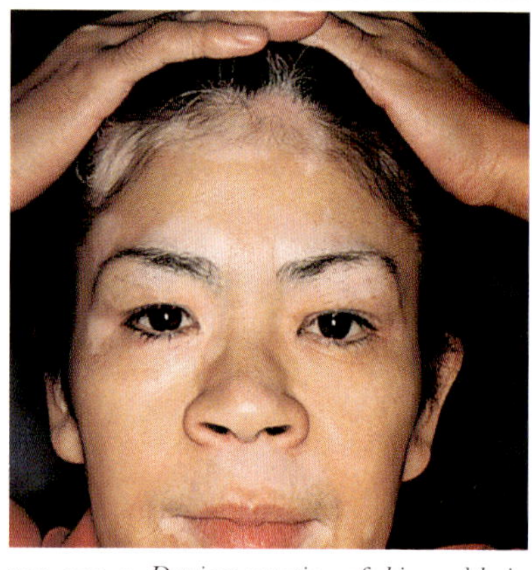

FIG. 100-2 *Depigmentation of skin and hair.*

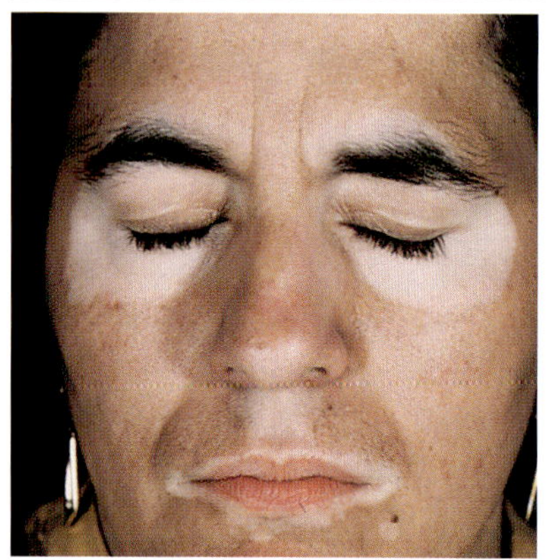

FIG. 100-3   *Bilateral, symmetrical zones of depigmentation.*

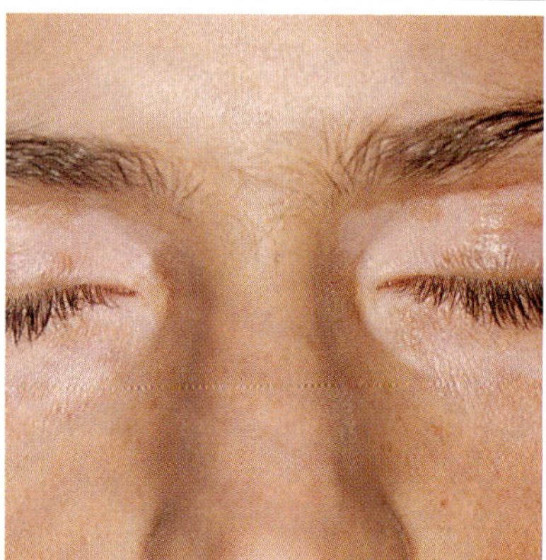

FIG. 100-4 *Bilateral, symmetrical depigmentation of skin of eyelids.*

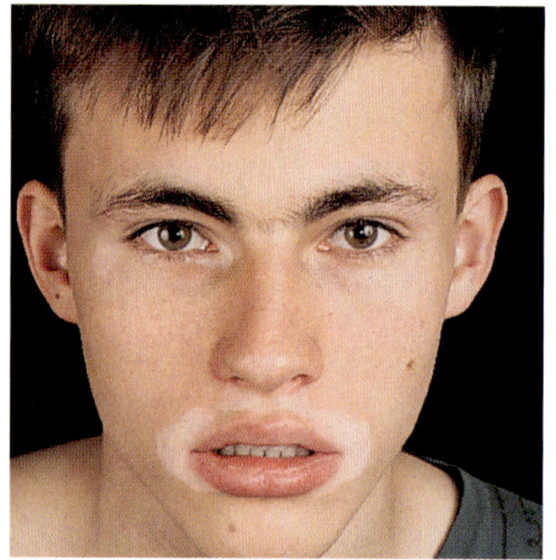

FIG. 100-5   *Perioral and juxtaocular depigmentation. The nevi on the face, including the ear, are of Miescher's type.*

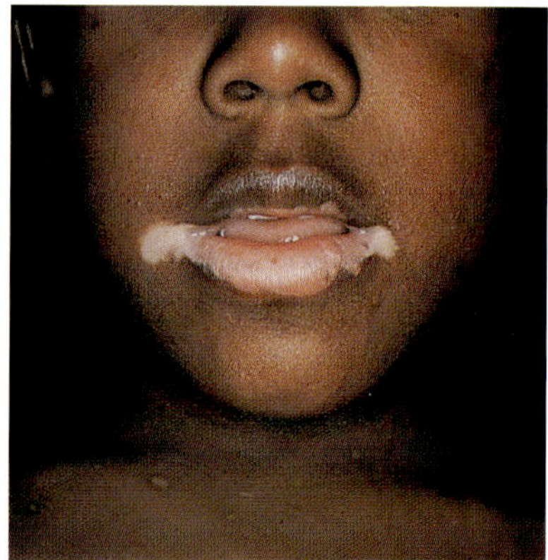

FIG. 100-6 *A patch of depigmentation across the lower lip and to a lesser extent the upper lip.*

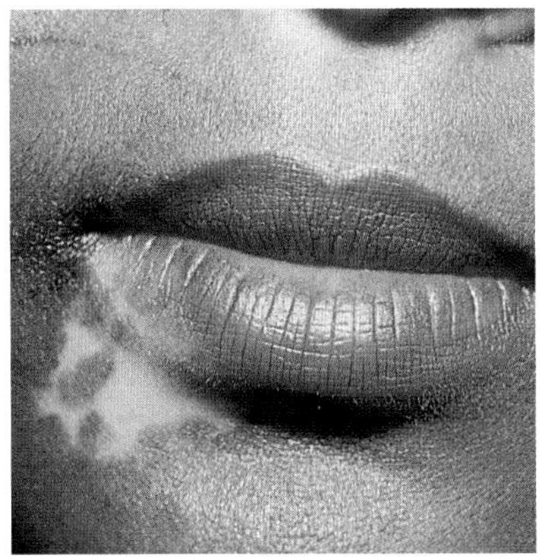

FIG. 100-7 *Patches of depigmentation.*

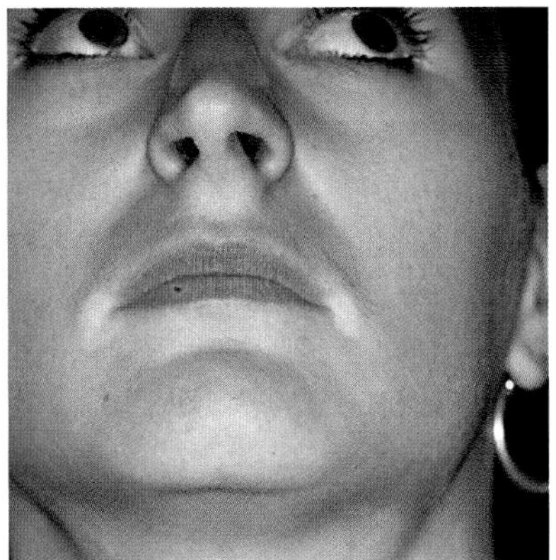

FIG. 100-8 *Depigmentation at the angles of the mouth.*

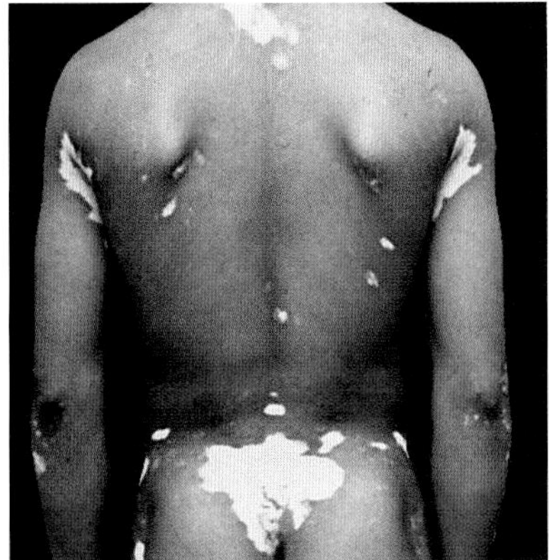

FIG. 100-9 *Bilateral, symmetrical depigmented macules and patches.*

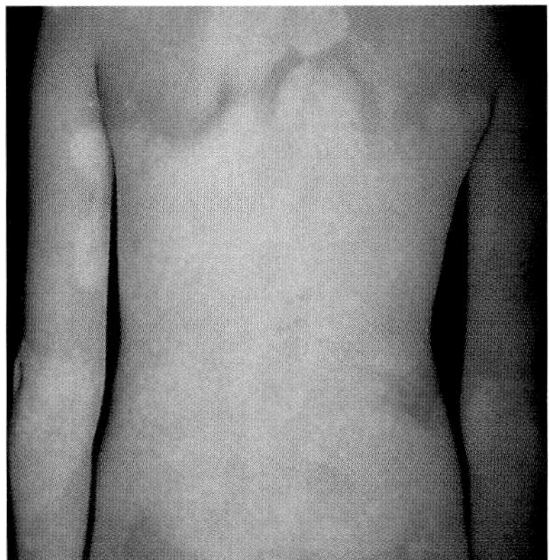

FIG. 100-10 *Widespread macules and patches of hypopigmentation.*

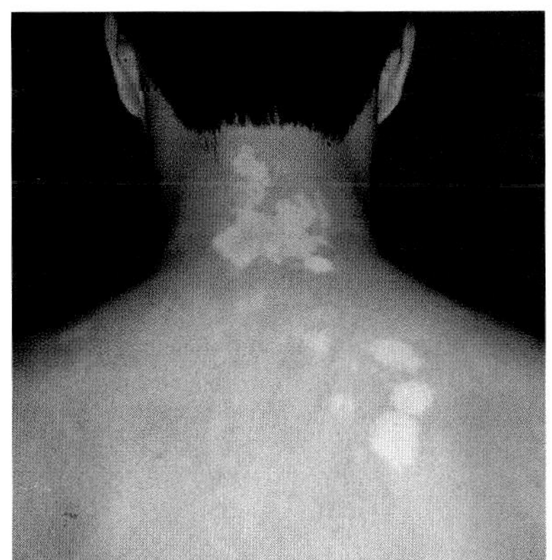

FIG. 100-11 *Patches of depigmentation.*

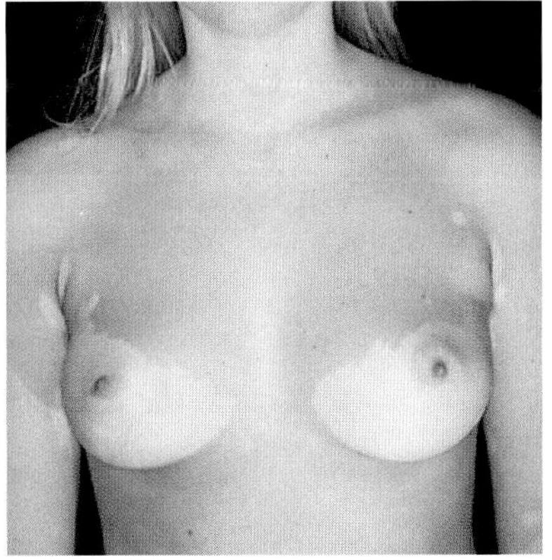

FIG. 100-12 *Bilateral symmetrical depigmentation.*

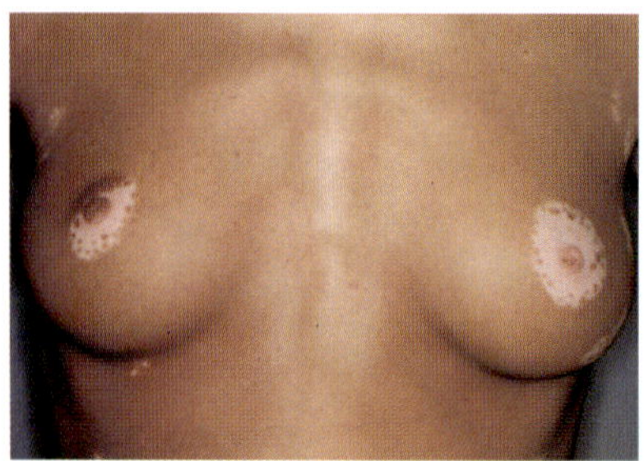

FIG. 100-13 *Depigmentation bilaterally and nearly symmetrically. In zones of depigmentation are tiny macules of repigmentation.*

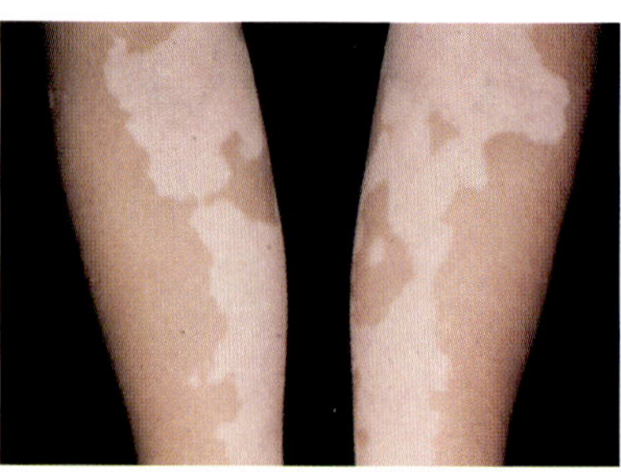

FIG. 100-14 *Bilateral, symmetrical, sharply circumscribed depigmented patches.*

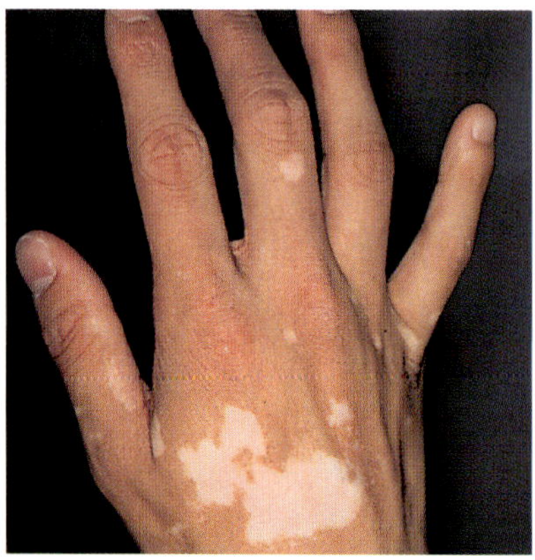

FIG. 100-15 *Macules and patches of depigmentation.*

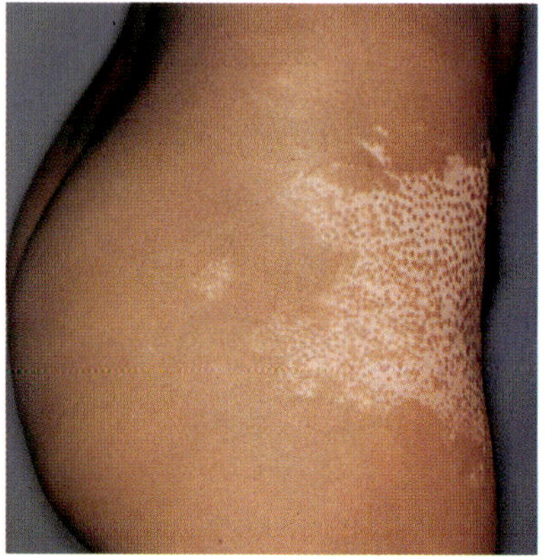

FIG. 100-16 *A patch of depigmentation with an ill-defined margin and numerous folliculocentric macules of repigmentation.*

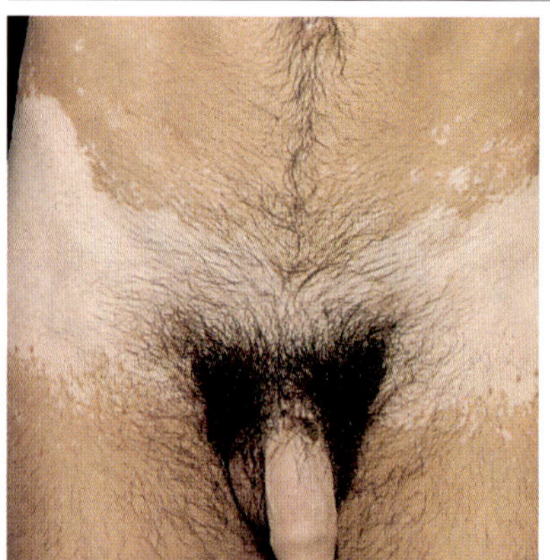

FIG. 100-17 *Macules and patches of depigmentation.*

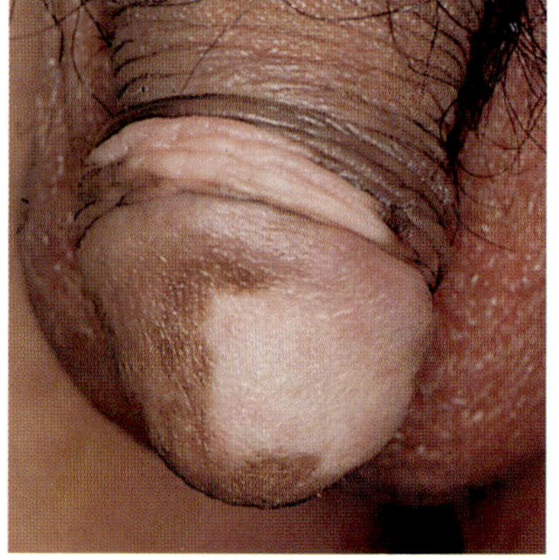

FIG. 100-18 *A hypopigmented, sharply circumscribed patch.*

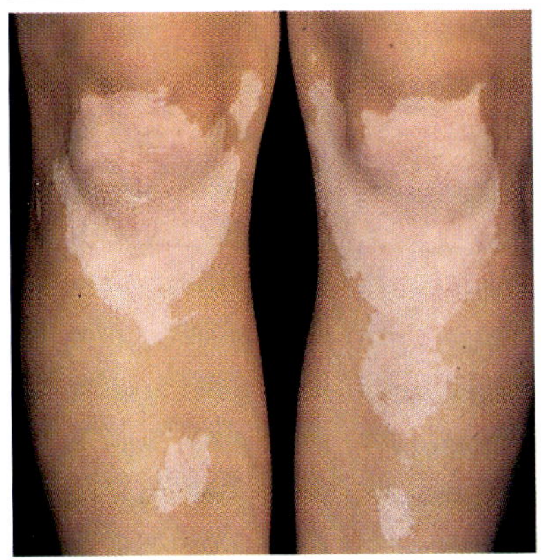

FIG. 100-19 *Patches of depigmentation in bilateral, symmetrical fashion.*

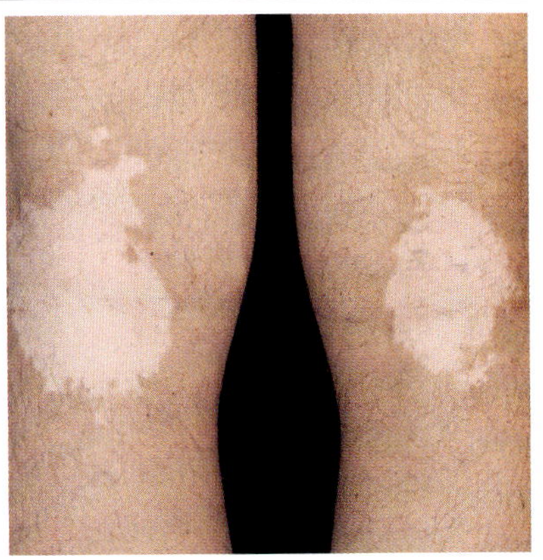

FIG. 100-20 *Zones of depigmentation.*

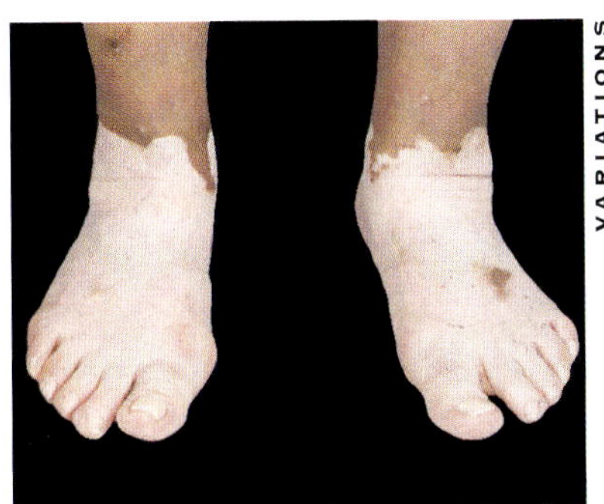

FIG. 100-21 *Depigmentation in sock-like distribution.*

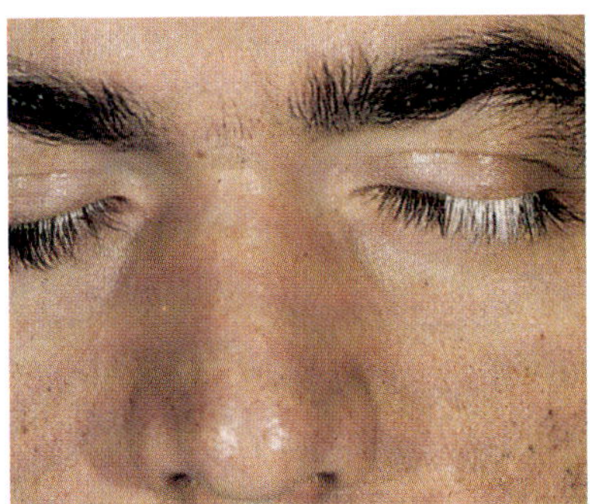

FIG. 100-22 *Depigmentation of hairs (poliosis) bilaterally.*

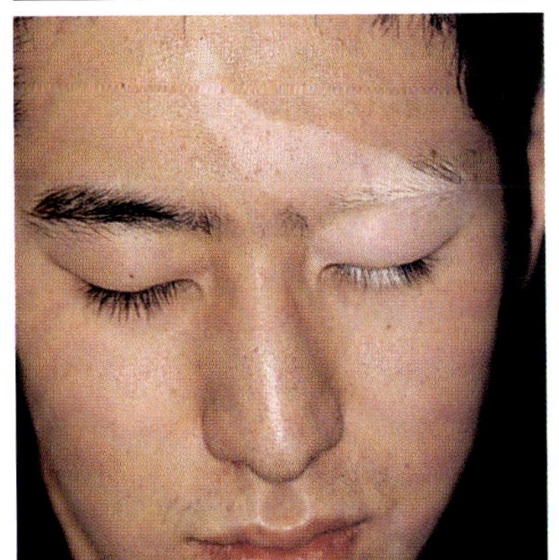

FIG. 100-23 *Depigmented patch in geographic shape involving the hair and the skin.*

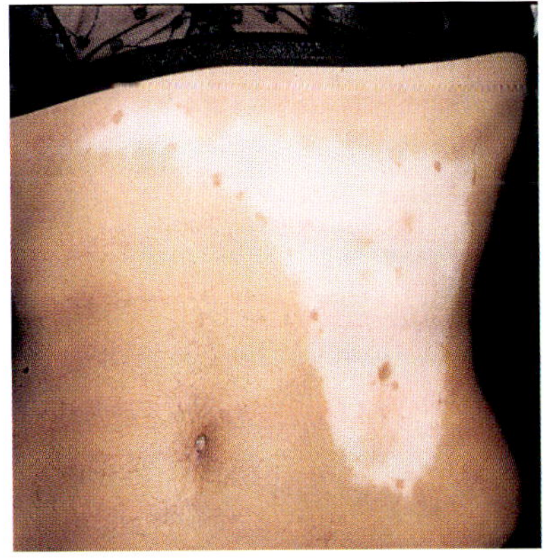

FIG. 100-24 *Depigmentation in segmental pattern.*

ADJUNCTIVE DIAGNOSTIC TESTS Studies of thyroid function may be performed in order to determine whether the gland is hyperactive, as sometimes is the case in persons with vitiligo.

COURSE Vitiligo usually begins as a pink macule that slowly whitens as it expands centrifugally. The macules of vitiligo tend to become patches of depigmentation. Once they have achieved a certain size, the patches of vitiligo may remain depigmented for a lifetime or repigment, seen at first as pigmented dots at sites of follicular ostia. Repigmentation occurs through the efforts of infundibular melanocytes, not follicular bulbar ones, that repopulate an epidermis that had been utterly devoid of melanocytes. In persons who are fortunate, there may be complete repigmentation.

INTEGRATION: UNIFYING CONCEPT Vitiligo is fundamentally an inflammatory process, beginning as it does with sparse superficial perivascular infiltrates of lymphocytes and with lymphocytes that also are present in the epidermis in company with slight spongiosis. At first, there is a full complement of melanocytes at the dermoepidermal junction, but, in time, the melanocytes disappear entirely from affected sites. When they disappear, no melanin is produced and none can be demonstrated by Fontana-Masson silver stain within the epidermis of vitiliginous lesions.

The cause of vitiligo is not known. Neither is it understood why some patients are able to become repigmented, and others are not. In certain cultures, like that of India, people with vitiligo are stigmatized because they are thought to be lepers. Leprosy in some patients is associated with hypopigmentation, but not with the depigmentation characteristic of vitiligo.

THERAPY Phototherapy (topical or systemic PUVA or UV-B) is the established treatment, but its efficacy is not consistent. New surgical methods for treatment include split-thickness and epidermal blister grafts.

XANTHOMAS

DEFINITION: Deposits of lipid in the skin and sometimes in subcutaneous tissues as a consequence often, but not always, of hyperlipidemia. The lipid deposits are expressed as yellowish papules and plaques, and nodules and tumors.

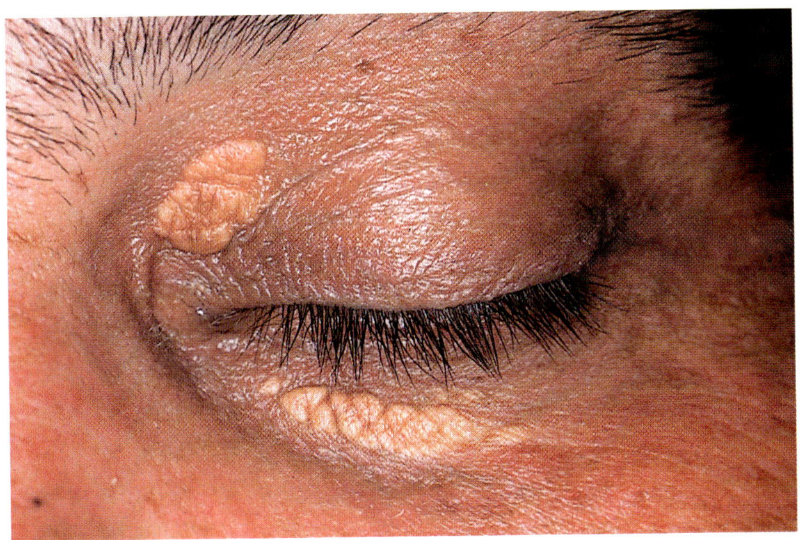

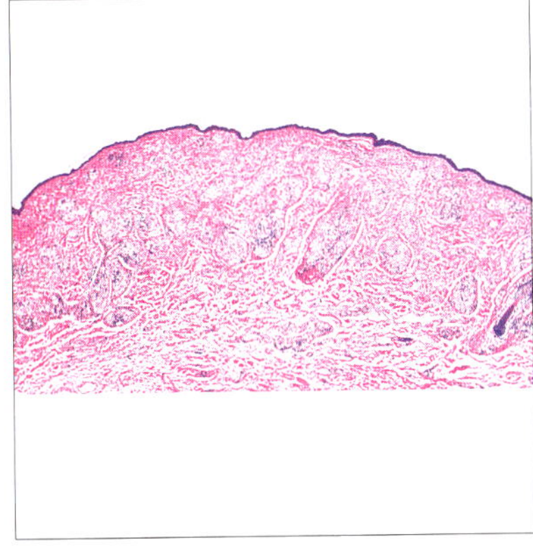

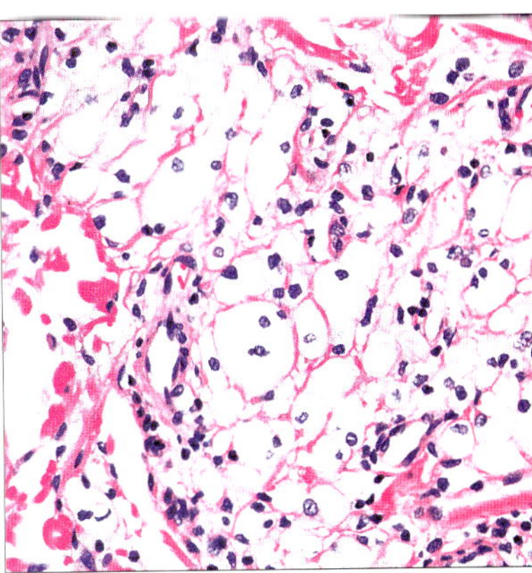

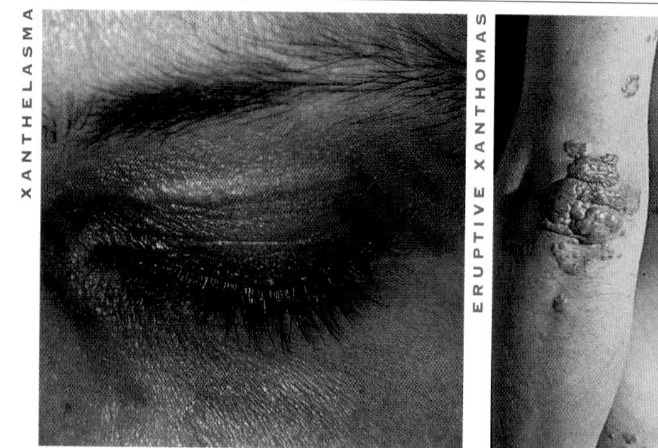

FIG. 101-1 *Plaque of xanthelasma.*

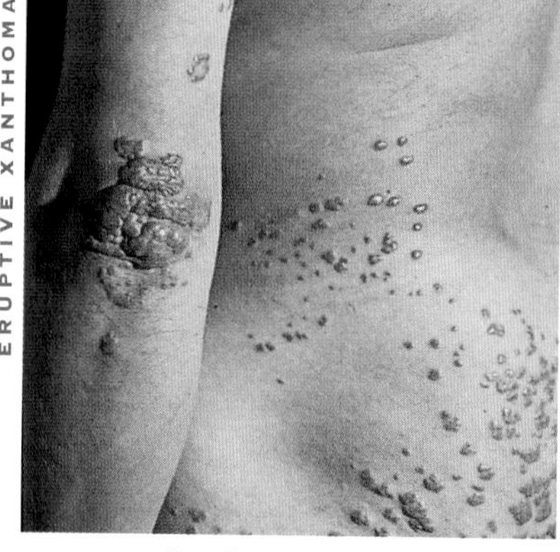

FIG. 101-2 *Papules, some of them in clusters.*

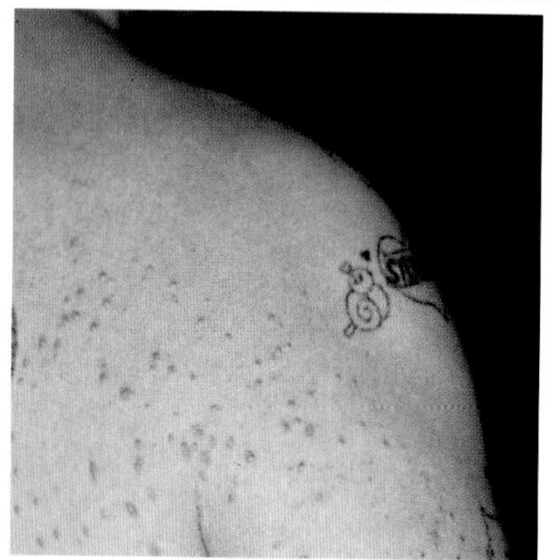
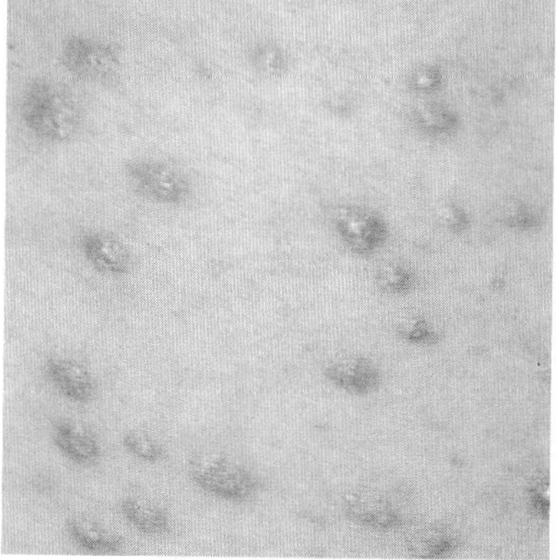

FIG. 101-3 (A, B) *Discrete acuminate papules in a patient with severe diabetes mellitus.*

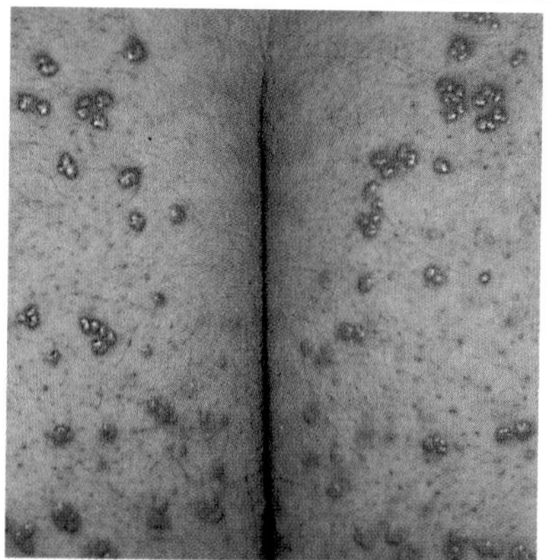

FIG. 101-4 *Smooth-surfaced yellow papules.*

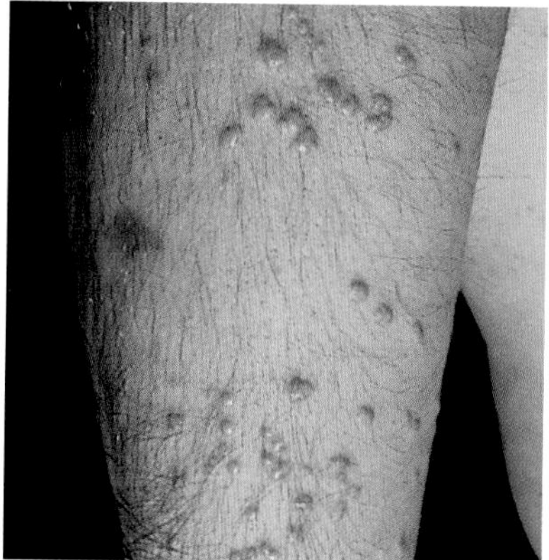

FIG. 101-5 *Globoid papules.*

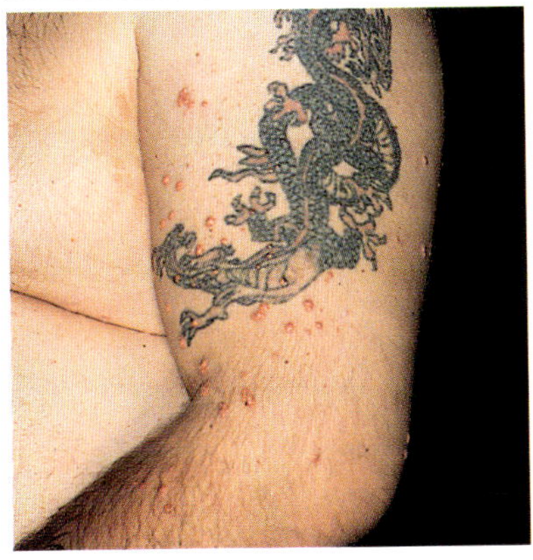

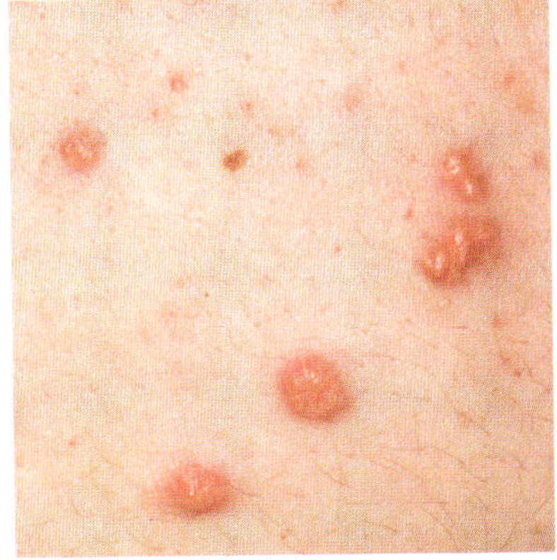

FIG. 101-6 (A, B) *Papules.*

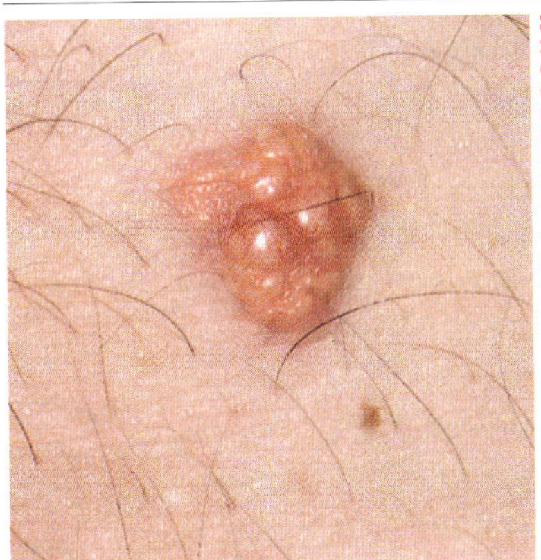

FIG. 101-6 (C) *A cluster of papules forms a nodule.*

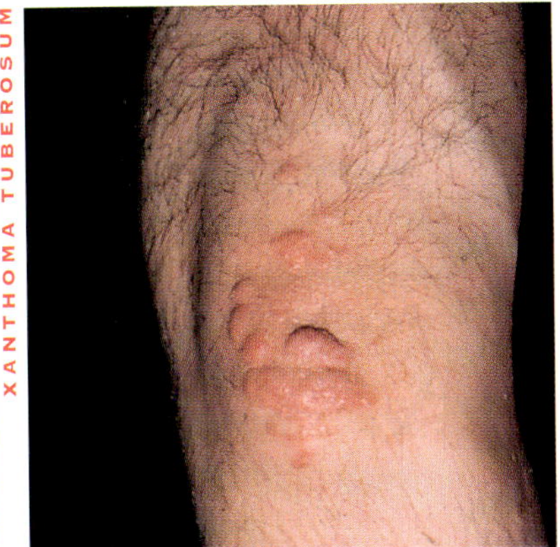

FIG. 101-7 *Papules and nodules of xanthoma tuberosum.*

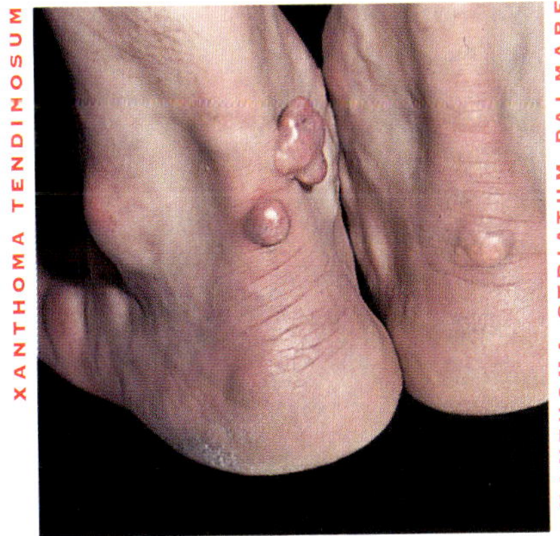

FIG. 101-8 *The lesions above the tendons are xanthoma tendinosum.*

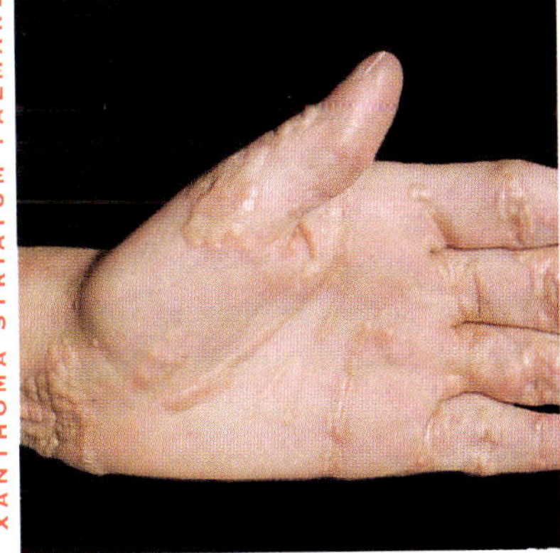

FIG. 101-9 *Papules positioned especially in creases in linear array (xanthoma palmare striatum).*

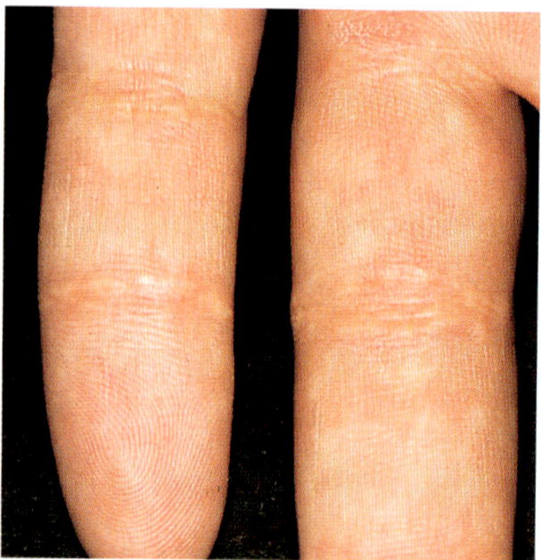

FIG. IOI-IO *Yellow papules in finger creases.*

ADJUNCTIVE DIAGNOSTIC TESTS Levels of serum lipids deserve to be assessed.

COURSE Xanthomas, whether they are papules of xanthoma palmare striatum, plaques of xanthelasma, or nodules and tumors of xanthoma tuberosum and tendinosum, tend to persist. Only eruptive xanthomas tend to involute and disappear completely. Some xanthomas, like striate xanthoma on a palm, remain small, whereas others, like papules of xanthoma tuberosum, tend to enlarge to become nodules and sometimes tumors.

INTEGRATION: UNIFYING CONCEPT Nearly all types of xanthomas result from lipid being deposited in the skin and being ingested there by macrophages. Not every xanthoma is a sign of hyperlipidemia. For example, xanthelasma may occur in persons who are normolipemic. Even in such cases though, meticulous workup nearly always reveals some disturbance in regard to the metabolism of lipids—lack of certain lipoproteins, for example. Xanthoma tuberosum and tendinosum occur in persons with familial hypercholesterolemia, xanthoma palmare striatum in persons with type III lipoproteinemia, plane xanthoma in persons who have an underlying lymphoproliferative disorder (or in persons who may be normolipemic), and eruptive xanthomas in those with a genetically transmitted lipoproteinemia. Biopsy of xanthomas reveals lipid-laden macrophages within the dermis and, in the case of xanthoma tuberosum and tendinosum, in the subcutis, too. Eruptive xanthomas are composed of abundant extracellular lipid within the dermis, around which foam cells are arranged in a palisade. In short, each type of xanthoma is diagnosable with specificity, clinically and histopathologically.

THERAPY The treatment depends on the status of the patient in regard to blood lipids. Abnormalities of serum lipoproteins should be addressed and lipoproteins reduced by systemic agents designed specifically for that purpose. Normolipidemic xanthomas may be excised or managed with laser surgery.

XANTHOGRANULOMA

DEFINITION A granulomatous inflammatory process that presents itself in children as multiple yellowish papules or nodules that often are associated

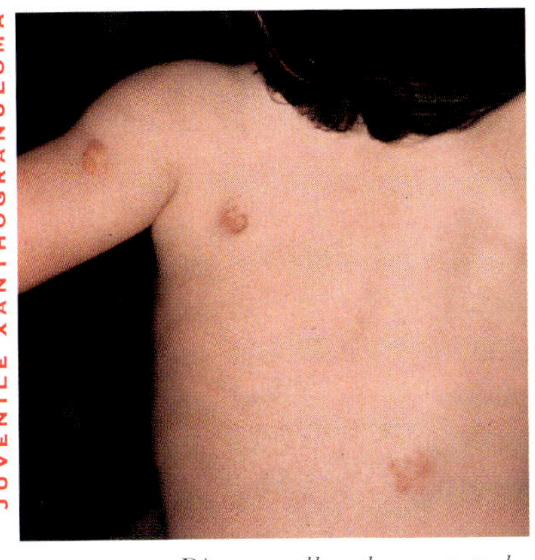

FIG. 101-11 *Discrete yellow-brown papules of xanthogranuloma.*

FIG. 101-12 *A papule.*

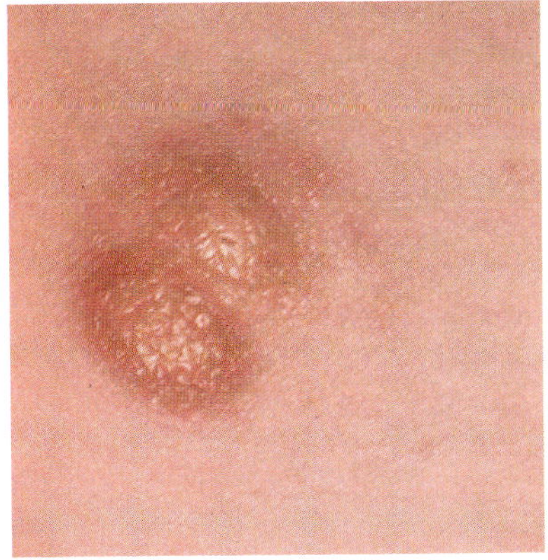

FIG. 101-13 *A cluster of small papules.*

with systemic involvement of eyes, liver, and testes. In adults it is usually a solitary lesion confined to the skin.

COURSE Xanthogranulomas that appear in children as papules that become nodules and in the course of months, involute without residuum. Xanthogranulomas in adults tend to achieve a certain size and to persist.

INTEGRATION: UNIFYING CONCEPT Juvenile xanthogranuloma is a systemic disease that, in addition to the skin, involves other organs such as the eye, testes, lungs, and heart. A fully-developed lesion of xanthogranuloma is made up of a dense, diffuse infiltrate of foam cells, many of which are multi-nucleate (Touton giant cells). The lipid-laden macrophages are joined by a mixture of inflammatory cells, among them neutrophils, eosinophils, and plasma cells. An early lesion, however, consists of sheets of histiocytes that contain hardly any lipid in their cytoplasm. It is easy to misdiagnose such a lesion histopathologically as a malignant neoplasm, e.g., a poorly differentiated carcinoma or a sarcoma. Late-resolving lesions of juvenile xanthogranuloma are associated with striking fibroplasia in addition to residual changes of foamy histiocytes. In brief, a xanthogranuloma is different from a true xanthoma, the former being fundamentally an inflammatory process and the latter being basically a deposit. Reticulohistiocytic granuloma and benign cephalic histiocytosis are merely morphologic variants of xanthogranuloma.

THERAPY Lesions in children resolve without treatment. A lesion in adults may be excised for reasons of cosmesis, but nothing really need be done about it.

INDEX

curettage, 220, 223, 398, 554, 567, 586
cyclophosphamide, 34, 100, 338, 452, 516
cystic
    acne, 114
    hamartomas, VII, XVI, 109–115, 427
cysts and cystic hamartomas, VII, XVI, 109–115

Dapsone, 100, 126, 131, 134, 234, 294, 300, 338, 593
Darier's disease, VII, XVI, 116–121, 177, 237, 275, 439, 484
deep
    fungal infections, VII, XVI, 122–126
    fungi, 122, 125
dermabrasion, 50, 121, 178, 223, 240, 530
dermatiaceous fungus, 123, 125
dermatitis herpetiformis, VII, XVII, 127–134
dermatofibroma, VII, 135–39
dermatofibroma with monster cells, 139
dermatofibrosarcoma protuberans, VII, 140–143
dermatofibrosis lenticularis disseminata, 178
dermatome, 252
dermatomyositis, VII, 144–149
dermatophytosis, VII, 150–158
dermatosis papulosa nigra, 219–220
dermoid cyst, 113
desmoplakin, 100
diffuse neonatal hemangiomatosis, 249
dilated pore of Winer, 112
dimple sign, 138
direct immunofluorescence, 33, 100, 102, 133, 335
distal
    onycholysis, 118
    type of onychomycosis, 156
drug eruptions, VII, XVI, 159–167
dyshidrotic dermatitis, VII, 168–172, 435
dystrophic epidermolysis bullosa, 180, 182–183

Eccrine
    gland, 114–115
    hidrocystoma, 113
    units, 211
ectasias, VIII, 241–251, 325
eczema herpeticum, 255–256
Ehlers-Danlos syndrome, 185, 422
electrocautery, 220, 223, 606, 637
electromyography, 147
electron microscopy, 183, 268
electrosurgery, 90
elephantiasis nostras, 189
emollients, 75, 103, 275, 551
eosinophilic folliculitis, 225
epidermal nevus, VII, XVI, 121, 173–178, 274, 438–439, 484
epidermolysis bullosa, VII, 179–85
    acquisita, 183–185
    letalis, 183
    simplex, 181–182, 184
epidermolytic hyperkeratosis, 121, 177, 274, 439, 484
epifocal patch test, 167
epiloia, 222
epithelioid histiocytes, 234, 294, 299, 303, 418, 535, 615

erosio interdigitalis candidomycetica, 105
eruption, IX, XXI, 103, 120, 160–161, 163–164, 166–167, 235, 237, 256, 462–463, 471, 475–479, 493, 638
erysipelas, VII, 186–189
erythema
    annulare centrifugum, VII, 190–193, 471, 505
    chronicum migrans, 91–93, 95–96
    contusiformis, 204
    induratum, 428, 430, 615
    multiforme, VII, 163, 194–200, 204, 516, 593
    nodosum, VII, 201–205, 299, 516, 593
erythroderma, 67–68, 75, 121, 160, 163, 177, 270, 274, 412–415, 439, 464, 473–474, 494, 497, 504, 509–512
eschars, 214, 216, 260, 399, 402–404, 546
etretinate, 50, 121
excision, 4, 77, 81, 89–90, 115, 139, 143, 178, 209, 220, 223, 240, 287, 320, 345, 368, 390–391, 423, 427, 521–522, 554, 586, 616, 630
extramammary Paget's disease, VII, 206–211

Fabry, angiokeratoma of, 250
factitious dermatitis, VII, XII, 74, 212–217
fibroid nodules, 95
fibromas, VIII, XVI, 218–220
fibroplasia, 16, 33, 77, 139, 517, 521, 539, 603, 615, 656
fibrosarcoma, 143
fibrosing septal panniculitis, 204
fibrosis, 16–17, 81, 126, 135, 139, 184–185, 242, 290, 350, 430
fibrous papule of the face and analogues of it, VIII, 221–223
fixed drug eruption, 163–164, 167
flagellation, 214
floret cells, 143, 320
focal
    acantholytic dyskeratosis, 121, 439, 484
    dermal hypoplasia, 178
    mucinosis, 114
follicular degeneration syndrome, 43
follicular hamartoma, 223
folliculitis and pseudofolliculitis, VIII, 224–228
folliculosebaceous cystic hamartoma, 115
folliculosebaceous-apocrine units, 211
Fordyce, angiokeratoma of, 248, 250
foreign body reaction, 228
fungus, 123, 125, 204, 607, 609–610
furuncle, 226
furunculosis, 226

Gamma globulin, 149
giant comedo, 112
giant-cell fibroblastoma, 143
glomangioma, 249
glomus tumor, 249
gluten-sensitive enteropathy, 131
Goltz syndrome, 178
Gottron's papules, 146, 148
granular deposits of IgA, 130
granuloma annulare, VIII, 229–234
granulomatous inflammation, 16–17, 81, 126, 135, 139, 234, 316, 430, 603, 615

A Clinical Atlas of 101 Common Skin Diseases *was written by A. Bernard Ackerman, Helmut Kerl, and Jorge Sánchez. Copy edited by Sarah Fitz-Hugh, Philadelphia, Pennsylvania. Cover and interior pages designed by Mary Jane Callister / Louise Fili Ltd, New York City. Production and general composition by John Matey, Hollis Digital Imaging Systems, Inc., Tucson, Arizona. Page composition by Wendy Voorhees, Painted Pony, Tucson, Arizona. Printed by R.R. Donnelley, Crawfordsville, Indiana, on 70 lb. Westvaco Sterling Web Gloss and set in Granjon and Copperplate 33BC. Published by Ardor Scribendi, New York City.*